Pediatrics Practical Essentials

Pediatrics Practical Essentials

Dr Anupama S, MD Pediatrics

Senior Resident, Government Medical College and Hospital -Thiruvallur,
Tamil Nadu, India

Dr R Nisha, MD Pediatrics, DNB, FPIC

Senior resident, Institute of Child Health and Hospital for Children, Egmore,
Tamil Nadu, India

Dr Sai Shiva G, MD Pediatrics, DM

Resident, Department of Pediatric Oncology, Regional Cancer Centre,
Thiruvananthapuram, Kerala, India

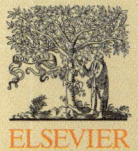

ELSEVIER

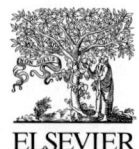

ELSEVIER

Reed Elsevier India Pvt. Ltd.
Registered Office: 818, 8th Floor, Indraprakash Building, 21, Barakhamba Road, New Delhi 110001
Corporate Office: 14th Floor, Building No. 10B, DLF Cyber City, Phase II, Gurgaon-122002, Haryana, India

First Printed in India 2023, Reprinted 2025

Sr Content Strategist: Mrinalini Bakshi
Content Project Manager: Supriya Barua Kumar
Sr Production Executive: Dhan Singh
Sr. Graphic Designer: Milind Majgaonkar

Typeset by GW India
Printed and bound at Balaji Art, Mumbai.

It gives me immense pleasure to write the foreword for this first edition of this book, *Pediatrics Practical Essentials*. This was a long felt need by the pediatric postgraduate students and fellows for a comprehensive book about clinical examination and presentation as a ready reference before the examinations. This is the first time that a practical book with FAQ format with vast discussion on long and short cases is prepared by young pediatricians. The authors have meticulously covered the requirement from basics to advanced concepts, which are essential for the case presentation and answering in the viva voce with confidence. This book extensively covers all aspects of history elicitation in a structured way for each case with appropriate explanations for the same. The case sheet format of presentation is a ready reference just before the examinations. The book has covered most of the MD and DNB clinical topics and has covered the difficult core topics including ECG, EEG, CT, and MRI in a simple way. The authors have taken care to include counseling and prognosis issues for each clinical case. I understand that a lot of hard work had gone into preparing this book with pictures to complement the learning resources.

This book will come "handy" in understanding the basic concepts and presenting cases with structured meticulous bedside approach.

I take this opportunity to congratulate Dr Anupama S, Dr R Nisha, Dr Sai Shiva G, and their team who have toiled hard to publish this first edition of *Pediatrics Practical Essentials*. I applaud their efforts and hope that the pediatric community will make best use of this educational resource for the benefit of acquiring rich knowledge.

Dr Poovazhagi V MD, DCH, PhD,
HOD and Professor of Pediatrics,
Department of Pediatric Intensive Care,
Institute of Child Health and Hospital for Children, Egmore,
Madras Medical College,
Chennai
Tamil Nadu, India

When postgraduate students enter the challenging and frantic realm of Pediatrics, they are called upon to apply themselves immediately to the direct care of children. For a pediatrician to deliver high-quality care, a mix of sound theory and accurate practical skills are essential. These skills can only be built on a base of thorough knowledge.

The term skills can range from accuracy in measuring blood pressure, to intubating, to effective and simple communication with the patient family and to handling complications.

Our team is delighted to introduce our first publication that aims to bridge the gap between skill and knowledge for pediatric postgraduate students. The purpose of this book is not only to help a postgraduate student for his or her examinations but also to efficiently and systematically arrive at a diagnosis and treat the condition. We strongly believe that this book will make a postgraduate clinically competent and theoretically sound.

This book, a first of its kind, is based on a FAQ (Frequently Asked Question) format which will help the student to face viva voce without fear. It covers both MD and DNB topics, OSCE especially on ECG, X-ray, EEG, CT/MRI. Each system covers long and short cases in depth from history elicitation to counseling and prognosis. Case sheet format at the beginning of each chapter acts as a ready reckoner for students before the examinations. For quick revision, each chapter has salient points in the form of Quick bites at the end. Overall, `it is a one-stop solution for students before their practical examinations.

We earnestly hope this book will help and guide all pediatric postgraduate students and lead them to become better physicians of tomorrow.

Anupama S
R Nisha
Sai Shiva G

ACKNOWLEDGEMENTS

I thank Professor Dr Poovazhagi who sowed the seeds for this book. Her teachings on history elicitation and clinical methodology stand to guide generations of students in systematic approach toward clinical case handling. Her constant encouragement drove us to coherently compile our thoughts into making this book.

I am grateful to Professor Dr Thangavelu for mentoring us in clinical methods, breaking down complex topics into simple methodologies by inspiring us to follow an algorithmic approach in clinical examination. I am especially thankful to him for demystifying difficult topics such as ECG, chest X-ray, and CT/MRI, which are among the essential learnings for OSCE examinations.

I thank Prof Dr Lakshmanaswamy for guiding us in the right direction when we approached him with our endeavor to write a book. He was instrumental in our journey of publishing this book.

I would also like to thank the professors for imbibing clinical knowledge which is the age old 'Golden Key' in diagnosing any disease, despite in an era of modern medicine where least importance is given for history elicitation and clinical examination.

I extend a very special thanks to my coauthors Dr R Nisha and Dr Sai Shiva G for their tremendous contribution to this book. While our team effort has created this book, their individualistic inputs on clinical approaches have made this treatise a holistic one.

I also acknowledge every reviewer of this book and all the contributors for their expert inputs and ideas.

I thank Dr Monisha for her constant support; with her deep insights, proofreading efforts, and illustrative help every chapter underwent a nuanced fine tuning.

I thank Dr Elayarani for her contribution to chapters on EEG, ECG, ETCO$_2$, Development, and Counseling, that cover difficult topics in the DNB practical examination which made this book unique.

I gratefully acknowledge the support received from the publishing team of RELX India Pvt. Ltd., especially, Nimisha Goswami (Director Content Strategy, India/SEA), Shabina Nasim (Head of Content Project Management – APAC), Supriya Barua (Content Project Manager) for technical support, ideas, and expert skills, which have ensured the high quality standards of this book.

I also thank Mr Rajesh Rajasekaran (Head, Education eProducts & Portfolio) of RELX India Pvt. Ltd. for his continued support throughout the journey of creating this book.

I also thank my family members who are my pillars of strength. Without my family's steadfast support, care, and motivation this book would have never materialized.

Finally, my heartfelt thanks to the Almighty for His blessings and guidance.

Anupama S

CONTRIBUTORS

Dr Arulganesh M, MD
Assistant Professor
Department of Pediatrics
Government Dharmapuri Medical College and Hospital
Dharmapuri, Tamil Nadu, India

Dr Dafni, MBBS
Thiruvallur Government Medical College and Hospital
Thiruvallur, Tamil Nadu, India

Dr Elayarani Elavarasan, DNB
Senior Registrar
Department of Pediatrics
Mehta Multispeciality Hospitals India Pvt Ltd
Chennai, Tamil Nadu, India

Dr Faiz, DNB
Junior Consultant
Department of Paediatrics
Cloud Nine Hospital, HRBR
Bangalore, Karnataka, India

Dr Ilakya Devadas, MBBS, DNB, FPEM
Senior Resident
Paediatric Emergency Services
Department of Paediatrics
Christian Medical College Vellore
Tamil Nadu, India

Dr Jahnavi M, DNB
Registrar, Pediatrics Emergency Department
Manipal Hospital, Old HAL Road
Bangalore, Karnataka, India

Dr Jana Priya Sugumar, DNB
PICU Registrar
Apollo Children's Hospital, Nungambakkam
Chennai, Tamil Nadu, India

Dr Jaya Karthika R, MD
Senior Resident
Department of Pediatricss
Government Vellore Medical College and Hospital
Vellore, Tamil Nadu, India

Dr Mahesh N, MD, DM (Neuro)
Senior Consultant Pediatric Neurologist
Chennai, Tamil Nadu, India

Dr Meenakshi N, MBBS
Government Medical College and Hospital -
Thiruvallur, Tamil Nadu, India

Dr A Monisha, MD, DNB
Senior Resident
Department of Pediatrics
Government Medical College and Hospital
Thiruvallur, Tamil Nadu, India

Dr Monisha P, MD, Fellowship in Neonatology (NNF)
Junior Consultant
Department of Pediatrics
R and R Hospitals
Chennai, Tamil Nadu, India

Dr S Naga Jyothi, DNB
Senior Resident
Department of Paediatrics
Dr Pinnamaneni Siddhartha Institute of Medical Sciences and
    Research Foundation, Chinoutapalli
Gannavaram, Andhra Pradesh, India

Dr Nishant Aravind, MBBS
Government Medical College and Hospital -
Thiruvallur, Tamil Nadu, India

Dr Priyadarshini S, DNB
DNB Resident
Department of Pediatrics
Mehta Multispeciality Hospitals India Pvt Ltd
Chennai, Tamil Nadu, India

Dr Ragul G, DNB
DNB Resident
Department of Pediatrics
Mehta Multispeciality Hospitals India Pvt Ltd
Chennai, Tamil Nadu, India

Dr R Ramya Devi, MBBS, DCH
Assistant Surgeon
Government Hospital Iluppur
Pudhukottai District, Tamil Nadu, India

Dr Ramya Selvam, MD
Registrar
General Pediatrics
Mehta Multispeciality Hospitals India Pvt Ltd
Chennai, Tamil Nadu, India

Dr Rekha GP, MD (DVL)
Assistant Professor
Department of DVL
Tagore Medical College and Hospital
Chennai, Tamil Nadu, India

Dr Sangkavi R, MBBS, MD
Resident (Final Year)
Chengalpattu Medical College Hospital
Tamil Nadu, India

Dr S Sathiya Priya, MD
Assistant Surgeon
City Police Hospital, Egmore
Chennai, Tamil Nadu, India

Dr Sivaranjani SC, MD
Assistant Professor
Department of Pathology
Government Thoothukudi Medical College
Thoothukudi, Tamil Nadu, India

Dr Vandana Kuniyedath Chalil, MBBS, DNB
Erlangen, Germany

Dr Annamalai Vijayaraghavan, MD, DCH
Consultant Pediatrician and Academic Coordinator
Mehta Multispeciality Hospitals India Pvt Ltd
Chennai, Tamil Nadu, India

Dr NC Gowrishankar, MD, DCH, DNB, FIAP
Pediatric Pulmonologist and Bronchoscopist
Head – Pediatrics, Operations and Quality
Mehta Multispeciality Hospitals India Pvt Ltd
Chennai, Tamil Nadu, India

Dr Nedunchelian K, MD, DCH, FIAP
Senior Consultant Pediatrician
Head – Research and Academics
Mehta Multispeciality Hospitals India Pvt Ltd
Chennai, Tamil Nadu, India

Dr Poovazhagi V, MD, DCH, PhD
HOD and Professor of Pediatrics
Department of Pediatric Intensive Care
Institute of Child Health and Hospital for Children, Egmore
Madras Medical College
Chennai, Tamil Nadu, India

Dr Thangavelu S, MD, DCH, DNB, MRCP (UK)
Senior Consultant and Director of Pediatrics
Department of Pediatrics
Mehta Multispeciality Hospitals India Pvt Ltd
Chennai, Tamil Nadu, India

Dr Vaishnavi Raman, MD, FPN (TNMGRU), FISPN
Senior Resident
Department of Pediatrics
ESI PGIMSR, KK Nagar
Chennai, Tamil Nadu, India

TABLE OF CONTENTS

Long Cases

Central Nervous System

1 Central Nervous System Examination

General Examination

1. Pallor − vasomotor collapse/intracranial bleeding/iron-deficiency anemia can cause cognitive dysfunction
2. Icterus − hepatic encephalopathy
3. Cyanosis − cyanotic congenital heart disease/CO_2 poisoning/central nervous system (CNS) depression
4. Generalized lymphadenopathy − SLE/TB/HIV/malignancies
5. Clubbing – syringomyelia and tertiary syphilis

Head-to-Foot Examination

Table 1.1 shows findings in head-to-foot examination in the CNS.

Higher Functions

Remember "COSSHMIB"
- C: Consciousness
- O: Orientation
- S: Sleep
- S: Speech and Language
- H: Handedness
- M: Memory
- I: Intelligence
- B: Behavior

C − CONSCIOUSNESS

Table 1.2 gives stages of consciousness.
Table 1.3 gives Glasgow Coma Scale (GCS).
Table 1.4 gives Full Outline of Unresponsiveness (FOUR) Score coma scale.
For older children and adolescents, Mini-Mental State Examination (MMSE) Scoring can be used for consciousness, orientation, and cognition assessment.

O − ORIENTATION

Orientation to time (ability to tell the day, month, and year), place (aware of the surroundings), person (identify mother), and self (ability to tell his or her name)

S − SLEEP

Any sleep disturbance (insomnia, parasomnias, or restless leg syndrome)

S − SPEECH AND LANGUAGE

- Any difficulty in fluency, word output, comprehension, repetition, naming, reading, writing, and copying
- Upper motor neuron lesion results in aphasia or dysphasia
- Lower motor neuron lesion results in dysarthria

H − HANDEDNESS

- Dominant hand is used for eating, combing, and writing
- It is tested indirectly as follows:
  - Ask the patient to kick a ball; observe the leg used.
  - Ask the patient to fold his or her arms across the chest. The dominant arm is placed anteriorly. When the patient stands at ease, dominant hand comes posteriorly.
  - Ask the patient to see through a hole; the dominant eye is used.

M − MEMORY

- Immediate memory − also called working memory (ability to reproduce random numbers, names, or objects told within a minute)

TABLE 1.1	Head-to-Foot Examination in Central Nervous System
Head-to-Foot Examination	**Findings**
Head	Shape, size, craniosynostosis, wide open fontanelles/bulging fontanelles, craniotabes, dilated scalp veins, bruit over the scalp, crack-pot resonance, alopecia, hypopigmented hair/localized swelling/bruises/depressed fracture
Face	Facial dysmorphism, facial asymmetry
Eyes	Pallor/icterus/phlycten/raccoon eyes/mongoloid slant/hypertelorism, canthal index (>38)/drooping of eyelids/nystagmus/strabismus/micropthalmia/cataract/chorioretinitis/cherry red spot/papilledema/optic atrophy, bushy eyebrow (Hurler syndrome), coloboma, telangiectasia, phlycten
Ears	Low-set ears/bat wing ear sign/Battle sign
Oral cavity	Tongue atrophy/uvula position/pharyngitis/tongue abnormal movements/dentition/ulcers, caries
Neck	Torticollis/short neck/low posterior hairline
Skin	BCG scar Neurocutaneous markers/erythematous rash/extensive mongolian spots/ichthyosis
Extremities	Wasting/pseudohypertrophy/contractures/bony deformities/pathological fractures
Spine	Kyphosis/scoliosis/tenderness/swelling/hairy patch/dimples − 5 mm deep and >25 mm from anal verge
Others	Naso Gastric (NG) tube/Ventriculo Peritoneal (VP) shunt/urinary bladder catheter

TABLE 1.2	Stages of Consciousness	
Term	**Description**	
Confusion	Disoriented to surroundings	
Lethargy	Difficulty to maintain aroused state	
Obtundation	Responds to stimuli other than pain	
Stupor	Responds only to painful stimuli	
Coma	Unresponsive to any type of stimuli, both internal and external	

Source: Adapted from Level of consciousness (GCS) (slideshare.net) – Slide 5

TABLE 1.3	Pediatric Glasgow Coma Scale (PGCS)

INFANTS	CHILDREN	ADULTS
Best eye opening 4 – Spontaneous 3 – Opens to verbal stimulus 2 – Opens to painful stimulus 1 – No response	**Best eye opening** 4 – Spontaneous 3 – Opens to verbal stimulus 2 – Opens to painful stimulus 1 – No response	**Best eye opening** 4 – Spontaneous 3 – Opens to verbal stimulus 2 – Opens to painful stimulus 1 – No response
Best verbal response 5 – Coos and babbles 4 – Irritable cry 3 – Cries to pain 2 – Moans to pain 1 – No response	**Best verbal response** 5 – Orientated 4 – Confused 3 – Inappropriate words 2 – Incomprehensible words 1 – No response	**Best verbal response** 5 – Orientated (person, place, time) 4 – Confused, disorientated 3 – Inappropriate words 2 – Incomprehensible words 1 – No response
Best motor response 6 – Spontaneous purposeful movement 5 – Localizes to pain 4 – Withdraws to pain 3 – Flexion (decorticate response) 2 – Extension (decerebrate response) 1 – No response	**Best motor response** 6 – Obeys commands 5 – Localizes to pain 4 – Withdraws to pain 3 – Flexion (decorticate response) 2 – Extension (decerebrate response) 1 – No response	**Best motor response** 6 – Obeys commands 5 – Localizes to pain 4 – Withdraws to pain 3 – Flexion (decorticate response) 2 – Extension (decerebrate response) 1 – No response

Source: Reproduced from Jerry Zimmerman, Alexandre T. Rotta. Fuhrman & Zimmerman's Pediatric Critical Care, Sixth Edition, Evaluation, stabilization, and initial management after trauma, Fig. 117.4, Philadelphia, Elsevier Inc., 2022.

TABLE 1.4	Full Outline of Unresponsiveness (FOUR) Score Coma Scale

Eye Response
4	Eyelids open or opened, tracking, or blinking to command
3	Eyelids open but not tracking
2	Eyelids closed but open to loud voice
1	Eyelids closed but open to pain
0	Eyelids remain closed with pain

Motor Response
4	Thumbs-up, fist, or "peace" sign
3	Localizing to pain
2	Flexion response to pain
1	Extension response to pain
0	No response to pain or generalized myoclonus status

Brain Stem Reflexes
4	Pupil and corneal reflexes present
3	One pupil wide and fixed
2	Pupil or corneal reflexes absent
1	Pupil and corneal reflexes absent
0	Absent pupil, corneal, and cough reflexes

Respiration
4	Not intubated, regular breathing pattern
3	Not intubated, Cheyne–Stokes breathing pattern
2	Not intubated, irregular breathing
1	Breathes above ventilatory rate
0	Breathes at ventilator rate or apnea

Source: Adapted from Robert Kliegman, Joseph St. Geme. *Nelson Textbook of Pediatrics*, 2-Volume, 21st Edition, Neurologic Emergencies and Stabilization, Table 85.1, Philadelphia, Elsevier Inc., 2020.

- Recent memory — also called short-term memory (ability to reproduce events/sentences that have been happened/spoken few minutes [5 minutes] back)
- Long-term memory – also called remote memory (ability to recall events happened long time [years] back)

I – INTELLIGENCE

Ability to reason, solve problems, think abstractly, and comprehend complex ideas

B – BEHAVIOR PROBLEMS

Any aggressiveness, temper tantrums, hyperactivity (ADHD), and autistic features

Seizures and Involuntary Movement

Differentiating features of seizures and involuntary movement are given in Table 1.5.

Cranial Nerves

OLFACTORY NERVE (CRANIAL NERVE I)

It can be tested only in older children (>5 years of age). In others, it can be mentioned that the test is not feasible.
- Before testing, rule out the obstructive lesions of nose.
- Test each nostril separately.
- Newborns respond by turning their heads toward the substance, alerting response, and withdrawal.

OPTIC NERVE (CRANIAL NERVE II)

Test the following.

Visual Acuity

Methods of visual acuity evaluation are given in Table 1.6.

Visual Field

- In an infant or a young child, field of vision is assessed by advancing a brightly colored object from behind the child's head into the peripheral visual field and noting when the child first looks at the object.
- In older children, confrontation method/perimetry is used.

Color Vision

- Ishihara's charts/Holmgren's wool method is used.

TABLE 1.6	Methods of Evaluating Visual Acuity	
Age	**Method of Testing**
Newborn	Optokinetic nystagmus — eye movement is in the direction of black and white stripes
Infancy	Red wool held at a distance of 25 cm from the eye — a 1-month-old baby follows the object at 90° and a 3-month-old baby follows at 180°
1–2 years	Ability to follow rolling white balls of various sizes
2–3 years	Card is held in front of the baby. A similar card is held by the examiner and a letter is pointed out. The child is asked to point out the similar letter in the card.
3–6 years	Modified or illiterate Snellen chart and illiterate E chart
>6 years	Snellen chart — distant vision Jaeger's chart — near vision

Pupils

- Size, shape, pupillary reflex, and menace reflex are noted.

Fundus Examination

- This examination is performed by holding ophthalmoscope close to the examiner's eye **and 12–18 inches away** from the infant's eyes.
- The other examination is red reflex test, which is performed in newborns. It is performed in a darkened room by using a direct ophthalmoscope.

OCULOMOTOR, TROCHLEAR, AND ABDUCENT NERVES (CRANIAL NERVES III, IV, AND VI)

Extraocular Movements

- Squint/strabismus
  - Hirschberg test: It is a screening test to check whether the child suffers from strabismus, and also to quantify strabismus. A flash light is shown in the center of the child's face and it is noted whether both sides (cornea and pupil) are at an equal distance from the light. Another name for Hirschberg test is corneal reflex test.
  - Technique
    Light is shown into the child's eye and the point from where the light reflects off the cornea is observed. If the child has normal ocular alignment, the light reflex lies slightly nasal from the center of the cornea (approximately 11 prism diopters — or 0.5 mm from the pupillary axis). In this test, light reflexes on both the corneas are compared. On the basis of where the light lands on the cornea, examiner can detect the following: abnormal eye turned out — exotropia; abnormal eye turned in — esotropia; abnormal eye higher than the normal one — hypertropia; or abnormal eye lower than the normal one — hypotropia.
    Fig. 1.1 shows Hirschberg test.
- Differentiating features of concomitant and incomitant squint are given in Table 1.7.
- Primary and secondary deviation: The deviation of squint eye is called primary deviation and when squinting eye

TABLE 1.5	Differentiating Features of Seizures and Involuntary Movements	
Features	**Seizures**	**Involuntary Movement**
Pattern	Tonic/clonic; chaotic	Stereotyped
Duration	Shorter	Longer
Loss of consciousness	Present	Absent
EEG	Abnormal	Normal
During sleep	Do not disappear	Disappear

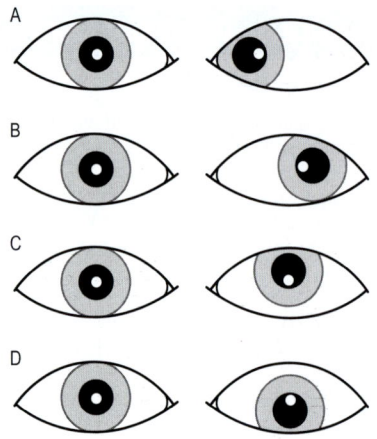

Fig. 1.1 Hirschberg test: (A) Esotropia (eye turned outward); (B) exotropia (eye turned inward); (C) hypertropia (eye turned upward); and (D) hypotropia (eye turned downward). *(Source: Reproduced from Michel Millodot. Dictionary of Optometry and Vision Science, Eighth Edition, Fig. S14, London, Elsevier Ltd, 2018.)*

TABLE 1.7	Differentiating Concomitant and Incomitant Squint	
Features	**Concomitant Squint**	**Incomitant Squint**
Presentation	Most common	Least common
Onset	Early childhood/gradual	Sudden
Deviation of eye	Primary deviation	Secondary deviation
Amount of gaze	Same in all directions	Varies with gaze position
Cause	Defective vision in one eye/change in accommodation/muscle maldevelopment	Muscle/nerve paralysis
Diplopia	Absent	Present
Extra Ocular Movements (EOM)	Normal	Restricted in affected muscle
Types	1. Convergent – two types: infantile and accommodative 2. Divergent – two types: intermittent and constant	3rd nerve – divergent squint, downward deviation and ptosis 4th nerve – head tilt toward opposite shoulder 6th nerve – convergent squint

Note: Pseudostrabismus– false appearance of squint seen in epicanthal fold.

is made to fix on an object by closing the normal eye, the normal eye deviates under cover – this is secondary deviation.

The following tests are used to differentiate between latent and manifest squint:
   a. Cover test is performed to differentiate between pseudostrabismus and manifest strabismus.
      • Normal eye is closed with an occluder.
      • It there is movement in the nonoccluded eye and that eye takes up fixation, it is manifest squint.
      • If there is no movement in the nonoccluded eye, it is pseudostrabismus (it is seen if the child has epicanthal fold).
   b. Cover–uncover test: To detect latent squint, each eye is covered separately one by one. If squint is present, the eye under cover will deviate as we are eliminating the fusion mechanism by occluding the other eye. On uncovering, the eye will move to normal position.
      Fig. 1.2 shows cover–uncover test.
- Differences between latent and manifest squint are given in Table 1.8.

Nystagmus

- Types
  1. Pendular
  2. Jerky
- Types based on the position of eye
  1. End-point nystagmus
  2. Fixation nystagmus
  3. Positional nystagmus

Ptosis

Check whether it is present or not.

Reflexes

- Direct and indirect light reflexes
- Accommodation reflex

Doll's Eye Movement

- Check for doll's eye movement in an unconscious child.

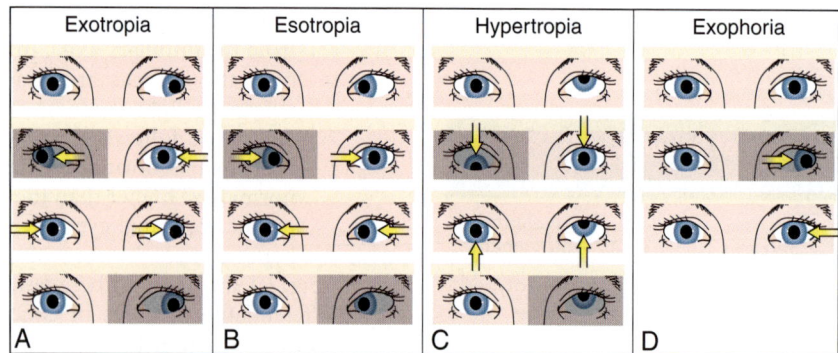

Fig. 1.2 Cover–uncover test. *(Source: Reproduced from Friedman, Neil J. Friedman, Roberto Pineda II. The Massachusetts Eye and Ear Infirmary Illustrated Manual of Ophthalmology, Fifth Edition, Appendix, Fig A.14, London, Elsevier Inc., 2021.)*

TABLE 1.8	Differences Between Latent and Manifest Squint	
Latent Squint		**Manifest Squint**
Not visible at rest		Visible at rest
Cover–uncover test – squint will manifest		Hirschberg test
Most common		Not common

TABLE 1.9	Motor Component of Facial Nerve	
Test		**Muscle Tested**
Ask the patient to frown		Frontal belly of occipitofrontalis
Ask the patient to tightly close the eyes		Orbicularis oculi
Ask the patient to blow the cheek		Buccinator
Ask the patient to whistle		Orbicularis oris
Ask the patient to show the teeth		Depressor angularis
Ask the patient to evert lower lip		Platysma

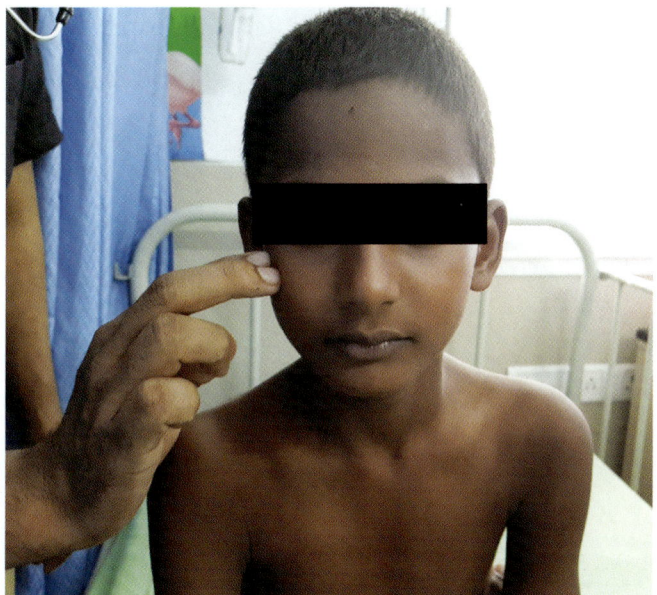

Fig. 1.3 Eliciting masseter reflex.

CRANIAL NERVE V

- Sensory component − sensations over the face
- Motor component − wasting of masseter and temporalis muscle, deviation of jaw on affected side on opening the mouth (Fig. 1.3)
- Reflexes − corneal, conjunctival, and jaw jerk

CRANIAL NERVE VII

- Sensory component − taste sensation on anterior two-thirds of tongue/Schirmer's test
- Motor component − look for facial asymmetry (Table 1.9)
- Reflexes − conjunctival, corneal, and stapedial reflex

CRANIAL NERVE VIII

- Vestibular component – it is tested by doll's eye movement and caloric testing (in older children).
  Caloric test: The patient is made to lie on the couch with his or her head elevated to 30° to bring the lateral semicircular canals into vertical plane. The patient is instructed to fix his or her eyes on a point in central gaze and the external ear is irrigated with water (air in ruptured tympanic) at 30°C and 44°C for 30–40 seconds. Response in normal ear (remember mnemonic COWS) will be as follows:
  - Cold water (30°C) − nystagmus away from ear being irrigated (opposite side)
  - Warm water (44°C) − nystagmus toward the ear under test (same side)
- Cochlear component− it is tested in older children by Rinne and Weber test as given in Table 1.10 (by using 512-Hz tuning fork)
- Murphy's sound localization method is used in infants and young children as shown in Fig. 1.4.

TABLE 1.10	Cochlear Component − Hearing Test			
Test	**Normal Ears**	**Conducting Deafness**	**Sensorineural Deafness**
Rinne test: Strike a tuning fork and place it on the mastoid process. When the patient ceases to hear, the fork is held near the external auditory canal. Normally, it is continued to be heard.	Air conduction (AC) > bone conduction (BC); Rinne test result is positive	BC > AC; Rinne test result is negative	AC > BC; Rinne test result is positive
Weber test: Vibrating fork is placed in the center of forehead or vertex of the head. Normally, the sound is heard equally in both ears.	Not lateralized	Lateralized to poorer ear	Lateralized to better ear
Absolute bone conduction: The patient's bone conduction is compared with the examiner's (meatus is occluded).	Same as examiner	Same as examiner	Reduced
Schwabach test: The patient's bone conduction is compared with the examiner's (meatus is not occluded).	Equal	Lengthened	Shortened

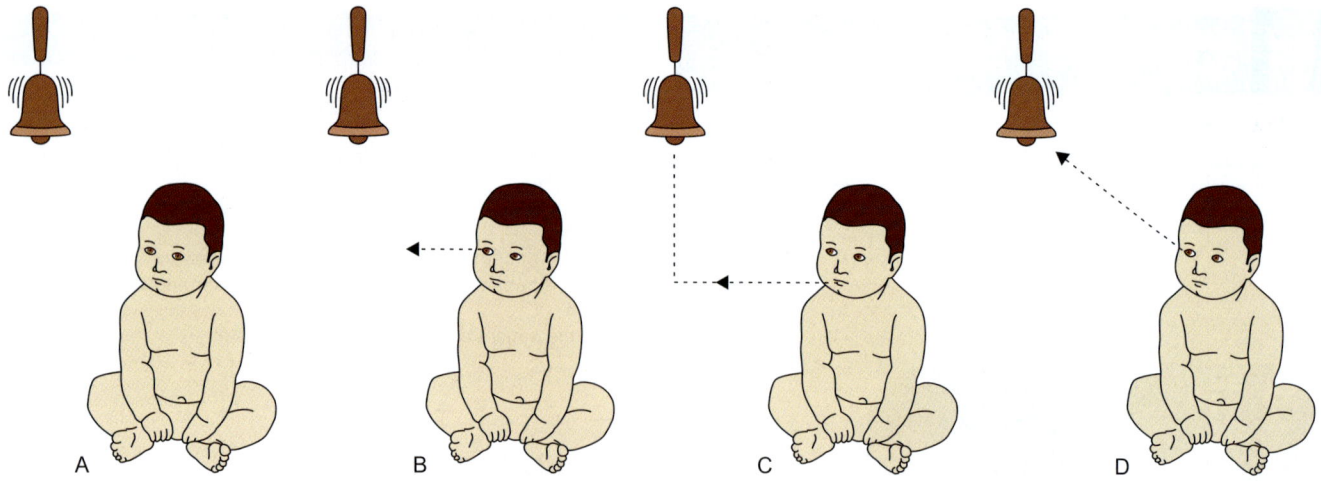

Fig. 1.4 (A–D) Localization of sound.

- Test is performed by ringing a bell at 45 cm away from the ear and away from the sight.
  - Newborn – startles or quietens
  - 3-month old – localizes in the same direction
  - 5- to 6-month old – looks downwards
  - 6- to 7-month old – looks upwards
  - 8- to 10-month old – looks diagonally</

CRANIAL NERVE IX

Check for gag reflex and taste sensation on the posterior one-third of tongue.

CRANIAL NERVE X

- Deviation of uvula to normal side
- Absence of elevation of soft palate on the affected side on saying "ahh"
- Bilateral lesions can produce dysphonia and impaired cough
- Pooling of secretions in oral cavity

SPINAL CRANIAL NERVE XI

- Look for prominence of sternocleidomastoid muscle.
- Check whether the patient is able to turn his or her head side-to-side.
- Check whether the patient is able to shrug the shoulders (Fig. 1.5).

CRANIAL NERVE XII

- Look for tongue movements.
- Check for wasting.
- Check for fasciculations.

Spinomotor System

POSTURE

Mention the posture of the child.

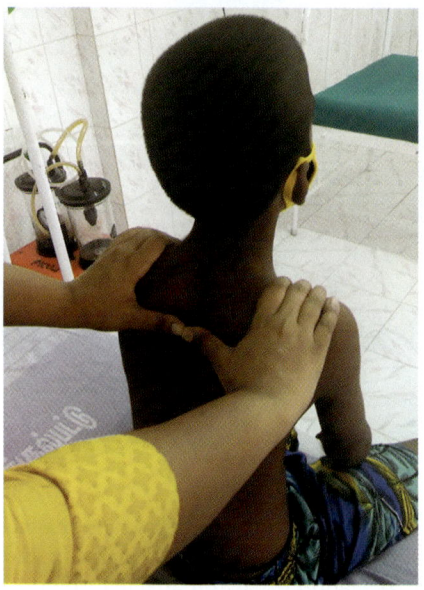

Fig. 1.5 Testing spinal accessory nerve.

BULK

- Look for wasting/pseudohypertrophy.

TONE

- Tone is defined as resistance to passive stretch of a muscle throughout its range of motion.
  a. Increased tone is of two types:
    - Spasticity: It is velocity dependent and has a sudden release after reaching a maximum (clasp-knife phenomenon).
    - Rigidity: It is velocity independent. Hypertonia is present throughout the range of motion.
  b. Decreased tone – flaccidity
    - In children up to the age of 2 years, check for
      - Active tone – pull to sit, vertical suspension, ventral suspension

TABLE 1.11	Ashworth's and Modified Ashworth's Classification – Grading of Spasticity

GRADE	DESCRIPTION
0	No increase in muscle tone
1	Slight increase in muscle tone, manifested by a catch and release or by minimal resistance at the end of the ROM when the affected part(s) is moved in flexion or extension
1+	Slight increase in muscle tone, manifested by a catch, followed by minimal resistance throughout the remainder (less than half) of the ROM
2	More marked increase in muscle tone through most of the ROM, but affected part(s) easily moved
3	Considerable increase in muscle tone, passive movement difficult
4	Affected part(s) rigid in flexion or extension

Source: Reproduced from Mary Patnaude. *Early's Physical Dysfunction Practice - Skills for the Occupational Therapy Assistant,* Fourth Edition, Assessment of Motor Control and Functional Movement, Fig. 6.2, St. Loius, Mosby Inc., 2022. (Credit- From Bohannon RW, Smith MB. Interrater reliability of a modified Ashworth scale of muscle spasticity. Phys Ther. 1987;67:206–207.)

  ◦ Passive tone − arm recoil sign, scarf sign, heel-to-ear test, popliteal angle, ankle dorsiflexion
  ◦ 180°, flip-flop maneuver
  For grading of spasticity, Ashworth's classification is used, which is given in Table 1.11.

POWER

- Power is a defined force of contraction that can be generated voluntarily by the muscle.
- The Medical Research Council scale for grading muscle strength is as follows:
  - Grade 0: No contraction
  - Grade 1: Flicker or trace of contraction
  - Grade 2: Active movement with gravity eliminated
  - Grade 3: Active movement against gravity
  - Grade 4: Active movement against gravity and resistance
  - Grade 5: Normal power
- Commonly, grade 4 is divided into 4−, 4, and 4+, denoting severe, moderate, and mild weakness, respectively, and some use 5− to signify minimal weakness.
- In children who are unable to cooperate, the best observed power is used. Power should not be tested in an unconscious child.
  Fig. 1.6A−S shows testing of power in children in upper and lower limbs.

COORDINATION

It should be tested only when the power is 3 or more.
  - Upper limb − finger-to-nose and finger-to-finger test, and dysdiadokokinesis.

- Fig. 1.7A and B shows finger-to-nose test and Fig. 1.8A and B shows dysdiadokokinesis.
- Lower limb − heel-to-knee test is shown in Fig. 1.9A and B, and tandem walking is shown in Fig. 1.10.

REFLEXES

- Reflex: A reflex is a consistent involuntary adaptive response to the stimulation of a sense organ. Reinforcement technique such as Jendrassik maneuver is used to elicit a reflex − clenching of teeth, flashing light in the eyes, and looking at the ceiling as shown in Fig. 1.11.
- Superficial reflex: Techniques for demonstrating superficial reflexes are given in Table 1.12.
- Deep tendon reflex: Root values of deep tendon reflex are given in Table 1.13.
- Grading of deep tendon reflex
  - Grade 0: Absent reflexes
  - Grade 1: Present (as normal ankle jerk)
  - Grade 2: Brisk (as normal knee jerk)
  - Grade 3: Exaggerated
  - Grade 4: Clonus
- Primitive reflex: For primitive reflexes, refer Chapter 2: Cerebral Palsy.

BABINSKI REFLEX

Normal Plantar Reflex

- When the lateral side of the sole of the foot is rubbed with a blunt instrument (which does not cause pain), three responses are seen:
  - Flexor − the toe curves downward and inward, the foot inverts
  - Extensor − the great toe (hallux) dorsiflexes, other toes fan out (Babinski sign)
  - No response
  Fig. 1.12 shows Babinski sign.

Reflexes Equivalent to Babinski Reflex When Upper Limb Is Injured or Amputated

Fig. 1.13A and B shows equivalent of Babinski sign in upper limb.
  - Hoffman reflex: Child's terminal phalanx of the middle finger is flicked downwards between the examiner's finger and thumb. The tips of the other fingers flex and the thumb flexes and adducts in states of hypertonia.
  - **Wartenberg reflex:** The patient supinates his or her hand, slightly flexing the fingers with thumb in abduction. The examiner pronates his or her hand and links his or her fingers with that of the patient's (Fig. 1.13B). On pulling each other:
    - Normal − thumb extends though phalanx; may flex slightly
    - Pyramidal lesion − thumb adducts and flexes strongly

Other Upper Limb Reflexes

- Klippel–Feil sign – involuntary flexion, opposition and adduction of the thumb on passive extension of fingers.
- Leri sign: On forcibly flexing the patient's wrist and finger when the forearm is kept supinated and slightly flexed, normally there is contraction of biceps and flexion of

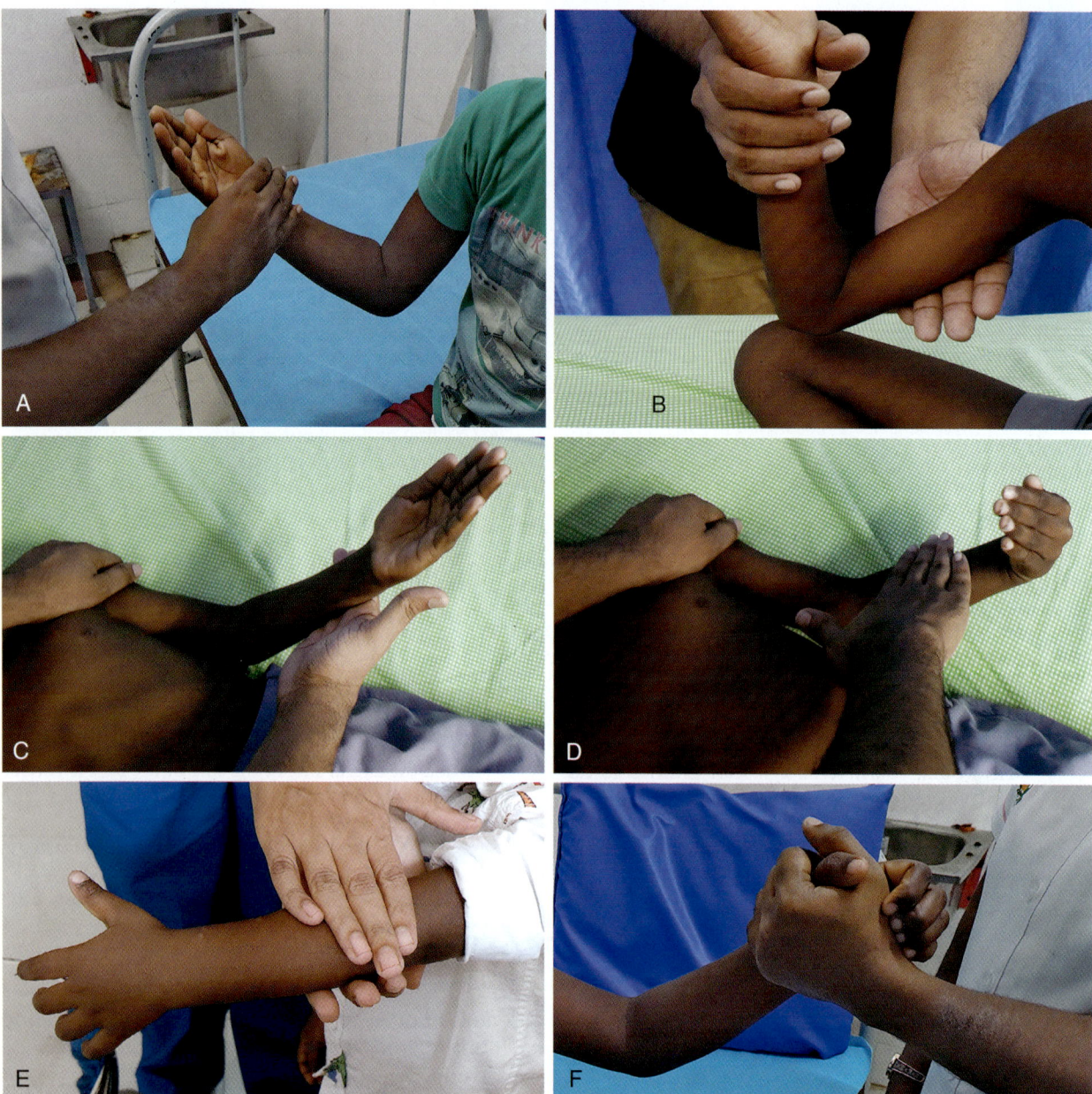

Fig. 1.6   (A) Testing biceps brachii by flexing the forearm against resistance. (B) Testing power of triceps against resistance. (C) Testing extensors of forearm against resistance. (D) Testing flexors of forearm against resistance. (E) Testing supinator – the posterior part of the proximal third of the radius is palpated in mid-position when the child's arm and forearm are in extension with the forearm in mid-position by actively resisting supination. (F) Testing brachioradialis by flexing the semipronated forearm with thumbs up.

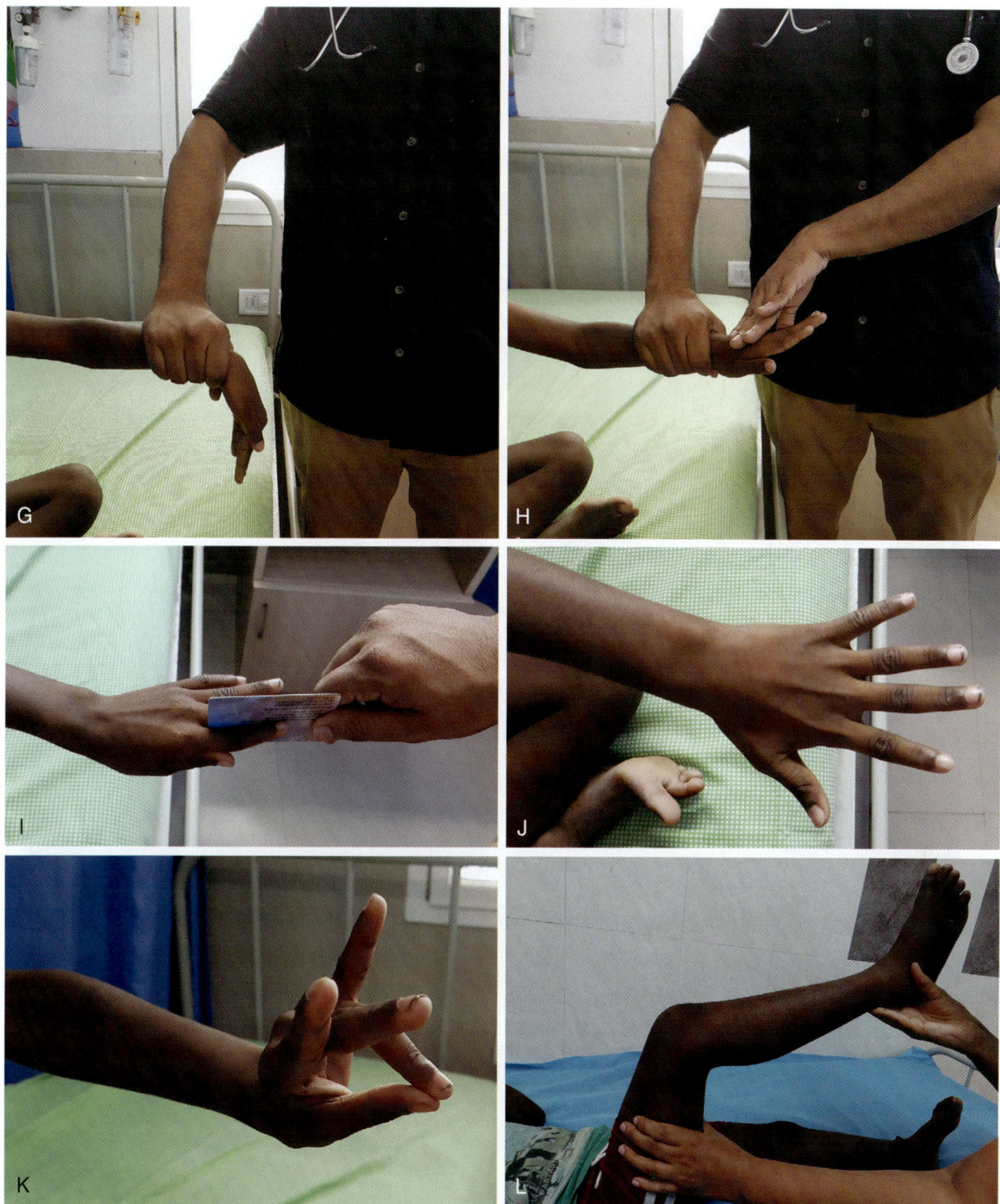

Fig. 1.6, cont'd (G) Testing flexors of wrist. (H) Extensor of wrist joint against resistance. (I) Testing adduction action of palmar interossei **(PAD)** of fingers. (J) Testing abduction by dorsal interossei of fingers **(DAB)**. (K) Testing opponens pollicis. (L) Testing flexors of hip joint.

Continued

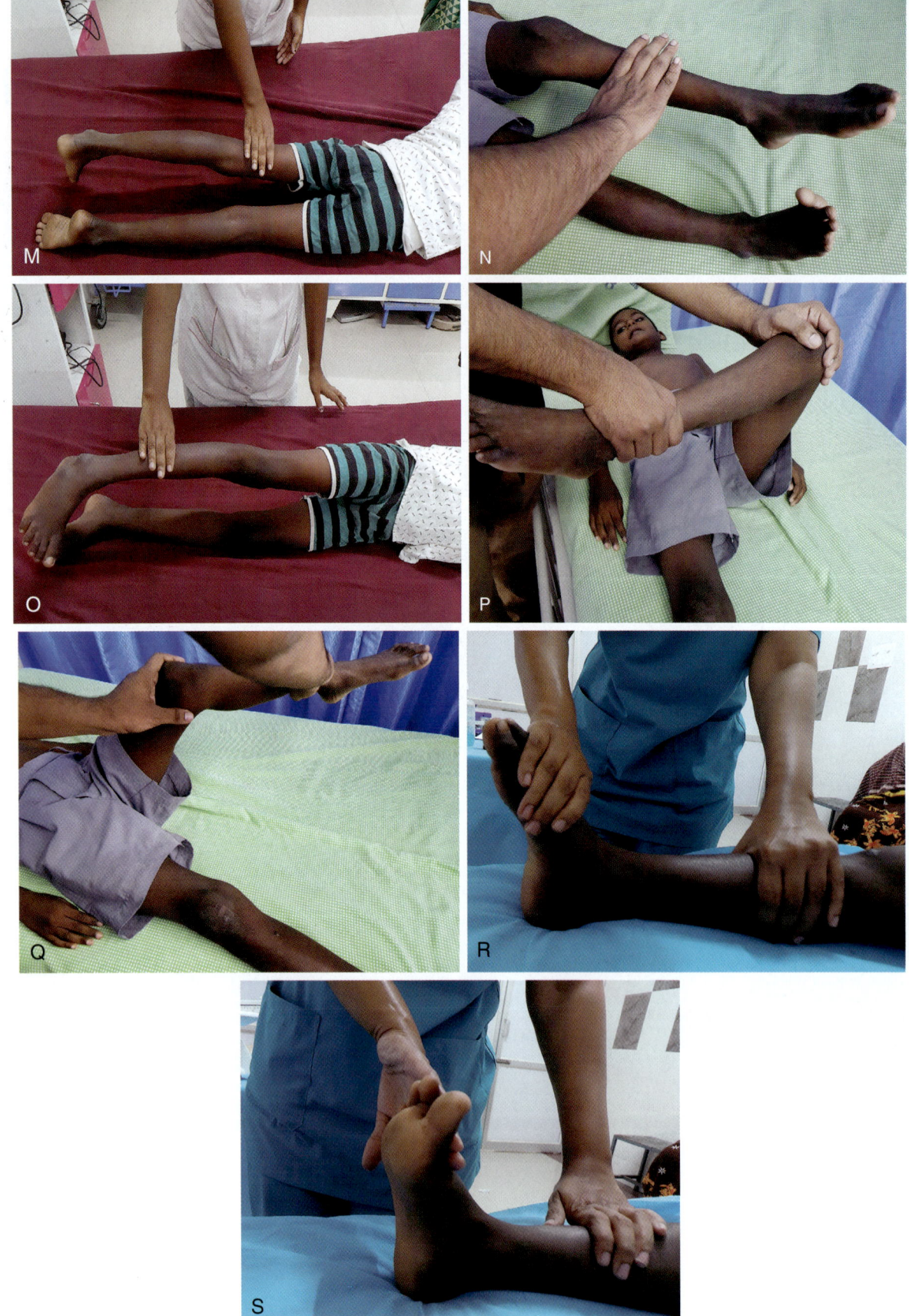

Fig. 1.6, cont'd   (M) Testing extensors of hip joint. (N) Testing flexion of knee joint. (O) Testing extension of knee joint. (P) Testing adduction. (Q) Abduction of knee joint. (R) Testing dorsiflexion of ankle joint. (S) Testing plantar flexion of ankle joint.

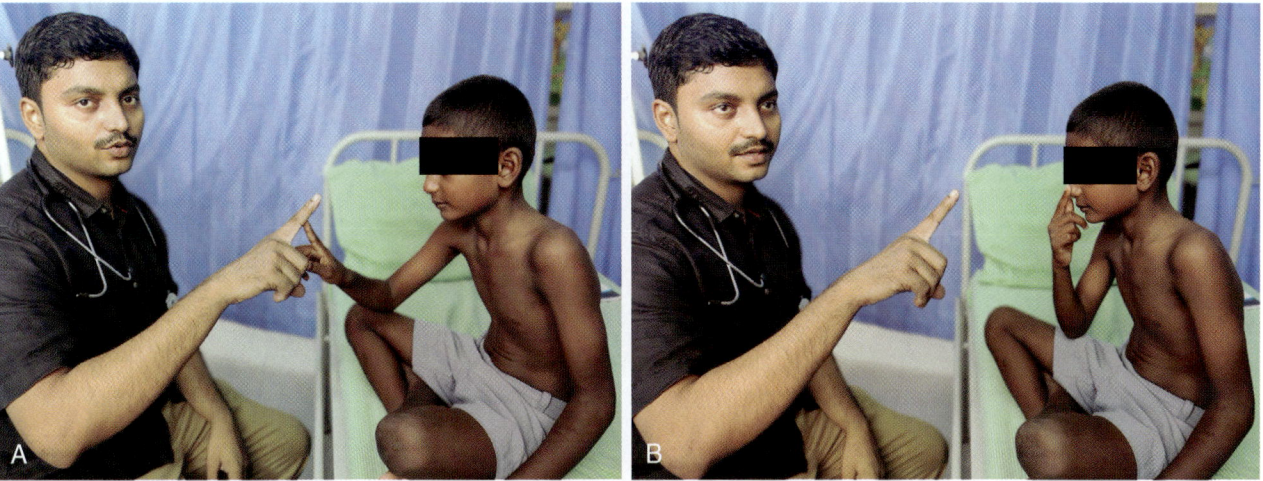

Fig. 1.7 (A and B) Finger-to-nose test (the child first touches the examiner's finger and then touches his nose).

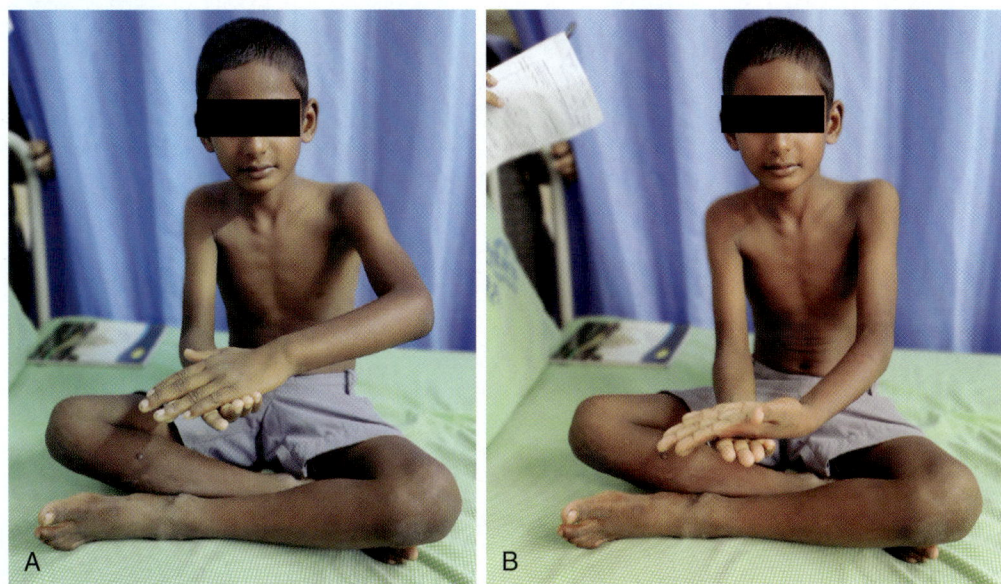

Fig. 1.8 (A and B) Dysdiadokokinesis.

elbow. This is absent in corticospinal tract lesion and is called Leri sign.

- Mayer sign: The patient's hand is held in examiner's hand, palm up, fingers slightly bent and thumb in slight flexion and abduction. Firm pressure on the proximal phalanges of third and fourth fingers flexing at the metacarpal joints causes adduction and opposition of thumb with flexion of metacarpophalangeal joints and extension at interphalangeal joints in normal individual. Absence of response is Mayer sign and indicates corticospinal lesion.

Reflexes Equivalent to Babinski Reflex When Lower Limb Is Injured or Amputated

- Gordon reflex: Squeezing or pinching calf muscle produces extensor plantar response in pyramidal tract lesion (Fig. 1.14A).

- Chaddock reflex: It refers to extensor response obtained on striking skin around the lateral malleolus in circular pattern (Fig. 1.14B).
- Oppenheim sign: Reflex is evoked by applying pressure on anteromedial aspect of tibia from above downward (Fig. 1.14C).
- Bing sign: Pinpricking of dorsum of the foot produces extensor reflex in pyramidal lesion.
- Gonda sign: Forceful snapping down of distal phalanx of second or fourth toe produces extensor response.
- Moniz sign: Forceful plantar flexion of the ankle produces extensor response in pyramidal lesion.
- Brissaud sign: When toe is absent or amputated, stroking of sole elicits contraction of tensor fascia lata which can be considered a part of plantar extensor response.

Fig. 1.14A–C shows equivalent of Babinski sign in lower limb.

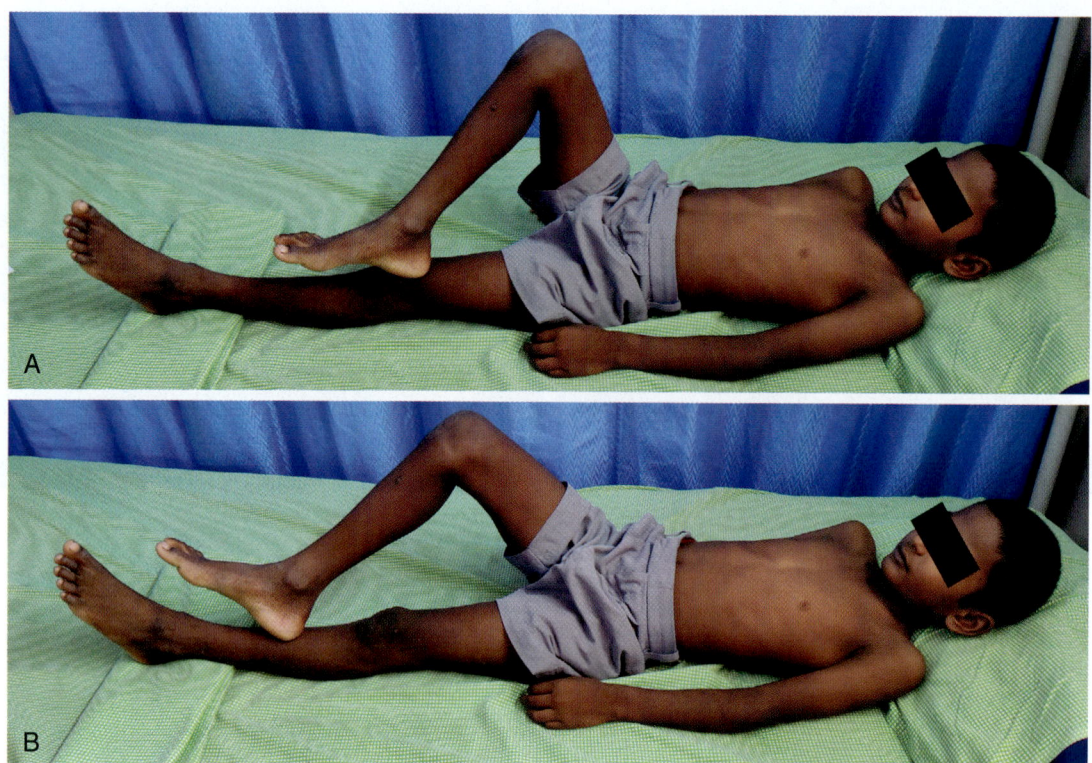

Fig. 1.9 (A and B) Heel-to-knee test.

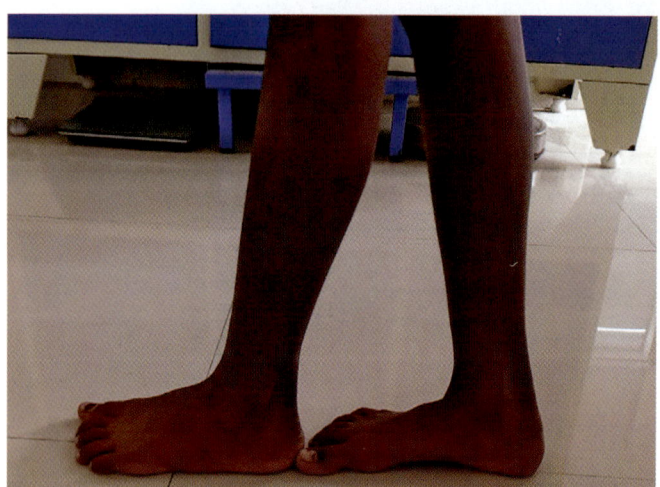

Fig. 1.10 Demonstrating tandem walking.

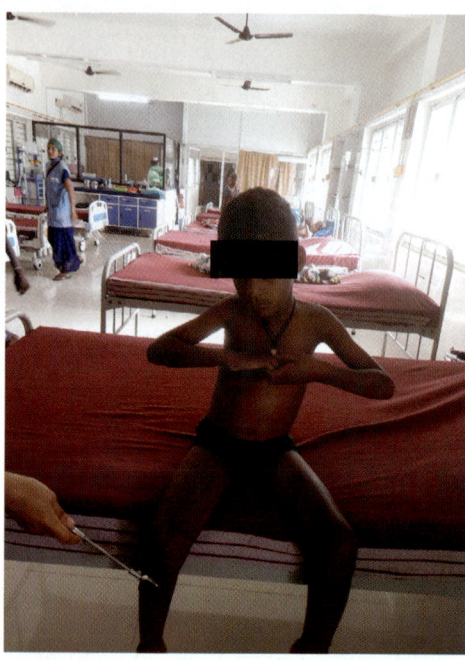

Fig. 1.11 Demonstrating Jendrassik maneuver.

Equivocal Babinski

To elicit a plantar reflex, patient has to be exposed from hip to toe.

1. Flexion of the hip or knee without movement of the toe.
2. Only extension of the great toe with or without movement of other toes.
3. Rapid and brief extension of toes at first, which is followed by flexion, and then again followed by extension.

Pseudo-Babinski Response

Babinski response obtained in the absence of pyramidal tract lesion is called pseudo-Babinski response. It is not associated with contraction of hamstring as in Babinski reflex and pressure on the base of the great toe can inhibit the withdrawal extensor response. The following responses are considered as pseudo-Babinski responses:

a. Voluntary withdrawal in overtly sensitive individual
b. Strong painful stimulus
c. Extrapyramidal lesion

TABLE 1.12	Eliciting Superficial Reflexes	
Superficial Reflex	**Segmental Level**	**Technique**
Corneal reflex	Afferent – 5th nerve Efferent – 7th nerve	When the patient looks in the opposite direction, corneal edge is touched with wisp of cotton
Conjunctival reflex	Afferent – 5th nerve Efferent – 7th nerve	Bulbar conjunctiva is touched with wisp of cotton
Pharyngeal reflex	Afferent – 9th nerve Efferent – 10th nerve	Posterior wall of pharynx is tickled
Palatal reflex	Afferent – 5th nerve Efferent – 10th nerve	Soft palate is tickled
Scapular reflex	Afferent: C4–C5 Efferent: Dorsal	Skin of the interscapular region is stroked
Abdominal reflex	T7–T11	Abdominal skin is stimulated in four quadrants
Cremasteric reflex	Afferent: Femoral nerve (L1, L2) Efferent: Genitofemoral nerve	Upper and inner part of thigh is stroked in a downward and inward direction
Plantar reflex	Afferent: Tibial nerve (S1, S2) Efferent: Tibial nerve	Knee is flexed and thigh is externally rotated; ankle joint is fixed and lateral side of sole is stroked till great toe

TABLE 1.13	Root Values of Deep Tendon Reflex
Deep Tendon Reflex	**Segmental Level**
Jaw jerk	Trigeminal nerve
Trapezius reflex	Spinal accessory nerve
Biceps jerk	C5–C6 musculocutaneous nerve
Supinator jerk	C5–C6 radial nerve
Triceps jerk	C6–C7 radial nerve
Finger flexion	C6–T1
Knee jerk	L2–L4 femoral nerve
Ankle jerk	S1 medial popliteal nerve
Adductor reflex	L2–L4 obturator nerve

CLONUS

- Definition

  It refers to a series of rhythmic involuntary muscular contraction induced by sudden passive stretching of a muscle or tendon. It is frequently seen in ankle, knee, and wrist. Sustained clonus is a sign of pyramidal tract lesion.

- Demonstration of clonus
  - Patellar clonus: The leg is extended and relaxed as shown in Fig. 1.15A. Method: The patella is grasped by the examiner between index finger and thumb and a sudden, sharp, downward thrust is executed.
  - Ankle clonus (Fig. 1.15B): Sharp dorsiflexion of the foot initiates stretch reflex in plantar flexors, provoking a reflex in dorsiflexors alternatively.

INVOLUNTARY MOVEMENTS

- Chorea (caudate): It refers to involuntary, continual, and irregular movements arising in the proximal joints and appearing to flit from one part to another.
  - Hypotonia
  - Darting tongue – involuntary protrusion and retraction of tongue
  - Pronator sign – palms facing outward when abducted above head
  - Milkmaid grip – milking action is perceived on holding the examiner's hand
  - Hung-up reflex – seen when eliciting knee jerk

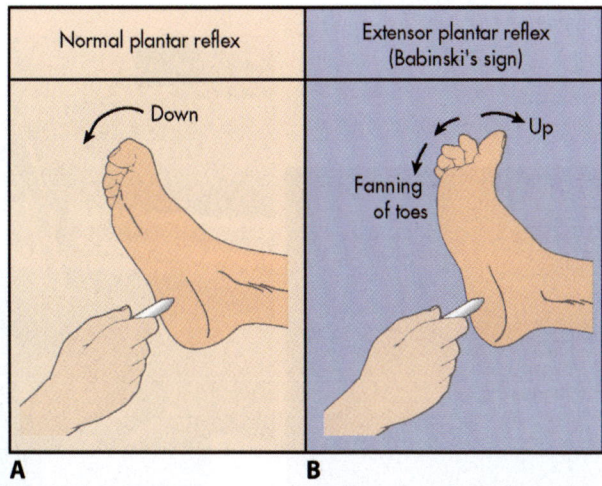

Fig. 1.12 Babinski sign. (*Source: Reproduced from* Harminder Singh, Itika Singh. *Fundamentals of Medical Physiology*, Figure 69-12, New Delhi, Elsevier India, 2018. [Source: Berne & Levy Principles of Physiology. 2006. Figure 9-16, Babinski's sign. A, The normal response to stroking the plantar surface of the foot. B, Babinski's sign (extensor plantar reflex) in a person with interruption of the corticospinal tract]).

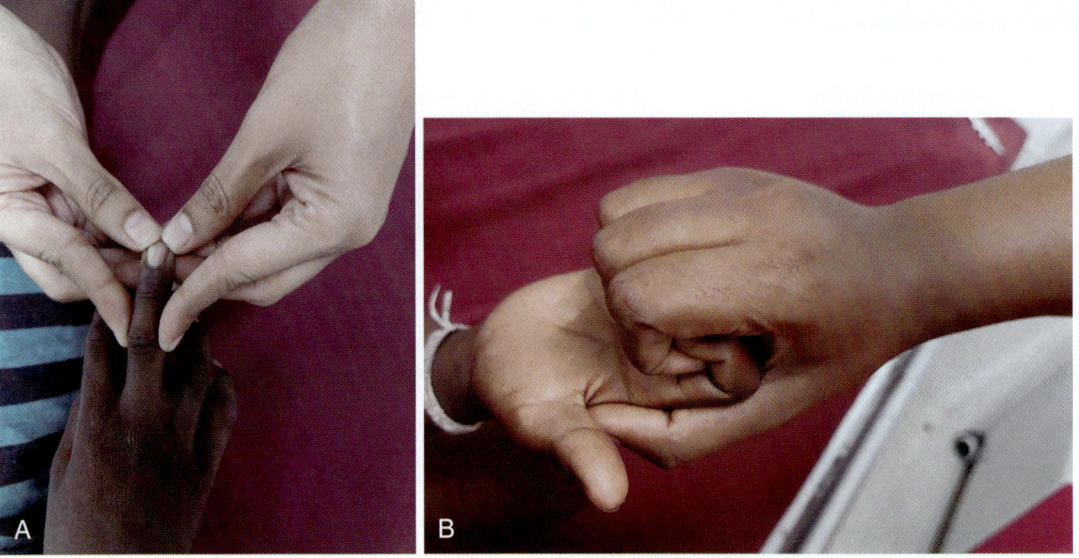

Fig. 1.13   (A) Eliciting Hoffman reflex. (B) Eliciting Wartenberg reflex.

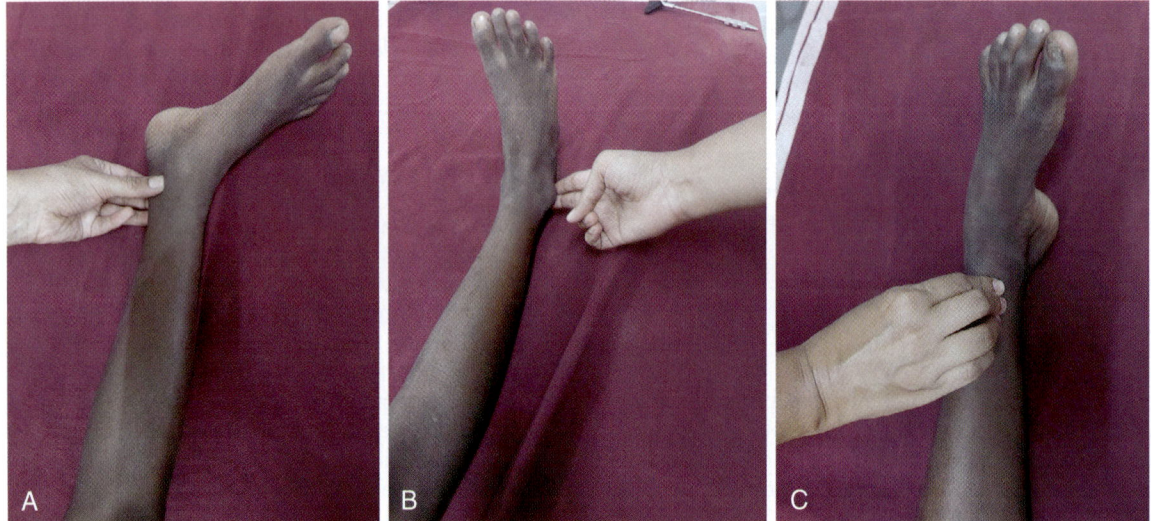

Fig. 1.14   (A) Gordon sign. (B) Chaddock sign. (C) Oppenheim sign.

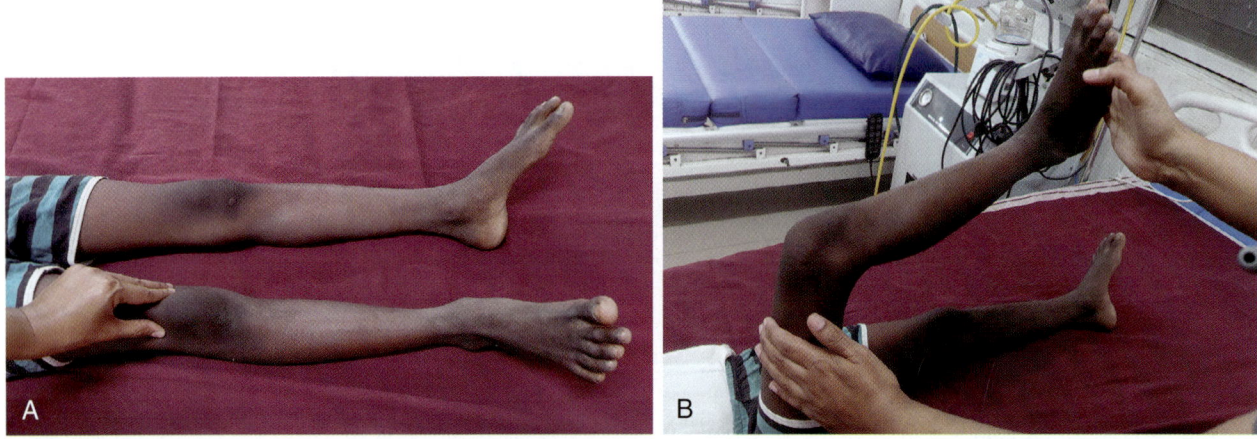

Fig. 1.15   (A) Eliciting patellar clonus. (B) Ankle clonus.

- Athetosis (putamen): It refers to slow writhing movement, most commonly involves wrist, fingers, and ankle.
- Hemiballismus (subthalamic nucleus): It refers to involuntary, high-amplitude flinging movement typically occurring proximally.
- Myoclonus: It refers to sudden, quick involuntary jerks of muscles.
- Tremor: It refers to oscillating, rhythmic movements about a fixed point or axis.
- Tics: It refers to involuntary, sudden, rapid, abrupt simple or complex movements or vocalization usually preceded by an urge that is relieved by carrying out the movement.
- Dystonia: It refers to intermittent and sustained muscle contraction that produces abnormal postures and movements of different parts of the body with twisting quality.
- Fibrillation: Rapid, irregular twitching of single muscle fibre (invisible).
- Fasciculation: Involuntary contraction and relaxation of single muscle fascicle or group of muscle fibers (visible, felt by the individual and palpable).
- Myokymia: Involuntary eyelid quivering or twitching, due to contraction by bundle of muscle fascicles.
- All involuntary movements disappear during sleep, except:
  - Spinal myoclonus
  - Periodic sleep movement

GAIT

The child is asked to walk in a straight line for at least 9 meters and then turn and walk back to the starting point, and the following points are noted:
- Posture of the body while walking
- Position and movement of the arm
- Arm swing
  - The distance between the feet both in forward and lateral directions
- The relative ease and smoothness of movement of the legs
- Regularity of the movement
- The ability to maintain a straight course
- The ease of turning and finally stopping

Sensory System

- Cortical sensation
  - Tactile localization
  - Tactile discrimination
  - Stereognosis
  - Graphesthesia
- Peripheral system: Check for the following sensations in each dermatome:
  - Fine touch
  - Crude touch
  - Pain
  - Temperature
  - Vibrations (by using 128-Hz tuning fork)
  - Joint sense (Fig. 1.16)
  - Position sense (Fig. 1.17)
- Joint sense
  It is tested on each side separately.
  - Ask the patient to close eyes.
  - It is tested from small joints. If the patient fails to identify, subsequently larger joints are tested.

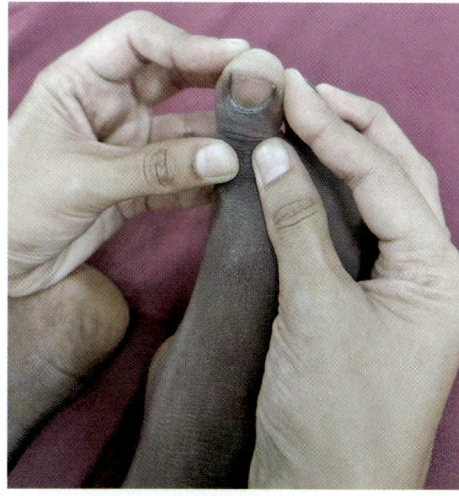

Fig. 1.16 Eliciting joint sense.

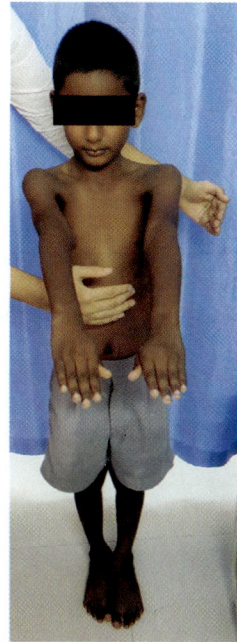

Fig. 1.17 Demonstrating Romberg sign – posterior column lesion (examiner should stand by the side of the child to prevent falling).

- Explain the patient which is up or down direction.
- The joint is fixed; the distal interphalangeal joint is moved up or down at 30° or side-to-side without touching the pulp of finger or adjacent toe or finger as shown in Fig. 1.16.
- Ask the patient to repeat the direction as instructed.
- Position sense (Romberg sign)
  Ask the patient to stand upright with feet together and eyes closed (Fig. 1.17). If the posterior column lesion is present, the patient sways and falls.

Cerebellar System

Look for the following:
- Dyssynergia: It refers to a difficulty in carrying out complex movements.

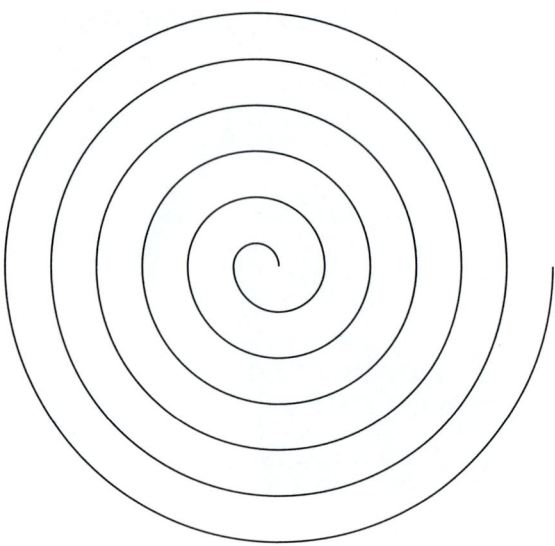

Fig. 1.18 Ask the patient to draw along the circle on the line to assess the cerebellar function.

- Dysmetria: It is the loss of ability to gauge the distance, speed, or power of movement.

It is clinically tested by asking the patient to follow the circle as shown in Fig. 1.18.

- Dysdiadochokinesia: It is the loss of ability to perform alternating movements smoothly and rapidly.
- Rebound phenomenon: Ask the patient to flex his or her elbow against the examiner's resistance. Then, suddenly let go of the patient's forearm. In case of cerebellar lesion, there is a loss of the "check reflex" because of failure of the ability to relax flexors of forearm. This may result in the patient striking his or her face with his or her hand.

- Hypotonia
- Ataxic gait
- Scanning speech
- Nystagmus
- Pendular knee jerk
- Intentional tremor
- Titubation

Signs of Meningeal Irritation

- Kernig sign: Ask the child to lie in supine position. Extension of flexed hip and knee causes painful spasm of hamstring muscle (Fig. 1.19).
- Brudzinski sign: It has two components:
  - Neck sign: Flexion of neck causes reflex flexion of knee and hip (Fig. 1.19).
  - Leg sign: Flexion of one limb causes flexion of the opposite limb.
- Benda sign: It is seen in TBM (Tuberculous meningitis).
  - Turning the head and chin of the child to one side causes upward and forward movement of the shoulder because of spasm of the trapezius muscle.
- Symphyseal sign: Abduction of leg and subsequent hip and knee flexion is seen when pressure is applied on the pubic symphysis.
- Cheek sign: When pressure is applied on the cheek below the zygoma, it leads to rising and flexion of forearm.
- Tache cerebrale: On stroking anywhere on the skin with a blunt object, there is raised red streak within 30–60 seconds (due to dilatation of superficial arterioles and capillaries).

Spine and Cranium

As described in general examination:
- Spine − tuft of hair, swelling, and hemangioma
- Cranium – head size (hydrocephalus) and shape

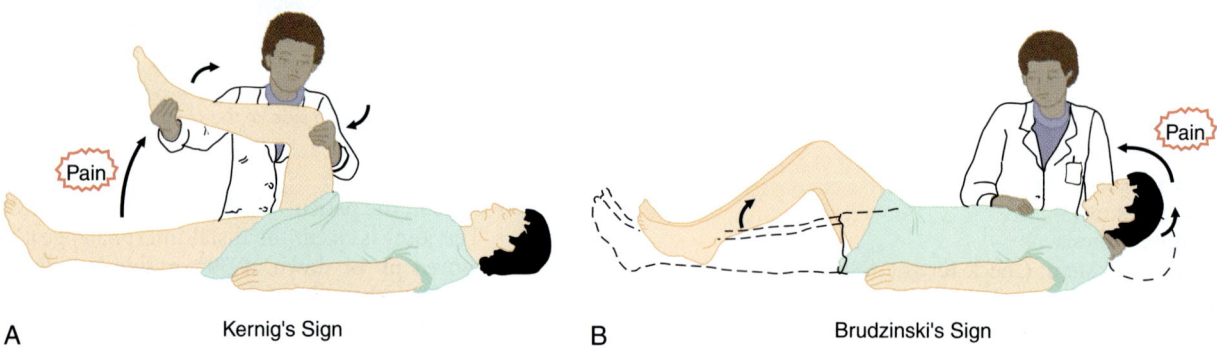

A   Kernig's Sign   B   Brudzinski's Sign

Fig. 1.19 Demonstration of meningeal signs. (Source: Reproduced from Malarvizhi S., Renuka Gugan. Black's Medical-Surgical Nursing: Clinical Management for Positive Outcomes, First South Asia Edition, Management of Clients with Cerebral Disorders, Figure 70–8, New Delhi, Elsevier India, 2019.)

Cerebral Palsy

Following introduction, seek permission from the caregiver and introduce yourself to the patient before history elicitation, and identify the case.

Name____Age____Sex____Consanguinity____Order of birth____Place____Informant____

Presenting Complaints and Duration

(To start with, a …-year-old child known to have neurological illness brought with the following complaints)

- Seizures
- Fever and fast breathing/breathing difficulty

History of Presenting Illness

- Seizures – seizure type (GTCS), number of episodes lasted for … minutes which the child used to have in the past, now admitted in the hospital and controlled with i.v. medication
- Fever – high grade, not associated with chills and rigors, associated with cough and cold or breathing difficulty
- Antenatal history taken first in any child with cerebral palsy (CP) because the child suffers from neurological problems since birth

Antenatal History

In CP, a detailed antenatal history is mandatory.

FIRST TRIMESTER

- Mother's age at marriage
- Birth order
- Conceived after how many years of marriage
- Spontaneous or induced conception
- Any abortion/medical termination of pregnancy/stillbirth/pregnancy confirmed by urine pregnancy test
- Registered and immunized
- History of hyperemesis
- Number of antenatal visits
- Immunization with TT/rubella vaccination
- Fever, rash, joint pain, and cervical swelling
- Any drug intake
- Irradiation exposure

SECOND TRIMESTER

- Quickening felt – 5 months
- Whether iron and folic acid taken regularly
- Antenatal scan
- Maternal weight gain
- Other complications in the antenatal period
    - Bleeding per vaginum
    - Twin gestation

- Eclampsia
- Maternal malnutrition
- Gestational diabetes, hypertension, anemia
- Chronic illness in the mother such as hypertension, diabetes, cardiac diseases, anemia, hypothyroidism, cardiac, any other systemic illnesses, and substance abuse

THIRD TRIMESTER

- History suggestive of urinary tract infection
- Any symptoms suggestive of chorioamnionitis (lower abdominal pain, foul-smelling discharge)
- Excessive bleeding
- Fetal movements
- Any monitoring done after hospital admission (CTG)

Natal History

- When did the labor pain start
- Rupture of membranes (duration from rupture of membranes to delivery)
- Induced/spontaneous onset of labor pain
- Progression of labor
- Place of delivery: Home/institutional
- Person conducting delivery: Trained/not trained (ANM)
- Duration of stages of labor
- Any history suggestive of precipitate labor
- Nature of delivery – natural/forceps/emergency or elective LSCS (indication/vacuum extraction)
- Difficult delivery
- Meconium staining or any fetal distress
- Breech/abnormal presentation

Immediate Postnatal History

- Cried immediately after birth and any resuscitative measures needed
- Preterm/post-term/term
- Birth weight – SGA/AGA/LGA
- Pale/cyanosis/pink
- Cry and activity – nil/excessive/normal
- Activity of child – normal/lethargic

Postnatal History

- Time when the feeding was initiated
- Breast milk flow and sufficient secretion present or not
- Any feeding or sucking difficulty
- Any prelacteal feeds
- Urine and meconium passed within 24 hours
- Any NICU admission for the following:
    - Birth asphyxia
    - Respiratory distress
    - Neonatal convulsions

- Jaundice/kernicterus – phototherapy or exchange transfusion done
- Any history of umbilical sepsis and umbilical catheterization
- Birth injuries
- Feeding difficulties
- Hypoglycemia

If there is a history of birth asphyxia, ask for the following 10 points:

1. Resuscitative measures at birth – duration/procedures such as bag and mask ventilation, intubation, chest compression, and adrenaline.
2. First seizure at … hours of life
   Were there any focal or subtle seizures or GTCS?
   How many anticonvulsants were required for seizure control?
   After how many hours did the seizure stop?
3. If the child is mechanically ventilated
   - How long (duration in days)
   - When weaning of ventilatory support started and CPAP, oxygen support given for how many days, and the child was in room air since when
   - Any history of neonatal shock and hypoglycemia
4. Feeding
   - I.v. fluid – how many days
   - Tube feed/paladai feed/expressed breast milk/direct breastfeeding and when it was initiated
   - How the sucking effort was
5. Any change in tone noted by the mother
   Flailness/slipping through the hand
   Lethargic
   Decreased spontaneous movements
6. Any CSF drawn (lumbar puncture)/neuroimaging done – USG cranium and MRI brain.
7. Any prescription of drugs for seizures at discharge.
8. Is the child on physiotherapy? Has the mother been familiar with physiotherapy?
9. At discharge – feeding, cry, and activity of the child.
10. Follow-up advice.

(Some examiners may expect developmental milestones; follow up the child till now and then obtain the central nervous system history.) You can present the development history after this or under a separate heading.

CENTRAL NERVOUS SYSTEM HISTORY

Higher Functions

- Whether the child recognizes the mother
- Interacts with the environment in the form of gestures/smile
- Obeys simple commands
- Is able to speak few words or makes inappropriate noise
- Handedness attained or not/when it was attained
- Sleep disturbance in the form of intermittent irritability or incessant cry in the night
- Behavioral problems – incessant cry, shouting, and hyperactivity

Cranial Nerve

- Ability to perceive light
- Ability to move eyeballs in all four directions
  (If nystagmus is present, ask for any abnormal jerky movement noted by the mother.)

- Ability to chew food
- Facial asymmetry, able to close both eyes while sleeping, drooling of saliva, and deviation of angle of the mouth
- Ability to hear and respond to sound
- Nasal twang of voice and nasal regurgitation
- Ability to move the head side to side
- Any deviation of the tongue on protrusion

Motor System

It starts as the mother notices the following:

- **Bulk:** Thinning of limbs (if so, unilateral or bilateral), both upper limb and lower limb in quadriparetic CP or upper limb and lower limb of one side in hemiplegic CP
- **Tone:** Stiffness noted by the mother in all limbs, symmetrical or one side involving upper limb/lower limb in the form of difficulty in changing diaper and cleaning the perineum
- Scissoring of legs when the child is held by the axilla or at rest
- **Power:** Ability to move limbs above the cot or whether it is only sideways or whether it is just some flickers only
- **Involuntary movement:** Which limb, smooth, rapid, jerky, forceful, and disappears during sleep

Cerebellar History

- Abnormal eyeball or head movement

Bladder/Bowel

- Able to express urinary or bowel needs in the form of gestures
- Needs assistance for toileting

Sensory

- Crying while giving vaccination or any i.m. injection

Autonomic

- History of flushing, sweating, and palpitation episodes

Spine and Cranium

- Cranium: Compared with sibling or peers, did the mother notice an abnormal head shape or size?
- Spine: Check for any swelling, tuft of hair, sinus, discharge, and abnormal curvature.

COMPLICATION HISTORY/COMORBID STATES

- Seizures
- Fever and breathing difficulty (aspiration pneumonitis)
- Fever, chills and rigors, and crying while passing urine (urinary tract infection)
- Bed sores, ulcer, and callosities
- Skeletal deformity/spine deformity
- Feeding difficulty

COURSE OF THE ILLNESS

Determine the age at which the child had seizures. Find out how the seizures started, whether they were associated with fever or meningeal signs, the number of drugs that the child is taking at present, compliance of anticonvulsant drugs, and whether the seizure type varied during the course of illness. Ask whether any lumbar puncture or imaging was performed and the number of times the child has been hospitalized since then. (For a child to have CP, he or she should not have progression of symptoms or loss of acquired milestones or any worsening during the period of infection or fever.) Now explain the current admission – the number of days of admission; explanation of the present seizure episode; improvement in or worsening of symptoms; on any drugs; compliance of the drug; on physiotherapy; and cause for the current admission (breakthrough seizures, Poor compliance of drug, and fever-provoked seizures).

Developmental History

Global Developmental Delay

Explain about the development quotient (DQ) for each domain and also average of all domains:

$$DQ = \frac{DA}{CA} \times 100$$

Dietetic History

Calorie gap, and type and consistency of food

Immunization History

Up to age according to the national immunization schedule or IAP schedule

Family History

- Consanguinity
- Similar illness in the family – any neurological problem
- Abortion
- Previous sibling death
- Visual or hearing problem in family

Socioeconomic History

According to the modified Kuppuswamy scale

Summary

A …-year-old male/female child born out of a consanguineous or non-consanguineous marriage with the following:
- Global developmental delay
- Early onset seizures
- With significant perinatal event
- Delayed milestones
- With or without involvement of vision and hearing
- Thinning and stiffness of all four limbs without sensory or cerebellar involvement
- In the background of no significant family history of similar illness
- Probably a central motor disease in the form of spastic quadriparetic or diplegic CP
- Probably due to perinatal insult
- Now with symptoms suggestive of aspiration pnuemonitis/urinary tract infection/breakthrough seizures
(At the end of the history, explain about the physiological, topographic, functional, and etiological classification of CP.)

General Examination

- Recognizing the mother and interaction
- Posture – lies along the cot with the elbows flexed and knee extended
- Pallor, icterus, cyanosis, clubbing, lymphadenopathy, and edema (PICCLE)
- Neurocutaneous markers (port-wine stain, adenoma sebum)
- Cortical thumb in upper limbs
- Any scissoring
- Contractures – elbow, knee, and ankle
- Any scar – tenotomy and contracture release
- Callosities
- Pathological fractures, dislocation of hips, and bony abnormality
- Any peripheral aid – tube feeds, feeding gastrostomy, baclofen pump, diapers, calipers, braces, and wheelchair
- Any limb length discrepancy
- BCG scar
- Assessment of the activities of daily living – brushing and using cup and spoon

Head-to-Foot Examination

- Head size – asymmetry (plagiocephaly), microcephaly, and loss of occipital hair
- Microcephaly – sutures (overriding/ridging of sutures and AF closed or opened)
- Receding forehead and prominent ears
- Abnormal shape of the skull – any occipital plagiocephaly due to positioning
- Scalp hair – whether sparse over the occiput, seborrheic dermatitis, and brittle hair
- Sutures overriding
- Ear – discharge
- Dysmorphic facies
- Eye – cataract, nystagmus, and squint
- Oral cavity – oral hygiene, dentition, and caries teeth
- Skin – bed sores and scar for surgeries
- Bony deformities – wind-swept deformity
- Signs of malnutrition

Vital Signs

(Always start with temperature assessment in vital signs examination.)
- Temperature
- PR – volume, regular, any specific character, any radio-femoral delay, and felt in all peripheral vessels
- RR – tachypnea and increased work of breathing
- BP
- SpO_2

Anthropometry

- Measure segmental length of each long bone from bony prominence in case of deformities and contractures where limb length is not measurable in standing or supine posture.

CNS Examination

HIGHER FUNCTIONS

1. Check whether the child is conscious, awake, and alert; recognizes the mother; interested in the surroundings; and interacts with the examiner.
2. Dexterity (handedness): Check with which hand the child receives a toy.
3. Comprehension: Test using a three-step command.
4. Language: Test by asking name; naming the common objects, body parts, alphabets, and numbers; reciting rhymes; and telling a story.
5. Cognition: Test by asking concepts such as big/small, tall/short, and open/close.
6. Sleep/behavioral disturbances: Observe whether the child displays aggressive behavior, crying, and hyperactivity.

CRANIAL NERVES (CN)

(Only whatever is feasible to check in a child with CP is mentioned here.)

- CN I: Tell that the first CN could not be tested.
- CN II: Check whether the child fixes and follows light/objects, pupil size, and reaction to light. Check the menace reflex – absent in cortical blindness. Perform examination of the fundi to look for optic atrophy.
  (Fundus is a must for an MD candidate; do not forget to tell in the examination.)
- CN III, IV, and VI: Check whether the child moves eyeballs in all four cardinal directions; also check for strabismus and ptosis.
- CN V: Check for pain sensation over the face, check whether the child is able to chew food, and also check for jaw jerk.
- CN VII: Check for the following:
  - Wrinkling of the forehead
  - Able to close eyes
  - Nasolabial fold
  - Deviation of angle of the mouth
  - Drooling of saliva
- CN VIII: Perform bedside testing by crackling of paper, using a rattle or bell.
- CN IX and X: Try to look when the child cries – palatal movement equal on both sides, uvula in midline, palatal arches, palatal and pharyngeal reflex, and speech (nasal twang).
- CN XI: Check whether the child is able to lift the head from a supine position and whether he or she turns the head on both sides.
- CN XII: Check for any deviation of the tongue and wasting.

MOTOR EXAMINATION

- Posture: Explain about the posture of the child as given in Table 2.1.
- Primitive reflex (don't forget to mention)
  - Rooting
  - Sucking
  - Glabellar tap
  - Plantar grasp
  - Asymmetric tonic neck response (ATNR)
  - Crossed extensor
  - Examining whether the child has postural reflex – parachute response
  - Involuntary movements – present in extrapyramidal CP or can be seen in any other CP (mixed type)
  - Gait – whether the child is able to walk independently

CEREBELLAR SIGNS

- Head nodding, nystagmus, gait abnormality, ataxia or imbalance, past pointing, and dysdiadochokinesia

AUTONOMIC SYSTEM

- Excessive sweating, tachycardia, and hypotension

SENSORY SYSTEM

- Sensations are intact in CP except in hemiplegic CP. Check for cortical sensations in the affected upper limb. If present, localize the level of lesion at the parietal lobe.

TABLE 2.1	Motor Examination		
Components		**Right**	**Left**
Bulk[a]		Normal	Normal
Tone		Hypertonia	Hypertonia
		Clasp knife spasticity	Clasp knife spasticity
Power (best observed power) Examine individual joints in upper and lower limbs – shoulder, elbow, hand grip, finger grip, hip, knee, ankle, toe grip		Grade 1–5/5	Grade 1–5/5
Reflexes			
Superficial reflexes (conjunctival, corneal, palatal, pharyngeal, abdominal, cremasteric in male children)		Present	Present
Plantar reflexes		Extensor	Extensor
Deep tendon reflexes[a] (jaw jerk, biceps, triceps, supinator, knee and ankle reflexes)		Exaggerated	Exaggerated
Clonus		Present	Present
a. Present when reflexes are exaggerated			
b. Can be absent if contracture present			

[a]Look for adductor spread of knee jerk, crossed extensor, and crossed adductor in the infant.

- Determine whether the child has the ability to appreciate touch or pain sensation, or you can mention that the child cried while giving an injection or vaccination.

SPINE AND CRANIUM

Microcephaly/plagiocephaly and any clues of spina bifida occulta

SIGNS OF MENINGEAL IRRITATION

Meningeal signs or signs of raised intracranial pressure

Other Systems

CARDIOVASCULAR SYSTEM

Apical impulse position, first and second heart sounds, and any murmur

RESPIRATORY SYSTEM

Respiratory rate, work of breathing/retraction, and any added sound

ABDOMINAL SYSTEM

- Any organomegaly

MUSCULOSKELETAL SYSTEM

Contractures/deformity/splints

Diagnosis

A child with central motor dysfunction probably CP in the form of spastic quadriparesis/global developmental delay/seizures/microcephaly/contractures/blindness/deafness, with level of disability Gross Motor Function Classification System (GMFCS) probably due to perinatal insult, now presenting with fever/aspiration pneumonitis/urinary tract infection/breakthrough seizures/nutritional status/other comorbid conditions – anemia and vitamin deficiency, if any

Diagnosis should include the following:
- Physiological – spastic
- Topographic – quadriplegic/diplegic CP
- Etiological – perinatal cause
- Anatomical – single/mixed
- Associated features – microcephaly and developmental delay (global)
- Other comorbid conditions – seizures, behavioral problems, ocular, hearing, etc.
- Complications – contracture, deformities, bedsores, and others such as nutritional status, respiratory infection, and urinary tract infection

Frequently Asked Questions

1. What is the significance of antenatal history in a child with CP?
   a. Fever, rash, cervical swelling, and arthralgia in the first trimester – suggestive of intrauterine infections
   b. Hyperemesis in the mother in the first trimester following which any barium study done in the mother might expose the baby to radiation
   c. Bleeding per vaginum in the second trimester – threatened abortion and antepartum hemorrhage
   d. Fever, lower abdominal pain, irritation while passing urine, increased frequency of urine, vomiting, and diarrhea – suggestive of urinary tract infection
   e. Fever, lower abdominal pain, and foul-smelling discharge – triad of chorioamnionitis

2. What are the intrauterine infections?
   TORCHES CLAP:
   - TO: Toxoplasmosis
   - R: Rubella
   - C: CMV
   - H: Herpes simplex
   - E: Enterovirus
   - S: Syphilis
   - C: Chickenpox
   - L: Lyme disease
   - A: AIDS
   - P: Parvovirus B19

3. What is PICME number?
   - Pregnancy and Infant Cohort Monitoring and Evaluation system (PICME) number in Reproductive and Child Health (RCH) is required to get birth certificates for the newborn.
   - All pregnant women should get registered under RCH to avoid discrepancies in the issue of birth certificate.
   - A 12-digit digital code RCH ID will be given to women.
   - The state government has made this ID mandatory for pregnant women from January 2018.

4. What is the dosage schedule of tetanus vaccination in pregnancy?
   - IAP: 27–32 weeks, one dose of Tdap, subsequent doses of Tdap in each pregnancy irrespective of the previous pregnancy
   - WHO: TT two doses, as soon as registration or 16–20 weeks, second dose 4 weeks after the first dose
   - Next pregnancy
     - <5 years: One booster dose
     - >5 years: Full two doses

5. Who is a registered mother?
   A registered mother is a woman whose name has been entered in the Eligible Couple Register, and after becoming pregnant her name has been transferred to the Antenatal Register and she has come for a minimum of four antenatal visits.

6. What is the safe radiation exposure in pregnancy?
   Table 2.2 shows the levels of radiation exposure and its effects.

7. What is the normal weight gain in pregnancy?
   Weight gain in pregnancy
   - BMI 18–25: 11–16 kg, which is the normal weight gain in pregnancy
   - BMI <18: 13–18 kg
   - BMI 25–30: 9–11 kg
   - BMI >30: 5–7 kg

8. What is the NCPP trial?
   Under the National Collaborative Perinatal Project (NCPP) trial, the major risk factors for CP include the following:
   1. Condition of the pregnancy itself – infection, trauma, drug reactions, or the progress of labor
   2. Environmental risk factors – socioeconomic condition/stress/medical care
   3. Biological factors – maternal age, and medical and reproductive history
   4. Genetic background of the parents
   5. Conclusion of the trial – events of labor and delivery are not major contributors to the occurrence of CP; most have origins before the onset of labor

9. When is quickening felt in the antenatal period?
   - Quickening is felt at 20 weeks in a primigravida, whereas it is felt at 16 weeks in a multigravida.

10. When does the fetal head engage in a primigravida and a multigravida?
    - In a primigravida, engagement of the fetal head occurs at 8 weeks prior to EDD, whereas in a multigravida, head engagement occurs at the onset of labor.

11. What are the stages of labor?
    First stage: Cervical effacement/true labor pain till full cervical dilatation of the cervix
    Second stage: Full cervical dilatation to delivery of the baby
    Third stage: Delivery of placenta
    Fourth stage: Contraction and retraction of the uterus and observation in the labor room

TABLE 2.2	Levels of Radiation Exposure and its Effects		
Gestational Age	**Threshold Dose (mGray)**	**Effects**
0–2 weeks	50–100	Death or no effect (all-or-none phenomenon)
2–8 weeks	200–250	Congenital anomalies (skeleton, eyes, genitals)
8–15 weeks	200–310	Severe intellectual disability (decreased IQ of 25 per 1000 mGray)
16–25 weeks	250–280	Severe intellectual disability
Throughout	10,000	Therapeutic abortion

TABLE 2.3	Stages of Labor and Duration	
Stages	**Primigravida**	**Multigravida**
First stage	12 hours	6 hours
Second stage	2 hours	30 min
Third stage	30 min	5–15 min

12. What is the duration of normal labor and what is prolonged labor?
    Stages and duration of labor are given in Table 2.3.
    • Prolonged labor: >16 hours
    • PROM – rupture of fetal membranes before the onset of labor
13. What is precipitate labor?
    Precipitate labor occurs when the first and second stages of labor complete within 2 hours.
14. What is the significance of APGAR score at birth?
    APGAR score per se does not indicate the developmental outcome.
    Early Apgar score decides whether the baby needs resuscitation or not.
    Extended Apgar score – at 10 and 20 minutes – predicts the neurodevelopment outcome later in life.
15. What are the eye findings seen in CP?
    • Strabismus
    • Nystagmus
    • Cataract – rubella
    • Cortical blindness
    • Myopia
    • Retrolental fibroplasia
    • Optic atrophy
16. What are the fundus changes in CP?
    Chorioretinitis with hydrocephalus: Toxoplasmosis
    Chorioretinitis with microcephaly with HSM: Cytomegalovirus infection
    Salt and pepper appearance: Rubella
17. What are the causes of long eyelashes?
    Infection: Tuberculosis and HIV
    Connective tissue: Dermatomyositis and systemic lupus erythematosus
    Allergic disorders: Allergic rhinitis and atopic dermatitis
    Syndromes: Cornelia de Lange syndrome, Hermansky–Pudlak syndrome, and Oliver–McFarlane syndrome
    Miscellaneous: Hypothyroidism and porphyria
18. *What are the early markers in CP?
    • Decreased spontaneous movements
    • Stereotyped abnormal movements
    • Constant fisting after 2 months of age
    • Reduced head circumference or fall in its growth
    • Delayed social smile
    • Primitive reflexes persisting beyond 6 months
    • Persistent asymmetric postural reflexes and delay in developmental milestones
    • Associated signs such as roving eyes, no visual following, nystagmus, persistent squint, and lack of auditory response also seen
(Sometimes the examiner might ask few questions on dentition as a part of general discussion.)

19. What are the causes for delayed dentition?
    • Protein–energy malnutrition
    • Rickets
    • Down syndrome
    • Cretinism
    • Osteogenesis imperfecta
    • Ectodermal dysplasia
20. When is a child said to have delayed dentition?
    If a child does not develop dentition >13 months, then he or she is said to have delayed dentition.
21. What is the dental formula for primary and secondary teeth?
    Dental formula
    Primary teeth: 2-1-0-2, total = 20
    Secondary teeth: 2-1-2-3, total = 32
22. Comment on the salient features of tooth eruption.
    a. Teeth in the upper jaw appear early than in the lower jaw except two – lower central incisors and second molar.
    b. Order of appearance = order of fall.
23. When do teeth start to fall?
    Time to start falling is 6 years.
24. What is the importance of tooth eruption in a child?
    Importance of teeth eruption
    Appearance of second molar = onset of puberty around 12 years
25. *How is development quotient calculated?

$$\text{Development quotient (DQ)} = \frac{\text{Average age at attainment}}{\text{Observed age at attainnment}} \times 100$$

Or

$$DQ = \frac{DA}{CA} \times 100$$

    DQ less than 70% is taken as developmental delay.
26. Is vaccination contraindicated in a child with CP?
    Vaccination is not contraindicated in a child with CP; however, if a neurodegenerative disorder is suspected, always ask the child to come for follow-up and assess the child for any neurodegeneration.
27. What is the significance of family history in a child with CP?
    • Family history of a neurological disorder points more toward a neurodegenerative or metabolic or chromosomal disorder.
28. *How is height measured in a child with CP with contracture?
    Height prediction in any child with CP can be done using segmental length as given in Table 2.4.
29. How is spasticity assessed in CP?
    Tone can be assessed by resting posture and passive and active tone (passive tone can be assessed by applying resistance to an extremity and measured by recording the angle formed at the joint by this movement, using a goniometer known as Amiel-Tison method as shown in Fig. 2.1).
    The following angles are measured:
    (i) Angle at the hip: Adductor angle
    (ii) Angle at the knee: Popliteal angle
    (iii) Angle at the ankle: Dorsiflexion angle (the angle is measured using a slow and a quick movement; a difference of fewer than 10° between the slow and the quick angle is considered as normal)

---

*Important question asked in the examination.

TABLE 2.4	Measurement of Segmental Length	
Segmental Measure	**Estimation Equation (cm)**	
MALES		
Ulna length	Height = (4.605 × UL) + (1.308 × A) + 28.003	
Forearm length	Height = (2.904 × FL) + (1.193 × A) + 20.432	
Tibial length	Height = (2.758 × TL) + (1.717 × A) + 21.818	
Lower leg length	Height = (2.423 × LL) + (1.327 × A) + 21.818	
FEMALES		
Ulna length	Height = (4.459 × UL) + (1.315 × A) + 31.485	
Forearm length	Height = (2.908 × FL) + (1.147 × A) + 21.167	
Tibial length	Height = (2.771 × TL) + (1.457 × A) + 37.748	
Lower leg length	Height = (2.473 × LL) + (1.187 × A) + 21.151	

A, age (years); FL, forearm length; LL, lower leg length; TL, tibial length; UL, ulna length.

Source: Gauld L, Kappers J, Carlin J, Robertson C. Height Prediction from Ulna Length. Dev Med Child Neurol. 2004;46:475–80.

The angles are expressed both as mean (SD) and as ranges. These ranges are then compared with those described by Amiel-Tison.

30. Which type of squint is seen in a child with CP?
    Nonparalytic (concomitant) squint is seen in a child with CP. It may be convergent or divergent.
31. What are the differences between paralytic and nonparalytic squint?
    Table 2.5 gives the differences between paralytic and nonparalytic squint.
32. *What is Critchley sign?
    Persistent cortical thumb is called Critchley sign. It is shown in Fig. 2.2.

Cortical thumb is normal up to 2–3 months of age, after which it should disappear.
33. What is commando crawl?
    Infants with diplegic CP, due to the involvement of both lower limbs, usually drag both lower limbs during creeping as if a soldier moves in a war zone instead of normal four-legged movements. This is called commando crawl as shown in Fig. 2.3.
34. *What is early hand preference?
    Preferential use of one upper limb for handling things and reaching for objects before 12 months of age is called definite early hand preference, which is a sign of hemiplegia.
35. Mention some methods for visual and mental assessment in children.
    Table 2.6 shows some methods for visual and mental age assessment.
36. How is hearing tested in young children?

1½–4 months	Ringing a bell at 15 cm	Observe for behavioral response, cessation of crying, ceasing limb movements
4–6 months	Striking a spoon on a cup at 45 cm	Infant should turn toward the sound
7–20 months	Using a rattle	Infant should locate the source of the sound
20–24 months	STYCAR toy chart	Use five to seven toys; on verbal command, the child should pick up the correct toy
Older children	Rinne, Weber, absolute bone conduction	

Age (months)	Adductor angle	Popliteal angle	Dorsiflexion angle	Scarf sign
0–3	40°–80°	80°–100°	60°–70°	Elbow not crossing the midline
4–6	70°–110°	90°–120°	60°–70°	Elbow crossing the midline
7–9	110°–140°	110°–160°	60°–70°	Elbow crosses beyond the axillary line
10–12	140°–160°	150°–170°	60°–70°	-

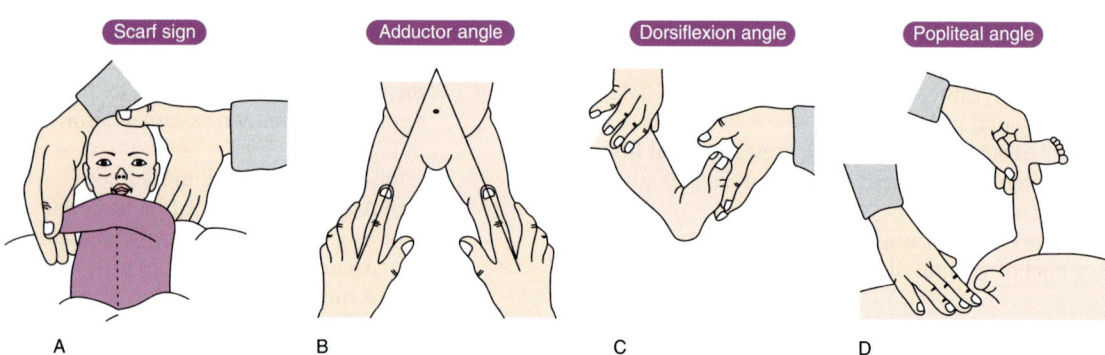

Fig. 2.1 Amiel-Tison method.

TABLE 2.5	Differences Between Paralytic and Nonparalytic Squint	
Paralytic Squint		**Nonparalytic Squint**
Diplopia+		No diplopia
Secondary deviation > primary deviation		Primary deviation = secondary deviation
Not maneuverable by doll's eye movement		Maneuverable by doll's eye movement

TABLE 2.6	Tests for Visual and Mental Age Assessment	
Age		**Method**
VISUAL ASSESSMENT		
Newborn		Optokinetic nystagmus/visual evoked potential
Infants		Following objects/light
1–3 years		Miniature toy test/picture test
3–6 years		E chart
>6 years		Snellen chart
Cover test		Strabismus
MENTAL ASSESSMENT		
Bayley Developmental Scale		Up to 42 months (three visits – first visit within 3 months)
Stanford–Binet Kamat Test		3–12 years
Wechsler Intelligence Scale		6–16 years

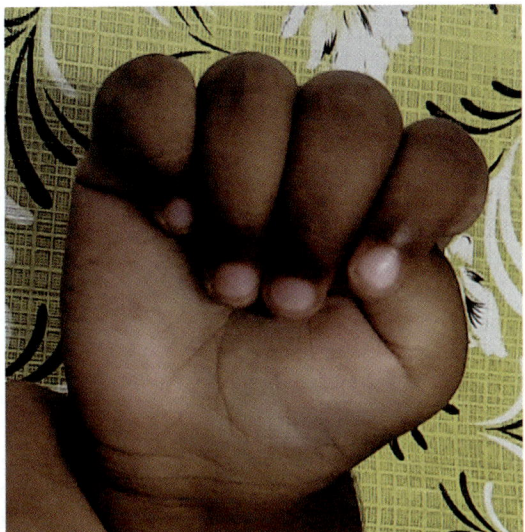

Fig. 2.2 Cortical thumb.

TABLE 2.7	Objective Hearing Assessments in Children	
Age		**Hearing Assessments**
Newborn		BERA
<5 months		Behavior observation audiometry
6 months to <2 years		Visual reinforcement audiometry
2–3 years		Play audiometry
>3 years		Audiometry

37. Mention some objective hearing assessments in children
    Table 2.7 gives some objective hearing assessments in children.
38. Name some indications for hearing assessment in children.
    1. Parental concern
    2. Family history of deafness
    3. NICU graduate
    4. TORCH infections
    5. Craniofacial anomalies
    6. Head trauma
    7. Post-meningitis and encephalitis
    8. Drugs – aminoglycosides, cisplatin, diuretics, and quinine
    9. Syndromes associated with deafness – Alport, Usher, Pendred, Waardenburg, Treacher Collins, and neuro-fibromatosis
39. How are dynamic and fixed contractures differentiated?
    Contracture is a condition of shortening and hardening of muscles, tendons, or other tissue, often leading to deformity and rigidity of joints. In dynamic contractures, there will be deformity of the joints; however, after physiotherapy, it may improve. In fixed contractures, when tendons are palpated, there will be cord-like thickening, which does not improve with physiotherapy – surgery is the only treatment.
40. What are the risk factors for CP?
    Flowchart 2.1 shows the risk factors for CP.
    Other risk factors are the following:
    • Maternal UTI – 40% risk with maternal UTI; with antibiotics, 11.5% risk; without antibiotics, 19% risk
    • Multiple pregnancy twins – 5–8 times risk for CP than singleton pregnancy; triplet – 20–47 times risk

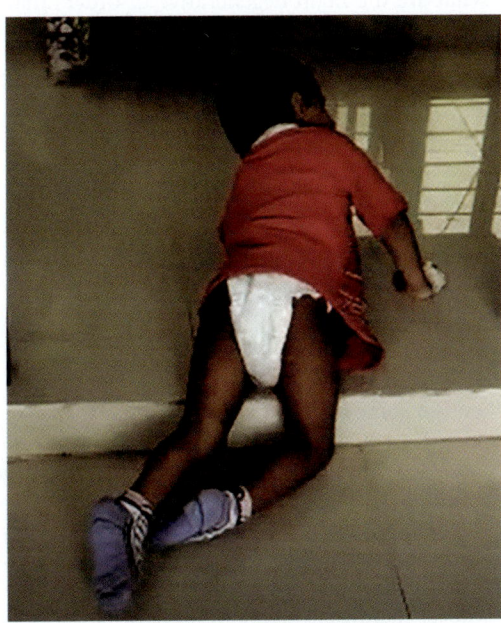

Fig. 2.3 Commando crawl.

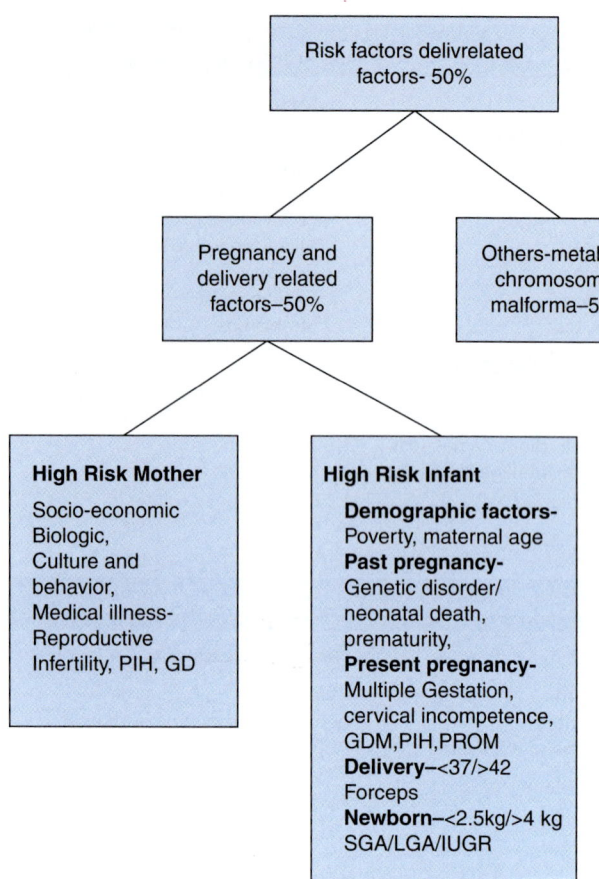

Flowchart 2.1 Risk factors for CP.

- CP in infertility treatment – 24% risk (increased incidence due to multiple gestation)
- Male with IUGR and birth weight <3rd percentile – 16 times more prone to CP
- Males with birth weight >97th percentile – four times more prone to CP
- Death of a twin in utero – 60 times more prone to CP of the surviving twin

41. Mention some major contributors in CP.
    Antenatal causes contribute to 90% of cases.
    Significant perinatal asphyxia is responsible for only 10% of cases.

42. Name few causes of acquired CP.
    - In majority of children, the cause is not known. Other causes include CNS infection (meningoencephalitis), hyperbilirubinemia, cerebrovascular accidents, and head injuries.

43. Mention some preventable causes of CP.
    - Prematurity
    - Maternal infection
    - Perinatal asphyxia
    - Hyperbilirubinemia
    - Better transport
    - Intraventricular hemorrhage – steroids

44. Mention some salient points in diagnosing CP at various stages.
    In severe and long-standing cases, the diagnosis is essentially clinical.

During evolving stages and for the diagnosis of mild cases, experience and repeated examinations over a period of time may be required.
Always exclude slowly progressive neurodegenerative disorders, neuromuscular disorders, spinal disorders, and other causes such as dyskinetic, hypotonic, and ataxic forms of CP.

45. Mention some points against the diagnosis of CP.
    - Regression of milestones
    - Progressive disease
    - Presence of organomegaly
    - Presence of dysmorphism
    - Positive family history

46. Mention some danger or red flag signs in CP.
    - Danger signs are the following:
      - Decrease in head circumference
      - Constant fisting >2 months
      - Delayed social smile
      - Persistent primitive reflexes >6 months
      - Obligate ATNR
      - Delayed postural reflexes
      - Persistent tone abnormalities
      - Persistent asymmetry in posture, movement, and reflexes

47. *What are CP impersonators?
    - CP impersonators are the following:
      - Hydrocephalus
      - Subdural hematoma
      - Dopa-responsive dystonia
      - Hypothyroidism
      - Inborn errors of metabolism

48. What are CP mimics?
    - CP mimics are the following:
      - Metabolic
        a. Treatable: Glutaric academia type 1
        b. Nontreatable: Lesch–Nyhan syndrome and Sjögren–Larsson syndrome
      - Muscular dystrophies
    - Mitochondrial disorders
    - Malformations

49. *What are the neurodegenerative disorders that resemble spastic CP?
    - Infantile Gaucher
    - Tay–Sachs disease
    - Familial spastic paraplegia
    - Glutaric aciduria type 1
    - Lesch–Nyhan syndrome
    - Niemann–Pick type C
    - Rett syndrome
    - Pelizaeus–Merzbacher disease

50. Name some differentials for ataxic CP.
    - Abetalipoproteinemia
    - Ataxia telangiectasia
    - Friedreich ataxia

51. Mention some differentials for dyskinetic CP.
    - GLUT 1 transporter deficiency

52. Name few differentials for nonprogressive disorders resembling CP.
    - Mental deprivation
    - Mental retardation
    - Malnutrition
    - Motor handicaps (spina bifida, myopathies)

53. *How is a child with CP investigated?
CP is a clinical diagnosis.
Investigations aid to:
    (a) Reveal possible etiology
    (b) Relate physical findings with neurological findings
    (c) Rule out similar conditions as DD
54. What is the role of neuroimaging in CP?
    • It is needed to:
        • Find out the etiology and extent of lesion
        • Find out the insult to the affected brain
    • CT
    Required when there are focal neurological signs, seizures, neurocutaneous markers, macrocephaly/microcephaly, and intrauterine infections
    • MRI
        • Picks up lesions missed by CT, e.g., neuromigrational disorders (lissencephaly/schizencephaly/agenesis/hypogenesis corpus callosum)
        • MRI sensitive than CT in early detection of periventricular leukomalacia and extent of lesions in the brainstem and basal ganglia (status marmoratus)
55. What is the role of ultrasonogram in CP?
    • Ultrasound in preterm: Periventricular leukomalacia
    • Extent: Correlates with prognosis
    • USG at birth in preterm
        • Parenchymal
        • Hemorrhagic (better prognosis)
        • Ischemic
        • More posterior the lesion – CP more likely
        • Better outcome for anterior lesions
        • Nonparenchymal (better prognosis), e.g., IVH
    • USG in term
        • Mainly due to HIE: Seen mainly in the thalamus, basal ganglia, and subcortical white matter
56. Mention some investigations for etiological workup in CP.
    a. Metabolic workup: When suggestive of IEM
    b. Skiagram skull: Craniosynostosis and intrauterine infections
    c. EEG: Location and extent of structural lesions and congenital malformations
    d. EMG: To rule out muscular pathology in rigid spastic children and as a guidance for physiotherapy
    e. Genetic evaluation
57. Name few screening tools used in CP.
Tools used in CP for the assessment of motor system are the following:
    • <6 months: Amiel-Tison angle
    • 6 months: Movement Assessment of Infant (MAI)
    • Alberta Infant Motor Scale (AIMS)
58. How is a child with CP evaluated?
    • Evaluation includes the following:
        1. Vision
        2. Hearing
        3. Thyroid function
        4. Evaluation of speech
        5. Metabolic screening – if the perinatal period was uneventful, positive family history
        6. Neuroimaging
        7. EEG – seizures

8. Specialist opinions for the assessment and management of comorbidities such as feeding difficulty, behavioral problems, dental problems, and contractures.
59. Enumerate the overall management in CP.
Management
    1. Multidisciplinary approach including physiotherapy, occupational therapy, speech therapy, and visual stimulation according to the needs of the patient
    2. Family-centered approach
    3. Management of spasticity and movement disorder
    4. Management of comorbidities – seizures, feeding difficulties, constipation, etc.
    5. Nutritional support
    6. Family support groups
    7. Management of intercurrent infections
60. What are the goals in the management of CP?
    • To minimize the disability
    • To promote independence and full participation in the society
    • To help target toward independence in activities of daily living and ability to go to school, earn a living, and have a social life

DISCUSSION ON CEREBRAL PALSY

61. *Define cerebral palsy.
CP is a diagnostic term used to describe a group of permanent (nonprogressive) disorders of movement and posture causing (changing motor) activity limitation that are attributed to nonprogressive disturbances (lesions or anomalies) in the developing fetal or infant brain often accompanied by disturbances of sensation, perception, cognition, communication, and behavioral and musculoskeletal problems (comorbid conditions) (Nelson, 20th edition).
62. What does the definition of CP imply?
The definition of CP further emphasizes the following points:
    a. CP is neither a disease nor a pathological or etiological entity.
    b. It comprises a heterogeneous group of clinical syndromes.
    c. It is nonprogressive/static encephalopathy (pathology is static, unlike progressive nature in degenerative disorders).
    d. The clinical pattern changes as the brain maturity continues throughout childhood.
    e. It is the central cause and not a spinal cause (spina bifida, etc.):
        (i) Cerebral cortex (spasticity)
        (ii) Cerebellum (ataxia)
        (iii) Basal ganglia (dyskinesia)
63. What is the prevalence of CP?
The overall prevalence of CP is 1.5–2.5 per 1000 live births.
The prevalence of various types of CP is as follows:
    • Spastic CP: 70%–80%
    • Diplegic CP: 50%
    • Quadriplegic CP: 30%
    • Hemiplegic CP: 20%

- Extrapyramidal CP: 10%–15%
- Ataxic and mixed CP: 5%–10%

64. What is the etiology in CP?
Multifactorial
65. Enumerate the causes of CP.
Table 2.8 gives the causes of CP.
Table 2.9 gives other causes of various types of CP.

66. Mention some pathological changes in the brain in CP.
Table 2.10 shows various pathological changes in CP.
67. Mention some clinical findings in CP.
Table 2.11 shows clinical features in each type of CP.
(FAQ 68–80 – discussion on HIE – might be asked during discussion on CP)

TABLE 2.8	Causes of CP			
Prenatal (Antenatal) (80%–90%)	**Perinatal (8%–10%)**	**Postnatal (10%)**	**Genetic Cause (2%)**	
a. Intrauterine infection b. Cerebrovascular accidents (PIH), IUGR, LBW c. Neural tube defects d. Genetic e. Migrational defects f. Cerebral malformation g. Other anatomical cerebral abnormalities h. Multiple gestation i. Physical trauma to mother	Perinatal asphyxia[a] due to: a. Prolonged labor b. Abnormal presentation c. Instrumental delivery d. Cesarean section	a. Neonatal – hyperbilirubinemia, sepsis, meningitis b. Intracranial hemorrhage c. Metabolic convulsions	a. Polymorphism in copy number variation (CNV), functional polymorphism in interleukin-6	

CP, cerebral palsy.
[a]Significant perinatal asphyxia – 10%.

TABLE 2.9	Other Causes of CP		
Spastic Quadriplegia	**Spastic Diplegia**	**Spastic Hemiplegia**	**Extrapyramidal**
TORCH infection Congenital malformation Lissencephaly	Spinal dysraphism Tumors of the spinal cord	Acquired hemiplegia Schizencephaly	Glutaric aciduria type 1 mitochondrial disorders
Early infantile leukodystrophy	Arginase deficiency, sulfite deficiency, molybdenum cofactor deficiency	Neurocutaneous • Sturge weber syndrome	Lesch nyhan syndrome
IEM • Aminoacidopathies • Organic acidemias • Urea cycledisorders	Hereditary spastic paraplegia		Neuronal ceroid lipofuscinosis
	Dopa-responsive dystonia		

CP, cerebral palsy.

TABLE 2.10	Pathological Changes in CP			
Newborn	**Lesion in Brain**	**Pathophysiology**	**Cause**	**Long Term**
Term	Watershed area	Bilateral necrosis of cortical and subcortical white matter	Decreased cerebral perfusion	Spastic quadriplegia (UL > LL)
Preterm	Periventricular region (descending fibers from cortex)	Bilateral necrosis of white matter	Infection, prematurity, perinatal hypoxia	Spastic diplegia (LL > UL)
Focal/multifocal ischemic necrosis	MCA (Middle Cerebral Artery) territory	Porencephaly/multiple encephalomalacia	Thromboembolic disorder (APLAS), inherited clotting factor deficiency, CNS malformation	Hemiplegic, quadriplegic CP
Status marmoratus	Basal ganglion	Selective neuronal necrosis/abnormal myelination/marbled appearance	Birth asphyxia	Dystonic CP

CP, cerebral palsy.

TABLE 2.11	Clinical Findings in CP		
Spastic CP	**Spastic Quadriplegia**	**Spastic Diplegia**	**Spastic Hemiplegia**
a. Most common, 70%–75% of cases b. Upper motor neuron signs Clasp knife hypertonia, exaggerated deep tendon reflexes, and extensor plantar response c. Severely disabled d. Majority have microcephaly, severe mental retardation, pseudobulbar palsy, growth failure, visual and hearing defects, seizures e. Hypertonia leading to arching of back and scissoring of legs frequent	a. All four limbs equally involved b. Hip subluxation or dislocation c. Delayed walking, toe walking because of tendo-Achilles contracture d. Arms are internally rotated, elbows extended or lightly flexed, and hands fisted e. Flexion contractures: Ankle, knee, elbow	a. Lower limbs involved more than upper limbs b. Minimal intellectual involvement c. Upper torso grows normally, whereas growth of lower limb is affected d. Characteristic of preterm babies with periventricular leukomalacia	a. Arm is more severely affected than leg b. Right-side involvement more common c. Paucity of movements and fisting of hand on affected side d. Definite hand preference in children younger than 12 months e. Arm held adducted, flexed, and internally rotated at the shoulder, with elbow flexed, forearm pronated, wrist flexed, and thumb adducted f. Leg held adducted, semiflexed at the knee and plantar flexed at the ankle g. In long-standing cases, asymmetry in the growth of limb may occur
Dyskinetic CP	**Ataxic CP**	**Hypotonic CP**	
a. Dystonic and choreoathetoid are the two forms b. Severe motor disability with persistent neonatal reflexes c. Asymmetric tonic neck response (ATNR) prominent d. Hypotonia with head lag, drooling, feeding difficulties e. Athetosis appears at 1 year of age f. Flaying of fingers, overflow movements, facial grimacing are prominent g. Exaggerated with intention and emotion h. Standing and walking is delayed i. Intelligence often preserved	a. Uncommon form b. Hypotonic and inactive, delayed walking c. Ataxic gait and wide-based gait d. Cerebellar signs present e. Ataxia may be associated with spasticity	a. Extremely rare b. Most cases are evolving form of dyskinetic or spastic CP c. Other causes to be excluded	

CP, cerebral palsy.

68. Define Hypoxic ischemic encephalopathy (HIE).
   According to the guidelines from AAP and ACOG, HIE is diagnosed when the following are present:
   • Profound metabolic or mixed acidemia (pH <7) in an umbilical artery blood sample if obtained
   • Persistence of and APGAR score of 0–3 for longer than 5 minutes
   • Neonatal neurological sequelae (coma, seizures, hypotonia)
   • Multiple organ involvement (kidney, liver, lungs, heart, intestines)
69. Name few new biomarkers in HIE.
   • Neuron-specific enolase
   • S100B
   • MRS – increased lactate and decreased *N*-acetyl aspartate peak
70. Mention some specific areas involved in a preterm/term child with HIE in MRI.
   HIE causes altered signal at the level of posterior limb of the internal capsule, thalamus, and basal ganglion. It occurs predominantly in the white matter in a preterm, and in watershed areas of the brain in a term child.

71. What are the early and late MRI findings in HIE in the newborn period?
   • Earliest (1–5 days): Persistent hypodense lesion in the occipital region
   • Later (10–14 days): Cystic encephalomalacia
72. Describe the findings in MRI brain in a preterm at 40 weeks suggestive of CP at 2 years of age.
   • Loss of volume of periventricular white matter, extent of cystic changes, ventricular dilation, and thinning of corpus callosum
73. Mention some newer modalities in HIE.
   1. Free radical scavengers – vitamin A, vitamin C, and allopurinol
   2. COX inhibitor – indomethacin
   3. NMDA receptor antagonist – MK 801 and magnesium
   4. Calcium channel blockers – flunarizine, nimodipine, and nicardipine
   5. Erythropoietin
   6. Decreased nitric oxide formation – nitroarginine
   7. Opioid antagonist – cannabinoid
   8. Whole body cooling
   9. Brain tonics – piracetam
   10. Stem cell transplantation

74. Name some predictors of poor outcome in HIE.
    - Intubation at resuscitation, poor APGAR <7, hypoglycemia, absence of sucking reflex >7 days, and mechanical ventilation> 5 days
75. Mention few ultrasound predictors of CP in newborn.
    USG findings of hypoechoic periventricular areas – a strong predictor of later motor dysfunction
76. What is status marmoratus?
    - Acute total asphyxia in the nucleus of basal ganglion in a full-term baby leads to scarring of the basal ganglion – maldevelopment of corpus striatum and nuclei of striae. It is the least common type of neuropathological variety. It is most common in term babies.
    - Cause includes altered myelination of putamen and caudate.
    - MRI shows bilateral hyperintensity in the thalamus.
    - Features of neuronal loss, gliosis, and hypermyelination are present.
    - Site: Lesion involves the basal ganglia (caudate nucleus and putamen).
77. Mention some pathological findings associated with preterm babies.
    Periventricular leukomalacia (PVL) and periventricular hemorrhagic venous infarcts (PHVI) are the pathological lesions associated with preterm babies.
78. Name few neuroprotective drugs to prevent neonatal problems.
    Two neuroprotective factors/drugs to prevent neonatal problems are antenatal steroids and magnesium sulfate.
79. Describe the role of $MgSO_4$ as a neuroprotective factor.
    a. Magnesium sulfate causes capillary stabilization.
    b. It prevents cytokine-mediated injury.
    c. It acts as an antioxidant.
80. Enumerate pathological and neuropathological association with four motor syndromes of CP.
    Table 2.12 gives pathological and neuropathological association with CP.
81. Name the classification system in CP and explain the components.
    Table 2.13 shows the INGRAM'S classification system.
82. Who discovered CP?
    - Sir John William Little discovered CP.
83. Who described the term cerebral palsy?
    - Sigmund Freud described the term CP.
84. What is the recent name for CP?
    Central motor dysfunction
85. Why is the term CP used after 2 years of age?
    - During the first 2 years of age, there is increased plasticity of newborn brain – one or the other site will compensate (due to increased neuronal circuit connections). As the age increases, plasticity of the brain decreases and illness will manifest, so the term CP requires established spasticity. When the clinical findings are evident to the degree that the child is unlikely to outgrow (i.e., if the findings are unequivocal or beyond doubt), then one can diagnose CP at any age. If there is a doubt, it is better to wait and review in subsequent visits. But

TABLE 2.12	Pathological and Neuropathological Association With CP			
Features	Spastic Diplegia	Spastic Quadriplegia	Hemiplegia	Extrapyramidal
Pathological association	Prematurity, ischemia, infections, endocrine, hemorrhages, LBW, kernicterus (athetoid)	Ischemia, infections, endocrine/metabolic, genetic, birth asphyxia, birth trauma, kernicterus (athetoid), congenital malformation	Thrombophilic disorders, infections, genetic, periventricular hemorrhagic infarction	Kernicterus, mitochondrial, genetic/metabolic
Neuropathology	Periventricular leukomalacia	Multicystic encephalomalacia, malformations, periventricular leukomalacia	Stroke in utero or neonatal	Basal ganglia – putamen, globus pallidus, thalamus

CP, cerebral palsy.

TABLE 2.13	Ingram's Classification			
Physiological	Topographic	Etiological	Functional GMFCS (Gross Motor Function Classification System)	Anatomical
Spastic	Monoplegia[a]	Prenatal	Level 1: Ambulatory in all settings	Cerebral
Athetoid	Paraplegia		Level 2: Walks without aides, but has limitations in community settings	Cerebellar
Ataxic	Hemiplegia	Perinatal	Level 3: Walks with aides	Extrapyramidal
Atonic	Triplegia[a]		Level 4: Wheelchair/adult assist	Mixed
Mixed	Quadriplegia			
Rigid	Diplegia	Postnatal	Level 5: Dependent on mobility	
Unclassified	Double hemiplegia			

[a]Very rare and may represent evolving forms.

intervention should never be delayed awaiting diagnosis and families should be informed that CP is a possibility.

86. Which is the overall most common type of CP?
Spastic diplegic CP (35%)

87. Which is the most common type of CP seen in preterm babies?
   - Spastic diplegic CP

88. Which are the most common types of CP seen in term babies?
   - Hemiplegic CP and quadriplegic CP

89. Give an example for CP with the maximum IQ disability.
   - Quadriplegic CP has the maximum IQ disability.

90. Give an example for CP with the least IQ disability.
   - Hemiplegic CP has the least IQ disability.

91. What are the causes of facial dysmorphism in CP?
   - Plagiocephaly
   - Down syndrome
   - Zellweger syndrome
   - Lowe syndrome

92. Mention few causes of incessant cry in CP.
   - Skin infection
   - Dental caries
   - GERD
   - Constipation
   - Joint contractures
   - Pathological fractures

93. Mention few early pointers suggestive of CP.
   a. Higher function – delayed milestones and seizures (newborn, early infancy)
   b. Reflex – rooting and sucking sluggish in the first week
   c. Persistence of grasp/Moro/ATNR
   d. Absent stepping in 2 months
   e. Movement – asymmetry/paucity of kicking/finger movement
   f. Decreased head circumference
   g. Development of hand preference <1 year (normal hand preference by 3 years of age)
   h. Excessive lethargy and irritability
   i. High-pitched cry
   j. Delayed social smile and poor head control
   k. Drags feet like commando sign/toe walking
   l. Bunny hopping – jumping while on knees (spastic diplegia)
      W-sitting: Adductor spasm. Hips cannot move out and remain adducted and internally rotated as seen in spastic diplegia but can be normal variant in dyskinetic CP as shown in Fig. 2.4.
   m. De Lange sign – scissoring in spastic diplegia (as shown in Fig. 2.5)
   n. Buttock crawl – spastic diplegia/quadriplegia

94. What are the pointers in CP?
Five "P":
   1. Progression of illness not present
   2. Persistence of primitive reflex
   3. Presence of pathological reflex
   4. Posture abnormalities
   5. Perinatal insult to the growing pain

95. Mention few soft neurological signs.
The following are the features of soft neurological signs:
   - Nonlocalizing neurological signs

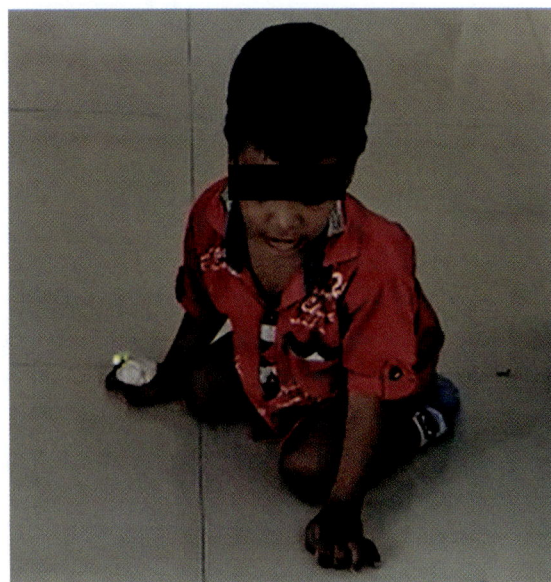

Fig. 2.4 W-sitting.

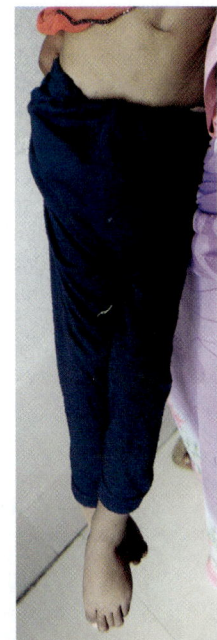

Fig. 2.5 De Lange sign.

   - Form of deviant performance on a motor/sensory test in the neurological examination that is abnormal for a particular age
   - Absence of certain signs at a particular age and presence of certain signs in an unexpected age
   - Examples: Abnormal finger-to-nose test, inability to identify right–left laterality, graphesthesia, and abnormal orientation in space

96. What are the late markers in CP?
   - Contractures
   - Skeletal deformities

97. Enumerate the ophthalmological findings in CP.
   - On clinical examination: Pupillary reflex present/absent menace because of cortical blindness

- Most common: Refractory error
- Others: Squint, vitamin deficiency, nystagmus, optic atrophy, chorioretinitis, cataract, and cherry red spot

98. Mention some causes of obesity in a child with CP.
    - Physical inactivity, sodium valproate therapy, and hypothyroidism
99. Enumerate the causes of dysarthria in CP.
    - Tongue spasm, oropharyngeal incoordination, and laryngeal spasm
100. Define wind-swept deformity.
    - Adduction contracture in one hip and abduction contracture in the other hip as shown in Fig. 2.6
101. Enumerate the causes of sudden hypotonia/areflexia in a child with CP.
    - Postictal state, sleep, and clonazepam therapy
102. *Enumerate the differentiating features of different types of CP clinically.
    Table 2.14 shows the salient features of different types of CP.
103. What is the most common cause of death in CP?
    - First cause: Respiratory cause (aspiration pneumonitis)
    - Second cause: Refractory seizures
104. What is the incidence of mental retardation in CP?
    - Quadriplegic CP: 30%–60%
    - Hemiplegic CP: 25%
105. How can one check for psuedobulbar palsy?
    - On throat examination, pooling of secretion is present and jaw jerk will be brisk.
106. What is the cause for adductor spasm in CP?
    - Increased tone in the antigravity muscle
107. Why does adductor alone go for spasm?
    The action of adductor is predominant because it is the strongest muscle in the lower limb.
108. What is the treatment for adductor spasm?
    - Adductor tenotomy
    - Obturator neurectomy

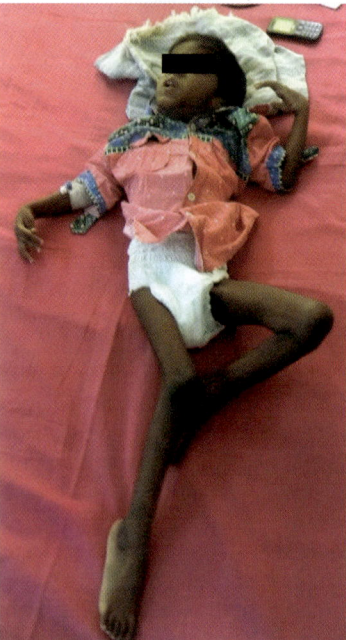

Fig. 2.6 Wind-swept deformity.

- Inj. botulinum toxin
- Fourth to eighth cranial nerves in preterm, CMV infection, and kernicterus

109. What are the causes for failure to thrive in CP?
    - Inadequate food intake
    - Recurrent vomiting
    - Aspiration
    - Hyperactive gag reflex
    - GERD
    - Spasticity – difficult chewing and swallowing
110. What are the causes of respiratory problem in a child with CP?
    Respiratory problem in a child with CP occurs with severe motor involvement:
    - Aspiration – due to pharyngeal incoordination
    - Upper airway obstruction
    - Respiratory muscle spasticity
    - Premature babies – bronchopulmonary dysplasia
111. What are the causes of bladder and bowel involvement in a child with CP?
    - Poor cognition
    - Poor communication skills
    - Decreased mobility
    - Neurogenic dysfunction
112. Enumerate the orthopedic problems in a child with CP.
    - Hip subluxation an d dislocation
    - Contractures
    - Scoliosis
113. What are the comorbid conditions in CP?
    - Central nervous system
      - Intellectual disability
      - Seizures
      - Behavioral problem
      - Learning disabilities
      - Communication problem/dysarthria
    - Cranial nerves
      - Visual impairment
      - Hearing problem
    - GIT
      - GERD
      - Teeth problems
      - Drooling
      - Oromotor dysfunction
      - Constipation
      - Bladder disturbance
    - Respiratory dysfunction
      - Aspiration pneumonitis
114. What are the causes of dental caries in CP?
    - Drooling of saliva
    - Poor mouth closure
    - Biting of teeth
    - Oral hypersensitivity
    - Gingivitis – anticonvulsant side effects
    - Dental malocclusion
    - Carbohydrate retention diet
    - Fluoride imbalance
115. What are the common cranial nerves involved in CP?
    - First most common: IX, X, XI, and XII nerves
    - Second most common: III, IV, and VI nerves
    - Third most common: Optic nerve
    - Cranial nerves IX and X: Exaggerated gag reflex

TABLE 2.14	Salient Features of CP			
Features	Atonic CP	Dyskinetic/Extrapyramidal CP		Ataxic CP
Tone	Hypotonia/ᵃForester sign+	Three stages: First, hypotonia; second, dystonia; third, hypertonia/involuntary movements		Hypotonia
Reflexes (DTR)	Exaggerated	Normal		Absent
Lesion	Frontal lobe	Basal ganglion		Cerebellum/brainstem
Plantar	Extensor	Flexor		Flexor
Others	Severe mental retardation	Choreoathetoid movement		Cerebellar signs

CP, cerebral palsy.
ᵃForester sign: When the child is lifted by axilla, there will be flexion of hips initially; later he or she will develop dystonia or spasticity as shown in Fig. 2.7.

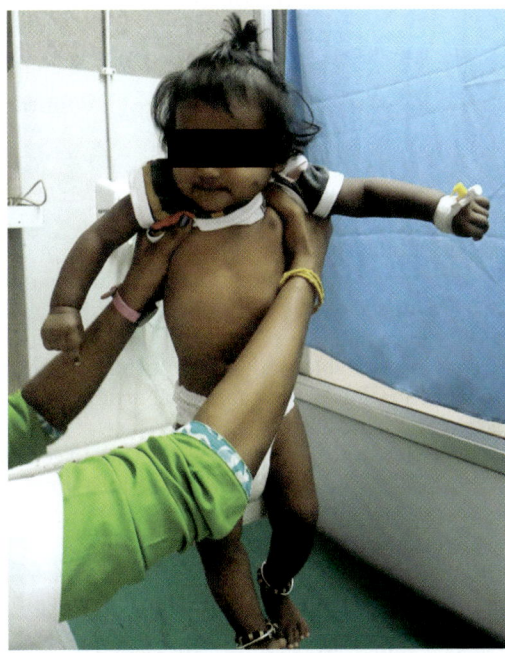

Fig. 2.7 Eliciting Forester sign.

116. Comment on the states of reflexes in CP.
   - Persistence of primitive reflexes
   - Nonappearance of maturational reflex
   - Appearance of pathological reflex
117. Why is there persistence of primitive reflex in CP?
   All primitive reflexes have a subcortical center; the cortex has an inhibitory region over the subcortical area. In CP, the cortex is affected so there occurs no subcortical inhibition by the cortex; hence, there is persistence of primitive reflex.
118. What is the equivalent of knee jerk in newborn?
   The equivalent of knee jerk in a newborn is adductor spread of knee jerk (hip adduction from the neonatal period to 8 months is considered normal); persistence after 8 months is considered abnormal.
119. Enumerate the complications of CP.
   - Sensory neural deafness
   - Chronic serous otitis media
   - Bulbar dysfunction
   - Dental caries
   - Kyphoscoliosis

   - Chest infection
   - Constipation
   - Dislocation
   - Malnutrition
120. How is constipation treated in a child with CP?
   - Increase of fluid and fiber intake
   - Use of commode and foot rest
   - Laxatives
   - Mineral oil to be avoided because laxative has the risk of aspiration and causing lipoid pneumonia
121. What are the comorbid conditions associated with CP? Table 2.15 gives the comorbid conditions in CP.
122. How are DQ and IQ assessed in children?
   Development quotient is assessed for children younger than 3 years and intelligence quotient for children older than 3 years.
   Normal is >85%.
   Table 2.16 gives the development quotient for children younger than 3 years.
   Table 2.17 shows the difference between intelligence quotient and development quotient.
123. What are the causes of feeding difficulties in a child with CP?
   - Because of tongue thrusting, pseudobulbar palsy, increased gag reflex, cricopharyngeal incoordination, and gastroesophageal reflux are the proposed causes

TABLE 2.15	Comorbid Conditions in CP		
Comorbid Conditions	Frequency	Remarks
Mental retardation	50–70	Most often in spastic quadriplegia and ataxic CP
Seizures	25–33	Most often in spastic hemiplegia and spastic quadriplegia; least often in dyskinetic CP
Hearing and speech problems	15–20	Most common in dyskinetic CP and spastic quadriplegia
Ocular	50–75	Refractory errors, strabismus (diplegia – Little disease)
Behavior problems	30–50	Stubborn, aggressiveness, lack of attention, and hyperkinetic behavior

CP, cerebral palsy.

TABLE 2.16	Development Quotient and Its Interpretation
DQ (%)	**Interpretation**
>85	Normal
70–85	Mild delay
<70	Severe delay

DQ, development quotient.

TABLE 2.17	Difference between Intelligence Quotient and Development Quotient	
Intelligence Quotient	**Development Quotient**	
Performance score	Questionnaire by the parent	
Performed by the child	Enquired to the parents	
For child older than 3 years	For child younger than 3 years	
Done by clinical psychologist	Done by pediatrician	

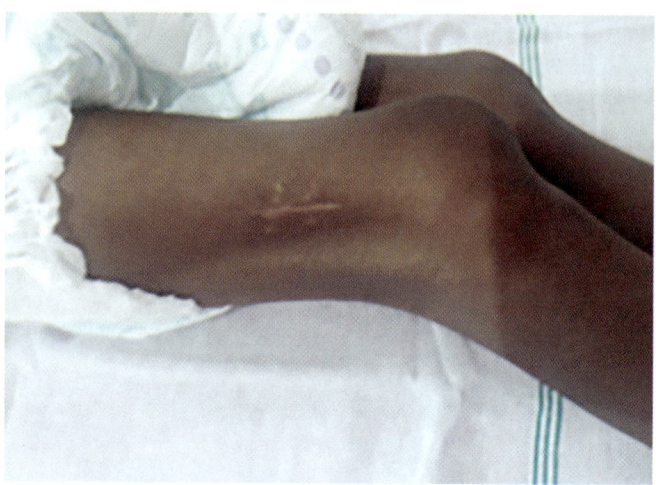

Fig. 2.8   Tendon release scar – for contractures.

of feeding problems in a child with CP. Diagnosis is done through videofluoroscopic barium studies to assess swallowing dysfunction.

124. How is swallowing difficulty managed in a child with CP?
    Management includes the following:
    • Adopting correct posturing during feeding
    • Small feed volume with increased frequency
    • Upright posture after meals
    • Thickening of feed
    • Antireflux drugs
    • Fundoplication
    • Gastrostomy feeding (last option)

125. Write a brief note on drooling.
    Common up to 1 year of age
    Uncommon in children older than 1 year (as the child starts talking, oropharyngeal coordination starts to occur)

126. What is the treatment for drooling?
    • The following are the treatment for drooling:
        • Nonsugar lollipops
        • Oromotor coordination exercise
        • Intraoral appliance
        • Anticholinergic drugs – glycopyrrolate
        • Inj. botulinum toxin (side effect, dental caries)
        • Salivary gland removal

127. What are the fields of mandatory referral in the evaluation of a child with CP?
    • Orthopedics – osteotomy
    • ENT – hearing
    • Ophthalmology – cataract
    • Physiotherapy/occupational therapy
    • Dentist – dental/oromandibular appliances/sialorrhea
    Fig. 2.8 shows tendon release scar for contractures.

128. What are the advantages of spasticity in a child with CP?
    • Preserves muscle bulk
    • Preserves bone density
    • Enables the child to stand

129. When should spasticity be treated?
    • When it affects the function of the limb
    • Developed contracture and deformities

130. Is CP preventable?
    CP is preventable and treatable but never curable. Genetic CP is preventable by abortion.

131. What is genetic CP?
    • 10%–14% of children with CP can have a genetic cause
    Causes of genetic CP include the following;
        a. Copy number variation (CNV) in genes
        b. Chromosome 2q24-25 mutation
        c. Interleukin-6 polymorphism
    Inheritance pattern includes the following:
        Parent with CP: Six times
    One sibling affected with CP: Nine times
    Twin with CP: 15 times

132. What is the role of a pediatrician in CP?
    Role of a pediatrician includes the following:
    • Head of the team
    • Early identification
    • To rule out other cause
    • Knows when to refer to whom
    • Drug prescription
    • To monitor the side effects of the drugs

133. What is family-centered approach?
    Parents, not only the mother but also the father, and siblings are taught how to work with a child in performing daily activities such as feeding, dressing, bathing, and playing. They are also taught about follow-up, physiotherapy, and occupational therapy.
    Main aims are the following:
    • To maximize the functional capacity of the child
    • To make him or her as independent as possible through a planned intervention program
    Involvement of the family is essential for the overall success in treating a child with CP.

134. What are interdisciplinary, transdisciplinary, and multidisciplinary approaches in CP?
    Fig. 2.9 shows the various approaches in CP.

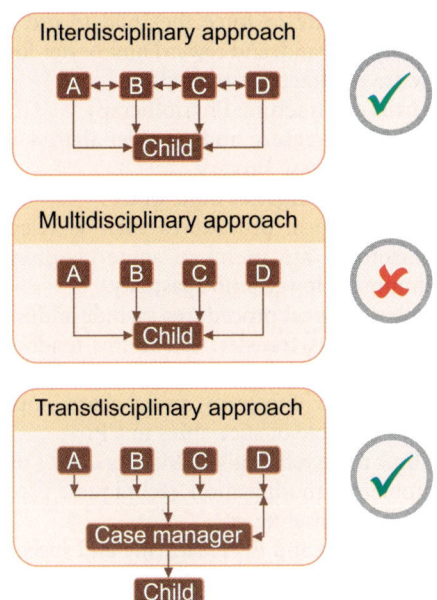

Fig. 2.9 Approach to CP.

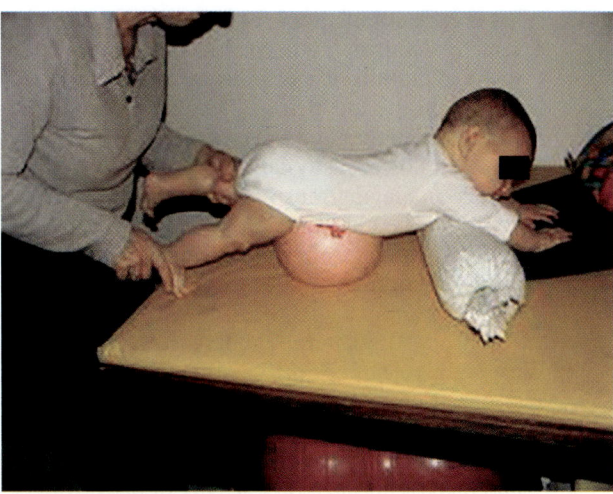

Fig. 2.10 Bobath method. *(Source: European Bobath Tutors Association - The Bobath Concept).*

135. What is the role of physiotherapy in CP?
Principles include the following:
- To improve function
- To abolish abnormal movements
- To promote normal movements
- To inhibit abnormal tone
- To decrease muscle tone in spasticity
- To inhibit primitive reflexes

Advantages are the following:
- Increases muscle strength
- Increases local muscle endurance
- Increases range of motion
- Prevents contractures and deformities

Components of physiotherapy are the following:
- Positioning – decreases stretch reflex
- Exercise – prevents contractures

136. Enumerate the physiotherapy techniques.
- There are several methods. There is no evidence to support the superiority of one over the other. Bobath technique is the most popular. However, an individualized approach according to the child's need is the best.
- Physiotherapy techniques include the following:
  A. Neurodevelopmental theory – Bobath method
    - To abolish abnormal reflexes (ATNR, etc.)
    - To handle the child with the use of key points and sensory stimulus
    - Techniques: Bobath, Vojta, Doman–Delacato, and Peto
  B. Proprioceptive neuromuscular facilitation (NF, Kabat method)
    - To reduce tone to facilitate movements with sensory stimulus
    - Techniques: Temple Fay and high-resistance exercises

The following are the physiotherapy techniques performed in a child with CP:
1. Bobath – neurofacilitation, kinesthetic by positioning the child in reflex inhibitory position as shown in Fig. 2.10

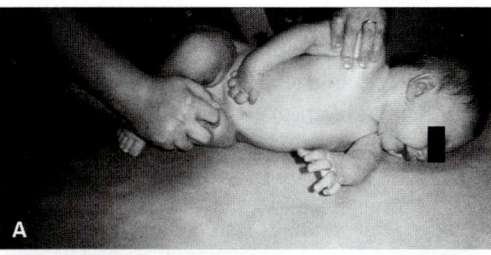

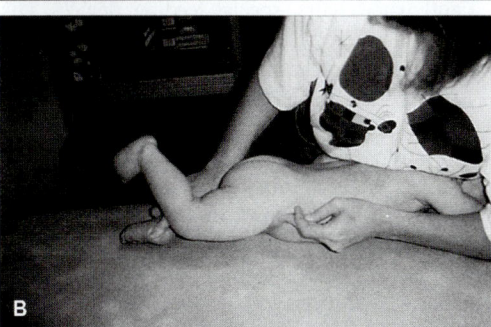

Fig. 2.11 Vojta method. *(Source: Reproduced from Hans-Michael Straßburg, Winfried Dacheneder, Wolfram Kreß. Entwicklungsstörungen bei Kindern: Praxisleitfaden für die interdisziplinäre Betreuung, 6. Auflage, Physiotherapie, Abb. 13.3, Munich, Urban & Fischer DEU, 2018.).*

2. Vojta – neurofacilitation, proprioceptive stimulation, inhibitive casting/bracing on the basis of reflex locomotion, and developmental kinesiology as shown in Fig. 2.11
3. Hippotherapy – horse riding
4. Temple Fay/patterning
5. Delicato method
6. Peto technique – conductive education in group for preparation of self-care
7. Ayers technique – sensory integration
8. Constrained induced (on immobilizing the normal limb, the child will use the affected limb)
9. Hyperbaric oxygen to revive the dormant neurons
10. Hydrotherapy – gravity elimination for better muscle function
11. Light/auditory stimulation

137. What is early stimulation?
    - Usually dendritic and synaptic proliferation occurs within 6 months of age. If there is lack of stimulation during this period, neuronal extinction occurs.
    - Early stimulation and intervention uses plasticity of the central nervous system:
        - Speech: Singing/musical toys/talking to the baby
        - Visual: Hanging a toy
        - Hearing: Songs/musical instruments
        - Tactile stimulation: Touching the baby with love and care
        - Sensory stimulation: Rubbing the baby gently

138. What is the role of occupational therapy in CP?
    The aim of occupational therapy is self-help in feeding and dressing, bathing, toilet training, with progressive development of intricate activities, fine motor activity, and increase in the motor activity of daily living. Occupational therapy consists of several components and these are taught one by one in the required sequence with training in sensory–perceptual–motor coordination.

139. What is home-based management program in CP?
    Parents are taught the correct method of handling and lifting the child and carrying out specific exercises as a part of multisensory stimulation as shown in Fig. 2.12.

140. What are the other therapies in CP?
    - Other therapies include electronic communication and orthopedic devices. CP also requires adaptive and mobility devices such as standing frames, walkers, tricycles and wheelchairs, special feeding devices, customized sitting, lowered toilet seats, and safety grab bars
    - For communication, Blissymbols, talking typewriters, electronic speech devices, and computers – artificial intelligence and computers for motor and language function – are required.
    - Occasionally splints, casts, and calipers may be required to maintain normal postures and to prevent deformity.

141. What is CIMT?
    Constraint-induced movement therapy (CIMT): Restrain the normal unaffected hand for 1–2 hours every day, motivate or force the child to use the affected paralyzed hand, and reward him or her for the same.

142. How are contractures treated?
    - Partial contracture: Physiotherapy
    - Fixed contracture and/or older than 4 years: Contracture release surgery

143. What are the surgeries done in CP?
    a. Neurosurgical procedures such as selective dorsal rhizotomy are useful in some children with predominant lower limb spasticity.
    b. Other surgical procedures include adductor neurectomy, psoas transfer, osteotomy, tendon tenotomy, salivary gland removal/Stensen duct removal, feeding gastrojejunostomy, and cochlear implant.

144. What is the role of specialties in CP?
    - Clinical psychologist: Management of behavior problems, modification techniques, psychotherapy, family counseling, etc.
    - Audiologist and ENT: Hearing and speech problems
    - Ophthalmologist: Corrective glasses, squint surgery, etc.

145. What are the electronic devices used in CP?
    - High-technology devices such as electronic feeding devices, computerized speech systems, and cochlear implants are the latest devices used in a child with CP.

146. What are the drugs used for spasticity?
    Table 2.18 shows the drugs used for spasticity.

147. What is the role of other drugs in CP?
    Other drugs have a limited role in the overall management.
    (a) Anticonvulsant drugs: Selection of an appropriate anticonvulsant drug important
    (b) Drugs used for dystonia: Haloperidol, reserpine, tetrabenazine, L-DOPA for dopa-responsive dystonia, benzodiazepine, and baclofen
    (c) For choreoathetoid: Haloperidol
    (d) Drugs for sleep disturbance: Melatonin (ramelteon), phenobarbitone, and nitrazepam
    (e) Other drugs: L-DOPA and trihexyphenidyl for extrapyramidal symptoms, methylphenidate for hyperactivity and aggressive behavior, atropine or benztropine for sialorrhea, and antireflux drugs for gastroesophageal reflux

148. How is a parent of a child with CP counseled?
    - Interaction of the doctor with the parents is very important.
    - Simple and honest explanations with emphasis on the positive aspects of the child should be provided.
    - When the child grows older, he or she needs appropriate schooling or special training according to his or her abilities.
    - The ultimate goals of management are the following:
        - To help the child to achieve his or her optimal developmental potential
        - To integrate him or her as a functional member in the society
    - Follow-up of the child should be performed.

149. How is a mother counseled regarding the prognosis about walking in a child with CP?
    - Sitting achieved by 2 years: 97% of children will walk.
    - Sitting achieved by 2–4 years: 50% of children will walk.
    - Sitting achieved by >4 years: 3% of children will walk.
    - Persistent ATNR and dystonia at 4 years of age: A child will never achieve ambulation.

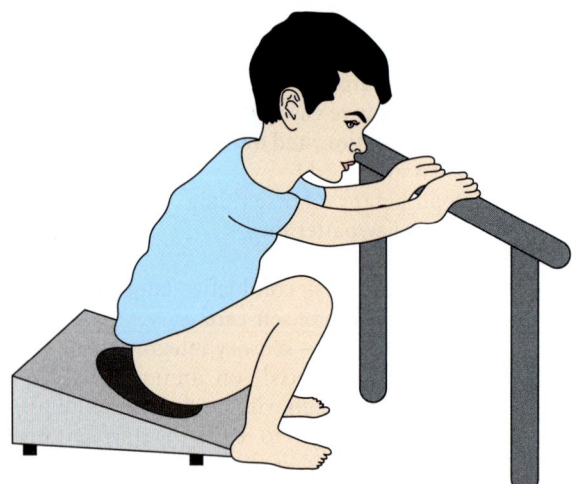

Fig. 2.12 Toileting for the child with CP.

150. How is the prognosis about walking explained with regard to the type of CP?
    - Hemiplegic CP: 100% of children walk by 2 years of age.
    - Diplegic CP: 90% of children walk by 4–7 years of age.
    - Quadriparetic CP: 15% of children walk; majority require total care.
151. What are the poor prognostic factors in a child with CP?
    - The following findings indicate poor prognosis in a child with CP:
        - No head control – 20 months
        - Persistent primitive reflex – 2 years
        - No sitting/floor mobility – 4 years
        - No walking – 7 years
152. What are the good prognostic factors in terms of ambulation in CP?
    - The child is 100% ambulant if he or she:
        - Sits by 2 years
        - Achieves independent crawling by 2–2.5 years
    - The child is 50% ambulant if he or she:
        - Sits by 3–4 years

TABLE 2.18	Drugs Used in CP		
Drug	**Action**	**Dose**	**Side Effects**
Diazepam	Potentiates GABA	1–10 mg (0.1–0.8 mg/kg/day) Three times a day	Sedation
Baclofen IT baclofen Baclofen infusion pump	Inhibits excitatory neurotransmitters at spinal cord	1.25–2.5 mg Two times a day 30–60 mg, every 6 h	Sedation, seizures Catheter kinking, disconnection, respiratory depression, coma
Tizanidine	Inhibits excitatory neurotransmitters	2–8 mg 2–3 times a day	
Dantrolene sodium		0.5 mg/kg/day – b.d.	
Botulinum toxin	Inhibits presynaptic release of acetylcholine	3–6 units/kg (once in 6 months, not less than 3 months; maximum dose per setting, 400 IU; and for each individual muscle, maximum 50 IU per muscle)	Muscle atrophy following repeated use
Selective dorsal rhizotomy	50% of posterior roots of spinal cord from L2 to S2 severed		Decreased sensation, neurogenic bladder

CP, cerebral palsy.

Quick Bites

- The most common cranial nerves involved in CP are cranial nerves IX, X, XI, and XII.
- Persistent cortical thumb is called Critchley sign.
- Commando crawl is seen in diplegic CP.
- The overall prevalence of CP is 1.5–2.5 per 1000 live births.
- CP is multifactorial in etiology.
- CP impersonators are hydrocephalus, subdural hematoma, dopa-responsive dystonia, hypothyroidism, and inborn errors of metabolism.
- Methods of treatment in CP are interdisciplinary, transdisciplinary, and family-centered approach.

3

Acute Hemiparesis

Following introduction, seek permission from the caregiver and introduce yourself to the patient before history elicitation, and identify the case.

Name____Age____Sex____Consanguinity____Order of birth____Place____Informant____

Presenting Complaints and Duration

- Paucity of movements of upper and lower limbs on one side of the body
- Seizures
- Deviation of angle of the mouth to one side

History of Presenting Illness

- Paucity of movement noticed by the mother on one side of the body while playing, not associated with loss of consciousness/seizures or diarrhea, vomiting, fever with rash, and ear discharge
- Nonprogressive weakness; however, help needed by the child for brushing and toileting, but weakness improving following hospitalization and treatment
- Seizures – focal or Generalised tonic clonic seizures (GTCS) lasting for 5 minutes, consciousness regained after few minutes associated with or without urination or defecation, and uneventful postconvulsive phase
- Drooling of saliva and slurring of speech
- Preferential use of hand present

CENTRAL NERVOUS SYSTEM HISTORY

Higher Functions

Altered level of consciousness, history of seizures – focal seizures, difficulty in speech, early handedness, sleep disturbance, altered behavior, and emotional disturbance

Cranial Nerve History

- Ability to perceive light
- Ability to move eyeballs in all four directions
- Ability to chew food
- Facial asymmetry, ability to close both eyes while sleeping, drooling of saliva, and deviation of angle of the mouth
- Ability to hear and respond to sound
- History of nasal twang of voice and nasal regurgitation
- Ability to move the head side to side
- Deviation of the tongue on protrusion

Motor System

- Difference in muscle bulk noted by the mother on one side of the body compared with on the other side, shortening of limbs on one side, and the smallness of the hand if a long standing history is present

- Floppiness/stiffness noted by the mother on one side of the body in the form of difficulty in changing a diaper of a young child
- Ability to move limbs; if able to move, whether it is above the cot or only sideways or just some flicker of movements only
- Abnormal posturing of the affected limb especially if walking
- Gait abnormality – the affected limb posture, dragging of one limb while crawling/creeping, history of not placing one heel/foot on the ground while standing, and position of the upper and lower limbs while walking depending on the motor ability
- Involuntary movements of the limb – proximal or distal, smooth, rapid, jerky, forceful, and absence during sleep

Cerebellar Features

- Swaying of the body
- Abnormal eyeball or head movement or tremors

Bladder/Bowel Disturbance

- Bladder/bowel control attained or not as age appropriate – whether needs assistance for toileting now or there is recent loss of bladder control or incontinence

Sensory Features

- History of perception of pain or crying while giving vaccination or any intramuscular injection and any history of loss of sensation in an older child

Autonomic Features

- Flushing, sweating, and palpitation episodes

Spine and Cranium

- Any abnormality in the head size noted by the mother compared with that of the sibling or peers
- Any swelling, tuft of hair, sinus, discharge, and abnormal curvature

HISTORY OF COMPLICATIONS

- Any history of headache or head banging, irritability, and vomiting – features suggestive of raised intracranial pressure
- History for pressure sores and contractures
- Fever, breathlessness, cough, and vomiting

ETIOLOGICAL HISTORY

- Intraoral pencil trauma
- Eye discharge/ear discharge
- Exanthematous fever
- Recent vaccination
- Leg ulcers, pain in fingers, bone pain, bleeding gums/skin bleeding, and blood transfusion

- Any bleeding disorder
- Pedal edema, abdominal distension, and puffiness of the face
- Diarrhea
- Cyanotic spell, breathlessness/suck–rest cycle, and palpitation
- Fever, joint pain, and rash
- Any surgery – prolonged immobilization
- Recurrent vomiting/convulsion
- Environmental exposure or living near plastic, glass, lead, and battery industries, and drug intake
- Chronic cough, weight loss, and prolonged fever
- Similar episodes before and their duration, and was on any drug prescribed for the same

PROGRESSION OF THE ILLNESS

- Static, improving, and worsening
- New neurological features
- Type of treatment received
- Whether on oral feeds or tube feeds
- If on any therapy for the illness

Past History

- Exanthematous fever
- Comorbid condition (heart disease/liver disease/renal/hematological disorder)
- Recent vaccination
- Similar episodes in the past
- Any medications

Antenatal History

- Antenatal ultrasound – any central nervous system (CNS) malformation
- Any history of drug intake – recreational drugs or therapeutic drugs (alcohol, cocaine, phencyclidine, antiepileptic drugs, antithyroid drugs, selective serotonin reuptake inhibitor [SSRI])
- Infections: Intrauterine infection, urinary tract infection, and exanthematous fever
- History of pregnancy induced hypertension, GDM, and decreased liquor (IUGR)

Birth History

- Breech delivery and history of instrumental delivery such as forceps delivery

Neonatal History

- Birth asphyxia, seizures, features of acute CNS infection (irritability, excessive lethargy), neonatal jaundice, infant of diabetic mother, and intrauterine growth retardation

Development History

- Congenital hemiparesis (yet to walk or stand)
- Acquired hemiparesis (after established standing or walk) – developmental delay, asymmetrical crawl, and early handedness

Dietetic History

As per 24-hour recall method – diet chart

Immunization History

Immunization – as per IAP/Universal Immunization schedule

Contact History

- History of tuberculosis
- Any history pertaining to any other system if relevant or if caregiver is concerned

Family History

Seizures, hemiparesis, tuberculosis, and bleeding tendency

Treatment History

History of medication intake – any treatment advised (drugs), physiotherapy, and aids

Socioeconomic History

According to the modified Kuppuswamy scale

Summary

A ...-year-old child with a history of paucity of movement on the _____ side of the body of duration ____ days with _____ onset, with deviation of angle of the mouth on the ____ side with or without seizures, probably a vascular event, probably a nonprogressive hemiplegia with or without facial nerve involvement, ICP features, and level of the lesion at probably the cortex or internal capsule or brainstem, would need examination findings to localize the site of lesion

General Examination

The child should be comfortable with the mother and examined in a lying posture:

- Consciousness: Eye contact, interaction with the examiner, and playful or dull looking
- Abnormal facies
- Obvious paucity of movement
- Wasting or shortening on one side (indicates chronic disease)
- Malnourishment
- Clubbing, cyanosis, and pallor
- Neurocutaneous marker – facial hemangioma (Sturge–Weber syndrome)
- Palpation of carotids – for any bruit
- BCG scar

Head-to-Foot Examination

- Head – head size, external injuries/bulging fontanelles, abnormal shape, cranial bruit, small head, large head, scar (surgery), Ventriculo peritoneal (VP) shunt, the absence of whorls, and hair loss (preferential lie)
- Face – raccoon eyes/batwing ear sign, discoloration in the face, and glaucoma

- Oral cavity – ecchymosis in the posterior pharynx, dental caries, high-arched palate, and capillary hemangioma looked for
- Eye/ear discharge/cataract/dislocation of lens
- Marfanoid features – tall stature, thumb sign, and wrist sign
- Neurocutaneous markers
- External markers of tuberculosis
- Markers of infective endocarditis
- Multiple bruises
- Petechiae
- Leg ulcers
- Wasting of limbs/nail dystrophy
- Bed sores
- Warm peripheries or cool peripheries
- Peripheral pulse felt

Vital Signs

1. Pulse rate – low volume or large volume
2. Blood pressure – hypotension or hypertension
3. Respiratory rate – the pattern of breathing can help localize the site of lesion
4. Temperature – raised (infection)

Anthropometry

Tall stature

Central Nervous System Examination

HIGHER FUNCTIONS

Ask for COSSHMIB (mnemonic):
- C: Consciousness (recognizes the mother)
- O: Orientation (interacts with the examiner, and orients to time, place, and person)
- S: Sleep
- S: Speech and Language
- H: Handedness (just hold a toy in front in one hand at a time and see with which hand the child reaches for the toy)
- M: Memory (by asking a simple question – what food the child had for breakfast, what was last night's dinner, and what is his or her father's name and home address)
- I: Intelligent quotient
- B: Behavior (any aggressiveness/sleep disturbance)

CRANIAL NERVES

- Cranial nerve I: Tell cranial nerve I could not be tested if the child is younger than 5 years; if the child older than 5 years and if there is no nasal block, conduct the test for olfactory nerve by using familiar smells with eyes closed
- Cranial nerve II: Ask for the following six points:
  A. Light perception
  B. Visual acuity
  C. Color vision
  D. Field of vision
  E. Direct and consensual light reflex
  F. Fundus
- Cranial nerves III, IV, and VI: Check for the movement of eyeballs in all four cardinal directions, strabismus, and ptosis
- Cranial nerve V: Check for the ability to perceive pain sensation over the face, able to chew food, and jaw jerk
- Cranial nerve VII
  - Wrinkling of the forehead present
  - Able to close eyes on both sides while sleeping
  - Absent nasolabial fold on the affected side
  - Deviation of the angle of the mouth to the normal side
  - Drooling of saliva
- Cranial nerve VIII: Ability to obey the mother's command and respond to the mother's call; response to sound – age appropriate
- Cranial nerves IX and X: Palatal movement – normal; uvula in the midline; palatal arches – normal; palatal and pharyngeal reflex – normal
- Cranial nerve XI: Ability to lift the head from a supine position and able to turn the head on both sides
- Cranial nerve XII: Any deviation of the tongue, fibrillation, or wasting

MOTOR SYSTEM

1. Explain about the posture of the child – posture of the affected limb seen in hemiparesis (flexion, adduction) with respect to the affected major joints
2. Bulk
   a. Reduced (any thinning/wasting) noted on the affected side
   b. Any growth arrest noted on the affected side – compare the nail size, thumb size, and hand size on both sides if the illness is of longer duration.
   c. Any leg length discrepancy – shortening of the limb or asymmetrical limb size on the affected side
3. Tone – hypertonia and clasp knife spasticity on the affected side
4. Power – reduced on the affected side
5. Reflexes
   - Superficial reflex – absent on the affected side; abdominal reflex retained
   - Deep tendon reflex – exaggerated on the affected side Plantar extensor on the affected side (plantar extensor till 2 years of age ideally till the child walks; however, asymmetry in any age is abnormal)
6. Involuntary movements – any choreic/dystonic movements while walking
7. Gait – circumduction gait/hemiplegic gait

CEREBELLAR SIGNS

- Head nodding, nystagmus, gait abnormality, ataxia or imbalance, past pointing, and dysdiadochokinesia

AUTONOMIC SYSTEM

- Excessive sweating, tachycardia, and hypotension

SENSORY SYSTEM

- Check for loss of cortical sensation – cortical sensory loss, two-point localization, two-point discrimination, stereognosis, graphesthesia, and hemisensory loss (depends on the level of the lesion).

SPINE AND CRANIUM

Any tuft of hair, swelling, and sacral dimple

SIGNS OF MENINGEAL IRRITATION

Present or not (Kernig/Brudzinski reflex)

Other System Examination

CARDIOVASCULAR SYSTEM

Apical impulse, murmur, and signs of congestive heart failure

RESPIRATORY SYSTEM

Any abnormal breathing pattern

ABDOMEN

Look for hepatosplenomegaly (metabolic cause).

MUSCULOSKELETAL SYSTEM

Any bony deformity and contractures

Diagnosis

A child with the following:
- Acute/chronic
- Nonprogressive/progressive
- Right or left hemiparesis
- Right or left UMN type of facial palsy
- Etiology – ischemia/hemorrhage/thrombosis (most common cause – idiopathic)
- Level of lesion – internal capsule (middle cerebral artery [MCA] territory), cortex, and subcortex level
- Signs of raised ICP +/−
- Nutritional status
- Other associated conditions – malnutrition and anemia

Frequently Asked Questions

1. What are the presenting complaints in a child with acute hemiparesis?

   Presenting complaints include the onset of illness, any preceding event, any associated illness, any underlying illness, and course – static, worsening, and recovery.

2. *List the significance of etiological history in a child with hemiparesis.

   Table 3.1 gives the etiological history in a child with hemiparesis.

3. What is the correlation between trauma and hemiplegia?

   a. Pencil injury: While keeping a pencil in the mouth, there occurs a tear in the intima of the vessel wall, leading to dissecting aneurysm, thrombus, and shedding of emboli; there may be a delayed appearance of the symptoms.

   b. Motor vehicle accidents/falls result in carotid artery injury at its bifurcation.

   c. Traction injuries to the neck as seen in athletes/gymnastics result in vertebral artery injury.

4. What is the relevance of antenatal history and hemiplegia?

   Table 3.2 gives the clues in antenatal history in a child with hemiparesis.

5. What are the risk factors for neonatal stroke?

   a) Infertility

   b) Primiparity

   c) Multiple gestations

6. What are the causes of neonatal stroke?

   a) Idiopathic, which is the most common

   b) Congenital heart disease

   c) Thrombotic placentopathy

   d) Prothrombotic disorders – protein C, protein S, and antithrombin III deficiency

   e) Antenatal cause – mother with collagen vascular disease, an autoimmune disorder, and antiphospholipid antibody syndrome (APLAS)

   f) Meningitis

7. *What are the early signs of hemiplegia in infancy?

   Asymmetric Moro, cortical thumb/Critchley sign, asymmetrical parachute, asymmetrical crawling, early hand preference (younger than 12 months), and normal swinging of the arm lost during walking/running

8. What are the clinical clues for hemiplegic CP on the basis of age?

   Table 3.3 gives the clinical clues in hemiplegia according to age.

9. How is family history important in a child with hemiplegia?

   a) Early onset of coronary heart disease

   b) Hyperlipidemia

   c) Metabolic homocystinuria and Mitochondrial encephalopathy Lactic Acidosis and Stroke like episodes (MELAS)

   d) Hemiplegic migraine

   e) Bleeding disorders

   f) Neurocutaneous syndromes

TABLE 3.1 Etiological History	
Etiology	**Significance**
Intraoral pencil trauma (popsicle injury/lollipop injury)	Carotid artery dissecting aneurysm – thrombosis
Trauma	Bleeding, injury
	TB meningitis – rupture of Rich focus in the brain
Eye discharge/ear discharge	a. Eye infection – orbital cellulitis (cavernous sinus thrombosis)
	b. Ear discharge – mastoiditis, brain abscess, cortical vein thrombosis
Exanthematous fever	Vasculitis
CNS infection	Vasculitis, thrombosis
Tuberculosis	Vasculitis, infarct, thrombosis
Diarrhea	Dehydration – hemoconcentration (thrombosis)
Thrombotic disorder – inherited thrombophilia	Thrombosis
Heart disease	First cyanotic spell: Tetralogy of Fallot (<2 years, thrombosis; >2 years, brain abscess)
	Second cyanotic spell: Features of heart failure – cardiomyopathy
	Third cyanotic spell: Acquired heart disease – rheumatic heart disease (atrial fibrillation)
Recent vaccination	Demyelination
Leg ulcers, pain in fingers, bone pain, bleeding gums	Sickle cell anemia – infarct
Any bleeding disorder	Intracranial bleeding
Pedal edema, abdominal distension, puffiness of face	Nephrotic syndrome – thrombosis
Fever, joint pain, rash	Systemic lupus erythematosus
Any surgery – prolonged immobilization	Deep vein thrombosis
Recurrent vomiting/convulsion	Metabolic cause – homocystinuria, sulfite oxidase deficiency (infarct)
Environmental exposure – plastic, glass, lead, battery industry	Lead encephalopathy
Chronic cough, weight loss, prolonged fever	Tuberculosis
Similar episodes in the past	Homocystinuria, moyamoya disease
Collagen vascular disease	Weakness of the vessel wall
Tonsillar abscess, retropharyngeal abscess	Inflammation of arterial wall

TABLE 3.2	**Antenatal History**
Etiology	**Relevance**
Antenatal – drug intake, infection, Pregnancy induced hypertension (PIH), intrauterine growth restriction (IUGR)	CNS malformation, infarct
Breech/forceps delivery	Carotid intimal tear
Neonatal history – asphyxia, CNS infection, IUGR	Infarct, vasculitis, polycythemia in IUGR – thrombosis

TABLE 3.3	**Clinical Clues in Hemiplegia**
Age	**Clinical Findings**
Newborn	Asymmetric Moro reflex as shown in Fig. 3.1
Infant	Upper limb: Inability to use, paucity of movements, early handedness, persistent fisting beyond 3 months, asymmetrical forward parachute
	Lower limb: Asymmetrical crawling, dragging of one foot
Older child	Abnormal posturing of the affected limb while walking, preferential lie, hair loss in a particular side, sensory disturbances on the affected side
	Upper limb: Thinning of the limb/smallness of the hand
	Lower limb: Not placing one heel/foot on the ground while standing

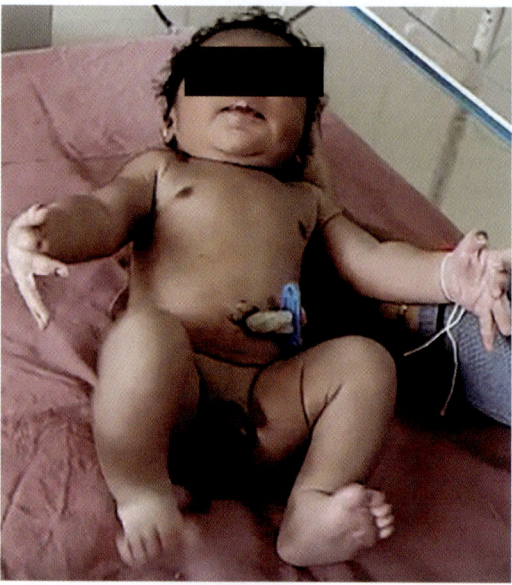

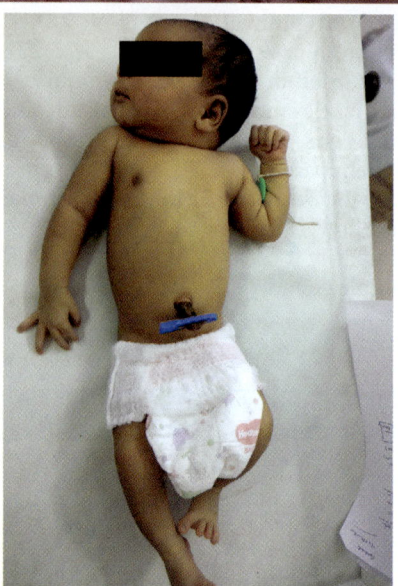

Fig. 3.1 Asymmetric Moro reflex.

g) Substance abuse in family members/socioeconomic status/parental harmony – for child abuse

10. What is the relationship between varicella vaccine and stroke?
    • The median interval between the chickenpox vaccine and the onset of neurological deficits is around 18 weeks.
    • Pathophysiology: Varicella vaccine–related vasculopathy and vessel-wall inflammation with secondary thrombosis may occur.

11. What is the correlation of limb pain in a child with hemiplegia?
    a) Sickle cell anemia (painful digits)
    b) Fabry disease (painful hands and feet)
    c) Deep vein thrombosis – pain in limbs
    d) Long bone fracture – embolism

12. What are the clinical clues in general examination in a child with hemiparesis?
    Table 3.4 gives the clues in general examination in a child with hemiparesis.

13. What is the significance of vital signs in a child with hemiparesis?
    Table 3.5 gives the significance of vital signs in a child with hemiparesis.

14. List the significance of head-to-foot examination in a child with hemiparesis.
    Table 3.6 gives the significance of head-to-foot examination in a child with hemiparesis.

15. What is the significance of anthropometry in a child with hemiparesis?
    Tall stature – Marfan syndrome and homocystinuria

16. What are the skeletal abnormalities seen in hemiplegia?
    a) Kyphosis
    b) Scoliosis
       Leg length discrepancy (Fig. 3.7 shows that the left leg is short; atrophic muscles are seen on the affected side)

TABLE 3.4	**Clues in General Examination**
Clinical Findings	**Relevance**
Pallor	Infective endocarditis
	Sickle cell anemia
	Hematological malignancies
	Bleeding disorder
	Autonomic instability
	Systemic lupus erythematosus (SLE)
Cyanosis	Cyanotic heart disease
Clubbing	Cyanotic congenital heart disease
	Infective endocarditis
	Suppurative lung disease
Generalized lymphadenopathy	SLE
	Tuberculosis
Pedal edema	Nephrotic syndrome
	Congestive heart failure

TABLE 3.5	Significance of Vital Signs	
Vital Signs	**Findings**	**Causes**
Pulse rate	Decreased volume	Hypovolemia
	Large volume	Left-to-right shunt
		Marfan syndrome
Blood pressure	Hypotension	Hypovolemic condition
	Hypertension	SLE
		Raised ICP
		Vasculitis
		Coarctation of aorta
		Thrombosis
Respiratory rate	Pattern of breathing	Localize the site of lesion
Temperature	Increased	Infections/malignancies

SLE, systemic lupus erythematosus.

17. What is the probable underlying etiology in a child with hemiparesis with seizures?
    Meningitis, trauma, homocystinuria, Sturge–Weber syndrome, and cerebral palsy
18. What is the percentage of intellectual impairment in a child with hemiparesis?
    Mental retardation is seen only in 33% of children with hemiparesis.
19. How common is a seizure in a child with hemiparesis?
    Seizures are common in about 25% of children with congenital hemiparesis, and 75%–90% of children with hemiparesis with Sturge–Weber syndrome.
20. What are the pointers toward cortical lesion?
    Table 3.7 gives the cortical signs and their method of elicitation.

TABLE 3.6	Significance of Head-to-Foot Examination
Head	Head size, external injuries/bulging fontanelles, abnormal shape, cranial bruit, small head, large head, scar (surgery), ventriculoperitoneal shunt, the absence of whorls, hair loss (preferential lie)
Face	Raccoon eyes/batwing ear sign, discoloration in the face, glaucoma
	Eye/ear infections
Oral cavity	a. Pharyngeal trauma – look for ecchymosis in posterior pharynx
	b. Dental caries
	c. High-arched palate (Marfan syndrome) – as shown in Fig. 3.2
	d. Capillary hemangioma – Sturge–Weber syndrome
Facial hemangioma	Sturge–Weber syndrome – facial hemangioma as shown in Fig. 3.3
Skin nodules/café au lait macule	Neurofibromatosis as shown in Fig. 3.4
External markers of tuberculosis	Scrofula, scrofuloderma as shown in Fig. 3.5, lupus vulgaris as shown in Fig. 3.6, phlycten, tinea versicolor, tuberculid, erythema nodosum, tuberculosis verrucosa cutis, lichen scrofulosorum
Markers of infective endocarditis	Rash, fingertip nodules, splinter hemorrhage
Signs of child abuse	Multiple bruises at various stages of healing
Petechiae	Bleeding disorders/connective tissue disorders/infection
Marfanoid features	Marfan syndrome, homocystinuria
Leg ulcers	Sickle cell anemia
Difference in thumb size or great toe size	Chronic insult/in utero insult
Wasting of limbs/nail dystrophy	Chronic illness
Cool peripheries	Congestive cardiac failure/hypovolemia
Warm peripheries	Autonomic instability/infection
Peripheral pulses – absent	Takayasu arteritis

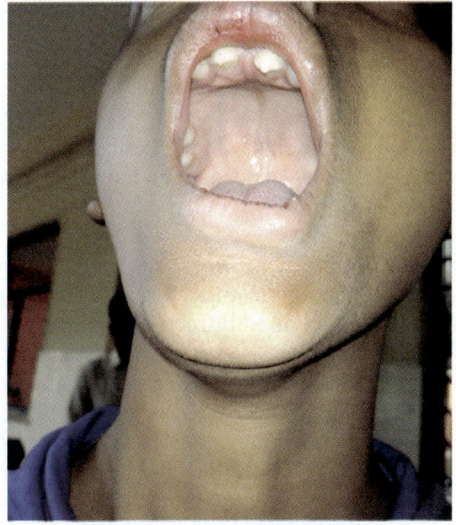

Fig. 3.2 High-arched palate as seen in Marfan syndrome (in a normal child, the posterior part of the hard palate is usually visualized when looked into an open mouth; in high-arched palate, the posterior part of the palate is not visualized).

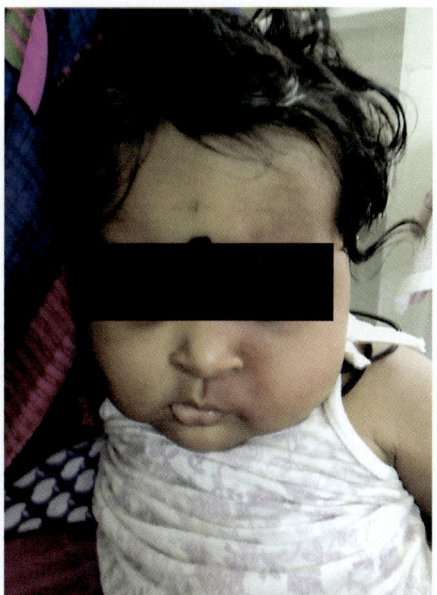

Fig. 3.3 Port-wine stain on left side of face.

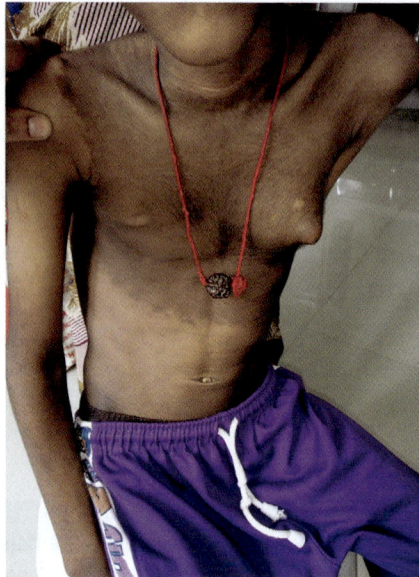

Fig. 3.4 Café au lait macule and plexiform neurofibroma in a child with neurofibromatosis type.

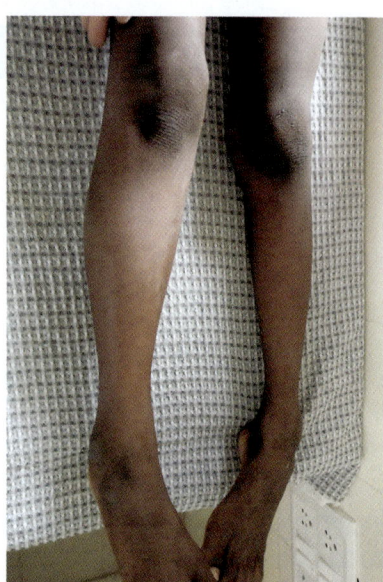

Fig. 3.7 Leg length discrepancy – left leg is shorter than right leg; muscles are atrophied on the affected side.

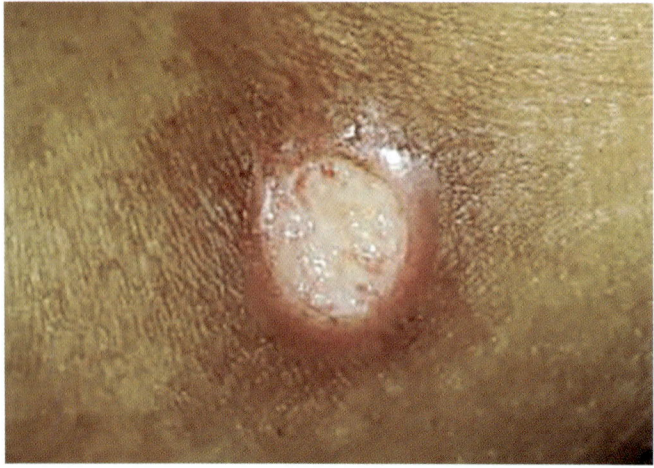

Fig. 3.5 Scrofuloderma seen in extrapulmonary tuberculosis – skin tuberculosis.

TABLE 3.7	Cortical Signs	
Dominant Cortical Signs	**How to Elicit the Signs?**
Apraxia	Inability to perform task or movements; child understands but unable to complete the skilled movements and gestures despite having the desire physical ability to perform – because of brain injury
Agraphia	Inability to write his or her name
Astereognosis	Inability to identify key or any objects in hand
Ideomotor apraxia	Inability to perform a complex motor task (ask the child to brush his or her teeth)
Nondominant cortical signs	Constructional apraxia – difficult to draw objects (ask the child to draw a clock)

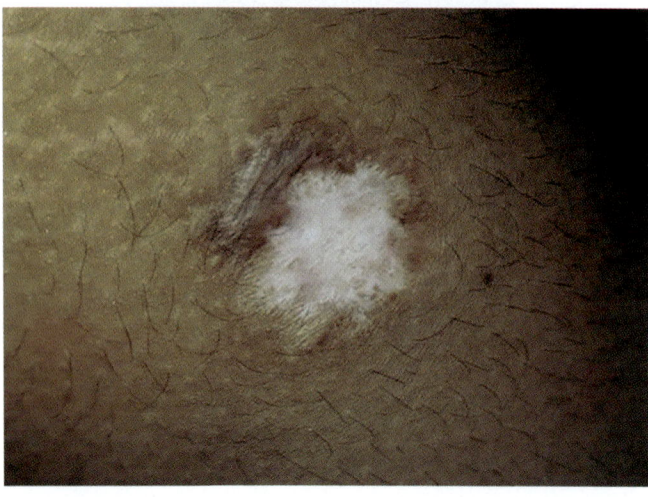

Fig. 3.6 Lupus vulgaris – seen in cutaneous tuberculosis.

21. *What are the eye signs seen in hemiplegia?
    a) Sturge–Weber – glaucoma and buphthalmos
    b) Optic atrophy
    c) Retinal angioma
    d) Homonymous hemianopia
    e) Lens dislocation: Homocystinuria – inferior-nasal
    f) Papilledema: Raised intracranial pressure
    g) Retinal bleeding: Retinal hemorrhages seen in trauma, bleeding disorder, leukemia, and infection
    h) Raccoon eyes: A base of the skull fracture
    i) Pallor: Iron-deficiency anemia and intracranial bleeding
    j) Cyanosis: Cyanotic congenital heart disease
    k) Proptosis: Tumor
22. How are eye position and site of lesion correlated in hemiplegia?
    Table 3.8 gives the correlation between eye position and site of lesion in hemiplegia.

TABLE 3.8	Level of Lesion and Its Corresponding Eye Position	
Level of Lesion	**Eye Position**	
Cerebral hemisphere	Deviated toward the side of the lesion	
Pontine lesion (P–P)	Deviated toward the paralyzed side	
Putamen	Loss of conjugate lateral gaze	
Thalamus	Loss of upward gaze + lateral gaze Unequal pupil	

23. What is the triad of retinitis pigmentosa?
    a. Arteriolar attenuation
    b. Waxy disk pallor
    c. Bone spicule retinal pigmentation
24. *Why is cranial nerve VII involved in hemiplegia?
    All the cranial nerve nuclei are supplied by pyramidal fibers of both sides except the lower part of cranial nerve VII which receives pyramidal fibers from the opposite side. Hence, the upper face receives fibers from the corticobulbar tract of both sides, whereas the lower face receives corticobulbar supply from the opposite side. Hence, the lower face is easily affected.
    *Questions related to facial nerve course in hemiparesis will be asked – kindly refer facial palsy chapter 26.
25. How is the leg length discrepancy demonstrated?
    Gross method: To demonstrate leg length discrepancy, flex the knee joint and check the level of both the knee joints by keeping a pen or pencil over both the knee joints and look for any difference in the level of the scale or pen as demonstrated in Fig. 3.8.
    Conventional method: Measure from the anterior superior iliac spine to the medial malleolus. Leg length difference of >1.5 cm is significant.
26. What are the clinical signs in hemiplegia?
    a) Hoover sign: It is used to differentiate organic and nonorganic paresis of the limb. When the child lies

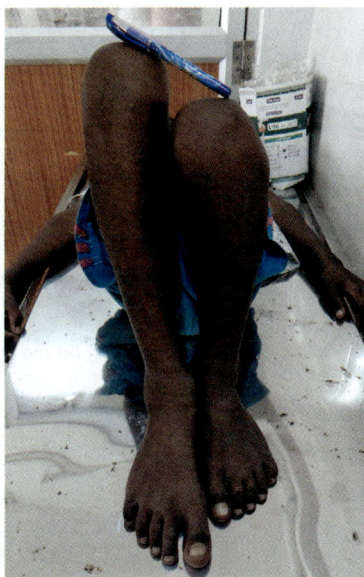

Fig. 3.8 Demonstration of leg length discrepancy.

supine, the examiner holds one hand under the heel of the normal limb and asks the child to flex the contralateral hip. The examiner should feel the normal limb to extend or exert pressure on the examiner's hand. This is based on the principle of synergistic contraction. Hoover sign is demonstrated in Fig. 3.9.
    b) Fog sign: It is used to identify subtle weakness. In case of a mild weakness, the child is asked to evert and walk at that time. The child will attain a hemiplegic posture then, to exhibit the weakness.
    c) Forest sign: Lift the child by the axilla; there will be flexion of the hips; later, the child will develop dystonia or spasticity.
    d) Grasset sign: There occurs normal contraction of the sternocleidomastoid on the paretic side.
27. What are the false localizing signs in a child with hemiplegia?
    a) Unilateral or bilateral III or VI nerve palsy
    b) Bilateral Babinski sign
    c) Bilateral grasp reflex
28. Why is abdominal reflex not lost in a child with hemiplegia as in an adult patient?
    Abdominal reflex is retained till late in infantile hemiplegia and cerebral diplegia, although the pyramidal tract is involved. This is because abdominal reflex is still a localized reflex in children.
29. What are the clinical clues for hemiplegic gait on the basis of age?
    • Infancy: Asymmetrical crawl, early handedness, and abnormal grasp looked for
    • Toddler: History of tiptoe walking, dragging gait, and involuntary movement while walking and running – dystonic posture
    • Childhood: Circumduction gait/hemiplegic gait
30. *Describe circumduction or hemiplegic gait.
    In this gait, the child throws his or her lower limb outwards and goes in a semicircle because of the weakness of dorsiflexion, leaning toward the opposite healthy side; the affected arm is adducted at the shoulder and flexed at the elbow and internally rotated. The lower limb is held in extension with plantar flexion at the foot and toes. Fig. 3.10 shows the circumduction gait.
31. What is the significance of other system examination in a child with hemiparesis?
    Table 3.9 gives the significance of other system examination in hemiparesis.
32. What is the correlation between hemiplegia and heart disease?
    Table 3.10 gives the correlation between heart disease and hemiplegia.
33. What is the pattern of involvement in the affected side in hemiparesis?
    • Motor involvement
      ∘ Affected: Upper limb > lower limb
      ∘ Recovery: Lower limb > upper limb > face
      ∘ Palm: Soft and supple palm
    • Posture
      ∘ Shoulder: Adducted, internally rotated
      ∘ Elbow, wrist, and fingers: Flexed as shown in Fig. 3.11A
      ∘ Lower limb: Extended, ankle equinus as shown in Fig. 3.11B

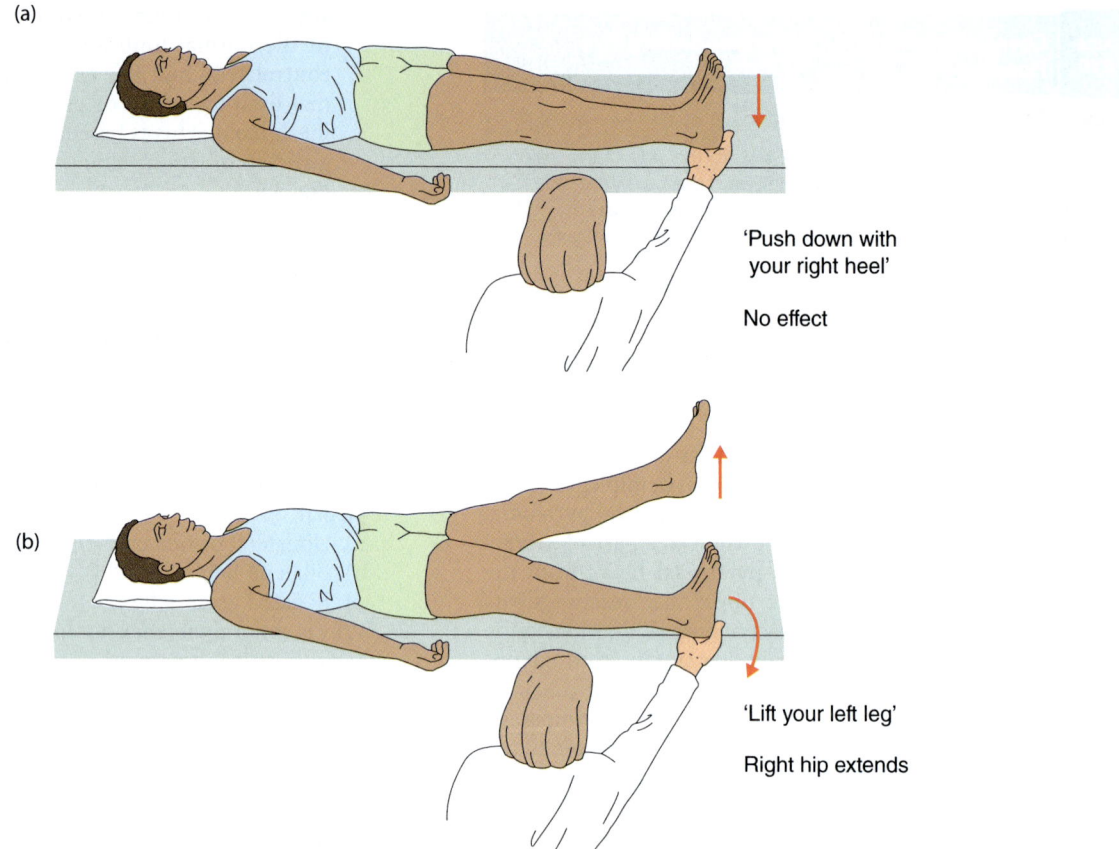

'Push down with your right heel'

No effect

'Lift your left leg'

Right hip extends

Fig. 3.9 Hoover sign. (a) The patient is unable to extend the hip and to press the heel into the bed on request. (b) The hip is extended involuntarily when the opposite leg is lifted off the bed. *(Source: Reproduced from Geraint Fuller, Mark Manford. Neurology, Third Edition, Functional disorders, Fig. 1, Edinburgh, Churchill Livingstone Ltd, 2010.)*

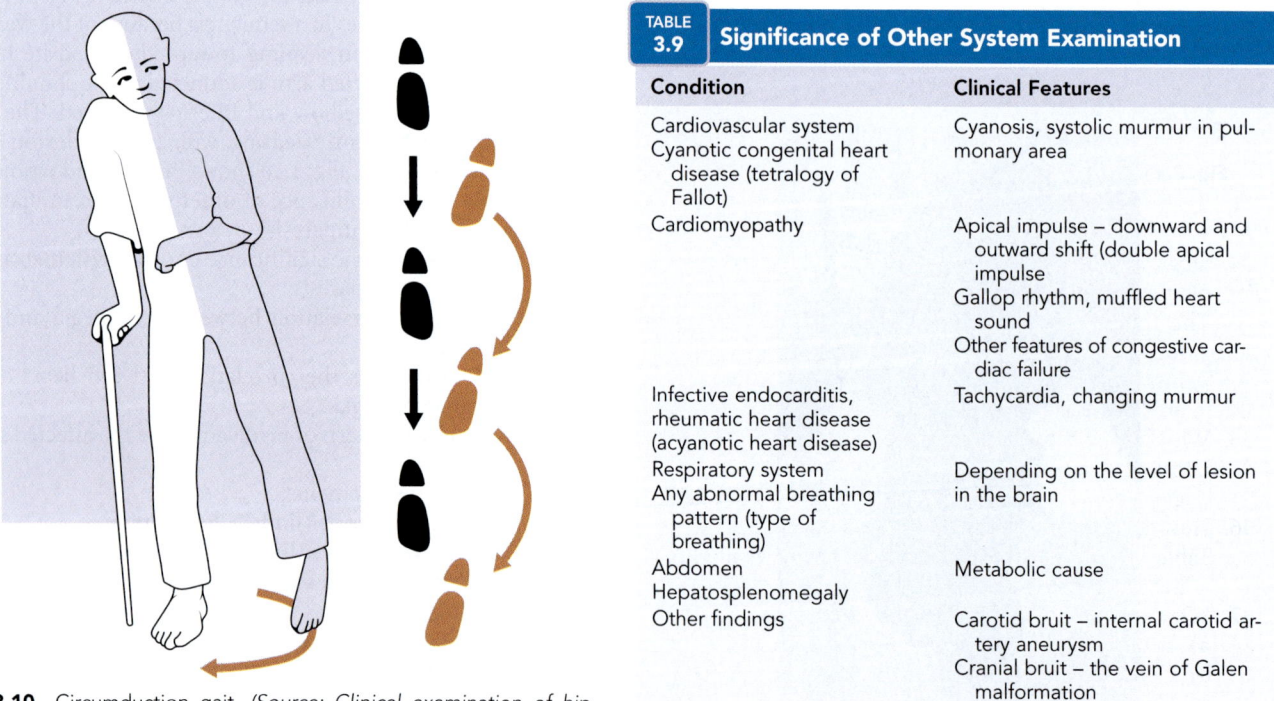

Fig. 3.10 Circumduction gait. *(Source: Clinical examination of hip (slideshare.net))*

TABLE 3.9	Significance of Other System Examination
Condition	**Clinical Features**
Cardiovascular system Cyanotic congenital heart disease (tetralogy of Fallot)	Cyanosis, systolic murmur in pulmonary area
Cardiomyopathy	Apical impulse – downward and outward shift (double apical impulse Gallop rhythm, muffled heart sound Other features of congestive cardiac failure
Infective endocarditis, rheumatic heart disease (acyanotic heart disease)	Tachycardia, changing murmur
Respiratory system Any abnormal breathing pattern (type of breathing)	Depending on the level of lesion in the brain
Abdomen Hepatosplenomegaly	Metabolic cause
Other findings	Carotid bruit – internal carotid artery aneurysm Cranial bruit – the vein of Galen malformation Renal bruit – renal artery stenosis

TABLE 3.10	Correlation Between Heart Disease and Hemiplegia	
Cyanotic Congenital Heart Disease		**Venous Infarct**
Cardiac abscess		Paradoxical embolism
Arrhythmia, left atrial myxoma, and mitral valve prolapse		Emboli
Cardiogenic shock, low perfusion		Watershed infarct

1. Internal rotation and adduction of the shoulder
2. Flexion at the elbow
3. Forearm pronation
4. Flexed wrist
5. Tight fist

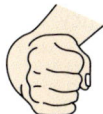
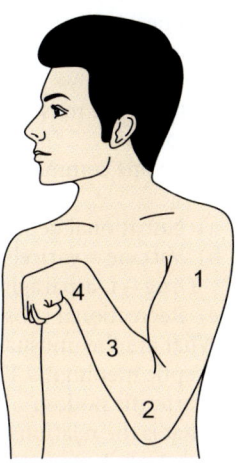

6. Clenched thumb

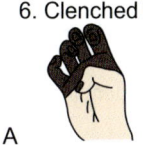

A

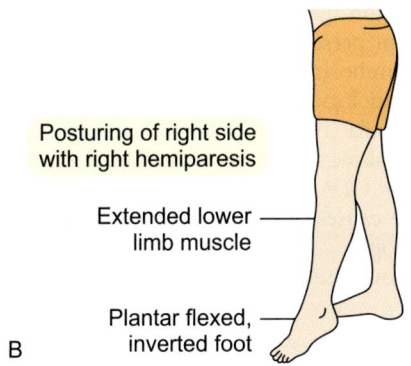

Posturing of right side with right hemiparesis

Extended lower limb muscle

Plantar flexed, inverted foot

B

Fig. 3.11 (A) Upper limb posture. (B) Lower limb posture.

34. How is thumb shortening on the hemiparetic side explained?
    The thumb has a large representation in the parietal lobe, so it is more affected and also represents in utero insult or chronic cause. Fig. 3.12 shows thumb shortening on the hemiplegic side.
35. Why is there unilateral clubbing in hemiplegia?
    Local autoimmune dysregulation is seen in the hemiplegic side because of chronic hemiplegia.
36. How is Erb palsy differentiated from hemiplegia?
    Table 3.11 gives the differences between Erb palsy and hemiplegia.
37. What are the complications associated with hemiplegia?
    a) Bedsores
    b) Contractures
    c) Convulsions
    d) Deep vein thrombosis

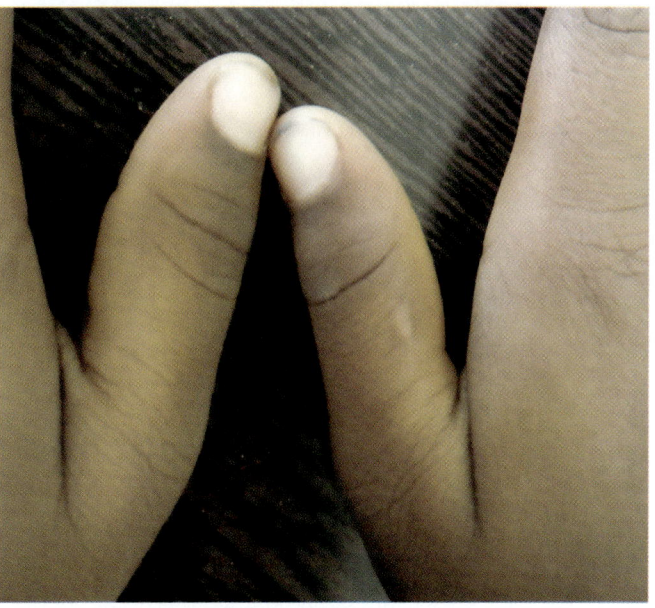

Fig. 3.12 Thumb shortening on hemiplegic side.

TABLE 3.11	Differences Between Erb Palsy and Hemiplegia	
Features	**Erb Palsy**	**Hemiplegia**
History	History of trauma, difficult labor	Usually picked up late – asymmetrical crawl, early handedness
Causes	Fractured clavicle, fractured humerus Brachial plexus injury	Hypoxic-ischemic encephalopathy (HIE) sequelae
Posture	Shoulder: Adducted Elbow: Extended Grasp reflex: Present Fig. 3.13 shows right Erb palsy	Shoulder: Adducted Elbow: Flexed Critchley thumb Fig. 3.14 shows hemiplegic limb

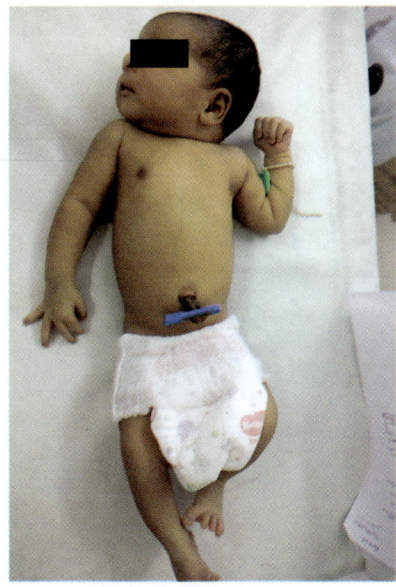

Fig. 3.13 Right Erb palsy.

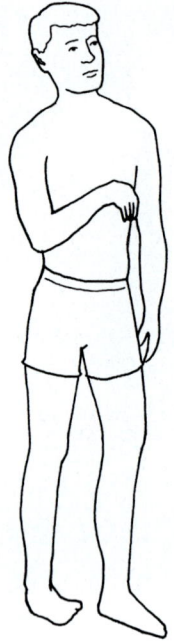

Fig. 3.14 Hemiplegic limb. *(Source: Reproduced from Mary Patnaude. Early's Physical Dysfunction Practice Skills for the Occupational Therapy Assistant, Fourth Edition, Neurotherapeutic Approaches to Treatment, Fig. 20.18, St. Loius, Mosby Inc., 2022.)*

e) Infection – bronchopneumonia and UTI
f) Joint deformity – fixed flexion deformity
g) Urinary tract infections

38. What are the differential diagnoses of stroke?
   a) Migraine
   b) Seizures
   c) Infections
   d) Demyelination
   e) Metabolic disturbances – hypoglycemia
   f) Watershed infarct by global hypoxic-ischemic encephalopathy

g) Hypertensive encephalopathy (posterior reversible leukoencephalopathy)
h) Inborn error of metabolism – neuroregression
i) Vestibulopathy
j) Acute cerebellar ataxia
k) Alternating hemiplegia of childhood

39. *What are stroke mimickers?
   a) Multiple sclerosis
   b) Hemiplegic migraine
   c) Cerebral tumor/abscess
   d) Head injury

40. Enumerate the causes of stroke.
   Flowchart 3.1 shows the causes of stroke.
   Table 3.12 shows the examples of various causes of stroke.

41. *What is the most common cause of stroke in children?
   Idiopathic

42. Name one common etiological association with hemiparesis.
   a) Nutritional deficiency – iron deficiency
   b) Vaccine – varicella
      Drug – L-asparaginase
   c) Recreational substance – cocaine

43. What are the unusual causes of stroke?
   Aseptic meningitis, Kawasaki disease, and infantile polyarteritis nodosa

44. What is the relationship between iron-deficiency anemia and stroke?
   (a) Rarely iron deficiency has been recognized as a significant cause of stroke in the adult or pediatric populations.
   (b) The common age group is around 6–18 months, and the patient presents with an ischemic stroke or venous thrombosis after a viral prodrome.
   (c) Three physiological mechanisms explaining iron-deficiency anemia (IDA) in childhood ischemic stroke are hypercoagulable state secondary to IDA, thrombocytosis secondary to IDA, and anemic hypoxia induced by IDA.

45. What are the causes of ischemic stroke on the basis of pathophysiology?
   Table 3.13 shows the causes of ischemic stroke.

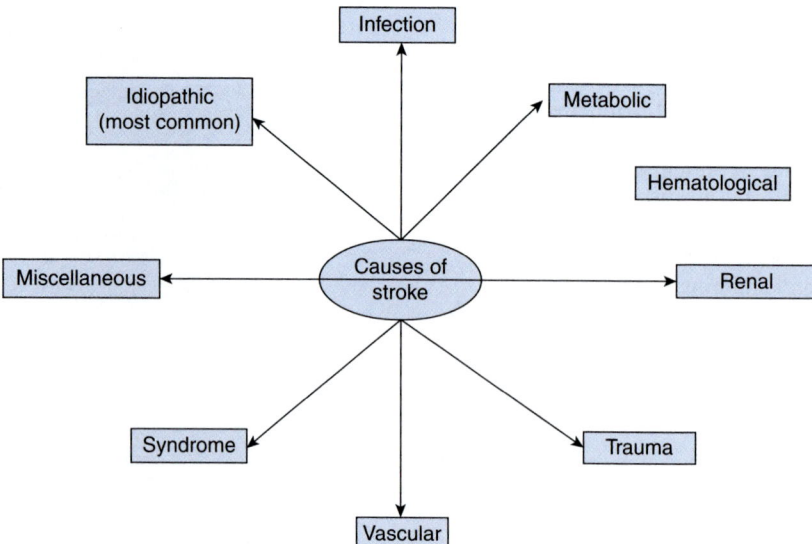

Flowchart 3.1 Causes of stroke.

TABLE 3.12	Various Examples of Each Cause of Stroke	
Infection	**Metabolic**	**Hematological**
Sepsis	Homocystinuria	Prothrombotic
Orbital cellulitis	Propionic acidemia	APLAS
ENT infection	MELAS	Protein C and protein S deficiency
Pharyngitis (Lemierre syndrome)		Write as Antithrombin III deficiency
Diarrhea		Sickle cell anemia
		ITP
Renal	**Trauma**	**Heart Disease**
Nephrotic syndrome	MCA – EDH	Congenital
Hemolytic uremic syndrome	Bridging vein – SDH	• Complex CHD
	SAH	• Coarctation of aorta
	Nonaccidental injury (NAI) – SDH	• Aortic stenosis
	Sports/gymnastic	• Left-to-right shunt with Valsalva maneuver
		• CCF – global cerebral ischemia
		Acquired heart disease
		• Rheumatic HD
		• Infective endocarditis
		• Myocarditis
		• Cardiomyopathy
Vascular	**Syndromes**	**Miscellaneous**
Post-varicella	Sturge–Weber syndrome	Lead/glass/battery
Moyamoya	PHACES	Drugs – L-asparaginase
Meningitis	Neurofibromatosis	Cocaine/OCP
SLE	Tuberous sclerosis	Lollipop stroke
Takayasu	Von Hippel–Lindau disease	Child abuse
AV malformation	Ataxia telangiectasia	Prolonged immobility
Aneurysm		
Hemangioma		
Fibromuscular dysplasia		

APLAS, antiphospholipid antibody syndrome; MCA, middle cerebral artery; SLE, systemic lupus erythematosus.

TABLE 3.13	Causes of Ischemic Stroke
Infections	Meningitis, encephalitis
Cardiovascular system	Rheumatic heart disease, septal defects, subacute bacterial endocarditis, arrhythmias, cardiomyopathies
Vasculitis	Immune vasculitis, moyamoya, fibromuscular dysplasia
Collagen vascular disease	Antiphospholipid antibody syndrome (APLAS)
Hematological	Antithrombin III deficiency, sickle cell anemia, polycythemia, thrombocytosis, leukemia, protein C and S deficiency
Metabolic	Organic acidemias, homocystinuria, mitochondrial disorders, Fabry disease
Trauma	Traumatic brain injury

46. What are the causes of hemorrhagic stroke?
   a. Coagulopathies
   b. Vascular malformations
   c. Tumors
   d. Hematological – leukemia, thrombocytopenia, and secondary to liver disorders
47. *What is the common association of stroke in Indian studies?
   • According to the AIIMS study in hemiplegia:
      • Ischemic stroke: 88% of cases (prothrombotic, cardiac, hyperlipidemia, homocystinuria)
      • Hemorrhagic stroke: 12% of cases

48. How does systemic lupus erythematosus cause hemiparesis?
   Thrombosis, infarction, and hemorrhage
49. What are the causes of chronic progressive hemiplegia?
   • Brain abscess
   • Arteriovenous malformation
   • Sturge–Weber syndrome
   • Tumor
   • Demyelinating disease – multiple sclerosis and adrenoleukodystrophy
50. What are the causes of recurrent hemiplegia?
   Remember as 4 M:
      a) Moyamoya disease (causes of moyamoya – primary and secondary [Down syndrome, Alagille syndrome, neurofibromatosis, fibromuscular dysplasia, tuberculosis, sickle cell])
      b) Metabolic – homocystinuria
      c) Migraine
      d) Multiple emboli
   Other causes of recurrent hemiplegia
      a) Todd paralysis
      b) Prothrombotic conditions
51. *What are the causes of transient hemiplegia?
   1. Transient ischemic attack
   2. Todd palsy
   3. Hemiplegic migraine
   4. Multiple sclerosis
   5. Hysterical hemiplegia

52. What are the causes of congenital hemiplegia?
    a) Prenatal/perinatal – birth asphyxia
    b) Vascular
    c) Preterm
    d) CNS malformation
53. What are the causes of paroxysmal hemiplegia?
    a) Hemiplegic migraine
    b) Todd paralysis
54. What are the causes of familial stroke?
    a) MELAS
    b) Fabry
    c) Sulfite oxidase deficiency
    d) Ornithine transcarbamylase deficiency
    e) Leigh syndrome
    f) Migraine
    g) Sickle cell anemia
    h) Hyperlipidemia
55. What is locked-in syndrome?
    • The child is aware of the surroundings.
    • There is no movement/communication.
    • Only vertical eye movement is possible.
    • The lesion is in the ventral pons.
56. What is one-and-a-half syndrome?
    • Seen in pontine lesion
    • Ipsilateral adduction defect in one eye and horizontal gaze-evoked nystagmus in the contralateral eye
    • Seen in internuclear ophthalmoplegia
57. What is internuclear ophthalmoplegia?
    • Internuclear ophthalmoplegia (INO) is an ocular movement disorder. In INO, there is conjugate lateral gaze palsy in one eye and ophthalmoplegia in the other eye as shown in Fig. 3.15. This is due to damage to the interneuron between two nuclei of cranial nerve VI and III (internuclear). This interneuron is called the medial longitudinal fasciculus (MLF).
    • This MLF is a nerve tract as shown in Fig. 3.16 that connects the oculomotor nucleus (cranial nerve III) of the ipsilateral side with the paramedian pontine reticular formation (PPRF) and cranial nerve VI of the contralateral pons. The INO is characterized by ipsilateral adduction deficit (partial or complete) in one eye with a contralateral, horizontal gaze-evoked nystagmus in the abducting eye.

58. What are the syndromes associated with hemiplegia?
    a. Sturge–Weber syndrome
    b. Neurofibromatosis
    c. Tuberous sclerosis
    d. Linear nevus syndrome
    e. PHACE syndrome
    f. Incontinentia pigmenti
59. What is congenital unilateral perisylvian syndrome?
    It refers to unilateral widening and verticalization of the Sylvian fossa associated with an abnormal ipsilateral perisylvian cortex. This leads to hemiplegia.
60. Name the hemiplegic syndromes according to the site of lesion.
    Table 3.14 gives the hemiplegic syndrome and its site of lesion.
61. How is a child with hemiparesis investigated?
    a) Complete blood count
       i. Raised total leukocyte count – infection
       ii. Polycythemia – dehydration and cyanotic heart disease
       iii. Anemia – sickle cell anemia/malignancy/bleeding disorders
       iv. Thrombocytopenia

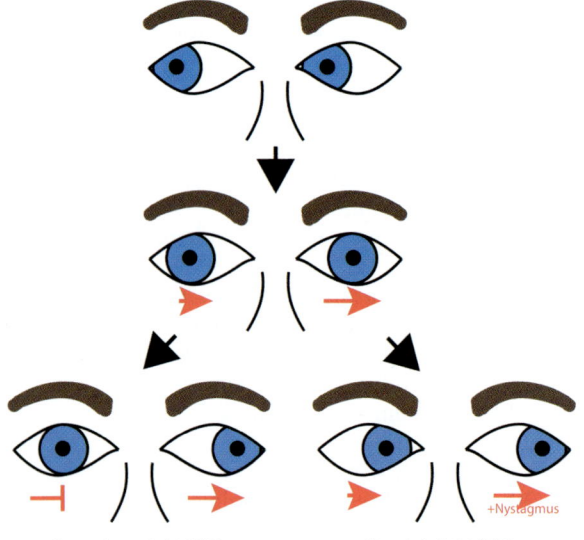

Fig. 3.15 Internuclear ophthalmoplegia (INO). The top image shows normal gaze to the right. With gaze to the left, the right eye lags behind the left (middle image) and may fail to adduct completely (bottom image). However, in milder INO only lag in the adducting eye will be evident. (*Source: Reproduced from Brad Frankum. Essentials of Internal Medicine, Third Edition, Neurology, Figure 19-18, Sydney, Churchill Livingstone AUS, 2015.*)

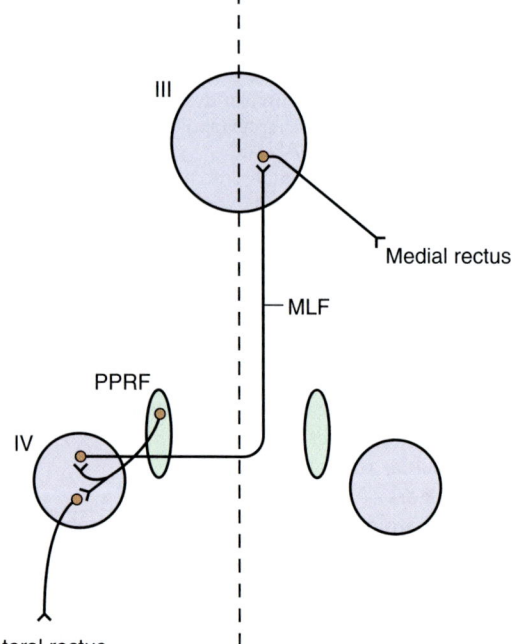

Fig. 3.16 Median longitudinal fasciculus (MLF) and paramedian pontine reticular formation (PPRF) nerve tract. (*Source: Supranuclear Control of Eye Movements | Ento Key.*)

TABLE 3.14	Hemiplegic Syndrome and Its Site of Lesion	
Level of Lesion	**Syndrome**	**Features**
Midbrain	Weber syndrome	Ipsilateral cranial nerve III palsy + contralateral hemiplegia
Pons	Benedikt syndrome	Weber + red nuclei lesion (ataxia, rigidity, tremor on opposite side)
	Raymond syndrome	Nerve VI + pyramidal tract
	Millard–Gubler syndrome	Nerve V + nerve VI + pyramidal tract
	Foville syndrome	Nerve VII + pyramidal tract + paramedian pontine reticular formation (median longitudinal fasciculus)
Medulla	Jackson	Nerves X and XII + pyramidal tract

b) Renal function test – abnormal in conditions causing global cerebral ischemia (hypovolemia) and nephrotic syndrome

c) Liver function test

d) Coagulation profile

e) Antinuclear antibodies

f) Cardiological workup – ECG, Echocardiogram, and chest X-ray

g) Prothrombotic workup – serum protein C, protein S, and antithrombin III levels

h) Metabolic workup – mitochondrial disorder (pyruvate, lactate)

i) Neuroimaging – MRI brain: Dyke–Davidoff–Masson sign (atrophic cerebral hemisphere secondary to brain insult with dilated ventricle [cystic changes with porencephalic cyst especially in the parietal lobe])

62. Mention few MRI findings in hemiplegia.
    a) Old infarct or gliosis
    b) Porencephalic cyst
    c) Schizencephaly
    d) Hemiatrophy
    e) Gyral calcification

63. How is a child with acute hemiparesis evaluated?
    Flowchart 3.2 gives the evaluation of a child with acute hemiparesis.

64. What are the contraindications for cerebral angiography?
    a. Complicated migraine
    b. Hemodynamic instability
    c. Allergic to contrast/dye
    d. Coagulopathy
    e. Severe intracranial hemorrhage

65. What is the initial line of management when a child presents with acute hemiparesis?
    a) Place the patient supine with the head end flat.
    b) Stabilize airway, breathing, and circulation.
    c) Maintain normothermia, euvolemia, normotension, and euglycemia (for children older than 2 years, no glucose-containing i.v. fluids unless hypoglycemic, and for children younger than 2 years, DNS fluid).
    d) Avoid hypoxia/hypercarbia – it can cause cerebral vasodilatation.
    e) Hypocarbia can cause cerebral vasoconstriction.
    f) Manage the raised intracranial pressure.

66. What are the indications for tissue plasminogen activator?
    a. Ischemic stroke
    b. No history of bleeding disorders, hypertension, major surgery in the past 14 days, and anticoagulant intake
    c. Patient presenting within 4.5 hours
    d. Age >2 years

67. What is the mechanism of action of tissue plasminogen activator (tPA)?
    • Blood clots are formed from the aggregation of activated platelets onto fibrin meshes. The breakdown of the fibrin meshes is achieved by plasmin. This plasmin

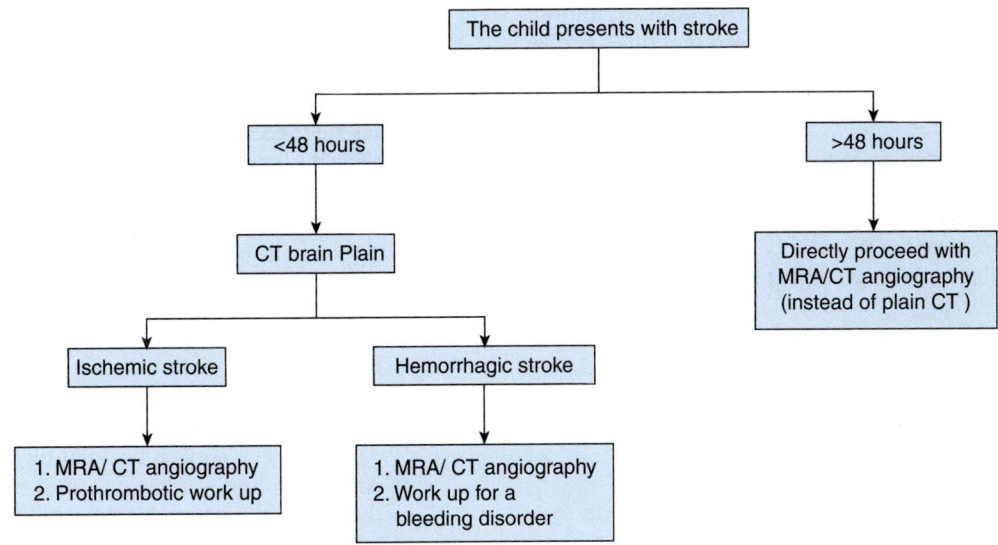

Flowchart 3.2 Evaluation of a child with acute hemiparesis.

cleaves fibrin, thus breaking down the meshwork of the clot. It is quickly inactivated by α_2-antiplasmin, an abundant inhibitor that restricts the action of plasmin because it is extremely short-lived. Thus, fibrinolysis is achieved by adequate generation of plasmin. Examples of PAs (plasminogen activators) are the tPA (tissue-type plasminogen activator) and the uPA (urokinase-type plasminogen activator).

68. How is tissue plasminogen activator administered?
    a. Dose is 0.9 mg/kg.
       (Administer 10% of the total dose over 5 minutes; remaining 90% dose is given as an infusion over 1 hour.)
    b. Watch for hypertension.
    c. This is followed by anticoagulants – aspirin/warfarin.
69. How is a child with hemorrhagic stroke managed?
    a. Stabilize the child.
    b. Refer the child for urgent neurosurgical intervention (burr hole drainage).
    c. Definitive repair of any vascular malformations is done after the child improves.
70. What is the supportive treatment given to a child with hemiparesis?
    a) Frequent suctioning of oropharyngeal secretions
    b) Frequent change of positions in the bed
    c) Nutritional support
    d) Physiotherapy
    e) Bowel and bladder care
71. How is hemiparesis caused by sickle cell anemia managed?
    • First-line management is the same – stabilize airway, breathing, and circulation (ABC).
    • When time-averaged mean maximum (TAMM) blood flow velocity is >200 cm/s by transcranial Doppler ultrasonography, transfusions are given to maintain target Hb 10 g/dL and target HbS <30% to prevent autotransfusion and volume overload.
    • Drug: Hydroxyurea is given.
72. What is the STOP trial in the management of stroke in sickle cell disease?
    Management of stroke in sickle cell disease
    a. Sickle cell disease was evaluated in the Stroke Prevention Trial in Sickle Cell Anemia (STOP trial).
    b. This randomized controlled trial done in children with sickle cell anemia revealed that there is 70% decrease in the incidence of stroke after elective transfusion compared with after standard transfusion.
73. What are the poor prognostic factors associated with hemiplegia?
    a) Age <3 years
    b) When presented with seizures
74. What are the neurological impairments seen in hemiplegia?
    Involuntary and hyperkinetic movement, behavioral problems, and seizures

DISCUSSION ON STROKE

75. What is the WHO definition of stroke?
    • WHO definition: Stroke is a clinical syndrome consisting of rapidly developing clinical signs of focal/global disturbance of cerebral function lasting more than 24 hours or leading to death with no apparent cause other than the vascular origin.
    • The definition of clinical stroke in the textbook by Fenichel is as follows: A focal neurological deficit lasting more than 24 hours, with neuroimaging evidence of abnormality in an established vascular territory.
76. What is the other name for hemiparesis?
    facio-brachio-crural paresis
77. *What is a transient ischemic attack (TIA)?
    TIA is a neurological deficit of <24 hours without neuroimaging abnormalities.
78. What is Todd paralysis?
    It is postictal paralysis that usually resolves completely without any deficit and lasts for few to 48 hours.
79. What are the types used in hemiplegia?
    Table 3.15 gives the types of hemiplegia.
80. What are the other types in stroke?
    a) Carotid/stuttering hemiplegia: It consists of a triad – visual disturbance, carotid bruit, and hemiplegia.
    b) Transient ischemic attack: It is a transient episode of focal neurological dysfunction caused by ischemia in the focal area in the brain or retina without infarction in the clinically relevant area of the brain or retina. Symptoms are resolved completely within 24 hours.
    c) Reversible ischemic neurological deficit (RIND): It lasts for >24 and <96 hours.
81. What is the pathophysiology in stroke and what is ischemic cascade system?
    Ischemic cascade is a series of events that take place following an ischemic insult to an organ.
    Flowchart 3.3 shows the ischemic cascade.
82. How does ischemia cause stroke in the child?
    Ischemia causes
    a) Reduction of blood flow to zero causes infarct in 4–10 minutes.
    b) Blood flow of 16 mL/100 g of brain tissue causes infarct in 1 hour.
    c) Blood flow of 20 mL/100 g of brain tissue causes ischemia but not infarct.
83. What is ischemic penumbra?
    It is the area of ischemic tissue surrounding the infarct region. If ischemia is not corrected, it can progress to infarct. Hence, it is the target area during revascularization.
84. What are the stages of hemiplegia?
    Table 3.16 shows the stages of hemiplegia.
85. What are the differences between thrombosis, embolism, and hemorrhagic stroke?
    Table 3.17 shows the differences between thrombosis, embolism, and hemorrhagic stroke.
86. How is hemiplegia classified?
    a) Anatomical – cortical, subcortical, internal capsule, brainstem, and cord
    b) Tone – spastic and flaccid
    c) Cause – primary and secondary
    d) Age of onset – congenital, infantile, and adult onset
    e) Artery involved – anterior carotid artery (ACA), middle cerebral artery (MCA), and posterior cerebral artery (PCA)

TABLE 3.15 Types of Hemiplegia	
Types of Hemiplegia	**Clinical Features**
Complete hemiplegia	UMN cranial nerve VII + hemiplegia
Incomplete hemiplegia	Hemiplegia without involvement of cranial nerve VII
Ipsilateral hemiplegia	Weakness on same side of a lesion
	Lesion below the level of the brainstem
Contralateral hemiplegia	Weakness opposite to the side of the lesion
	Lesion above the level of the brainstem
Crossed/contralateral hemiplegia	At brainstem level
	Ipsilateral LMN cranial nerve palsy + contralateral hemiplegia
Brachial monoplegia	Upper limb paralysis
Crural monoplegia	Lower limb paralysis
Cruciate hemiplegia at the level of decussation	Brachial monoplegia of one side + contralateral crural monoplegia
Bibrachial	Paralysis of both upper limbs
Bilateral hemiplegia	Paralysis of all four limbs
Triplegia	Three limbs involved – both upper limbs + one lower limb
Cord hemiplegia	Lesion below medulla but above C5 segment
	Posterior column involvement on the same side
	Spinothalamic on the opposite side
	Cranial nerves are spared
Stuttering hemiplegia	Stroke in evolution is a progressive worsening in the neurological deficit interspersed with transient improvements followed by a fully evolved stroke

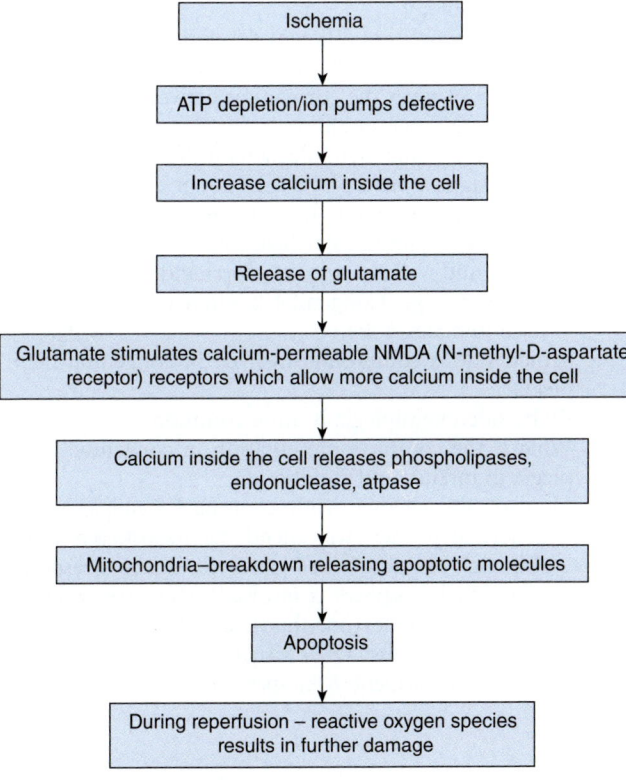

Flowchart 3.3 Ischemic cascade.

TABLE 3.16 Stages of Hemiplegia		
Stage of Neuronal Shock	**Stage of Recovery**	**Stage of Residual Paralysis**
First stage	Second stage	Final/third stage
Few hours/days to 2–3 weeks	After 3–4 weeks	Following recovery
Drowsy/coma	Following order:	Classical hemiplegic gait
Hypotonia	Face – earliest to recover	
DTR – absent		
Plantar – no response	UL - first flexor	
	LL - first extensor	
	Dorsiflexor of foot	
	Finger movement difficult to recover	

Note:
UL - Upper limb
LL - Lower limb

89. How is the level of lesion in stroke localized?
Table 3.20 shows the level of lesion and stroke.
90. *What are watershed areas of the brain?
a) They are vulnerable border zones between the anterior cerebral artery (ACA), middle cerebral artery (MCA), and posterior cerebral artery (PCA).
b) They are prone to ischemia in global hypoperfusion.
c) Watershed areas are the bilateral parasagittal area of the cortex (between ACA and MCA), the bilateral parieto-occipital region of the cortex (between MCA and PCA), and the subcortical white matter (between lenticulostriate branch and MCA) as shown in Fig. 3.17.
91. What is lacunar infarction?
Lacunar infarcts are 3 mm to 2 cm in diameter. They are small or deep infarcts due to occlusion of perforating/penetrating arteries in the brain substance. They occur because of atherothrombotic/lipohyalinotic occlusion of penetrating arteries.

87. What are the clinical clues in a child with hemiparesis to identify the type of artery involved?
Table 3.18 shows the clinical clues to identify the type of artery involved in a child with hemiparesis.
88. How is stroke classified on the basis of a clinical course?
Table 3.19 shows the classification of stroke on the basis of the course of clinical illness.

TABLE 3.17	Differences Between Thrombosis, Embolism, and Hemorrhagic Stroke		
Features	Thrombosis	Embolism	Hemorrhage
Cause	Vessels (vasculitis, systemic lupus erythematosus, meningitis, encephalitis, postinfection, cerebral abscess), CNS infection Hematological – hypercoagulable (nephrotic syndrome, proteins C and S, sickle cell disease)	Cardiac (cyanotic congenital heart disease, acyanotic congenital heart disease, arrhythmia) Infective endocarditis Septic emboli from the abscess	A bleeding tendency, trauma, arteriovenous malformation, aneurysm
Onset	Subacute	Acute	Catastrophic
Time of onset	Immediately after waking up	Precipitated by exertion	
Progression	Stepladder	Maximal at onset	
Prognosis	Good	Poor	Poor
History of TIA	Present	Absent	Absent
History of headache/neck pain	Absent	Absent	Present
Loss of Consciousness	Only if large areas are involved	Unusual	Present

TIA, transient ischemic attack.

TABLE 3.18	Clinical Clues to Identify the Type of Artery Involved in a Child With Hemiparesis		
ACA/Heubner Artery	MCA/Charcot's Artery	PCA	
Spastic UL Flaccid LL	Flaccid UL/spastic LL Face and arm affected	Visual defect Loss of color recognition	
Cortical sensory loss + Urinary incontinence	Cortical sensory loss + Wernicke's aphasia	Memory loss Loss of naming of objects	

ACA, anterior carotid artery; MCA, middle cerebral artery; PCA, posterior cerebral artery.

TABLE 3.19	Course of Stroke in a Child			
	ACUTE ONSET		CHRONIC ONSET	
Nonprogressive	Progressive	Nonprogressive	Progressive	
1. Vascular 2. Infection – meningitis, encephalitis 3. Trauma – concussion, contusion	1. Cerebral abscess 2. Tumor 3. SDH, EDH, ICH	1. Posttraumatic 2. Postmeningitic sequelae 3. Postencephalitic sequelae	1. SOL, cerebral abscess 2. NDD adrenoleukodystrophy 3. Sturge–Weber syndrome 4. Moyamoya disease	

92. What is congenital hemiplegia?
    Congenital hemiplegia occurs as a result of a prenatal/perinatal or early postnatal problem (<28 days after birth).
93. What is the pathophysiology in congenital hemiplegia?
    Pathophysiology
    Insult can occur at different developmental stages during pregnancy/birth causing congenital hemiplegia.
    Table 3.21 gives the correlation between age of insult and CNS manifestations.
94. *Why is congenital hemiplegia identified late?
    Clinical signs of hemiplegia may not be evident until the child is old enough to use the affected limb. The child may show signs such as being slower to crawl, pull to stand, and walk, or may develop hand dominance at a very early age. Congenital hemiplegia is more common in males, 1.4:1.
95. Which side is commonly involved in congenital hemiplegia?
    Right-sided hemiplegia is more common.
96. What is the common presentation in congenital hemiplegia in infancy and childhood?
    Most of the children with congenital hemiplegia have a normal IQ and will attend the mainstream school. Although language is well preserved usually (irrespective of which hemisphere is involved), there are significant learning difficulties (one-third), seizures (common [25%–30%]), strabismus (17%), visual impairment (17%), and hearing impairment (8%); speech is normal.

TABLE 3.20	Level of Lesion and Stroke				
Cortex	Subcortex	Internal Capsule	Brainstem	Spinal Level (Below Medulla, Above C5)
Monoparesis	Monoplegia/hemiplegia	Dense (complete) hemiplegia	Crossed hemiplegia	Incomplete hemiplegia
Speech affected	No dysphagia	Global aphasia	Dysarthria	-
Seizure +	No seizures	Seizures +/−	Cerebellar symptoms +	-
Cortical type of sensory loss	-	Hemisensory loss	Multiple cranial nerve involvement	No cranial nerve involvement
Spatial disorganization, release reflex	Homonymous hemianopia	UMN type of facial palsy	Horner syndrome	-

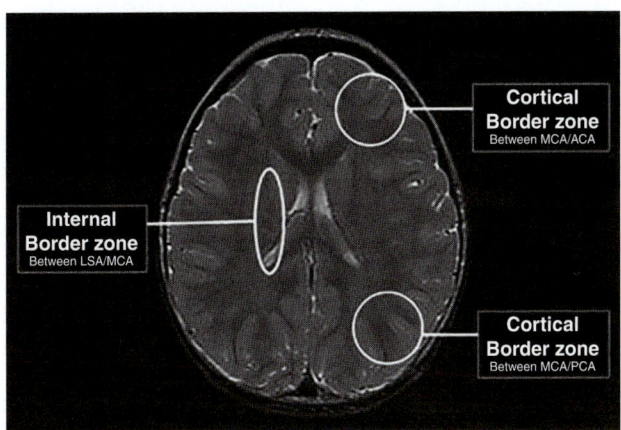

Fig. 3.17 Watershed areas in brain. *(Source: Review article: The role of hypotension in perioperative stroke | SpringerLink.)*

TABLE 3.21	Age of Insult and CNS Manifestations
Age	**Manifestation**
Early pregnancy	Cerebral malformations
24–34 weeks (either during pregnancy or after a preterm birth)	Periventricular lesions
Just before or around the time of a term birth	Cortical infarctions

TABLE 3.22	Neuroimaging Findings in Congenital Hemiparesis
Age of Onset	**CNS Manifestations**
First trimester	Brain malformations (migrational abnormalities) (18%)
Second trimester, especially in preterm	Periventricular white matter lesions (71%)
Third trimester, common in term	Perinatal arterial infarction (30%)
Term	Brain malformation, infarcts, and hemorrhage
Preterm	Perivascular hemorrhagic infarcts
Neonatal infarct	1. Resuscitation of hypotension 2. Multiartery infarct – congenital heart disease, disseminated intravascular coagulation, polycythemia 3. Carotid artery damage during a difficult delivery

97. Enumerate the clinical clues in congenital hemiplegia.
    a) Arms and legs show spasticity on the affected side.
    b) Growth arrest is apparent after 6 months of paresis.
    c) Sensory abnormalities are seen in affected limbs in 60% of children.
    d) Epilepsy is a common feature but mental retardation is not common.
98. How are neuroimaging findings correlated in congenital hemiparesis?
    Neuroimaging findings in congenital hemiparesis are given in Table 3.22.
99. What is the treatment strategy in congenital hemiplegia?
    a) Treatment is only to maximize efficiency.
    b) The arm can be very often ignored by the child, so early awareness of its use and encouragement of the use of the affected limb is important. This should be combined with the improvement of efficiency.

c) Develop an awareness of the affected side and make both sides to look symmetrical.
d) It is essential to include the weaker side in everyday activities and play, to make your child as ambidextrous as possible.
e) Children with hemiplegia are encouraged to develop better use of their weaker side through involvement in their chosen sports and hobbies, as they get older.
f) Prevent fixed deformity.
g) Provide support for families.
h) Offer surgical treatments – to correct deformities or to improve limb function.
i) Provide medical treatment for spasticity – baclofen and diazepam.
j) Botulinum toxin is used for spastic limbs.
100. What is infantile hemiplegia?
    This condition may be noted at birth or develop in the first 6 months of life – often an abrupt onset. It is probably caused by a cerebrovascular accident in utero or in the perinatal period. It occurs more often in boys than in girls and it affects the right side of the body twice as often as the left.
101. What are the differences between congenital and acquired hemiplegia?
    Table 3.23 gives the differences between congenital and acquired hemiplegia.
102. What are the differences between infantile and adult hemiplegia?
    Table 3.24 gives the differences between infantile and adult hemiplegia.

TABLE 3.23	Differences Between Congenital and Acquired Hemiplegia	
Features	**Congenital Hemiplegia**	**Acquired Hemiplegia**
Higher functions (seizures)	Less common	More common
Language aphasia/dysphasia (if right hemiplegia)	Absent	Present
Homonymous hemianopia	Present	Less common
UMN facial involvement	Absent	Present
Abdominal reflex	Retained	Lost
Cortical sensory loss	More common	Less common
Involuntary movements	Les common	More common
Vasomotor changes	More common	Less common

TABLE 3.24	Differences Between Infantile and Adult Hemiplegia	
Features	**Infantile Hemiplegia**	**Adult Hemiplegia**
Site of lesion	Cortex/subcortex	Internal capsule
Higher functions	Seizures: Common Speech: Not affected	Seizures: Uncommon Speech: Affected (dysphasia)
Abdominal reflex	Retained	Lost
Differential involvement	Upper limb > lower limb	Upper limb = lower limb
Growth retardation	Shortening of limbs Hemiatrophy	No shortening
Autonomic/sensory loss	Common	Less common

TABLE 3.25	Differences Between Organic and Psychogenic Hemiplegia	
Clinical Findings	Organic Hemiplegia	Psychogenic Hemiplegia
Parts affected	The entire half of the body, upper face spared	Sparing of face, tongue, sternomastoid
Tone	Spasticity present	Variable tone
DTR	Exaggerated	Normal
Abdominal reflexes	Absent	Normal
Babinski sign	Present	Absent
Gait	Circumduction	Bizarre gait with dragging of the foot
Hoover sign	Present	Abnormal
Hemianesthesia	Not common	More common – extends exactly to the midline

103. What are the differences between organic and psychogenic hemiplegia?
Table 3.25 gives the differences between organic and psychogenic hemiplegia.
104. What is moyamoya disease?
   a) Definition: Progressive narrowing of the intracranial portion of an internal carotid artery, usually in the distal branches of the internal carotid artery
   b) Pathophysiology: Gradual progressive obliterative arteriopathy of the internal carotid artery
   c) Causes
      a. Primary: Idiopathic
      b. Secondary: Down syndrome, Alagille syndrome, neurofibromatosis, sickle cell anemia, and fibromuscular dysplasia
      c. Usually, anterior cerebral artery affected and the posterior cerebral artery spared
   d) Clinical features: Mostly in the subcortical area and carotid bruit present
   e) Investigation: CT angiography (puff of smoke appearance [moyamoya meaning tiny vessels looking like smoke in angiography])
   f) Treatment
      a. Medical: T. aspirin 5 mg/kg/day
      b. Surgical: Anastomosis of the superficial temporal artery with dural venous sinuses
105. What is alternating hemiplegia of childhood?
   a) Onset – 18 months of age
   b) Alternating between one side of the body and the other (hemiplegia on the affected side completely resolves and reappears on the other side)
   c) Choreoathetoid and dystonic posturing observed on the hemiparetic side

   d) Paroxysmal disturbances such as tonic/dystonic attacks, nystagmus, and dyspnea during the attacks
   e) Immediate disappearance of all symptoms on going to sleep, with recurrence after 10–20 minutes of awakening in long-lasting bouts; regression of symptoms with sleep and reappearance on awakening
   f) Evidence of developmental delay, mental retardation, other neurological abnormalities including choreoathetosis, dystonia, or ataxia
   g) Differential diagnoses: Moyamoya and dystonic posturing
106. Enumerate CNS vasculitis.
Diagnostic criteria for CNS vasculitis: Childhood primary angiitis of CNS (cPACNS)
   a) Newly diagnosed focal deficit/psychiatric illness in a child younger than 18 years

      i. +

   b) Angiographic/histological evidence of vasculitis

      1. In the absence of

   c) Systemic underlying condition
   d) MRI – vessel stenosis (arteriolar constriction – beaded appearance)
107. What are the types of CNS vasculitis?
Table 3.26 gives the various types of CNS vasculitis.
108. How is a child with CNS vasculitis managed?
   • Treatment: Antithrombotic agent and high-dose corticosteroid in pulses
   • Immunosuppressive therapy: I.v. cyclophosphamide and inj. mycophenolate mofetil
   • Prognosis: Appropriate therapy – two-third with no neurological deficit
109. Which neurocutaneous syndrome is commonly associated with hemiparesis?
Sturge–Weber syndrome
110. What are the clinical manifestations of Sturge–Weber syndrome?
The most common clinical manifestations are port-wine stain on the face (cutaneous angioma) and epilepsy, which is seen in 80% of patients. Other features are glaucoma, buphthalmos, and intracranial calcification. Fig. 3.18 shows port-wine stain and buphthalmos seen in a child with Sturge–Weber syndrome.
111. Why is there a color change (port-wine stain) in Sturge–Weber syndrome?
Port-wine stain color change in Sturge–Weber syndrome is due to overabundance of capillaries.
112. What do the tram-track lines in CT brain indicate in Sturge–Weber syndrome?

TABLE 3.26	Various Types of CNS Vasculitis			
Primary CNS Vasculitis (Primary Angiitis of CNS [PACNS])		Secondary CNS Vasculitis	Antibody-Mediated Encephalitis
Large/medium vessel	Small vessel	Present with neuropsychiatric manifestation	Intracellular or cell surface antigen
Two types – progressive and nonprogressive	Usually progressive	Cause: Infection Systemic vasculitidis	
Presents as hemiplegia	Presents with seizures	Connective tissue disorder Lymphomas	
Angiography: Abnormal	Angiography: Normal, detected by brain biopsy		

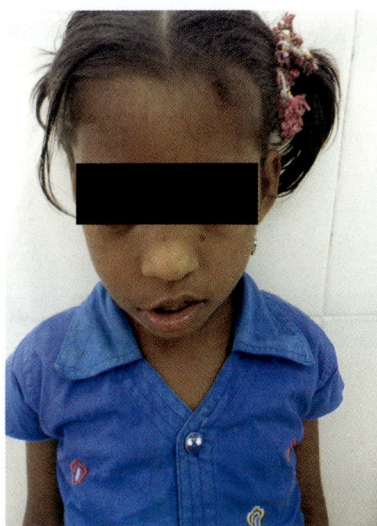

Fig. 3.18 Port-wine stain and buphthalmos on right side of face seen in Sturge–Weber syndrome.

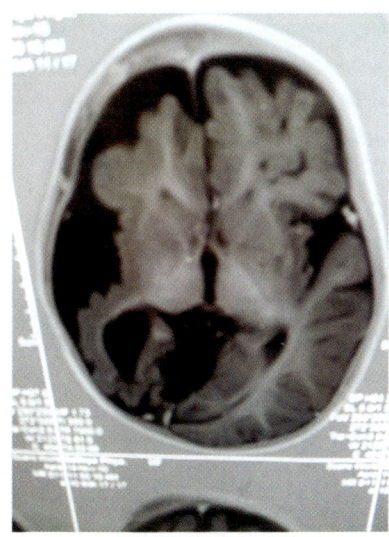

Fig. 3.20 Hemiatrophy of the right frontal and parietal regions seen in long-standing Sturge–Weber syndrome.

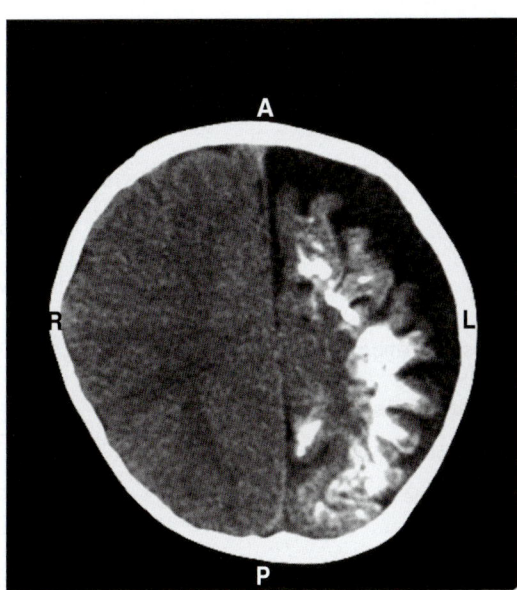

Fig. 3.19 Subcortical calcification along the left frontal, parietal, and occipital lobes depicting tram-track-like appearance. *(Source: Reproduced from Rohini Nadgir, David Yousem, David Yousem et al. Neuroradiology: The Requisites, Third Edition, Congenital Disorders of the Brain and Spine, Figure 9-51, Philadelphia, Mosby Inc., 2010.)*

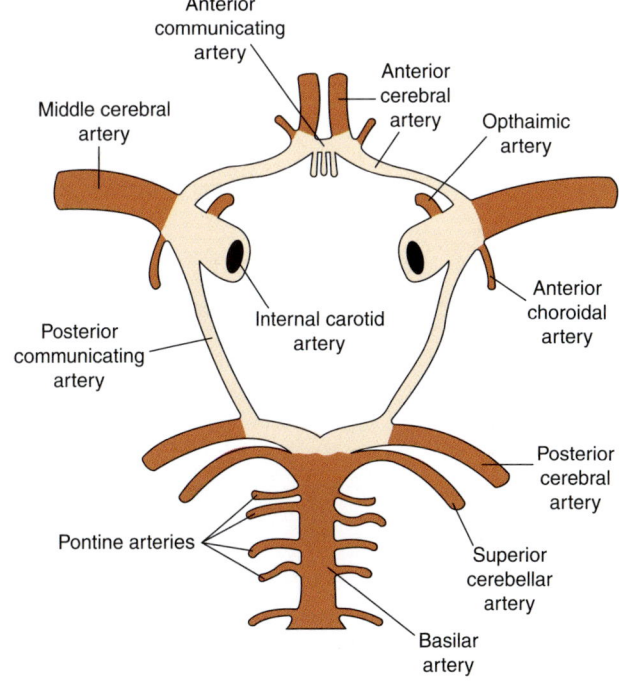

Fig. 3.21 Schematic representation of circle of Willis. *(Source: https:// www.google.co.in/imgres?imgurl5https%3A%2F%2Fupload. wikimedia.org%2Fwikipedia%2Fcommons%2Fthumb%2F2%2F2e%2FC ircle_of_Willis_en.svg%2F1200px-Circle_of_Willis_en.svg.png&imgre furl=https%3A%2F%2Fen.wikipedia.org%2Fwiki%2FCircle_of_Willis&tb nid=64zZIyNOAQsR6M&vet=12ahUKEwi5n6DEu9_uAhUZaSsKHWq4B wMQMygAegUIARDSAQ..i&docid5ko5Ue57wG-dC4M&w= 1200&h=1911&q=circle%20of%20willis&hl=en&ved=2ahUKEwi 5n6DEu9_uAhUZaSsKHWq4BwMQMygAegUIARDSAQ.)*

These are parallel lines of calcification that resemble the sulcal folds of the parietal–occipital lobe as shown in Fig. 3.19.

Fig. 3.20 shows hemiatrophy of the frontal and parietal regions depicting a long-standing disease.

DISCUSSION ON ANATOMY OF BRAIN

113. What is the circle of Willis?
   Fig. 3.21 gives the schematic representation of the circle of Willis. The circle of Willis consists of the following:
   - Anteriorly: Anterior cerebral artery (left and right) and anterior communicating artery
   - Posteriorly: Posterior cerebral artery (left and right)
   - Laterally: Posterior communicating artery (left and right)
   - Internal carotid artery (left and right)
   The middle cerebral artery supplying the brain is not considered part of the circle of Willis.

114. Enumerate the blood supply in each surface of the brain.
   Table 3.27 gives the blood supply in each surface of the brain.

TABLE 3.27	Blood Supply in Each Surface of the Brain		
Anterior Cerebral Artery		**Middle Cerebral Artery**	**Posterior Cerebral Artery**
• Medial surface of the cerebrum • Superior border of the frontal and parietal lobes • Precentral lobule • Movement of the lower limb • Micturition and defecation		• Most of the anterolateral surface of the cerebral hemisphere • Motor/sensory/speech area	• Occipital lobe • Inferior and medial temporal lobes • Visual cortex

TABLE 3.28	Blood Supply of Internal Capsule			
Internal Capsule	**Anterior Limb**	**Genu**	**Posterior Limb**	**Retrolentiform Part**
Upper half	MCA (lenticulostriate branch)	MCA (lenticulostriate branch)	MCA (lenticulostriate branch)	Anterior choroidal artery
Lower half	ACA (recurrent branch – Heubner)	ACA + direct branch from the internal carotid artery	Anterior choroidal artery (a branch of the internal carotid artery)	Anterior choroidal artery

ACA, anterior carotid artery; MCA, middle cerebral artery.

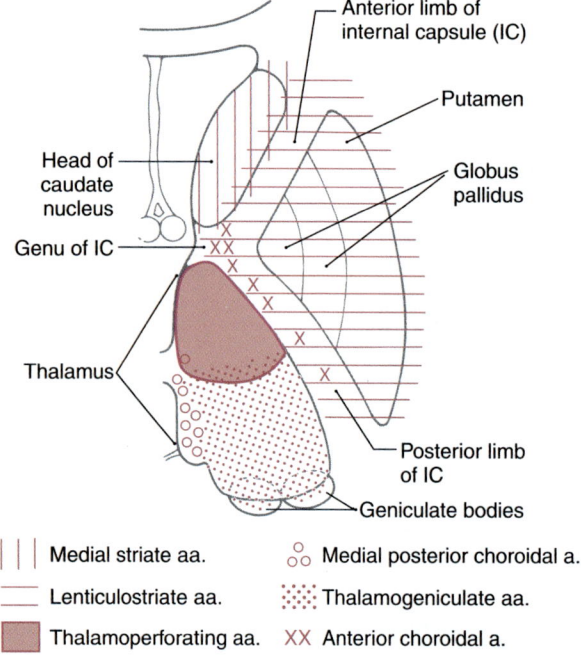

Fig. 3.22 Schematic representation of blood supply of internal capsule. (*Source: Reproduced from Duane E. Haines, Gregory A. Mihailoff. Fundamental Neuroscience for Basic and Clinical Applications,* Fifth Edition, The Diencephalon, Fig. 15.17, *Philadelphia, Elsevier Inc., 2018.*)

115. Discuss the blood supply of the internal capsule.
     Table 3.28 gives the blood supply of the internal capsule.
     Fig. 3.22 gives the schematic representation of blood supply of the internal capsule.
116. Trace the pyramidal tract.
     Fig. 3.23 gives the schematic representation of the pyramidal tract.
     Pyramidal tract:
     • Cortex: About 50% of the corticospinal tract originates from the primary motor cortex (Betz cells). Additional fibers arise from the premotor, supplementary motor, somatomotor cortex, cingulate gyrus, and parietal lobe.
     • Corona radiata is a white matter sheet which consists of corticospinal, corticopontine, and corticobulbar tracts.
     • The internal capsule contains ascending and descending axons from the cerebral cortex.

• Medulla oblongata: About 80% of the corticospinal fibers decussate or cross the midline at the level of the lower part of the medulla oblongata called the anterior corticospinal tract and 10% remain on the same side and another 10% decussate as they exit the spinal cord.
117. What are Brodmann areas in the brain?
     Fig. 3.24 shows Brodmann area in the brain.
     • 3, 1, and 2: Primary somatosensory area
     • 4: Primary motor area
     • 6: Premotor area/supplementary motor area
     • 17: Primary visual cortex
     • 18: Secondary visual cortex
     • 41 and 42: Primary auditory area
     • 44 and 45: Broca's area (inferior frontal gyrus – pars opercularis and pars triangularis)
     • 22: Superior temporal gyrus (Wernicke's area)

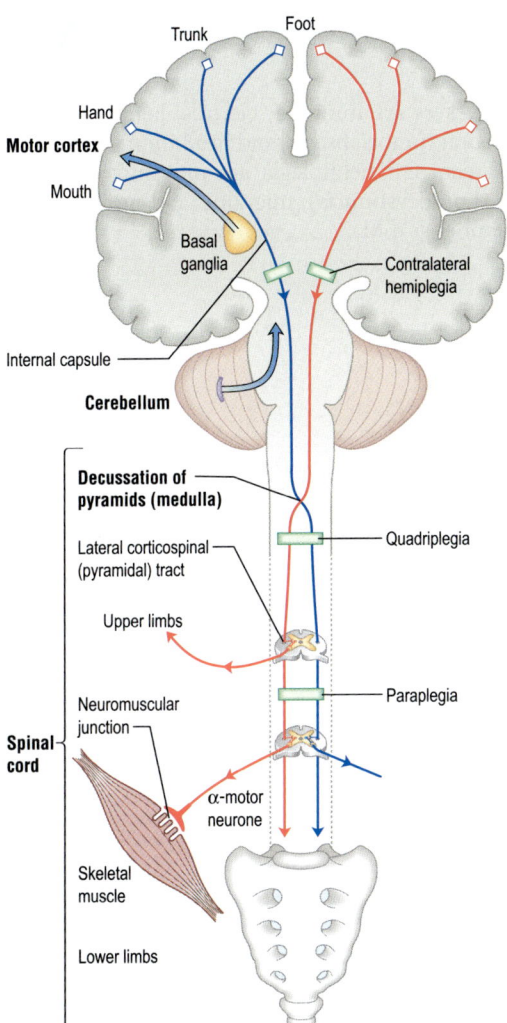

Fig. 3.23 Pyramidal tract. *(Source: Reproduced from Nicola Zammitt, Euan Sandilands. Essentials of Kumar & Clark's Clinical Medicine, Seventh Edition, Neurology, Fig. 17.1, Oxford, Elsevier Ltd, 2022.)*

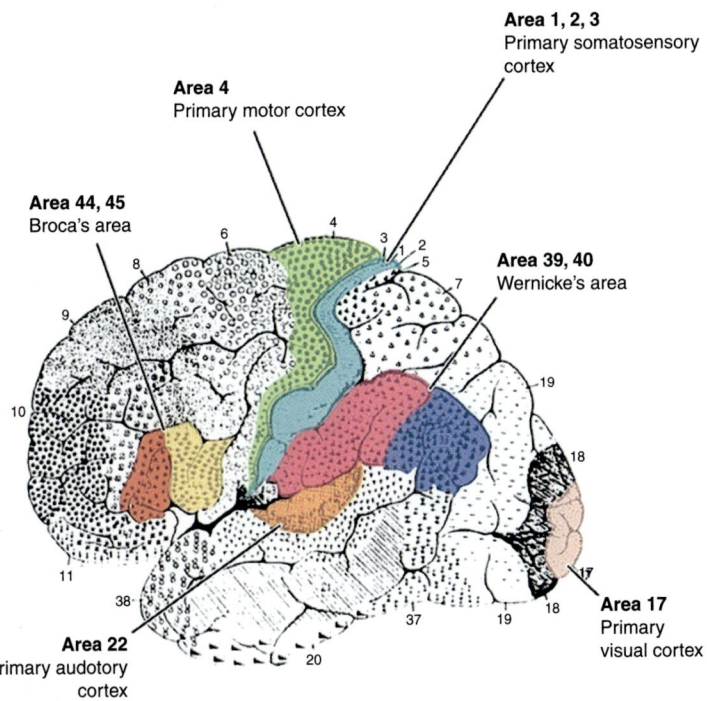

Fig. 3.24 Brodmann classification system. *(Source: The Brodmann Areas ~ Retrain the Brain: Neurofeedback Therapy (krishnak97.blogspot.com.))*

Quick Bites

- The most common cause of acute hemiparesis in a child is idiopathic.
- Another name for hemiparesis is fasciobrachiocrural paresis.
- Todd paralysis is postictal paralysis, which usually resolves completely without any deficit and lasts for few to 48 hours.
- Stroke mimickers are multiple sclerosis, hemiplegic migraine, cerebral tumor/abscess, and head injury.
- Causes of recurrent hemiplegia are moyamoya disease, metabolic (homocystinuria), migraine, and multiple emboli (remember as 4 M).

Acute Flaccid Paralysis

Following introduction, seek permission from the caregiver and introduce yourself to the patient before history elicitation, and identify the case.

Name____Age____Sex____Consanguinity____Order of birth____Place____Informant____

Presenting Complaints and Duration

- Difficulty in walking and fall by buckling

History of Presenting Illness

(Elicit the presenting illness as a story.)

The child was apparently normal ————- days back, and went to bed normally; the following morning, the mother noticed that the child had difficulty in walking on getting up from the bed, but went to school on day 1; however, the child had difficulty in climbing the school bus/van, and had difficulty in walking and running in school as evident by frequent falls. On day 2, the child did not go to school, and needed assistance for wearing clothes and bathing. On day 3, the mother noticed that the child had difficulty even in getting up from the bed and also needed assistance for using toilet and eating.

- Flailness/floppiness of both lower limbs which was gradual in onset and progressive, and initially involved lower limb followed by upper limb which was bilateral, symmetrical, and ascending in nature, as noticed by the mother
- Fever at onset or not, girdle pain, irritability, tingling sensation, and any seizures
- Any fluctuation/diurnal variation in weakness
- Bladder and bowel involvement in the form of retention of urine/constipation
- Profuse sweating, flushing, and palpitation
- Breathing difficulty

CENTRAL NERVOUS SYSTEM HISTORY

Higher Functions

- Recognizes the mother, obeys commands, altered sensorium, seizures, slurring of speech, early handedness, sleep disturbance, or altered behavior

Cranial Nerve History

- Ability to perceive light
- Ability to move eyeballs in all four directions and abnormal eyeball position
- Ability to chew food
- Facial asymmetry, able to close both eyes while sleeping, drooling of saliva, and deviation of angle of the mouth
- Ability to hear and respond to sound
- Nasal twang of voice and nasal regurgitation
- Ability to move the head side to side

- Any deviation of the tongue on protrusion
- Gait abnormality – waddling gait
- Involuntary movements

Cerebellar Features

- Swaying of the body
- Walking in a straight line
- Abnormal eyeball or head movement or tremors

Bladder/Bowel Disturbance

- Ability to perceive sensation of fullness of the bladder and able to void fully

Sensory Features

- History of perception of pain or crying while giving vaccination or any intramuscular injection, tingling sensation, and numbness

Autonomic Features

- Flushing, sweating, and palpitation episodes

Spine and Cranium

- Swelling/pain at the back and head size

COMPLICATION HISTORY

Bed sores, respiratory failure, and urinary tract infection

ETIOLOGICAL HISTORY

- Precipitating factors such as exertion and carbohydrate loading
- Diarrhea
- Preceding illness such as GI-Gastrointestinal infection, URI-Upper respiratory tract infection
- Diurnal variations and ocular involvement
- Breathlessness
- Swallowing difficulty, nasal regurgitation, and nasal twang
- Clumsiness of activities
- Walking followed by buckling
- Tripping while walking
- Sensory system involvement – able to appreciate dress on the body
- Bladder and bowel involvement
- Fever at the time of onset of weakness
- Fever 2 weeks prior to the onset of weakness
- Pain and paresthesia (peripheral neuropathy)
- Intramuscular injection
- Tonsillectomy
- Spinal trauma
- Recent vaccination
- Pica and abdomen pain
- Dog bite and rabies vaccine

- Ptosis, abnormal eyeball position, and breathing difficulty
- Travel in the past (35 days)
- Exanthem – varicella
- Exposure to paint or glass industry near the house and sewage disposal in socioeconomic status
- Drug (steroid and gentamicin, vincristine intake) and toxin – organophosphorus compound
- Honey ingestion/corn syrup
- Pain and change in color of the urine

Course During Hospitalization

Determine whether the child's symptoms have improved or worsened; take complete treatment history (if given any intravenous infusion – IVIG) including lumbar puncture, imaging, ventilation, and physiotherapy, and check how far the child has recovered.

Past History

- Similar illness in the past
- Intensive care unit admission
- Diarrhea
- Fever with sore throat
- Upper respiratory tract infection/pneumonia
- Recent travel
- Exanthematous fever
- Surgery – tonsillectomy
- Intramuscular injections

Antenatal History/Birth/Postnatal History

- Drug intake in the mother (congenital Guillain–Barré syndrome [GBS])
- Any NICU admission

Developmental History

Any development delay

Dietetic History

Any feeding problem

Immunization History

Detailed history about OPV – where given (government or private sector), how many doses, whether IPV given, pulse polio vaccination, recent vaccination – influenza vaccine, and when last polio vaccine was given (to rule out vaccine-associated paralytic polio [VAPP])

Contact History

Any history of contact with tuberculosis

Family History

Father's occupation – construction worker, gardener (soil dust containing botulinum spores), and similar illness in the neighborhood (polio infection)

Socioeconomic History

Sanitation (polio), drinking water, waste disposal, and exposure to lead or glass industries

Summary

A …-year-old female/male child presented with a history of acute onset of bilateral, symmetrical ascending paralysis with no history of fever at onset and absence of fluctuation in weakness or periodicity with normal higher functions, with cranial nerve involvement in the form of deviation of angle of the mouth/expressionless facies and regurgitation of feed, with or without breathing difficulty, flailness of both lower limbs, no involuntary movements, absence of bladder and bowel involvement, and absent sharp sensory level, probably a child with acute flaccid paralysis (AFP) and to proceed further with examination.

General Examination

- Consciousness and orientation
- Posture (frog leg posture)
- Both eyes partially opened or closed
- Pallor
- Edema
- Scar
- Bed sores
- Whether the child is on any oxygen support/mechanical ventilation, NG tube, central line, or any VP-ventriculoperitoneal shunt mentioned

Head-to-Foot Examination

- Head (occipital region) – tick bite
- Eyes – ptosis, hyperpigmentation, or violaceous patch over the eyes (dermatomyositis)
- Hydration status (dehydration can be because of diarrhea or excessive sweating because of autonomic dysfunction/poor oral intake)
- Tonsillitis/bull neck – diphtheria
- Skin rash
- Knuckle pigmentation (vitamin B12 deficiency)
- Bite marks
- Spine swellings/tenderness over the spine
- Gibbus and spine hematoma

Vital Signs

- Temperature – any fever
- Pulse rate – tachycardia or bradycardia
- Respiratory rate/pattern of breathing
- Blood pressure – hypotension or hypertension
- SpO_2 – polio; and GBS – postural variation of vital signs

Anthropometry

Check height/weight/weight for height/BMI.

Central Nervous System Examination

HIGHER FUNCTIONS

- Altered sensorium, seizures, speech disturbance, handedness, and sleep disturbance

CRANIAL NERVES

- Cranial nerve I: Ability to perceive smell in both nostrils
- Cranial nerve II: Papilledema and features of optic atrophy or optic neuritis
- Cranial nerves III, IV, and VI: Ptosis, strabismus, and nystagmus
- Cranial nerve V: Pain sensation over the face, able to chew food, and jaw jerk
- Cranial nerve VII
  - Wrinkling of the forehead present
  - Able to close eyes on both sides while sleeping
  - Absent nasolabial fold on the affected side
  - Deviation of angle of the mouth to the normal side
  - Drooling of saliva present
- Cranial nerve VIII: Ability to hear sound on both sides
- Cranial nerve IX
  - Uvula in midline
  - Palatal arches and pharyngeal arches normal
  - Palatal and pharyngeal reflex normal
- Cranial nerve XI
  - Ability to lift the head from a supine position
  - Whether turns the head on both sides
- Cranial nerve XII
  - Any deviation of the tongue
  - Fibrillation or wasting

TABLE 4.1	Motor System Examination	
Motor System Examination	Right	Left
Bulk	Upper limb: Normal Lower limb: Normal	Upper limb: Normal Lower limb: Normal
Tone	Upper limb: Hypotonia Lower limb: Hypotonia	Upper limb: Hypotonia Lower limb: Hypotonia
Power	Shoulder joint: 3/5 Elbow: 3/5 Wrist: 3/5 Finger grip: Weak Neck muscle: Weak Trunk: Weak Hip joint: 2/5 Knee joint: 2/5 Ankle joint: 2/5 Toe grip: Weak	Shoulder joint: 3/5 Elbow: 3/5 Wrist: 3/5 Finger grip: Weak Neck muscle: Weak Trunk: Weak Hip joint: 2/5 Knee joint: 2/5 Ankle joint: 2/5 Toe grip: Weak
Superficial reflexes	Normal	Normal
Plantar	No response	No response
Deep tendon reflexes#	Biceps: Absent Triceps: Absent Supinator: Absent Knee jerk: Absent Ankle jerk: Absent	Biceps: Absent Triceps: Absent Supinator: Absent Knee jerk: Absent Ankle jerk: Absent

#Always perform reinforcement maneuver (Jendrassick maneuver or Jendrassick equivalent) before commenting on absent deep tendon reflex.

MOTOR SYSTEM

- Motor examination as given in Table 4.1
- Posture: Lies along the cot with the shoulder adducted and internally rotated; elbow and wrist extended; and hips, knee, and ankle extended
- Check for any clawing of hands present
- Stance and gait: Waddling gait (mention about gait only when the child walks independently)
- Involuntary movements: Ataxia

CEREBELLAR SYSTEM

- Nystagmus and head nodding

AUTONOMIC SYSTEM

Profuse sweating, tachycardia or bradycardia, and hypotension or hypertension

SENSORY SYSTEM

Test for sensation on both sides and mark if there is a sharp sensory level.

SPINE AND CRANIUM

Spinal tenderness, straight leg raising test +, tripod sign, head drop, gibbus, and hematoma

SIGNS OF MENINGEAL SIGNS

- Three fingerbreadth test (to assess meningismus [GBS])

Other System Examination

CARDIOVASCULAR SYSTEM

- Tachycardia or bradycardia

RESPIRATORY SYSTEM

Pattern of breathing and any respiratory distress

ABDOMEN

- Distended bladder (in polio and transverse myelitis) and fecal mass (loaded rectum) in GBS

Diagnosis

A child with AFP with/without cranial nerve involvement with quadriparesis with/without bulbar weakness, probably GBS with a Hughes disability score of ———— with or without complications, nutritional status, and other comorbid conditions – anemia and vitamin deficiency, if any

Frequently Asked Questions

1. How is the onset of illness described in AFP?
   - Onset – acute/gradual
   - Duration – for how many days
   - Progressive or nonprogressive
   - Ascending/descending
   - Bilateral/symmetrical/asymmetrical
   - Proximal/distal
   - Rate of progression of weakness
2. List the significance of etiological history in AFP.
   The clinical features and its relevant etiology are given in Table 4.2.
3. What is the significance of onset of symptoms and AFP?
   - Immediate: Trauma and vascular etiology – hematoma and hemorrhage
   - Minutes to hours: Snake bite, electrolyte disturbance, and periodic paralysis
   - Hours to days: Spinal tumor, GBS, and lead poisoning
4. What is the significance of place of living and AFP?
   - Rural areas: Snake bite and OPC poisoning
   - Urban areas: Plastic and paint industry (lead exposure)
5. What are the precipitating factors for periodic paralysis?
   Exertion and carbohydrate load – lead to high insulin because of carbohydrate intake that causes low potassium in blood which is the precipitating factor for periodic paralysis.
6. Why does exertion cause periodic paralysis?
   Exertion causes sympathetic stimulation resulting in stimulation of beta-2 receptors that results in shift of potassium into the cell causing hypokalemia.
7. What is the significance of fever and AFP?
   - Fever at the time of onset of weakness: Polio
   - Fever 2 weeks prior to the onset of weakness: GBS
8. What is the significance of buckle and triple while walking ?
   History of buckling while walking seen in GBS, but tripping while walking seen in hereditary motor sensory neuropathy
9. What does pain in AFP indicate?
   Myalgia is seen in polio and paresthesia is seen in GBS. Other causes include viral myositis, pain with cramps (mitochondrial myopathy), and localized backache (Pott spine).
10. What is the importance of recent travel in AFP?
    Polio, Japanese encephalitis, and west Nile virus infection can occur with travel to the endemic regions.
11. What is pseudoparalysis?
    Pseudoparalysis means that there is restriction of movements because of pain, but there is no weakness, nuchal rigidity, and CSF pleocytosis.
12. What are the causes of pseudoparalysis?
    (Remember as skin to bone)
    - Boils
    - Hematoma
    - Abscess
    - Trauma
    - Fracture
    - Toxic synovitis
    - Osteomyelitis
    - Septic arthritis
    - Others: Scurvy and congenital syphilis
13. List the significance of past history in AFP.
    History related to past illness is given in Table 4.3.

TABLE 4.2	Etiological History in AFP
Clinical Features	**Etiology**
Preceding illness such as GI infection, URI	Guillain–Barré syndrome
Diarrhea	Hypokalemic paralysis
Diurnal variations and ocular involvement	Myasthenia gravis
Breathlessness, swallowing difficulty, nasal regurgitation, nasal twang	Bulbar involvement in polio, GBS
Clumsiness of activities	Ataxia in Miller Fisher
Sensory system involvement	Transverse myelitis
Bladder and bowel involvement	
Intramuscular injection	Traumatic neuritis and provocation paralysis in polio
Tonsillectomy	Any surgery or trauma – exposure of the nerve endings to poliovirus
Recent vaccination	GBS and VAPP
Pica, abdomen pain	Lead poisoning
Dog bite – rabies vaccine	GBS
Ptosis, abnormal eyeball position	Snake bite
Exanthema	Varicella
Psychiatric behavior, abnormal color of urine	Acute intermittent porphyria
Pain, change in color of the urine	Rhabdomyolysis
Paint, glass, plastic industry near the house	Lead exposure
Sewage disposal	Poliovirus
Drug (steroid and gentamicin, vincristine intake), toxin – OPC	Affect neuromuscular junction
Honey ingestion/corn syrup	Botulinum toxin – botulism
Abdominal pain, change in color of the urine	Porphyria

AFP, acute flaccid paralysis; GBS, Guillain–Barré syndrome; VAPP, vaccine-associated paralytic polio.

TABLE 4.3 Past History in AFP

Etiology	Past History
Chronic inflammatory demyelinating polyneuropathy, myasthenia gravis	Similar illness as mentioned previously
Critical illness neuropathy	Critical care admission or critical illness in the past
Guillain–Barré syndrome	Diarrhea, fever 2 weeks back
Diphtheria	Fever with sore throat
Mycoplasma infection causing AIDP	Upper respiratory tract infection/pneumonia
Polio, Japanese encephalitis, west Nile fever	History of recent travel
AIDP	Exanthematous fever
Provocative polio	Surgery – tonsillectomy
Traumatic neuritis	Intramuscular injection

AFP, acute flaccid paralysis; AIDP, acute inflammatory demyelinating polyneuropathy.

TABLE 4.4 Clinical Clues in Examination in AFP

Clinical Features	Cause
Altered sensorium	Polio, porphyria, lead poisoning/Miller Fisher variant
Signs of dehydration	Diarrhea or excessive sweating because of autonomic dysfunction/poor oral intake
Tonsillitis/bull neck	Diphtheria
Skin rash/hyperpigmentation	Dermatomyositis, vitamin B12
Bite marks	Snake bite, tick bite
Spine swellings/tenderness	Gibbus and spine hematoma
Anemia	Lead poisoning, vitamin B12 deficiency, porphyria

AFP, acute flaccid paralysis.

14. **What are the causes of recurrent weakness?**
Familial periodic paralysis, myasthenia gravis, multiple sclerosis (may initially present as GBS), polymyositis, and rarely recurrent GBS (10%)

15. **What is the significance of antenatal history in AFP?**
History of drug intake – sulfasalazine in the mother causes congenital GBS.

16. **What is the significance of family history in GBS?**
Father: Construction worker, gardener (soil dust containing botulinum spores), and similar illness in the neighborhood (lead poisoning, polio outbreak)

17. **What is the significance of immunization history in a child with AFP?**
Give a detailed immunization history – OPV – how many doses were given; when it was last given whether it was given in a private or government setup; whether the child received any pulse polio immunization; and whether any influenza vaccine was given.

18. **Is there any contraindication for vaccine in a child who was treated for GBS in the past?**
There is no contraindication in receiving vaccine with a past history of GBS. However, the vaccine has to be deferred till 3–11 months after administration of IVIG.

19. **What is the significance of environmental history in AFP?**
Poor sanitation, drinking impure water, improper waste disposal, and exposure to lead factory or glass industries can cause polio.

20. **What are the clinical clues in examination in AFP?**
Examination clues are discussed in Table 4.4.

21. ***What is the significance of vital signs in AFP?***
- Temperature – fever, which suggests polio/secondary infections such as UTI and aspiration pneumonia
- Tachycardia or bradycardia – autonomic instability in GBS
- Respiratory rate – bradypnea and pattern of breathing
- Blood pressure – hypertension or hypotension for autonomic instability in GBS
- SpO$_2$ and postural variation of vitals – polio and GBS

22. **What are the differentials if AFP is associated with seizures?**
GBS with hypertensive encephalopathy due to autonomic imbalance, lead poisoning, and ADEM, which can present with seizures

23. **What are the differentials if a child with suspected AFP presented with altered sensorium?**
Altered sensorium seen in polio, porphyria, lead poisoning, and Miller Fisher variant

24. **Which is the most common cranial nerve involved in GBS?**
Bilateral LMN type of facial nerve palsy is common in GBS.

25. **How is bifacial weakness in children checked?**
Only history can reveal bilateral facial weakness. There is no clue in examination also. Ask the mother whether the child sleeps with both eyes partially closed (if it is present recently after the onset of illness, it is suggestive of bifacial weakness).

26. **What is the significance of fundus examination in a child with AFP?**
Fundus in GBS – papilledema (Miller Fisher variant, autonomic instability in GBS); optic atrophy – multiple sclerosis

27. **What is the differential for a child with ptosis + proximal weakness + hearing and cardiac defect?**
Mitochondrial myopathy

28. **What are the possible differentials if a child refuses to walk suddenly along with weakness?**
Acute cerebellar ataxia and GBS are the close possible differentials for acute onset of weakness + difficulty in walking.

29. **What are the clinical clues in cranial nerve examination in AFP?**
   a. Bilateral LMN facial palsy (bilateral forehead wrinkles absent, bilateral nasolabial fold absent, only able to distinguish by asking the mother whether the child sleeps with both eyes fully closed or partially opened recently)
   b. External ophthalmoplegia because of the involvement of cranial nerve VI in Miller Fisher variant of GBS
   c. Optic neuritis, papilledema, and optic atrophy – Miller Fisher variant of GBS

30. **Which reflex is last to disappear in GBS?**
Ankle jerk is the last reflex to disappear in GBS.

31. **What is the significance of plantar reflex in AFP?**
Lost early in neuropathies
Preserved until late in myopathies

Present throughout (no change), neuromuscular junction pathology

Plantar – no response in GBS

32. What is the order of recovery of muscle strength or appearance of reflex in GBS?

The first muscle that is involved is the last to recover.

33. Which type of GBS is associated with clawing of hand?

Acute motor and sensory axonal neuropathy (AMAN) is associated with claw hand and carries a poor prognosis.

34. What are the clinical clues in the examination of spine in AFP?

Spinal tenderness and straight leg raising test seen in radiculopathy, tripod sign in polio, head drop in polio, gibbus in tuberculosis, and hematoma in spinal trauma

35. How are power of the neck and truncal weakness checked?

Neck muscle: Ask the child to lift the neck (flex and extend the neck against resistance).

Trunk: Ask the child to get up from supine position and turn side to side.

36. How is neck stiffness assessed in a child?

Ask the child to flex the neck and measure the distance between the chin and the neck using three finger widths.

37. What is the significance of examination of other systems in AFP?

Cardiovascular: Tachycardia or bradycardia (autonomic manifestation – GBS, acute porphyria)

Respiratory: respiratory distress (for aspiration), and respiratory effort (for respiratory muscle weakness)

Abdomen: Distended bladder in polio and transverse myelitis

Loaded rectum (fecal mass – constipation) in GBS

38. *What are the differential diagnoses of AFP?

Differential diagnoses:

1. GBS
2. Acute transverse myelitis
3. Traumatic neuritis
4. Poliomyelitis

39. What are the distinguishing features of different causes of AFP?

The different causes of AFP are discussed in Table 4.5.

40. What are the investigations performed in AFP?

1. AFP surveillance
2. CBC and CRP – to rule out infection
3. Serum electrolytes – hypokalemic periodic paralysis
4. Serum creatinine kinase – myopathies
5. Lumbar puncture – CSF (albuminocytological dissociation)
6. Nerve conduction study – GBS
7. Electromyography – acute denervation of muscle
8. Muscle biopsy – normal or denervation atrophy
9. MRI spine – to rule out other cause
10. Serology of *Campylobacter*/*Helicobacter pylori*
11. Stool culture for bacteria or virus

TABLE 4.5 Different Causes of AFP

Features	Polio	GBS	Traumatic Neuritis	Transverse Myelitis
Etiology	Poliovirus types 1, 2, 3	Delayed hypersensitivity immunological reaction	Trauma	Usually unknown, multiple viruses
Onset of paralysis	24–48 h	Few hours to 10 days	Few hours to days	Few hours to days
Fever at onset	High, always present at the onset of paralysis, disappears later	Not common	Can present before, during, and after flaccid paralysis	Rarely present
Cranial nerve involvement	Only when bulbar or bulbospinal involvement	Often present, Miller Fisher syndrome	Absent	Absent
Respiratory insufficiency	Only when bulbar or bulbospinal involvement	In severe cases	Absent	Absent
Flaccid paralysis	Acute, proximal > distal asymmetrical	Acute, distal symmetrical	Acute, affecting only one limb Asymmetrical	Usually involving lower limb Symmetrical
Muscle tone	Reduced or absent in the affected limb	Global hypotonia	Reduced or absent in the affected limb	Lower limb – hypotonia
Deep tendon reflex	Decreased or absent	Globally absent	Decreased to absent	Absent in lower limb early, later hyperreflexia
Autonomic	Dysautonomia	Frequent blood pressure alterations, sweating, flushing, and fluctuation in body temperature	Rare	Hypothermia in affected limb
CSF WBC	WBC: Highly elevated	WBC: <10	WBC: Normal	WBC: Normal
Protein	Protein: Normal	Protein: High	Protein: Normal	Protein: Slightly elevated
Bladder dysfunction	Absent	Transient	Never	Present
Nerve conduction study at 3rd week	Anterior horn cell disease	Abnormal demyelination	Abnormal suggestive of axonal damage	Normal or decreased
EMG at 3 weeks	Abnormal	Normal depending on recovery	Normal depending on recovery	Normal
Sequelae: 3 months to 1 year	Severe asymmetrical atrophy of muscles, later skeletal deformities	Symmetrical atrophy of distal muscle mass	Affected limb – moderate atrophy	Flaccid diplegia, atrophy after years

AFP, acute flaccid paralysis; GBS, Guillain–Barré syndrome.

41. What are the clinical clues for mitochondrial myopathies?

Proximal muscle weakness, exercise intolerance, encephalopathy (seizures, stroke-like episode, ataxia), hearing defect, eye (cataract, progressive external ophthalmoplegia + optic atrophy), cardiac (heart block, cardiomyopathy), and endocrine (diabetes, stunted growth)

FAQ ON AFP SURVEILLANCE

42. *Define AFP.

AFP is defined as a sudden onset of weakness or floppiness of <4-week duration involving any part of the body in an apparently normal child younger than 15 years or of any age in whom polio is suspected.

43. Explain the term AFP.
   • Acute: Rapid progression or short, brief duration
   • Flaccid: Floppy or soft and yielding to passive stretching at any time during illness
   • Paralysis: Loss of motor strength

44. Why is age <15 years included in the definition of AFP?

Poliomyelitis occurs predominantly in children younger than 15 years. Polio is unlikely in children older than 15 years.

45. Define the terms paralysis, paresis, and plegia.
   • "Paralysis" means loss of voluntary muscle contraction due to interruption of neuronal pathways from the cerebral cortex to the muscle fiber.
   • "Paresis" means mild weakness and plegia means severe muscle weakness.

46. List the causes of AFP according to the level of lesion.

Table 4.6 gives the different causes of AFP pertaining to the level of lesion.

47. What is the first step in the management of a child with AFP?

Any child with AFP should undergo AFP surveillance.

48. *What is AFP surveillance?

Definition: It is defined as the ongoing and systematic collection, analysis, interpretation, and dissemination of data about cases of a disease, used as a basis for planning, implementing, and evaluating disease prevention and control activities. Surveillance refers to collection of data for action, which includes the following:
   • Data: Timely, precise, and core data
   • Action: Immediate, focused, and appropriate

49. What are the types of AFP surveillance?

There are two types – active and passive.

50. What is active surveillance?

TABLE 4.6	Different Causes of AFP According to the Level of Lesion
Spinal cord level	*Compressive* a. Traumatic myelopathy b. Vertebral fractures c. Extradural hematoma d. Spinal epidural abscess e. Spinal intradural abscess f. Pott spine g. Discitis *Noncompressive* a. Acute transverse myelitis b. Neuromyelitis optica c. Multiple sclerosis d. Systemic inflammatory disorders
Anterior horn cell	Poliovirus Non-polio enterovirus *Mycoplasma* Japanese encephalitis, vaccine-derived paralytic polio, rabies, varicella
Peripheral nerves/ roots	Guillain–Barré syndrome CMV polyradiculopathy Porphyria Post-diphtheritic polyneuropathy Lyme borreliosis Drugs such as vincristine Vasculitic neuropathy Critical illness neuropathy
Neuromuscular junction	Myasthenia gravis Organophosphorus poisoning Snake envenomation Drugs such as aminoglycosides Botulism Tick paralysis Hypermagnesemia
Muscle	Polymyositis Viral myositis Toxic myopathies Hypokalemic/hyperkalemic periodic paralysis Hypomagnesemia, hypokalemia

AFP, acute flaccid paralysis.

Active surveillance is when DIO collects data by regular visits from the following:

1) Hospitals
2) Health workers
3) Anganwadi workers
4) TBA

51. What is passive surveillance?
Routine weekly reporting by the reporting unit is passive surveillance.

52. How is an unreported case followed up?
- If the child got admitted in the hospital: Collect stool sample immediately.
- If the child is not admitted in the hospital: The child should be investigated at his or her residence.

53. What is the rate of reporting of AFP in a district?
- At least 1 case of AFP per year reported for every 1 lakh population of children younger than 15 years

54. What is the background rate of reporting AFP in India?
"Background" rate of AFP from other parts of the India: Each district reports at least 2 cases per 1 lakh population of children younger than 15 years.

55. What are the steps in AFP surveillance?
Flowchart 4.1 shows the steps in AFP surveillance.

56. Mention the selection criteria for children for AFP surveillance.
Any children younger than 15 years with syndrome of AFP are selected for surveillance.

57. How is a child with AFP investigated?
- Step 1: Case verification – DIO/SMO (District Immunisation officer/ Station medical officer) personally sees whether the case it meets the AFP case definition (steps in verification include history of the index case, physical examination of case, filling the case information form [CIF], and determining travel history of the child and family).
- Step 2: Adequate two stool specimens are collected 24 hours apart, both within 14 days of paralysis onset.
- Step 3: Specimens arrive at a WHO-accredited lab in good condition (adequate volume [>8 g], good condition for transportation of stools: no leakage, no desiccation, ice pack present, appropriate documentation [lab request form]).

58. How is a hot case identified?
The characteristic signs and symptoms of a "hot case" are the following:
a. Any children younger than 15 years with a history of fever at the onset of paralysis + asymmetrical proximal patchy paralysis
b. Any children younger than 5 years with rapidly progressive paralysis leading to bulbar involvement and death

59. What is the importance of stool sample in a child with AFP?
The highest yield of virus is from stool, and the other samples for virus yield are CSF, throat, and blood but they have only a low yield.

60. What is the preferred method for collection of stool sample?
Before collecting stool specimens from contacts, ensure that the child has not received OPV within the last 30 days.
- Stool collected in a sterile container – preferred method
- Rectal tube – less preferred method
- Limitations on rectal tube collection (see figure 4.1) are the following:
  a) Lower virus isolation rates
  b) Smaller volume for backup test

61. Enumerate the procedure for collection of a stool sample.
a. Stool specimens should be collected within 14 days of the onset of paralysis.
b. If missed, they can be collected up to a period of maximum 60 days from the onset of paralysis.
c. Two stool samples should be collected at an interval of 24 hours because of intermittent shedding of the virus.
d. Specimens should be collected before outbreak response immunization (ORI).
e. Explain the process of collection to the child/parent/guardian.
f. Stools are collected in a dry, clean, wide-mouthed, leak-proof, preferably transparent, plastic, or glass container of 30−60 mL size with a screw on cap which tightens securely – not essential to be a sterile one. In the absence of such a container, any clean and dry container may be used but prevention of leakage during transport has to be ensured.
g. The container should have a waterproof label with the following:
  a. Name of the patient
  b. EPID (Electronic portal imaging device number) } *Written in indelible ink*
  c. Specimen number
h. Identification of the case, labeling of the sample, and date of collection should be pasted.
i. Collect the fresh stool from the child's diapers, or get the child to defecate onto a clean paper.
j. Approximately 5−8 g, i.e., adult thumb size, is adequate quantity for necessary lab tests and backup should be kept for repeat tests.
k. Do not collect up to the brim of the container. Laxatives should not be used.
l. In case of a critically ill child, the sample can be collected using rectal tubes as shown in Fig. 4.1.
m. Do not collect specimen if the onset is >2 months; instead, perform a 60-day follow-up.

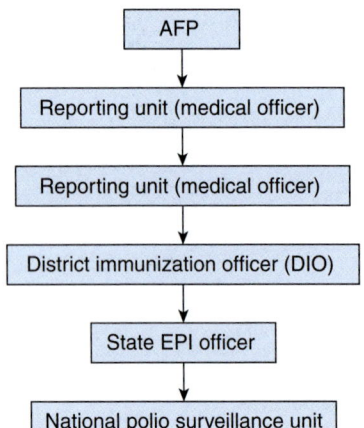

Flowchart 4.1   Steps in acute flaccid paralysis (AFP) surveillance.

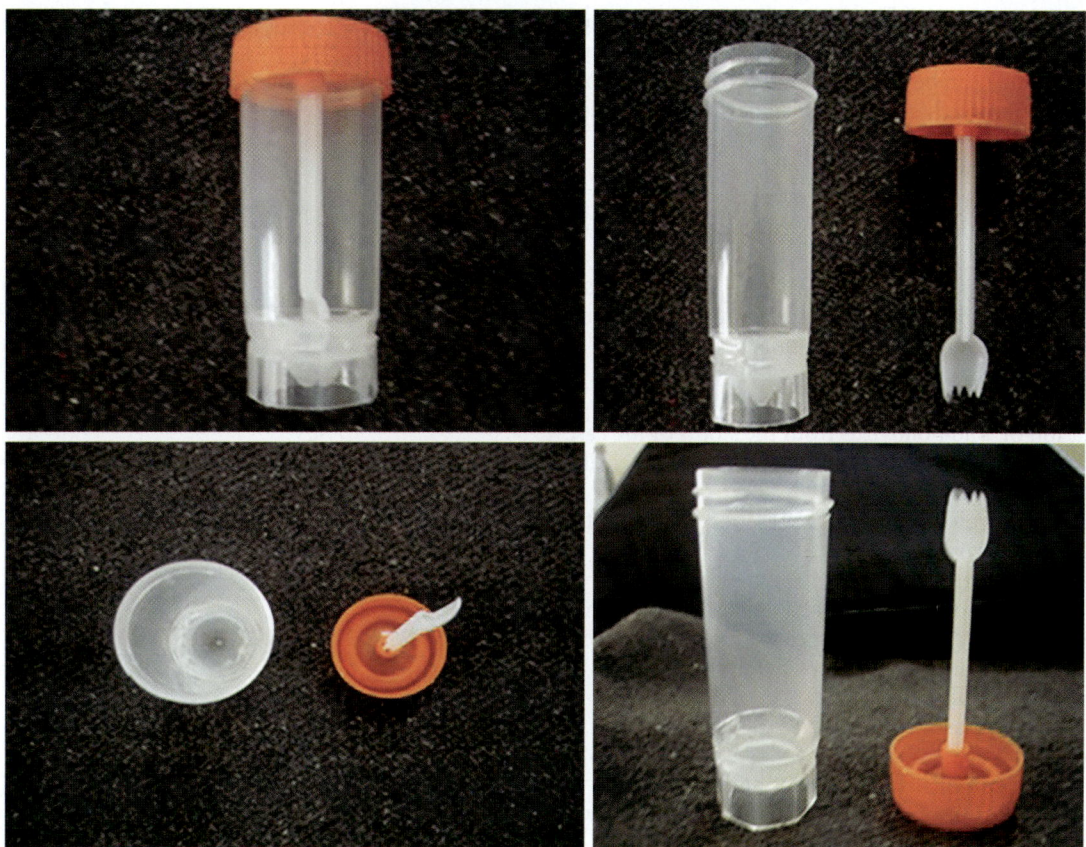

Fig. 4.1   Rectal tube.

n. Properly filled Laboratory Referral Form (LRF) should accompany specimens to the assigned laboratory.

62. How is a stool specimen transported and stored?
    - The specimen container should be packed in a plastic sealed bag.
    - Where possible, both specimens from one case should be packed in a single carrier.
    - Temperature should be <8°C – stool carrier/vaccine carrier having four fully frozen ice packs at −20°C. *Label/paint with different colors.*
    - If delay is >2 hours, keep the specimen in a deep freezer.
    - There should be provision of replacement of ice in case of delay.

63. What are the qualities of a good sample?
    Two specimens at least 24 hours apart collected within 14 days of the onset of paralysis; each specimen of adequate volume (8–10 g), arrived at a WHO-accredited laboratory in good condition with no desiccation and no leakage, with adequate documentation and evidence that cold chain maintained was during transit

64. *What is reverse cold chain?
    a. The specimen should be stored at 2–8°C.
    b. The sample should reach the laboratory within 72 hours of dispatch.
    c. If this is not possible, the specimen must be frozen at −20°C and then shipped frozen.
    d. The stool shipment carriers should not be mixed with vaccine carries. If this is unavoidable, the stool specimen should be sealed in two to three layers of plastic bags and carefully separated from the vaccines or other medicines.
    e. If contamination of vaccine carrier with stool specimen is suspected, the vaccine carriers should be disinfected with 1% sodium hypochlorite solution for a contact period of 30 minutes.

65. What is contact stool collection?
    Contact stool specimen should be collected from all "hot AFP cases" with inadequate specimen.

66. How are contacts of AFP cases selected?
    Five children younger than 5 years living in and around the residence of the index case are selected for contact stool specimen. One stool specimen should be collected from each contact child.

67. How are stool specimen results reported?
    The presence of wild poliovirus in any one of the five contacts suggests that the index case is infected with wild poliovirus. Any index AFP case with one or more contacts testing positive for wild poliovirus is classified as "confirmed polio."

68. How is poliovirus isolated?
    - Two types of cell lines are available – RD cell line and L20B cell line.
    - RD cell line favors the growth of all enteroviruses, whereas L20B cell line favors the growth of only poliovirus.
    - About 1 g of stool is disinfected with 10 suspensions of chloroform and phosphate-buffered saline and then the sample is inoculated in cell lines.

- Normally the cytopathological effect (CPE) is expected within 7 days of inoculation; if negative after 7 days, the specimen can be watched for another 7 days also.
- If CPE is observed only in RD cell line, then it is passed into L20B cell line for confirmation of poliovirus.
- If no CPE is observed in L20B cell line also, then it can be declared as non-polio enterovirus.

69. When should non-polio enterovirus infection be suspected clinically?

When weakness is associated with pain, fever at onset with meningeal signs, asymmetric weakness, and early bladder involvement, suspect non-polio enterovirus infection.

70. What is confirmed polio?
- Isolation of wild poliovirus from the stools of the case
- Residual neurological sequelae at 60 days after the onset of paralysis
- Residual neurological sequelae present at 60 days after the onset of paralysis
- Death before follow-up
- Patient lost before follow-up could determine whether compatible residual neurological sequelae were present at 60 days after the onset of paralysis

71. Describe the virological classification of AFP cases.

The virological classification of AFP cases is described in Flowchart 4.2.

72. How is the result of stool specimen interpreted?

The interpretation of stool specimen is given in Flowchart 4.3.

73. What is the significance of 60-day follow-up?
- *Significance of 60-day follow-up*
  - Should not be performed before the 60th day
  - Residual weakness# looked for
  - Thorough cranial nerve examination
  - All data in CIF cross-checked
  - Changes notified to NPSU
    #Even minimal limping/wasting/asymmetrical skin folds means that residual weakness is present.
- The 60-day follow-up is required for the following:
  - All cases with inadequate stool specimens
  - All cases with wild poliovirus isolated with adequate stool specimens
  - All cases with vaccine poliovirus isolated even if stool specimens were adequate

Virological Classification of AFP Cases

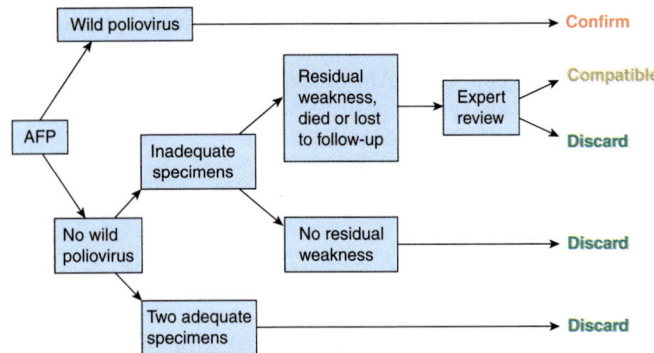

Flowchart 4.2 Virological classification of acute flaccid paralysis (AFP) cases.

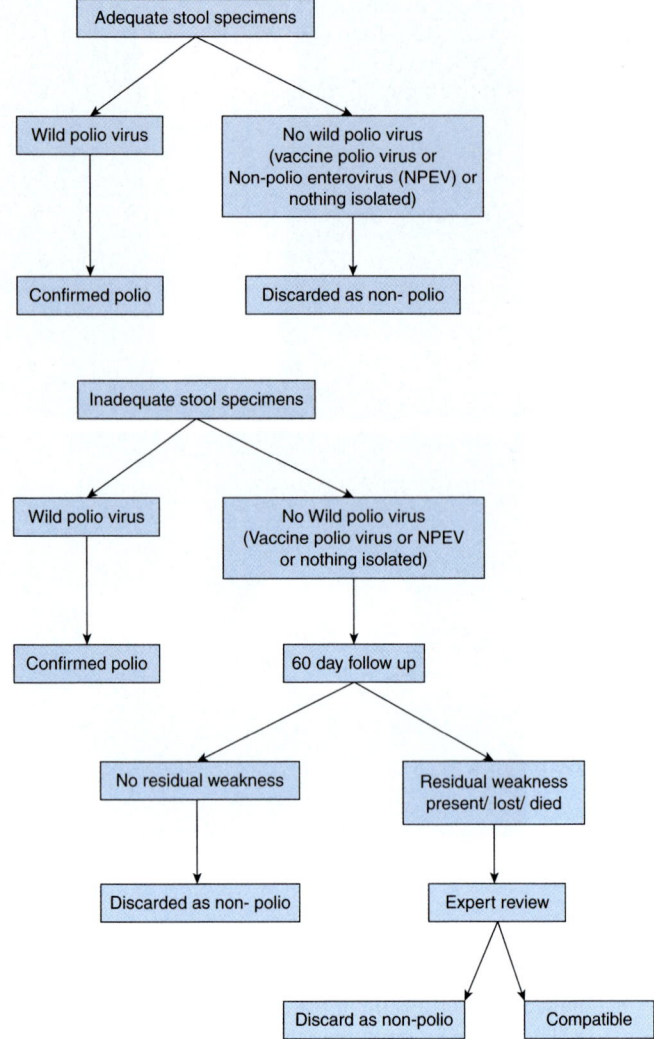

Flowchart 4.3 Stool specimen and its interpretation.

- *The 60-day follow-up not required for cases with adequate stool specimens in whom no poliovirus (wild or vaccine) was isolated*

74. What are the samples to be preserved in a child who died of polio?
- Stool
- Intestinal content
- Spinal cord biopsy

75. How is a polio outbreak managed?
- Collect stool sample.
- Outbreak response immunization (ORI) contains the following components:
  - Rural: Entire village
  - Urban: Municipal ward – 500 children younger than 5 years
  - Immunization procedure
  - Single-dose OPV to all children aged 0–5 years irrespective of the number of doses received previously

76. *What is outbreak response immunization (ORI)?

ORI is performed in case of the following:
1. Reported AFP case fits the definition.

Note: AFP is not because of trauma.
2. Outbreak control begins immediately and not after stool reports.

77. What is active case search during an outbreak?
    - Active case search is conducted by the following:
      - Door-to-door search
      - Strategic points – temples, preschools, schools, hospitals, clinics, and drug stores
      - Urban centers – pediatricians/neurologists contacted

78. What are the program surveillance indicators in AFP?
    - Sensitivity of AFP surveillance is assessed by the following:
      - Monitoring reported rate of AFP/100,000 children
      - Younger than 15 years – at least 2 cases of AFP/ 100,000
      - Weekly negative reporting
      - Monthly negative reporting
      - Percentage of two stool samples collected within 2 weeks after the onset of paralysis – should be at least 80% higher

79. How long should AFP surveillance be continued?
    - Three years after the last confirmed case, which is a requirement for certification.

FAQ ON POLIOMYELITIS

80. Define polio.
    A case of poliomyelitis is defined as any child younger than 15 years with acute flaccid paralysis (including Guillain–Barré syndrome) or any person with paralytic illness at any age when polio is suspected.

81. What are the three serotypes in polio?
    - Poliovirus 1, 2, and 3

82. *Mention the names of three serotypes of polioviruses.
    Type 1: Brunhilde virus
    Type 2: Lansing virus
    Type 3: Leon virus

83. Mention the family to which poliovirus belongs.
    a. Picornaviridae family
    b. Enterovirus

84. Describe the morphology of poliovirus.
    a. RNA virus
    b. Nonenveloped

85. *What type of poliovirus causes epidemics?
    Type 1 followed by type 3

86. What is the cause of vaccine-associated paralytic polio (VAPP)?
    Type 2 virus

87. What are the unique features of poliovirus?
    The poliovirus is not soluble in ether or other lipid solvents, because of a lack of lipid envelope. It survives extremes of pH; hence, it can successfully infect the gastrointestinal tract. Once excreted, the poliovirus can survive outside the human body for days at room temperature, for weeks in a refrigerator, and for many years at freezing temperatures. Poliovirus infection can cause lesions of neuronal destruction in the spinal cord and medulla.

88. When was the last polio case reported in India?
    January 13, 2011, in West Bengal

89. *When was India declared polio free?
    India was declared polio free on March 27, 2014.

90. Describe the paralysis in polio.
    a. Rapidly progressive (complete paralysis attained within 72 hours of the onset of paralysis)
    b. Proximal patchy
    c. Asymmetrical paralysis.
    d. With fever and spasm at the time of onset of paralysis
    e. Residual paralysis after 60 days
    f. Absence of sensory loss

91. What are the types in polio?
    Flowchart 4.4 provides a schematic representation of polio and its types.

92. *Mention **some signs in polio**.
    a. *Tripod sign:* It is otherwise called "Amoss sign." It is a condition in which the child sits with hands leaning backward because of the spasm of back muscles as shown in Fig. 4.2.

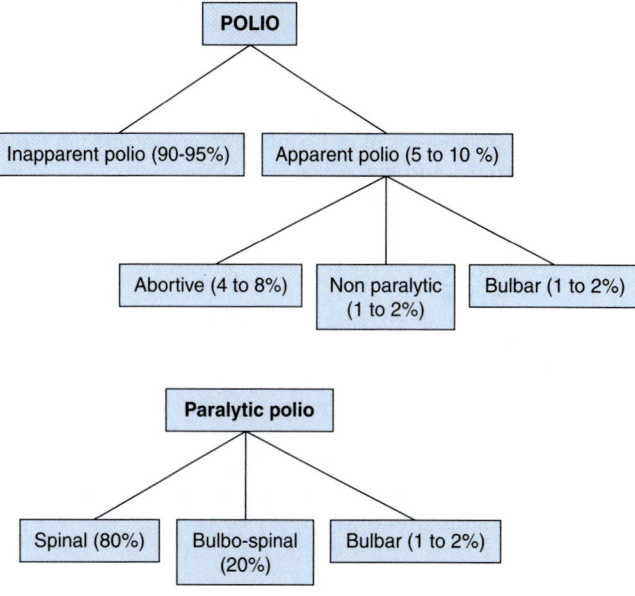

Flowchart 4.4   Different types of polio.

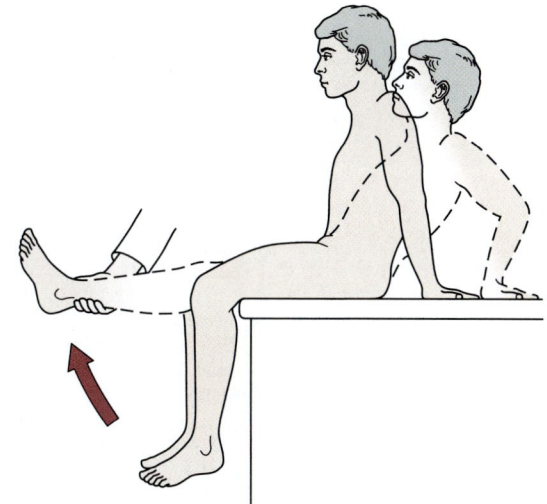

Fig. 4.2   Tripod sign. The child's knees and hips are flexed, the neck extended, the back arched lordotically, and the arms brought back in a plane posterior to the pelvis to support the thorax. (Source: Reproduced from David J. Magee, Robert Manske. *Orthopedic Physical Assessment*, Seventh Edition, Hip, Fig. 11.100, St. Louis, Saunders, 2021.)

b. *Rope sign:* It is an acute angulation between the chin and the larynx because of the weakness of hyoid muscles. The hyoid bone is pulled posteriorly causing narrowing of the hypopharyngeal inlet.

c. *Head drop* in polio is elicited by placing the hands under the child's shoulders and raising the trunk. In polio, the head will drop.

93. What is kiss-the-knee test in polio?

Kiss-the-knee test: When the child is asked to sit up and kiss the knees, the knees will be sharply drawn up because of stiffness of the spine.

94. What are the clues in history in a child with polio?

- Any surgery such as tonsillectomy – provocation paralysis
- Any strenuous exercise, pregnancy, immune deficiency, injury, and i.m. injections – provocation paralysis
- Factors favoring the transmission such as inadequate vaccination, overcrowding, and poor sanitation
- The rate of progression of weakness, symmetrical/asymmetrical
- Fever and myalgia at the time of onset of paralysis

95. Describe the pathogenesis in polio.

The pathogenesis of polio infection is described in Flowchart 4.5 and Fig. 4.3.

96. What is the course of poliovirus infection?

The course of poliovirus infection is described in Fig. 4.4.

- The incubation period is usually between 7 and 14 days.
- The poliovirus may be found in the blood of patients from the 3rd day after exposure.
- The virus is regularly present in the throat and in the stools before the onset of illness.
- It may persist in the stools up to 12–17 weeks.
- In individuals with paralysis, the virus can be detected in the feces for several weeks and sometimes months after onset.

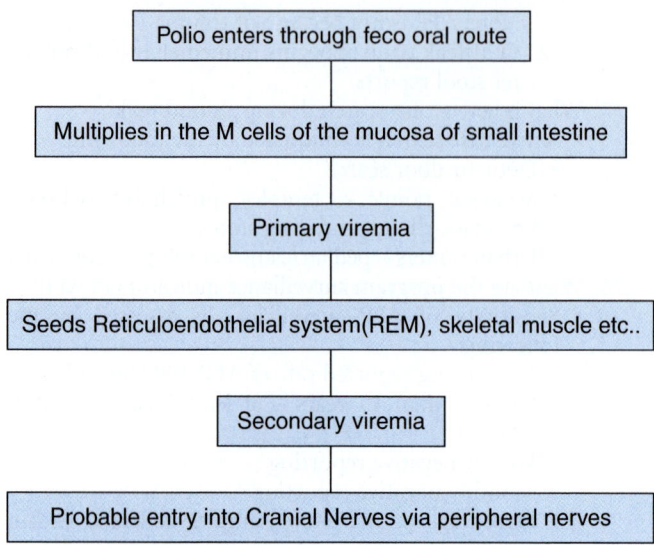

Flowchart 4.5 Pathogenesis in polio.

97. What are the clinical features of paralytic polio?

- There occurs acute onset of fever up to 39°C.
- Muscle pain (relieved by motion), paresthesia, spasms, and fasciculations are present.
- Paralysis occurs following the 1st to 2nd days.
- It is a flaccid paralysis with absent stretch reflexes that were initially hyperactive.
- The hallmark sign of this paralysis is its asymmetric distribution: Proximal muscles of the extremities tend to be involved more than the distal muscles, and the legs are more commonly affected than the arms.
- Progression of paralysis usually lasts for 2–3 days and ends when the patient becomes afebrile.

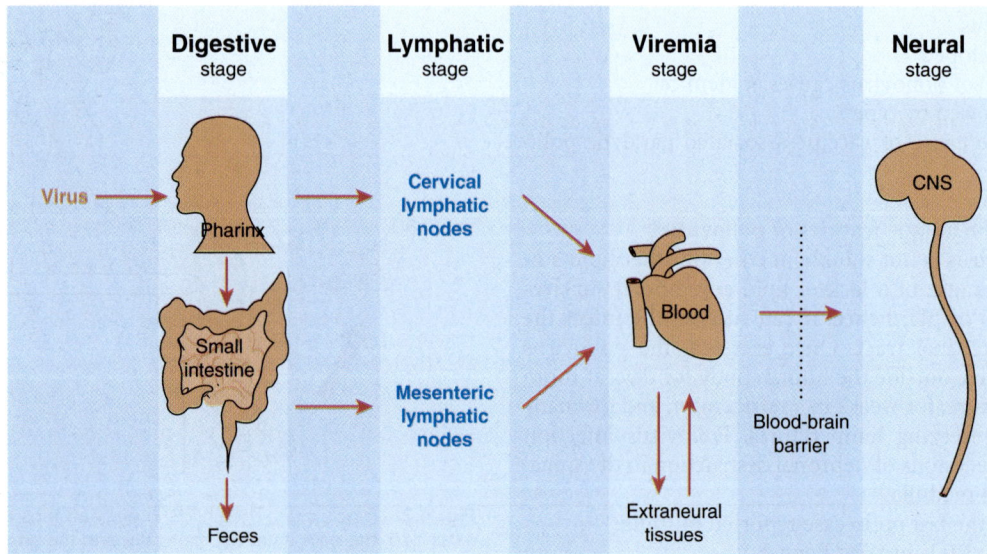

Fig. 4.3 Pathogenesis of polio. (*Source:* Based on Poliovirus, Pathogenesis of Poliomyelitis, and Apoptosis. February 2005. Current Topics in Microbiology and Immunology 289:25-56)

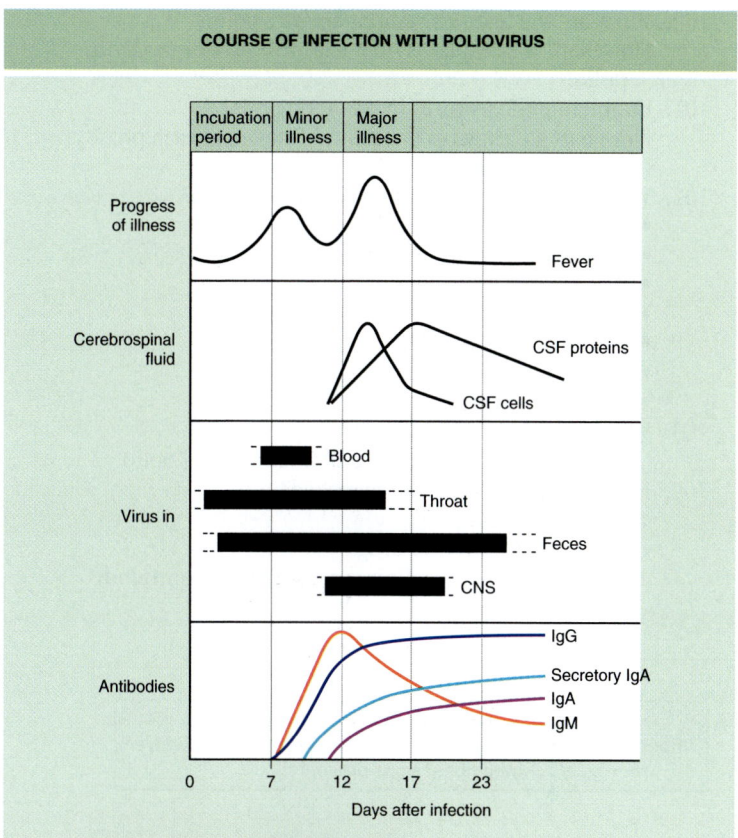

Fig. 4.4 Course of poliovirus infection. (Source: *Reproduced* from Jonathan Cohen, William Powderly. *Infectious Diseases,* Second Edition, Enteroviruses: Polioviruses, Coxsackie viruses, Echoviruses and Enteroviruses 68–71, Figure 213.7, Mosby, 2004.)

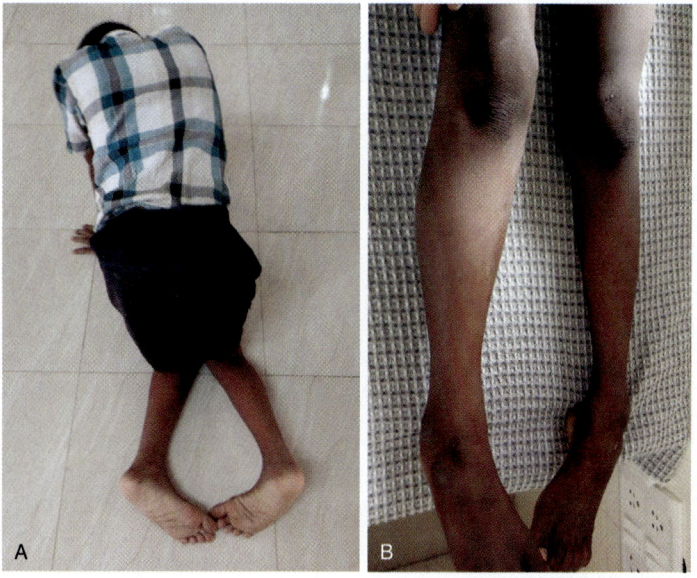

Fig. 4.5   (A) Paraparesis. (B) Asymmetrical weakness of both lower limbs.

- Sensory loss is extremely rare and should suggest another diagnosis, possibly GBS.
- Fig. 4.5A and B depicts paralytic polio.

98. What are the clinical features of inapparent polio?
   Clinical features are the following:
   a. Fever, malaise, anorexia, and headache
   b. Complete recovery
   c. No neurological sequelae

99. What is the clinical course in abortive polio?
   The course of abortive polio is described in Flowchart 4.6.

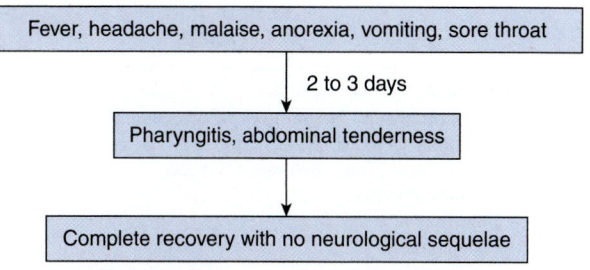

Flowchart 4.6   Course of abortive polio.

100. What are the features of nonparalytic polio?
   Flowchart 4.7 explains the features of nonparalytic polio.
101. Enumerate the features in paralytic polio?
   Flowchart 4.8 explains the clinical features in each phase of paralytic polio.
102. What are the clinical features in bulbar polio?
   - Nasal twang and regurgitation
   - Inability to swallow
   - Pooling of secretions
   - Absence of cough
   - Deviation of the palate
   - Vital center involvement
   - Rope sign present
103. What is bulbospinal polio?
   Combination of features of bulbar and spinal polio
104. How is a child with polio managed?
   a. Supportive care
   b. No specific antiviral drugs
   c. Intramuscular injections and surgeries contraindicated

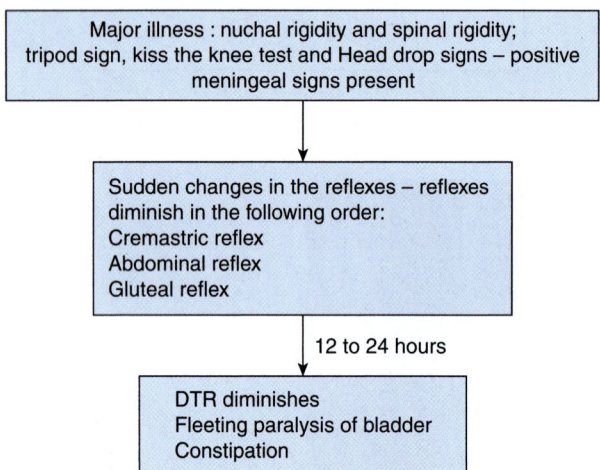

Major illness : nuchal rigidity and spinal rigidity; tripod sign, kiss the knee test and Head drop signs – positive meningeal signs present

↓

Sudden changes in the reflexes – reflexes diminish in the following order:
Cremastric reflex
Abdominal reflex
Gluteal reflex

↓ 12 to 24 hours

DTR diminishes
Fleeting paralysis of bladder
Constipation

Flowchart 4.7   Features of nonparalytic polio.

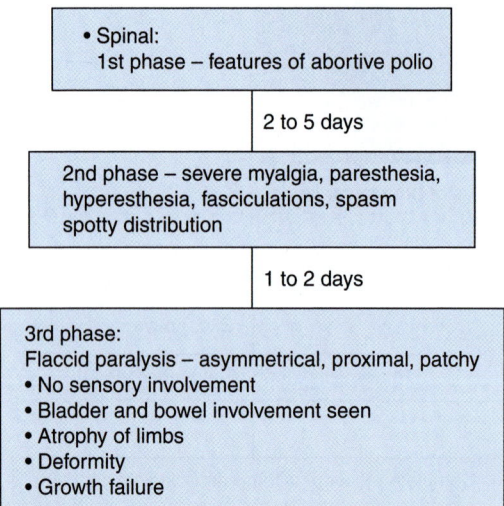

- Spinal:
  1st phase – features of abortive polio

↓ 2 to 5 days

2nd phase – severe myalgia, paresthesia, hyperesthesia, fasciculations, spasm spotty distribution

↓ 1 to 2 days

3rd phase:
Flaccid paralysis – asymmetrical, proximal, patchy
- No sensory involvement
- Bladder and bowel involvement seen
- Atrophy of limbs
- Deformity
- Growth failure

Flowchart 4.8   Clinical features in each phase of paralytic polio.

d. For abortive polio: Analgesics, sedatives, bed rest, and nutrition care
   e. For nonparalytic polio: Analgesics, hot packs once in 2–4 hours for 15 minutes, firm bed, and positioning – supine with hips slightly flexed, knees straight, and feet at right angle to legs
   f. For paralytic polio
   - Proper positioning
   - Change in position every 3–6 hours
   - Gentle physiotherapy after the pain has disappeared
   - Hot fomentation for spasm
   - Bladder and bowel care
   - High fluid intake
   - Additional salt
   - Monitoring for bulbar weakness
   - Monitoring of vital signs
105. What are the acute complications in polio?
   - Acute gastric dilatation
   - Melena
   - Hypertension
   - Hypercalcemia
   - Nephrocalcinosis
   - Acute pulmonary edema
106. What are the features of bulbar involvement in polio?
   - Pooling of secretions
   - Inability to effectively swallow (offer a cup of water to the child and ask him or her to drink; see whether the child can effectively swallow)
   - Diminishing single breath count
   - Subcostal/intercostal retractions
   - Seesaw breathing
   - Shoulder abduction palsy (C5 involvement)
107. What is the 60-day follow up in a child with AFP?
   - It is performed for the cases of AFP with isolation of wild or vaccine poliovirus from stool specimen and for the cases in whom adequate stool specimen could not be obtained because of some reason or the other.
   - It is performed to determine the presence or absence of residual paralysis.
   - It is performed between the 60th and the 90th day.
   - First, the AFP case has to be verified.
   - Determine whether the weakness is static or progressed.
   - Look for the atrophy and skin folds.
   - The tone and the reflexes have to be checked.
   - Measure all the body circumferences.
108. What is non-polio AFP?
   - If wild poliovirus is not isolated from adequate stool sample
   - If the stool sample is adequate, whether it is polio or non-polio AFP and is compatible with the results of 60-day follow up
   - If no residual paralysis on 60-day follow up, then called non-polio AFP
109. What are the key strategies in polio eradication?
   There are four key strategies for polio eradication as follows:
   1. Achieve highest coverage levels through routine immunization program (achieving the primary doses of OPV as per schedule for all children younger than 1 year).

2. Implement nation-wide mass immunization campaigns (pulse polio immunization).
3. Strengthen surveillance of AFP.
4. Conduct "mop-up" vaccination campaigns.

110. *What are mass immunization campaigns?
Mass immunization campaigns: On these days, all target children younger than 5 years should be given a dose of OPV irrespective of their previous immunization to interrupt the final chain of transmission of wild poliovirus. The concept is sudden replacement of wild poliovirus with the shedded vaccine virus so that the wild poliovirus gets gradually knocked off. It is usually conducted in the months of January and March every year (low transmission of virus during those months). (Note: The terms mass immunization campaign, pulse polio, National Immunization Day [NID], and supplementary immunization activity [SIA] are all the same.)

111. What are mop-up campaigns?
If a polio case is detected, then door-to-door, child-to-child verification of immunization is performed to break the final chain of transmission. This is called mop-up campaign.

112. What is ring immunization or outbreak response immunization?
Once a case of polio is identified, one dose of OPV has to be given for all children in the age group of 0–59 months irrespective of their previous immunization. This covers about 500 children or 5 km radius in rural areas and this has to be completed within 1 week.

113. Define VAPP.
VAPP is defined as those cases of AFP who have residual weakness 60 days after the onset of paralysis and those in whom vaccine-related poliovirus but not wild poliovirus is isolated in stool samples.

114. What are the types of VAPP?
- Recipient VAPP: Vaccine recipient within 4–40 days of receiving OPV
- Contact VAPP: Contact of the vaccine recipient

115. What is the cause of VAPP?
It occurs because of loss of attenuating mutations and reversion to neurovirulence during replication of the vaccine virus in the gut. It may occur in the vaccine recipient within 4−40 days of receiving the OPV or because of contact with the vaccine recipient.

116. What is the incidence of VAPP in India?
- The overall incidence of VAPP in India is 1 per 4.1–4.6 million doses.
- The incidence of VAPP is 1 per 2.8 million (following the first dose) and 1 per 13.9 million of subsequent dose recipients.

117. What are the risk factors for VAPP?
First dose of OPV and B-cell immunodeficiency

118. Does the risk of VAPP increase with subsequent dose of polio vaccine?
The first dose of OPV causes an increased risk of VAPP compared with subsequent dose of OPV. This lower risk on subsequent dose may be attributed to lower take of vaccine (because only the vaccine that takes up can cause VAPP), birth dose of OPV, maternal antibodies, and early immunization with OPV.

119. What is the causative virus for VAPP?
VAPP is caused by type 3 poliovirus.

120. What is VDPV?
It occurs because of the mutation and recombination in the human gut and is 1%–15% divergent from the parent vaccine virus. In addition to this, it is also transmissible and capable of causing outbreaks.

121. *What are the differences between VAPP and VDPV?
Table 4.7 gives the differences between VAPP and VDPV.

122. What is polio switch?
The switch from trivalent OPV (tOPV) to bivalent OPV (bOPV) is called polio switch. The type 2 component of tOPV causes more than 90% of vaccine-derived polioviruses (VDPVs) and 40% of vaccine-associated paralytic polio (VAPP). It also interferes with the immune response to poliovirus types 1 and 3 in tOPV.

123. *Why was polio switch recommended by WHO?
Type 2 polio was eradicated from India by 1999. Since then, no wild polio type 2 was reported from our country. But the number of VAPP by type 2 poliovirus was on the rise. This scenario was seen all over the world where trivalent OPV was used. Hence, WHO decided to switch over from trivalent OPV to bivalent OPV.

124. Why was bivalent OPV introduced?
VDPV is caused mainly by poliovirus type 2; in bOPV, only type 1 and type 3 strains are present, thereby decreasing the chance of VDPV associated with type 2 virus.

125. What are the components of bivalent OPV?
Bivalent OPV consists of type 1 and type 3.

126. When did polio switch take place in India?
Switch from trivalent to bivalent OPV was on April 25, 2016.

TABLE 4.7	Differentiating Features of VAPP and VDPV	
Features	**VAPP**	**VDPV**
Definition	Because of loss of attenuating mutations and reversion to neurovirulence during replication of the vaccine virus in the gut	Because of the mutation and recombination in the human gut, consists of 1%–15% divergent from the parent vaccine virus
Types	a. Recipient VAPP: Vaccine recipient within 4–40 days of receiving OPV b. Contact VAPP: Contact of the vaccine recipient	a. cVDPV: VDPV with evidence of virus circulation in the population causing two or more paralytic cases b. iVDPV: VDPV in an immunodeficient person c. aVDPV: VDPV of ambiguous origin isolated from the environmental sources or evidence of circulation not established
Transmissible	Not transmissible	Transmissible
Outbreaks	Does not cause	Cause outbreaks

VAPP, vaccine-associated paralytic polio; VDPV, vaccine-derived polioviruses.

127. When was India declared free of tOPV?

India was declared free of tOPV on **May 9, 2016**, National Validation Day.

128. What are the types of VDPV?

Types of VDPV are as follows:
- **cVDPV:** VDPV with evidence of virus circulation in the population causing two or more paralytic cases
- **iVDPV:** VDPV in an immunodeficient person
- **aVDPV:** VDPV of ambiguous origin isolated from the environmental sources or evidence of circulation not established

129. What are the risk factors for outbreak because of cVDPV?

Risk factors include drop in immunization coverage, high population densities, tropical conditions, and previous eradication of wild virus.

130. Why was IPV introduced following polio switch?

IPV reduces the risks associated with the withdrawal of OPV type 2. In case of outbreaks, it interrupts the transmission of the disease with the use of monovalent OPV type 2 and by boosting immunity to poliovirus types 1 and 3.

131. What are the differentiating factors in IPV and OPV?

The differentiating factors between IPV and OPV are given Table 4.8.

132. *What is the current polio immunization schedule in Universal Immunization Programme (UIP)?

In most of the southern states, fractional IPV 0.1 mL is given intradermally during the 6th and 14th weeks along with pentavalent vaccine, whereas in the northern states, one dose of IPV 0.5 mL is given along with pentavalent vaccine at the 14th week or the first contact afterwards.

133. *What is the current IAP recommendation (2018) on polio vaccine?
- Ideally IPV should replace OPV as early as possible.
- The best option is three doses of intramuscular IPV in primary series.
- Alternatives are as follows:
  a. Two doses of intramuscular IPV instead of three doses are given starting at 8 weeks with an interval of 8 weeks between the two doses (in India, these are given at 6 weeks because primary immunization schedule starts at 6 weeks).
  b. If IPV is not feasible or available, the child is given three doses of bOPV. The child should be referred for two fractional doses of IPV at a government facility at 6 and 14 weeks, or should be offered at least one dose of intramuscular IPV either standalone or as a combination vaccine at 14 weeks.

134. *What is post-polio syndrome?
- It refers to a group of disorders experienced by childhood poliomyelitis sufferers, typically starting 30–40 years after the initial onset.
- It is diagnosed when there is a new history of decreased muscle strength, weakness, and atrophy in an asymmetrical distribution compatible with previous polio attack, along with electrophysiological findings of acute denervation superimposed with chronic denervation – reinnervation in the absence of another neuromuscular cause.
- This delayed syndrome is thought to be a consequence of gradual natural deterioration of motor neurons that survived the initial episode.

   The weakness can be in already affected muscles or in the muscles previously thought to be unaffected. Effects include new-onset muscle weakness, pain, atrophy, and fatigue.
- The new symptoms are often accompanied by fasciculation or additional atrophy.
- It is not an infectious process; it occurs because of the failure of the oversized motor units created during the recovery process of poliomyelitis.
- Affected patients do not shed the virus.
- No single examination or lab test can definitely diagnose this condition.
- Different studies show that complications occur in 20%–30% of previously paralyzed patients because of late motor neuron deterioration.

135. How does immunity occur following poliovirus infection?
- Exposure to poliovirus initiates a complex process that eventually results in both humoral (systemic) and mucosal (local) immunity.
- An important barrier for inhibiting person-to-person transmission is mucosal immunity.
- It provides lifelong immunity against the disease, but is limited to the particular type of poliovirus involved (type 1, 2, or 3).
- Thus, infection with one type does not protect against infection with the other two types. IgM and IgG antibodies are detected in the serum as early as 1–3 days following natural infection but disappear after 2–3 months.
- Replication of poliovirus in the epithelium of the pharyngeal and intestinal mucosa produces local antibody (secretory IgA is dominant) and mucosal immunity to poliovirus.
- But the resulting local immunity is not absolute and a large dose of poliovirus can replicate in the oropharynx and in the intestine even in the presence of secretory IgA.
- Individual protection against paralytic poliomyelitis is provided by IgG antibody which neutralizes polioviruses in the serum.
- Maternally derived type-specific poliovirus antibodies are protective against polio, and children with higher levels of maternal antibodies have lower seroconversion rates.

136. What are the risk factors for severe polio disease?
- Pregnancy
- Immunoglobulin deficiency
- Intramuscular injection and other trauma
- Tonsillectomy

TABLE 4.8	Differentiating Factors Between IPV and bOPV	
IPV	**bOPV**
Inactivated vaccine	Live attenuated vaccine
Injectable form – intramuscular or intradermal	Oral form
Trivalent	Bivalent
Types 1, 2, 3	Types 1 and 3

FAQ ON GUILLAIN–BARRÉ SYNDROME

137. Define GBS.

It is an acute, frequently severe, and fulminant polyradiculoneuropathy that is autoimmune in nature characterized by the rapidly progressing paralysis, areflexia, and albuminocytological dissociation. It is otherwise called the Landry's ascending paralysis.

138. What is the incidence of GBS?
- It occurs in all age groups but is rare in those younger than 1 year.
- Incidence is 0.3–1.3 per 100,000 per year.

139. What are the risk factors for GBS?
- Risk factors include upper respiratory/gastrointestinal infections 10−14 days preceding the onset of paralysis. Common organisms include the following:
- GIT: *Campylobacter jejuni, Helicobacter pylori*
- RS: *Mycoplasma*
- Others: Cytomegalovirus, Lyme disease, and *Haemophilus influenzae* (Miller Fisher variant), and HIV
- Undercooked poultry, unpasteurized milk, and contaminated water

140. What are the vaccines associated with GBS?

Vaccines: Tetanus toxoid, typhoid, influenza, OPV, rabies, and conjugated meningococcal vaccine

141. What are the drugs causing GBS?

Drugs: Captopril, d-penicillamine, gold, and streptokinase

142. What are the subtypes in GBS?

Variants of GBS are as follows:
- Acute inflammatory demyelinating polyneuropathy (AIDP) – most common
- Acute motor axonal neuropathy (AMAN)
- Acute motor sensory axonal neuropathy (AMSAN)
- Acute sensory neuropathy
- Acute pandysautonomia
- Cervicobrachiopharyngeal
- Bibrachial
- Occulopharyngeal
- Ropper's variant (bilateral cranial nerve VI and VII palsy)
- Distal limb variant

143. What are the regional variants in GBS?
- Fisher syndrome – serum antibodies GQ1b and GT1a positive
- Oropharyngeal – GT1a positive

144. What is overlap syndrome?

Fisher/Guillain–Barré overlap syndrome – positive for all antibodies (GM1, GD1, GQ1, GalNac-GD1a)

145. What are the clinical clues in GBS?
- Bilateral progressive symmetrical flaccid ascending paralysis
- Areflexia or hyporeflexia
- Weakness progressing over days to weeks
- No persistent bladder/bowel involvement
- No sharp sensory level

146. *What are the factors to assess respiratory weakness in a child with GBS?

Clinical parameters useful in the assessment of respiratory weakness in children with AFP are the following:
- Respiratory rate: Tachypnea and use of accessory muscles
- Pooling of secretions: Use a tongue depressor to look into the mouth for pooling of secretions
- Swallowing dysfunction: Ask the child to take a sip of water and check whether he or she is able to swallow
- Weak cough
- Reduced speech volume
- Single breath count
- Chest rise and abdomen rise
- Diaphoresis and tachycardia

147. *What are the infections associated with GBS?
- GIT – *Campylobacter jejuni*
- Respiratory – *Mycoplasma*
- Infectious mononucleosis, Lyme disease, cytomegalovirus, and *Haemophilus influenzae* (Miller Fisher syndrome)

148. *What are Asbury diagnostic criteria in GBS?
A. Asbury criteria
- *Diagnostic features*
  Symmetrical, ascending flaccid paralysis
  With areflexia or hyporeflexia
- *Supporting features*
  Progression of symptoms over days to weeks
  Relative symmetry
  Bilateral facial weakness
  Mild/no sensory involvement
  Recovery in 2–4 weeks after progression ceases
  Autonomic dysfunction
  Absence of fever at the time of onset of weakness
  Typical CSF findings
  Nerve conduction study showing demyelinating neuropathy
- *Features that exclude the diagnosis*
  Abnormal metabolism of porphyrin
  Recent diphtheria
  Diagnosis of botulism, myasthenia, toxic neuropathy, or poliomyelitis
  Pure sensory without weakness
- *Features causing doubt in the diagnosis*
  Persistent bladder and bowel dysfunction
  Severe pulmonary dysfunction
  Minimal weakness at onset
  Fever at the time of onset of weakness
  Marked asymmetry of the weakness
  Bladder or bowel dysfunction at onset
  Rise in mononuclear cells in CSF

149. What are Brighton's diagnostic criteria in GBS?

Brighton's criteria: Six parameters are considered in this:
1. Bilateral and flaccid weakness
2. Decreased or absent DTR
3. Monophasic interval between onset and nadir of weakness between 12 hours and 28 days
4. Electrophysiological study consistent with GBS
5. CSF: Cytoalbuminologic dissociation
6. Absence of alternative diagnosis

Level 1: All six parameters are present (highest diagnostic significance).

Level 2: Either CSF or NCS findings should be present; all other four are positive.

Level 3: Neither CSF nor NCS is suggestive of GBS.

Level 4: All are not suggestive of GBS except for no other possible alternate diagnosis (lowest significance).

TABLE 4.9	Neurophysiological Criteria for AIDP, AMSAN, and AMAN	
AIDP	**AMSAN**	**AMAN**
1/4 in two nerves Or 2/4 in one nerve 1. Motor conduction velocity <90% LLN 2. Distal motor latency >110% ULN 3. pCMAP/dCMAP ratio <0.5 4. F-response latency >120% ULN	None of AIDP except 1/4 (one out of four) in one nerve + dCMAP <10% LLN + Sensory action potential amplitude <LLN	None of AIDP + 1/4 (one out of four) in one nerve + dCMAP <10% LLN + Sensory action potential amplitude – normal

AIDP, acute inflammatory demyelinating polyneuropathy; AMAN, acute motor axonal neuropathy; AMSAN, acute motor sensory axonal neuropathy; CMAP, compound muscle action potential; LLN, lower limit of normal; ULN, upper limit of normal.

150. What are the neurophysiological criteria for AIDP, AMSAN, and AMAN?
    The neurophysiological criteria are given in Table 4.9. Conduction velocity reduced in one or two nerves is the main feature in all types.
151. What are the CSF criteria in GBS?
    1. Elevated CSF protein >45 mg/dL (maximum protein levels reaches by 4–6 weeks)
    2. Normal opening pressure
    3. Fewer, <10 mononuclear cells ± pleocytosis (lymphocytes <100)
152. Mention some numericals in GBS.
    • GBS is an ascending paralysis with symmetrical involvement. However, asymmetrical involvement is seen in 9% of cases.
    • Reflexes can be normal in 10% of cases.
    • GBS progresses up to 2–4 weeks, reaches maximum weakness in 4-week duration, plateaus for weeks to months, and then recovers.
    • Twenty-five per cent of cases of GBS need mechanical ventilation.
    • Bulbar involvement/bifacial weakness (shown in Fig. 4.6) is seen in 50% of cases.
    • Sensory involvement is seen in 20% of cases.
    • Autonomic dysfunction is seen in 75% of cases.
    • Mortality is <5%.
    • Relapse rate is 5%–10%.
    • Residual deformity is seen in 10% of cases.
    • Urinary involvement is seen in 20% of cases.
    • Preceding URI/GIT is seen in 65% of cases.
    • Meningismus is seen in 50%–80% of cases.
153. What is the correlation between antibodies and infection in GBS?
    Majority of the children have infection prior to the onset of weakness, which is progressive and reaches its maximum within 4 weeks; antiganglioside antibody levels decrease over time. The correlation between antiganglioside antibodies and GBS infection is given in Fig. 4.7.
154. What is the triad of Miller Fisher syndrome?
    • Triad of Miller Fisher (3 A's): Ataxia, areflexia, and acute external ophthalmoplegia
155. Which cranial nerve is involved in Miller Fisher type of GBS?
    Cranial nerve VI is the most common cranial nerve involved in Miller Fisher variant.

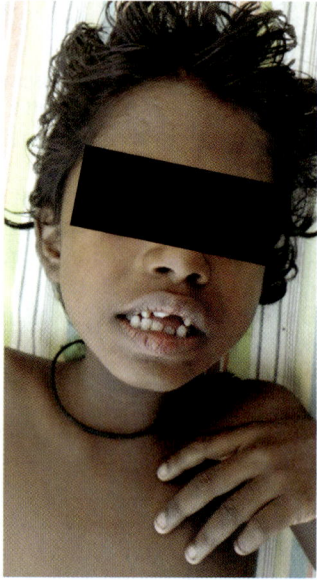

Fig. 4.6 Bifacial weakness in GBS.

156. What are the clinical features in Miller Fisher syndrome?
    • Cranial nerve VI palsy
    • Papilledema
    • Optic neuritis
    • Distal paresthesia
    • Urinary incontinence/retention
    • Differential diagnosis: Bickerstaff encephalitis
157. What are the clinical clues in autonomic dysfunction?
    Autonomic dysfunction, one of the poor prognostic factors, is seen in 75% of cases of GBS.
    • Excessive sweating
    • Tachycardia/bradycardia (more common)
    • Postural hypotension (more common)/hypertension
    • Occasional asystole
    • Shock
158. *What are the differentials in a child with AFP with severe autonomic involvement?
    a. Porphyria
    b. Botulism
159. What are the salient features of GBS caused by *Campylobacter jejuni* infection?
    GBS caused by campylobacter jejuni has a regional distribution, severe presentation usually seen in China,

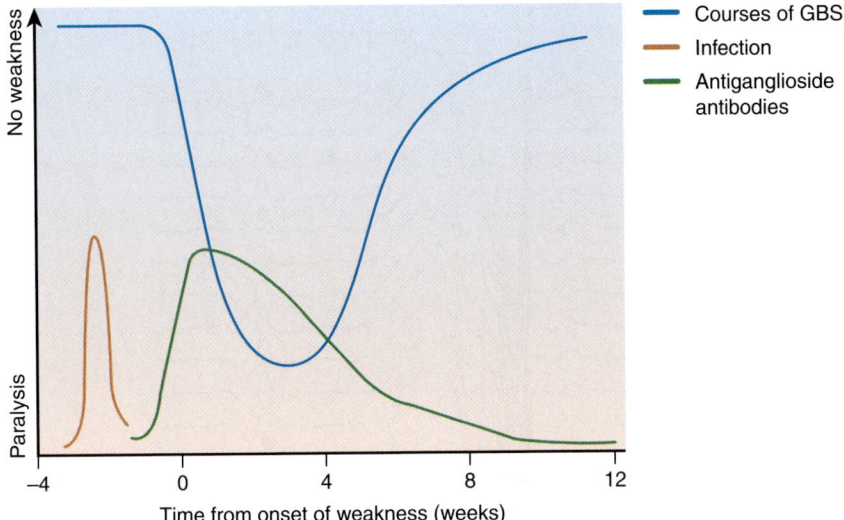

Fig. 4.7 Correlation between antibodies and infection in GBS. *(Source: Van Doorn PA, Ruts L, Jacobs BC. Clinical features, pathogenesis, and treatment of Guillain–Barré syndrome. The Lancet Neurology. 2008 Oct 1;7(10):939-50.)*

requires ventilatory support has high risk for mortality, late recovery, mostly AMAN type; antibodies against GM1 and GD 1A are usually positive in these children.

160. What is congenital GBS?
- Absence of maternal neuromuscular disease
- Neonate with general hypotonia, weakness, and areflexia
- Fulfillment of all CSF and electrophysiological criteria
- General improvement in the first few months
- No residual disease by 1 year of age
- History of ulcerative colitis and intake of prednisone and mesalamine (sulfasalazine) noted in such mothers

161. How is a child with GBS investigated?
    a. Serum electrolytes are determined to rule out dyselectrolytemia.
    b. CSF analysis is performed during the 2nd week of illness.
       It shows elevated proteins and <10 WBCs/mm³. This is called the albumin cytological dissociation and is diagnostic of GBS.
    c. Bacterial and viral cultures are usually negative.
    d. MRI spine: Findings include enhancement of cauda equina, intrathecal nerve roots, and cranial nerve roots with gadolinium contrast; MRI spine also helps to rule out other spinal pathology.
    e. Nerve conduction study is normal in the early phase of the disease except for the F-wave latencies which peak by 2 weeks of illness (F waves are called foot waves) as given in Fig. 4.8.
    f. Serum antibodies against GM1 and GD1 are usually seen in axonal type rather than in demyelinating type.

162. What is the significance of serum antibodies in GBS?
    Antibodies are positive in the following:
    a. *Campylobacter jejuni* – GM1 and GD1a
    b. Miller Fisher variants – GQ1b and GT1a

163. What are the indications for MRI spine in a child with suspected GBS?
    Indications include the following:
    i. Asymmetrical weakness
    ii. Early bladder involvement
    iii. Sensory level
    iv. Upgoing plantars

164. Why is CSF analysis performed in the 2nd week of illness?
    Albuminocytological dissociation is formed because of antigen–antibody complex and it takes around 7–10 days to destroy the blood–brain barrier. That is why it is performed in the 2nd week.

165. *What is the cause of albuminocytological dissociation in GBS?
    It is an inflammatory process and not an infectious process. Hence, the cell counts remain normal or only slightly elevated rather than proteins getting elevated.

166. What are the possible differentials if the cell count is elevated in the CSF in a child with suspected GBS?
    Differentials include HIV and Lyme disease.

167. What is critical illness neuropathy or myopathy?
    It occurs in 25%–45% of critically ill children with severe illness. It occurs as a complication of severe illness that causes apoptosis of motor and sensory axons. Clinical features include predominant lower limb weakness and respiratory muscle weakness in the form of difficult weaning. Long-term sequelae include decrease in the quality of life and decreased exercise capacity.

168. *What is the disability score used in GBS?
    It is called the Hughes disability score:
    0: Healthy
    1: Minor symptoms but capable of running
    2: Able to walk 5 m across an open space without support but not able to run
    3: Able to walk 5 m across an open space with support
    4: Bedridden/chair bound
    5: Requires assisted ventilation
    6: Dead

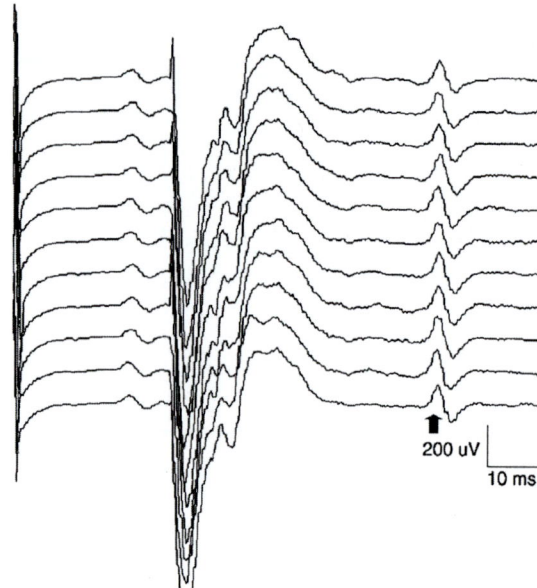

Fig. 4.8   Nerve conduction study in GBS – abnormality in F-wave response (prolongation, absence, or infrequency of F wave). (Source: Reproduced from Steve Vucic, Matthew C. Kiernan, David R. Cornblath and Guillain-Barré syndrome: An update, *Journal of Clinical Neuroscience*, 16: 733–741.)

169. What is the significance of Hughes disability score in GBS?

    Hughes disability score of >2 or inability of the child to walk unaided for 10 m is an indication for IVIG in GBS.

170. What is the management of a child with GBS in the emergency room?
    a. Respiratory care
    b. Management of bulbar weakness
    c. Management of cardiovascular instability
    d. Management of electrolyte disturbance if any
    e. To rule out other etiology – snake bite (look for fang marks) and trauma (spinal cord pathology)

171. How is a child with GBS treated?
    a. Stabilization of airway, breathing, and circulation
    b. Careful monitoring for bulbar involvement and planning for elective intubation
    c. Pain management in the initial phase
    d. Bladder/bowel care
    e. Nutrition (NG tube feeding if the patient is not able to swallow/fluid and electrolyte management)
    f. Suctioning of oropharyngeal secretions
    g. Physiotherapy from day 1
    h. Monitoring pulmonary function (breathing pattern, serial single breath count, spirometry)
    i. Parent counseling
    j. Monitoring vital signs for autonomic dysfunction (twice-daily blood pressure monitoring, continuous ECG monitoring)
    k. *IVIG*, which is the drug of choice in GBS (it is given at a dose of either 400 mg/kg/day for 5 days or 1 g/kg/day for 2 days)
        • If there is no improvement, the second course of IVIG is planned.
        • If there is no further improvement, **plasmapheresis** is planned.
    l. No role of steroids in GBS except in chronic inflammatory demyelinating polyradiculoneuropathies (CIDP) in which they are given as i.v. high-dose pulsed methylprednisolone
    m. Treatment of underlying infection not necessary as it is self-limiting

172. What is the role of IVIG in GBS?
    a. Targeted attack on Schwann cell membrane and myelin by antibodies prevented by blockage of Fc receptor on macrophage
    b. Regulation of anti-idiotypic or anti-cytokine auto-antibodies in the pooled immunoglobulin
    c. In B cell, upregulation of inhibitory Fc gamma receptor 11B
    d. Downregulation of B-cell activating factor and complement cascade
    e. High concentration of circulating immunoglobulin causing breakdown of IgG

173. What is plasmapheresis?
    It is performed to remove antibodies in treating autoimmune conditions. In this method, plasma from the body is removed by withdrawing blood, separating it into plasma and cells, and the cells are transfused back into the bloodstream.

174. Enumerate plasmapheresis.
    • Plasmapheresis is performed at a rate of 25−50 mL/kg/cycle EOD × 6 cycles. Each cycle is followed by FFP transfusion or 5% human albumin.

175. What are the complications associated with IVIG administration?
    Complications: Thrombocytopenia, anaphylaxis, and deep vein thrombosis

176. What is the contraindication for IVIG administration?
    IgA deficiency

177. What are the complications of plasmapheresis?
    • Sepsis

- Hypocalcemia
- I.v. inaccessibility
- Dysautonomia
- Arrhythmia – long QT

178. What are Erasmus criteria and what are they for?

The Erasmus GBS Outcome Score (EGOS) given in Table 4.10 helps in predicting the likelihood of recovery from GBS at 6 months. Three clinical characteristics are assessed including age, diarrhea preceding the GBS, and MRC sumscore at 2 weeks into the disorder. EGOS helps to counsel about the prognosis.

Total score (1–7) = ___

Score <3-very likely to walk independently at 6 months
>5- 50% unable to walk independently at 6 months

179. What is the clinical course of GBS?
   a. Gradual onset
   b. Rapid progression up to 2 weeks in 80% of cases and 4 weeks in 97% of cases
   c. Plateau in 1–28 days
   d. Maximal weakness reached within 4 weeks
   e. Bulbar weakness seen in 50% of cases
   f. Beginning of spontaneous recovery in 2–3 weeks
   g. Improvement always opposite to the direction of spread of weakness (bulbar weakness recovers first followed by lower limb power)
   h. Good prognosis
   i. Possibility of acute relapse in 7% of children

180. What are the sequelae in GBS?

Permanent axonal loss in some children with or without clinical signs, chronic neuropathy, and easy fatiguability

181. What are the findings in nerve conduction study?

The patients are normal in the first few days, but later develop conduction block and F-wave latency. Conduction block indicates good outcome.

182. What are the poor prognostic features in GBS?
   - Age less than 1 year
   - High disability score
   - Apopleptic palsy
   - Cranial nerve involvement

- Axonal type
- Low MRC scale score
- Unable to walk/bladder involvement at the time of presentation
- Prolonged duration of ventilation
- Severe autonomic involvement
- Maximum weakness at the time of presentation
- Poor outcome with sequelae – cranial nerve involvement, intubation, and maximum disability at the time of presentation

183. What is the order of recovery in GBS?
   - Bulbar weakness recovers first and lower limb weakness recovers last.
   - Tendon reflexes are the last to recover.
   - The first muscles to be involved are the last to recover and vice versa.

184. *What is the incidence of recurrent GBS?

Ten per cent of patients can have recurrent GBS.

185. *Comment on the mortality in GBS.
   - The overall mortality rate is around 5%.
   - Three features that predict the overall mortality are cranial nerve involvement, intubation, and maximal disability at the time of presentation.

186. What is Froin syndrome?

It is the coexistence of xanthochromia, high protein level, and marked coagulation of CSF with normal cell count. It occurs because of blockage of CSF pathway in the spine because of tumor/abscess/meningeal irritation.

187. What are the differential diagnoses of Froin syndrome?
   - Spinal tumor
   - Meningitis
   - Abscess in the spine
   - Ependymoma in the spine

188. What is Queckenstedt's maneuver?
   - It is a clinical test to diagnose spinal stenosis.
   - The patient is placed in lateral decubitus position.
   - Lumbar puncture is performed.
   - Opening pressure is measured.
   - Both jugular veins are compressed by the clinician's assistant which leads to an increase in the intracranial pressure.
   - If the anatomy is normal, intracranial pressure will be reflected as a rapid rise in the pressure within 10–12 seconds.
   - In case of spinal stenosis, there will be only a slow response – hence a positive Queckenstedt's maneuver.

FAQ ON ACUTE TRANSVERSE MYELITIS

189. What are the salient features of transverse myelitis?
   - Acute onset
   - Ascending weakness
   - Sharp sensory level
   - Bladder and bowel involvement
   - Can be symmetrical or asymmetrical

190. What are the clinical clues in transverse myelitis?
   - Hypotonia, absent reflexes, and mute plantar in the acute state but after a few weeks the child develops spasticity, brisk reflexes, and upgoing plantar
   - Sensory deficit
   - Bladder involvement

TABLE 4.10	Erasmus GBS Prognosis Score	
Prognostic Factor	**Characteristics**	**Score Points**
1. Age (years)	<40	0
	>40	1
2. Diarrhea within 4 weeks before GBS symptoms	No diarrhea	0
	Diarrhea present	1
3. Degree of disability at 2 weeks into illness	a. Minor symptoms, able to run	1
	b. Can walk unassisted but cannot run	2
	c. Needs walker to walk	3
	d. Bed or chair bound	4
	e. On ventilator even briefly	5

GBS, Guillain–Barré syndrome.

191. What are the clinical findings in early and late stages of transverse myelitis?

Table 4.11 gives the clinical findings in early and late stages of transverse myelitis.

192. What are the diagnostic criteria in transverse myelitis?

The Transverse Myelitis Consortium Working Group (TMCWG) criteria are as follows:
- Presence of sensory, motor, or autonomic dysfunction attributable to spinal cord level
- Bilateral signs or symptoms not necessarily symmetrical
- Progression to nadir less than 21 days
- Exclusion of extra-axial compressive pathology by MRI spine

193. What are the differentials if a child has relapsing–remitting demyelinating disorders?
- About 75% of children with ATM have longitudinal extensive myelitis (LETM >3 spinal segments).
- Serum aquaporin-4 antibodies should be performed in all children with LETM to rule out neuromyelitis optica spectrum disorders.
- Ophthalmic examination and MRI brain screening are performed in such children.

194. Comment on the CSF in transverse myelitis.

It is mostly normal. Sometimes it may show lymphocytic pleocytosis.

195. How is a child with transverse myelitis managed?

Give methylprednisolone at a dose of 10−30 mg/kg/day for 5 days followed by oral prednisolone 1–2 mg/kg/day for 2 weeks and then taper and stop in 2–4 weeks.

196. What is the outcome in transverse myelitis?

Outcome is guarded because about 40%–50% of children tend to have persistent motor and bladder dysfunction.

197. What are the poor prognostic features in transverse myelitis?
- Maximal weakness reached within 24 hours
- Severe impairment at the time of presentation
- Delay in the initiation of treatment
- Prolonged duration of impairment
- Elevated proteins in CSF
- Secondary infections such as urinary tract infections

FAQ ON TRAUMATIC NEURITIS

198. What are the clinical features in traumatic neuritis?
- Acute onset
- Sciatic nerve injury – most common
- Monoparesis
- History of i.m. injection in that limb (sciatic neuropathy because of intramuscular injection in the gluteal region is the commonest form)
- Absent knee jerk and preserved ankle jerk
- Asymmetrical involvement, sensory deficits, and lack of CSF pleocytosis, which favors the diagnosis of traumatic neuritis

199. How is a child with traumatic neuritis managed?

Management is only supportive care.

FAQ ON DIPHTHERITIC POLYNEUROPATHY

200. What are the clinical features of diphtheritic polyneuropathy?
- It begins 3–4 weeks following the primary infection.
- Descending paralysis begins with paralysis of the soft palate and postpharyngeal and laryngeal muscles, causing difficulty in swallowing and nasal quality of voice.
- Cranial neuropathies characteristically occur in the 5th week.
- Symmetrical neuropathy occurs 10 days to 3 months after oropharyngeal infection.
- Motor deficits and diminished DTR occur.

201. What are the causes of descending paralysis?
- Botulism
- Poliomyelitis
- Diphtheria

202. What are the other differentials for diphtheritic polyneuropathy?

The close differential for diphtheritic polyneuropathy is descending GBS and its distinguishing features are given as follows:
- Even CSF findings will be similar to those of diphtheritic polyneuropathy.
- The only way to distinguish is by serological diagnosis and even that will be negative if the patient has received antitoxin during the primary infection.
- Antitoxin in the primary infection is effective only when it is given within 48 hours.

203. What is the prognosis in diphtheritic polyneuropathy?

Recovery is usually slow but complete.

204. What is the role of corticosteroids?

Corticosteroids do not decrease the incidence of complications and are not recommended.

205. What are the distinguishing features of other differential diagnoses of AFP?

The findings in other differentials of AFP are given in Table 4.12.

TABLE 4.11	Clinical Findings in Early and Late Stages of Transverse Myelitis	
Features	**Early Stages**	**Late Stages**
Type of paralysis	LMN type – flaccid	UMN type – spastic
Tone	Decreased	Increased
Deep tendon reflex	Areflexia	Hyperreflexia
Babinski sign	Negative	Positive

TABLE 4.12	**Distinguishing Features of Other Differentials of Acute Flaccid Paralysis**

Conditions	Clinical Findings	Onset of Paralysis	Progression of Paralysis	Sensory Signs/ Symptoms	Diminished or Absent DTR	Residual Paralysis	Pleocytosis
Poliomyelitis	Paralysis	Incubation period (7–14 days) 4–35 days	24–48 h, proximal > distal, asymmetric	No	Yes	Yes	Aseptic meningitis PMN (Polymorphonuclear Neutrophils)
Non-polio enterovirus	Paralysis	As in polio	same as above	No	Yes	Yes	same as above
Guillain–Barré syndrome	Preceding infection, LMN, facial palsy	Hours to 10 days	Acute symmetric ascending (days to 4 weeks)	Yes	Yes	+/−	No
Acute traumatic sciatic neuritis	Acute, asymmetrical	Hours to 4 days	Complete, affected limbs	Yes	Yes	+/−	No
Acute transverse myelitis	Acute, symmetrical hypotonia in lower limbs	rapidly progressive	Hours to days	Yes	Yes (early)	Yes	Yes
Spinal cord compression	Paralysis	Complete	Hours to days	Yes	Yes	+/−	+/−
Neuropathies, *Corynebacterium diphtheriae*	Palatal paralysis, blurred vision	Incubation period 1–8 weeks, paralysis 8–12 weeks after illness	–	Yes	Yes	–	+/−
Clostridium botulinum	Abdominal pain, diplopia, ptosis, mydriasis	Incubation period 18–36 h	Symmetric, rapid, descending	+/−	No		No
Tick-borne paralysis	Ocular symptoms	Incubation period 5–10 days	Acute, symmetric, ascending	No	Yes		No
Myasthenia gravis	Diplopia/ptosis, dysarthria Fatiguability Weakness		Multifocal	No	No	No	No
Disorders of muscle (Polymyositis)	Autoimmune disease	Chronic	Weeks to months	No	Yes	No	No
Viral myositis	Proximal > distal	Subacute	Hours to days	No	No	No	No
Hypokalemic periodic paralysis		Respiratory muscles Proximal limb	Postprandial Sudden onset	No	Yes	+/−	No

Quick Bites

- Tripod sign, rope sign, and head drop sign are seen in poliomyelitis.
- Type 1 followed by type 3 poliovirus causes polio epidemics.
- Type 2 virus causes vaccine-associated paralytic polio (VAPP).
- Polio switch from trivalent to bivalent OPV was on April 25, 2016.
- India was declared polio free on March 27, 2014.
- Acute motor and sensory axonal neuropathy (AMAN) is associated with claw hand and carries a poor prognosis.

- Bilateral LMN type of facial nerve palsy is common in GBS.
- Cranial nerve VI is the most common cranial nerve involved in Miller Fisher variant.
- The triad of Miller Fisher (3 A's) includes ataxia, areflexia, and acute external ophthalmoplegia.
- Ten percent of patients can have recurrent GBS.
- The overall mortality rate in GBS is around 5%.
- Hughes disability score is used to assess the severity in GBS and the need of IVIG.

5

Floppy Infant

Following introduction, seek permission from the caregiver and introduce yourself to the patient before history elicitation, and identify the case.

Name____Age____Sex____Consanguinity____Order of birth____Place____Informant____

Presenting Complaints and Duration

- Delayed milestone
- Flailness/floppiness of all four limbs and limpness noticed since birth
- Recurrent respiratory tract infection

History of Presenting Illness

- Not attained age-appropriate milestone (head holding achieved or not)
- Flailness noticed by the mother while handling, which was gradual in onset, progressive, bilateral, and symmetrical
- Repeated cough/cold/fever/breathlessness
- Constipation

CENTRAL NERVOUS SYSTEM HISTORY

Higher Function History

- Alert, recognizes the mother, seizures, speech, early handedness, and behavior or sleep disturbance

Cranial Nerve History

- Ability to perceive light and history of white eye
- Any history of drooping of eyelids, ability to move eyeballs in all four directions, or restriction of eyeball movement
- Ability to chew food and difficulty in opening the jaw
- Ability to close both eyes while sleeping, drooling of saliva, deviation of angle of the mouth, lack of facial expression, and facial asymmetry
- Ability to hear and respond to sound
- History of nasal twang of voice, nasal regurgitation, choking while feeding, weak cry, and difficulty in swallowing
- Ability to move the head side to side
- Abnormal movement or twitching in the tongue

Motor System

- Posture (the lower limb always lies along the cot with knees by the side [frog-like posture]; thinning of muscles noted by the mother on both extremities/chest/face; floppiness noted by the mother in the form of slipping from hands; while lifting the child by the axilla, the child hanging like a rag doll or dangling of legs present [as compared with in the previous sibling])
- Ability to move legs above the cot and ability to kick around the bed or paucity of spontaneous movement or unable to bear weight on legs or always keeps the lower limb by the side of the cot/unable to raise the arm, however able to move fingers/toes
- Any history of twitching noticed by the mother over the body
- Any history of involuntary movements

Cerebellar Features

- Abnormal eyeball or head movement or tremors

Bladder/Bowel Disturbance

- History of urinary incontinence or dribbling and constipation

Sensory Features

- History of perception of pain or crying while giving vaccination

Autonomic Features

- Flushing, sweating, and palpitation episodes

Spine and Cranium

- Any abnormality in the head size noted by the mother compared with in a sibling or peers
- Any swelling, tuft of hair, sinus, discharge, and abnormal curvature

HISTORY OF COMPLICATIONS

- Fever, breathlessness, cough, vomiting (recurrent aspiration because of poor swallowing, pliable chest), bed sores/skin ulcers, and failure to thrive

ETIOLOGICAL HISTORY

- Easy fatiguability on repeated using of the muscle, drooping of eyelids, and periodicity or diurnal variation
- Seasonal variation – worsens during winter
- Corn syrup/honey intake (infant)/prelacteal feeds
- Suck–rest cycle/breathing difficulty/fatigue while feeding
- Flushing/sweating/palpitation/postural hypotension/arrhythmias
- Upper abdomen distension and early morning convulsions with breathlessness
- Obesity
- White eye
- Abnormal chest deformity
- Pigmentation of skin
- Joint hyperextensibility, clubfoot, and joint contracture
- Drug intake
- Failure to thrive

Past History

- Previous admission for recurrent respiratory tract infection

Antenatal History

- History of decreased fetal movements
- Drug exposure (lithium/phenytoin/carbamazepine)
- Polyhydramnios (poor swallowing)
- Delayed onset of labor/prolonged labor (poor fetal movements)
- Cesarean section (malpresentation)

Birth History

Breech presentation, cesarean section (formal presentation), history of birth asphyxia, and poor breathing effort

Neonatal History

Postdated, IUGR, history of limpness, feeding difficulties (poor suck), drooling or pooling of secretions, breathlessness/abnormal breathing pattern, decreased spontaneous movement, weak cry, abnormal posture/contractures, convulsions in the neonatal period, neonatal hyperbilirubinemia, and dribbling of urine/leaky stools or constipation

Development History

Delay in predominant motor milestone

Dietetic History

As per 24-hour recall method

Immunization History

According to IAP or Universal Immunization schedule

Family History

Delayed milestones, history of death in infancy in sibling, ptosis, or easy fatigability in the mother

Treatment History

Any NG tube feeding and drugs

Socioeconomic History

According to the modified Kuppuswamy scale

Summary

A …-month-old child with a history of delayed milestones and flailness noted by the mother, with absence of periodicity or diurnal variation, with normal higher functions, with breathing difficulty/nasal regurgitation and low-volume cry, with abnormal movement noted in the tongue with flailness of all four limbs, in the background of no significant perinatal event suggestive of a floppy child now admitted with a history of fever or breathing difficulty

General Examination

- Posture – pithed frog position
- Paucity of movement or any involuntary movement

- Contractures/scar
- Bed sores/ulcers
- Bony deformity – scoliosis
- Any accessories – NG tube, oxygen support, gastrostomy, and tracheostomy

Head-to-Foot Examination

- Head – size and loss of hair in the occipital area/occipital flattening
- Face – dysmorphic facies, expressionless facies, and tented, inverted V mouth
- Eyes – cataract, ptosis, squint, and absent tears
- Tongue – fasciculation
- Chest deformity/scoliosis
- Skin – increased laxity (Ehlers–Danlos syndrome)
- Joints – arthrogryposis
- Genitalia – testis (palpable on both sides)

Vital Signs

Temperature
Pulse rate
RR – breathing pattern and evidence of respiratory distress
Blood pressure

Anthropometry

Any features of malnutrition

Central Nervous System Examination

HIGHER FUNCTIONS

Conscious, alert looking, recognizes the mother, speech, and sleep disturbance

CRANIAL NERVES

- Perceives light, direct and consensual light reflex, and fundus normal
- Ptosis, moves eyeballs in all four cardinal directions, and strabismus
- Pain sensation over the face, able to chew food, and jaw jerk
- Wrinkling of the forehead present
- Ability to close eyes on both sides while sleeping
- Absent nasolabial fold on the affected side
- Deviation of the angle of the mouth to the normal side
- Drooling of saliva present
- Hearing normal
- Palatal movement normal, uvula in the midline, and any pooling of secretions present
- Palatal arches normal, and palatal and pharyngeal reflex normal
- Ability to lift the head from supine position
  Whether turns the head on both sides
- Fibrillation or wasting, myotonia, and tongue fasciculations

MOTOR SYSTEM

- Attitude/posture – frog-like posture
- Motor examination findings as given in Table 5.1

TABLE 5.1 Findings in Motor System Examination		
Motor System Examination	**Right**	**Left**
Bulk	Wasting	Wasting
Tone (all four limbs)[a]	Hypotonia	Hypotonia
Power	Proximal > distal	Proximal > distal
Superficial reflexes	Normal	Normal
Plantar	Flexor	Flexor
Deep tendon reflexes	Absent	Absent

[a]180° flip test.

- Completion of motor system examination with the examination of the mother for myotonia or myopathic features
- Gait – wide based
- Involuntary movements – no

CEREBELLAR SIGNS

- Head nodding, nystagmus, gait abnormality, ataxia or imbalance, past pointing, and dysdiadochokinesia

AUTONOMIC SYSTEM

- Excessive sweating, tachycardia, and hypotension

SENSORY SYSTEM

Touch/temperature/pain sensation

SPINE AND CRANIUM

Any tuft of hair, swelling, and sacral dimple

SIGNS OF MENINGEAL IRRITATION

Present or not (Kernig/Brudzinski reflex)

Other System Examination

ABDOMEN

Hepatomegaly and palpation of fecal mass

CARDIOVASCULAR SYSTEM

Apical impulse – cardiomegaly, murmur, and abnormal heart sounds

RESPIRATORY SYSTEM

Breathing pattern and respiratory distress

MUSCULOSKELETAL EXAMINATION

Contractures, hip dislocation, and arthrogryposis

Diagnosis

A …-month-old child with gradually progressive/static quadri-paresis since birth, decreased fetal movements, no mental retardation, no significant prenatal/perinatal events, generalized hypotona, areflexia, and fasciculations; most probable diagnosis – spinal Muscular atrophy, type …, nutritional status; other co-morbid conditions – anemia and vitamin deficiency if any

Frequently Asked Questions

1. How are neuromuscular disorders classified depending on the age of onset?

   The age of onset of disease and neuromuscular disorders are given in Table 5.2.

2. List the significance of etiological history in a floppy infant.

   Etiological history and its significance are given in Table 5.3.

3. What are the possible complications in a floppy infant?
   a. Recurrent aspiration (poor swallowing)
   b. Pliable chest – recurrent respiratory tract infection
   c. Cardiac failure in cardiomyopathy
   d. Failure to thrive – because of chronic cough, feeding difficulty, and breathlessness
   e. Bed sores and skin ulcers
   f. Constipation

4. Why does malpresentation occur in a child with a neuromuscular disorder?

   In a fetus with a neuromuscular disorder, breech delivery/malpresentation requiring cesarean section is higher because turning requires adequate fetal mobility.

5. What are the clues in antenatal, natal, and neonatal histories in a floppy infant?

   Table 5.4 gives the clues in antenatal, natal, and neonatal history elicitation.

6. How is family history significant in a floppy infant?
   • Family history of sibling death seen in spinal muscular atrophy (SMA), congenital myotonic dystrophy, and congenital myopathy
   • Mother – easy fatiguability (maternal myasthenia) and myopathic facies (congenital myotonic dystrophy)

7. Enumerate the clues in the examination in a floppy infant.

   Table 5.5 gives the examination clues in a floppy child.

8. Describe frog-like posture and jug handle posture.

   Pithed frog position (Fig. 5.7A): Upper limb – shoulder adducted (external rotation – jug handle appearance; internal rotation – frog-like); elbow and wrist flexed; lower limb flexed; hip flexed and externally rotated, knee flexed, and ankle dorsiflexed

   Jug handle posture (Fig. 5.7B): Frog-like posture with internal rotation

9. What is the importance of vital signs in a floppy infant?
   • Temperature: Increased in familial dysautonomia
   • Heart rate: Tachycardia and slow and irregular rhythm (cardiomyopathy – Pompe disease, mitochondrial disease)
   • Respiratory rate: Breathing pattern (paradoxical breathing – the abdomen goes in on inspiration [Normal Respiration: chest wall goes in on inspiration and out on expiration])
   • Blood pressure: Increased (familial dysautonomia)

TABLE 5.2 Classification of Neuromuscular Disorders and the Age of Onset

Congenital-Onset Motor Disorder	Early Onset to Childhood-Onset Motor Disorder	Childhood-Onset to Adulthood-Onset Motor Disorder	Adult-Onset Motor Disorder
Congenital muscular dystrophy (CMD) with merosin deficiency	Duchenne muscular dystrophy	Becker muscular dystrophy	Limb–girdle types 1A, 1C, 2L
CMD with abnormal glycosylation of dystroglycan a. Walker–Warburg b. Muscle eye brain disease c. CMD type 1 C	Emery–Dreifuss muscular dystrophy	Fascioscapula humeral dystrophy	
CMD with rigid spine syndrome type 1	Limb–girdle muscular dystrophy with lamin AC deficiency	Emery–Dreifuss muscular dystrophy with Merlin	
Ullrich syndrome	Limb–girdle muscular dystrophy with calpain deficiency	Limb–girdle type 2 except 2A, 2L	

TABLE 5.3 Etiological History

Etiology	History
Myasthenia gravis	Periodicity – diurnal variation, fatiguability on repeated using of the muscle, drooping of eyelids
Myotonic muscular dystrophy	Seasonal variation – worsens during winter
Botulinum toxin	Corn syrup/honey intake/prelacteal feeds
Pompe disease (cardiomyopathy)	Suck–rest cycle/breathing difficulty/fatigue while feeding
Familial dysautonomia	History of flushing/sweating/palpitation/postural hypotension/arrhythmias
Drug intake	Drugs causing weakness: Vincristine, captopril, chloroquine, phenobarbitone in porphyria, penicillamine, aminoglycoside
Myotonic dystrophy	White eye – cataract
Ehlers–Danlos syndrome	Joint hyperextensibility, clubfoot
Adrenoleukodystrophy	Pigmentation

TABLE 5.4	Antenatal, Natal, and Neonatal Histories
Presenting Complaints	**History**
Antenatal	Decreased fetal movements
	Polyhydramnios
	Malpresentation
Gestation age	Postdated (because of unengagement of the head)
Cesarean section	Malpresentation
Prolonged labor	Birth asphyxia (inadequate fetal movement)
	Respiratory distress
Birth weight	IUGR
Hypotonia	Respiratory distress/abnormal breathing pattern – seesaw breathing
Diet history	Feeding problems
	Ask for the total duration to finish the feed in one breast (normally 15–20 min; if the child takes more than 30 min, it is prolonged)
	Sucking – poor suck/prolonged sucking is because of lack of a tight seal of lips, fatiguability, regurgitation of feed, fasciculation of tongue
	Neuromuscular disorder, congenital myasthenia syndromes
Abnormal posture	Pithed frog – hypotonia
Cryptorchidism	Weak abdominal muscle (abdominal muscle contraction is required for normal descent of testis into the scrotal sac)
Arthrogryposis	Fetal immobilization
Hypotonia	Joint dislocation – congenital dislocation of the hip
Spinal muscular atrophy	Hyperalert look
Head size	Hydrocephalus (Arnold–Chiari malformation)
Cry	Weak cry – neuromuscular disorder
	Fatiguable cry – congenital myasthenia syndrome
	Hoarse cry – hypothyroid
Myelomeningocele	Urine – dribbling of urine (palpable bladder), leaky stools (patulous anus)
Hypothyroid	Constipation

TABLE 5.5	Clinical Clues in the Examination in a Floppy Infant
Cause	**Clinical Clues**
Hypothyroid	Coarse facies (Fig. 5.1)
Trisomy 21/Zellweger syndrome	Down facies
Glycogen storage disorder (Pompe disease)	Doll-like facies
Myotonic muscular dystrophy	Inverted V-shaped upper lip (Fig. 5.2)
	Temporal scalloping
Nemaline rod myopathy	Dolichocephaly, open mouth, expressionless facies, hanging jaw (Fig. 5.3)
Myasthenia gravis, mitochondrial myopathy	Ptosis (Fig. 5.4)
Ehlers–Danlos syndrome	Hyperextensibility of joints (Fig. 5.5)
Lowe, mitochondrial disorder	Cataract, squint
Familial dysautonomia	Absent tears
Tongue	Fasciculation – SMA
	Protruding tongue – hypothyroidism, Down syndrome
	Absent fungiform papillae –Pompe disease
	Big tongue – DMD
Cutis laxa	Hyperelasticity of skin (Fig. 5.6)

10. How is tone assessed in children?
    Tone in children is assessed in three ways:
    1. Resting posture: Postural tone is achieved by prolonged contraction of antigravity muscles in response to low-intensity stretch because of gravity. The spontaneous posture of the baby is observed when he or she lies undisturbed.
    2. Passive tone: It is evaluated by applying certain maneuvers to the infant while he or she remains passive at rest. The maneuvers are performed slowly, gently, and just to the point of discomfort.
    3. Active tone: Check for the active movement of the child.
11. *What is 180° flip maneuver? How is it demonstrated?
    The 180° flip examination is used to assess gross motor in infants of 2–10 months of age.
    • Lying supine (assess the posture adopted, abnormal ATNR, involuntary movements with CP, paucity of movements for hemiplegia) as shown in Fig. 5.8A

_____

*Important question asked in the examination.

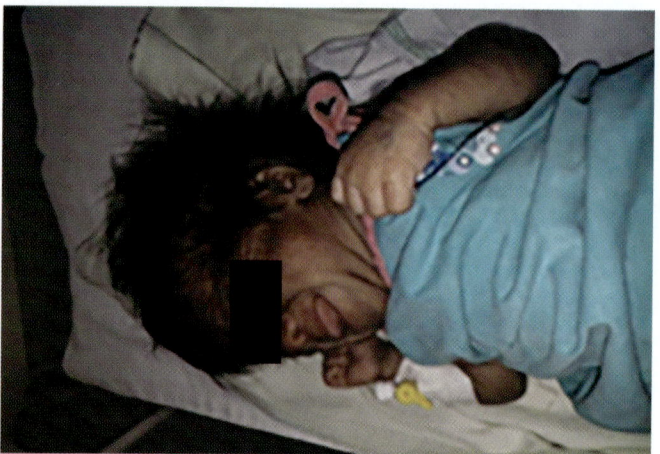

Fig. 5.1 Coarse facies in hypothyroidism.

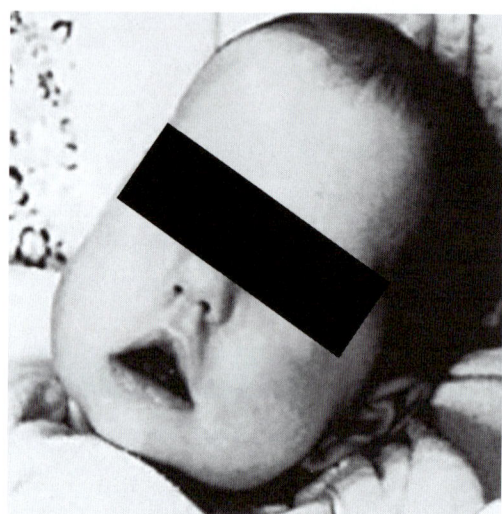

Fig. 5.2 Inverted lip in myotonic muscular dystrophy. *(Source: Nelson, 20th edition, Chapter 609.3, Fig. 609-4.)*

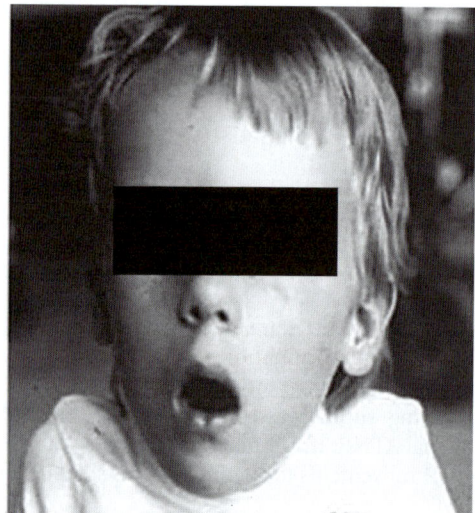

Fig. 5.3 Open mouth because of weak masseter in nemaline rod dystrophy. *(Source: Nelson, 21st edition, Chapter 626, Fig. 626.6, p. 3265.)*

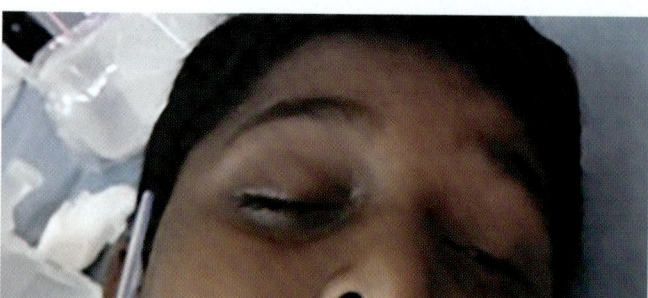

Fig. 5.4 Ptosis in myasthenia gravis.

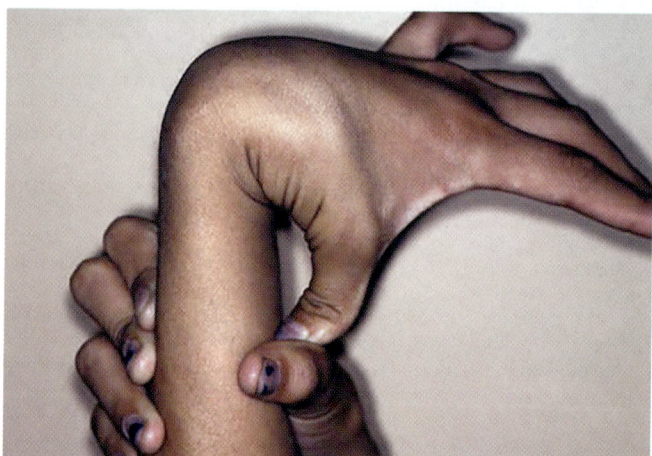

Fig. 5.5 Hyperextensible joints. *(Source: Nelson, 21st edition, Chapter 679, Fig. 679.5, p. 3529.)*

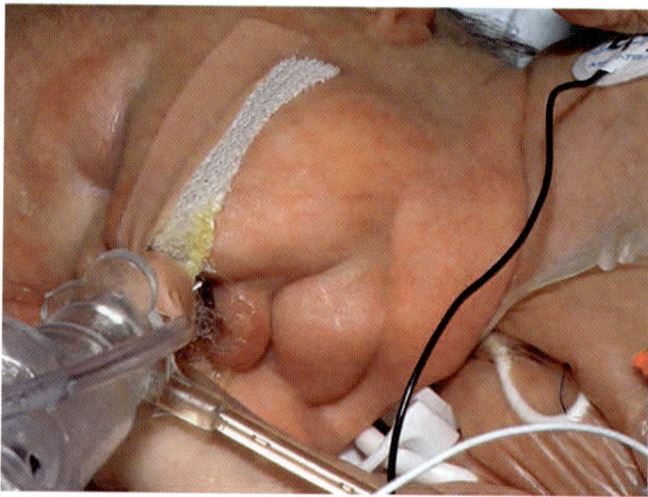

Fig. 5.6 Cutis laxa. *(Source: Nelson, 21st edition, Chapter 678, Fig. 678.8, p. 3521.)*

- Pull to sit (assess head lag and grasp) as shown in Fig. 5.8B
- Sitting (assess sitting ability [head and trunk control], and then perform lateral propping, back straight or rounded) as shown in Fig. 5.8C
- Vertical suspension (weight bearing) by holding under axillae (observe for any scissoring of lower limbs or hypotonia) as shown in Fig. 5.8D

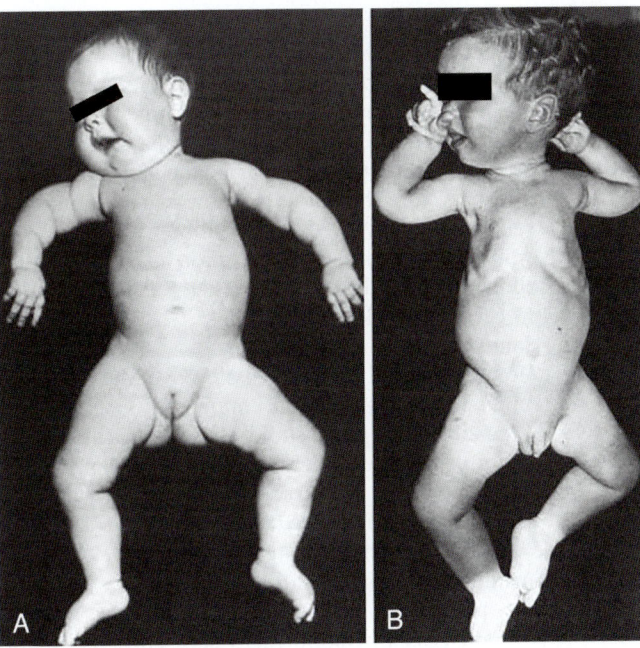

Fig. 5.7 (A) Pithed frog position. (B) Jug handle position. *(Source: Nelson, 21st edition, Chapter 625, p. 3246, Fig. 625.1.)*

- Ventral suspension (assess any arching of the back) as shown in Fig. 5.8E
- Prone position (to detect arching of the back, ability to raise the head and trunk above the horizontal plane) as shown in Fig. 5.8F

12. What is scarf sign?

Scarf sign is used to assess tone in a floppy child. Put the child in supine position, head in midline, and hold one of the infant's hands and try to put it around the neck as far as possible around the opposite shoulder. Observe how far the elbow goes across the body. In a floppy infant, the elbow easily crosses the midline as seen in Fig. 5.9.

13. What is rag doll appearance?

A floppy child resembles a rag doll because there is hypotonia of all four limbs.

14. What are the differentials in a floppy child with tachypnea?

1. Recurrent respiratory tract infection – SMA and atonic cerebral palsy
2. Cardiac – Pompe disease, mitochondrial disorder, and congenital myotonic dystrophy
3. Paradoxical breathing – SMA
4. Bell-shaped chest/splayed lower ribs – SMA

15. What are the differentials in a floppy child with expressionless facies?

1. Congenital myotonic dystrophy
2. Myasthenia gravis
3. Congenital myopathy

16. What are the differences between myopathic facies and myotonic muscular dystrophy facies?

Table 5.6 gives the differences between myopathic and myotonic muscular dystrophy facies.

17. What are the clinical clues in a floppy child for identification of the cause?

Table 5.7 gives the clinical clues in diagnosing a floppy child.

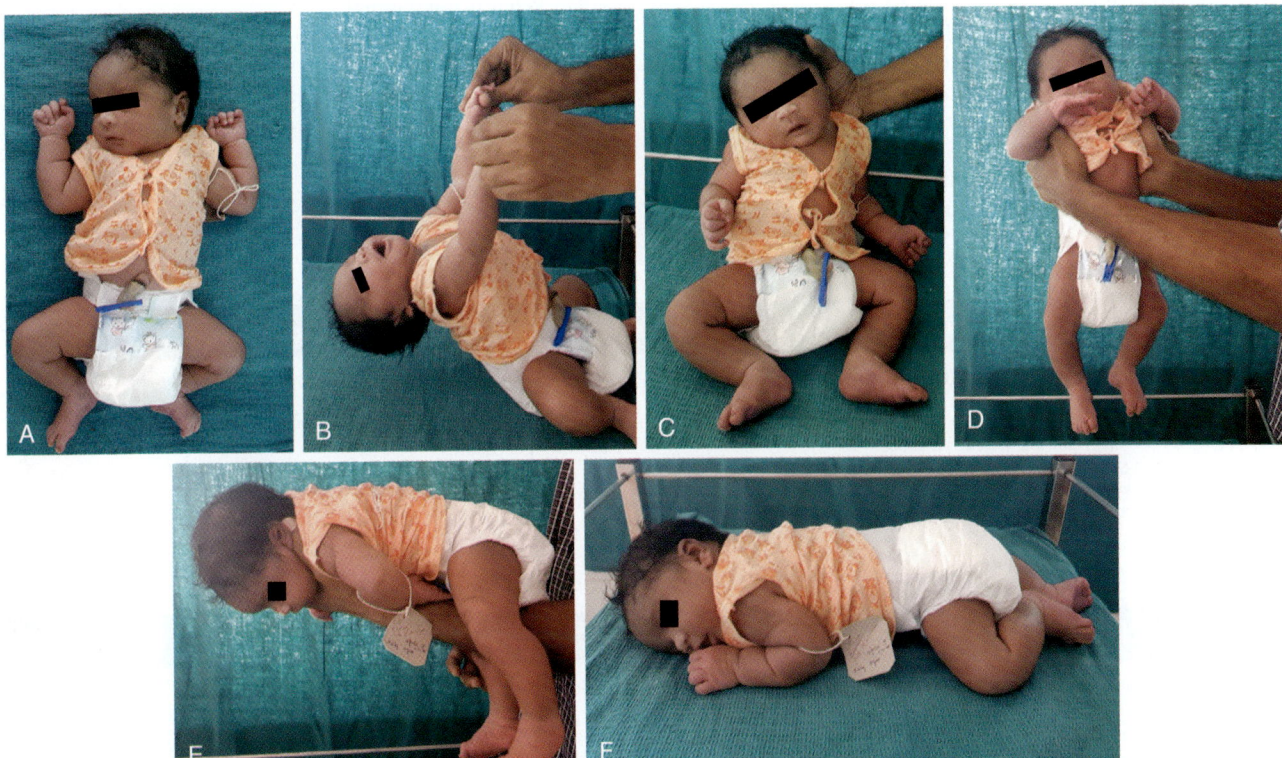

Fig. 5.8 (A) Flexed at elbow, hip, and knee. (B) Pull to sit maneuver. (C) Sitting maneuver. (D) Vertical suspension maneuver. (E) Ventral suspension maneuver. (F) Prone position.

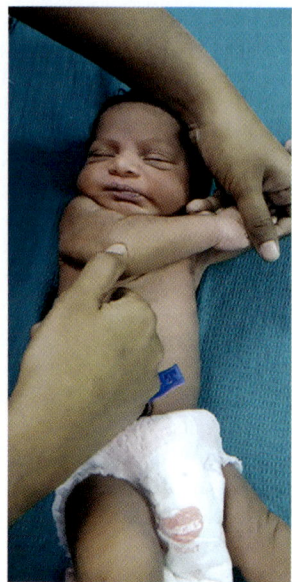

Fig. 5.9 Scarf sign maneuver – baby in supine position, head in midline, and elbow drawn across the opposite shoulder.

18. Describe the gait in myopathy.
    a. Waddling gait and myopathic gait (because of proximal muscle weakness of the pelvic girdle muscle)
    b. Trendelenburg gait – abductor weakness (gluteus medius and minimus are affected): Normal side, hip in a higher position; affected side, hip low (Fig. 5.10A and B)
19. *How can one differentiate between fibrillation and fasciculation?
    Table 5.8 gives the differences between fibrillation and fasciculation.
20. Demonstrate fasciculation clinically.
    Fasciculation is demonstrated clinically by sudden tap over the deltoid/biceps or seen in the tongue when the tongue is examined inside the mouth.
21. What is myotonia?
    The phenomenon of impaired relaxation of a muscle after forceful voluntary contraction is called myotonia.

It is commonly seen in hands and eyelids. It is due to repetitive depolarization of the muscle membrane and characterized on electrophysiological studies by waxing and waning rhythmical discharges.
22. What are the clinical features of myotonia?
    These include difficulty in releasing the handgrip after a handshake, unscrewing a bottle top, or opening the eyelids if the eyes are shut forcefully.
    Myotonia shows impaired relaxation of hand muscle following forceful contraction (Fig. 5.11).
23. *How can one check for myotonia?
    1. Handshaking
    2. Percussion myotonia – percussion over the tongue
       Percussion over the thenar eminence
       Percussion over the deltoid muscle (watch for the dimple to appear [because of delayed relaxation of the muscle] as shown in Fig. 5.12)
    3. The child asked to look up (watch for sudden downward eye movements showing lid lag)
    4. Inability to release a holding object
24. What is pseudomyotonia or myotonia-like reaction?
    It is characterized by abnormally slow contraction and relaxation in response to mechanical or electrical stimulation seen in hypothyroidism due to slow reaccumulation of calcium in the endoplasmic reticulum and in the disengagement of thin actin and thick myosin filaments.
25. What are the distinguishing features between myotonia and pseudomyotonia?
    Table 5.9 gives the differences between myotonia and pseudomyotonia.
26. What is polyminimyoclonus?
    Fine movements of fingers in SMA
27. What is myokymia?
    • Involuntary eyelid muscle contraction, lower eyelid > upper eyelid
    • Pathological – facial myokymia and neuromyotonia
    • Treatment – Warm compression and a decrease in caffeine
28. What is neuromyotonia?
    • Another name: Isaac syndrome

TABLE 5.6	Differences Between Myopathic Facies and Myotonic Muscular Dystrophy Facie
Myopathic Facies (Expressionless Facies)	**Myotonic Muscular Dystrophy (MMD)**
Dolichocephaly	Narrow head, scalloped/concave temporalis muscle
High arched palate ± cleft	High arched palate
Mouth – open, downturned corners of the mouth	Thin cheeks, inverted V upper lip
Bilateral ptosis	

TABLE 5.7	Clinical Clues in Diagnosing Floppy Child
Floppy child with predominant face involvement	Congenital myotonic dystrophy Myasthenia gravis
Floppy child with predominant upper limb involvement	Spinal muscular atrophy (proximal > distal)
Floppy child with predominant lower limb	Myelomeningocele
Floppy child with predominant distal limb	Myotonic muscular dystrophy
Floppy child with normal movement	Connective tissue (Ehlers–Danlos syndrome, Marfan syndrome, osteogenesis imperfecta)

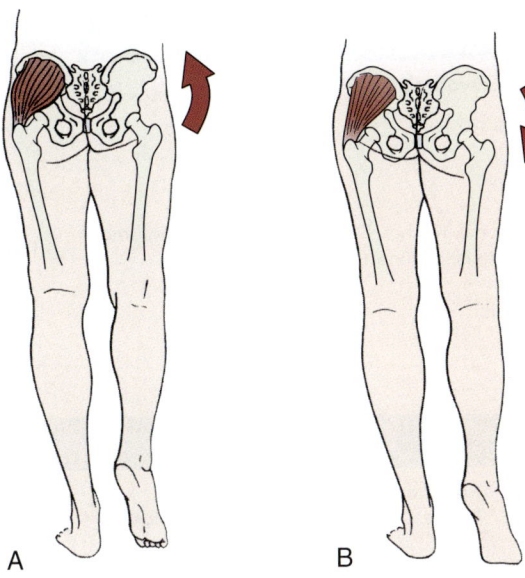

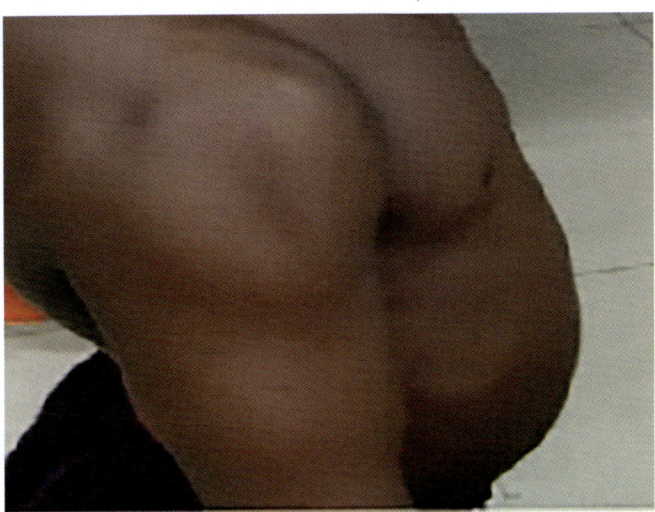

Fig. 5.12 Percussion myotonia.

Fig. 5.10 Trendelenburg gait : A) Back view of a person standing on one leg shows normal level of right hip (curved upward arrow). B) Back view of a person standing on one leg shows right hip dropping to one side (curved downward arrow) suggestive of hip abductor weakness. (Source: Reproduced from David J. Magee, Robert Manske. *Orthopedic Physical Assessment*, Seventh Edition, Hip, Fig. 11.98, St. Louis, Saunders, 2021.)

TABLE 5.8	Differences Between Fibrillation and Fasciculation	
Fibrillations	**Fasciculation**	
Individual muscle fiber is affected	Groups of muscle fiber are affected	
Denervation hypersensitivity of single muscle fiber	Underlying active degeneration of group of muscle fibers	
Fine	Coarse	
Not detectable (under the skin)	Visible by the naked eye	
Only through electromyography/USG		
Delivered by myofibril	Delivered by the motor unit	
Fibrillation potential – small amplitude, short duration	Fibrillation potential – larger and longer in duration	

- Pathophysiology: Autoreactive antibodies – voltage-gated potassium/chloride channelopathies on motor nerve which causes peripheral nerve hypersensitivity
- Three causes: Acquired, 80%; others, hereditary and paraneoplastic syndrome
- Clinical features: Muscle cramps, stiffness, myotonia-like symptoms – slow relaxation, walking difficulties, fatigue, and fasciculation
- Diagnosis: Electromyography (EMG) and typical myotonic discharge which has a waxing and waning quality – dive bomber sound
- Treatment: Anticonvulsants – phenytoin, plasma exchange, and IVIG

29. What is warm-up phenomenon in neuromyotonia?
    Myotonia typically occurs after a period of rest and decreases with continuing exercise, referred to as the warm-up phenomenon.
30. What are the differential diagnoses for fasciculation?
    Anterior horn cell, spinal muscular atrophy, benzodiazepine withdrawal, organophosphorous poisoning, and neuromuscular involvement – myasthenia, snake bite, and magnesium deficiency
31. *How are various neuromotor disorders differentiated?
    Table 5.10 gives the clinical features of various neuromuscular disorders.
32. How can one differentiate between SMA and atonic CP?
    Table 5.11 gives the differences between SMA and atonic CP.
33. *How are neuropathy and myopathic weakness differentiated?
    Table 5.12 gives the clinical features of neuropathy and myopathic weakness.
34. Describe the clinical features suggestive of motor unit disorders.
    Alert-looking child, weak cry, poor suck, motor weakness, paucity of movement, muscle atrophy, fasciculation, absent deep tendon reflex, failure of movement by postural reflexes, normal sensation, absence of other organ dysfunction, winging of the scapula, paradoxical breathing, and normal CPK

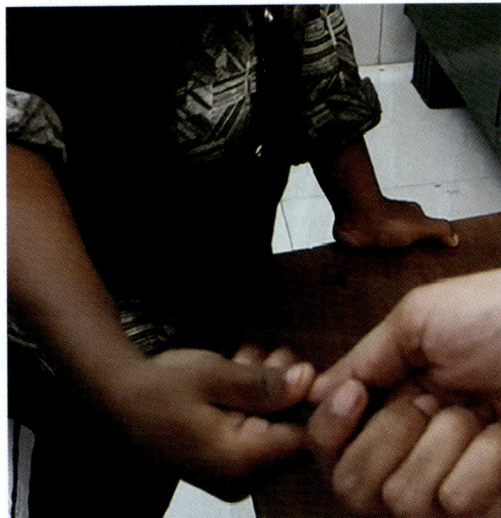

Fig. 5.11 Myotonia – hand muscle.

TABLE 5.9   Differences Between Myotonia and Pseudomyotonia

Features	Myotonia	Pseudomyotonia (Hypothyroid)
Percussion myotonia	Usual	Occasional
Grasp myotonia	Usual	Rare
Stiffness	Common	Common
Warm-up phenomenon	Common	Absent
Muscle enlargement	Usual	Occasional (Kocher–Debré–Semelaigne syndrome)
Delay in relaxation after tendon reflex	Rare	Characteristic (hung-up knee jerk)
Response to quinine and procaine	Usual	None
EMG	Repetitive firing	Irritability

EMG, electromyography.

TABLE 5.10   Clinical Features of Various Neuromuscular Disorders

Features	Central	Motor Neuron	Peripheral Nerve	NMJ	Muscle
Weakness	Central hypotonia; proximal > distal	Proximal > distal	Distal > proximal	Proximal = distal	Proximal > distal
Muscle atrophy	−	++++	+	−	++
Fluctuating	−	−	−	+++	−
Weakness/diurnal variation	−	−	−	++	−
Sensory changes	−	−	Lost	−	−
DTJ	Brisk	Absent	Decreased	Diminished	Normal

TABLE 5.11   Differences Between SMA and Atonic CP

SMA	Atonic CP
No higher function affected	Seizure +, MR +
No seizures, no MR, no speech delay	
Development – predominant motor delay (alert looking, social smile normal)	Gross delay
Fasciculations +	No fasciculations
Reflexes – absent	Reflexes – retained and brisk
No associated microcephaly or macrocephaly	Microcephaly ±

35. Describe the features of neuropathic disorder.
    Predominant distal weakness, sensory disturbance, trophic ulcers, abnormal nerve conduction study, and normal EMG
36. What are the possible differentials in a floppy infant with higher function involvement?
    • Floppy infant + normal higher function: SMA
    • Floppy infant + seizures: Mitochondrial disorder
    • Floppy infant + mental retardation: Syndromic child (Down syndrome) and atonic cerebral palsy
37. What are the possible differentials if the weakness improves with physiotherapy?
    If the weakness improves with physiotherapy, it is central hypotonia.
    Motor unit disorder (lower motor neuron disorder) does not improve with physiotherapy.
38. What are the differentials in an alert-looking infant with feeding difficulty?
    a. Congenital myotonic dystrophy
    b. Transient myasthenia and genetic myasthenic syndromes
    c. Familial dysautonomia

d. Prader–Willi syndrome
e. SMA
Fig. 5.13 shows a hyperalert-looking infant in spinal muscular atrophy (SMA).

39. Describe the distinguishing features of disorders of the motor system.
    Table 5.13 gives the clinical features and various disorders of the motor system.
40. List the causes of central motor hypotonia and peripheral motor hypotonia.
    Table 5.14 gives the various causes of central and peripheral motor hypotonia.
41. What is anticipation and in which condition is it seen?
    • Anticipation is a phenomenon that is passed on to the next generation in which the symptoms of the genetic disorder become apparent at an earlier age with each generation and also an increase in severity of symptoms is noted.
    • Causes: These include myotonic muscular dystrophy, Friedreich ataxia, and fragile X syndrome.
42. What are the stepwise investigations done in a floppy child?
    Table 5.15 gives the stepwise investigations in a floppy child.
43. What is the role of EMG in a myopathic child?
    a. To exclude other neuromuscular disorder (neuromuscular junction disorder, neuropathies)
    b. To confirm the diagnosis of certain myopathies in which motor units with characteristic morphology and recruitment pattern are identified
    c. To identify target muscle for biopsy
44. What are the problems to be anticipated in a floppy infant undergoing muscle biopsy?
    The anesthetist should be informed of the full picture.
    1. Muscle relaxants avoided because they can lead to profound and prolonged weakness
    2. Risk of malignant hyperthermia

TABLE 5.12	Clinical Features of Neuropathy and Myopathic Weakness	
Clinical Features	**Neuropathy**	**Myopathy**
Distribution of wasting and weakness	All are distal > proximal except SMA – proximal > distal	All are proximal > distal except myotonic muscular dystrophy – distal > proximal
DTR	Lost early	Preserved till late
Fasciculation	Characteristic	Absent
Sensory disturbance	Yes	No
Fatiguable weakness	Yes	No
Myotonia	Absent	Present
Myalgia	Yes	Yes

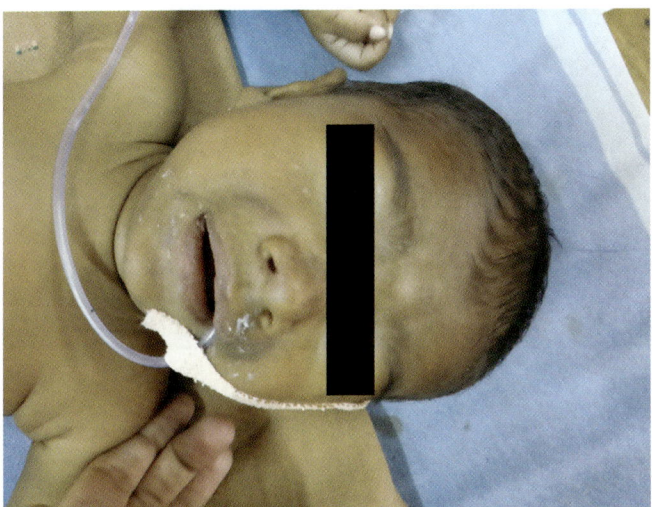

Fig. 5.13 Hyperalert look in a child with SMA.

45. What are the muscle biopsy findings in a child with myopathy?
    a. Nemaline rod myopathies: Rod-like inclusion bodies
    b. Myotubular myopathy: A row of central nuclei within the core of cytoplasm
    c. Congenital muscle fiber-type disproportion (CMFTD): Disproportion in size and relative ratios of histochemical fiber types

DISCUSSION ON SPINAL MUSCULAR ATROPHY

46. *What are the types of SMA?
    • Type 1 (acute infantile or Werdnig–Hoffmann)
      ○ Onset: Birth to 6 months
      ○ Extraocular muscle (EOM) not affected and facial movements not affected or minimal
      ○ Alert child and no cerebral involvement
    • Type 2 (chronic infantile – Dubowitz disease)
      ○ Onset: 6–18 months
      ○ Most common form presenting as motor delay
    • Type 3 (chronic juvenile, Kugelberg–Welander)
      ○ Onset: After 18 months
    • Type 4 (adult onset)
47. *Which neurons and muscles are spared in SMA?
    Cranial nerves III, IV, and VI and sacral spinal cord innervating the striated muscle of urethral and anal sphincters are spared; diaphragm is involved in the last.
48. What is the SMN1 gene?
    The SMN1 gene codes for the survival of motor neuron (SMN) protein. It also provides instructions for making the SMN protein. The SMN protein is found throughout the body, with high levels in the spinal cord.
49. Explain the pathophysiology behind SMA.
    The SMN1 gene arrests the apoptosis of motor neuroblasts. Spinal muscular atrophies occur when there is failure of stoppage of physiological apoptosis of

TABLE 5.13	Features of Various Disorders of the Motor System	
Causes	**Examples**	**Clinical Features**
Central causes	a. Chromosomal disorder (Down syndrome, Prader–Willi, Turner syndrome, Marfan syndrome) b. IEM (metabolic myopathy – Pompe disease), peroxisomal (Zellweger) c. Chronic nonprogressive disorder (cerebral dysgenesis, perinatal asphyxia)	No alertness, lethargy, poor feeding, central/axial hypotonia, neonatal seizures, hyperactive reflexes, mental retardation
Motor neuron	Spinal muscular atrophy	Generalized weakness that spares the diaphragm, facial muscle, pelvis, sphincters, fasciculation
Nerves	Peripheral neuropathy	Distal muscle group involved, weakness with wasting
Neuromuscular junction	Myasthenia syndromes, botulism	Bulbar (cranial nerve, facial nerve involvement), oculomotor muscles exhibit a greater degree of involvement
Muscle	Congenital myopathies Metabolic myopathies Congenital muscular dystrophy Congenital myotonic dystrophy	Weakness is prominent Proximal > distal Hypoactive reflexes Joint contractures

TABLE 5.14	**Various Causes of Central and Peripheral Motor Hypotonia**		

Floppiness Without Weakness (Floppy + Strong − Cerebral Hypotonia)	Floppiness With Weakness (Floppy + Weak − Motor Unit Disorders)	Combined Central and Motor Unit Hypotonia

A–I (mnemonic)
  A: Atonic CP (fisting of hands, movement through postural reflexes, scissoring on ventral suspension, normal or brisk reflexes)
  B: Birth trauma, benign congenital hypotonia
  C: Chromosomal disorder
  D: Down syndrome
  E: Endocrine (hypothyroid)
  F: Familial dysautonomia
  G: Genetic defect (Lowe, familial dysautonomia)
  H: Hypoglycemia
  I: IEM (organic acidemia, GSD, peroxisomal disorders, Pompe, infantile GM1 gangliosidosis)
Others
  Non-neurological – chronic illness (CHD, RTA, CRF, malnutrition deprivation, CF, celiac)
  Increased laxity – osteogenesis imperfecta, Ehlers–Danlos, and Marfan syndrome
	1. Anterior horn cells – SMA
	2. Peripheral nerves – HMS1 familial
	3. NM junction – infantile myasthenia, transitory myasthenia gravis, infantile botulism
	4. Muscles – congenital myopathies, congenital myotonic dystrophy
		Pompe disease, mitochondrial disorders Hypoxic ischemic encephalomyelopathy, perinatal hypoxia secondary to motor unit disorders

TABLE 5.15	**Stepwise Investigations in a Floppy Child**

Investigations	Findings
Step 1: CPK	The first step before electromyography (EMG) and muscle biopsy (CPK raised in dystrophies, normal or low in myopathies, neuropathies) False positive: CPK will increase after a muscle biopsy False negative: Low CPK seen when steroid is given
Step 2: EMG	Polyphasic; short-duration, low-amplitude motor unit action potential
Step 3: Nerve conduction study	To rule out whether neuropathy is suspected
Step 4: Molecular study – SMN gene	Confirmatory
Others: Muscle biopsy	Done, if SMN1 gene is negative
CT, MRI	HIE, cerebral malformation
Karyotype	Down syndrome
Fish methylation studies	Prader–Willi syndrome, very long chain fatty acid disorder (VLCFA), Zellweger syndrome

SMN, survival of motor neuron.

neuroblasts because of which the process of cell death continues to occur beyond the fetal period.

50. What is the molecular genetics involved in SMA?

About 95% of children with SMA carry mutations that delete a section called exon 7 in both the copies of SMN1 gene. Therefore, little or no SMN protein is made. In about 5% of people with SMA, one copy of the SMN1 gene has a deletion of exon 7 and the other copy has a different mutation that disrupts the production or function of the SMN protein. Around 65 mutations in the SMN1 gene cause SMA. SMN1 gene deletion or mutation in SMN1 exon 7 is homozygously absent in 94% of patients with clinically typical SMA.

51. What are the variants of SMA?

Table 5.16 gives the variants of SMA.

52. How is a child with SMA managed?

No medical treatment is able to delay the progression. Supportive care includes physiotherapy, vigorous treatment of respiratory infection, feeding (NGT or

TABLE 5.16	**SMA and Its Variants**

Variant	Major Features
SMA with respiratory distress type 1 (SMARD1)	Autosomal recessive Mild hypotonia + weak cry/progressive distal weakness + respiratory distress (diaphragmatic paralysis)
Pontocerebellar hypoplasia type 1	Likely autosomal recessive Arthrogryposis + bulbar deficit early + extraocular defects + cognitive deficit
X-linked infantile SMA with bone fractures	X-linked Lethal course Arthrogryposis + congenital bone fractures + respiratory failure
Congenital SMA with predominant lower limb involvement	Nonprogressive but have severe disability Arthrogryposis + hypotonia + weakness with distal lower limb weakness early

gastrostomy), keeping ideal weight, annual flu vaccine, pneumococcal vaccine, and Hib vaccine.

53. What are the newer drugs approved by FDA to treat a child with SMA?

Nusinersen (Spinraza) was approved by FDA in 2016 for SMA. Another drug is ataluren, which is an antisense oligonucleotide to treat the mutations in chromosome 5q.

54. What are the recent advances in SMA?

The FDA-approved gene therapy for children with SMA younger than 2 years is Zolgensma – adeno-associated virus. It is a vector-based gene therapy that delivers a fully functional copy of the human SMN1 gene into the target motor neuron cells.

DISCUSSION ON OTHER CAUSES OF MOTOR UNIT DISORDERS

55. What are the salient features of congenital myopathy?

These include early onset, nonprogressive, perinatal or neonatal presentation with significant family history, normal CPK, ECG, EMG, and NCS. Diagnosis is by muscle biopsy.

56. What is the course of congenital myopathies?

They are mostly hereditary and nonprogressive with a good outlook for a normal life span.

57. What are the types of congenital myopathies?

Four types (all have neonatal hypotonia + weakness):

1. Central core
2. Congenital muscle fiber-type disproportion – extraocular muscle (EOM) affected
3. Myotubular myopathy – EOM affected, ptosis, and facial involvement
4. Nemaline rod myopathy (most common variant) – typical facies (dolichocephalic head), high arched palate, and facial weakness

58. What is the pathophysiology in congenital myopathy?

A possible defect in genetic mutation in the muscle formation causing the maturational arrest of fetal muscle in the myotubular stage is the basic pathophysiology in congenital myopathy.

59. How is congenital myopathy confirmed?

Diagnosis is by muscle biopsy followed by electron microscopy findings which show disorganized triads and focal loss of myofilaments. Immunohistochemistry reveals desmin and vimentin positive.

60. What is hereditary motor sensory neuropathy (HMSN)?

It refers to a group of perinuclear neuropathies of hereditary origin. Clinical features include predominant motor involvement and enlarged thickened nerves with sensory and autonomic manifestations later.

61. What are the other names for HMSN?

Other names are Charcot–Marie–Tooth and peroneal muscular atrophy.

62. What are the clinical features of HMSN?

Age of presentation (adolescent or adult), progressive, foot drop (initial symptom), pes cavus, wasting of muscles of the leg, weak dorsiflexors (stork leg or inverted champagne bottle appearance), sensory involvement (pain, numbness), and trophic ulcers

63. What are the types of HMSN?

The following are the types of HMSN:

- HMSN I (Charcot–Marie–Tooth disease 1) – hypertrophic *demyelinating* neuropathies (the most common HSMN)
- Hereditary neuropathy with liability to pressure palsies (HNPP; tomaculous neuropathy) – severely hypertrophic *demyelinating* neuropathy
- HSMN II (Charcot–Marie–Tooth disease 2) – *axonal* neuropathies
- HSMN III (Dejerine–Sottas disease) – severe hypertrophic *demyelinating* neuropathies with onset in infancy
- HMSN Type 4 (infantile Refsum disease) – progressive motor and sensory involvement, ichthyosis, progressive hearing loss, and retinitis pigmentosa

64. Enumerate the salient features of other muscular disorders.

Table 5.17 gives the clinical features of other muscular disorders.

TABLE 5.17	Clinical Features of Other Muscular Disorders

Disease	Clinical Features
Metabolic myopathies	• Types: Primary or secondary. • Carnitine deficiency (lipid storage myopathy). • Mitochondrial disease. • Fatty acid oxidation disease.
Familial dysautonomia	• Floppy child with absent deep tendon jerk + temperature instability, absent tears, absence of fungiform papillae (most striking feature). • The absence of fungiform papillae in the tongue is a major diagnostic, almost pathognomonic feature for familial dysautonomia or type III of hereditary sensory and autonomic neuropathy.
Benign congenital hypotonia	• Not a disease, descriptive term for undiagnosed nonprogressive hypotonia, diagnosis of exclusion. • Normal or mild delay in motor development that improves later. Early hypotonia since birth, active movements of limbs, normal DTJ. • Good prognosis, improves well with physical therapy, no contractures. • Normal lab: Muscle enzymes, EMG, nerve conduction velocity (NCV), histology. Problems: recurrent shoulder dislocation, excessive spine mobility can lead to stretch injury, nerve compression.
Arthrogryposis multiplex congenita	• Not a disease, a descriptive term in which there are numerous congenital contractures.
Zellweger syndrome	• One of three peroxisome biogenesis disorders associated with impaired neuronal migration, brain maldevelopment, hypomyelination. • Progressive loss of hearing and vision. • Craniofacial abnormalities (such as a high forehead, hypoplastic supraorbital ridges, epicanthal folds, midface hypoplasia, and a large fontanel). • Eye abnormalities. • Hepatomegaly, renal cysts, chondrodysplasia punctata (punctate calcification of the cartilage in specific regions of the body). • Newborn may present with profound hypotonia (low muscle tone), seizures, apnea, and an inability to eat. • Patients with Zellweger syndrome show elevated very long chain fatty acids in their blood plasma.
Botulism	• <6 months with intake of canned food, honey. Other causes: Outdoor construction workers and family gardeners may bring the spores in the cloth contaminated by soil. • Clinical features: 5Ds Dysphagia Dysarthria Dysphonia Diplopia Dilated pupils • Recovery by 2–3 months.

Quick Bites

- Alert, floppy, and normal perinatal period – SMA
- Perinatal events, floppy, brisk reflexes, and higher functions affected – atonic CP
- Decreased fetal movements, SGA/IUGR, undescended testis, funnel/bell-shaped chest, generalized hypotonia, motor delay, and severe mental retardation – myopathy
- Syndromic facies with hypotonia – Down syndrome
- All myopathies are proximal weakness except myotonic dystrophy
- All neuropathies are distal weakness except spinal muscular atrophy
- Floppy child with absent DTJ, temperature instability, absence of fungiform papillae, and absent tears – familial dysautonomia
- Flat facies, flat occiput, high forehead, upward slanting of palpebral fissures, hypertelorism, epicanthal folds, and anteverted nares – Zellweger syndrome
- Hypotonia, obesity, almond-shaped eyes, thin upper lip, narrow bifrontal diameter of the skull, strabismus, hyperphagia, undescended testes, hypogonadism, small hands and feet, and mental retardation – Prader–Willi syndrome (PWS)
- Cataract, rickets, and hypotonia – Lowe syndrome
- Elongated face, large/protruding ears, flat feet, and large testis – fragile X syndrome

6

Neurodegenerative Disorders

Following introduction, seek permission from the caregiver and introduce yourself to the patient before history elicitation, and identify the case.

    Name____Age____Sex____Consanguinity____Order of birth____Place____Informant____

Presenting Complaints and Duration

- Loss of acquired developmental milestones
- Any history of seizures

History of Presenting Illness

- Mention that the child was apparently normal till ... age, and then mention whether there was any precipitating event – fever/vomiting/diarrhea/altered sensorium at the onset of symptoms.
- Describe the order of milestones lost by the child in the mother's words and explain what the child is able to do now.
- For example, a 10-month-old female child was apparently normal till 2 months back, when she developed a cough and coryza for 1 week, for which she was prescribed oral medications, not associated with fever or altered sensorium at that time following which the mother noticed that the child was not able to grasp objects in hand, which the child was able to do previously, and not able to reach for objects. Now for the past 2 months, there is a progressive loss of acquired milestones in the order of loss of social smile, not interested in the surroundings, and not able to sit with support, followed by not recognizing the mother. However, the child now has partial head control.

CENTRAL NERVOUS SYSTEM HISTORY

Higher Functions

- History of seizures/change in seizure type, deterioration of higher mental functions, change in personality, behavior or deterioration in school performance, and social withdrawal

Cranial Nerve

- Ability to perceive light/diminution of vision
- Ability to move eyeballs in all four directions/squint/abnormal eyeball movement
- Ability to chew food
- Facial asymmetry, ability to close both eyes while sleeping, drooling of saliva, and deviation of angle of the mouth
- Ability to hear and respond to sound/hyperacusis
- Nasal twang of voice and nasal regurgitation
- Ability to move the head side to side
- Any deviation of the tongue on protrusion/twitching

Motor System

a. Any thinness noted by the mother on extremities
b. Floppiness (slipping through hands)/stiffness noted by the mother in the form of difficulty in changing a diaper

c. Ability to move limbs above the cot or able to move only sideward or whether there are just some flickers of movements
d. Any abnormal posturing of the affected limb while walking
e. Any gait disturbance
f. Involuntary movement if present – which limb is involved, smooth, rapid, jerky, forceful movement, which disappears during sleep or not, clumsiness in activity
g. Increased startle response
h. Abnormal eyeball or head movement and imbalance while walking

Cerebellar Features

- Abnormal eyeball or head movement or tremors

Bladder/Bowel Disturbance

- History of urinary incontinence or dribbling and constipation

Sensory Features

- History of perception of pain or crying while giving vaccination

Autonomic Features

- Flushing, sweating, and palpitation episodes

Spine and Cranium

- Any abnormality in the head size noted by the mother compared with in sibling or peers
- Any swelling, tuft of hair, sinus, discharge, and abnormal curvature

COMPLICATIONS HISTORY

a. Headache, blurring of vision, and vomiting (signs of raised ICP)
b. Others: Failure to gain weight/feeding difficulties/aspiration/recurrent infections/contractures/sleep disturbances/bed sores

ETIOLOGICAL HISTORY

- Acute febrile event (fever with seizures/altered sensorium prior to the onset)
- Recent trauma
- Abnormal increase in head size
- Recurrent seizures
- Abnormal odor/skin/hair changes
- Exposure to toxins (lead)
- Abdominal distension/jaundice/failure to gain weight
- Frequent fall/bed sores
- Behavior/poor scholastic performance
- Abnormal hand writhing movement
- Abnormal head position (torticollis)/early morning headache

- Failure to gain weight//skin changes/edema/social withdrawal
- Tingling sensation/numbness/trophic ulcers in the foot

Past History

- Exanthematous fever, previous hospitalization (vomiting, failure to thrive – inborn error of metabolism), and acute CNS infection followed by neuroregression – post-meningitic sequelae)

Antenatal/Natal and Postnatal History

Antenatal/natal history
- Recurrent abortion
- Fever with rash with cervical swelling (TORCH infections)
- Increased fetal movements

Postnatal history
- Onset of symptoms in the newborn period, neonatal jaundice, and seizures in the newborn period

Development History

Mention about the milestones achieved by the child and loss of milestones in the order of disappearance (language, motor, hearing, and vision).

Describe how the onset was (gradual or acute, any precipitating event) and milestones at present.

Dietetic History

- Feeding difficulties

Immunization History

- Up to age according to Universal Immunization schedule or IAP

Contact History

- Any history of contact with TB

Family History

Sudden infant death syndrome, previous sibling with developmental delay with similar complaints, and previous sibling death

Treatment History

History of medication intake – any treatment advised (enzyme replacement, bone marrow transplantation)

Environmental History

Glass or paint industry near the house

Socioeconomic History

According to the modified Kuppuswamy scale

Case Summary

A ...-year-old child with progressive loss of acquired milestones with or without seizures, with or without cranial nerve involvement, with or without weakness/stiffness of all four limbs, with or without skin or hair involvement, and with or without family history; probably a neurodegenerative disorder with gray or white matter disease or both; would like to proceed further with examination

General Examination

Posture/sensorium/pallor/icterus/cyanosis/clubbing/pedal edema/generalized lymphadenopathy

Head-to-Foot Examination

- Head: Appears small/big in size
- Facial dysmorphism
- Hair: Hypopigmented
- Skin: Mongolian spots (persistent or large Mongolian spots), hyperpigmentation, and angiokeratomas
- Eye: Cloudy cornea, cataract, retinitis pigmentosa, cherry red spots, optic atrophy, nystagmus, telangiectasia, and macular degeneration
- Ear: Hearing loss
- Exaggerated startle response
- Hernia (inguinal/umbilical hernia)
- Joint stiffness/dysostosis

Vital Signs

Check for temperature, pulse rate, respiratory rate, blood pressure, and SpO$_2$.

Anthropometry

- Height: Short stature
- Weight: Failure to gain weight
- Head circumference: Microcephaly/macrocephaly
- Weight/height for a child younger than 5 years or BMI if the child is older than >5 years

Examination of Central Nervous System

HIGHER FUNCTIONS

- Seizures/change in seizure type; deterioration of higher mental functions; mental retardation; change in personality, behavior, or school performance – regression in language skills; and social withdrawal

CRANIAL NERVE

- Poor visual acuity, cloudy cornea, cataract, fundus – retinitis pigmentosa, cherry red spots, optic atrophy, nystagmus, telangiectasia, and macular degeneration
- Squint and nystagmus
- Ability to chew food
- Facial asymmetry, loss of nasolabial fold, and deviation of angle of the mouth
- Hearing loss and hyperacusis

- Palatal movement normal, uvula in the midline, and any pooling of secretions present
- Palatal arches normal, and palatal and pharyngeal reflex normal
- Ability to lift the head from supine position and whether turns the head on both sides
- Fibrillation or wasting, myotonia, and tongue fasciculations

MOTOR SYSTEM

- Bulk: Thinness/wasting of limbs
- Tone: Stiffness/flaccidity
- Power: On both sides
- Reflexes: Deep tendon reflex exaggerated in white matter disease
- Plantar extensor in white matter disease
- Others: Increased startle response/persistent primitive reflex
- Involuntary movement: Clumsiness of activity (chorea) and hand writing movement (Rett syndrome)
- Gait: Imbalance and abnormal posture while walking

CEREBELLAR SYMPTOMS

- Head nodding, nystagmus, gait abnormality, ataxia or imbalance, past pointing, and dysdiadochokinesia

AUTONOMIC SYSTEM

- Excessive sweating, tachycardia, and hypotension

SENSORY SYSTEM

- Peripheral neuropathy – tingling/numbness/ulcers over the foot

SPINE AND CRANIUM

- Abnormal increase in the head size

SIGNS OF MENINGEAL IRRITATION

Present or not (Kernig/Brudzinski reflex)

Other Systems

CARDIOVASCULAR SYSTEM

- Pansystolic murmur and features of congestive heart failure

ABDOMEN

- Hepatosplenomegaly

RESPIRATORY SYSTEM

- Effortless tachypnea

Diagnosis

A child with loss of acquired milestones, with or without seizures, with or without cranial nerve involvement – hearing or visual disturbance, spasticity or flaccidity, with or without complications, and predominantly gray or white matter or both – probable etiology being a neurodegenerative disorder, nutritional status, and other comorbid conditions (anemia, vitamin deficiency if any)

Frequently Asked Questions

1. What is the salient history that should be elicited in neurodegenerative disorders (NDD)?
   a. Age of onset of illness/till what age the child was normal
   b. Type of onset – rapid or gradual
   c. Course of illness – progressive/nonprogressive or static
   d. Any precipitating factors – fever with seizures, toxin (exposure), vomiting, or diarrhea
   e. Previously how the child was and the current condition of the child – photograph or videography of the child at earlier ages

2. What is the significance of etiological history in neurodegenerative disorders?
   (Remember as A–G.)
   A: Abdominal distension and jaundice (metabolic cause presenting with organomegaly, hypothyroidism)
   B: Behavioral problems – inconsolable cry and bony deformity (Farber disease)
   C: Coarse facies – thick lips and tongue (mucopolysaccharides)
   D: Posture (exception P for D) (opisthotonus – Gaucher, Niemann–Pick, Krabbe)
   E: Early morning lethargy (glycogen storage disorder)
   F: Fever (hyperpyrexia)
   G: Growth retardation/failure to thrive (IEM)
   Others
   a. Skin
      Dry skin/abnormal skin swelling: Fabry disease
      Eczema: Biotinidase deficiency
   b. Pica: Lead poisoning
   c. Head size: Increasing – hydrocephalus
   d. Smell of urine: IEM
   e. Hair changes: Hypopigmented lesion – phenylketonuria, Menkes kinky hair, and tyrosinemia
   f. Acute febrile event (fever with seizures)/altered sensorium prior to the onset: Post-meningitic sequelae
   g. Trauma prior to the onset – post-traumatic sequelae
   h. Recurrent seizures – epileptic encephalopathies
   i. Exposure to toxin (heavy metals such as mercury) – encephalopathy
   j. Frequent falls/bed sores – peripheral neuropathy
   k. Behavior/poor scholastic performance – Wilson disease and adrenoleukodystrophy
   l. Abnormal hand writhing movement – Rett syndrome
   m. Abnormal head position (torticollis)/early morning headache – CNS tumor/mass
   n. Failure to gain weight//skin changes/edema/social withdrawal – severe acute malnutrition

3. What is the significance of antenatal/neonatal history in a neurodegenerative child?
   a) Recurrent abortion – TORCH infections, HIV, and syphilis
   b) Increased fetal movements – glycine encephalopathy (nonketotic hyperglycinemia) and Krabbe disease
   c) Onset of symptoms in the newborn period – galactosemia, phenylketonuria, maple syrup urine disease, urea cycle disorders, nonketotic hyperglycinemia, and Alexander disease

4. What is the significance of age of onset of neurodegenerative disorders?
   The age of onset of neurodegenerative disorders is given in Table 6.1.

5. *What are the clues in the examination in a neurodegenerative child?
   Table 6.2 gives the clinical clues in examination in a neurodegenerative child.

6. What are the specific skin findings seen in neurodegenerative disorders?
   a. Seborrheic dermatitis and eczema – biotinidase deficiency (seborrheic dermatitis shown in Fig. 6.8 and eczema is shown in Fig. 6.9)
   b. Hyperpigmentation – adrenoleukodystrophy
   c. Hair changes – Menkes kinky hair and biotinidase
   d. Photosensitivity – Cockayne syndrome
   e. Fair and blonde – PKU as shown in Fig. 6.10
   f. Ichthyosis – Sjögren–Larsson syndrome, Refsum disease as shown in Fig. 6.11, Zellweger disease, and biotinidase disease
   g. Peau d'orange skin – carbohydrate deficiency
   h. Pellagra – Hartnup disease

7. *Define neuroregression.
   Neuroregression is defined as follows: "a previously healthy child begins to deteriorate, losing already attained skills with progressive loss of speech, hearing, vision, and muscle strength for more than 3 months."

TABLE 6.1	Age of Onset of Neurodegenerative Disorders
Age of Onset	**Neurodegenerative Disorders**
Neonatal (<1 month)	• Generalized GM1 gangliosidosis • GSD type I • Neonatal adrenoleukodystrophy • Mucolipidosis type II • Alexander disease
Early infantile (1–12 months)	1–3 months • Infantile neuronal ceroid lipofuscinosis (NCL) • GSD type II (Pompe) 3–6 months • Gaucher • Niemann–Pick • Krabbe • Canavan disease 3–12 months • Lesch–Nyhan syndrome • Pelizaeus–Merzbacher disease
Late infantile (1–4 years)	• Hurler • Metachromatic leukodystrophy • Neuroaxonal dystrophy • Leigh disease • Others: GM2 gangliosidosis, Niemann–Pick type C
Late childhood (5–15 years)	4–8 years • Juvenile form of NCL • Sanfilippo 5–10 years • Adrenoleukodystrophy • Hunter

TABLE 6.2	Clinical Clues in Examination
Clinical Features	**Disease**
Macrocephaly	CATS (pneumonic) – Canavan disease, Alexander disease, Tay–Sachs disease, Sandhoff disease as shown in Fig. 6.1, glutaric aciduria type 1
Microcephaly	Krabbe disease, neuronal ceroid lipofuscinosis, phenylketonuria, metachromatic leukodystrophy, Rett syndrome, HIV disease
Facial dysmorphism	Inclusion cell disease, GM1 gangliosidosis, Menkes disease, mucopolysaccharides, Zellweger disease as shown in Fig. 6.2
Hair changes	Menkes disease, mucopolysaccharides, biotinidase deficiency (shown in Fig. 6.3), Cockayne disease
Skin changes	a) Large/persistent Mongolian spots – Hunter disease, Hurler disease, GM1 gangliosidosis (shown in Fig. 6.4), mannosidosis, Niemann–Pick diseases b) Hyperpigmentation (ALD) (shown in Fig. 6.5) c) Angiokeratosis – Fabry disease shown in Fig. 6.6, mucolipidosis, fucosidosis
Eye changes	a) Corneal opacity – Lowe syndrome, GM1 gangliosidosis, and mucopolysaccharidoses b) Cataract – Fabry disease, galactosemia, homocystinuria, Lowe syndrome, Myotonic dystrophy, Lowe syndrome, Zellweger disease, galactosemia c) Keyer – Fleischer (KF) ring – Wilson Disease as shown in Fig. 6.7 d) Retinitis pigmentosa – abetalipoproteinemia, Mucopolysaccharidoses (MPS), Refsum disease, Zellweger syndrome, Neuronal Ceroid Lipofuscinosis (NCL), Cockayne syndrome, Hallervorden–Spatz disease, Kearns–Sayre syndrome e) Cherry red spots: GM1 gangliosidosis, Niemann–Pick disease types A and B, Tay–Sachs disease, sialidosis, Wolman disease, Krabbe disease, metachromatic leukodystrophy f) Optic atrophy – Canavan disease, globoid cell leukodystrophy, metachromatic leukodystrophy Pelizaeus–Merzbacher disease, GM2 gangliosidosis – juvenile type g) Nystagmus: Ataxia telangiectasia, Gaucher disease types 2 and 3, Kearns–Sayre syndrome, Niemann–Pick disease type C, Pelizaeus–Merzbacher disease h) Macular degeneration – neuronal ceroid lipofuscinosis i) Retinal degeneration – NCL
Exaggerated startle response	Tay–Sachs disease, Krabbe disease
Deafness	MPS, ALD, mitochondrial disorders, peroxisomal disorders
Hyperacusis	Krabbe disease, TAy-sachs disease
Hepatosplenomegaly	MPS, GM1 gangliosidosis, Gaucher disease, Niemann pick disease
Hernia	MPS, GM1 gangliosidosis
Peripheral neuropathy	Metachromatic leukodystrophy (MLD), Krabbe disease, mitochondrial disorders
Hydrocephalus/raised intra-cranial pressure	MPS, Alexander disease
Cardiac	Cardiomyopathy, valvular disease (MPS)
Joint stiffness/dysostosis	Joint stiffness/dysostosis (MPS)
Short stature	Lesch–Nyhan syndrome

NCL, neuronal ceroid lipofuscinosis.

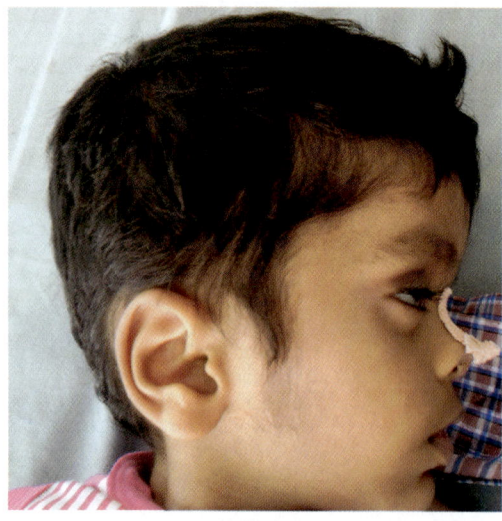

Fig. 6.1 Macrocephaly – Sandhoff disease.

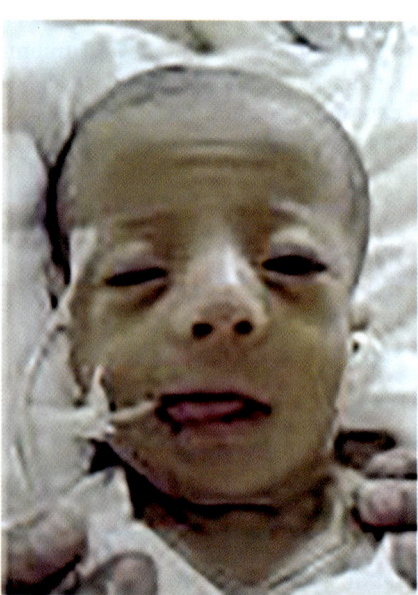

Fig. 6.2 Facial dysmorphism: Zellweger disease – high forehead, shallow supraorbital ridges, anteverted nares, and mild micrognathia. *(Source: Nelson, 21st edition, p. 746, Fig. 104.3.)*

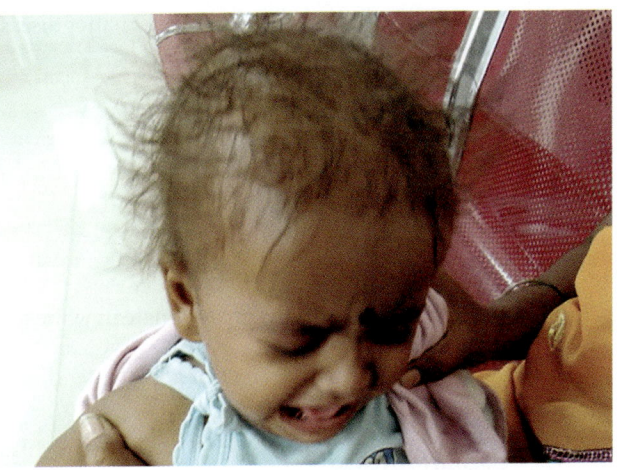

Fig. 6.3 Alopecia – biotinidase deficiency.

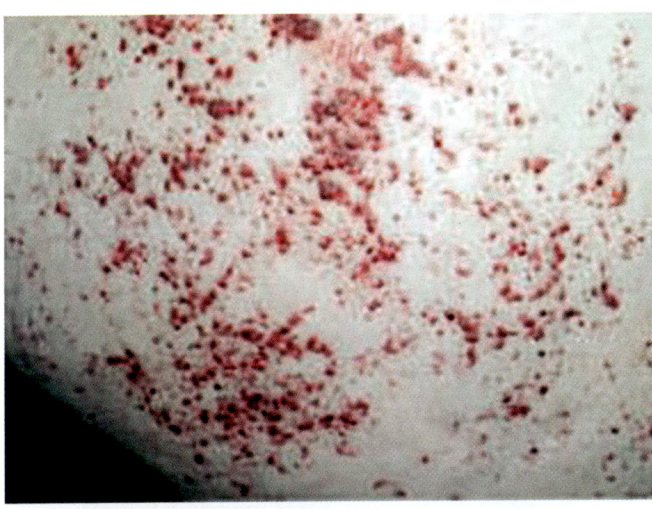

Fig. 6.6 Angiokeratomas – Fabry disease. Mostly seen in "bathing trunk area" – in between umbilicus and knee – large, dark red, and nonblanchable. *(Source: Nelson, 21st edition, p. 774, Fig. 104.19.)*

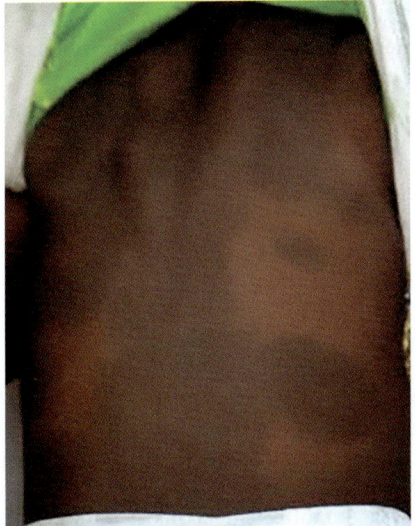

Fig. 6.4 Large Mongolian spots – GM1 gangliosidosis.

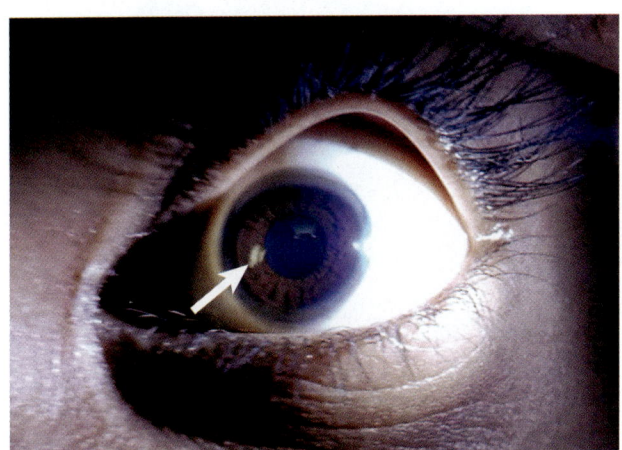

Fig. 6.7 KF ring – Wilson disease.

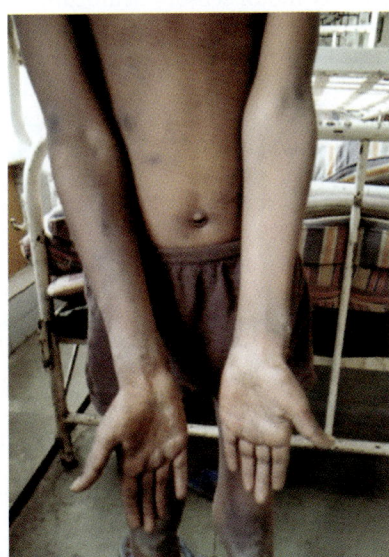

Fig. 6.5 Hyperpigmentation – adrenoleukodystrophy.

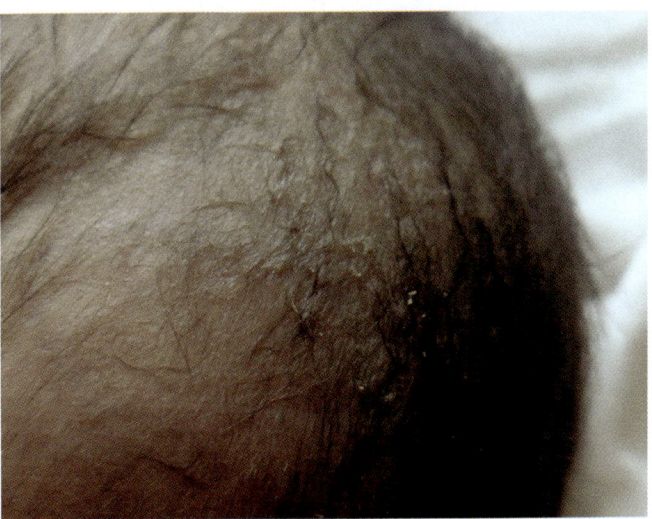

Fig. 6.8 Seborrheic dermatitis.

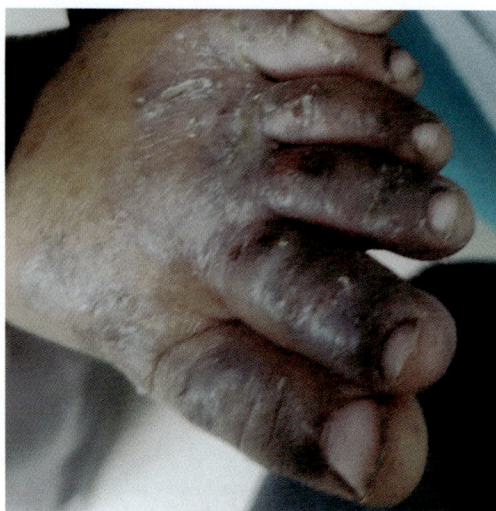

Fig. 6.9 Eczema.

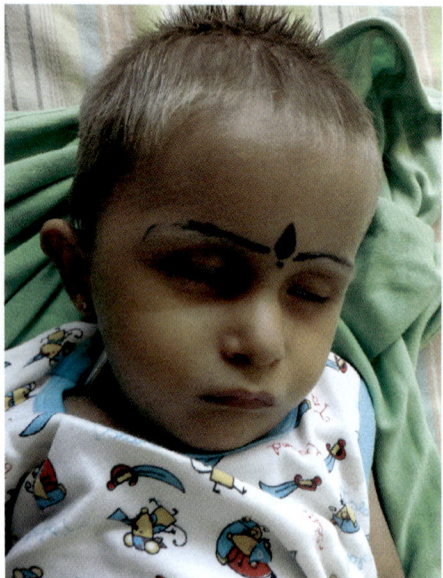

Fig. 6.10 PKU – fair and blonde.

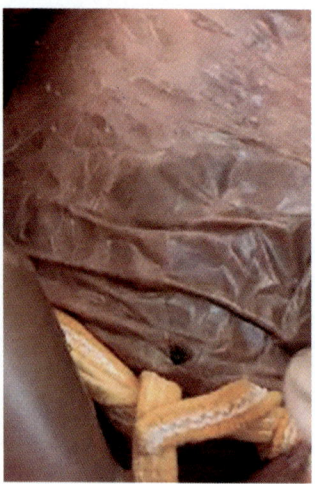

Fig. 6.11 Ichthyosis.

8. What are the early and late signs of white matter disease?
   - Early signs
     - Spasticity/Babinski
     - Peripheral neuropathy
     - Vision decline
     - Optic nerve atrophy
     - Ataxia
   - Late signs
     - Cognitive decline
     - Seizures
   - Upper motor neuron signs predominate in white matter disease.

9. *What are the early and late signs of gray matter disease?
   - Early signs
     - Behavior change
     - Cognitive decline
     - Seizures
     - Vision decline
     - Retinal degeneration
   - Late signs
     - Spasticity/Babinski

10. Enumerate the neurological features associated with neurodegeneration.
    - Developmental arrest – regression
    - Seizures (infantile spasms, myoclonus)
    - Gradual development of spasticity
    - Dementia
    - Visual and/or auditory deterioration
    - Extrapyramidal signs
    - Cerebellar signs
    - Macrocephaly/microcephaly
    - Speech problems
    - Psychiatric problems

11. *Name some neurodegenerative diseases (NDD) that present with acute encephalopathy.
    MSUD, organic acidemia, urea cycle disorder, and non-ketotic hyperglycinemia

12. What are the differentials of self-mutilation?
    a. Lesch–Nyhan syndrome
    b. Tyrosinemia
    c. Riley–Day syndrome
    d. Hereditary motor sensory neuropathy

13. What are the other specific features seen in NDD?
    a. Autistic behavior – Phenylketonuria (PKU)
    b. Pseudobulbar features – Gaucher disease, GM 1 gangliosidosis
    c. Extrapyramidal features
    d. Ataxia – Leigh disease
    e. Movement disorder – Huntington disease, Wilson disease, glutaric acidemia, Mitochondrial encephalopathy lactic acidosis, and Stroke-like episodes syndrome, Lesch–Nyhan, and Hallervorden–Spatz
    f. Hyporeflexia + extensor plantar – Krabbe disease and Metachromatic leukodystrophy (MLD)
    g. Pendular nystagmus – Pelizaeus-Merzbacher disease (PZD) and Leigh disease
    h. Rigidity/opisthotonus/tonic spasm – Krabbe disease and Gaucher disease
    i. Intermittent hyperventilation – Leigh disease and congenital lactic acidosis
    j. Pancytopenia – organic acidemia, isovaleric acidemia, propionic acidemia, Gaucher disease, and methylmalonic acidemia

k. Renal – Lowe disease, wilson disease, Von gierke disease, fabry disease

l. Pulmonary involvement – Niemann pick disease type B and lysinuric protein intolerance

14. What are the other systemic clues in neurodegenerative disorders?

Systemic findings
- Failure to thrive
- Alopecia
- Abnormal hair
- Hepatomegaly/hepatosplenomegaly
- Cardiomyopathy
- Skin changes
- Bone marrow depression

15. What are IEM presenting as neurodegeneration in school-going children?
   a. Wilson disease
   b. SSPE
   c. X-linked adrenoleukodystrophy
   d. Batten disease – neuronal ceroid lipofuscinosis (NCL)
   e. Niemann pick disease type C

16. What are the causes of intractable seizures of a newborn?
   a. Pyridoxine deficiency
   b. Nonketotic hyperglycinemia
   c. Biotinidase deficiency
   d. GLUT1 transporter deficiency
   e. Sulfite oxidase deficiency
   f. Molybdenum cofactor deficiency

17. What is the importance of other system examination in neurodegenerative disorders?
   a. Cardiovascular system: Pansystolic murmur (because of mitral regurgitation), cardiomyopathy and congestive heart failure (seen in mitochondrial disease), and mucopolysaccharidoses
   b. Abdomen: Hepatosplenomegaly – Mucopolysaccharidoses
   c. Respiratory system: Effortless tachypnea – an inborn error of metabolism

18. What are the possible differentials in a child with a neurodegenerative disorder?
   a) Post-meningitic sequelae
   b) Hydrocephalus
   c) Neurodegeneration
   d) Psychiatric illness – Attention Deficit Hyperactive Disorder and autism
   e) Space-occupying lesion – tumor and abscess
   f) Chronic CNS infection – HIV, slow viral disease, prion disease, and SSPE
   g) Epileptic encephalopathy
   h) Acquired – hypothyroidism

19. *What is the stepwise approach in neurodegenerative disorders?

Step 1: Symptoms suggestive of the neurodegenerative disorder
Step 2: Gray matter or white matter involvement
Step 3: Ruling out other remediable causes (hydrocephalus, hypothyroidism)
Step 4: Clues in MRI brain

20. What are the conditions that mimic a neurodegenerative disorder?

Hydrocephalus, hypothyroidism, epileptic encephalopathy, lead encephalopathy depression, and repeated trauma

TABLE 6.3	Clues in MRI	
Areas Involved (Hyperintensity in MRI)[a]	**Disease**
Anterior part	Alexander disease
Posterior part	Adrenoleukodystrophy
Anterior + posterior + subcortical U fibers involved	Krabbe disease, canavan disease
Anterior + posterior with sparing of subcortical U fibers	Metachromatic leukodystrophy, Pelizaeus–Merzbacher disease (PMZ)
Garland appearance	Adrenoleukodystrophy
Tigroid appearance	PMZ
Tiger eye appearance	Hallervorden–Spatz disease
Giant panda sign	Wilson disease
Double panda sign	Leigh disease, Wilson disease

[a]MRI pictures of neurodegenerative disorder are given in Chapter 55.

TABLE 6.4	Clinical Differences Between Gray and White Matter Diseases	
Gray Matter	**White Matter**
M: Mental decline	S: Spasticity
M: Macular degeneration	O: Optic atrophy
C: Convulsions	A: Ataxia
	P: Peripheral neuropathy
Examples	
GM1, GM2, MPS	MLD, ALD, PMZ
Lowe syndrome, Zellweger syndrome	Canavan disease, Alexander disease, Krabbe disease
Sialidosis, mucosidosis, fucosidosis	
Niemann–Pick disease	
Gaucher disease	

21. *What are the clues in MRI in a neurodegenerative disorder?

Table 6.3 gives the clues in MRI in a neurodegenerative disorder.

22. What is the hallmark of neurodegenerative disorders?

Regression with progression

23. What are the nonmetabolic/noninherited causes of developmental regression?
   a) Hydrocephalus
   b) Post-traumatic/post-meningoencephalitic sequelae
   c) Epileptic encephalopathies
   d) Subacute sclerosing panencephalitis (SSPE)
   e) Slow virus disease

24. *What are the clinical clues to differentiate gray and white matter diseases?

The clinical differences between gray and white matter diseases are given in Table 6.4.

25. What are the differentiating points between gray and white matter diseases?

Table 6.5 gives the overall differences between gray and white matter diseases.

26. Which neurodegenerative disorder presents with heart disease?

Valvular heart disease – MPS 1, 2, 4, and 6; Fabry disease (valvular incompetence); cardiomyopathy/CCF – Friedreich

TABLE 6.5	Overall Differences Between Gray and White Matter Diseases	

Gray Matter Lesions	White Matter Lesions
1. Age *Younger than 1 year to infancy:* Fructose intolerance, galactosemia, glycogen storage disorder, Gaucher disease, Niemann pick disease type A, GM1 and GM2 gangliosidosis, Zellweger disease, phenylketonuria, Maple syrup urine disease (MSUD), biotinidase deficiency, Menkes disease *1–5 years:* Rett syndrome, neuronal ceroid lipofuscinosis, MPS types 1 and 2, mitochondrial encephalopathies *Older than 5 years:* Ataxia telangiectasia, Huntington's chorea	*Younger than 1 year to infancy:* Alexander disease, Krabbe disease, PMD *1–5 years:* Metachromatic leukodystrophy *Older than 5 years:* Adrenoleukodystrophy, multiple sclerosis, Schilder disease
2. Gender Females: Rett syndrome Males-X-linked recessive disease – Hunter disease, Fabry disease	Males: Menkes kinky hair, ALD, PMD
3. Initial presentation Seizures; regression of social, language, and cognitive functions	Long tract signs – motor regression, rigidity, visual and hearing loss, feeding difficulty
4. Macrocephaly MPS, GM2 gangliosidosis	MLD, Alexander disease, canavan disease (also remember MAC for macrocephaly)
5. Microcephaly NCL, Rett syndrome	Krabbe disease, PMD Normal head size – ALD, MLD
6. Peripheral neuropathy Farber disease, Niemann pick disease type C	Krabbe disease, MLD
7. MRI Gray matter disease – cerebral atrophy Tiger eye appearance in Hallervorden–Spatz disease	*Areas Involved (Hyperintensity in T2W)* / *Disease* Anterior part / Alexander Posterior part / Adrenoleukodystrophy Anterior + posterior + subcortical U fibers involved / Krabbe disease, Canavan disease Anterior + posterior with sparing of subcortical U fibers / Metachromatic leukodystrophy, Pelizaeus–Merzbacher disease

NCL, neuronal ceroid lipofuscinosis.

ataxia; mitochondrial disease; and heart block – Kearns–Sayre syndrome

27. *What is cherry red spot?

It is a dull red spot in the center of the macula (fovea) surrounded by a grayish white halo. The grayish white halo is because of accumulation of lipids in the ganglion cell layer. Because the fovea does not have ganglionic cell, it transmits the underlying choroid vessels – bright red color – and hence the central part looks red and is called the cherry red spot. This is shown in Fig. 6.12A and B.

28. What are the causes of cherry red spot?

Tay–Sachs disease, Sandhoff disease, GM1, Niemann–Pick, Farber, and sialidosis

Note: Not seen in Fabry disease and Gaucher disease

29. *What are the nonmetabolic causes of cherry red spot?

Retinal artery ischemia and ocular contusion

30. What are the causes of angiokeratomas?

Fabry disease and GM1 gangliosidosis, galactosialidosis, fucosidosis, and mannosidosis

31. Give examples of neurodegenerative disorders that present with myoclonic seizures.

Neuronal ceroid lipofuscinosis, sialidosis, Schindler disease, GM1 gangliosidosis, Gaucher types 2 and 3, and fucosidosis

32. What are the neurodegenerative disorders that present with hydrops fetalis?

Gaucher, Niemann–Pick, GM1 gangliosidosis, Wolman, and sialidosis

33. Give examples of gray matter diseases with organomegaly.

GM1, Gaucher, Niemann–Pick disease, Farber, sialidosis, and fucosidosis

34. Give examples of gray matter diseases without organomegaly.

GM2, NCL, Menkes kinky hair disease, and Rett syndrome and Alpers syndrome

35. Give examples of neurodegenerative diseases (NDD) with dysmorphic facies.

Zellweger disease, GM1 gangliosidosis, MPS, and Lowe syndrome

36. Give examples of NDD with corneal opacity.

Lowe syndrome, GM1, and MPS – except Hunter

37. Give examples of NDD with deafness.

Friedreich ataxia, Refsum disease, and mitochondrial disease

38. Give examples of NDD with bone marrow findings.

Gaucher disease – Gaucher cell/ghost cell/wrinkled paper appearance as shown in Fig. 6.13A

Niemann–Pick disease – sea-blue histiocyte/vacuolated histiocyte as shown in Fig. 6.13B

GM1 gangliosidoses – Farber disease (foamy histiocyte)

39. Enumerate the specific enzymes deficient in each neurodegenerative disease.

Table 6.6 gives the diseases and their specific enzyme deficiency.

40. How is a child with a neurodegenerative disorder investigated?

a. Blood
   • Complete blood count
   • Blood glucose and ketone bodies
   • Serum electrolytes
   • Serum calcium
   • Anion gap
   • Aminotransferases

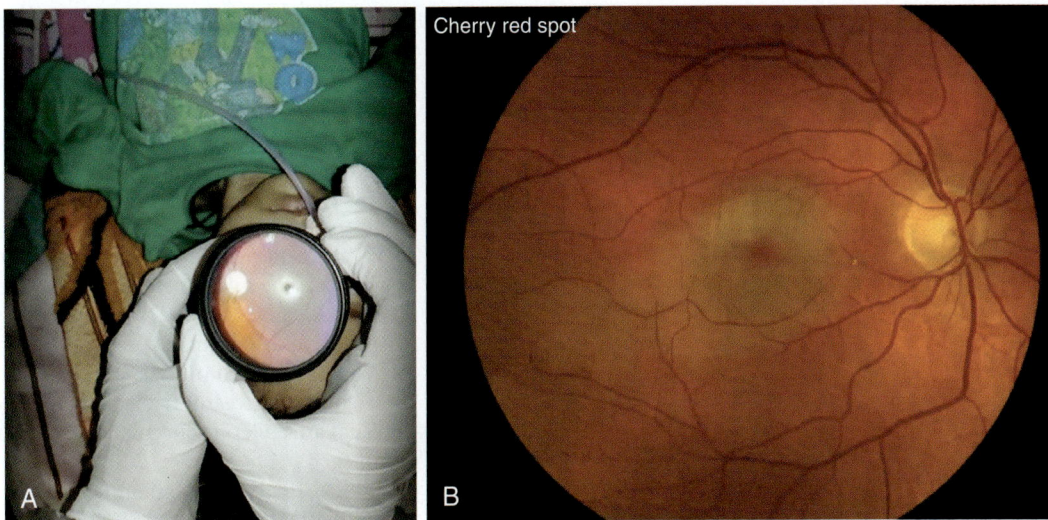

Fig. 6.12 (A) Fundoscopic examination using direct ophthalmoscope. (B) Cherry red spot.

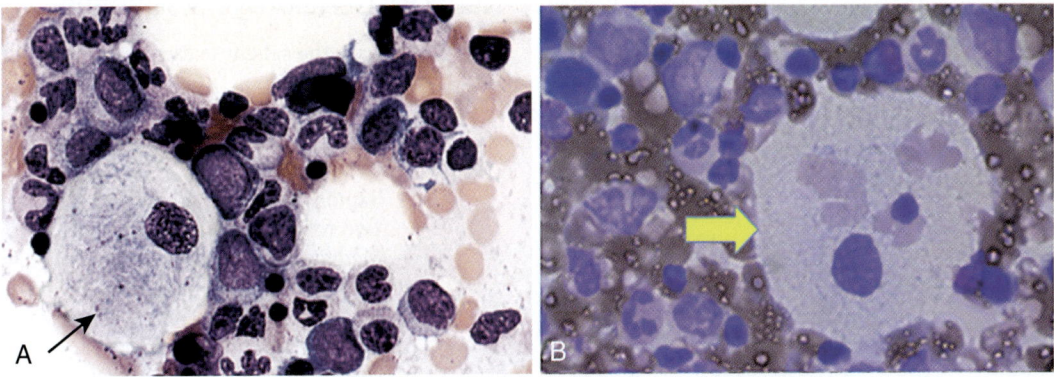

Fig. 6.13 Gaucher cell. (A) Arrow head shows crumpled tissue paper appearance. (B) Arrow head shows sea-blue histiocytes – finely vacuolated cytoplasm. *(Source: (A) Reproduced from Theodore O'Connell, Ryan Pedigo. USMLE Step 1 Secrets in Color, Fifth Edition, Genetic and metabolic disease, Figure 11.7, New Delhi, Elsevier Inc., 2023. (Credit line - From Goljan E. Rapid Review Pathology. 4th ed. Philadelphia: Elsevier; 2013, Fig. 14-15A.). (B) (Source: Reproduced from Magdalena Cerón-Rodríguez, Edgar Ricardo Vázquez-Martínez, Constanza García-Delgado et al and Niemann-Pick disease A or B in four pediatric patients and SMPD1 mutation carrier frequency in the Mexican population, Annals of Hepatology, 18: 613–619.)*

- Lactic acid and pyruvic acid (mitochondrial disease, Alper syndrome)
- Ammonia (ornithine transcarbamylase [OTC] deficiency)
- b. Urinalysis: Color, odor, ketones, pH, and metabolites
- c. Neuroimaging
- d. Chromosomal analysis – chromosomes 1 and 16 – neuronal ceroid lipofuscinosis; chromosomes 6 – Lafora disease (progressive myoclonus epilepsy)
- e. Electrophysiological studies – electroencephalogram (EEG), electroretinogram (ERG), and visual evoked potential (VEP)

41. Enumerate the findings in EEG and other electrophysiological studies suggestive of NDD.
   - Findings in electroencephalogram (EEG) suggestive of NDD
     - Diffuse cortical and subcortical gray matter involvement – bilateral synchronous paroxysmal discharges
     - White matter disease – continuous nonparoxysmal slow-wave activity
     - Both gray and white matter diseases – bilateral synchronous paroxysmal discharges with a marked increase in slow-wave activity
     - Infantile NCL – slow reduction in amplitude after infancy with high-voltage complexes induced posteriorly with photic stimulation
     - Infantile neuroaxonal dystrophy – diffuse fast (beta-wave) of moderate amplitude after 2 years of age
     - Alper disease (progressive neuronal degeneration) – multiple spikes superimposed on lateralized slow waves (predict liver involvement)
   - Electroretinogram (ERG): Low or extinguished ERGs in peroxisomal disorder
   - Visual evoked potential (VEP): Can see abnormality in the anterior visual pathway, optic nerve, and chiasma
     Points to remember:
     - Abnormal VEP and absent ERG seen in GM2 gangliosidosis
     - Normal VEP and abnormal ERG in retinitis pigmentosa
   - Other investigations performed in NDD
     - Brainstem auditory evoked potential
     - Somatosensory evoked potential
     - Nerve conduction velocity
     - Electromyogram
     - Enzyme activity/assay

TABLE 6.6	**Defective Enzymes and Diseases**
Disease	**Defective Enzyme**
Pompe disease	Alpha-glucosidase
Gaucher disease	Beta-glucosidase
Fabry disease	Alpha-galactosidase
GM1 gangliosidosis	Beta-galactosidase
Sialidosis	Sialidase
NCL	Infantile: infantile- palmitoyl-protein thioesterase enzyme (CLN1 disease) late infantile- TTP1-tripeptidyl peptidase1 (CLN2 disease)
Niemann pick disease	Sphingomyelinase
GM2 gangliosidosis	Hexosaminidase A – Tay-sach disease Hexosaminidase A and B – Sandhoff disease
Farber disease	Ceramidase
Wolman disease	Acid lipase
Menkes disease	Copper-transporting P-type ATPase
Krabbe disease	Galactocerebroside beta-galactosidase
MLD	Aryl sulfatase
ALD	Mutation in the glial fibrillary acid protein gene
Canavan disease	Aspartoacylase
Adrenoleukodystrophy	Mutation in the ABCD gene needed for peroxisomal transport of VLCFA
PMD	Mutation in lipid protein needed for myelin formation

NCL, neuronal ceroid lipofuscinosis.

TABLE 6.7	**Clues in Urine Odor**
Inborn Error of Metabolism	**Urine Odor**
Glutaric acidemia type 2	Sweaty feet odor
Hawkinsinuria	Swimming pool odor
Isovaleric acidemia	Sweaty feet
Maple syrup urine disease	Maple syrup
Hypermethioninemia	Boiled cabbage
Multiple carboxylase deficiency	Tomcat urine
Phenylketonuria	Mousy or musty odor
Trimethylaminuria	Rotting fish
Tyrosinemia	Boiled cabbage, rancid butter

42. Give some examples of diseases with late onset of diminished vision.

    Late onset of low vision seen in NCL, mitochondrial disease, Hunter, Refsum disease, and MPS IV

43. What are the clues in urine odor in neurodegenerative diseases?

    Table 6.7 gives the clues in urine odor.

44. What is urine metabolic screening?

    Table 6.8 gives the details of urine metabolic screening.

45. What are the clues in urine analysis in a neurodegenerative disorder?
    a. Urine metabolic screening: Positive in Hurler phenotype
    b. Urine reducing substance: Positive in galactosemia
    c. Urine metachromatic granules: Positive in MLD and negative in Krabbe disease
    d. Urine N-acetylaspartate: Positive in Canavan disease and negative in Alexander

46. What are the neurodegenerative disorders that can be treated with enzyme supplementation/other specific therapy?
    Table 6.9 gives the specific management of neurodegenerative disorders.

47. What is Lorenzo oil?
    4:1 ratio of glycerol trioleate and glycerol triuricate

48. What are epileptic encephalopathies? Mention few points on each.
    Table 6.10 gives the salient features of epileptic encephalopathy.

DISCUSSION ON SOME OF THE NEURODEGENERATIVE DISORDERS

49. What are the salient features of Krabbe disease?
    Krabbe disease
    - Also called globoid cell leukodystrophy
    - Cause: Galactosylceramide beta-galactosidase enzyme deficiency
    - Rapidly progressing demyelinating disorder of infancy
    - Two forms – juvenile and adult forms
    - Median age of onset: 4 months (1–7 months)
    - Starts with irritability and hyper-reactive to stimuli – exaggerated startle reflex as shown in Fig. 6.14 and progresses to hypertonia
    - Unexplained low-grade fever
    - Psychomotor arrest and regression
    - In 2–4 months, opisthotonus and loss of all milestones
    - Tendon reflexes depressed and later disappear
    - Startle myoclonus seen and later seizures developed
    - Blindness before 1 year of age
    - Several forms: Globoid dystrophy, infantile spasm syndrome, and focal neurological deficit
    MRI
    - Diffuse demyelination of cerebral hemispheres
    - Motor nerve conduction velocity – prolonged
    - Absent enzyme activity in lymphocytes and cultured fibroblasts – establishes the diagnosis
    Treatment
    - Hematopoietic stem cell transplantation

TABLE 6.8	**Urine Metabolic Screening**				
Test	**Reagent**	**Urine**	**Color Change**	**Disease**
Benedict's	Benedict's reagent (2 mL)	0.2 mL	Green	Galactosemia
Ferric chloride	2 drops	1 mL	Apple green – greenish brown	PKU Histidinemia
Cetrimide	6 drops	1 mL	White	Sanfilippo disease
Cyanide nitroprusside	Sodium hydroxide + sodium cyanide + sodium nitroprusside	2 mL	Violet	Homocystinuria
2,4-Dinitrophenylhydrazine (DNPH)	10 drops	1 mL	Yellow	MSUD

TABLE 6.9	Neurodegenerative Disorders and Their Specific Management	
Neurodegenerative Disorder	**Enzyme Replacement/Management**	
Gaucher disease	Velaglucerase and taliglucerase	
Niemann – Pick disease type B	Completed phase 1 trial (no approved drugs) – histone deacetylase inhibitor (HDACi)	
Niemann Pick disease type C	Vorinostat – crosses the blood–brain barrier and into brain tissue of mice in phase 1/2 trial	
Fabry disease	Fabrazyme	
Mucopolysaccharidoses	MPS 1 – Aldurazyme MPS 2 – Elaprase MPS 3 – Naglazyme	
Pompe disease	l-Carnitine	
Krabbe disease, MLD, ALD	Bone marrow transplantation	
Menkes kinky hair	Copper sulfate	
Mitochondrial myopathies	Nicotinamide (riboflavin, l-carnitine, CoQ10)	
Wilson disease	d-Penicillamine, zinc acetate, liver transplantation	
Refsum disease	Reduction of phytanic acid intake (dairy products, green vegetables, meat, fish)	

TABLE 6.10	Epileptic Encephalopathy				
Features	**West Syndrome**	**Dravet Syndrome**	**Lennox–Gastaut Syndrome**	**Landau–Kleffner Syndrome**	**Progressive Myoclonic Epilepsy of Infancy**
Age	2–12 months	<1 year	2–10 years	1–5 years	<1 year
Triad	a. Epileptic spasm b. Developmental regression c. Dysrhythmia (high voltage, slow, chaotic background with multifocal spikes)	a. Multiple seizure types b. Initial normal EEG, later slow and generalized spikes c. Hypotonia/unsteady gait	a. Developmental delay b. Multiple seizure type c. EEG: 1- to 2-Hz spike and slow waves, polyspike burst in sleep + slow background in wakefulness	Benign childhood epilepsy with centro-temporal spike + language impairment (auditory agnosia) + temporal discharge in sleep	Severe myoclonic seizures (sleep myoclonus) + burst suppression in EEG + Lafora inclusion bodies
Treatment	ACTH/steroid West syndrome + tuberous sclerosis – vigabatrin	Valproic acid, benzodiazepine, ketogenic diet Newer agent – stiripentol Contraindicated – lamotrigine	Sodium valproate, topiramate	Nocturnal diazepam therapy Steroid Speech therapy	Valproic acid, clonazepam

EEG, electroencephalogram.

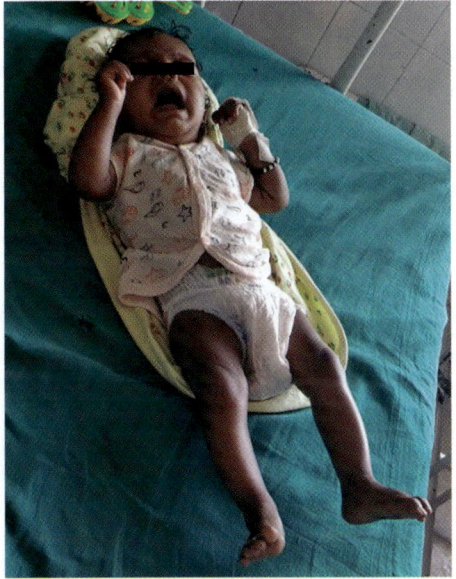

Fig. 6.14 Krabbe disease – exaggerated startle reflex.

50. What are the salient features of Leigh disease?
Leigh disease
  - Subacute necrotizing encephalopathy; neurogenic muscle weakness, ataxia, and retinitis pigmentosa (NARP)
  - Autosomal recessive transmission
  - Abnormality in mitochondrial energy generation
  - Primarily affects neurons of the brainstem, thalamus, basal ganglia, and cerebellum
  - Onset: 3–12 months of age
  - Lactic acidosis with intercurrent illness
  - Psychomotor regression with hypotonia, spasticity, movement disorders (including chorea), cerebellar ataxia, and peripheral neuropathy
  - Hypertrophic cardiomyopathy
  - Stability interspersed with episodes of deterioration
  - Death by 2–3 years of age
Diagnosis
  - Raised lactate levels in blood and CSF – more so with 60 minutes after a glucose load test
  - MRI brain: Bilateral hyperintense signal abnormality in the brainstem and/or basal ganglia

Treatment
  * Supportive – sodium bicarbonate; anticonvulsants; baclofen, tetrabenzene, and baclofen for dystonia

51. What are the salient features of Alexander disease?
Alexander disease
  * Mutation gene encoding NADH
  * Autosomal dominant
  * Pathological hallmark – Rosenthal fibers (rod-shaped or round bodies stain red with H&E and black with myelin stain) appearing as granules in the cytoplasm of astrocytes
  * Infantile (71%), juvenile, and adult forms
  * Onset: Any time after birth to early childhood
  * Psychomotor arrest and regression
  * Spasticity, seizures, and no optic atrophy
  * Increase in head size
  * Death by the 2nd or 3rd year
MRI (four out of five findings)
  * Extensive cerebral white abnormalities with frontal predominance
  * Periventricular rim of decreased intensity on T2-weighted images and increased signal on T1-weighted images
  * Abnormalities in the thalamus and basal ganglia
  * Brainstem abnormalities (midbrain and medulla)
  * Contrast enhancement of one or more of the following areas: ventricular, periventricular rim, frontal white matter, optic chiasm, fornix, basal ganglia, thalamus, dentate nucleus, and brainstem
Treatment
  * Supportive

52. What are the salient features of adrenoleukodystrophy?
Adrenoleukodystrophy
  * X-linked recessive
  * Start of symptoms usually by age 4–10 years
  * Loss of previously acquired neurological abilities, hyperactivity, seizures, and ataxia
  * Adrenal gland failure (Addison type)
Diagnosis
  * VLCFA is detected.
  * MRI shows white matter abnormalities.
Treatment
  * Dietary restriction of VLCFA, ±Lorenzo oil, and bone marrow transplantation

53. What are the salient features of metachromatic leukodystrophy?
Metachromatic leukodystrophy
  * Autosomal recessive inheritance
  * Onset: 12–24 months (infantile) or 4–12 years (juvenile)
  * Deficiency in arylsulfatase A
  * Accumulation in lipid sulfatide in the myelin sheath, brain, and peripheral nerve
  * Cognitive function affected initially, followed by motor difficulties and dysarthria
Treatment
  * Symptomatic and bone marrow transplantation

DISCUSSION ON MUCOPOLYSACCHARIDES

54. Mention some salient features of various types of mucopolysaccharides.
Table 6.11 gives the salient features of various types of mucopolysaccharides.

55. What are the clinical, radiological, and biochemical findings in a child with MPS?

TABLE 6.11	Salient Features of Various Types of Mucopolysaccharides		
Types	**Enzyme Defect**	**Clinical Features**	**Salient Points**
Type I Hurler Prototype of all MPS	Alpha-L-iduronidase	Coarse facies Hurler phenotype Eye: Corneal clouding, retinal degeneration, glaucoma Ear: Combined Sensory neural hearing loss (SNHL) + conductive hearing loss Central nervous system (CNS): Hydrocephalus, no IQ disability Cardiovascular system (CVS): Aortic valve disease, OSA, organomegaly – HSM	Inguinal hernia at birth
Type II Hunter (X-linked)	Iduronate sulfate sulfatase	Classical phenotype Chronic diarrhea Spastic paraplegia	Newborn – extensive Mongolian spots
Type III Sanfilippo (four types-A to D) Most common	type IIIA-Heparan-S-sulfamidase type IIIB-N-Acetyl-alpha-D glucosaminidase type IIIC-Acetyl-CoA-glucosaminide N acetyltransferase type IIID-N-Acetylglucosamine-6 sulfate sulfatase	Severe CNS involvement No HSM Behavior problem	No organomegaly
Type IV (two types-A and B)	type IVA-N-Acetylgalactosamine-6-sulfate sulfatase type IVB-beta-Galactosidase	Short trunk, dwarfism Triad – mild corneal opacity, genu valgum, kyphosis Normal intelligence	Atlantoaxial dislocation Dysostosis multiplex
Type VI Maroteaux–Lamy disease	Arylsulfatase B	Similar to Hurler	Spinal cord compression (thickening of dura)
Type VII Sly	Beta-glucuronidase	Nonimmune fetal hydrops	Granulocytic inclusion in leukocytes
Type IX	Hyaluronidase 1	Nodular periarticular masses	Mild dysostosis

MPS can be diagnosed under three categories:

A. Clinical

Hurler phenotype

1. Large head
2. Mental retardation
3. Hypertelorism
4. Flat nasal bridge
5. Deafness
6. Thick lips
7. Large tongue
8. Umbilical hernia
9. Stiff joints
10. Corneal clouding
11. Short stature

Fig. 6.15 shows the Hurler phenotype.

Fig. 6.16A–D shows a child with type 2 MPS – Hunter syndrome.

B. Radiological

Skeletal survey

First, pelvic X-ray; second, DL spine AP and lateral view; third, X-ray of both hands AP; and fourth, skull

Classical X-ray findings in MPS

Seen in all type of MPS

- **X-ray pelvis**
  - Round iliac wings
  - Narrow ileum with inferior part tapering
  - Shallow acetabular fossa
  - Underdeveloped medial portion of proximal femoral epiphysis
  - Femoral neck valgus position
- **X-ray spine**
  - Platyspondyly with anterior beaking and posterior scalloping of vertebral bodies
- **X-ray hands**
  - Metacarpals are short and show proximal hypoplasia or tapering.
  - Bullet shaped phalanges
- **X-ray skull**
  - J-shaped sella (Fig. 6.17)
- **Chest X-ray ribs**
  - Paddle-shaped ribs/oar-like ribs in Hurler (thick anteriorly and thin posteriorly)

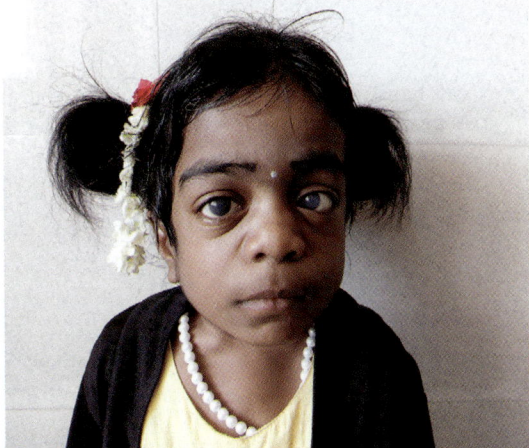

Fig. 6.15 Hurler syndrome – corneal opacity, hypertelorism, flat nasal bridge, and thick lips.

- Earliest findings: Thick ribs

Fig. 6.18A–F shows the X-ray of MPS – Hurler syndrome.
- Other radiological features of MPS are as follows:
  1. Trabeculated diaphysis of long bones and irregular metaphysis
  2. Abnormal spacing of teeth – dentigerous cyst

C. Biochemical testing
- Urine metabolic screening: Cetrimide test – for glycosaminoglycans
- Quantitative analysis: By tandem mass spectroscopy (type-specific profile: tissue source, cultured fibroblast; and leukocytes, measurement of lysosomal enzymes)

56. *Give examples of Hurler phenotype.
   a. GM1 gangliosidosis
   b. Sialidosis
   c. Fucosidosis
   d. Mannosidosis
   e. Cretinism
   f. MPS
   g. Multiple sulfatase deficiencies

57. *Discuss the salient features seen in x-ray of pelvis of a Down syndrome child.
   a. Mickey mouse appearance (broad and flared iliac wings) flat acetabulum, reduced acetabular angle resulting in abnormal ilial index seen in Down syndrome as shown in Fig. 6.19

58. What are the X-ray findings in mucolipidosis (I-cell disease)?
   - Periosteal cloaking – diaphysis widening
   - Vertebrae – inferior beaking
   - Metacarpal proximal tapering

59. How is a child with MPS managed? Mention the complications of the treatment given.
   Treatment
   - Enzyme replacement therapy is available for MPS 1, 2, and 6 (Aldurazyme, Elaprase, Naglazyme); type 4 is in preclinical trial.
   - However, there is no change in mental retardation because these enzymes do not cross the blood–brain barrier.
   - Definitive therapy is bone marrow transplantation.
   - Treatment of complications
     1. For valve regurgitation – valve replacement
     2. Corneal opacity – keratoplasty
     3. Hydrocephalus – VP shunt
     4. Morquio (AT dislocation) – spine stabilization

60. What are the antenatal screenings available for MPS?
   Antenatal screening includes carrier screening for Hunter, and chorionic villous sampling and amniotic fluid analysis for MPS types 1, 2, and 6.

61. Mention some salient points of each type of MPS.
   - All autosomal recessive except Hunter disease (X-linked)
   - Common organs involved in MPS – eyes, ear, skeletal, mentation, and cardiac
   - MPS with inguinal hernia at birth – Hurler disease
   - MPS with excessive Mongolian spots – Hunter disease
   - No mental retardation – Morquio disease, Maroteaux–Lamy, and scheie disease
   - No corneal clouding in Hunter but retinal degeneration occurs
   - Middle constriction of metacarpal maintained in Morquio but lost in Hurler described as bullet shaped

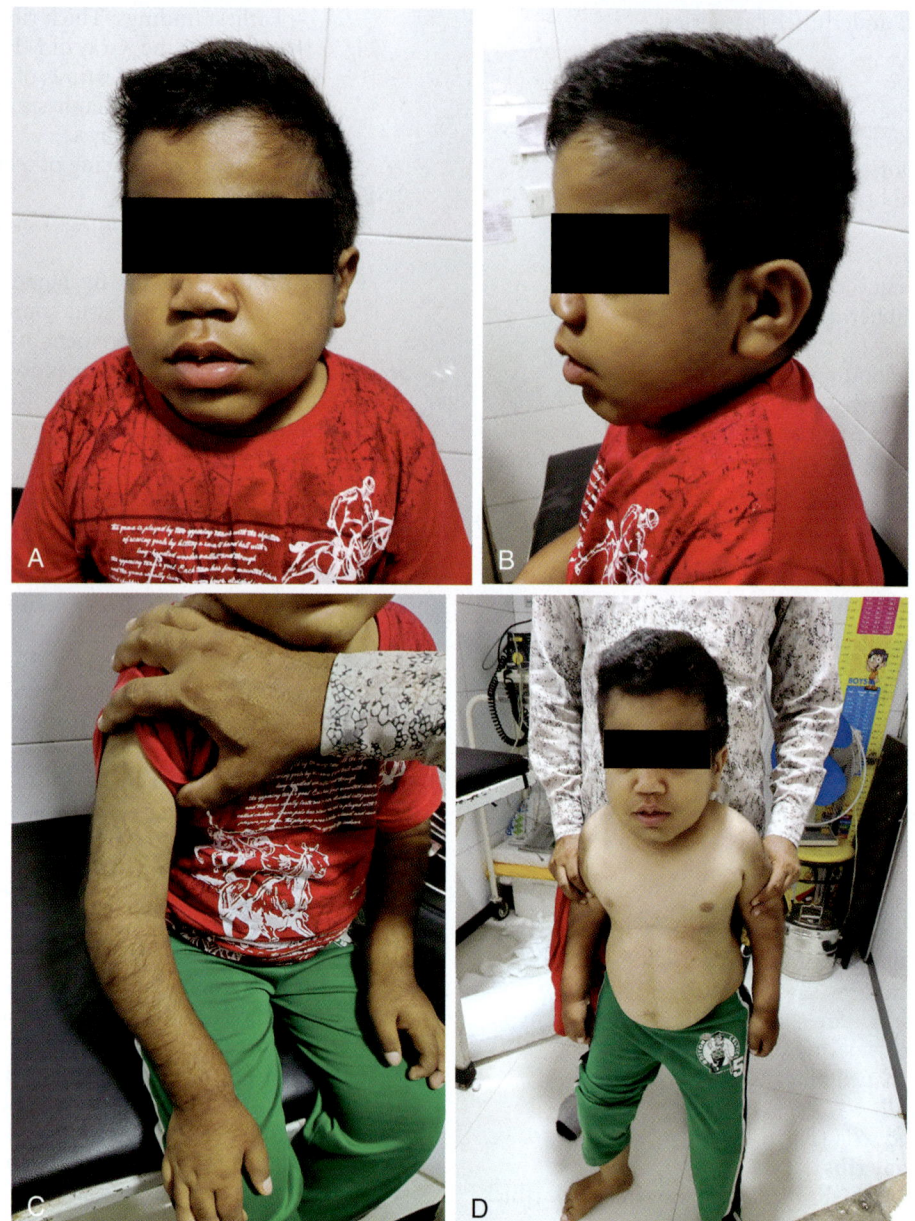

Fig. 6.16   (A–D) MPS – Hunter syndrome. (A) Flat nasal bridge, thick lips, and hypertelorism. (B) Large head. (C) Stiff joints. (D) Short stature.

- Classical radiography – Morquio disease and Hurler types
- Anterior beaking of body of vertebra seen in Morquio disease and inferior beaking in Hurler disease
- Seizures common in MPS 1, 2, and 3
- Retinal degeneration and hydrocephalus common in types 1 and 2
- Severe CNS involvement, no organomegaly, hirsutism, and hyperactive behavior – Sanfillipo disease
- Instability of odontoid process/atlantoaxial dislocation seen in Morquio disease
- Fetal hydrops seen in type 6 (Sly)
- No hearing impairment in type 4
- Most common type: First, type 3; second, types 1 and 2
- No hepatosplenomegaly – Morquio and Sanfilippo

- X-ray hand – bullet-shaped metacarpal (because of loss of middle constriction) in Hurler; and middle constriction maintained in Morquio
- Triad of Morquio (type 4) – corneal opacity, kyphosis, and genu valgum

DISCUSSION ON INBORN ERRORS OF METABOLISM

62. How are inborn errors of metabolism classified?
    a) Carbohydrate disorders
    b) Fatty acid oxidation disorders
    c) Protein disorders – aminoacidopathies, organic acidemias, and urea cycle disorders
    d) Mitochondrial disorders

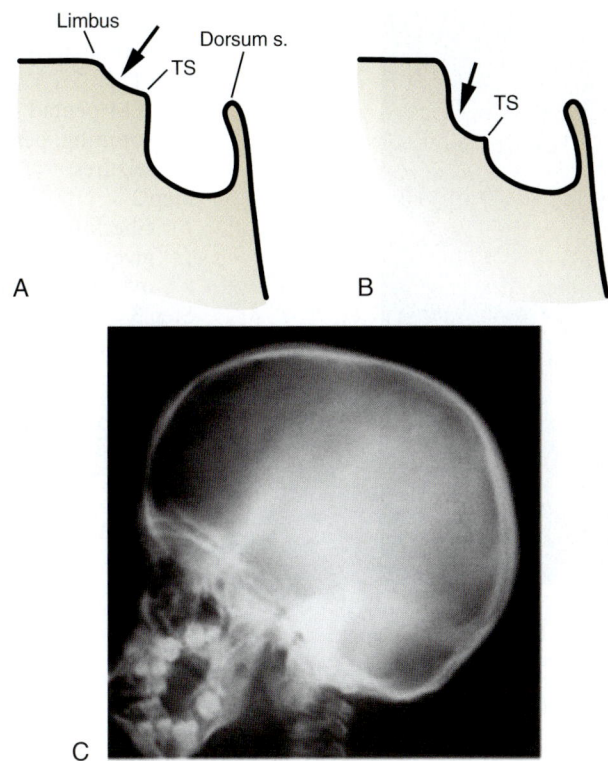

Fig. 6.17 Schematic representation of (A) normal J-shaped sella and (B) abnormal J-shaped sella. The limbus and tuberculum sella (TS) and the chiasmatic groove (arrow) are more vertically aligned with the tuberculum positioned more inferiorly in abnormal J shaped sella. (C) X-ray picture of abnormal J shaped sella. *(Source A and B: Reproduced from Peter Som, Hugh Curtin. Head and Neck Imaging, Fifth Edition, Pathology of the Central Skull Base, FIGURE 13-6, Philadelphia, Mosby, 2011.) (Source C: Reproduced from Lee A. Grant, Nyree Griffin. Grainger & Allison's Diagnostic Radiology Essentials, Second Edition, Congenital Skeletal Anomalies, u005010-022af, London, Elsevier Ltd, 2019.)*

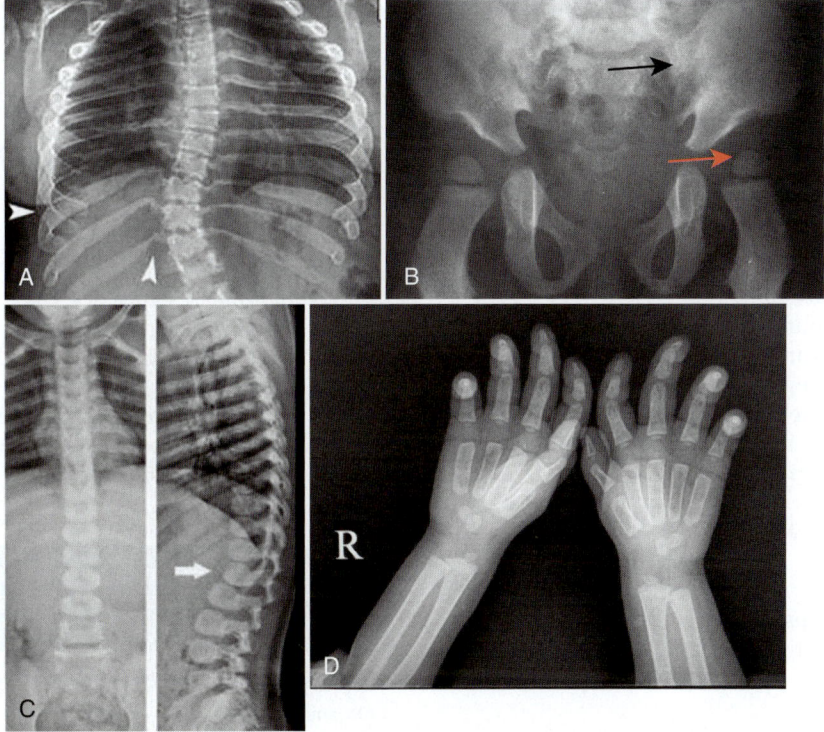

Fig. 6.18 (A) Oar-like ribs (white arrows shows ribs tapered proximally and wider distally). (B) Black arrow-round iliac wings with inferior tapering, poorly developed acetabulum, red arrow - underdeveloped medial portion of proximal femoral epiphysis (C) X-ray spine – arrowhead, flat and rounded vertebral bodies (platyspondyly). fig 6.17 (D) X ray hand -bullet shaped phalanges. *(Source: (A) Imaging findings of mucopolysaccharidoses: a pictorial review. Insights into Imaging volume 4, pages 443–459 (2013). (B) Source: Reproduced from John Taylor, Tudor Hughes, Donald Resnick. Skeletal Imaging: Atlas of the Spine an Extremities, Second Edition, Pelvis and Symphysis Pubis, FIGURE 6-15, St. Louis, Saunders, 2011. (C) Imaging findings of mucopolysaccharidoses: a pictorial review | Insights into Imaging | Full Text (springeropen.com).*

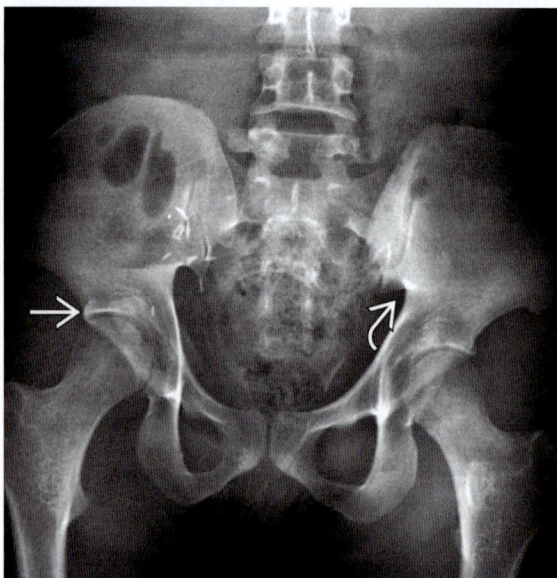

Fig. 6.19 X-ray pelvis – Down syndrome shows Mickey mouse appearance- broad iliac wings, horizontal acetabular roofs, underdeveloped femoral heads, a narrow sacrosciatic notch. *(Source: Reproduced from Kirkland Davis, Donna Blankenbaker. ExpertDDX: Musculoskeletal, Second Edition, Dwarfism With Horizontal Acetabular Roof, Elsevier Inc., 2018.)*

63. What are the categories of IEM on the basis of the substrate?
    1. Carbohydrate: Hypoglycemia, metabolic acidosis, and lactic acidosis
    2. Fatty acid oxidation disorder: Hypoglycemia
    3. Aminoacidopathies: Some presenting with metabolic acidosis
    4. Organic acidemias: Hyperammonemia and metabolic acidosis
    5. Urea cycle disorder: Hyperammonemia
    6. Mitochondrial disorders: Lactic acidosis and hypoglycemia
64. What is IEM pentad?
    - IEM pentad
       - Sudden-onset lethargy
       - Refusal of feeds
       - Intractable vomiting
       - Intractable seizures
       - Intractable hypoglycemia
65. When should IEM be suspected?
    - History – parental consanguinity
    - Family history – neonatal death
       - Similar illness in siblings
       - Developmental delay
    - Clinical
       - Encephalopathy
       - Effortless tachypnea
       - Recurrent vomiting
       - Cardiomyopathy
       - Dysmorphism
    - Lab
       - Metabolic acidosis
       - Hyperammonemia
       - Hypoglycemia
       - High lactate

66. What is the stepwise management of IEM?
    Stepwise management in IEM
    Step 1
       - IEM pentad – lethargy, refusal to feed, persistent vomiting, persistent hypoglycemia, and persistent seizures
    Step 2
       - Check for pH, ketones, and ammonia. Table 6.12 gives the findings in organic acidemia, fatty acid oxidation disorder, and urea cycle disorder.
    Step 3
       - If all three normal (pH, ketones, ammonia – normal)

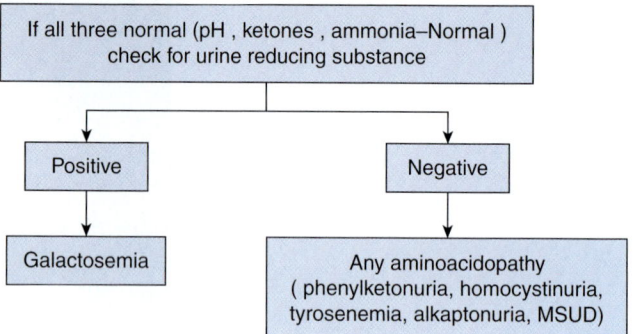

Step 4
       - Urine odor as given in Table 6.7
67. What are the four I's to be remembered in acute encephalopathy?
    Infection, injury, intoxication, and IEM
68. What are the neurological manifestations of IEM?
    - Common: Acute encephalopathy and seizures
    - Other features: Abnormal tone, floppy child, lethargy, coma, and seizures
69. What are IEM that present with seizures at onset?
    - Urea cycle disorders
    - Amino acid metabolism disorders
    - Organic acidemias
    - Gangliosidoses
    - Mitochondrial disorders
    - Pyridoxine deficiency
    - Biotinidase deficiency
    - Nonketotic hyperglycinemia
70. What are IEM that present with jaundice?
    - Causes
       - Infants: Tyrosinemia and galactosemia (cataract, convulsions)
       - Older children: Wilson

TABLE 6.12	Laboratory Findings in Organic Acidemia, Fatty Acid Oxidation Disorder, and Urea Cycle Disorder		
Disease	**pH (Acidosis)**	**Ammonia**	**Ketones**
Organic acidemia	+++	+++ (increased 500)	+++
Fatty acid oxidation disorder	+++	++ (increased 200)	–
Urea cycle disorder	–	+++ (increased 1000)	–

71. What are IEM that present with organomegaly?
    - Renomegaly – isease (GSD type I), Zellweger syndrome, and tyrosinemia
    - Hepatomegaly – galactosemia, glycogen storage disorders, and tyrosinemia
    - Hepatosplenomegaly – Niemann pick disease, gaucher disease, and mucopolysaccharidoses
72. What are IEM that present without organomegaly?
    Metachromatic leukodystrophy, neuronal ceroid lipofuscinosis, krabbe disease, fabry disease
73. What are IEM that present with skin and hair abnormalities?
    - Perioral eruption – multiple carboxylase deficiency
    - Increased pigmentation – adrenoleukodystrophy
    - Decreased pigmentation of hair – PKU
    - Alopecia – multiple carboxylase deficiency
    - Kinky hair – Menkes disease
74. What are IEM that present with eye involvement?
    - Cataract – galactosemia, Zellweger, and homocystinuria
    - KF ring – Wilson disease
    - Heterochromia iris/Retinitis pigmentosa (RP) – Zellweger disease
    - Cherry red spot – Niemann pick disease, krabbe disease, MLD, farber disease, GM1 ganliosidosis, GM2 gangliosidosis and Wolman disease
75. Give examples of X-linked IEM.
    X-linked recessive (all IEM have autosomal recessive inheritance)
    A. Fabry disease
    B. Hunter syndrome
    C. Menkes disease
    D. Lesch–Nyhan syndrome
    E. Ornithine transcarbamylase deficiency
76. What are IEM that present in school-age children?
    a. Wilson disease
    b. Subacute sclerosing panencephalitis
    c. Niemann–Pick type C
    d. X-linked adrenoleukodystrophy
    e. Batten disease
77. What are IEM with normal mentation?
    Gaucher type 1, Fabry disease, Niemann–Pick B, and Wolman disease
78. What are IEM that present with peripheral neuropathy?
    MLD, Krabbe, and Niemann–Pick disease
79. What are IEM that present with acute cardiogenic failure?
    - Pompe disease
    - Fatty acid oxidation (FAO) disorders
    - Mitochondrial cytopathy
80. What are the clinical presentations of fatty acid oxidation defect?
    1. Skeletal and cardiac muscles: Hypotonia, weakness, cardiomyopathy, and failure
    2. Reye-like episodes of hypoketotic hypoglycemia, hyperammonemia, hepatic failure, and encephalopathy
    3. Sudden Infant Death Syndrome (SIDS)
    4. Hemolysis, elevated liver enzymes, and low platelets (HELLP) syndrome (mothers of the affected fetus may develop acute fatty liver of pregnancy or HELLP syndrome)
81. What are the clues in examination and lab in IEM?
    - Hyperammonemia + metabolic acidosis + skin lesions: Multiple carboxylase (biotinidase) deficiency
    - Hyperammonemia + metabolic acidosis + progressive dystonia + retinal hemorrhage + intracranial hemorrhage (mimics child abuse): Glutaric acidemia type 1
    - IEM with dysmorphism/hypotonia: Zellweger syndrome
    - IEM with unusual facies (cherubic facies): GSD type I
    - Uncontrollable hiccup: Nonketotic hyperglycinemia
    - Neutropenia and thrombocytopenia: Propionic acidemia
    - Acute hepatic dysfunction: Tyrosinemia
82. What are IEM that present with dysmorphic facies?
    - Zellweger syndrome: High forehead, large Anterior fontannelle, hypoplastic supraorbital ridges, epicanthal folds, broad nasal bridge, high-arched palate, and deformed ear lobes
    - Lysosomal storage disease: Coarse facial features at birth in mucolipidosis II and GM1 gangliosidosis; develops with age in MPS
    - Homocystinuria: Long face and lanky body habitus (Marfanoid phenotype)
    - Smith–Lemli–Opitz syndrome: Cleft palate, Congenital heart disease (CHD), hypospadias, polydactyly, and syndactyly
83. What are the points to be remembered in diagnosing IEM?
    - High ammonia and metabolic acidosis: Organic acidemia
    - High ammonia and no acidosis: Urea cycle disorder
    - Normal ammonia and no acidosis: Amino acid disease
    - Hypoglycemia, no ketonuria, myopathy, and cardiomyopathy: Fatty acid oxidation defect
    - Lactic acidosis, ammonia normal or mild rise, and hypoglycemia±: Mitochondrial disorder
    - Hypoglycemia and lactic acidosis: Carbohydrate disorder
84. What are IEM that present with metabolic acidosis?
    - Organic acidemia: Methylmalonic acidemia, propionic acidemia, isovaleric acidemia, glutaric acidemia, and biotinidase deficiency
    - Carbohydrate: Hereditary fructose intolerance and GSD types I and III
    - Fatty acid oxidation defect: Medium-chain acyl carnitine deficiency
85. What are IEM that present with hyperammonemia?
    - Systemic illness: Preterm, valproate, liver disease, and Reye syndrome
    - Urea cycle disorders (metabolic alkalosis)
    - Organic acidemias (metabolic acidosis)
    - Fatty acid oxidation defects (hypoglycemia)
86. What are IEM that present with hypoglycemia?
    - With ketonuria: Glycogen storage disorder (GSD) type 1
    - With ketonuria + high lactate: Neoglucogenesis defects
    - With no ketonuria + high fatty acid: Fatty acid oxidation defect
87. What are IEM that present with stroke or stroke-like illness?
    a. MELAS
    b. Homocystinuria
    c. Organic acidopathies
    d. OTC deficiency
88. What are the levels of investigations in IEM?
    Levels of investigations in IEM
    Level I
    Complete blood count (CBC), Arterial blood gas (ABG), liver function test, renal function test, and urine ketones

Level II
   • Ammonia, lactate, and pyruvate
Level III
      1. Plasma amino acids (quantitative)
      2. Urine organic acids (qualitative)
      3. Plasma acylcarnitine profile

89. What are the laboratory features in IEM?
   Table 6.13 gives the laboratory features in IEM.

90. What are the samples that should be taken in a child with suspected IEM who dies before the diagnosis?
   a. A total of 5 mL plasma separated from heparinized blood frozen at −70°
   b. Serum collected without anticoagulant
   c. Whole blood refrigerated at 4° for leukocyte separation and DNA
   d. Urine suprapubic tap at 2–8°
   e. Needle liver biopsy
   f. Other samples – skin (for fibroblast culture), muscle, and brain

91. What are the clues in MRI brain to identify IEM?
   • Glutaric acidemia I – basal ganglion changes
   • MSUD – white matter changes
   • Methylmalonic acidemia – abnormalities in the globus pallidus

92. How is hyperammonemia treated?
   1. Emergency: Avoid catabolism, high-carbohydrate feeds only, and 10% dextrose intravenous ornithine transcarbomylase deficiency (OTC) or without intravenous insulin
   2. Drugs
      a. Sodium benzoate i.v./oral 250 mg/kg stat
      b. I.v. carnitine
      c. I.v. antibiotics
      d. Oral metronidazole and lactulose
      e. Arginine and sodium phenylbutyrate
      f. Carbaglu
   3. Hemofiltration and hemodialysis
   4. Cerebral edema treated
   5. Avoid the following:
      a. Valproic acid
      b. Prolonged fasting or starvation
      c. Intravenous steroids
      d. Excessive protein/undue restriction
      e. Illness and dehydration
      f. Bone fractures or excessive bruising
      g. Any physiological or psychological stress

93. What is the crisis management in IEM?
   a. Maintain ABCs, respiratory failure, shock, and seizures.
   b. IVF: 1.5 × maintenance – D 10 1/2 NS with appropriate potassium without causing overload. Avoid Ringer lactate (lactic acidosis).
   c. Monitor glucose (target – 120–180 mg); add insulin infusion.
   d. If acidosis is present, treat with bicarbonate infusion (60 mEq/L).
   e. Avoid steroid (to avoid catabolism), valproate (increases ammonia), and mannitol (ineffective).
   f. Recognize and correct acidosis, hypoglycemia, and cerebral edema.
   g. Monitor vitals, ammonia, glucose, electrolytes, RFT, and LFT.
   h. Give antibiotics to control sepsis and production of OA from intestinal bacteria.
   i. The patient is kept NPO for 48 hours. Stop all proteins and offending sugars.
   j. The patient is reintroduced to a low-protein diet or specific diet.
   k. Eliminate toxins:
      i) Na benzoate 250 mg/kg loading followed by three divided doses
      ii) Arginine infusion
      iii) Sodium phenyl acetate
      iv) L-Carnitine 100 mg/kg i.v. Q 8 hourly
      v) Lactulose
      vi) Carbaglu
      vii) If no decrease in 8 hours, hemodialysis or Peritoneal dialysis started
   l. Vitamins and cofactors
      • Pyridoxine – for pyridoxine-responsive seizures and homocystinuria
      • Folic acid – for folinic acid–responsive seizures
      • Hydroxycobalamin: 1 mg/day intramuscular for methylmalonic acidemia
      • Biotin – for biotinidase deficiency and multiple carboxylase deficiency
      • Thiamine – for MSUD and glutaric aciduria
      • Riboflavine – for MSUD and glutaric aciduria
      • Nicotinamide – for Hartnup disease
      • Carnitine – for carnitine deficiency

94. What modifications should be done in the diet in specific IEM?
   Table 6.14 shows the diet modifications in IEM.

TABLE 6.13	**Laboratory Features in IEM**					
Findings	Amino Acid Disorder	Organic Acidemia	Urea Cycle Disorder	Carbohydrate Disorder	Fatty Acid Disorder	Mitochondrial Disease
Metabolic acidosis	±	++	−	±	±	±
Respiratory alkalosis	−	−	+	−	−	−
Hyperammonemia	±	+	++	−	±	−
Hypoglycemia	±	±	−	+	+	±
Ketonuria	P	P	P	P	A	P
High lactate	±	±	−	+	±	++

Note: P-present
A-absent

TABLE 6.14	Diet Modifications in IEM
Disorder	**Diet**
Fructose intolerance	Avoid fruit juices
Pyruvate dehydrogenase deficiency	High fat, low carbohydrate
Organic acidemias	High carbohydrate, low protein and fat
Beta-oxidation defects	High-carbohydrate, low-fat diet; continuous feeding, avoid fasting
Ketolysis defect	Low fat, low protein, carnitine supplementation
Long-chain fatty acid deficiency	Medium-chain triglycerides
Purine and pyrimidine metabolism	Avoid nuts, nonvegetarian

Approach to IEM

Flowchart 6.1 gives the approach to metabolic acidosis.
Flowchart 6.2 gives the approach to organic acidemia.
Flowchart 6.3 gives the approach to a child with lactic acidosis.
Flowchart 6.4 gives the approach to a child with hypoglycemia.
Flowchart 6.5 gives the approach to a child with hyperammonemia.
Flowchart 6.6 gives the overall approach to metabolic disorder.

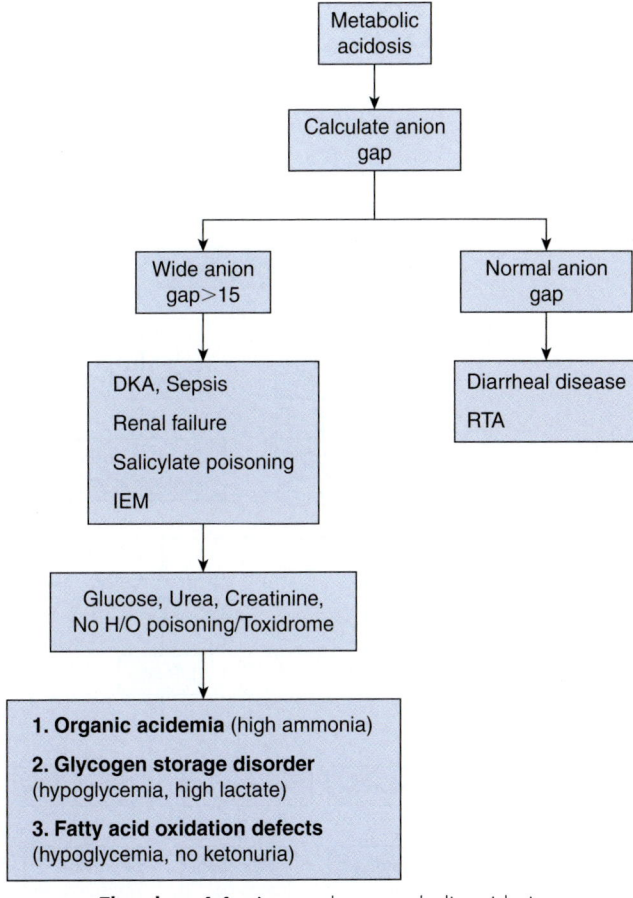

Flowchart 6.1 Approach to metabolic acidosis.

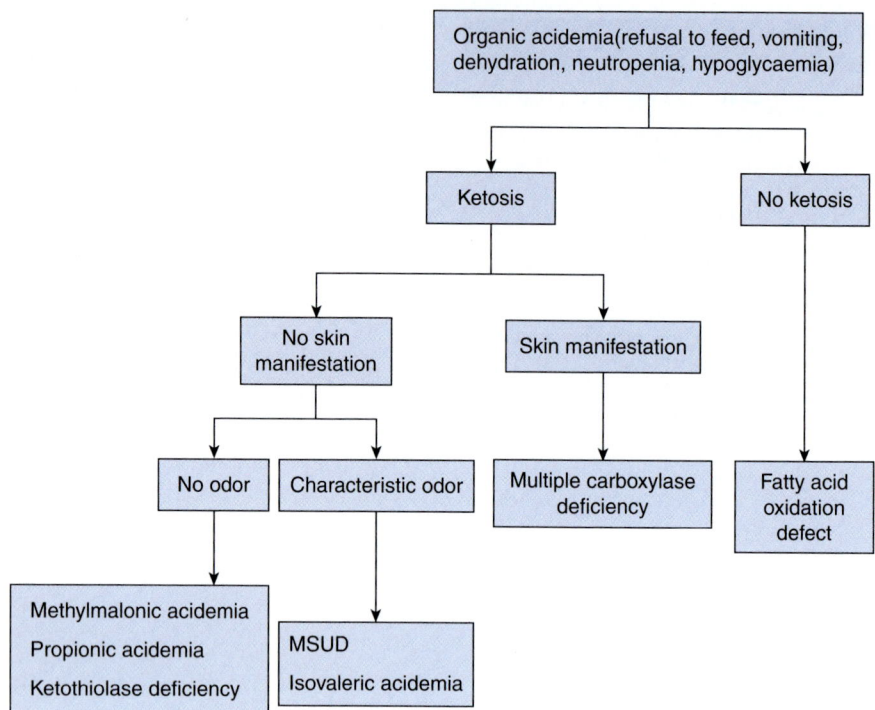

Flowchart 6.2 Approach to organic acidemia.

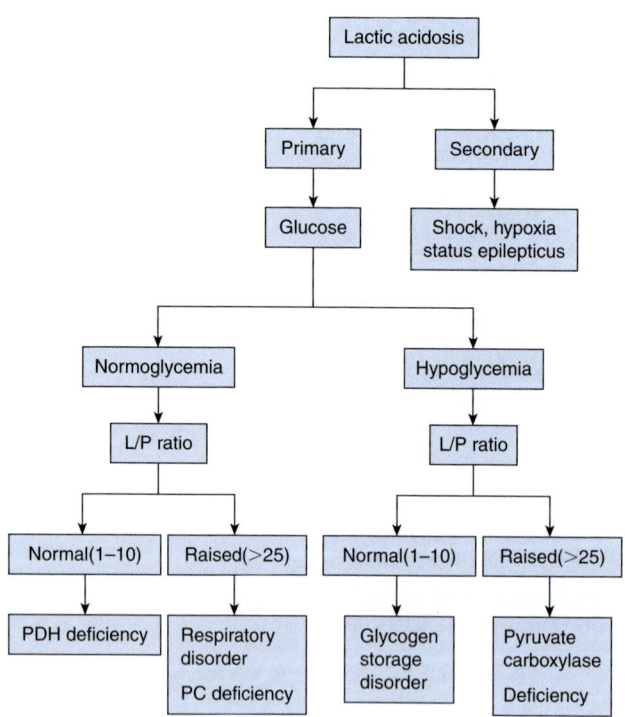

Flowchart 6.3 Approach to lactic acidosis.

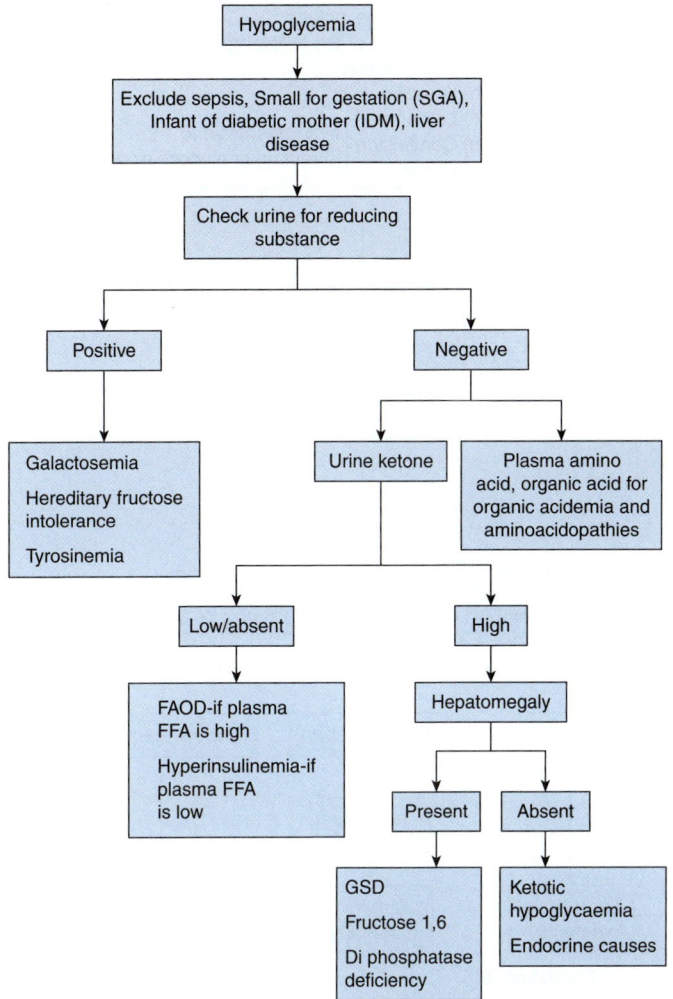

Flowchart 6.4 Approach to hypoglycemia.

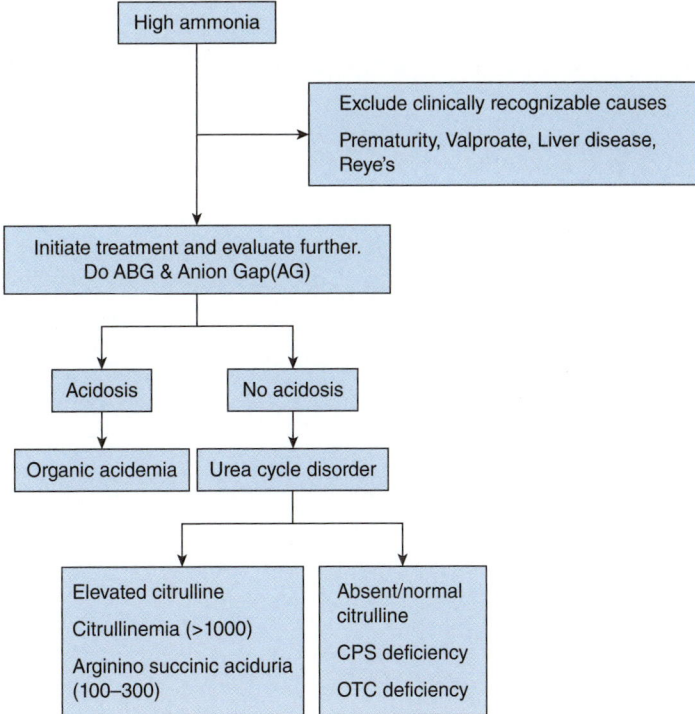

Flowchart 6.5 Approach to hyperammonemia.

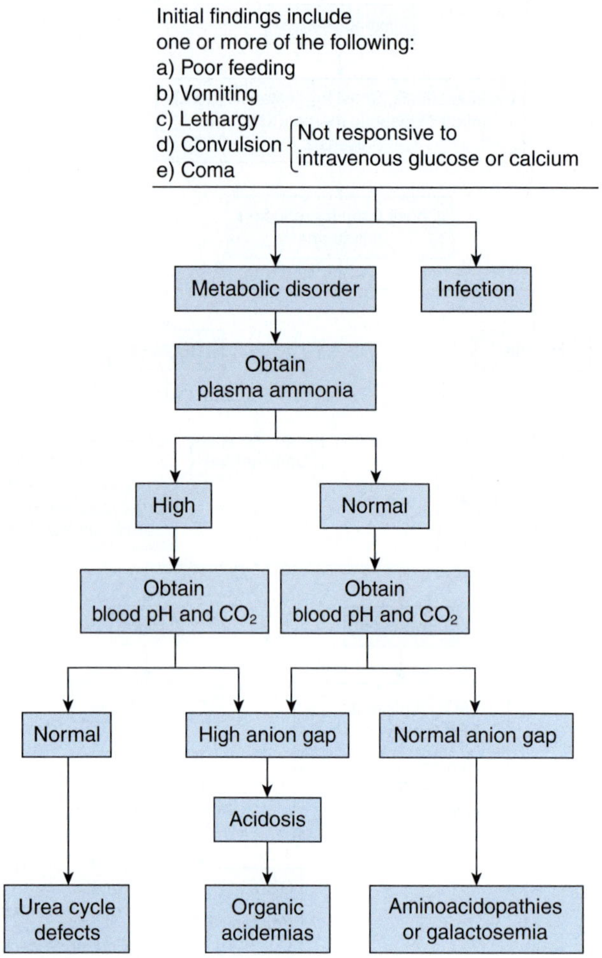

Initial findings include
one or more of the following:
a) Poor feeding
b) Vomiting
c) Lethargy
d) Convulsion
e) Coma
Not responsive to
intravenous glucose or calcium

Metabolic disorder

Infection

Obtain
plasma ammonia

High

Normal

Obtain
blood pH and CO_2

Obtain
blood pH and CO_2

Normal

High anion gap

Normal anion gap

Acidosis

Urea cycle
defects

Organic
acidemias

Aminoacidopathies
or galactosemia

Flowchart 6.6 Overall approach to metabolic disorder.

Quick Bites

1. NDD with macrocephaly: Canavan disease, Alexander disease, Sandhoff, and Tay–Sach (CATS – pneumonic)
2. Cherry red spot seen in all lysosomal storage disorders except Fabry and Gaucher diseases
3. Central nervous system + peripheral nervous system involvement seen in metachromatic leukodystrophy and Krabbe disease
4. Enzyme replacement therapy: Gaucher disease, Neimann–Pick types B and C, and MPS 1, 2, and 3
5. High ammonia + metabolic acidosis + ketones positive: Organic acidemia
6. Very high ammonia + no acidosis: Urea cycle disorder
7. Normal ammonia + no acidosis: Amino acid disease
8. Hypoglycemia + no ketonuria + myopathy + cardio-myopathy: Fatty acid oxidation defect
9. Lactic acidosis + normal or mild rise ammonia ± hypo-glycemia: Mitochondrial disorder
10. Hypoglycemia + lactic acidosis: Carbohydrate disorder

7 Postmeningitic Sequelae

Following introduction, seek permission from the caregiver and introduce yourself to the patient before history elicitation, and identify the case.

Name____Age____Sex____Consanguinity____Order of birth____Place____Informant____

Presenting Complaints and Duration

- Loss of an acquired milestone
- Seizures

History of Presenting Illness

(Narrate like a story: The mother noticed the loss of acquired milestones around ...... months of age. Initially, the child was able to sit with support; gradually over few weeks, the child was not able to sit with support, and now the child has partial head control. Previously, the child was able to talk in monosyllables, but now the child is able to only vocalize or coo.)

- Seizures – generalized tonic–clonic convulsions, lasting for few minutes controlled with medication associated with fever
- Explain the current admission – how many days, improved or worsening, on any drugs, on physiotherapy, and any surgery done

CENTRAL NERVOUS SYSTEM HISTORY

Higher Functions

- Whether the child recognizes the mother
- Interacts with the environment in the form of gestures/smile
- Whether obeys simple commands
- Able to speak few words or makes inappropriate noise
- Early hand preference
- Sleep disturbance in the form of intermittent irritability or incessant cry in the night
- Aggressive behavior

Cranial Nerves

- Cranial nerve II: Check the ability to perceive light
- Cranial nerves III, IV, and VI: Check the ability to move eyeballs in all four directions and any abnormal jerky movements
- Cranial nerve V: Check the ability to chew food
- Cranial nerve VII: Check facial asymmetry, ability to close eyes while sleeping, drooling of saliva, and deviation of angle of mouth
- Cranial nerve VIII: Check the ability to hear and respond to sound
- Cranial nerves IX and X: Check nasal twang of voice and nasal regurgitation
- Cranial nerve XI: Check the ability to move the head side to side

- Cranial nerve XII: Look for any deviation of the tongue on protrusion

Motor System

The mother noticed the following:

- Thinning of limbs, and if so, whether unilateral or bilateral, and upper limb or lower limb
- Stiffness/flailness noted by the mother in all limbs, symmetrical or one-side upper limb/lower limb in the form of difficulty in changing diaper, and scissoring of legs when the child is held by the axilla or at rest
- Ability to move limbs above the cot or whether it is only sideways or just some flickers
- Involuntary movement – which limb, smooth, rapid, jerky, forceful, and disappears during sleep

Cerebellar Features

- Abnormal eyeball or head movement or tremors

Bladder/Bowel Disturbance

- History of urinary incontinence or dribbling and constipation

Sensory Features

- History of perception of pain or crying while giving vaccination

Autonomic Features

- Flushing, sweating, and palpitation episodes

Spine and Cranium

- Any abnormality in the head size noted by the mother compared with in a sibling or peers
- Any swelling, tuft of hair, sinus, discharge, and abnormal curvature

COMPLICATION HISTORY

- Seizures
- Fever and breathing difficulty (aspiration pneumonitis)
- Fever, chills, rigors, and crying while passing urine (urinary tract infection)
- Bed sores, ulcer, and callosities
- Skeletal deformity/spine deformity
- Feeding difficulty

ETIOLOGICAL HISTORY

- Fever, head banging, vomiting, seizures, and abnormal posturing
- Altered behavior and personality changes
- Prodromal symptoms – flu-like illness and diarrhea (dehydration – thrombosis)

- Fever with rash and vesicles
- Any epidemic of encephalitis-like illness in the neighborhood
- Recent – travel
- Trauma and pica eating
- Ear discharge
- Other concurrent systemic illness (cardiac, pneumonia)
- Dysentery
- Oral thrush and skin infection
- Bed sores, constipation, and skin ulcers

Rule out other differential diagnoses:
- History suggestive of regression of milestones
- Increasing head size/gait abnormalities
- Evidence of raised intracranial pressure – headache and irritability
- Failure to thrive/malnutrition
- Seizures/regression of milestones/writhing or involuntary movement of hands

Past History

Elicit the course of illness and the following history in the past admission:
- Fever with seizures
- How many days the seizure persisted
- Controlled with how many drugs
- Whether ventilated or not
- Duration of hospital stay
- Any imaging done – what the results were
- Any fluid drained from the back (lumbar puncture)
- Whether the mother was informed of brain fever
- Any neurological deficit/milestone regression prior to discharge (at the time of discharge, whether the neurological status was the same as prehospital or with loss of milestones)
- Whether the mother was advised to continue anticonvulsant drugs or physiotherapy, or any hearing assessment advised
- Whether the child is recovering now or has static neurological status

Antenatal/Natal/Postnatal

- Neonatal sepsis and meningitis

Development History

Start from the newborn period milestones achieved prior to illness, and then loss of acquired milestones postillness, and at present what the development age is,

Dietetic History

Malnutrition

Immunization History

Hib and pneumococcal vaccine

Contact History

Any history of contact with TB

Family History

Seizure disorder and previous infant/child deaths

Treatment History

History of medication intake – for seizures

Environment History

Any epidemic of illness – seen in encephalitic syndrome

Socioeconomic History

According to the modified Kuppuswamy scale

Case Summary

A ...-year-old child, normal till ... of age, had fever with seizures suggestive of central nervous system (CNS) infection in the past following which the child had loss of acquired milestones, seizures, stiffness of all four limbs, and spastic quadriparesis, in the background of normal neonatal/family history; would like to think in terms of postmeningitic/postencephalitic sequelae and proceed further with examination.

General Examination

- General appearance – eye contact and interacts with the surroundings
- Attitude (in the mother's lap, decorticate/decerebrate pithed frog, dystonic posture)
- Malnourished
- Any oxygen support, i.v. fluid, and NG tube feeding
- Bed sores, skin ulcers/skin changes, and contractures
- Neurocutaneous marker

Head-to-Foot Examination

- Head
  - Size: Microcephaly/craniosynostosis
  - Hydrocephalus: Crackpot resonance if anterior fontanelle is closed
  - VP shunt: Scar looked for in the abdomen (if the shunt is present, look for any infection at the site – redness, warmth surrounding skin erythema, pain, shunt function – by proximal or distal occlusion)
- Eyes: Cataracts or retinopathy (secondary to congenital infections), visual field deficits, strabismus, and sunset sign
- Hearing: Any impairment
- Oral cavity: Dental caries and drooling
- BCG scar: Mantoux if done previously

Vital Signs

- Check for temperature, pulse rate, respiratory rate, blood pressure, and SpO_2.

Anthropometry

Height/length, weight, weight/height, or BMI
Head circumference – microcephaly/macrocephaly and hydrocephalus

Central Nervous System Examination

HIGHER FUNCTIONS

- COSSHMIB
  - C: Consciousness – awake and alert
  - O: Orientation – interacts with the mother or examiner (to time, place, person)
  - S: Sleep
  - S: Speech and Language – any inappropriate noises or inappropriate words
  - H: Hand preference
  - M: Memory – what the child had in the morning and afternoon
  - I: Intelligence
  - B: Behavior – excessively aggressive

CRANIAL NERVES

(Only whatever is feasible to check in a child with CP is mentioned here.)

- Cranial nerve I: Tell that cranial nerve I could not be tested
- Cranial nerve II
  Six points
  - A. Light perception
  - B. Visual acuity
  - C. Color vision
  - D. Field of vision
  - E. Direct and consensual light reflex
  - F. Fundus
- Cranial nerves III, IV, and VI: Moves the eyeball in all four cardinal directions, strabismus, and no ptosis
- Cranial nerve V: Pain sensation over the face, able to chew food, and jaw jerk
- Cranial nerve VII
  - Wrinkling of the forehead
  - Able to close eyes
  - Nasolabial fold
  - Deviation of the angle of the mouth
  - Drooling of saliva
- Cranial nerve VIII: Deafness
- Cranial nerves IX and X: Nasal regurgitation, palatal movement, and uvula in the midline
  Palatal arches, palatal and pharyngeal reflex, and speech – nasal twang
- Cranial nerve XI: Able to lift the head from supine position
  Whether turns the head on both sides
- Cranial nerve XII: Any deviation of the tongue, fibrillation, or wasting

MOTOR EXAMINATION

- Explain about the posture of the child
- Examination of motor system as given in Table 7.1
- Involuntary movements – hand writhing movement or pill rolling movement (Rett syndrome)
- Gait if ambulant

CEREBELLAR SYMPTOMS

- Head nodding, nystagmus, gait abnormality, ataxia or imbalance, past pointing, and dysdiadochokinesia

TABLE 7.1	Motor System Examination	
Components	**Right**	**Left**
Bulk	Normal	Normal
Tone	Hypertonia Clasp knife spasticity	Hypertonia Clasp knife spasticity
Power (best observed power) Tell individual joint in upper and lower limbs – shoulder, elbow, hand grip, finger grip, hip, knee, ankle, toe grip	Grade 1–5/5	Grade 1–5/5
Reflexes		
Superficial reflexes	Present	Present
Deep tendon reflexes	Exaggerated	Exaggerated
Plantar	Extensor	Extensor
Clonus (can be absent if contracture present)	Present	Present

AUTONOMIC SYSTEM

- Excessive sweating, tachycardia, and hypotension

SENSORY SYSTEM

- Ability to appreciate touch and pain sensation

SPINE AND CRANIUM

- Any swelling in the back (describe the swelling)
- Head size – small in size/hydrocephalus/flattened on one side (asymmetrical plagiocephaly)

SIGNS OF MENINGEAL IRRITATION

- Present or not (Kernig/Brudzinski reflex) and signs of raised ICP

Intra Cranial Pressure (ICP)

CARDIOVASCULAR SYSTEM

Apical impulse position, S1 and S2, and any murmur

RESPIRATORY SYSTEM

Respiratory rate, any chest retractions, and any added sound

ABDOMINAL SYSTEM

Any organomegaly

MUSCULOSKELETAL SYSTEM

Contractures/deformity/splints

Diagnosis

A child with spastic quadriparesis, probably postmeningitic/encephalitic sequelae with or without hydrocephalus, developmental regression, and other comorbid conditions – seizures, behavioral problems, ocular, hearing problems with or without complications, Lower respiratory tract infection (LRI), Urinary tract infection (UTI), breakthrough seizures, nutritional status, and others including anemia and vitamin deficiency if any

Frequently Asked Questions

1. What are the clinical manifestations of acute bacterial meningitis?
   Acute bacterial meningitis occurs in two forms:
   a. Sudden onset and rapid progression (less common)
   b. Subacute form and gradual progression (more common)
2. What are the seizure types seen in bacterial meningitis?
   The most common seizure types are Generalised tonic clonic seizures (GTCS) (80%) and focal seizures (20%).
3. How does acute encephalitis syndrome present?
   Acute encephalitis presents as altered sensorium and involuntary movements with rapid progression of the disease.
4. What are encephalopathy and encephalitis?
   Encephalopathy is a clinical syndrome in which pathology is not present per se in brain (symptoms secondary to severe systemic illness), whereas in encephalitis there occurs inflammation in the brain and pathological features (both clinical and imaging markers) are present.
5. What are the signs of raised ICP?
   Headache, vomiting, blurring of vision, lateral gaze palsy (involvement of cranial nerve VI), and papilledema are the signs of raised ICP.
6. What are the initial manifestations of papilledema?
   Enlargement of the blind spot may be the first manifestation but does not affect the vision but long-standing papilledema can cause blindness.
7. How does diarrheal disease cause encephalopathy?
   Diarrhea causes dyselectrolytemia which in turn causes encephalopathy. Other causes include rotavirus-associated encephalopathy and *Shigella dysenteriae* encephalopathy.
8. Mention few points about *Shigella* encephalopathy.
   Shigella encephalopathy is defined as any child with shigellosis (stool culture positive for *Shigella*) having disorientation, drowsiness, confusion, convulsion, or coma. All the four species (*S. dysenteriae*, *S. flexneri*, *S. boydii*, and *S. sonnei*) can cause *Shigella* encephalopathy; however, *S. dysenteriae* is toxin-mediated, whereas other species do not produce toxin but cause encephalopathy by inflammatory cytokines. Ekiri syndrome is a severe form of *Shigella* encephalopathy characterized by rapidly developing seizure and coma with only mild colitis.
9. What are the differential diagnoses for postmeningitic sequelae?
   a. Neurodegenerative disorder
   b. Hydrocephalus
   c. Malnutrition
   d. Demyelinating disorder
   e. Rett syndrome
   f. Tumors
   The rest of the discussion is mainly on meningitis and encephalitis.
10. *What is the etiology of acute pyogenic meningitis?
    Table 7.2 gives the causative agents of acute pyogenic meningitis.

_____ .

*Important question asked in the examination.

TABLE 7.2	Causative Agents of Acute Pyogenic Meningitis
Age Group	**Causative Organisms**
0–1 month	Early: Group B streptococci, *E. coli*, *Klebsiella* Late: *E. coli*, *Klebsiella*, *Enterobacter*, *Staphylococcus*
1–3 months	Most common, *Streptococcal pneumoniae*; second most common, meningococci; third most common, Hib; fourth most common, Gram-negative organism
3 months to 5 years	Pneumococci, meningococci, Hib
Older than 5 years	Pneumococci, meningococci
Immunocompromised	Gram-negative, fungal

11. What are the causes of aseptic meningitis?
    - Aseptic meningitis is cerebrospinal fluid (CSF) culture-negative for an organism but there are protein and sugar abnormalities.
    - Causes of aseptic meningitis
      A. Infectious causes
         a. Viruses: Enterovirus, arbovirus, measles, mumps, rubella, Cytomegalo virus (CMV) and Ebstein Barr virus (EBV)
         b. Bacteria: Mycobacterium Tuberculosis, *Bartonella*, *Brucella*, *Rickettsia*, *Mycoplasma*, and *Chlamydia*
         c. Fungi: *Coccidioides*, *Cryptococcus*, and *Candida*
         d. Parasites: *Angiostrongylus*, Gnathostomata, *Toxocara*, *Trichinella*, *Acanthamoeba*, and Plasmodium
      B. Postinfectious: Vaccine – rabies and influenza
      C. Demyelinating/allergic encephalitis
      D. Systemic/immunological mediated
      E. Malignancy
      F. Drugs: NSAIDs, carbamazepine, and antibiotics – ciprofloxacin
12. What are the risk factors for meningitis?
    Table 7.3 gives the risk factors associated with meningitis.
13. What is the pathophysiology behind bacterial meningitis?
    Pathophysiology
    1. Bacteremia
    2. Contiguous spread – mastoiditis, sinusitis, and orbital cellulitis
    3. Viral meningitis – increased permeability, perivascular cuffing, and necrosis
    4. Physiology of cerebral injury is due to toxins
14. What are the complications seen in meningitis?
    a. Increased Intra cranial pressure (ICP): Cerebral edema, hydrocephalus, subdural effusion, and secondary abscess formation
    b. Cerebral injury: Hypoxia, toxin, and cerebritis
    c. Hydrocephalus: Communicating, basal exudates (most common); noncommunicating, gliosis and fibrosis of aqueduct of Sylvius
    d. Focal neurological deficit
    e. Sensory neural deafness – more common with pneumococci and second Hib (mainly because of cochlear

TABLE 7.3	Risk Factors Associated With Meningitis
Risk Factors	**Features**
Host: a. Age	Young age group
b. Immunodeficiency	B cell: Bacteria T-cell defect: *Listeria* Terminal complement deficiency: Meningococci
c. Anatomical defect	Functional and anatomical asplenia
d. Malnutrition	Decreased immunity
e. Condition with CSF leak	1. CSF otorrheac 2. Vestibulocochlear fistula 3. Traumatic CSF leak 4. Lumbar dural sinus 5. CSF shunt
Agent	Organisms as mentioned previously
Environment	Overcrowding, poor socioeconomic status

CSF, cerebrospinal fluid.

infection and direct inflammation); deafness caused by another organism (not known)
f. Cranial nerve palsy
g. SIADH
h. Subdural effusion
i. Subdural/intracranial abscess
j. Stroke
k. Neurodevelopment impairment
l. Pericarditis, arthritis, and DIC – secondary to menin-gococcal meningitis

15. When should subdural effusion be suspected in a child with meningitis?
a. Increase in head size
b. Bulging AF
c. Signs of raised ICP
d. Seizures
e. Prolonged fever

16. *What is acute encephalitis syndrome (AES)?
Acute encephalitis syndrome is defined as a person of any age, at any time of year with the acute onset of fever and a change in mental status and/or new onset of seizures.

17. What are the causative organisms in acute encephalitis?
• Overall most common cause of viral meningoen-cephalitis: Enterovirus
• Second common cause: Human herpes virus (HSV type 1)
• Third common cause: Dengue
• Fourth common cause: Measles
• Fifth common cause: Mumps
• Sixth common cause: Chikungunya

18. Give examples of neurotropic viruses and their sites of involvement in the brain.
Neurotropic viruses
1. Rabies: Brainstem/spinal cord
2. Arbovirus: Japanese B encephalitis (JE) – basal ganglion
3. West Nile/dengue virus: Bilateral thalamus
4. Varicella: Cerebellum

19. What is the most common cause of sporadic encephalitis?
HSV type 1 is the most common cause of sporadic en-cephalitis.

20. What is the most common cause of chronic meningitis?
• Tubercular meningitis (TBM) is the most common cause of chronic meningitis.

21. What are the possible differentials when movement dis-order is associated with CNS infection?
• First: Viral encephalitis
• Second: Autoimmune encephalitis
• Third: TBM

22. How is JE infection confirmed?
• Laboratory-confirmed JE: A suspected case that has been lab confirmed (IgM JE-positive or JE PCR-positive)
• Probable JE: A suspected case that occurs in geo-graphic areas close to a lab-confirmed case of JE

23. What is the most common complication of mumps en-cephalitis?
Deafness caused by the nerve VIII involvement because of mumps encephalitis is the most common complica-tion. The second most common complication includes gonadal involvement (orchitis and oophoritis).

24. What is postmeningitic sequela?
It refers to a residual disability which persists after the termination of acute or subacute illness in a previ-ously normal child. Clinically, there should be no signs of acute infection (fever, meningeal signs). The exact duration of the sequela is arbitrary, usually 2–4 weeks.

25. What are the features of postmeningitic or postencepha-litic sequelae?
1. Intellectual impairment
2. Loss of acquired milestone
3. Motor weakness
4. Visual and hearing defects
5. Psychiatric manifestations
6. Epilepsy
7. Extrapyramidal movements

26. How can one differentiate between acute meningitis and acute encephalitis?
Usually, when a child presents in an acute condition, it is difficult to come to a conclusion; however, in acute meningitis, there is predominant cranial nerve in-volvement, focal deficit, and seizures, whereas in acute encephalitis, altered sensorium, extrapyramidal symp-toms, and rapid progression of the disease will be the predominant presentation.

27. *How can one differentiate between postmeningitic and postencephalitic syndromes?
Table 7.4 gives the differences between postmeningitic and postencephalitic syndromes.
Note: Hydrocephalus is not a complication of posten-cephalitis sequelae.

28. How is a child with suspected meningitis investigated?
a) To rule out bacteremia: CBC, CRP, and blood culture (blood culture positivity seen in 80%–90% of children)
b) Renal function test: Urea and creatinine elevated in a patient with hypotension
c) Serum electrolytes: Low sodium – SIADH
d) CSF analysis638910
e) Imaging

29. What are the indications for lumbar puncture to deter-mine acute CNS infection?
a. Any meningeal sign
b. Any fever with seizures <6 months

TABLE 7.4	Differences Between Postmeningitic and Postencephalitic Syndromes	
Features	Postmeningitic Syndrome	Postencephalitic Syndrome
Age	Any age Tubercular meningitis (TBM): Rare in children younger than 6 months	Any age
Onset	Acute: Bacterial Subacute and gradual: TBM	Acute and rapid
Seasonal variation/ epidemic	No	Yes
Hydrocephalus	Yes	No
Brain affected	Meninges, cranial nerve, cortex	Cerebellum, extrapyramidal system, hypothalamus
Optic atrophy/ multiple cranial nerve involvement	Yes	No
Mental retardation	Less common	More common
Behavioral problem	Less common	More common
Decerebrate/ decorticate rigidity	Less common	More common
Sequelae	Hydrocephalus Cranial nerve palsies	Minimal brain dysfunction ADHD Short attention span

c. Any febrile seizures within the duration of 6 months to 1 year in a patient whose vaccination status is not known or who is not immunized with Hib or pneumococcal vaccine

30. What are the indications for repeat lumbar puncture in a child diagnosed with acute CNS infection?
   a. Gram-negative meningitis
   b. Drug-resistant meningitis
   c. HSV PCR-positive to show a decrease in titer

31. What are the contraindications for lumbar puncture?
   1. Hemodynamic instability
   2. Suspected posterior fossa mass
   3. Impending herniation/midline shift in CT
   4. Raised ICP (to perform imaging before lumbar puncture)
   5. Skin infection in the local area
   6. Platelet count <20,000
   7. Any bleeding disorder

32. *What are the indications for imaging before performing a lumbar puncture?
   1. In an unconscious child
   2. Raised ICP itself not a contraindication but papilledema caused by supratentorial space-occupying lesion

33. *How is the cerebrospinal fluid (CSF) analyzed bedside following lumbar puncture?
   - CSF should be analyzed within 30 minutes of CSF tap.
   - There is a decrease in CSF neutrophils by 50% within 2 hours of collection.
   - Macroscopy: Check the opening pressure (using manometer), color, blood stain, turbidity, and cobweb coagulum formation.

- Microscopy: Take a drop of CSF and stain it with Leishman stain and look under a high-power microscope.
   1. Cells: Neutrophils and lymphocytes can be identified.
   2. Ameba with darting movement can be identified.
   3. Normal CSF:plasma glucose ratio is 0.7.
   4. Normal pH is 7.28–7.32.

34. What are the features of normal CSF?
   Normal CSF
   a) Clear and colorless
   b) Opening pressure: 50–175 mm Hg
   c) Specific gravity: 1.006–1.009
   d) Glucose: 40–80 mg/dL
   e) Total protein: 15–45 mg/dL
   f) Lactate: Less than 35 mg/dL
   g) CSF leukocytes (white blood cells): 0–5/mm^3 (adults and children); up to 30/mm^3 (newborns)
   h) Differential: 60%–80% lymphocytes; 30% monocytes; 2% other
   i) Gram stain: Negative and culture sterile
   j) No red blood cells
   k) Opening pressure
      - 250 mm H_2O: Intracranial pressure (nonobese)
      - >280 mm H_2O: Obese children
      - <60 mm H_2O: Intracranial hypotension
   l) Glucose: 60% peripheral blood glucose (because of enzymatic inhibition rather than actual bacterial consumption of the glucose)

35. Mention some differentials of lymphocytes in CSF in a child with meningitis.
   1. Viral meningitis
   2. TBM
   3. Autoimmune encephalitis
   4. Medicamentous (IVIG, INH)
   5. Carcinomatous
   6. Chemical
   7. Intrathecal methotrexate, anesthetic agent

36. What are the viruses that cause an increase# in polymorphonuclear neutrophils in CSF?
   1. Eastern equine encephalitis
   2. Lymphocytic choriomeningitis
   #Even early phase of viral encephalitis can have an increase in PMN.

37. What are the viruses that cause a decrease in sugar level in CSF?
   1. Mumps
   2. Lymphocytic meningitis
   3. HSV

38. What are the parameters that are altered in traumatic CSF tap?
   - Protein and glucose are altered.
   - Diagnosis is confirmed by Gram stain and culture is not altered.

39. *What are the CSF findings in a traumatic tap?
   To identify a traumatic tap, measure cell counts in three consecutive tubes of CSF. If the number of RBCs is relatively constant, then the count is attributed to a traumatic tap.
   In a traumatic tap, there is an artificial increase of WBCs in CSF (i.e., increase by 1 WBC in CSF for every 500–1000 RBCs in CSF). The correction factor is accurate as long as the peripheral WBC count is not extremely high or low. In addition, there is an increase

in 1 mg/dL of CSF protein for every 750 RBCs. Fig. 7.1A–C shows three consecutive samples of traumatic lumbar puncture.

40. How is CSF rhinorrhea identified?
    CSF rhinorrhea
    1. Clinitest or Dextrostix test
       If Dextrostix-positive, it is CSF.
    2. Beta-2 transferrin in CSF identified by electrophoresis indicates CSF rhinorrhea.
41. *How is blood-stained CSF identified?
    Target sign/halo sign: When CSF mixed with blood is collected on a tissue/filter paper, a central darker region is formed by blood and the peripheral lighter region is formed by CSF. This is called halo sign.
    Fig. 7.2 shows target sign.
42. What is the significance of CSF lactate?
    1. <25 mg/dL: Viral
    2. 25–35 mg/dL: TBM
    3. >35 mg/dL: Acute bacterial infection

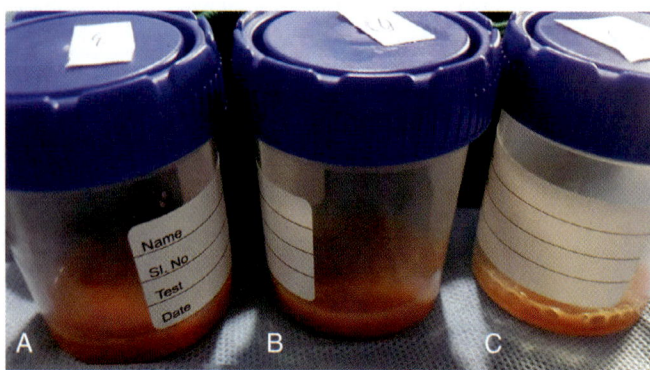

Fig. 7.1 (A–C) Clearing of hemorrhagic fluid from containers A to C suggestive of traumatic CSF tap.

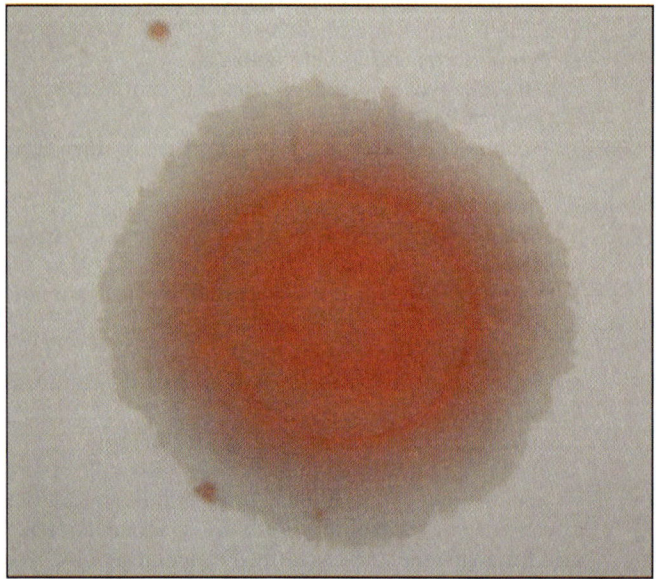

Fig. 7.2 Target sign – the central darker region is formed by blood and the peripheral lighter region is formed by CSF. (Source: Reproduced from Ravi Sunder, Kevin Tyler and Basal skull fracture and the halo sign, *CMAJ* 185(5): 416.)

43. What is the IgG index in CSF analysis?
    It is calculated as follows:

    $$\text{CSF IgG index} = \frac{\text{CSF IgG/serum IgG}}{\text{CSF albumin/serum albumin}}$$

    • Normal value, <0.7, indicates an intact blood–brain barrier (BBB).
    • Increase in CSF IgG without a concomitant increase in CSF albumin suggests local production of IgG which is seen in multiple sclerosis and SSPE.
44. What is the CSF albumin index?

    $$\text{CSF albumin index} = \text{CSF albumin (mg/dL)/} \\ \text{Serum albumin (g/dL)}$$

    A value <9 indicates intact BBB and there is no sign of CNS infection.
45. What are the other inflammatory markers of bacterial meningitis in CSF?
    1. CRP >100 mg/dL
    2. Increased TNF
    3. Increased interleukin-1
    4. Increased lactate
46. What are the CT/MRI findings in acute CNS infection?
    a) TBM: Basal exudates and communicating hydrocephalus
    b) Ring lesion: Tuberculoma and neurocysticercosis
    c) Focal ischemia
    d) Basal ganglia enhancement: Japanese encephalitis
    e) Frontotemporal hemorrhagic infarct: HSV encephalitis
    f) Brainstem involvement: Rabies encephalitis
47. What are the indications for repeat imaging in a child?
    1. Raised ICP or worsening of clinical condition
    2. To look for complication – hydrocephalus, subdural effusion, and abscess
48. How is a child with acute encephalitis syndrome managed?
    Table 7.5 gives the stepwise management in acute encephalitis syndrome.
49. What is the antibiotic dosage given in meningitis?
    • Ampicillin 300 mg/kg/day in three divided doses; maximum dose 8 g/day
    • Cefotaxime 300 mg/kg/day in three divided doses; maximum dose 12 g/day
    • Ceftriaxone 100 mg/kg/day b.d.; maximum dose 4 g/day
    • Vancomycin 60 mg/kg/day in three divided doses; maximum 4 g/day if pneumococci resistance >25% to third-generation cephalosporins in the population
50. How is HSV encephalitis treated?
    CSF HSV-positive: 21 days of i.v. acyclovir (newborn, 20 mg/kg/dose three times a day; or children, 10 mg/kg/dose t.d.s. or 400 mg/m²), every 8 hours till repeat CSF shows negative PCR
51. What are the other preferred antibiotics in a child with beta-lactam allergy?
    Vancomycin + rifampicin
52. *What is the role of corticosteroids in meningitis?
    a. Reduce the cytokine-mediated inflammatory cascade
    b. Reduce the edema formation
    c. Reduce the sensorineural hearing loss caused by Hib
53. What are the dose and duration of steroids in meningitis?
    • Dose: 0.15 mg/kg/dose every 6 hours for 48 hours given to all children with acute meningitis older than 6 weeks of age

TABLE 7.5	Management in Acute Encephalitis Syndrome
Steps	**Management**
Step 1 *Rapid assessment and stabilisation*	ABC (Maintain Airway, Breathing- oxygen if required, Circulation-fluid boluses, inotropes) Treat fever, hypothermia, Treat ongoing seizures (benzodiazepines followed by phenytoin) Identify signs of cerebral herniation and raised intracranial pressure (ICP)
Step 2 *Clinical evaluation*	History and examination
Step 3 *Investigations*	Blood/serum Cerebrospinal fluid MRI brain Throat or nasopharyngeal swab
Step 4 *Empirical treatment (if CSF cannot be done or patient is sick)*	Ceftriaxone and vancomycin (if streptococcal pneumonia organism prevalence in community >25%) Acyclovir (in suspected sporadic viral encephalitis) Artesunate (Stop if peripheral smear and RDT (rapid diagnostic test) are negative)
Step 5 *Supportive care*	Maintain hydration Euglycemia, Treat fever, Head end elevation 15 to 30 degree (in case of raised ICP) Treat seizures with anticonvulsants Steroids (Pulse dose) if Acute demyelinating encephalomyelitis (ADEM) is suspected
Step 6 *Prevention and treatment of complications*	*Complications:* Aspiration pneumonia, nosocomial infections, coagulation disturbances *Nutrition:* Early feeding *Physiotherapy*, postural change to prevent bed sores and exposure keratitis *Psychological* support to patient and family

- Maximum benefit: <1–2 hours before antibiotic initiation but may be effective if given concurrently or soon after the first dose

54. What is the total duration of antibiotics in different meningitides?
    1. Meningococci: 5–7 days
    2. *Haemophilus influenzae*: 7–10 days
    3. Pneumococci/pyogenic meningitis: 10–14 days
    4. Gram-negative bacilli: 3 or 2 weeks after CSF is sterile
    5. If no organism detected, and cell protein and glucose suggestive of meningitis (culture-negative bacilli): 7–10 days
    6. *Listeria*: 14–21 days

55. What are the clinical signs to assess the improvement in a child with meningitis?
    a. Decline in fever spikes
    b. Decrease in irritability/meningeal signs

56. What are the changes seen in CSF after the initiation of antibiotics?
    1. CSF becomes sterile in 24–48 hours.
    2. Protein and cell count does not change for 2–3 weeks.
    3. CSF sugar will become normal in 48–72 hours.

57. For a traumatic tap, 1 mg of protein can be reduced for how many RBCs?
    For a traumatic tap, 1 mg of protein can be reduced for 1000 RBCs.

58. Enumerate the CSF findings in various CNS infections. Table 7.6 gives the CSF findings in various CNS infections.

59. What are the drugs causing raised intracranial pressure? Withdrawal of drugs nalidixic acid, nitrofurantoin, and corticosteroids causes raised intracranial pressure

60. What are the endocrine causes of raised ICP? Hypothyroidism, hyperthyroidism, and hypoparathyroidism are the endocrine causes of raised ICP.

61. How is raised intracranial pressure managed?
    1. Head-end elevation to 25–30°
    2. Correction of hypoxia
    3. Controlled hyperventilation to maintain PCO_2 between 35 and 40 mm Hg
    4. Normothermia
    5. Euglycemia
    6. Sedation with barbiturates preferred – neuroprotective factors
    7. Seizure control
    8. Hyperosmolar treatment
       a. Mannitol 0.5–1 g/kg/dose t.d.s.
       b. Hypertonic saline 5 mL/kg/dose

62. How long should anticonvulsants be continued in a child with acute CNS infection?
    Duration of anticonvulsants
    - Only with acute CNS infection without any sequelae: 3 months
    - Any child with seizures with focal deficit or mental retardation or imaging abnormality: 2 years

63. What is the overall prognosis in acute CNS infection?
    1. Highest mortality for pneumococcal meningitis
    2. Poor prognosis – age <6 months
    3. Seizures beyond 4 days of disease onset
    4. Coma at presentation
    5. Focal signs at presentation
    6. Follow-up of a child with audiological screening

64. What are the preventive measures performed in meningococci meningitis and *Haemophilus influenzae* meningitis?
    a. Vaccine
    b. Prophylaxis: Drugs
       - Meningococci: Rifampicin 20 mg/kg/day in two divided doses for 2 days
       - *Haemophilus influenzae*: Rifampicin 20 mg/kg/day in two divided doses for 4 days

TABLE 7.6	CSF Findings in Various CNS Infections			
Condition	Leukocytes (mm³)	Protein (mg/dL)	Glucose (mg/dL)	Others
Normal	<5 lymphocytes	20–45	>50% or 75% of serum glucose	–
Acute bacterial meningitis[a]	100–10,000, PMNs predominate (turbid)	100–500	Decreased, usually <40% or 50% of serum glucose	Organism seen in Gram stain or culture
Partially treated meningitis	5–10,000, mononuclear cells predominate if treated for a prolonged period	100–500	Normal or decreased	CSF sterile The antigen can be detected by PCR
Viral meningoen-cephalitis	<1000 cells, mononuclear cells predominate	50–200	Normal	HSV encephalitis and enterovirus by PCR of CSF
TBM	10–500 PMNs early but lympho-cytes predominate throughout	100–3000	<50	*M. tuberculosis* detected by PCR of CSF or by culture of CSF
Fungal meningitis	5–500, mononuclear cells predominate	25–500	<50	Yeast: CSF Cryptococcal antigen: PCR

CNS, central nervous system; CSF, cerebrospinal fluid; TBM, tubercular meningitis.
[a]Amebic encephalitis similar to acute bacterial meningitis picture; mobile amebas are seen in CSF by hanging drop method.

FAQ ON TUBERCULAR MENINGITIS

65. What is the common age group in TB meningitis?
The most common age group is 9 months to 4 years.
66. What are the different forms of neurotuberculosis?
A. Intracranial
TBM
Tubercular encephalopathy
Tubercular vasculopathy
Space-occupying lesion:
a. Tuberculoma
b. Tubercular abscess
B. Spinal
1. Pott spine and Pott paraplegia
2. Tubercular arachnoiditis
3. Nonosseous spinal tuberculoma
4. Spinal meningitis
67. Enumerate the pathogenesis in Tuberculous meningitis (TBM).
• Rich and McCordock proposed the pathogenesis of CNS tuberculosis.
• Pathogenesis in TB meningitis
a. Hematogenous spread of TB from primary lesion by bacteremia to meninges causes the mycobacteria to multiply in Rich focus multiply in Rich focus.
b. Bacteria then enter a quiescent phase.
c. When a stimulus comes, such as Auto - immune response or trauma, it ruptures and clinical manifestations will appear.
68. Which is the common site involved in TB meningitis?
The most common site is the brainstem.
69. Which cranial nerve is more commonly involved in TBM?
The most common cranial nerve involved is cranial nerve VI.
70. Discuss the pathophysiology in TBM.
Flowchart 7.1 gives the pathophysiology in TBM.
71. What are the stages in TBM?
British Medical Council staging of TBM
• Stage 1: Prodromal stage – nonspecific and lasts for 2–3 weeks
• Stage 2: Meningeal irritation – signs of meningitis, cranial nerve palsy, raised intracranial pressure, and communicating hydrocephalus

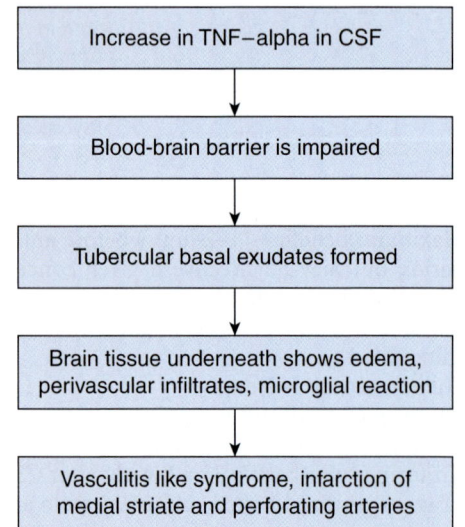

Flowchart 7.1 Pathophysiology in tubercular meningitis.

• Stage 3: Diffuse or local cerebral involvement – convulsion, coma, and paralysis
72. What is the most common seizure type seen in TBM?
The most common type of seizures in TBM is GTCS followed by focal followed by involuntary movements.
73. What is the ratio of incidence of TBM in BCG-vaccinated and unvaccinated children?
The ratio of occurrence of TBM in BCG-vaccinated and unvaccinated children is 1:3.
74. What are the complications seen in TBM?
1. Hydrocephalus (suspect when long time to recover, seizures not controlled with antiepileptic drugs, increasing head size, failure to improve, CSF pressure)
2. Infarct
3. Vasculitis
4. Adhesions – permanent cranial nerve involvement
75. What is the order of improvement in TBM?
The order of improvement is as follows:
• First: Regaining consciousness and control of convulsions

- Second: Focal/cranial nerve improvement
- Third: Decrease in CSF cell count and CSF protein

76. What are the sequelae of TB meningitis?
    1. Immediate sequelae: Hydrocephalus, thrombosis of cerebral vessels, TB arachnoiditis, and cranial nerve involvement
    2. Delayed sequelae: Hemiplegia, intellectual impairment, and optic atrophy

77. What are the CSF findings suggestive of TBM?
    a. CSF: Predominant lymphocytic reaction (60–400 white cells per mL)
    b. Protein 0.8–4 g/L
    c. CBNAAT sensitivity 40% but 80%–100% specific
    d. Smear acid-fast bacilli (AFB)-positive
    e. AFB culture and sensitivity

78. What does cobweb formation in TBM indicate and what is its significance?

    Coagulum formation (cobweb) is because of high fibrin and protein content in CSF. Allow the CSF sample to stand overnight and examine the sample in the morning for fibrin clot. The clot is delicate and it is because of marked rise in CSF protein. It may have entrapped tubercle bacilli which could be demonstrated microscopically by staining for acid-fast bacilli. Fig. 7.3 shows cobweb formation in TB meningitis.

79. What are the findings in CT brain in TBM?
    a. Exudates in the basal cistern or Sylvian fissure (spider leg appearance)
    b. Hydrocephalus
    c. Infarcts
    d. Gyral enhancement
    e. Tuberculoma – seen in 16% of cases

80. What is the significance of Mantoux and chest X-ray in TBM?
    - TST: Nonreactive in 50% of cases
    - CXR: Normal in 20%–50% of cases

81. What is the treatment for TBM?
    - CAT 1: All new cases

Intensive phase (daily regime): 6 months – HRZE + continuation phase HRE
    H: Isoniazid
    R: Rifampicin
    Z: Pyrazinamide
    E: Ethambutol

82. What is the total duration of TBM treatment?
    - Intensive phase: No extension
    - Continuation phase: Can extend up to 12 months

83. What is the role of steroids in TBM?
    Steroids improve the survival rate and neurological outcome.

84. What is the dose of steroids used in TBM?
    T. prednisolone 2–4 mg/kg/day for 4 weeks, tapered over 1–2 weeks

85. What are the neurological complications of anti-tuberculosis drugs (ATT)?
    Complications of the drugs
    1. Ethambutol: Optic neuritis
    2. Streptomycin: Sensory neural deafness

86. *What is paradoxical phenomenon in TBM?
    When the child is started on ATT and the compliance is good, after improvement for the initial 10 days, the child later will have worsening of symptoms because of immune reconstitution inflammatory syndrome (IRIS) and this is called paradoxical phenomenon in TBM.

87. What is IRIS?
    IRIS is due to disordered immune recovery leading to a dysregulated immune response to an antigen and resultant exaggerated inflammatory features within a milieu of proinflammatory cytokines.

88. *How can one differentiate between pyogenic meningitis and TBM?
    Table 7.7 gives the differences between pyogenic meningitis and TBM.

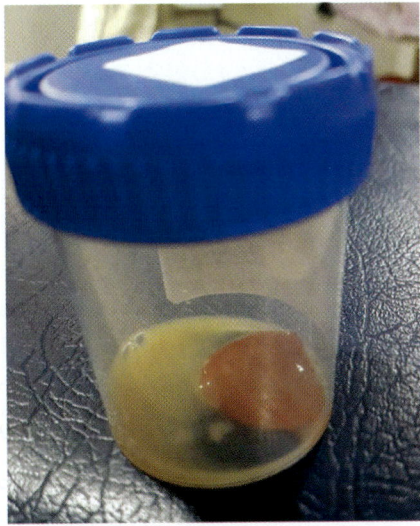

Fig. 7.3 Cobweb formation in TB meningitis in CSF.

TABLE 7.7	Differences Between Pyogenic Meningitis and Tubercular Meningitis	
Features	**Pyogenic Meningitis**	**Tubercular Meningitis**
History		
Onset	Acute	Chronic
Altered sensorium/seizures	May be present	More common
Fever	High grade	Low grade
Clinical features		
Focal deficit	Less common	More common
Cranial nerve involvement	Less common	2, 3, 4, 6, and 7 more involved
CSF		
Appearance	Purulent	Straw colored
Predominant cell	Neutrophils	Lymphocytes
Protein	40–60 mg/dL	>60 mg/dL
Globulins (normal beta-globulin > gamma-globulin)	Normal	Gamma-globulin > beta-globulin
LDH	Isozyme 5 increased	Isozyme 3 increased
Chloride	Normal – mild increase	Decreased because of vomiting
Magnesium	CSF > serum level	CSF = serum level
Complications Hydrocephalus	+	++++

CSF, cerebrospinal fluid.

89. What are the differences between tuberculoma and neurocysticercosis?

    Table 7.8 gives the differences between tuberculoma and neurocysticercosis.

90. Mention the salient features of HSV encephalitis.
    a) Focal seizures/focal deficit
    b) Speech and language impairment
    c) CSF: RBC in CSF
    d) Predominant mononuclear cell
    e) MRI: Temporal lobe abnormalities/frontotemporal hemorrhagic infarct
    f) EEG: PLEDS/bilateral independent periodic lateralizing epileptiform discharges (BiPLEDS) in EEG – HSV encephalitis
    g) Increase in mortality by 75% if not treated with acyclovir
    h) Recurrence: 45%
    i) Sequelae: Behavioral problems
    j) Can trigger autoimmune encephalitis

91. Mention few important features of Japanese encephalitis.
    • Japanese encephalitis
       a. Zoonotic disease
       b. Natural host: Amplifier host
       c. Reservoir: Birds
       d. Vector: *Culex tritaeniorhynchus*
       e. Stages
          Stage 1: Prodromal illness (2–3 days)
          Stage 2: Acute stage (3–4 days)
          Stage 3: Subacute stage (7–10 days)
          Stage 4: Convalescence (4–7 weeks)

    f. Characteristic features: Altered level of consciousness, rapid progression, and rapidly changing CNS features (hyperreflexia followed by hyporeflexia/plantar that changes)
    g. CSF: Mild pleocytosis
    h. Case fatality rate: 24%–42%
    i. Prognosis
       Recovery: 1/3
       Sequelae: 1/3
       Death: 1/3

92. Enumerate some features of brain abscess.
    • Age group: 4–8 years
    • Causes: Embolization from congenital heart disease (right-to-left shunt), endocarditis, meningitis, chronic otitis media, mastoiditis, sinusitis, and orbital cellulitis
    • Most common organism: *Streptococcus milleri* group
    • CSF: Sterile (WBC and protein can be mildly elevated)
    • MRI: Diagnostic of choice – ring-enhancing lesion on contrast
    • Empirical: Vancomycin, metronidazole, and third-generation cephalosporins used for 4–6 weeks
    • No need for surgery if:
       ○ Abscess size <2 cm
       ○ Short duration, <2 weeks
       ○ No signs of ICP
       ○ Child neurologically intact
    • Surgery indicated if:
       ○ Encapsulated capsule
       ○ Abscess size >2.5 cm
       ○ Signs of raised ICP
       ○ Multiloculated/location in the posterior fossa

TABLE 7.8	Differences Between Tuberculoma and Neurocysticercosis	
Features	**Tuberculoma**	**Neurocysticercosis**
Causative organism	*Mycobacterium tuberculosis*	*Taenia solium*
Size	>2 cm	<2 cm
Number	Multiple	Mostly single or multiple
Wall thickness	Thick walled	Thin walled
Calcification	Yes	No
Edema	Less	More
Location	Posterior fossa infratentorial	Gray–white matter junction
CNS features	Meningitis/cranial involvement+	Focal seizures
T2 MRI	Hypointensity with surrounding enhancement (ring-enhancing lesion) Midline shift	Hyperintensity with hypointense scolex Ring enhancement depends on the stages of NCC Escobar's pathological stages 1. Vesicular: Viable parasite with intact membrane, therefore no host reaction 2. Colloidal vesicular: Parasite dies within 4–5 years, cyst fluid turbid (symptomatic stage) 3. Granular nodular: Edema decreases, cyst retracts 4. Nodular calcified: End stage/quiescent, no edema
MRS	Lipid peak	Amino acid peak (decreased *N*-acetylaspartate) Increased choline:creatinine ratio >1
Treatment	CAT 1: ATT – HRZE + HRE, can extend up to 12 months T. prednisolone: 1–2 mg/kg/day 4–6 weeks and taper	Before starting treatment, get ophthalmological evaluation performed to rule out cysticercus in the eye; when albendazole is started, live scolex die and produce an inflammatory reaction and can cause optic neuritis and blindness Prior to albendazole, give steroids for 3 days and start on albendazole dose 15 mg/kg/day in two divided doses for 28 days

CNS, central nervous system.

93. What are the salient features of eosinophilic meningitis?
    a) Ten or more eosinophils per cubic millimeter
    b) Organisms: *Angiostrongylus cantonensis* and *Gnathostoma spinigerum*
    c) Fever, peripheral eosinophilia, vomiting, and creeping skin eruption
    d) Treatment: Only supportive
    e) Prognosis good (70% of patients recover without sequelae)
94. Enumerate some features of autoimmune encephalitis.
    a. Most common age: Younger than 1 year to adults
    b. In children older than 12 years, 80% females; younger than 2 years, 40% boys
    c. Prototype: Anti-NMDA receptor antibodies; other types, anti-VGKC antibodies and limbic encephalitis
    d. Causes: Precipitating event, infection/postinfection; most common, *Mycobacterium*, HSV 1 and 2, and influenza
    e. Clinical features
       a. Orofacial dyskinesia
       b. Psychiatric manifestations
       c. Autonomic dysregulation
    d. Language and social behavior affected
    f. Abnormal movement – choreoathetoid movement
    g. Diagnosis
       a. MRI brain: Nonspecific
       b. CSF pleocytosis and increase in protein
       c. EEG: Extreme delta brush
    h. Definitive: CSF 85% and serum anti-NMDA receptor antibody 100% sensitive
    i. Management as given in Table 7.9

TABLE 7.9	Management in Autoimmune Encephalitis	
First Line		**Second Line**
1. I.v. methylprednisolone 30 mg/kg 3–5 days + 2. IVIG 2 g/kg – 2 days; taper 1–2 mg/kg – 6–12 weeks (combined methylprednisolone + IVIG)		1. Rituximab/plasmapheresis if no or partial improvement 2. Refractory or severe cases: I.v. pulse cyclophosphamide three to four cycles monthly 3. Concurrent treatment: Status epilepticus/psychosis

Quick Bites

- For every 750 RBCs in CSF, there is 1 mg/dL rise in protein in CSF.
- For every 500–1000 RBCs in CSF, there is an increase by 1 WBC in CSF.
- Cobweb formation is seen in TBM.
- The most common cause of viral meningoencephalitis is enterovirus.
- The most common cause of sporadic encephalitis is HSV type 1.
- Rich and McCordock proposed the pathogenesis of central nervous system tuberculosis.

Paraplegia

Introduce yourself before history elicitation, get permission from the caregiver, and identify the case.

Name____Age____Sex____Consanguinity____Order of birth____Place____Informant____

Presenting Complaints and Duration

- Weakness/refusal to stand or walk
- Gait disturbances
- Sensory deficits
- Loss of bladder or bowel control

History of Presenting Illness

WEAKNESS

- Onset: Acute (minutes to hours)/subacute (days to months)/chronic (3 or more months)
- Progression: Rapidly progressive/slowly progressive/nonprogressive/gradually improving
- Distribution: Limbs involved, symmetrical/asymmetrical, ascending/descending, and proximal/distal
- Whether associated with history suggestive of hypertonia (feeling of tightness)/hypotonia (feeling of slipping through fingers)/changes in tone

GAIT DISTURBANCES

- Clumsiness of gait
- Limping
- Crossing of legs (scissoring) while walking
- Toe walking
- Frequent falls

SENSORY DEFICITS

- Hyperesthesia/paresthesia (numbness/tingling/pins and needles)
- Numbness in the lower limbs
- Numbness in the perineum
- Ability to appreciate cold and warm objects
- Trophic ulcers
- Whether dissociative anesthesia present (pain and temperature lost and touch is preserved)
- Sharp/shooting pain/pricking with pins and needles/radiating down a limb or trunk exacerbated by coughing/sneezing/straining (Suggestive of root or radicular pain)

BLADDER/BOWEL DISTURBANCES

- Whether able to appreciate sense of bladder filling
- Urgency/increased frequency
- Hesitancy/overflow incontinence/urinary retention
- Urinary retention – painful/painless
- Bowel – constipation/incontinence

- Whether catheterized or requires clean intermittent catheterization.

CENTRAL NERVOUS SYSTEM HISTORY

Higher Function History

Altered sensorium, seizures, speech, early handedness, and behavior or sleep disturbance

History for Cranial Nerve Involvement

- Ability to perceive and differentiate smell
- Ability to perceive light
- Any history of drooping of eyelids, ability to move eyeballs in all four directions, or restriction of eyeball movement
- Ability to chew food and difficulty in opening the jaw
- Ability to close eyes while sleeping, drooling of saliva, deviation of angle of the mouth, lack of facial expression/frowning, and facial asymmetry
- Ability to hear and respond to sound.
- History of nasal twang of voice, nasal regurgitation, choking while feeding, weak cry, and difficulty in swallowing
- Ability to move the head side to side and shrugging of shoulder
- Abnormal movement or twitching in the tongue

Motor System

- Posture
- Thinning of muscles as noted by the mother on both lower limbs
- Ability to turn to side while lying/ability to get up from lying to sitting position
- Ability to get up from sitting to standing position
- Ability to raise the arm above the shoulder/buttoning shirt or mixing food with fingers/ability to wear slippers without difficulty
- Abnormal/involuntary movement

Cerebellar Involvement

Abnormal or involuntary movement/slurring of speech/frequent falls/incoordination of movements/abnormal movements of eyes, past pointing, and ataxic or broad-based gait

Bladder/Bowel Disturbance

Urinary incontinence or dribbling and constipation

Autonomic Nervous System

Abnormal sweating/postural hypotension/bladder and bowel disturbances (as discussed earlier)

Sensory Features

History of perception of pain or crying while giving vaccination, and perception of touch and temperature variation

Spine and Cranium

- Any abnormality in the head size noted by the mother compared with in sibling or peers
- Any swelling, tuft of hair, sinus, discharge, and abnormal curvature

COMPLICATION HISTORY

- History of recurrent urinary tract infection
- Constipation or fecal impaction
- Contractures
- Foot deformities
- Bed sores
- Mobile/immobilized
- Inability to perform activities of daily living – by self or requires help

ETIOLOGICAL HISTORY

- Falls/road traffic accident/child abuse
- Loose stools or viral upper respiratory illness prior to weakness
- High-grade fever/back pain
- History suggestive of root pain
- Chronic back pain without fever
- Swelling in the back/discharge/hair along the back
- Low-grade fever/cough >2 weeks, weight loss, back pain, weakness, and family history of tuberculosis
- Viral fever and vaccination history
- Loss of vision
- Rashes over the face/rash in a dermatomal pattern
- Ingestion of poison/insect bite
- Failure to thrive/chronic vomiting/diarrhea/skin hyperpigmentation
- Birth trauma/history of prematurity/umbilical artery catheterization
- Family history of progressive paraplegia

Past History

Look for the history of tuberculosis/similar complaints in the past/seizures/surgery.

Antenatal/Neonatal/Postnatal History

History suggestive of antenatal insult to the brain/investigations in favor of open neural tube defects/folic acid intake/preterm delivery/birth trauma/suggestive of hypoxic ischemic encephalopathy/NICU stay/umbilical artery catheterization

Developmental History

Check whether only motor developmental delay is present or other domains are also affected.

Dietetic History

Determine whether any protein–calorie gap is present. Check for the presence of evidence of malnutrition. Check how feeding is done – by self/through nasogastric tube/Percutaneous endoscopy gastrostomy. Ask what the consistency of feeds is.

Immunization History

Check whether vaccination up to date.

Family History

Look for the history of tuberculosis/progressive spastic paraplegia in other family members.

Treatment History

Confirm whether undergoing any physiotherapy/taking any medications for the spasticity.

Socioeconomic History

Note the socioeconomic class and per capita income.

Summary

Miss/Master _____, aged _____, _____ born to consanguineous/nonconsanguineous marriage, is brought with history of weakness of lower limbs since _____, rapidly/slowly/nonprogressive, with/without gait disturbances, with/without sensory disturbances, with/without root/radicular pain, with/without bowel or bladder disturbances, with/without cranial nerve (CN) involvement, with/without other CNS involvement with the etiological history suggestive of _____, and with/without any complications and functional status.

General Examination

Posture of the child and nutritional status
Pallor/icterus/clubbing/cyanosis/lymphadenopathy/edema

Head-to-Foot Examination

Head: Shape/dysmorphic/plagiocephaly/anterior fontanelle
Face: Dysmorphism
Eye: Optic neuritis/telangiectasia/signs of malnutrition or vitamin deficiency
Chest: Chest deformities/paradoxical respiration
Skin: Café au lait/neurofibromas/BCG scar/trophic ulcers/bed sores/Mantoux test
Limbs: Foot deformities/pes cavus (foreshortening of the foot)/stunted growth of limbs
Spinal myoclonus (dermatomal distribution)
Anus: Patulous anus

Anthropometry

Weight, height/length, weight for height/BMI, head circumference, Mid Upper Arm Circumference (MUAC), and chest circumference (last three in patients younger than 5 years)

Vital Signs

Temperature, pulse rate, respiratory rate (important for ruling out any respiratory muscle involvement), blood pressure (to look for postural hypotension), and SpO_2

CNS Examination

HIGHER FUNCTIONS

Look for COSSHMIB (mnemonic):

C: Consciousness – recognizes the mother

O: Orientation – interacts with the examiner and orients to time, place, and person

S: Sleep

S: Speech and language

H: Handedness (just hold a toy in front of one hand at a time and see with which hand he or she reaches for the toy)

M: Memory – by asking a simple question (what food the child had for breakfast, what the last night's dinner was, and what the child's father's name and home address are)

I: Intelligence quotient

B: Behavior – any aggressiveness/sleep disturbance

CRANIAL NERVES

CN I: Tell that CN I could not be tested if the child is younger than 5 years; if the child is older than 5 years, test for olfactory nerve by using familiar smells with eyes closed and ensuring that there is no nasal block

CN II: Six points:

A. Light perception

B. Visual acuity

C. Color vision

D. Field of vision

E. Direct and consensual light reflex

F. Fundus – choroid tubercles

CN III, IV, and VI: Check the movement of eyeballs in all four cardinal directions, strabismus, and ptosis

CN V: Check the ability to perceive pain sensation over the face, ability to chew food, and jaw jerk

CN VII

- Check whether the ability to wrinkle the forehead is present
- Check whether the child is able to close eyes on both sides while sleeping
- Check whether there is absence of nasolabial fold on the affected side
- Check the deviation of the angle of the mouth to the normal side
- Check whether drooling of saliva is present

CN VIII: Check the ability to obey the mother's command and respond to the mother's call, and response to sound (age appropriate)

CN IX and X: Check the palatal movement (normal), uvula in the midline, palatal arches (normal), and palatal and pharyngeal reflexes (normal)

CN XI: Check the ability to lift the head from a supine position and ability to turn the head on both sides

CN XII: Look for any deviation of the tongue, fibrillation, or wasting

MOTOR SYSTEM

1. Posture: Flexion in the hips and knees and dorsiflexion of both feet
2. Bulk: May be atrophied in lower limbs
3. Tone: Hypertonia present in lower limbs in spastic paraplegia/flaccid in spinal shock
4. Power: Decreased in both lower limbs
5. Reflexes
   - Superficial reflex: Normal
   - Deep tendon reflex: Exaggerated deep tendon reflexes in spastic paraplegia/diminished or absent in spinal shock.

EXTRAPYRAMIDAL SYSTEM

- Abnormal movement present or not
- Coordination of movements
- Gait abnormality

SENSORY SYSTEM

Assess on both sides and compare; repeat according to dermatomal segment to comment on the level of involvement. Sensory examination is very important in a patient with paraplegia; hence, keep practicing.

Superficial Sensations (Lateral Spinothalamic Tract)

- Light touch
- Pain
- Temperature

Deep Sensations (Posterior Column)

- Proprioception
- Vibration (use 128 Hz)
- Sense of joint position
- Deep pain
- Romberg sign

Cortical Sensations

- Two-point discrimination
- Stereognosis
- Graphesthesia
- Sensory inattention

CEREBELLAR SIGNS

Assess for coordination of movements as well as involuntary movements including titubation, nystagmus, dysarthria, dysmetria, dysdiadochokinesia, rebound phenomenon, hypotonia, pendular knee jerk, and ataxia.

AUTONOMIC NERVOUS SYSTEM

Abnormal areas of sweating/generalized flushing

Blood pressure measured in supine position and in sitting/standing position (postural hypotension)

SPINE AND CRANIUM

Vertebral defects: Kyphosis/scoliosis/gibbus

Neurocutaneous markers: Café au lait spot and neurofibromas

Tuft of hair, sinus opening, mass, pigmentation, and capillary hemangioma

Palpable bladder and anal sphincter: Assess the tone

Craniovertebral anomalies

MENINGEAL SIGNS

Neck stiffness, Kernig sign, and Brudzinski sign

Other Systems

RESPIRATORY

Chest expansion/respiratory muscle involvement/features suggestive of tuberculosis

CARDIOVASCULAR

Murmur, cardiomegaly, and features of congestive cardiac failure

ABDOMEN

Determine whether any hepatosplenomegaly is present. Palpate the bladder, and check whether it is catheterized.

MUSCULOSKELETAL SYSTEM

Especially vertebrae – any deformity

Diagnosis

A child with the following:
- Lower motor neuron dysfunction
- Paraparesis/paraplegia
- Acute, subacute, or insidious (slowly progressive)
- Anatomical level (vertical level) – vertebral level, sensory level, motor level, and reflex
- Location of the lesion (horizontal level) – intramedullary or extramedullary (whether extradural or intradural)
- Etiology (compressive/demyelination/infective/vascular/congenital/others)
- Complications
- Functional classification
- Nutritional status and other comorbid conditions – anemia and vitamin deficiency if any

Frequently Asked Questions

1. Define paraplegia.

   Weakness or paralysis of both the lower limbs, possibly the trunk, without involvement of the upper limbs.

2. Enumerate the classification of paraplegia.

   Flowchart 8.1 shows the classification of paraplegia.

3. *What are the differential diagnoses for spinal paraplegia?

   Table 8.1 gives the differential diagnoses for spinal paraplegia.

4. Give examples of intracranial causes of paraplegia.

   Hydrocephalus, parasagittal meningioma, sagittal sinus thrombosis, unpaired anterior cerebral artery occlusion, acute demyelination, cerebral palsy, brain tumor, and multiple sclerosis.

5. What does the clumsiness of gait suggest about the onset of paraplegia?

   It is the feature of a slowly progressive disorder. On the other hand, refusal to stand or walk is suggestive of an acute process.

6. List the significance of the onset of the disease to identify the etiology in paraplegia.

   Flowchart 8.2 shows the differential diagnosis of paraplegia according to the onset of the disease.

7. Which viral infections and vaccines can act as triggers in demyelinating disorders?
   - Viral infections: Influenza, Epstein–Barr virus, cytomegalovirus, varicella, enterovirus, measles, mumps,

---

*indicates important questions asked in examination

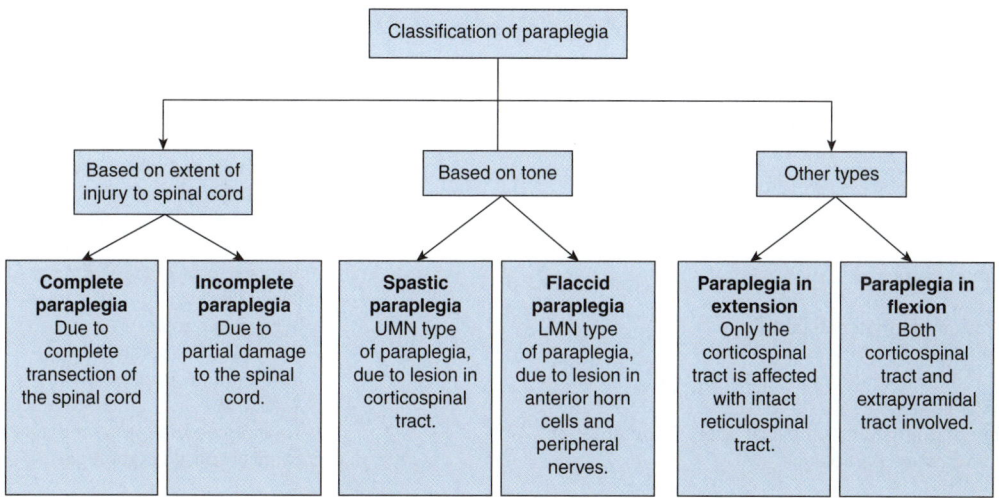

Flowchart 8.1 Classification of paraplegia.

TABLE 8.1	**Differential Diagnoses for Spinal Paraplegia**					
Compressive		**Demyelination**	**Infection**	**Vascular**	**Congenital**	**Others**
EXTRADURAL		• Transverse my-elitis	• Tuberculosis	• Cord infarction	• Myelomenin-gocele	**DEGENERATION**
• Trauma (concussion, epidural hematoma, fracture dislocation)		• Devic disease	• Discitis	• Spinal artery occlusion	• Tethered cord	• Spinocerebellar ataxia
• Gibbus		• Multiple scle-rosis	• Polio	• Dissecting aneurysm	• AV malforma-tion	• Familial spastic paraplegia
• Disk prolapse		• Encephalomy-elitis	• Herpes zos-ter myelitis	of aorta	• Arachnoid cyst	• Motor neuron disease
• Metastasis				• Bleeding AVM	• Atlantoaxial dislocation	**METABOLIC**
• Epidural abscess					• Caudal regres-sion syndrome	• Adrenoleukodys-trophy
INTRADURAL					• Chiari malfor-mation	• Argininemia
Extramedullary	**Intramedullary**					• Krabbe disease Toxic Immunological (post-vaccine)
• Schwannoma	• Primary cord Neoplasms					Physical (electro-cution and irradiation)
• Neurofibroma	• Syringomyelia					Nutritional (vitamin B12 deficiency)
• Meningioma	• Hematomyelia					
• AV malforma-tions						

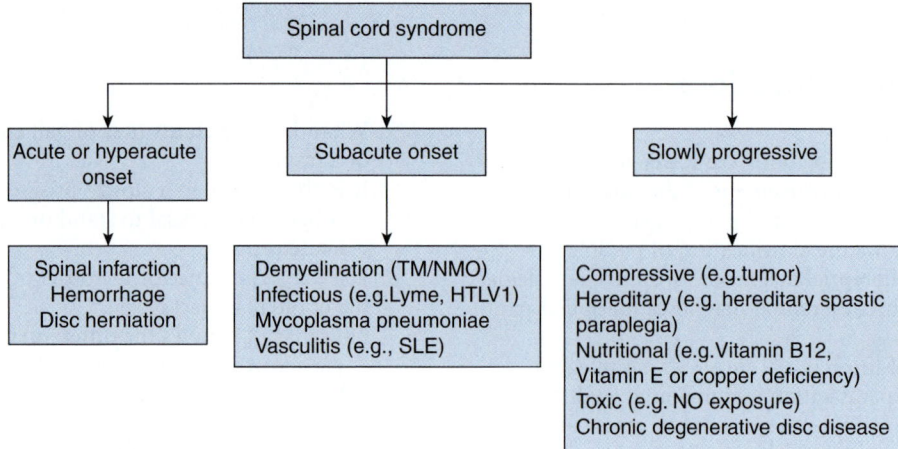

Flowchart 8.2 Differential diagnosis of paraplegia according to onset of disease.

TABLE 8.2	Significance of Etiological History in Paraplegia
History	**Etiology**
Falls, road traffic accident/child abuse	Trauma
Loose stools or viral upper respiratory illness prior to weakness	Acute demyelinating neuropathy
High-grade fever/back pain	Epidural abscess/diskitis
History suggestive of root pain	Epidural lesions
Chronic back pain without fever	Arachnoid cysts/AV malformations
Swelling in the back/discharge/hair along the back	Spinal dysraphism
Low-grade fever/cough >2 weeks, weight loss, back pain, weakness, family history of tuberculosis	Pott spine, tuberculous osteomyelitis of spine
Viral fever, vaccination history	Transverse myelitis/ADEM
Loss of vision	Devic disease
Rashes over face/rash in dermatomal pattern	SLE/herpes zoster
Ingestion of poison/insect bite	Lathyrism/tick paralysis
Failure to thrive/chronic vomiting/diarrhea/skin hyperpigmentation	IEM/immunosuppression
Past history of similar complaints	ADEM/MS
Birth trauma/history of prematurity/umbilical artery catheterization	Trauma/cerebral palsy/neonatal cord infarction
Family history of progressive paraplegia	Familial spastic paraplegia

rubella, herpes simplex, and other organisms, e.g., *Mycoplasma pneumoniae.*
- Vaccines: Rabies, smallpox, measles, mumps, rubella, Japanese encephalitis B, pertussis, diphtheria, polio, tetanus, and influenza.

8. *List the significance of etiological history in paraplegia. Table 8.2 gives the significance of etiological history in paraplegia.

9. What is the importance of CN examination in paraplegia?
   - CN II affected in Devic disease
   - CN VII affected in Guillain–Barré syndrome
   - CN X/XI/XII affected in high cervical cord lesion

10. What are the causes of spastic paraplegia?
   - Congenital causes: Cerebral palsy and Chiari malformation
   - Trauma: Spinal cord transection
   - Degenerative disorders: Devic disease
   - Hereditary disorders: Familial spastic paraplegia, adrenoleukodystrophy, Krabbe disease, Pelizaeus–Merzbacher disease, and Sjögren–Larsson syndrome
   - Compressive lesions of the spinal cord
   - Infectious disorders
   - Poisoning: Lathyrism

11. What is the posture of the lower limbs in a child with spastic paraplegia?
   There occurs flexion in the hips and knees and dorsiflexion of both feet (the resultant posture seems like crouching). Occasionally extreme spastic extension is seen at the knees and feet typically in an equinovarus posture.

12. Describe the gait seen in spastic paraplegia.
   - Infants: Scissoring gait (because of increased adductor tone)
   - Slow, short steps, and toes scuffed with each step ahead
   - Weight deliberately shifted from one foot to another (because the patient is unstable)

13. What are the features of a spinal cord disorder?
   Clear-cut sensory and motor levels, mixed upper motor neuron (UMN) and LMN findings, and bladder or bowel involvement

14. Name some spinal cord disorders associated with scoliosis.

These include neural tube defects, spinal cord tumors, degenerative disorders, and weakness of paraspinal muscles of one side. If scoliosis is seen in girls before puberty or boys at any age, it should raise the suspicion of a spinal cord disorder or a neuromuscular disease.

15. What is the difference between paraplegia in flexion and paraplegia in extension?
    - *Paraplegia in flexion:* It is more seen in complete lesion of the spinal cord, higher level of lesion, and prolonged fixation of the paralyzed limb in adduction and flexion. Both pyramidal tract and extrapyramidal tract are involved; therefore, there is increased tone in flexors than in extensors.
    - *Paraplegia in extension:* It is more seen in incomplete lesions of the spinal cord, lower level of spinal lesion, and elimination of nociceptive stimuli. Only the pyramidal tract is involved with an intact extrapyramidal tract; hence, tone is increased in antigravity muscles.

16. What is spinal myoclonus and its significance?

Spinal myoclonus refers to brief and irregular contractions of a small group of muscles that persist even during sleep. It occurs in the dermatome affected, thereby helping to localize the site of lesion.

Cause includes irritation of motor neurons and interneurons by the lesion.

17. What is hereditary spastic paraplegia and its mode of inheritance?

Hereditary spastic paraplegia is a heterogeneous group of genetic disorders with the predominant presentation being progressive spastic paraplegia.

Inheritance is as follows: autosomal dominant, 70%; and autosomal recessive, 25%.

TABLE 8.3	Differences Between Compressive Lesions and Noncompressive Lesions	
Features	Compressive Lesions	Noncompressive Lesions
Onset	Subacute/slowly progressive	Acute
Symmetry	Asymmetrical	Symmetrical
Bladder and bowel involvement	Early	Late
Root pain	Present	Absent
Zone of hyperesthesia	Present	Absent, may be present in transverse myelitis
Upper level of sensory loss	Present	Absent, may be present in transverse myelitis
Flexor spasm	Present	Absent

18. How can one differentiate between compressive lesions and noncompressive lesions?

Table 8.3 gives the differences between compressive lesions and noncompressive lesions.

19. *Trace the ascending sensory tracts with the help of a diagram.

Fig. 8.1 gives the cut section of spinal cord showing the ascending tracts.

Table 8.4 gives the ascending sensory tracts with the respective sensations.

Fig. 8.2 shows the spinothalamic tract.

Fig. 8.3 shows the posterior column tract and Fig. 8.4 shows the spinocerebellar tract.

20. *How is the lesion in paraplegia localized?

Fig. 8.5 shows the localization of lesion in paraplegia.

Presentation according to level of involvement

Table 8.5 gives the clinical features of paraplegia according to the level of involvement.

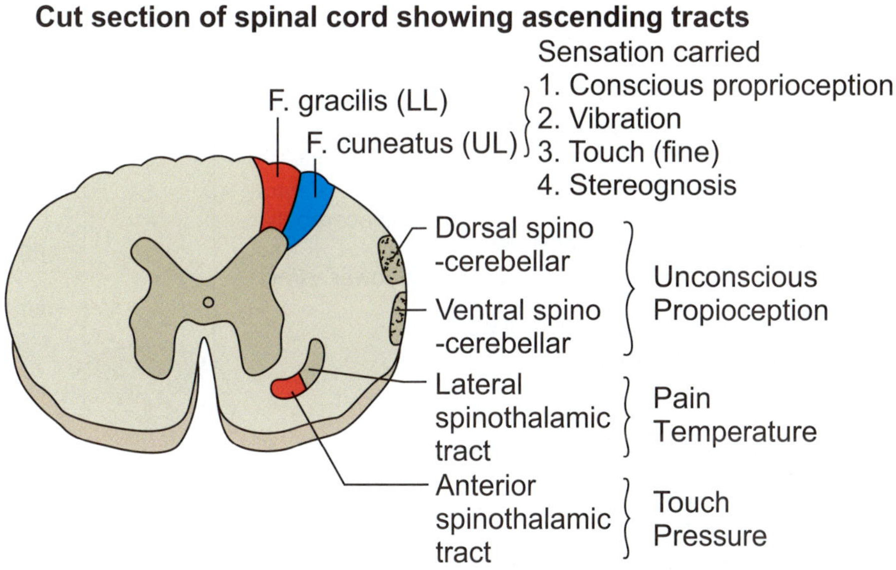

Cut section of spinal cord showing ascending tracts

Fig. 8.1 Cut section of spinal cord showing the ascending tracts.

TABLE 8.4	Ascending Sensory Tracts With the Respective Sensations	
Ascending Sensory Tracts	**Sensation Carried**	
Anterior spinothalamic tract	Touch, pressure	
Lateral spinothalamic tract	Pain, temperature	
Dorsal/posterior column tract	Conscious proprioception, vibration, fine touch, stereognosis	
Spinocerebellar tracts	Unconscious proprioception except for upper limb	
Cuneocerebellar pathway (through the fasciculus cuneatus of the posterior column)	Unconscious proprioception for upper limb	

Posterior column tract

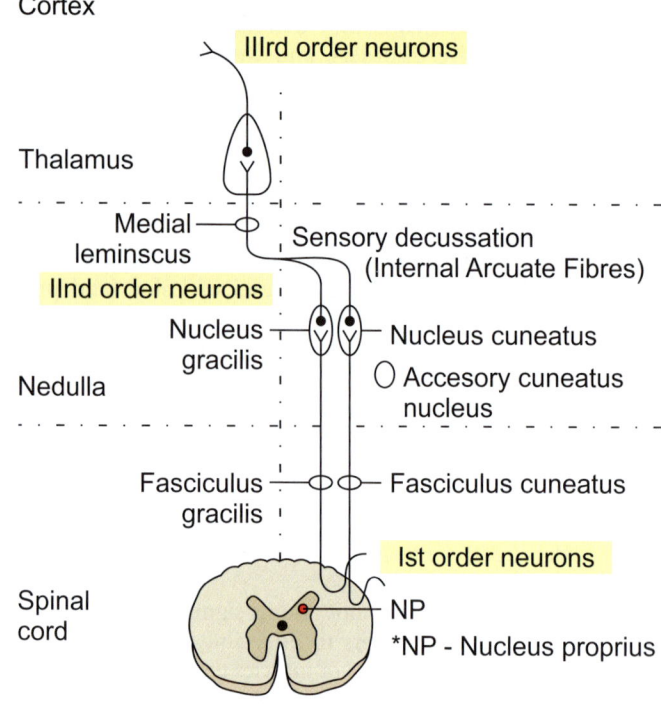

Fig. 8.3 Posterior column tract.

Spinothalamic tract

Anterior ST tract: Touch and pressure
Lateral ST tract: Pain and temperature

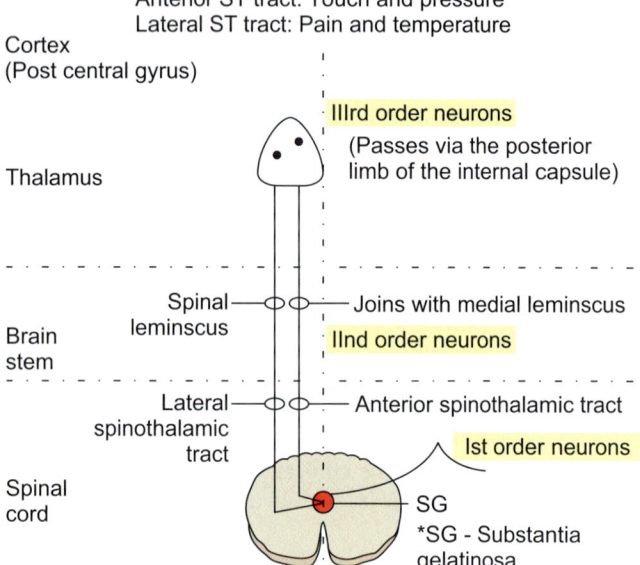

Fig. 8.2 Spinothalamic tract.

Spinocerebellar tract (Unconscious proprioception)

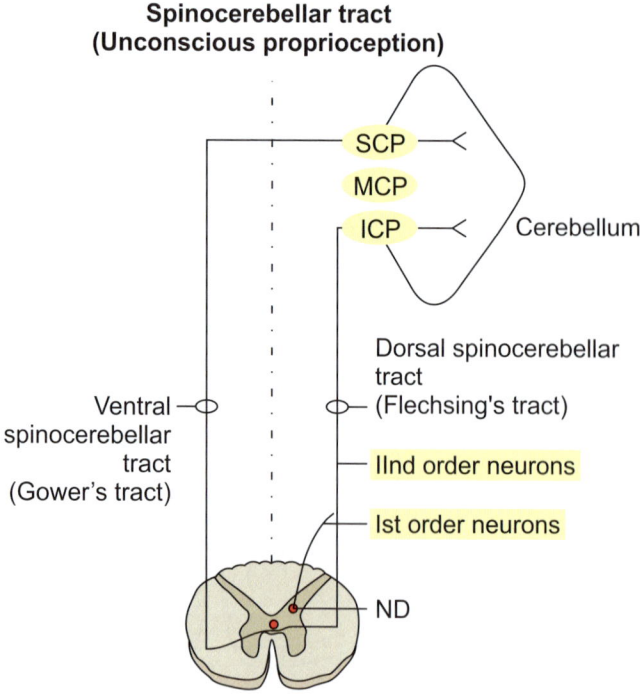

SCP - Superior cerebellar peduncle
MCP - Middle cerebellar peduncle
ICP - Inferior cerebellar peduncle
ND - Nucleus dorsalis

Fig. 8.4 Spinocerebellar tract.

Flowchart 8.3 gives the localization of spinal lesion.
- Vertebral level
  The level of spinal tenderness/deformity can help find the spinal level.
  Table 8.6 gives the localization of the spinal level according to the vertebral level.
- Motor level
  Table 8.7 gives the localization of the motor level according to the clinical presentation.
- Sensory level
  Table 8.8 gives the localization of the sensory level.
  Rule of 3 is as follows: C3, nape of neck; T3, axilla; L3, knee; and S3, perianal.
  Dermatomes are not random! Here is an easy way to remember the dermatomes. Fig. 8.6 shows an easy way to remember the distribution of dermatomes in the body.
- Reflex level

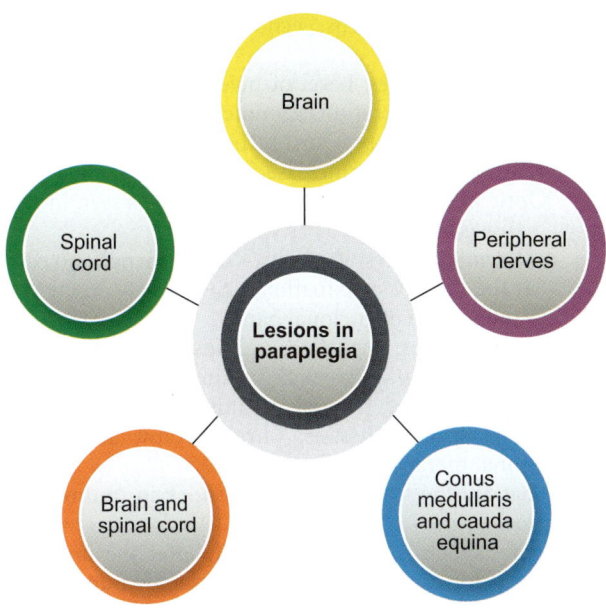

Fig. 8.5 Localization of lesion in paraplegia.

Table 8.9 shows the reflexes with corresponding levels. Clinical features at various levels of involvement are shown in Table 8.10.

21. State the differences between extradural and intradural lesions.

Table 8.11 gives the differences between extradural lesions and intradural lesions.

22. *Enumerate the differences between intramedullary and extramedullary causes of paraplegia.

Table 8.12 gives the differences between intramedullary and extramedullary lesions.

23. How can one differentiate between conus medullaris and cauda equina syndrome?

Table 8.13 gives the differences between conus medullaris and cauda equina syndrome.

24. List the common clinical syndromes associated with spinal paraplegia.

Table 8.14 shows the common clinical syndromes associated with spinal paraplegia.

Figs 8.7–8.9 show Brown–Séquard, central cord, and anterior cord syndromes.

25. Up to what age is toe walking considered normal? What is the differential diagnosis for isolated toe walking?

- Toe walking is normal up to 2 years.
- Differential diagnoses for pathological toe walking are the following:
  - Spinal cord lesions – e.g., tethered cord syndrome

TABLE 8.5 Clinical Features of Paraplegia According to Level of Involvement

Cerebral Cortex	Brainstem	Spinal Cord	Peripheral Nerves
• Seizures • Loss of cortical sensation • Increased intracranial tension • Early bladder involvement – uninhibited bladder (sudden and uncontrolled evacuation, no residual urine) • Upper motor neuron (UMN) features – hypertonia, brisk deep tendon reflexes, plantar extensor	• Cranial nerve dysfunction • Involvement of vital centers (decreased BP, respiratory abnormalities, arrhythmias) • UMN features	• Extramedullary versus intramedullary • Level of lesion in spinal cord • Mixed UMN and LMN features (usually exaggerated reflexes except for spinal shock) • Dermatomal sensory loss • Bladder and bowel involvement	• Symmetrical distal sensory impairment • Symmetrical distal weakness and wasting • Loss of deep tendon reflexes distally • Nerve thickening may be present • Higher mental functions, cranial nerves, bladder, and bowel spared

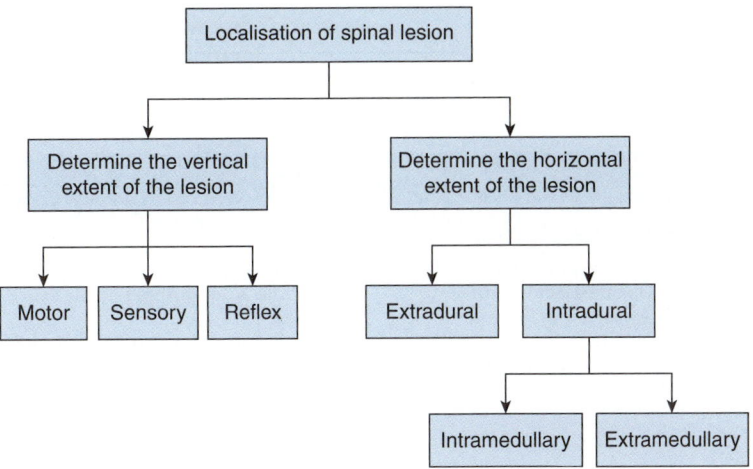

Flowchart 8.3 Localization of spinal lesion.

- Arginase deficiency
- Autism
- Idiopathic

26. What are the predisposing factors, clinical features, diagnosis, and management of transverse myelitis?
    - *Predisposing factors:* Infections (viral – hepatitis A, mumps, varicella, herpes simplex, mumps, Epstein–Barr virus, echovirus) and autoimmune process
    - *Clinical features:* Level of myelitis – usually thoracic, sensory demarcation, asymmetric leg weakness, filling of the bladder present but not emptying voluntarily, and possibility of increased or reduced DTR

    Optic neuritis with transverse myelitis is seen in Devic disease.
    - *Diagnosis:* MRI spine/brain – signal change and edema at the level of myelination; CSF study – raised WBC, protein, and oligoclonal bands
    - *Management:* High-dose steroids (i.v. methylprednisolone 20 mg/kg/day with maximum 1 g/day) for 3–5 days, followed by oral prednisolone for 4–6 weeks, IVIG, plasmapheresis, physiotherapy, and occupational therapy

27. What are the features of spinal shock in trauma to the spinal cord?

    Spinal shock is seen immediately after the injury and lasts for usually 1 week in infants and young children and up to 6 weeks in adolescents. In spinal shock, there is flaccid weakness of the limbs below the level of lesion associated with loss of deep tendon reflexes and superficial reflexes.

28. What is the order of recovery in spinal trauma following spinal shock? In addition, what is mass reflex?
    - Superficial reflexes return first → plantar becomes extensor → massive withdrawal reflexes → DTR return and become exaggerated.
    - Mass reflex: Very small stimulation of the foot/leg causes dorsiflexion of the foot, flexion at the knees, adduction of the thighs, contractions of the abdomen, sweating, piloerection, and emptying of the bladder and bowel.

29. What is the immediate management in case of trauma to the spinal cord?
    - Surgical reduction if fracture dislocation
    - Immobilization
    - Steroids to prevent neurological morbidity – i.v. MPS 30 mg/kg for the first 8 hours after injury followed by 4 mg/kg/h for 23 hours

30. What are the causes of paraplegia in a child with Pott spine?

    It can be because of cold abscess, granulation tissue, necrotic debris/sequestrum from bone involvement or disk tissue, vascular thrombosis of spinal arteries, and granulomatous mass causing compression effect.

TABLE 8.6	Localization of Spinal Level According to Vertebral Level	
Vertebral Level	**Spinal Level**	
Cervical	Add 1	
T1–T6	Add 2	
T7–T9	Add 3	
T10	L1, L2	
T11	L3, L4	
T12	L5	
L1	Sacral and coccygeal	

TABLE 8.7	Localization of Motor Level According to Clinical Presentation	
Motor System Examination	**Interpretation**	**Localization of Lesion**
UMN signs present in both upper and lower limbs	Lesion is before the point where LMN leaves the spinal cord to innervate the upper limbs	Probably C1–C5 (high cervical cord)
UMN signs in both lower limbs but LMN signs in both upper limbs	Lesion is at the point where the spinal nerves innervating the upper limbs leave the CNS	Probably C5 to T2
UMN signs in the lower limbs with normal findings in the upper limb	Lesion is in the spinal cord above the point where the nerves innervating lower limb leave the spinal cord and below the region of cord innervating the upper limbs	Probably T2 to L1
LMN signs in both lower limbs without any other signs	Lesion is in the region of spinal cord that innervates the lower limbs	Probably L1 to S2

UMN, upper motor neuron.

TABLE 8.8	Localization of Sensory Level			
Cervical	**Thoracic**	**Lumbar**	**Sacral**	
C1: No cutaneous supply	T1: Ulnar aspect of forearm	L1: Inguinal ligament	S1: Sole of feet, little toe, Achilles tendon and strip of skin above it	
C2: Occiput, earlobe, angle of jaw	T2: Ulnar aspect of arm	L2: Middle anterior thigh	S2: Posterior calf and thigh	
C3: Supraclavicular fossa	T3: Axilla	L3: Knee	S3: Ischial tuberosity	
C4: Tip of shoulder	T4: Nipple	L4: Medial aspect of leg, medial malleolus	S4, S5: Perianal area	
C5: Upper outer border of arm	T4–T12: Thorax to abdomen	L5: Lateral aspect of leg		
C6: Lateral lower arm (radial border)	T10: Umbilicus			
C7: Middle finger				
C8: Little finger, ulnar aspect of hand				

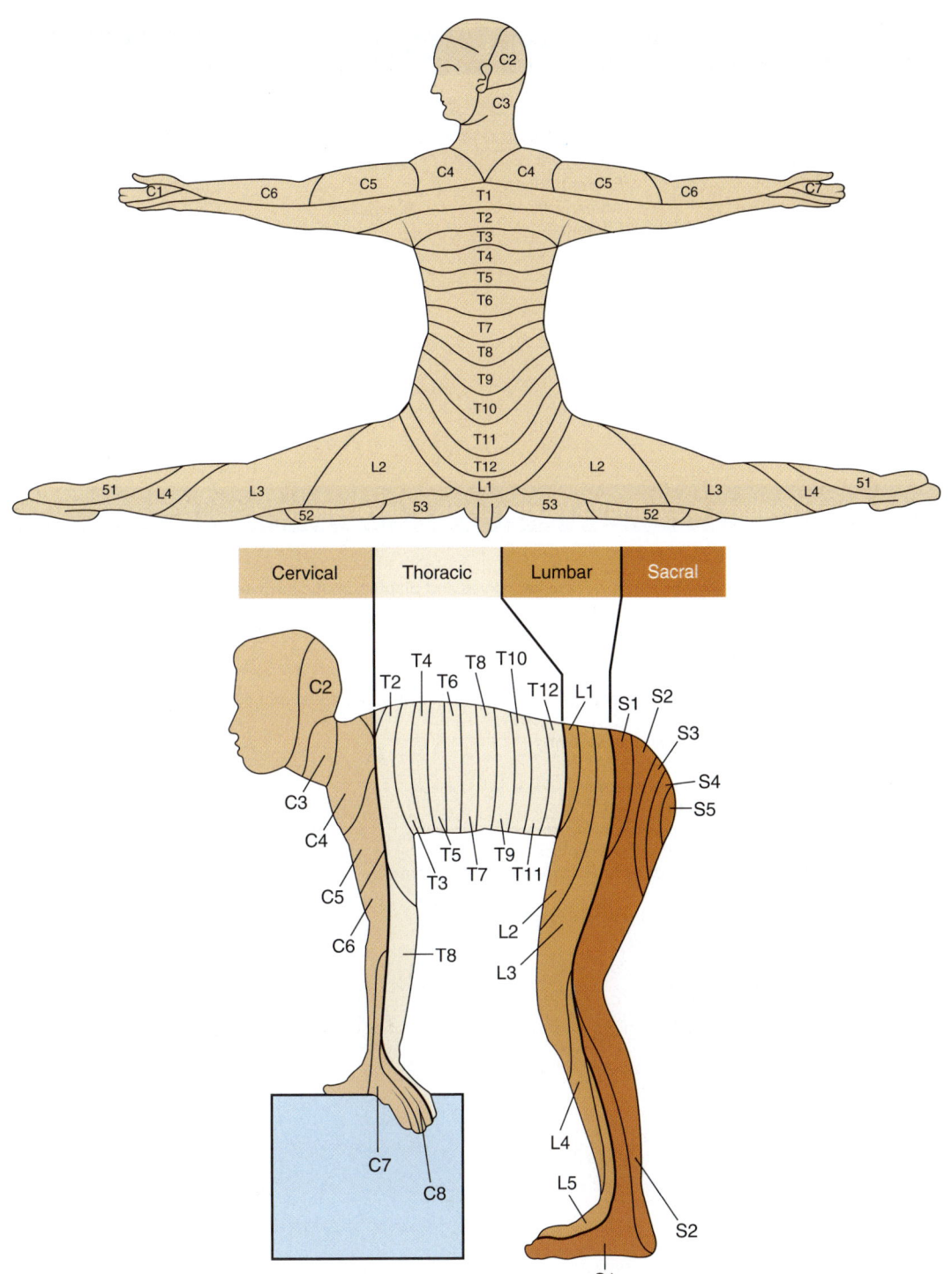

Fig. 8.6 Dermatomal distribution. *(Source: Koeppen & Stanton: Berne and Levy Physiology, 6th edition. Copyright 2008 by Mosby).*

31. Discuss the radiological features of Pott spine and its treatment.

Radiological features
  - Earliest sign: Narrowing of the intervertebral disk space
  - Erosion of the adjacent surfaces of the vertebral bodies
  - Collapse of the vertebral bodies and diminished intervertebral space
  - Bony fusion
  - Kyphosis

Management
  - Complete bed rest and immobilization
  - Antituberculous therapy
  - Surgical decompression: Anterolateral decompression, anterior decompression with spinal fusion, and costotransversectomy

TABLE 8.9	Reflexes With Corresponding Levels			
SUPERFICIAL REFLEXES			**DEEP TENDON REFLEXES**	
Reflex	**Root Value**		**Reflex**	**Root Value**
Corneal, conjunctival	Afferent: V Efferent: VII		Jaw jerk	Afferent: V Efferent: V
Palatal, pharyngeal	Afferent: IX Efferent: X		Biceps jerk	C5, C6
Abdominal	T7–T12		Supinator	C5, C6
Cremasteric	L1, L2		Triceps	C6, C7
Bulbocavernosus	S2–S4		Knee jerk	L2, L4
Anal	S4, S5		Ankle jerk	S1, S2
Plantar	L5–S2			

TABLE 8.10	Summary of Clinical Features According to Various Levels of Involvement
Cord Segment	**Clinical Features**
C3–C4	Quadriplegia with paralysis of lower cranial nerves and diaphragmatic involvement
C5	Quadriplegia Biceps and supinator reflexes lost or decreased Exaggerated triceps reflex Inverted supinator reflex
C7	Paraplegia with weakness of triceps and extensors of wrist and fingers, other upper limb muscles spared Absent triceps reflex
C8–D1	Spastic paralysis of trunk and lower limbs Horner syndrome may be present Upper limb tendon reflexes normal Lower limb reflexes exaggerated
D6	Spastic paralysis of muscles of abdomen and lower limbs Upper abdominal superficial reflexes lost Upper limb tendon reflexes normal, lower limbs exaggerated
D9–D10	Spastic paraplegia Upper abdominal superficial reflexes spared Lower abdominals lost
D12–L1	Spastic paraplegia Abdominal reflexes present Cremasteric reflex lost
S1–S2	Flexion of hip, adduction of thigh, extension at knee, dorsiflexion of foot normal, all other movements in lower extremity weak Knee jerks present, ankle jerks lost Plantar reflexes lost
S3–S4	No paraplegia Retention of urine and feces Anal and bulbocavernosus reflexes lost Deep tendon jerks normal

TABLE 8.11	Differences Between Extradural Lesions and Intradural Lesions	
Features	**Extradural Lesions**	**Intradural Lesions**
Causes	Vertebral tumors, extradural abscess	Glioma, astrocytoma
Local pain	Present	Absent
Local tenderness	Present	Absent
Root pain	Present	Absent

TABLE 8.12	Differences Between Intramedullary and Extramedullary Lesions	
Features	**Extramedullary Lesions**	**Intramedullary Lesions**
Location	Found arising from outside or inside the dura	Found arising from the substance of the cord
SYMPTOMS		
Weakness	Asymmetrical	Symmetrical
Initial symptom	Weakness	Sensory loss
Pain	Early root pain, radiating	Late, burning
Paresthesia	Rare, late presentation	Occurs in all stages
Sensory level	Level ascends with progression	Level descends with progression
SIGNS		
Motor system	LMN signs at the level of lesion, UMN signs below and appear early. Pyramidal tract involvement is early	Long segment involvement of LMN, UMN signs appear late. Pyramidal tract involvement is late
Sensory involvement	Sacral sensations are lost early	Sacral sparing present. Dissociative anesthesia present
Bladder and bowel	Late involvement	Early involvement
Trophic changes	Not marked	Marked

UMN, upper motor neuron.

TABLE 8.13	Differences Between Conus Medullaris and Cauda Equina Syndrome
Conus Medullaris	**Cauda Equina**
Most distal bulbous part of spinal cord	Tapering end of spinal cord that continues as the filum terminale distal to the end of spinal cord resembling horse tail
Mild symmetric weakness	Marked, asymmetric weakness
Symmetric bilateral sensory loss	Unilateral, asymmetric
Bilateral symmetrical saddle anesthesia	Saddle anesthesia may be present
Dissociative sensory loss may be present	Dissociation of sensations absent
Knee jerks preserved but ankle jerks may be diminished (because of extension of lesion to S1–S2)	Both knee and ankle jerks may be absent
Bladder involvement early	Bladder involvement late

TABLE 8.14	Common Clinical Syndromes Associated With Spinal Paraplegia		
Brown–Séquard Syndrome	**Central Cord Syndrome**	**Anterior Two-Third Syndrome**
• Because of functional hemisection of the spinal cord • Ipsilateral weakness (pyramidal tract) • Ipsilateral loss of joint position and vibratory sense (posterior column) • Contralateral loss of pain and temperature (spinothalamic tract) below the level of the lesion • Segmental signs (radicular pain or muscle atrophy or loss of DTR – U/L)	• Because of disorder of gray matter, nerve cells, and the spinothalamic tracts crossing near the central canal (e.g., trauma, syringomyelia, tumors) • Arm weakness out of proportion to leg weakness (in lesions of the cervical cord) • Dissociated sensory loss – loss of pain and temperature (in cape distribution over shoulders, lower neck, and upper trunk) but intact light touch, joint position, and vibration	• Because of extensive disease of the spinal cord with sparing of the posterior columns (e.g., thromboembolism of anterior spinal artery) • All motor, sensory, and autonomic functions are lost below the level of lesion with the exception of vibration and joint position which are intact

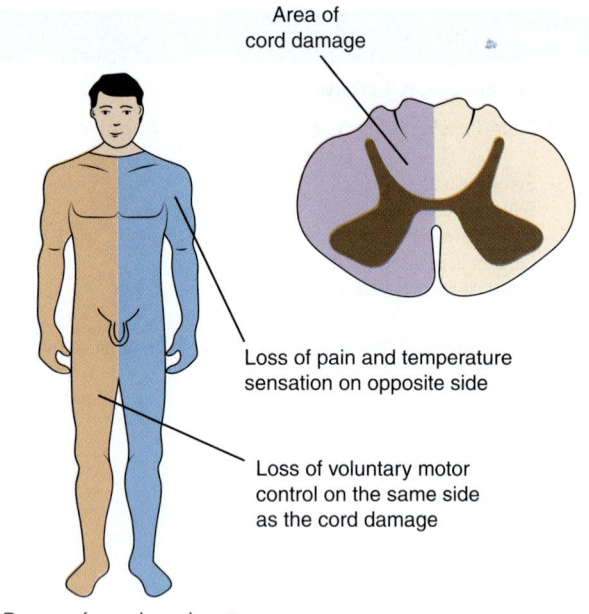

Area of
cord damage

Loss of pain and temperature
sensation on opposite side

Loss of voluntary motor
control on the same side
as the cord damage

Brown-séquard syndrome

Fig. 8.7   Brown–Séquard syndrome. *(Source: Based on Saadia Shams; Abdul Arain: Brown Sequard Syndrome. Copyright © 2021, StatPearls Publishing LLC).*

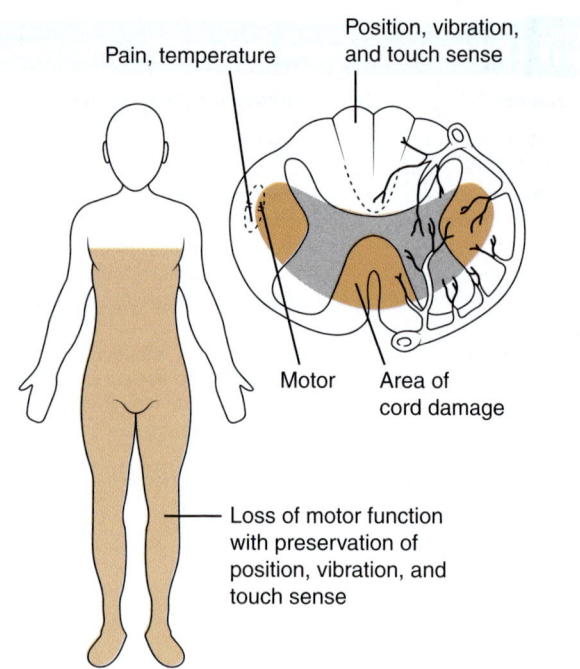

Pain, temperature

Position, vibration,
and touch sense

Motor   Area of
cord damage

Loss of motor function
with preservation of
position, vibration, and
touch sense

Fig. 8.9   Anterior cord syndrome. *(Source: Redrawn from Ignatavicius and Workman: Medical-surgical Nursing Critical Thinking for Collaborative Care, 2002. Elsevier).*

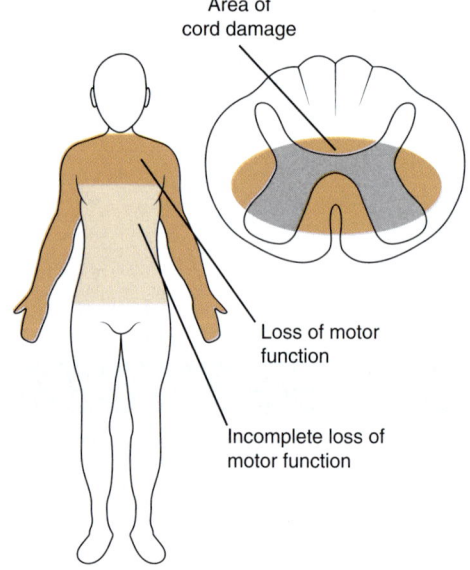

Area of
cord damage

Loss of motor
function

Incomplete loss of
motor function

Fig. 8.8   Central cord syndrome. *(Source: From Ignatavicius and Workman: Medical-surgical Nursing Critical Thinking for Collaborative Care, 2002. Elsevier).*

32. *What are the types of neurogenic bladder?
    Table 8.15 gives the various types of neurogenic bladder. Other types of bladder are the following:
    - Sensory/atonic bladder: It occurs because of selective destruction of sensory fibers between the bladder and the spinal cord or afferent tract to the brain seen in lesions with peripheral neuropathy and cauda equina, and in diabetes. This is similar to an areflexic bladder but voluntary micturition is intact here.
    - Motor/deafferented bladder: It occurs because of destruction of parasympathetic motor innervation of the bladder. It is seen in polio, peripheral neuropathy, trauma, and cauda equina lesions. There is usually painful retention of the bladder.
    - Detrusor sphincter dyssynergia: It occurs because of incoordination between the detrusor and the sphincter seen in lesions at the suprasacral spinal cord. In this, voiding is obstructed, resulting in urinary retention and increased residual urine.

33. What are the investigations to be done in paraplegia?
    Table 8.16 gives the level of investigations in paraplegia.

34. Discuss the treatment modalities including recent advances in paraplegia.
    Table 8.17 gives the various treatment modalities in paraplegia.

35. Discuss the common congenital causes of paraplegia – clinical features, associations, diagnosis, and management.
    Table 8.18 shows the congenital causes of paraplegia.

TABLE 8.15	Types of Neurogenic Bladder		
Type of Bladder	**Cortical Bladder**	**Hyper-Reflexic Bladder**	**Areflexic Bladder**
Level of lesion	Above the level of pons	Between sacral spinal cord and brainstem	In the sacral portion of the spinal cord with interruption of the reflex arc
Cause	Demyelination, frontal lobe tumors, cerebrovascular accidents	Trauma to spinal cord, transverse myelitis	Cauda equina lesions, conus medullaris lesions Injury to sacral roots/pelvic nerve
Features	• Detrusor hyper-reflexia (urge incontinence) • No residual urine • Loss of social inhibition	• Sudden emptying • Incomplete evacuation • Difficulty in initiating micturition • Low-volume contracted bladder	• Dribbling incontinence • Significant residual urine • Difficulty in initiating micturition • Loss of bladder sensation • Atonic large bladder
Other names	Uninhibited bladder, spastic bladder	Reflex neurogenic, automatic bladder, spinal bladder, UMN bladder, contractile bladder	Autonomous bladder, hypotonic bladder, LMN bladder, detrusor areflexia, denervated bladder, acontractile bladder

UMN, upper motor neuron.

TABLE 8.16	Level of Investigations in Paraplegia
Level I	• Complete blood count • Serum electrolytes (potassium level) • Serum calcium • ESR • X-ray spine
Level II	• CSF study • MRI • Electromyogram (EMG) • Nerve conduction study • Antinuclear antibody (ANA), dsDNA • Vitamin B12, folic acid levels
Level III	• Genetic testing • Myelography

TABLE 8.17	Treatment Modalities in Paraplegia		
	Specific Treatment[a]	**Supportive Treatment**	**Surgical Treatment**
	• Surgical decompression • High-dose steroids • Antibiotics • Plasmapheresis • Intravenous immunoglobulin (IVIG) • Chemotherapy • Irradiation • Embryonic stem cell therapy (recent)	• Physiotherapy • Bladder and bowel care • Assist devices • Orthotics • Wheel chairs • Prevention of complications • Psychological support	• Surgical decompression • Surgical stabilization

[a]Trauma: Surgical decompression and high-dose steroids; infective cause: antibiotics; Demyelination and autoimmune disease: high dose steroid, plasmapheresis and IVIG; malignancy: chemotherapy and irradiation.

TABLE 8.18	Congenital Causes of Paraplegia			
Cause	**Clinical Features**	**Associations**	**Diagnosis**	**Management**
1. Arachnoid cyst	• Single/multiple • Usually thoracic • Radicular pain and paraplegia	Neurofibromatosis – type 2	MRI brain/spine – cyst looks similar to CSF	Shunting if symptomatic
2. Chiari malformations	• Headache • Insidious onset • Oropharyngeal dysfunction • Scoliosis • Headache, neck pain • Weakness • Sensory loss	Type 1: Associated with hydrosyringomyelia Type 2: 50% of cases, associated with hydrocephalus, respiratory distress	MRI brain: To see the posterior fossa and cervical cord CT: To look for any bony abnormalities	Posterior fossa decompression, Ventrivulo peritoneal (VP) shunt
3. Spinal dysraphism (spina bifida cystica, meningocele, meningomyelocele)	• Hydrocephalus • At birth: Flaccid legs, dislocated hips, arthrogryposis • Thoracic lesions: Spastic paraplegia, spastic bladder, level of sensory loss • Conus medullaris lesion: Flaccid paraplegia, lumbosacral sensory loss, distended bladder with overflow incontinence	Chiari malformations	• EMG: To look for distribution of segmental dysfunction • Cranial USG: In newborns • MRI brain: To look for malformations of brain	Surgical closure VP shunt

TABLE 8.18	Congenital Causes of Paraplegia—cont'd			
Cause	**Clinical Features**	**Associations**	**Diagnosis**	**Management**
4. Tethered spinal cord (anchoring of conus medullaris to the base of vertebrae by thickened filum terminale, lipoma, dermal sinus, or diastematomyelia)	• External signs of spinal dysraphism • Clumsiness of gait • Stunted growth • Deformity of foot or leg • Bladder/bowel dysfunction • Scoliosis • Exaggerated DTR, plantar extensor	Spina bifida occulta, diastematomyelia (bifid spinal cord)	• X-ray of spine • MRI spine: Essential feature is a low-lying conus medullaris (If it extends below L2–L3 interspace in children older than 5 years, it is abnormal)	Surgical correction of the tethering
5. Arteriovenous malformation	• Insidious onset • Subacute or chronic pain • Subarachnoid hemorrhage • Paraplegia • Loss of bladder control	Usually uncommon in childhood	• MRI spine: To distinguish intramedullary from dural and extramedullary locations of the malformations • Arteriography: To show the extent and feeding vessels	Surgical management
6. Atlantoaxial dislocation	• Acute/slowly progressive depending on age • Mostly quadriplegia, sometimes paraplegia	Mucopolysaccharidosis (especially Morquio syndrome) Klippel–Feil syndrome, Down syndrome, and other chromosomal anomalies	• Flexion X-ray: To assess the separation between the dens and the anterior arch of C1 • MRI spine: To see the relationship between cord and subluxing bones	Surgical stabilization, spinal decompression

EMG, electromyogram.

Quick Bites

1. In any child presenting with predominant lower limb involvement with a clear-cut level of lesion, dermatomal sensory involvement, or features of bladder and bowel disturbances or root pain, have a strong suspicion for paraplegia and try to elicit the etiology.

2. The most common type is spastic paraplegia, which has upper motor neuron features in the lower limb. The most common level of lesion is at the thoracolumbar level.

3. Never forget to examine the sensory system and palpate for the bladder in a patient with paraplegia, which gives a clue for diagnosis and level of involvement.

4. Do not forget to include the functional classification in the diagnosis because this sums up the current status of the child and how it affects his or her daily living.

5. Have a basic understanding of the anatomy of ascending tracts while studying paraplegia without which it may be difficult to understand the level of lesion.

Ataxia

Following introduction, seek permission from the caregiver and introduce yourself to the patient before history elicitation, and identify the case.

Name____Age____Sex____Consanguinity____Order of birth____Place____Informant____

Presenting Complaints and Duration

- Swaying while walking
- Frequent falls

History of Presenting Illness

- Swaying while walking
- Inability to walk/unsteadiness while walking/increasing difficulty in walking
- Frequent falls
- Onset: Acute/intermittent/gradual
- Progressive or nonprogressive
- Static/improving/worsening
- Abnormal hand movements or fine movements of hands (tremors)
- Unsteadiness in reaching out and holding objects in one hand or both hands
- Change in handwriting and scholastic performance
- Seizures and dizziness
- Abnormal eye movements/abnormal head movements (opsoclonus/nystagmus)
- Tingling sensation/numbness/decreased perception of pain over the legs (peripheral neuropathy)

CENTRAL NERVOUS SYSTEM HISTORY

Higher Functions

Higher function impairment (history of seizures, speech problems – dysarthria, memory, emotional lability, scholastic backwardness)

Cranial Nerve History

- Ability to perceive light
- Any drooping of eyelids, ability to move eyeballs in all four directions, or restriction of eyeball movement
- Ability to chew food and difficulty in opening the jaw
- Ability to close both eyes while sleeping, drooling of saliva, deviation of angle of the mouth, lack of facial expression, and facial asymmetry
- Ability to hear and respond to sound
- Nasal twang of voice, nasal regurgitation, choking while feeding, weak cry, and difficulty in swallowing
- Ability to move the head side to side
- Abnormal movement or twitching in the tongue

Motor System

- Stiffness/flailness (age of onset – acute [noticed recently] or chronic [noticed in one limb or both the limbs over a period of time])
- Gait abnormalities – high stepping gait/walking in cloud/broad-based gait
- Any involuntary movements

Cerebellar Features

- Abnormal eyeball or head movement or tremors

Bladder/Bowel Disturbance

- Urinary incontinence or dribbling and constipation

Sensory Features

- Perception of pain or crying while giving vaccination and feeling the ground while walking

Autonomic Features

- Flushing, sweating, and palpitation episodes

Spine and Cranium

- Any abnormality in the head size noted by the mother compared with sibling or peers
- Any swelling, tuft of hair, sinus, discharge, and abnormal curvature

COMPLICATION HISTORY

- Headache, vomiting, convulsions, unconsciousness, and altered sensorium (increased ICT)

ETIOLOGICAL HISTORY

- Recent febrile illness with/without exanthem and GIT illness
- Recent immunization
- Drugs (piperazine citrate, anticonvulsants, streptomycin, antihistamines), toxins, and drug abuse (cocaine, heroin, phencyclidine)
- Early morning headache and vomiting/behavioral changes/unconsciousness/altered sensorium
- Trauma
- Otorrhea/tinnitus
- Mental retardation/regression of milestones
- Diarrhea/fat malabsorption
- Visual impairment
- Symptoms suggestive of liver disease
- Repeated episodes
- Eye redness/skin changes
- Extrapyramidal abnormalities, breathing abnormalities, and ptosis

- Constipation/lethargy/mental retardation
- Photosensitivity reactions/abdominal pain/psychosis/urine color change on standing
- Chronic cough/weight loss
- Increasing head circumference

Past History

- Similar episodes in the past
- Recent exanthematous fever
- Recent vaccination

Birth History

History of birth asphyxia (ataxic cerebral palsy)

Developmental History

Any regression of milestones

Dietetic History

According to 24-hour recall method

Immunization History

Recent immunization (live virus injection – MMR, varicella, flu vaccine)

Contact History

Koch's contact (tuberculoma)

Family History

Similar complaints in the family and episodic/self-limiting episodes

Socioeconomic History

According to the modified Kuppuswamy scale

Summary

A ...-year-old child with inability to walk/unsteadiness while walking/frequent falls, which was acute/intermittent/gradual in onset, progressive or nonprogressive, and static/improving/worsening
  Associated with/without abnormal head/eye movements, with/without similar episodes in the past, with/without history of recent vaccination/exanthematous fever, and with/without significant family history; probably ataxia; would proceed with examination to localize the site of lesion (posterior column/vestibular/cerebellar) and etiology

General Examination

- Posture
- Sick looking or not
- Sensorium
- Nutritional status
- Ichthyosis
- Neurocutaneous markers – hemangioma and telangiectasia
- Skeletal – pes cavus and scoliosis

Head-to-Foot Examination

- Skull shape: Occiput – flat
- Anterior fontanelle: Bulging or flat
- Eyes: Cataract
- Pallor
- Tendon xanthomas: cerebrotendinous xanthomatosis

Vital Signs

- Temperature
- Pulse rate
- Respiratory distress (irregular jerky breathing – Joubert syndrome)
- Blood pressure – hypertension (raised ICP)
- SpO_2

Anthropometry

- Any short stature

Central Nervous System Examination

HIGHER FUNCTIONS

Speech – staccato/dysarthria and seizures/mental retardation (cerebellar malformation, mitochondrial disease, inborn errors of metabolism)

CRANIAL NERVES

- Cranial nerve I: Tell that cranial nerve I could not be tested if the child is younger than 5 years; if the child is older than 5 years, test for the olfactory nerve by using familiar smells with eyes closed and ensuring that there is no nasal block
- Cranial nerve II: Six points:
  A. Light perception
  B. Visual acuity
  C. Color vision
  D. Field of vision
  E. Direct and consensual light reflex
  F. Fundus
- Cranial nerves III, IV, and VI: Movement of eyeballs in all four cardinal directions, strabismus, and ptosis
- Cranial nerve V: Ability to perceive pain sensation over the face, able to chew food, and jaw jerk
- Cranial nerve VII
  - Wrinkling of the forehead present
  - Able to close eyes on both sides while sleeping
  - Absent nasolabial fold on the affected side
  - Deviation of the angle of the mouth to the normal side
  - Drooling of saliva
- Cranial nerve VIII: Ability to obey the mother's command, respond to the mother's call, and response to sound age appropriate
- Cranial nerves IX and X: Palatal movement normal, uvula in the midline, palatal arches normal, and palatal and pharyngeal reflexes normal
- Cranial nerve XI: Ability to lift the head from a supine position and able to turn the head on both sides
- Cranial nerve XII: Any deviation of the tongue, fibrillation, or wasting

MOTOR EXAMINATION

- Posture: Describe the posture of the child
- Tone: Hypotonia (cerebellar lesion)
- Power: Usually normal
- Reflexes
  - Hyporeflexia (pendular – knee-jerk) (metachromatic leukodystrophy, Friedreich ataxia, abetalipoproteinemia)
  - Absent (Miller Fischer variant)
  - Brisk (ataxic CP)
- Gait: Wide-based gait

CEREBELLAR SIGNS

- Titubation (head movement sidewards, bobbing or swaying of the head and trunk/head nodding – moving the head forward and backward)
- Upper limbs: Tone (hypotonia), past pointing, Gordon Holmes rebound phenomenon, intention tremor, postural holding test, dysdiadochokinesia, dysmetria, and finger-to-nose and finger-to-finger tests
- Truncal ataxia
- Lower limbs: Wide-based gait, tandem walking, Romberg's test, pendular knee-jerk, Heel knee test and toe-to-finger test

AUTONOMIC SYSTEM

- Excessive sweating, tachycardia, and hypotension

SENSORY SYSTEM

Numbness/tingling sensation, trophic ulcer, foot drop, absent Deep tendon reflex, atrophic foot, and wasting of muscles (signs of peripheral neuropathy)

SPINE AND CRANIUM

Any tuft of hair, swelling, and sacral dimple

SIGNS OF MENINGEAL IRRITATION

Present or not (Kernig/Brudzinski reflex)

MUSCULOSKELETAL SYSTEM

Any bony deformity and contractures

Other System Examination

ABDOMEN

Hepatosplenomegaly (Wilson) and malabsorption (abetalipoproteinemia)

CARDIAC

Cardiomyopathy - Friedreich ataxia and mitochondrial disorder

RESPIRATORY SYSTEM

Sinopulmonary infection – ataxia telangiectasia

Diagnosis

A ...-year-old male/female child with acute or chronic/progressive or nonprogressive/recovering or worsening/bilateral or right/left-sided truncal or axial ataxia with/without any other central nervous system deficits (motor/sensory), with/without raised intracranial tension, and with/without malnutrition/trophic changes, probable etiology being ——-, and cerebellar/vestibular/peripheral neuropathy – posterior column, nutritional status, and other comorbid conditions – anemia and vitamin deficiency if any

Frequently Asked Questions

1. List the clues in history for etiology in a child with ataxia.
   Table 9.1 gives the clues in etiological history in a child with ataxia

2. *What is the significance of recent immunization in a child with ataxia?
   Following immunization, demyelination (ADEM can present as ataxia)

3. What are the differentials if there is intermittent ataxia precipitated by infection and drugs?
   Metabolic causes: Aminoacidopathies, urea cycle disorder, and mitochondrial cytopathies are associated with intermittent ataxia.

4. What is the significance of family history in a child with ataxia?
   Similar illness in family members: Episodic ataxia type (1–7) and inherited ataxia

5. What are the neurocutaneous syndromes associated with ataxia?
   Ataxia telangiectasia and Von Hippel–Lindau disease are the neurocutaneous syndromes associated with ataxia.

6. What are the differentials if a child with ataxia presented with skeletal deformity?
   Skeletal deformities such as pes cavus (Fig. 9.2) and scoliosis (as shown in Fig. 9.3) are seen in Friedreich ataxia and ataxia with vitamin E deficiency.

7. What are the differentials if ataxia is associated with a short stature?
   Mitochondrial disease, ataxia telangiectasia, and abetalipoproteinemia

8. *What is the significance of ocular examination in a child with ataxia?
   Table 9.2 gives the significance of ocular examination.

9. What are the skin findings in a child with ataxia?
   a. Ichthyosis: Refsum disease
   b. Alopecia and dermatitis: Biotinidase deficiency
   c. Telangiectasia over pinna and bulbar conjunctiva: Ataxia telangiectasia
   d. Skin and tendon xanthoma (as shown in Fig. 9.4A), ataxia with vitamin E deficiency, and cerebrotendinoxanthomatosis (Fig. 9.4B shows eruptive xanthoma over the face)

10. What is the significance of cranial nerve examination in ataxia?
    • Cranial nerve II: Fundus examination – retinitis pigmentosa, papilledema, and optic atrophy
    • Cranial nerves III, IV, and VI: Oculomotor apraxia and nystagmus/opsoclonus
    • Cranial nerve VIII: Deafness

11. *What is oculomotor apraxia?
    Oculomotor apraxia consists of absence or defect of controlled, voluntary, and purposeful eye movement, difficulty in moving the eyes horizontally, and moving the eyes fast. The main difficulty is in saccade initiation, but there is also impaired cancellation of the vestibulo-ocular. Patients have to turn their head to compensate for the lack of eye movement initiation

---

*Important question asked in the examination.

TABLE 9.1	Clues in Etiological History
Etiology	**History**
Cerebellitis	Recent febrile illness with/without exanthem, GIT illness
	Most common: Viral – chickenpox, enteroviruses, coxsackie, influenza; bacteria – enteric fever, *Mycoplasma*, *Legionella*
Demyelination	Recent immunisation, infection
Drug intake	Drugs such as piperazine citrate, anticonvulsants, streptomycin, antihistamine
Drug abuse	Drugs such as cocaine, heroin, phencyclidine
Posterior fossa tumor	Early morning headache, vomiting/behavioral changes/unconsciousness/altered sensorium
Vestibulitis	Otorrhea/tinnitus
Neurometabolic disorders – sphingolipidoses/Marinesco–Sjögren syndrome	Mental retardation/regression of milestones
Benign paroxysmal vertigo, stroke, migraine	Dizziness
Abetalipoproteinemia	Diarrhea/fat malabsorption
Refsum disease	Visual impairment
Wilson disease	Jaundice, neuropsychiatric manifestations
Epilepsy/basilar artery migraine	Repeated episodes
Ataxia telangiectasia	Eye redness – telangiectasia of eyes as shown in Fig. 9.1/skin changes
Mitochondrial disease	Extrapyramidal abnormalities, breathing abnormalities, ptosis
Hypothyroidism	Constipation/lethargy/mental retardation
Concussion, posterior circulation stroke	Trauma, fall
Porphyria	Photosensitivity reactions/abdominal pain/psychosis/urine color change on standing
Tuberculosis	Chronic cough/weight loss
Hydrocephalus	Increasing head circumference

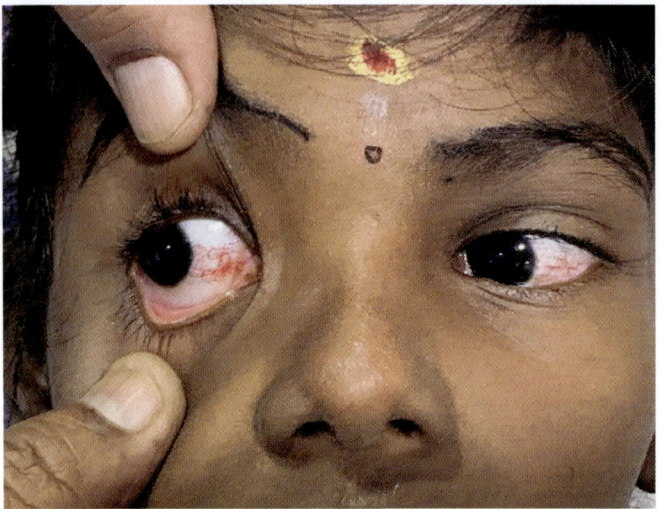

Fig. 9.1 Telangiectasia of eyes.

TABLE 9.2	**Significance of Ocular Examination**
Clinical Features	**Etiology**
Pigmentary retinopathy	Congenital disorder of glycosylation, Refsum disease, abetalipoproteinemia
Optic atrophy	Friedreich ataxia
Aniridia	Gillespie syndrome
Cataract	Marinesco–Sjögren syndrome
Oculomotor apraxia	Joubert syndrome, ataxia telangiectasia, ataxia with oculomotor apraxia types 1 and 2
Retinal dystrophy	Mevalonate kinase deficiency
Opsoclonus (dancing eyes)	Opsoclonus-myoclonus-ataxia syndrome (paraneoplastic syndrome) – occult neuroblastoma
Ophthalmoplegia	Miller Fisher variant of Guillane barre syndrome (GBS)

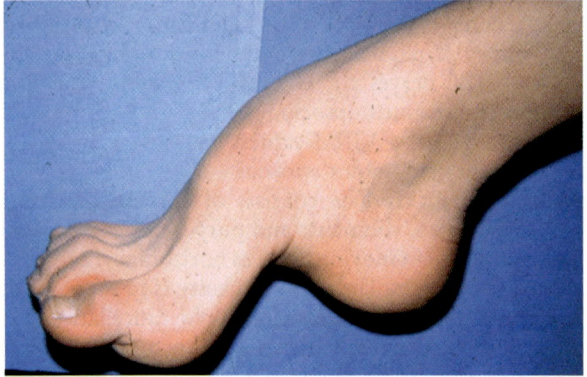

Fig. 9.2 Pes cavus – Friedreich ataxia. (*Source: Reproduced from Bradley and Daroff's Neurology in Clinical Practice, Eighth Edition. Proximal, Distal, and Generalized Weakness, Fig. 28.3, (c) 2022, Credit line - From Krause, F.G., Guyton, G.P. Mann's surgery of the foot and ankle, In: Coughlin, M.J., Saltzmanand, C.L., Anderson, R.B. (Eds.), Mann's Surgery of the Foot and Ankle, ninth ed. pp. 1361–1382. Copyright © 2014 by Saunders, an imprint of Elsevier Inc. Published by Elsevier.*)

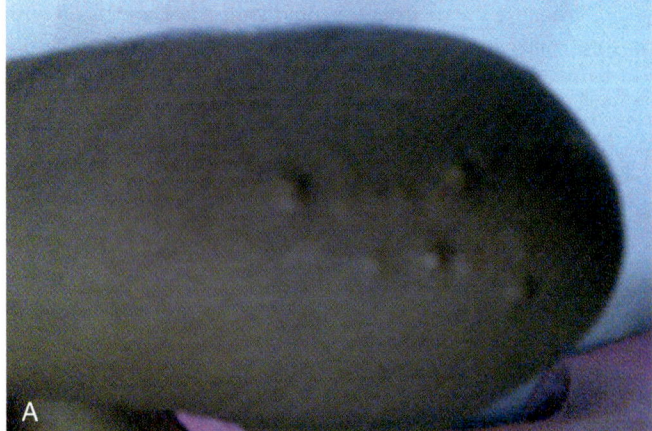

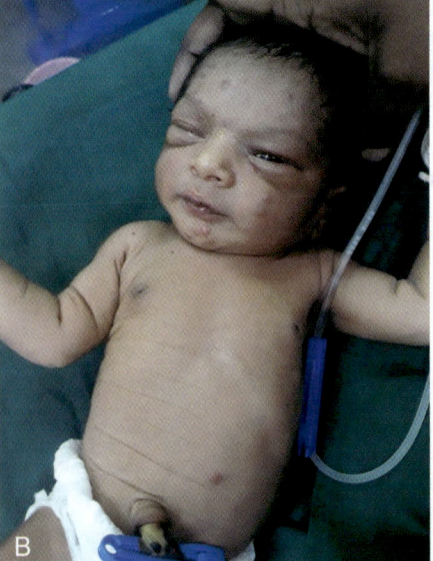

Fig. 9.4 (A) Tendon xanthoma. (B) Eruptive xanthoma over the face.

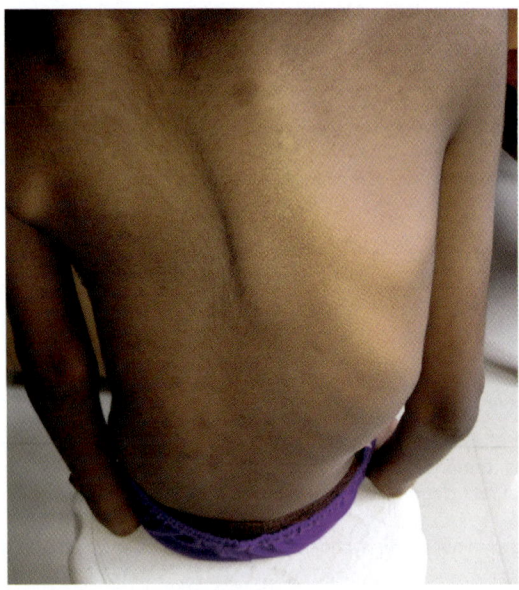

Fig. 9.3 Scoliosis.

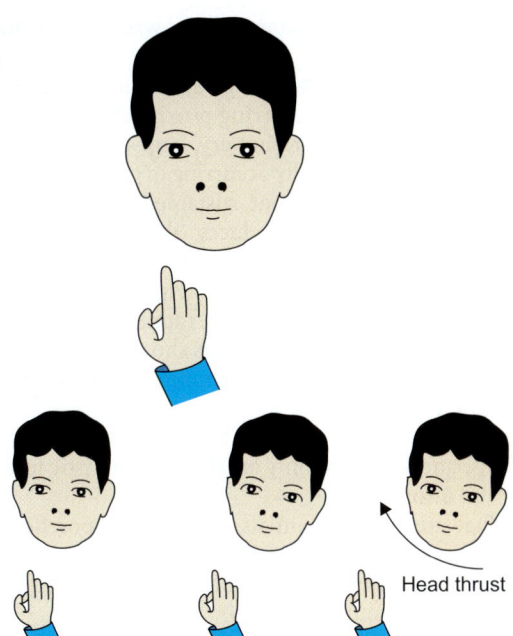

Fig. 9.5 Schematic representation of oculomotor apraxia. (*Source: Rami Shasha, MD, FRCSC on Twitter: "Oculomotor Apraxia as seen in Joubert Syndrome #ophthalmology #optometry #art #drawing #medicine #joubert https://t.co/hSjKqJyJW7"/Twitter*)

to follow an object or see objects in their peripheral vision, but they often exceed their target. The schematic representation of oculomotor apraxia is as shown in Fig. 9.5.

Fig. 9.6A–C demonstrates oculomotor apraxia – the child turns her head from midline to periphery rather than tracing the finger with her eyes.

12. What are the diagnostic criteria for opsoclonus myoclonus syndrome?

Three out of the following four supportive findings should be present:

a. Opsoclonus

b. Myoclonus and/or myoclonus

c. Behavioral changes/sleep disturbance

d. Tumorous condition and/or presence of antineuronal antibodies

13. What are the differentials if a child with ataxia presents with endocrine abnormality?

a. Diabetes + ataxia: Friedreich ataxia

b. Hypogonadism in females + ataxia: Spinocerebellar ataxia (SCA; infantile onset)

c. Marinesco–Sjögren syndrome

14. What are the causes of ataxia with deafness?

Friedreich ataxia, mitochondrial disorder, Refsum disease, and infantile onset of spinocerebellar ataxia

15. What is the significance of other system examination in a child with ataxia?

a) Abdomen: Hepatosplenomegaly (Wilson) and malabsorption (abetalipoproteinemia)

b) Cardiac

- Friedreich ataxia: Cardiomyopathy
- Abetalipoproteinemia: Cardiomegaly and arrhythmia
- Mitochondrial disease: Cardiomyopathy

c) Respiratory system: Sinopulmonary infection (ataxia telangiectasia)

16. How is a child with ataxia investigated?

Investigations are done mainly to identify the etiology.

a. Peripheral smear: Acanthocytes

b. For all children with acute/intermittent ataxia: Urine and/or serum toxin screening – drugs (cocaine, heroin, phencyclidine)

c. For congenital ataxia for malformation and demyelination: Imaging studies and MRI brain (better visualization of the posterior fossa and the cerebellum)

d. MRI abdomen: Pheochromocytoma

e. Vitamin E levels: Abetalipoproteinemia and ataxia with vitamin E deficiency

f. Nerve conduction: Peripheral neuropathy

g. Should carry out investigations to rule out neuroblastoma (urinary Vanillylmandelic acid (VMA)

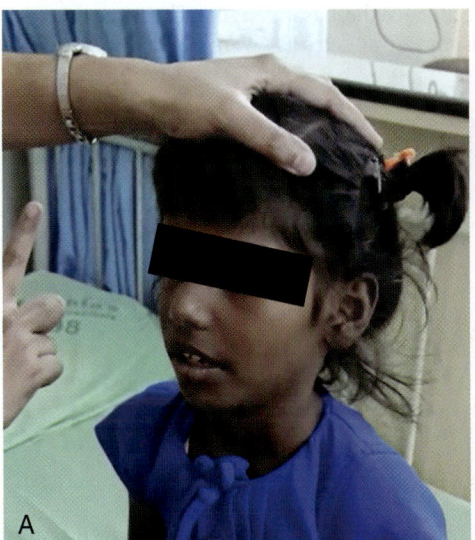
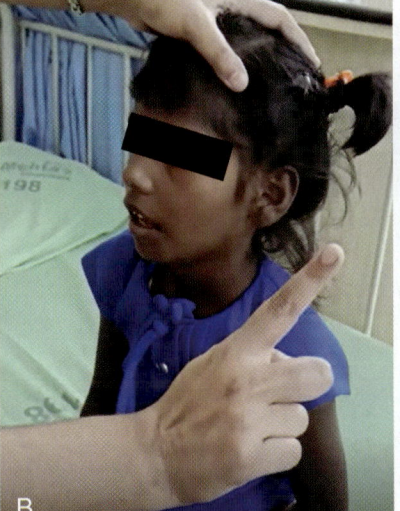
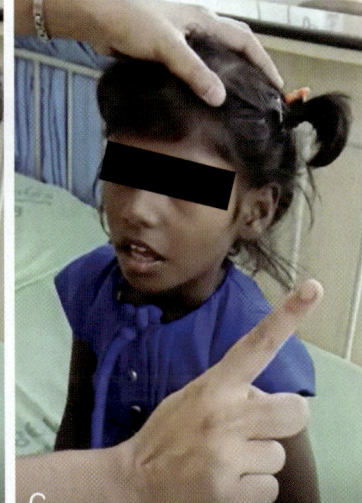

Fig. 9.6   (A) Head in midline. (B) Finger in the periphery. (C) Head thrust – child moves her head rather than tracing the finger with her eyes.

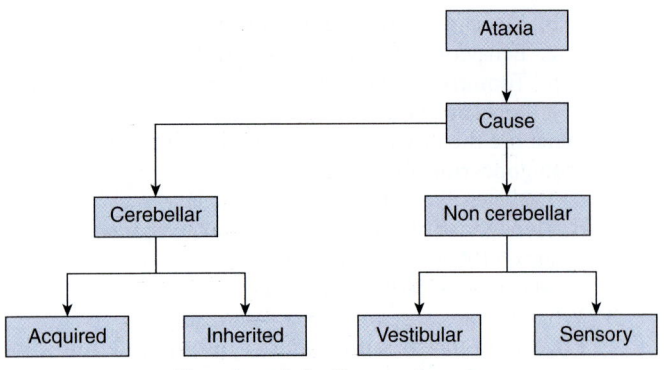

Flowchart 9.1 Causes of ataxia.

level, radioactive isotope scan- metaiodobenzyl-guanidine (MIBG scan), CT chest, abdomen, etc.)

h. Metabolic: Serum lactate, pyruvate, ammonia, and ketones

17. *Define ataxia.

Ataxia is defined as the inability to make smooth, accurate, and coordinated movements usually because of dysfunction of the cerebellum, the sensory pathway of the spinal cord, or a combination of these.

18. What are the causes of ataxia?

The causes of ataxia are given in Flowchart 9.1.

19. How is ataxia classified depending on the onset?

Ataxia: Acute, intermittent, and chronic

20. *What are the causes of acute ataxia in children

Table 9.3 gives the causes of acute ataxia.

21. What are the causes of intermittent ataxia?

Table 9.4 gives the causes of intermittent ataxia.

22. What are the causes of congenital ataxia?

Table 9.5 gives the causes of congenital ataxia.

23. What are the causes of inherited ataxia?

Table 9.6 shows the causes of inherited ataxia.

24. Name one common cause of each type of ataxia.

a. Acute: Postinfectious cerebellar demyelination

b. Intermittent: Inborn error of metabolism

c. Inherited: Friedrich ataxia

25. *What are the other movement disorders seen in childhood?

a. Chorea: Involuntary, irregular, continuous or movement fragments with variable rate and direction that occur unpredictably and randomly

b. Athetosis: Involuntary, slow, writhing, continuous movements

c. Ballism: Involuntary, large-amplitude, flinging movements typically occurring proximally

d. Hemiballismus: Involuntary, large-amplitude, flinging movements typically occurring in one-half of the body

e. Dystonia: Intermittent, sustained involuntary muscle contracture that produces abnormal posture and movements of different parts of the body with a twisting quality as shown in Fig. 9.8

f. Tics: Involuntary, sudden, rapid, abrupt, repetitive, nonrhythmic movements as shown in Fig. 9.9, which can be simple or complex motor movements or phonic vocalization

26. What are the characteristic features of tics?

Urge and suppressibility are the characteristic features of tic disorder.

27. What are the differentials if there is hyporeflexia with extensor plantar seen in a child with ataxia?

Abetalipoproteinemia, Friedreich ataxia, and metachromatic leukodystrophy

28. *What are acanthocytes?

RBCs with irregular circumferential pointed projection because of alteration in the cholesterol:phospholipid ratio are called acanthocytes (as shown in Fig. 9.10) and are seen in abetalipoproteinemia.

29. How are acanthocytes differentiated from burr cells?

Burr cell has a regular distribution of projections or serrations along the surface of the RBC, whereas acanthocytes have an irregular distribution of projections as shown in Fig. 9.11.

30. What are the causes of acanthocytes?

1. Liver disease
2. Vitamin E deficiency
3. Congenital abetalipoproteinemia (triad – fat malabsorption + neuromuscular abnormalities + retinitis pigmentosa)
4. Neuroacanthocytosis

31. What is neuroacanthocytosis?

Neuroacanthocytosis is a range of genetic syndromes with mutations with varied clinical features but primarily producing neurodegeneration of the brain, specifically the basal ganglia. There are four types of neuroacanthocytes as given in Table 9.7.

TABLE 9.3	Causes of Acute Ataxia	
Causes of Acute Ataxia	Clinical Features	Diagnostic Clues
Infectious and postinfectious: Varicella, coxsackie B, Epstein-Barr virus (EBV), influenza A and B	Sensorium: Normal Gait and truncal ataxia	Cerebrospinal fluid (csf): Mild pleocytosis Negative cultures MRI brain: Normal or mild nonspecific changes
Acute disseminated encephalomyelitis (ADEM)	Altered sensorium + seizures + meningism symptoms	MRI brain: Multifocal, patchy, subcortical white matter demyelination in the cerebrum, cerebellum, basal ganglia, brainstem
Drugs: Anticonvulsants, antihistamines	In an unsupervised toddler or adolescent because of drug abuse, lethargy + confusion + nystagmus	Serum toxin screening
Miller Fischer variant of GBS	Triad: Ataxia, ophthalmoplegia, and areflexia	CSF: cytoalbuminological, serum GQ1b antibody positive
Opsoclonus-myoclonus-ataxia syndrome Neuroblastoma	Irritability rapid chaotic multidirectional ocular movements, truncal ataxia	USG/CT: Tumor of posterior mediastinum or adrenals

TABLE 9.4	Causes of Intermittent Ataxia	

Causes of Episodic Ataxia	Metabolic Causes of Ataxia
Types 1–7 Types 1, 2, 7 • Childhood onset • AD inheritance • Stress and physical exertion are triggers • In between the attacks, the child is normal	1. Maple syrup urine disease 2. Biotinidase deficiency 3. Organic acidemia 4. Urea cycle disorder 5. Mitochondrial disease 6. Refsum disease

TABLE 9.5	Causes of Congenital Ataxia	

Disease	Clinical Features	MRI Findings
Joubert syndrome and related disorders	Episodic hyperpnea Oculomotor apraxia Facial dysmorphism Retinal dystrophy	Molar tooth sign Keyhole sign Triangular 4th ventricle
Chiari malformation	Dizziness/headache worsened by coughing Lower cranial nerve palsy	1. Herniation of cerebellar tonsil 2. Herniation of lower brainstem with myelomeningocele 3. With occipital encephalocele 4. Cerebellar agenesis
Dandy–Walker malformation	Large head – occipital prominence, excessive sleepiness, nystagmus	Agenesis of the vermis, cystic dilation of the 4th ventricle, enlarged posterior fossa
Gillespie syndrome	Aniridia, dysmorphism, hypotonia, mental retardation	Vermian hypoplasia, cerebral atrophy

TABLE 9.6	Causes of Inherited Ataxia	

Disease	Clinical Features	Diagnostic Clues
Friedreich ataxia	SNHL + Optic atrophy + Hypertrophic cardiomyopathy + Skeletal abnormality (pes cavus, kyphoscoliosis) + Impaired position and vibration sense + Peripheral neuropathy (shown in Fig. 9.7) + Hypoactive knee and ankle reflex with extensor plantar + Diabetes	MRI spine – thinning of cervical spinal cord Nerve conduction study – axonal neuropathy DNA mutation analysis
Ataxia telangiectasia	Telangiectasia (bulbar conjunctiva, pinna, soft palate) Recurrent sinopulmonary infection Immune deficiency Increased incidence of lymphoreticular malignancies	Increased serum alpha-fetoprotein >10 ng/mL, high carcinoembryonic antigen Decreased IgA, IgE, IgG2
Abetalipoproteinemia (Bassen–Kornzweig syndrome)	Malabsorption + Hyporeflexia with extensor plantar + Cardiomegaly Arrhythmia + Retinitis pigmentosa	Cerebellar atrophy in MRI Peripheral smear – acanthocytes Low LDL, VLDL, triglycerides
Refsum disease	Night blindness, cataract, peripheral neuropathy, deafness Ichthyosis	High phytanic acid in the blood
Spinocerebellar ataxia	Peripheral neuropathy, deafness Optic atrophy Primary hypogonadism in females	Cerebellar and brainstem atrophy

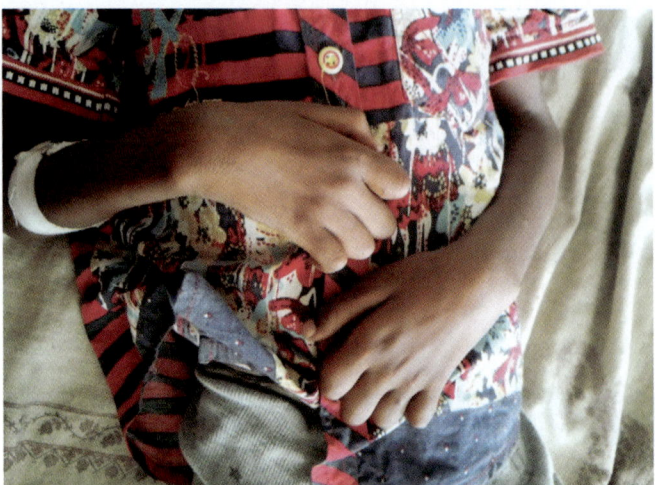

Fig. 9.7   Peripheral neuropathy in Friedreich ataxia.

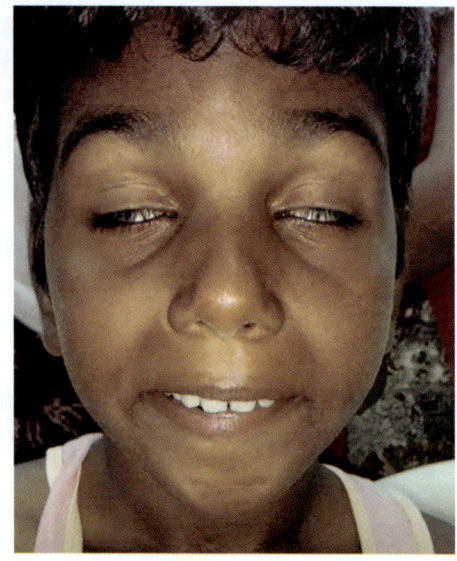

Fig. 9.9   Complex tic – eye blinking + facial grimace.

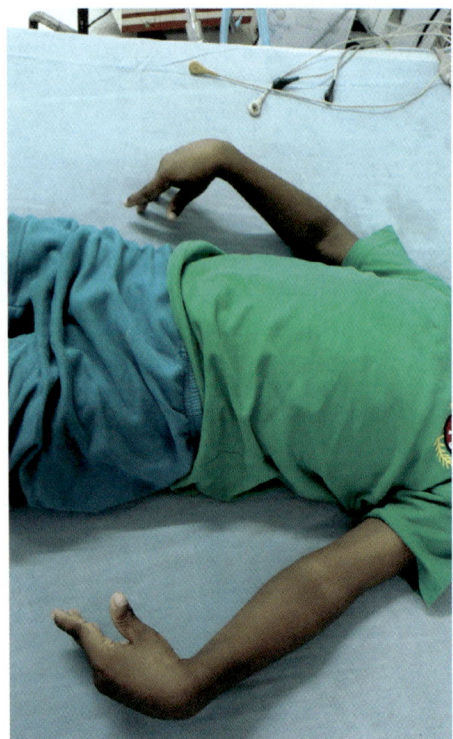

Fig. 9.8   Dystonia in the upper limb.

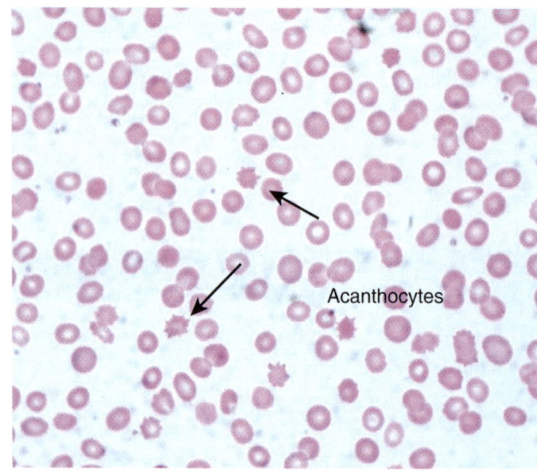

Fig. 9.10   Acanthocytes. Arrowhead, irregular circumferential pointed projections. *(Source: Acanthocytosis Article (statpearls.com)).*

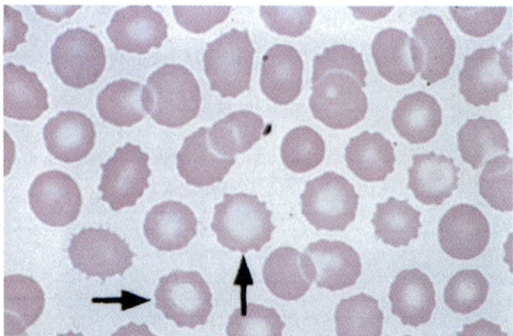

Fig. 9.11   Burr cell. Arrowhead shows regular projections along the surface of RBC. *Source:* Reproduced from *USMLE Step 2 Secrets, Sixth Edition. Hematology, Fig. 17.13, © 2022, Credit line - From Hoffman R, et al. Hematology: Basic Principles and Practice. 5th ed. London: Churchill Livingstone; 2008 [fig. 156-1]. Published by Elsevier.*

TABLE 9.7	Types of Neuroacanthocytes	
Disease	**Inheritance**	**Clinical Features**
Chorea acanthocytes	Autosomal recessive Altered Lyn kinase activity with increased tyrosine phosphorylation	Dystonia, chorea, and progressive cognitive and behavioral changes and seizures; peripheral smear – >3% acanthocytes, MRI – caudal atrophy
McLeod syndrome	X-linked recessive Mutations in the *XK* gene encoding the Kx blood type antigen, one of the Kell antigens	Movement disorder, peripheral neuropathy, cognitive impairment, and psychiatric symptoms; arrhythmia and dilated cardiomyopathy
Pantothenate kinase–associated neurodegeneration	An autosomal recessive condition caused by mutations in *PANK2*	Dystonia, dysarthria, spasticity, retinopathy
Huntington disease-like-2	An autosomal dominant condition caused by mutations in *JPH3*	Similar to Huntington disease (chorea, dementia, behavioral changes)

Quick Bites

1. Diabetes + pes cavus + peripheral neuropathy + posterior column involvement: Friedrich ataxia
2. Characteristic features of tic disorder: Urge and suppressibility
3. Most common cause of acute ataxia: Postinfectious cerebellar demyelination
4. Most common cause of intermittent ataxia: Inborn error of metabolism
5. Most common cause of inherited ataxia: Friedrich ataxia

Cardiovascular System

10 Cardiovascular System Examination

General Examination

- General appearance: Whether alert, active/irritable (hypoxic irritability), interested in the surroundings, recognizes the mother, and comfortable on the mother's lap/dyspneic at rest
- Mentioned whether the child is under oxygen support/nasogastric feed/intravenous line
- Pallor/icterus/cyanosis/clubbing/lymphadenopathy/edema
- Any external markers of congenital heart disease/infective endocarditis

Head-to-Foot Examination

- Dysmorphic facies
- Sweating on the forehead
- Eyes: Plethora, icterus, fundus examination, cataract, and aortic regurgitation signs
- Oral cavity: Any dental caries
- Chest and spine deformity
- Skin: Look for peripheral rashes of infective endocarditis
- Any external markers of infective endocarditis/peripheral signs of aortic regurgitation

Vital Signs

- Temperature: Measured in the axilla using a digital thermometer
- Pulse rate: Rate, rhythm, volume, character, condition of the vessel wall, felt in all peripheries, and any radioradial or radiofemoral delay
- Respiratory rate: Rate, pattern of breathing, and any accessory muscles involved
- Blood pressure: Both upper and lower limb blood pressure; also mention the side and position of the patient during measurement
- Jugular venous pressure: Raised or not

Anthropometry

- Length (younger than 2 years)/height (older than 2 years) (cm)
- Weight (kg)
- Weight for length/height – up to 5 years; body mass index – older than 5 years
- Mid-arm circumference from 12 to 59 months of age
- Head circumference up to 5 years of age
- Upper segment:lower segment ratio

Cardiovascular System Examination

INSPECTION

- Tracheal position
- Chest wall shape and symmetry – any deformities
- Apical impulse – side and position with respect to nipples
- Precordial bulge
- Engorged veins over the chest wall
- Visible pulsations – aortic, pulmonary, epigastric, suprasternal, and carotid areas
- Neck veins – engorged or not
- Scars and sinuses over the chest
- Inspection of the back – any visible pulsations

PALPATION

- Confirm tracheal and apical impulse position by palpation
- Apical impulse – mention the side, felt in which intercostal space and position with respect to the midclavicular line, and character
- Thrill – location and timing (systolic or diastolic)
- Parasternal heave – with grading
- Palpable heart sounds
- If dilated veins are present, find the direction of flow of blood
- Palpation of the back – any thrill

PERCUSSION

- Method of percussion
  - Right heart border
    Start from the right 2nd intercostal space, go downward up to liver dullness, and then go one space above and then proceed medially. Normally, the right heart border corresponds just lateral to the sternal border.
  - Left heart border
    Start percussing from the left 4th intercostal space, and then percuss laterally up to the midaxillary line. Usually, the left heart border corresponds to the apical impulse.

AUSCULTATION

- Generally, the order of auscultation is mitral, tricuspid, aortic, and pulmonary.
- Another method is to start with the area where maximum findings are heard. For example, I would like to start with the mitral area and then proceed with the other areas because maximum findings are in the mitral area.
- Findings in each area should include the following:
  - First and second heart sounds
  - Murmur: Timing (systolic or diastolic), grading, pitch, character, quality, conduction, and variation with respect to position and respiration
  - Mitral area: Left 5th intercostal space in the midclavicular line (corresponds to the apical beat)
  - Tricuspid area: Left 4th intercostal space just lateral to the lower end of the sternum

- Aortic area
  - First aortic area: Right 2nd intercostal space close to the sternum
  - Second aortic area or Erb's area: Left 3rd intercostal space close to the sternum
- Pulmonary area: Left 2nd intercostal space close to the sternum
- Gibson's area: Left 2nd intercostal space away from the sternum
- Other areas: Carotids, supraclavicular region, infraclavicular region, axillary region, and back (interscapular and infrascapular regions)

DIAGNOSIS

(Example)
- Cyanotic: Cyanotic congenital heart disease with reduced/increased pulmonary blood flow with/without CCF/PHT/infective endocarditis in sinus rhythm
- Acyanotic: Acyanotic congenital heart disease, probably small/moderate/large ventricular septal defect with/without congestive cardiac failure/pulmonary hypertension/infective endocarditis in sinus rhythm
- Acquired heart disease, probably rheumatic in origin with mild/moderate/severe mitral regurgitation with/without congestive cardiac failure/pulmonary hypertension/infective endocarditis in sinus rhythm

Frequently Asked Questions

1. How is clubbing graded?

   Grading of clubbing
   I. Softening and fluctuation of the nail bed
   II. Obliteration of the Lovibond angle (normal angle is <165°) – Schamroth sign
   III. Parrot beak appearance due to increased convexity of the nail fold; drumstick appearance due to thickening of the whole distal finger
   IV. Hypertrophic pulmonary osteoarthropathy (HPOA)

2. *Define clubbing. What is the time taken for it to develop?
   - Clubbing refers to selective bulbous enlargement of the distal portion of the distal phalanx because of proliferation of the subungual connective tissue. It appears in the index finger first.
   - Time taken for the clubbing to develop is as follows:
     - Lung abscess: 2 weeks
     - Infective endocarditis: 3 weeks
     - Cyanotic heart disease: 6 months
     - Bronchiectasis: 1 year

3. Enumerate the theories in clubbing.

   Theories in clubbing
   i. *PDGF mediated:* Normally megakaryocytes enter the pulmonary circulation where they are broken down and hence do not interact with the vascular endothelium. In case of reduced pulmonary circulation, megakaryocytes interact with the vascular endothelium, form plugs, and get activated to produce PDGF, which in turn leads to connective tissue proliferation and causes clubbing.
   ii. *Vagal stimulation:* Afferent nerves from the lungs to the brainstem cause reflex vasodilation. Vagotomy has helped to decrease symptoms in patients with lung carcinoma.
   iii. *Hypoxic theory:* It explains clubbing in heart diseases that results in the formation of arteriovenous fistula, which in turn causes shunting of blood.
   iv. *Tumor necrosis factor (TNF) and hepatocyte growth factor* cause connective tissue proliferation.
   v. *Hormonal theory:* Certain lung diseases elaborate hormones, which causes vasodilation in the distal limb, e.g., growth hormone, parathormone, estrogen, prostaglandin, and bradykinin.
   vi. *Ferritin:* Ferritin gets oxidized during pulmonary circulation. In conditions with reduced pulmonary blood flow, reduced ferritin is increased, which causes AV anastomosis and hypertrophy of the terminal phalanx. The ferritin enters the systemic circulation and causes vasodilation because it escapes degradation.

4. Define cyanosis. What are its types?

   Cyanosis refers to bluish discoloration of the skin and mucous membrane because of an increased quantity of reduced hemoglobin of >5 g/dL or 30% of total Hb or PaO_2 less than 85% or because of abnormal hemoglobin pigments in the blood perfusing these areas.

Types:

Central Cyanosis	Peripheral Cyanosis
a) Reduced Hb is >5 g/dL	Sluggish blood flow to the affected parts
b) Sites: Soft palate, tongue, oral mucosa, nail bed, and ear lobes	Sites: Tips of the fingers and toes, palms and soles
c) Extremities will be warm	Extremities will be cold
d) Cyanosis may not improve with oxygen	Cyanosis improves with oxygen
e) PaO_2 is <85%	PaO_2 is 85%–100%
f) Warmth has no effect	Warmth improves cyanosis
g) Clubbing present	Clubbing absent
h) Polycythemia is present	Polycythemia is absent
i) Causes: Decreased atmospheric oxygen; high altitude; obstructive lung diseases such as asthma; ventilation–perfusion mismatch; foreign body obstruction; interstitial pneumonia; right-to-left cardiac shunts – TOF (Tetralogy of Fallot) TGA (Transposition of Great Arteries) TA (Truncus Arteriosus) TAPVC (Total Anomalous Pulmonary Venous Connections), and Eisenmenger complex; abnormal Hb such as methemoglobinemia (>1.5 g%)	Causes: Hypothermia, shock

Fig. 10.1A shows central cyanosis and Fig. 10.1B shows peripheral cyanosis – soles.

5. List the external markers of congenital cardiac defects.
   Table 10.1 gives the external markers of congenital cardiac defects.

6. Discuss the cardiac defects associated with antenatal use of certain drugs.
   Table 10.2 gives the antenatal drug usage and associated cardiac defects in babies.

7. Name some maternal conditions associated with congenital cardiac defects.
   Table 10.3 gives the maternal conditions and their associated congenital cardiac defects.

8. Grade pedal edema in heart disease.
   Fig. 10.2 shows the various grades of pedal edema.
   1+: 2 mm of depression; barely detectable; immediate rebound
   2+: 4 mm of depression; a few seconds to rebound
   3+: 6 mm of depression; 10–12 seconds to rebound
   4+: 8 mm of depression; > 20 seconds to rebound

9. What are the external markers of infective endocarditis?
   - Elevated temperature
   - Tachycardia
   - Embolic phenomena: Roth spots (fundus examination), petechiae, splinter nail bed, hemorrhages, Osler nodes (pulp of the fingers), and central nervous system or ocular lesions
   - Vascular phenomena: Conjunctival hemorrhages and Janeway lesions (palms)

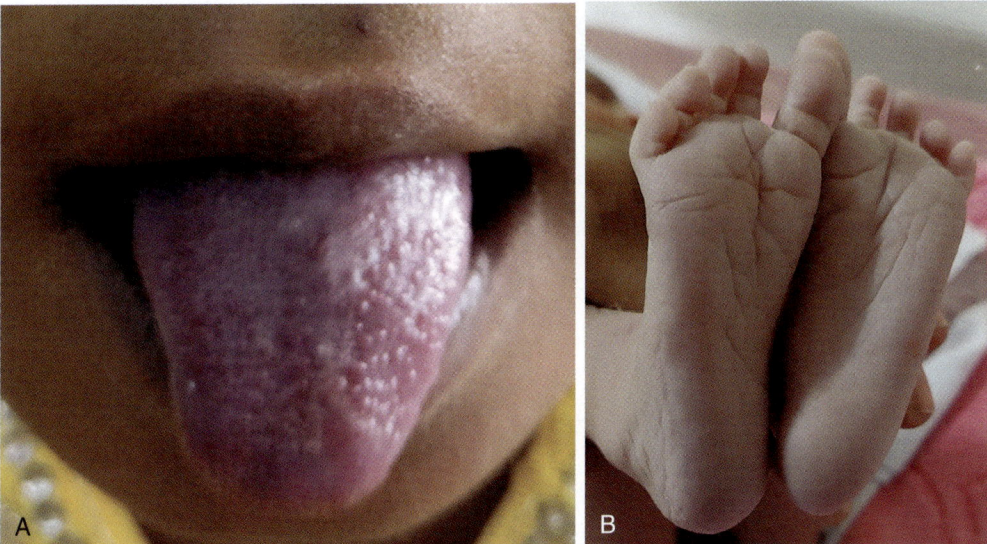

Fig. 10.1 (A) Central cyanosis. (B) Peripheral cyanosis – soles.

TABLE 10.1 External Markers of Congenital Cardiac Defects		
External Markers	**Syndrome**	**Associated Cardiac Defect**
Elfin facies	William syndrome	Supravalvular aortic stenosis, pulmonary artery stenosis
Mongoloid facies, single palmar crease, hypotonia, mental retardation	Down syndrome	Endocardial cushion defects, ventricular septal defect, patent ductus arteriosus
Hypertelorism, short philtrum, downslanting eyes, T-cell defect, hypocalcemia	DiGeorge syndrome	Interrupted aortic arch, truncus arteriosus, ventricular septal defect, patent ductus arteriosus, tetralogy of Fallot
Chondrodystrophic dwarfism, polydactyly, short distal limbs, neonatal teeth, bell-shaped chest	Ellis–Van Creveld syndrome	Atrial septal defect
Webbed neck, cubitus valgus, short stature	Turner syndrome	Coarctation of aorta
Absent radii, normal thumb, thrombocytopenia	TAR syndrome (thrombocytopenia with absent radius)	Atrial septal defect
Arachnodactyly, subluxation of lens, tall stature	Marfan syndrome	Aortic aneurysm, aortic regurgitation, mitral regurgitation

TABLE 10.2 Antenatal Drug Usage and Associated Cardiac Defects in Babies	
Drugs	**Cardiac Defects**
Sodium valproate	Coarctation of aorta, hypertrophic left heart syndrome, aortic stenosis, pulmonary atresia, ventricular septal defect
Hydantoin	Pulmonary stenosis, ventricular septal defect, atrial septal defect, patent ductus arteriosus, coarctation of aorta
Alcohol	Ventricular septal defect, patent ductus arteriosus, atrial septal defect, tetralogy of Fallot
Trimethadione	Transposition of great vessels, tetralogy of Fallot, hypertrophic left heart syndrome
Lithium	Atrial septal defect, Ebstein anomaly
Estrogen	Ventricular septal defect, tetralogy of Fallot, transposition of great vessels
Progesterone	Tetralogy of Fallot
Thalidomide	Tetralogy of Fallot, ventricular septal defect, atrial septal defect, truncus arteriosus
Amphetamines	Ventricular septal defect, patent ductus arteriosus, atrial septal defect, transposition of great vessels, and tetralogy of Fallot
Indomethacin	Intrauterine closure of ductus arteriosus
Vitamin D	Supravalvular aortic stenosis
Vitamin A	Conotruncal anomalies, tetralogy of Fallot, pulmonary atresia, truncus arteriosus, transposition of great vessels

10. Define pulse.

Pulse is defined as the waveform felt by the finger generated by the left ventricular systole that traverses the arterial tree in a peripheral direction at a rate faster than that of a blood column.

11. *What is called trisection method?
- It is the method of palpating pulse.
- For example, while palpating the radial pulse, the forearm should be in a semiprone position with the wrist slightly flexed. Use the pulp of the fingers to palpate the pulse.
- Palpate the pulse using three fingers, i.e.:
  - Index finger: To dampen the effect of pulsations from nearby vessels (obliterating finger)
  - Middle finger: To note the rate, rhythm, character, volume, and condition of the vessel wall (palpating finger)
  - Ring finger: To fix the radial artery (emptying finger)

TABLE 10.3	Maternal Conditions and Their Associated Congenital Cardiac Defects	
Maternal Conditions	**Cardiac Defects**
Diabetes	Asymmetrical septal hypertrophy, transposition of great vessels, ventricular septal defects, patent ductus arteriosus
Phenylketonuria	Tetralogy of Fallot, ventricular septal defect, atrial septal defect, patent ductus arteriosus, coarctation of aorta
Rubella	Pulmonary artery stenosis, patent ductus arteriosus, ventricular septal defect, atrial septal defect
Systemic lupus erythematosus	Congenital heart blocks
Mumps	Endocardial fibroelastosis

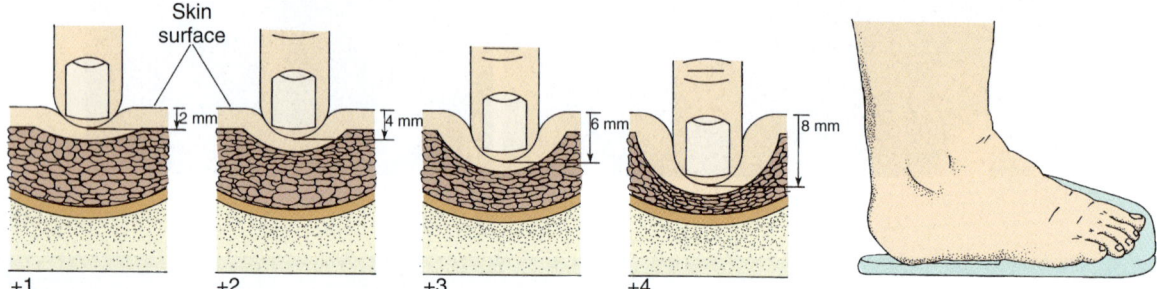

Fig. 10.2   Various grades of pedal edema. *(Source: Reproduced from Holly K. Stromberg. Medical-Surgical Nursing: Concepts and Practice,* Fifth Edition, *Fluids, Electrolytes, Acid-Base Balance, and Intravenous Therapy, Fig. 3.5, St. Louis, Saunders, 2023.)*

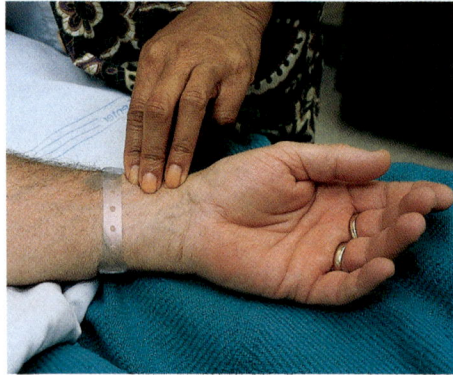

Fig. 10.3   Trisection method of palpating radial pulse. *(Source: Reproduced from Anne Perry, Patricia Potter, Wendy Ostendorf. Nursing Interventions & Clinical Skills, Seventh Edition, Health Assessment, STEP 4g(2), St. Louis, Mosby, 2020.)*

Fig. 10.3 shows the trisection method of palpating the radial pulse.

12. Discuss cardiac palpation.

    Application of hand in cardiac palpation is shown in Fig. 10.4.
    - Pulse: To palpate pulses
    - Metacarpophalangeal joint: To palpate thrill
    - Base of the palm: To palpate parasternal heave

13. Enumerate the palpable peripheral pulses and their surface anatomy.
    - Superficial temporal: Anterior to the ear as it crosses the temporal bone's zygomatic process
    - Carotid: Against the anterior tubercle of the transverse process of the 6th cervical vertebra (Chassaignac tubercle)
    - Brachial: In cubital fossa, medial to the biceps tendon
    - Radial: Palmar aspect of the wrist between the flexor carpi radialis tendon and the radius

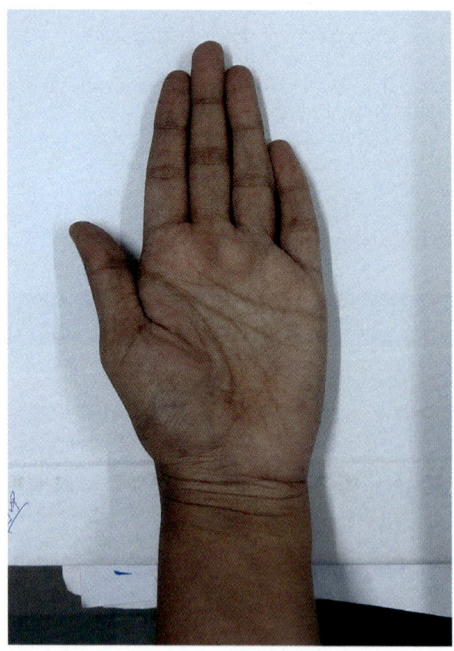

Fig. 10.4   Application of hand in cardiac palpation.

- Femoral: Below the inguinal ligament, midway between anterior superior iliac spine and pubic symphysis (not pubic tubercle)
- Popliteal: The knee flexed before palpating, in midline, on the popliteal side of the lower end of the femur
- Posterior tibial: 1 cm posterior and inferior to the medial malleolus between the flexor digitorum longus and the flexor hallucis longus
- Dorsalis pedis: Lateral to the extensor hallucis longus over tarsal bones

14. Describe various types of pulse and give examples for each.

    Fig. 10.5A to F gives various types of pulse and examples in each.

15. Define blood pressure.

    The lateral force exerted by blood column per unit area of the vascular wall that is expressed in millimeters of mercury

16. *How is the correct cuff size to measure the blood pressure chosen?

    • The inflatable bladder should cover at least two-thirds of the length of the upper arm.
    • The inflatable bladder should cover 80%–100% of the arm circumference.

    Table 10.4 shows the appropriate cuff size in children according to age.

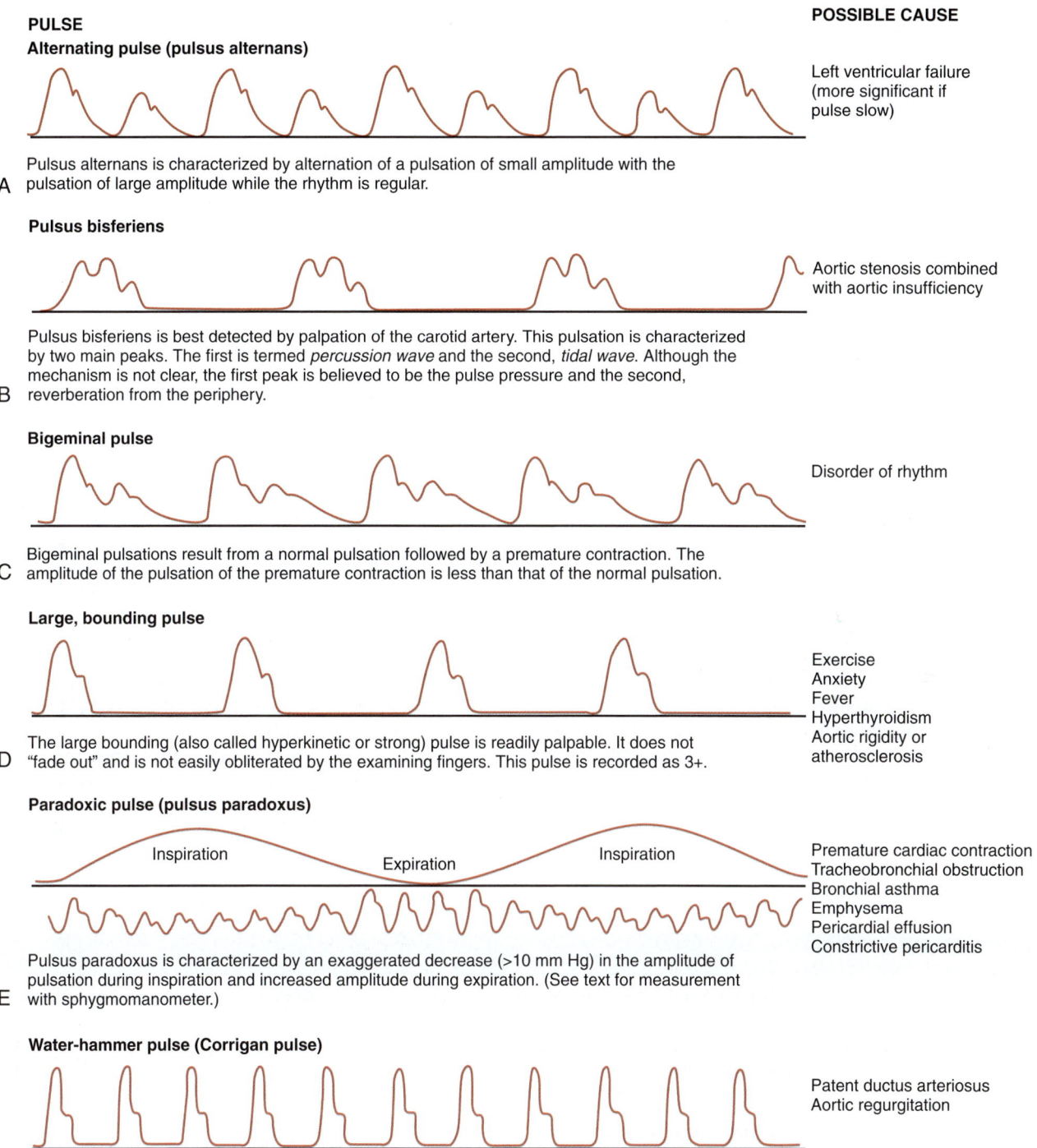

PULSE

POSSIBLE CAUSE

Alternating pulse (pulsus alternans)

Left ventricular failure (more significant if pulse slow)

A Pulsus alternans is characterized by alternation of a pulsation of small amplitude with the pulsation of large amplitude while the rhythm is regular.

Pulsus bisferiens

Aortic stenosis combined with aortic insufficiency

B Pulsus bisferiens is best detected by palpation of the carotid artery. This pulsation is characterized by two main peaks. The first is termed *percussion wave* and the second, *tidal wave*. Although the mechanism is not clear, the first peak is believed to be the pulse pressure and the second, reverberation from the periphery.

Bigeminal pulse

Disorder of rhythm

C Bigeminal pulsations result from a normal pulsation followed by a premature contraction. The amplitude of the pulsation of the premature contraction is less than that of the normal pulsation.

Large, bounding pulse

Exercise
Anxiety
Fever
Hyperthyroidism
Aortic rigidity or atherosclerosis

D The large bounding (also called hyperkinetic or strong) pulse is readily palpable. It does not "fade out" and is not easily obliterated by the examining fingers. This pulse is recorded as 3+.

Paradoxic pulse (pulsus paradoxus)

Premature cardiac contraction
Tracheobronchial obstruction
Bronchial asthma
Emphysema
Pericardial effusion
Constrictive pericarditis

E Pulsus paradoxus is characterized by an exaggerated decrease (>10 mm Hg) in the amplitude of pulsation during inspiration and increased amplitude during expiration. (See text for measurement with sphygmomanometer.)

Water-hammer pulse (Corrigan pulse)

Patent ductus arteriosus
Aortic regurgitation

F The water-hammer pulse (also known as collapsing pulse) has a greater amplitude than expected, a rapid rise to a narrow summit, and a sudden descent.

Fig. 10.5 (A) Normal pulse. (B) Collapsing pulse. (C) Hypokinetic pulse. (D) Pulsus parvus et tardus. (E) Hyperkinetic pulse. (F) Pulsus bisferiens. (*Source: Reproduced from Jane Ball, Joyce Dains, John Flynn et al. Seidel's Guide to Physical Examination: An Interprofessional Approach, Tenth Edition, Blood Vessels, FIG. 16.9, St. Louis, Elsevier Inc., 2023.*)

TABLE 10.4	Cuff Size According to Age	
Age (Year)	**Width of the Bladder (cm)**	
<1	2.5	
1–5	5.0	
6–10	10.0	

17. List the precautions to be taken while measuring the blood pressure.
    - Cuff size should be appropriate.
    - Blood pressure apparatus should be at the level of the upper arm.
    - The lower end of the cuff should end 2–3 cm above the cubital fossa.
    - The patient should not be anxious.
18. Discuss the formula for pulse pressure and mean arterial pressure.

$$Pulse\ pressure = Systolic\ pressure - Diastolic\ pressure$$

$$Mean\ arterial\ pressure = Diastolic\ pressure + one\text{-}third\ pulse\ pressure$$

19. Define hypertension.
    Systolic or diastolic blood pressure ≥95th percentile for that age, sex, and height on ≥3 occasions
20. Classify hypertension.
    As per AAP guidelines (2019), Table 10.5 gives classification of hypertension.
    - **Prehypertension**
        - Systolic or diastolic blood pressure between 90th and 95th percentiles
    - **Stage 1 hypertension**
        - Blood pressure between 95th and 99th percentiles plus 5 mm Hg
    - **Stage 2 hypertension**
        Blood pressure above the 99th percentile plus 5 mm Hg
21. Explain the importance of jugular venous pressure.
    Jugular venous pressure is an indirect measure of central venous pressure and reflects the pressure in the right atrium.
22. Why is the right internal jugular vein preferred?
    The internal jugular vein is preferred because of the following reasons:
    - It has no valves.

- It has a fixed course.
- It does not go through any muscular plane.
- It is in direct communication with the right atrium.
- It is located between the two heads of the sternocleidomastoid and is located easily.

23. *How is jugular venous pressure measured?
    - The patient should be kept at 45° with the head and neck supported.
    - Turn the head to left.
    - If JVP is raised, the pulsations are seen in the neck.
    - The upper level of pulsations in the internal jugular vein is noted. Fig. 10.6A demonstrates the method to note the highest point of venous pulsation.
    - The vertical distance between the sternal angle that is zero point and the upper border of the oscillating column is measured.
    - This is done by drawing a transverse line over the upper border of the oscillating column.
    - Another horizontal line is drawn at the level of the sternal angle.
    - The vertical distance between both the horizontal lines measures the venous pressure as shown in Fig. 10.6B.
    - It is said to be elevated if the distance is more than 3 cm.
    - Central venous pressure = 5 + JVP (the right atrium is 5 cm above the sternal angle).
    - The normal central venous pressure is 5–9 cm H_2O or 7 mm Hg.
24. Enumerate the waves in JVP.
    - "a" wave: It is a positive wave that is produced because of the right atrial contraction.
    - "c" wave: It is also a positive wave that occurs because of the closure of the tricuspid valve and bulging of the same into the right atrium during ventricular systole.
    - "x" wave: It is a negative wave that occurs because of the relaxation of the right atrium.
    - "v" wave: It is a positive wave that occurs because of the filling of the right atrium with the tricuspid valves closed.
    - "y" wave: It is a negative wave that occurs because of the opening of the tricuspid valve and rapid emptying into the right ventricle.
    Fig. 10.7 shows the waves in jugular venous pressure.
    (**Mnemonic:** Function at waveforms – ASK ME)
25. Discuss the abnormalities in jugular venous pressure.
    Table 10.6 shows the abnormalities in jugular venous pressure.

TABLE 10.5	Classification of Hypertension	
Classification	**Children Aged 1–12 Years (Percentile Based)**	**Adolescents (13–19 years) (mm Hg Based)**
Normotensive	<90th percentile	<120/<80
Elevated BP (previously called prehypertension)	≥90th to <95th percentile or 120/80 mm Hg to <95th percentile (whichever is lower)	120/<80 to 129/<80
Stage 1 hypertension	≥95th to <95th percentile +12 mm Hg or 130/80 to 139/89 mm Hg (whichever is lower) **Previous Stage 1 hypertension** Blood pressure between 95th and 99th percentiles plus 5 mm Hg	130/80 to 139/89
Stage 2 hypertension	≥95th percentile +12 mm Hg or ≥140/90 mm Hg whichever is lower **Previous Stage 2 hypertension** Blood pressure above 99th percentile plus 5 mm Hg	≥140/90

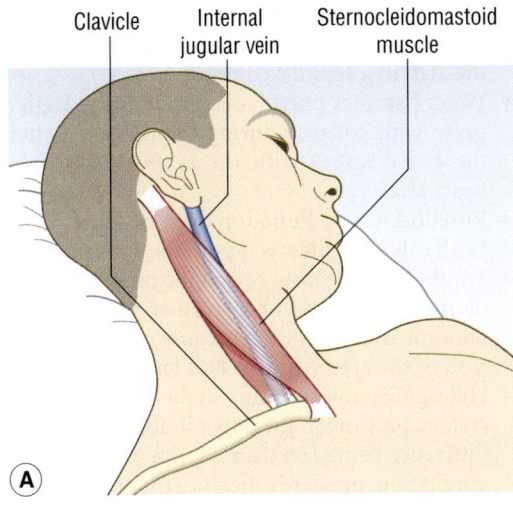

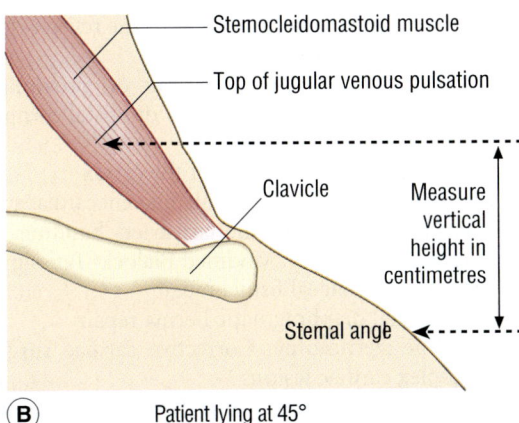

Fig. 10.6 (A) To mark the highest point of jugular venous pulsation. (B) Measurement of jugular venous pressure. *(Source: Reproduced from Tim Hall. PACES for the MRCP: with 250 Clinical Cases, Third Edition, Cardiovascular and nervous system, Figure 3.2, Oxford, Churchill Livingstone, 2013.)*

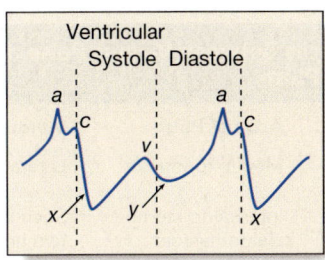

Fig. 10.7 JVP waves. A, atrial filling; S: systole; K, klosed tricuspid; M, maximal atrial filing; E: emptying of atrium. *(Source: Reproduced from Brian Walker, Nicki R Colledge, Stuart Ralston. Davidson's Principles and Practice of Medicine, Twenty-Second Edition. Cardiovascular disease, Oxford, Churchill Livingstone, 2014.)*

Kussmaul sign: It refers to paradoxical rise in JVP during inspiration seen in constrictive pericarditis.

26. How can one differentiate a venous pulse from an arterial pulse?

Table 10.7 shows the differences between a venous pulse and an arterial pulse.

27. What is called Trail sign?

It is the undue prominence of the clavicular head of the sternocleidomastoid on the side to which the trachea is deviated as shown in Fig. 10.8.

28. List the sites for visible pulsations and their associated conditions.
   • Suprasternal notch: Pulsations are seen in the following conditions:
     Aortic lesions
     Aneurysm of arch of aorta
   • Epigastric pulsations: Seen in the following conditions:
     Thin individuals
     Abdominal aorta aneurysms
     Pulsations of the liver in CCF with tricuspid regurgitation
     Right ventricular hypertrophy
     Tricuspid stenosis

TABLE 10.6	Abnormalities in Jugular Venous Pressure	
JVP	**Mechanism**	**Conditions**
Large a wave	Obstruction to tricuspid valve	Tricuspid stenosis Right atrial myxoma
	Noncompliant right ventricle	Pulmonary stenosis Pulmonary hypertension
Canon a wave	Right atrium contracts against the closed AV valve	Complete heart block Ventricular tachycardia
Abnormal x descent	Decreased x descent	Tricuspid regurgitation
	Increased x descent	Pulmonary regurgitation Atrial septal defect Anomalous pulmonary venous connection
Large v wave	Excess filling of right atrium	Atrial septal defect Total anomalous pulmonary venous connection Tricuspid regurgitation
	Poor right atrial compliance	Constrictive pericarditis Right atrial myxoma
Abnormal y descent	Decreased y descent	Tricuspid stenosis Right atrial myxoma
	Increased y descent	Tricuspid regurgitation Constrictive pericarditis Right heart failure

TABLE 10.7	Differences Between Venous Pulse and Arterial Pulse	
Features	**Arterial Pulse**	**Venous Pulse**
In relation to sternocleidomastoid	Medial to muscle	Lateral to the muscle
Site	Internal to sternocleidomastoid	Seen between the two heads of sternocleidomastoid
Palpation	More felt than seen	More seen than felt
Number of waves	Single	Multiple
Variation	Does not vary	Varies with posture, respiration, and pressure over the liver
Obliteration	Cannot be obliterated	Can be obliterated by pressure
Level	No upper level	Has a definite upper level
Wave pattern	Dominant outwards	Dominant inwards

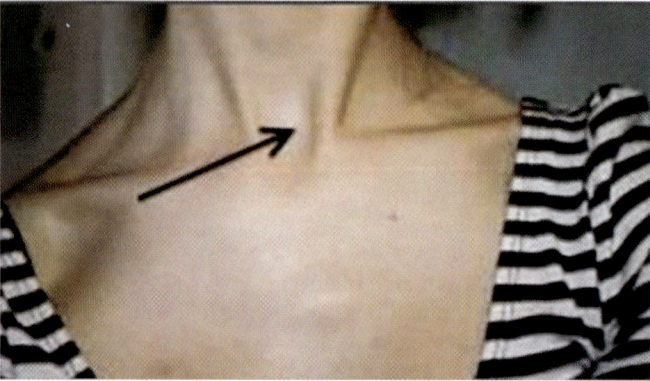

Fig. 10.8   Trail sign. *(Source: Clinical Examination of RS (slideshare.net))*

29. What is tracheal tug?
    - The aneurysm of the arch of aorta may be associated with tracheal tug.
    - Tracheal tug is the pull of the trachea into the thoracic cavity with every systole in cases with aortic aneurysm.
30. What is Suzman sign?
    Visible pulsation over the scapula with the patient bending forward because of the collaterals in a case of coarctation of aorta is called Suzman sign.
31. List the peripheral signs in aortic regurgitation.
    - de Musset sign: Nodding of the head with each cardiac contraction
    - Corrigan sign: Dancing carotids
    - Lighthouse sign: Flushing of the face with each cardiac cycle
    - Landolfi sign: Rhythmic constriction and dilatation of pupils with heartbeats and not related to the light reflex
    - Becker sign: Retinal artery pulsations
    - Muller sign: Pulsatile uvula
    - Oliver Cardarelli sign: Pulsations of the larynx
    - Quincke sign: Alternate flushing and blanching in the nail bed

- Locomotor brachii: Prominent pulsations in the brachial artery seen in the medial aspect of the arm, with the arm in a semiflexed position
- Water hammer pulse (collapsing pulse): High-volume pulse with collapse during the diastole better felt in the radial artery with the arms elevated above the heart level
- Rosenbach sign: Pulsation over the liver
- Gerhardt sign: Enlarged pulsatile spleen
- Traube sign: Hearing of systolic murmur with the bell of the stethoscope on proximal compression of the femoral artery, which is because of the sudden distension of the artery (pistol shot femorals)
- Hill sign: Systolic pressure in the lower limb more than systolic pressure in the upper limb, the normal pressure difference being less than 20 mm Hg, but in aortic regurgitation, pressure difference more than 20 mm Hg
- Durozeiz murmur: Diastolic murmur heard with the diaphragm of the stethoscope on compressing the femoral artery distally because of the reverse direction of the blood flow
- Durozeiz sign: Systolic murmur on proximal compression and diastolic murmur on distal compression of the femoral artery
- Dennison sign: Pulsations of the cervix

32. *Discuss the scars associated with different cardiac surgeries.
    - Left thoracotomy: Pulmonary artery banding
    - Right thoracotomy: Modified Blalock–Taussig shunt
      Tracheoesophageal fistula repair
      Congenital diaphragmatic hernia repair
    - Midline sternotomy: Corrective cardiac surgery for complex cardiac lesions
    - Posterolateral thoracotomy: PDA ligation and division
      Coarctation of aorta
      Blalock–Taussig shunt
    - Anterior thoracotomy: Pericardiectomy for pericardial effusion
    - Submammary scar: Atrial septal defect repair
      Fig. 10.9A and B shows the scars associated with various cardiac surgeries.
33. Define apical impulse.
    Apical impulse is defined as the lowest and outermost definite cardiac impulse which gives maximum thrust to the palpating finger.
34. What is the position of apical impulse with respect to age?
    Table 10.8 shows the position of apical impulse according to age.
35. How can one palpate for apical impulse?
    The following steps show the correct method of palpation of apical impulse:
    - Step 1: Use two hands flat on the chest – to rule out dextrocardia.
    - Step 2: Feel the apical impulse with the flat hand over the left side of the chest.
    - Step 3: Use the ulnar border of the palm to further locate the apical impulse.
    - Step 4: Use the index and middle fingers to further locate the apical impulse.
    - Step 5: Use the tip of the middle finger to point the apical impulse.
    Fig. 10.10A–E shows the steps involved in locating the apical impulse.

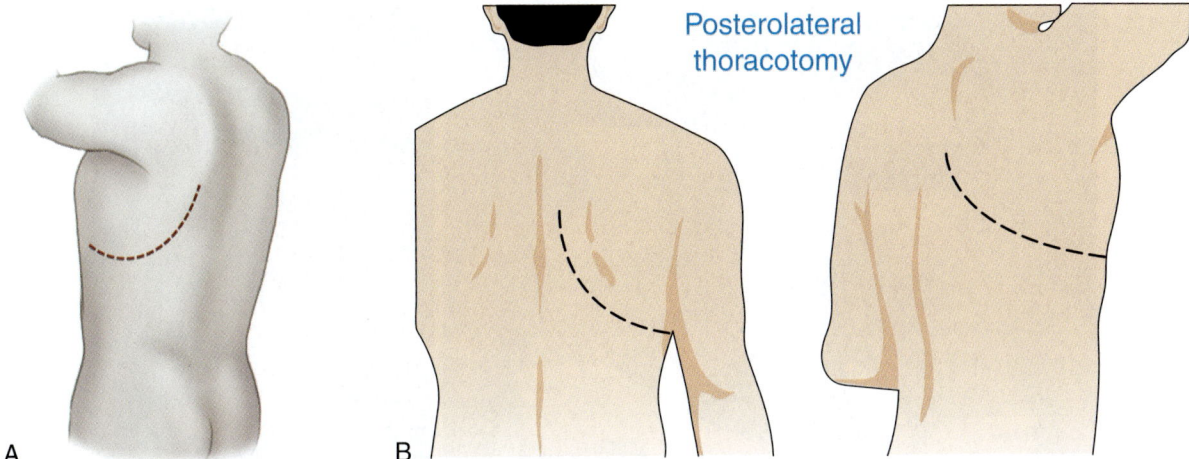

Fig. 10.9 (A) Left thoracotomy (1), right thoracotomy (2), left upper chest (3), median sternotomy (4), and anterior thoracotomy (5). (B) Posterolateral thoracotomy. (*Source: Reproduced from Ellen Hillegass. Essentials of Cardiopulmonary Physical Therapy, Fifth Edition, Cardiovascular and thoracic interventions, Figure 13.1, St. Louis, Elsevier Inc., 2022.*)

| | Position of Apical Impulse | Relation to |
| TABLE 10.8 | **Position of Apical Impulse According to Age** | |

Age	Position of Apical Impulse	Relation to Midclavicular Line
Newborn	Left 3rd intercostal space	Lateral to midclavicular line
Infancy	Left 3rd intercostal space	Lateral to midclavicular line (1 cm)
1–4 years	Left 4th intercostal space	Lateral to midclavicular line
4–8 years	Left 5th intercostal space	At the midclavicular line
>8 years	Left 5th intercostal space	Medial to midclavicular line

36. How can one differentiate between heaving and hyperdynamic apical impulses?
    Table 10.9 shows the differences between heaving and hyperdynamic apical impulses.
37. In which area is tapping apical impulse heard?
    Mitral stenosis
38. List the causes of absent apical impulse.
    - Obese children
    - Apical impulse behind the ribs
    - Pleural effusion
    - Pericardial effusion
    - Emphysema
    - Pneumothorax
    - Hydropneumothorax
39. *What is parasternal heave? In which condition is it seen?
    Parasternal heave is detected by placing the base of the hand over the left parasternal area. In the presence of heave, the heel of the hand is lifted off the chest for each systole (another method is by placing a pen or a pen cap over the parasternal area and look for lifting off the object as shown in Fig. 10.11). It is seen in right ventricular enlargement and left atrial enlargement.
40. How is the parasternal heave graded?
    Table 10.10 shows the grading of parasternal heave.

41. What is Dressler's grading of parasternal heave?
    - Grade 1: Visible
    - Grade 2: Sustained
    - Grade 3: Not sustained
42. How is precordial prominence looked for?
    Precordial prominence is seen in long-standing cardiac diseases because of chamber hypertrophy. One should look into the anterior chest wall – looking into the precordium by standing from the foot end of the patient, bending down so that the examiner's eye is at the level of chest wall as shown in Fig. 10.12.
43. Explain the percussion of the heart border.
    It can be skipped in the examination. But it is always good to know.
    - Left heart border
      ○ Start from the 4th and 5th intercostal spaces in the midaxillary line and come medially toward the apical beat.
      ○ Dullness usually corresponds to the apical beat.
    - Right heart border
      ○ Start from the 2nd intercostal space at the midclavicular line, percuss downwards up to the liver dullness, and then go one space above the liver dullness in the midclavicular line and proceed medially toward the sternal border.
    Fig. 10.13 shows the important areas in percussing the heart border.
44. Name the structures forming the right and left borders of the heart.
    - Right border
      Superior vena cava
      Aortic arch
      Right atrium
      Right ventricle
    - Left border
      Pulmonary bay
      Aortic knuckle
      Left atrial appendage
      One-third of the left ventricle

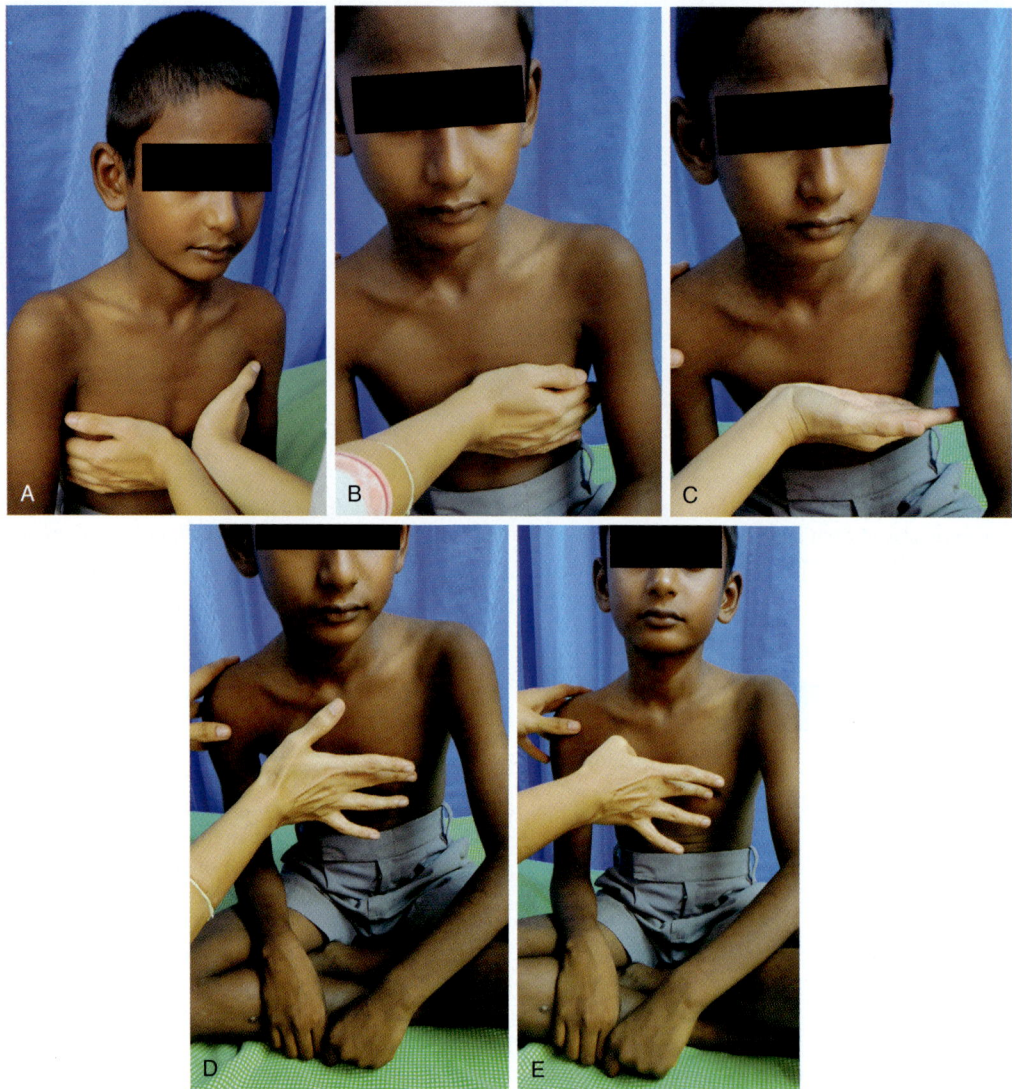

Fig. 10.10 (A) Step 1: Use two hands flat on the chest – to rule out dextrocardia. (B) Step 2: Feel the apical impulse with flat hand over the left side of the chest. (C) Step 3: Use ulnar border of the palm to further locate the apical impulse. (D) Step 4: Use index and middle fingers to further locate the apical impulse. (E) Step 5: Use tip of the middle finger to point the apical impulse.

TABLE 10.9	Differences Between Heaving and Hyperdynamic Apical Impulses	
Features	**Heaving Impulse**	**Hyperdynamic Impulse**
Site	Normal	Shifted downward and outward
Duration	More than two-thirds of the systole Sustained thrust	Less than two-thirds of the systole Ill-sustained thrust
Intercostal space	Felt in one intercostal space	Felt in more than one intercostal spaces
Pathological changes	Concentric hypertrophy due to pressure overload	Dilatation of the ventricle due to the volume overload
Causes	Aortic stenosis Hypertension Coarctation of aorta	Mitral regurgitation Aortic regurgitation VSD PDA

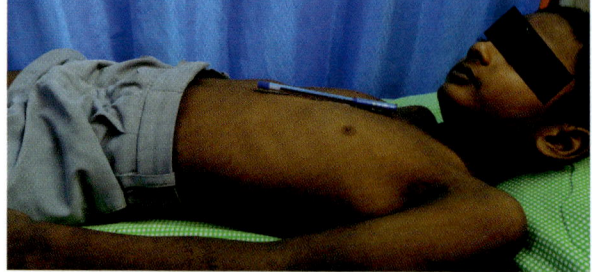

Fig. 10.11 Parasternal heave – place a pen or pen cap over the parasternal area and look for the lifting of the object.

TABLE 10.10	Grading of Parasternal Heave	
Grade	**Examination Findings**	
I	Only visible, not palpable	
II	Visible, palpable, and obliterable	
III	Visible, palpable but not obliterable	

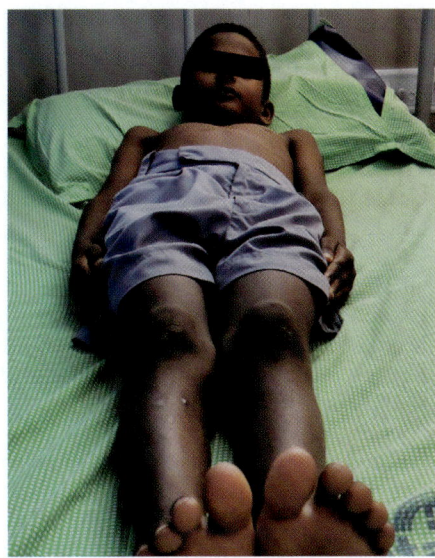

Fig. 10.12 Precordial prominence – inspection.

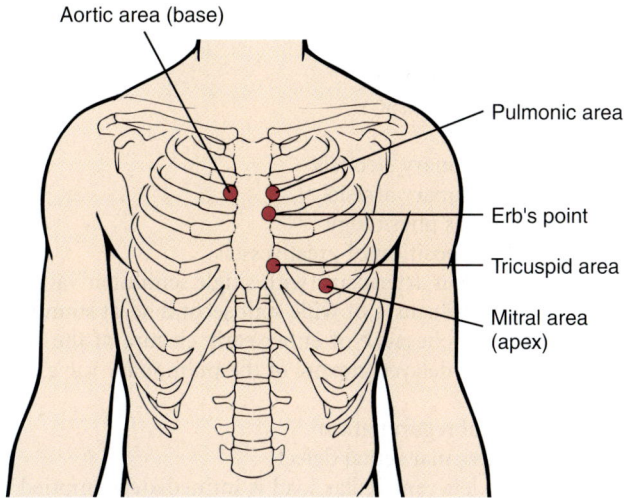

Fig. 10.14 Areas of auscultation. (*Source: Reproduced from Susan deWit. Medical-surgical nursing: concepts & practice, First edition, The Cardiovascular System, Figure 17-10, St. Loius, Saunders, 2009.*)

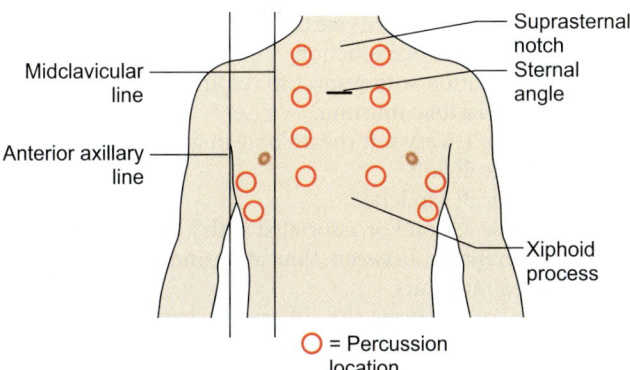

Fig. 10.13 Heart border percussion. (*Source: https://courses.minia.edu. eg/Attach/14828percussion_and_auscultation_of_the_chest.pdf, p. 8.*)

- **Base of the heart**
  Both the atria, mainly the left atrium
- **Inferior surface** is formed by two-thirds of the left ventricle.
- **Apex** is formed by the left ventricle.
- The **posterior-most** chamber is the left atrium.
45. List the areas of auscultation.
    - Mitral area: Left 5th intercostal space in the midclavicular line (corresponds to the apical beat)
    - Tricuspid area: Left 4th intercostal space just lateral to the lower end of the sternum
    - Pulmonary area: Left 2nd intercostal space close to the sternum
    - First aortic area: Right 2nd intercostal space close to the sternum
    - Second aortic area (Erb's area): Left 3rd intercostal space close to the sternum (early diastolic murmur of aortic regurgitation and pansystolic murmur of ventricular septal defect are best heard here)
    - Gibson's area: Left 2nd intercostal space away from the sternum (continuous murmur of patent ductus arteriosus is best heard here)
    Fig. 10.14 shows the areas of auscultation.

46. What is the reason for occurrence of the first heart sound?
    The first heart sound occurs because of the closure of the atrioventricular valves (mitral and tricuspid valves) and is best audible at the apex.
47. When is the first heart sound said to be loud?
    When the first heart sound of the aortic area is louder than the A2 of the aortic area, it is called loud S1.
48. What are the causes of soft S1?
    - Mitral regurgitation
    - Tricuspid regurgitation
    - Calcified mitral stenosis
    - Aortic regurgitation
    - Prolonged PR interval (digitalis overdose)
    - Myocarditis
    - Pericardial effusion
    - Conditions with muffled heart sounds such as emphysema and obesity
49. What are the causes of loud S1?
    - Mitral stenosis
    - Tricuspid stenosis
    - High-output states such as ASD, VSD, and PDA
    - Atrial myxoma
    - Short PR interval
50. What is the reason for occurrence of the second heart sound?
    - The second heart sound occurs because of the closure of aortic and pulmonary valves and it marks the beginning of diastole.
51. Discuss the causes of soft and loud second heart sounds.
    - **Soft S2**
      - Soft A2 – calcified aortic stenosis
      - Soft P2 – calcified pulmonary stenosis
    - **Loud S2**
      - Loud A2
        Systemic hypertension
        Aortic aneurysm
      - Loud P2
        Pulmonary hypertension
        Pulmonary arterial dilatation

52. List the causes of single S2.
    - Absent A2
      - Aortic stenosis
      - Aortic atresia
    - Absent P2
      - Pulmonary stenosis
      - Pulmonary atresia
      - Fallot's physiology
      - Transposition of great vessels
      - Truncus arteriosus (with single semilunar valve)
53. Explain the causes of wide split second heart sound.
    - It occurs because of either early closure of the aortic valve or delayed closure of the pulmonary valve.
    - Early A2
      - Mitral regurgitation
      - Ventricular septal defect
        The left ventricular load is immediately emptied either into the left atrium or into the right ventricle.
    - Delayed P2
      - Pulmonary stenosis (right ventricular volume is emptied slowly)
54. What is fixed split second heart sound?
    - In a normal individual, during inspiration, there occurs increased venous return. Hence, the closure of pulmonary valve is delayed when compared with that of the aortic valve. Hence, the second heart sound is split as A2P2. But during expiration, both the valves close simultaneously and hence a single S2 is heard.
    - But if the second heart sound is split during inspiration and expiration, it is called "fixed split."
    - Causes
      - Atrial septal defect
      - Right bundle branch block
      - Total anomalous pulmonary venous connection
      - Right ventricular failure
55. List the causes of reverse splitting of S2.
    - **Early P2**
      - Wolff–Parkinson–White syndrome
    - **Delayed A2**
      - Severe aortic stenosis
      - Hypertrophic obstructive cardiomyopathy
      - Systemic hypertension
      - Large PDA
      - Left bundle branch block
56. What is the reason for occurrence of the third heart sound?
    - It occurs because of the initial passive filling of the ventricles.
    - It is normal in children and athletes.
    - Pathological causes of S3
      - High-output states such as ASD, VSD, and PDA
      - Regurgitant lesions such as mitral regurgitation, aortic regurgitation, and tricuspid regurgitation
      - Hypertrophic obstructive cardiomyopathy
      - Constrictive pericarditis
      - Systemic hypertension
      - Pulmonary hypertension
57. What is the reason for occurrence of the fourth heart sound?
    - It occurs because of the emptying of the atrium into the noncompliant ventricle.
    - It is always pathological.
    - Causes

    - Systemic hypertension
    - Pulmonary hypertension
    - Ventricular failure
    - Hypertrophic obstructive cardiomyopathy
58. Explain the grading of systolic murmur.
    - Levine and Freeman's grading
      - Grade 1: Very soft (heard in a quiet room)
      - Grade 2: Soft, but easily audible
      - Grade 3: Moderately loud but no thrill
      - Grade 4: Loud murmur with thrill
      - Grade 5: Very loud with thrill and the murmur will be heard with the stethoscope placed barely over the chest
      - Grade 6: Loud with thrill and is heard with the stethoscope even off the chest wall
59. How can one describe a murmur?
    A murmur has to be described in the following headings:
    - Site – where it is heard maximum
    - Timing – whether systolic or diastolic
    - Intensity – as per the Levine and Freeman's grading
    - Pitch – whether high pitched or low pitched
    - Quality – whether soft/harsh/blowing/rough/vibratory/humming (generally the murmurs because of obstructive lesions are rough [AS, PS]; the murmurs because of regurgitation [M] are blowing in nature)
    - Radiation/conduction
    - Variation with respect to respiration/posture
60. Grade diastolic murmur.
    - Grade 1: Very soft (heard only in good circumstances)
    - Grade 2: Soft
    - Grade 3: Moderate
    - Grade 4: Loud or associated with a palpable thrill
61. *Differentiate between clinically conducted and transmitted murmurs.
    Table 10.11 shows the differences between conducted and transmitted murmurs.
62. Name two conducted murmurs.
    The ejection systolic murmur of aortic stenosis is conducted to the apex and axilla.
    The pansystolic murmur of mitral regurgitation is conducted to the axilla and back.
    (Usually, the murmurs from the pulmonary and the tricuspid valves are localized.)
63. Explain innocent murmur.
    - Innocent murmurs are otherwise called benign or functional murmurs. They are murmurs that occur in the absence of any anatomical or physiological abnormalities of the heart and the circulation. They can occur in conditions such as fever, anemia, or any high-output states.
    - Features
      - Asymptomatic
      - No cyanosis

TABLE 10.11	Differences Between Conducted and Transmitted Murmurs	
Conducted Murmur		**Transmitted Murmur**
Same intensity		Decreased intensity
Same duration		Same duration

TABLE 10.12	Differences Between Innocent Murmur and Organic Murmur	
Features	**Innocent Murmur**	**Organic Murmur**
Site	Localized	Diffuse
Timing	Usually systolic	Can be systolic or diastolic
Quality	Soft and short	Rough and blowing
Thrill	Absent	Present
Structural defect	No evidence of valvular lesion	Evidence of valvular lesion present
Age	Usually present in children	Any age group

- Normal pulses
- Normal heart sounds
- Systolic murmur of grade ≤3/6 with no radiation or transmission
- Normal ECG
- Normal chest X-ray

64. How can one differentiate between an innocent murmur and an organic murmur?

   Table 10.12 shows the differences between an innocent murmur and an organic murmur.

65. What is Still's murmur?
   - It is a type of innocent murmur.
   - It is a soft, short, low-pitched, musical murmur heard in the mid-systole in the area between the lower left sternal border and the apex with a grade of 2–3/6 and no radiation.
   - It is common in those older than 3 years.
   - Chest X-ray, ECG, and echocardiography will be normal.

66. What is venous hum?
   - It is a type of innocent murmur.
   - It is a continuous murmur with a loud diastolic component heard best with the bell of the stethoscope on the neck and the upper chest.
   - It is heard best in the supraclavicular area with the child in sitting posture with the head turned to one side.
   - It disappears on lying down.
   - The hum is because of the kinking of large veins (jugular veins) at the transverse process of the atlas.
   - Hence, any change in the posture that relieves the kinking of the vessels obliterates the hum.

67. What is de carvallo sign?
   - All right-sided murmurs accentuate during inspiration and all left-sided murmurs accentuate during expiration.
   - This is because during inspiration, there is an increase in venous return because of negative intrathoracic pressure and there is an increased flow through the right side of the heart. At the same time, the flow to the left side of the heart is decreased. The vice versa happens during expiration.

11

Approach to Congenital Heart Diseases

1. How can one differentiate between respiratory and cardiac causes of distress?

   In a child who presents with distress, it is important to know whether it is because of cardiac cause or respiratory cause.

   Table 11.1 shows the differences between respiratory and cardiac causes of cyanosis.

2. What is hyperoxia test and what is its significance?

   Hyperoxia test

   It helps to differentiate between cyanosis caused by cardiac disease and that caused by pulmonary diseases. If central cyanosis is confirmed by arterial PaO_2, the test can be performed by giving 100% oxygen through a plastic hood (oxyhood) for 10 minutes. In pulmonary causes, the arterial PaO_2 exceeds 100 mm Hg. In heart diseases with significant right-to-left shunt, arterial PaO_2 does not exceed 100 mm Hg and the rise is not more than 10–30 mm Hg.

Approach to Cyanosis

PULSE OXIMETRY SCREENING TEST FOR CYANOTIC CONGENITAL HEART DISEASES

- American Academy of Pediatrics (AAP) recommends four-limb saturation screening between 24 and 48 hours before discharge.
- Criteria for positive screening
  1. Any oxygen saturation measuring <90%
  2. Oxygen saturation <95% in the right hand and either foot on three measures, each separated by 1 hour
  3. >3% absolute difference in oxygen saturation between the right hand and foot on three measures, each separated by 1 hour
- Critical congenital heart disease (CCHD): Pulse oximetry screening helps in diagnosing seven CCHDs:
  1. Hypoplastic left heart syndrome
  2. Pulmonary atresia
  3. Tetralogy of Fallot
  4. Total anomalous pulmonary venous return
  5. D-Transposition of great arteries
  6. Tricuspid atresia
  7. Truncus arteriosus
- Other CCHDs that may not be detected in pulse oximetry screening include the following:
  1. Coarctation of aorta
  2. Double outlet right ventricle
  3. Ebstein anomaly
  4. Interrupted aortic arch
  5. Single ventricle
  6. L-Transposition of great arteries

STEPWISE APPROACH TO CYANOSIS

- Step 1
  - Take a chest X-ray to see whether the lung fields are plethoric or oligemic.
- Step 2
  - If the lung fields are plethoric, auscultate to note the type of murmur.
- Step 3
  - If the lung fields are oligemic, take an ECG to see the axis deviation.

(ECG reading is dealt with in a separate topic.)

Flowcharts 11.1 and 11.2 show the approach to cyanotic congenital heart diseases. Flowcharts 11. 3 to 11. 5 show various classification of congenital heart disease.

Classification of Congenital Heart Diseases

TABLE 11.1	Differences Between Respiratory and Cardiac Causes of Cyanosis	
	Respiratory Causes	Cardiovascular Causes
Retractions	More	Comparatively less, predominantly subcostal
Hyperoxia test	PaO_2 improves	PaO_2 does not improve
Chest X-ray Cardiac size Lung fields	Generally normal Infiltrations/ pneumonia +	Cardiomegaly +/− Plethora/oligemia +
ECG	Generally normal	Right/left-axis deviation +

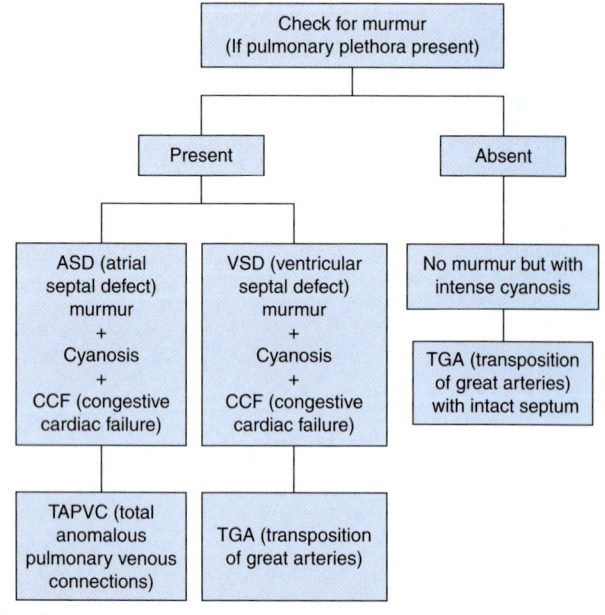

Flowchart 11.1 Approach to cyanotic congenital heart diseases (based on clinical findings-murmur and cyanosis).

184

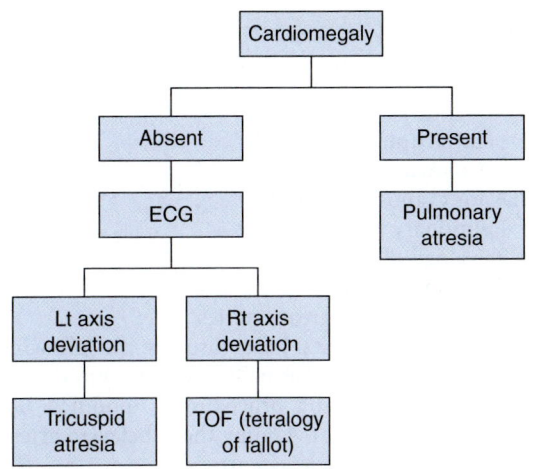

Flowchart 11.2 Approach to cyanotic congenital heart diseases (based on chest x-ray and ECG).

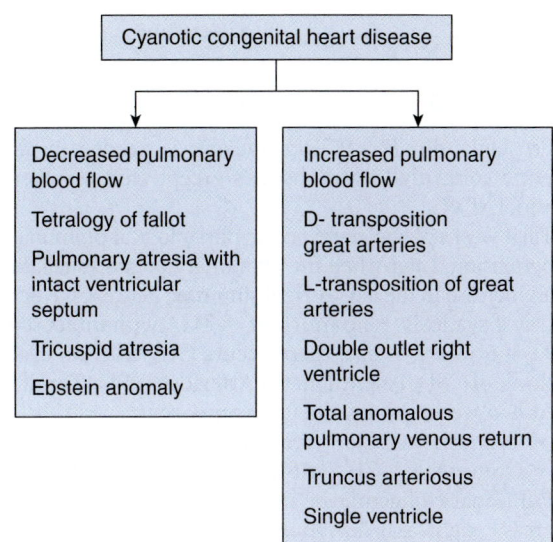

Flowchart 11.5 Classification of cyanotic congenital heart diseases.

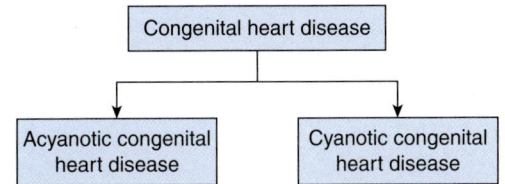

Flowchart 11.3 Classification of congenital heart diseases.

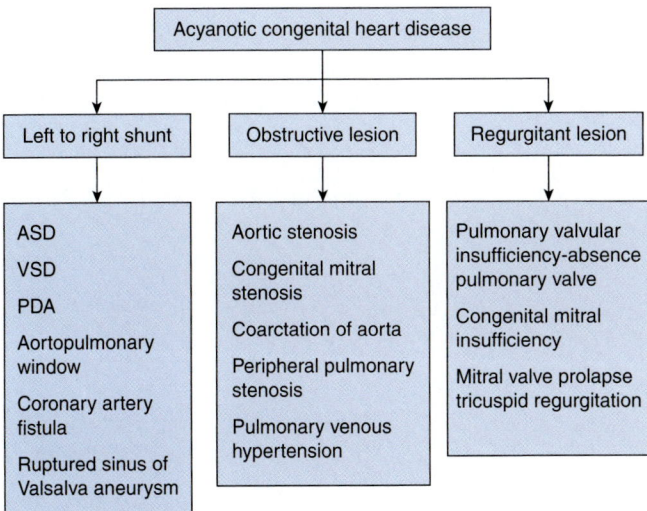

Flowchart 11.4 Classification of acyanotic congenital heart diseases.

Quick Bites

- Prostaglandin E1 (PGE1) infusion is needed in all cyanotic congenital heart diseases except truncus arteriosus and TAPVC.
- Till 4 weeks of age, there occurs physiological pulmonary hypertension. Later when the pulmonary pressures fall, there is an increase in the left-to-right shunting; hence, CCF occurs.
- Day 4 cyanosis + no murmur = TGA with intact septum.
- At 4–6 weeks of age, there occurs CCF with no cyanosis; think of VSD, Patent Ductus Arteriosus (PDA), and ASD.
- At 4–6 weeks of age, the following occur:
  - Cyanosis + CCF + VSD murmur = TGA with VSD
  - Cyanosis + CCF + ASD murmur = TAPVC
- Pulmonary oligemia + cyanosis + ESM in pulmonary area + right-axis deviation + normal sized heart = TOF.
- DDs for shock on day 4 (left-sided outflow tract obstruction)
  - Hypoplastic left heart syndrome
  - Critical aortic stenosis
  - Interrupted aortic arch
  - Coarctation of aorta
- DDs for cyanosis on day 4
  - Pulmonary atresia
  - Tetralogy of Fallot
  - Tricuspid atresia
  - Transposition of great arteries
- For cyanotic congenital heart diseases, the following procedures are performed as palliative procedures:
  - At birth: Lifesaving procedure – modified Blalock–Taussig (BT) shunt (joining the subclavian artery with the ipsilateral subclavian artery)
  - Four months: Hemi-Fontan surgery – pulmonary artery + superior vena cava
  - Four years: Fontan surgery – pulmonary artery + inferior vena cava

Tetralogy of Fallot

Following introduction, seek permission from the caregiver and introduce yourself to the patient before history elicitation, and identify the case.

Name____Age____Sex____Consanguinity____Order of birth____Place____Informant____

Presenting Complaints and Duration

- Breathing difficulty

History of Presenting Illness

- Cyanotic spell – history of crying while feeding/defecation/incessant or inconsolable cry (more predominant in the morning), followed by deep and rapid breathing without significant subcostal recession, followed by deepening of bluish discoloration of the lips and tongue, and later gasping respiration or anoxic seizures or limpness
- Bluish discoloration of the nails and tongue present since…months of age
- Feeding difficulty, suck–rest–suck cycle, forehead sweating, decreased urine output, and presacral edema
- Holding of breath before the episode
- Recurrent respiratory tract infections
- Inadequate weight gain
- Fever with altered sensorium/focal seizures/incessant cry/weakness of limbs
- Diarrhea/focal deficits
- Fever with rashes in the extremities

COURSE DURING HOSPITALIZATION

The child was admitted with breathlessness and hence was put in the knee-chest position and started on oxygen and i.v. medications, and was on i.v. fluids for…days and on NG tube feeding; the child has improved with oxygen requirement through mask/stable in room air.

Past History

- Similar episodes (history of cyanotic spell) and the number of episodes so far
- Whether frequency increased or decreased (indicates collateral development) and started on any oral medication (oral propranolol)
- Any previous hospitalizations
- Whether advised about any surgery
- Oral drugs and when they were started

Antenatal History

Important points not to be missed are the following:
- Mother's age at conception (tetralogy of Fallot [TOF] incidence is high in elderly mothers, also in patients with Down syndrome associated with TOF)
- Any drug ingestion (carbamazepine, trimethadione, thalidomide, sex hormones, alcohol, hydantoin, retinoic acid)
- Any illness such as phenylketonuria
- Irradiation and history of IU infections
- Immunization in pregnancy
- Any ultrasound or fetal Echocardiogram suggestive of heart disease

(Remember five "I"s not to be missed in AN (Antenatal) history are ingestion, illness, irradiation, immunization, and infections.)

Natal and PN History

- Term/preterm
- Whether cried at birth
- Detailed feeding history
- Breathing pattern
- Any history of lethargy and poor feeding/frequent aspiration/vomiting
- Whether bluish discoloration was noted at birth
- History of convulsions (DiGeorge syndrome because of hypocalcemia)
- Whether advised for surgery at that time
- History of prolonged jaundice (Alagille syndrome)

Developmental History

Developmental delay in case of Down and Trisomy 18 syndrome

Dietetic History

Failure to thrive (as suggested earlier)

Immunization History

- It is important to know whether the child has been receiving selective vaccines (killed) (e.g., in DiGeorge syndrome, live vaccines are not given because of T-cell dysfunction).
- In addition, in conditions such as polysplenia/asplenia, vaccines for capsulated organisms should be given.

Contact History

Tuberculosis and measles

Family History

Similar illness in the family

Socioeconomic History

According to the modified Kuppuswamy scale

Summary

A…-year-old male/female child with a history suggestive of cyanotic spell with previous similar episodes, with no symptoms suggestive of CCF and no recurrent lower respiratory tract infection (LRI), probably cyanotic congenital heart disease – tetralogy of Fallot

General Examination

- Awake, active, and comfortable on the mother's lap
- On oxygen support
- Conjunctiva congested (never say pallor)
- Not icteric
- Clubbing of grade
- Central cyanosis +
- No lymphadenopathy
- No edema
- No external markers of heart disease/infective endocarditis

Head-to-Foot Examination

- Head size
- Dysmorphic facies – any conotruncal facies (hypertelorism, bloated eyelids, small palpebral fissure, fish mouth, deformed ears) and Down facies
- Eyes: Congested conjunctiva (polycythemia), Ruth spots (infective endocarditis), cataract (Down syndrome), Coloboma Iris, (CHARGE syndrome) posterior embryotoxon (Alagille), retinitis pigmentosa (Laurence–Moon–Biedl), and hypertelorism
- Ear deformities: Goldenhar syndrome and CHARGE
- Oral cavity: Dental caries especially in children older than 2 years
- Chest deformities such as absence of pectoralis major in Poland syndrome
- Any joint abnormalities: Gouty arthritis (a complication of TOF) and TAR-thrombocytopenia with absent radius syndrome
- Nail changes: Clubbing
- Syndactyly and brachydactyly (Poland syndrome)
- Skin bleeds (coagulopathy – a complication of TOF)
- External genitalia – normal (CHARGE)

Vital Signs

- Temperature – fever in case of brain abscess
- Pulse rate – rate, rhythm, volume of pulse, condition of the vessel wall, and whether felt in all peripheries (rate, rhythm, and volume are expected to be normal in TOF)
- Respiratory rate
- Blood pressure – upper and lower limbs
- Saturation in all four limbs
- JVP – usually normal in TOF

Anthropometry

Weight, height/length, BMI, and weight/height

Cardiovascular System

INSPECTION

- Trachea
- Chest wall symmetry/any chest anomalies (Poland syndrome)
- Apical impulse seen is usually normal in position according to age
- Precordial bulge – yes or no
- Increased precordial activity – yes or no
- Visible pulsations – yes or no
- Any scars/sinuses
- Inspection of the back – pulsation and scars (surgery – BT shunt)

PALPATION

- Tracheal position confirmed
- Apical impulse position confirmed (expected to be normal)
- Any thrill
- Parasternal heave
- Palpable heart sounds
- Palpation at the back

PERCUSSION

The left heart border corresponds to the apex, and the right heart border corresponds to the right sternal margin.

AUSCULTATION

- Started with the pulmonary area because the auscultatory findings are more in the pulmonary area
- Pulmonary area – S1, normal, single second heart sound heard
- Left 3rd and 4th spaces (upper left sternal border): Ejection systolic murmur of grade…best heard with the diaphragm of the stethoscope with the child leaning forward during inspiration
- Mitral area, tricuspid, and aortic – S1 and S2 normal, no murmur
- No VSD murmur (pansystolic murmur) in TOF because VSD in TOF is nonrestrictive

Other System Examination

- Give importance to the central nervous system to rule out focal deficits (hemiparesis) and features of raised ICP.
- In addition, palpate the abdomen to palpate the liver (midline liver) and polysplenia.

Diagnosis

A child with congenital cyanotic heart disease with decreased pulmonary flow, probably Fallot physiology – TOF with hypercyanotic spell with no IE/focal deficits in sinus rhythm

Frequently Asked Questions

1. Mention few points favoring the diagnosis of TOF.
   - Most common cyanotic congenital heart disease
   - History of cyanosis from 6 months of age onwards
   - History of cyanotic spell
   - No history suggestive of congestive cardiac failure (CCF), recurrent respiratory tract infections, and failure to thrive
   - Normal pulse and normal Jugular venous pressure (JVP)
   - No precordial prominence
   - No parasternal heave
   - Second heart sound single and loud in the pulmonary area
   - Ejection systolic murmur heard in the pulmonary area
2. How common is TOF?
   Five per cent to 10% of all congenital heart diseases
3. Describe the embryology in TOF.
   - Anterocephalad malalignment of the infundibular (outlet) septum with the muscular (trabecular) septum is the hallmark of TOF. This is the cause of right ventricular outflow tract obstruction, overriding of aorta, and a high VSD.
   - Arrested development of bulbus cordis results in malformation of the root of the pulmonary artery and its valves, leading to infundibular or valvular stenosis.
   - Incomplete rotation of the spiral septum is responsible for the dextroposition and overriding of the aorta.
   - Failure of the aortic septum to meet the interventricular septum inevitably results in a high interventricular septum.
   - Fig. 12.1 shows the embryology in TOF.
4. Enumerate the components of TOF.
   The four components of TOF are the following:
   - Valvular/infundibular pulmonary stenosis (stenosis/severity: pulmonic, 10%; subpulmonic, 45%; combination, 30%; pulmonary atresia, 15%)
   - Large, membranous (subaortic) VSD

   - Dextroposition of aorta and hence the aorta overrides both the ventricles because of the position of the ventricular septum
   - Right ventricular hypertrophy (concentric) not a developmental abnormality but is because of the altered hemodynamics caused by the above-mentioned malformations
   - Remembered as HAPI (hypertrophy of right ventricle (RV), aorta overriding, pulmonary stenosis, infundibular VSD)

   Fig. 12.2 shows the components of TOF.
5. What is Fallot's physiology?
   Ventricular septal defect with pulmonary stenosis
6. Explain the reason for a child with TOF presenting with cyanosis at birth.
   Right ventricular outflow tract obstruction is severe enough. The degree of cyanosis and the age of the first presentation depend on the degree of pulmonary outflow tract obstruction. Or it can also be because of an extreme form of TOF that is pulmonary atresia.
7. *What is pink Fallot?
   It may be because of mild/moderate RVOT obstruction such as in acyanotic or pink TOF.
   Presentation in pink TOF is as follows:
   - No cyanosis
   - Congestive cardiac failure (predominant VSD symptoms, features of left-to-right shunt)
   - Recurrent respiratory tract infections
   - Precordial bulge because of right ventricular hypertrophy
   - Predominantly left-to-right shunt because of less severe pulmonary stenosis
   - Only ventricular septal defect (VSD) murmur heard
   - ECG – biventricular hypertrophy
   - Extreme Fallot – severe pulmonary stenosis and pulmonary atresia

---

*Important question asked in the examination.

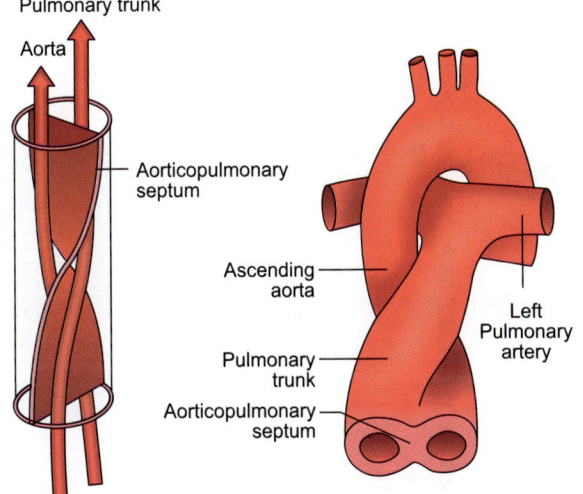

Fig. 12.1 Spiral septum shifted to right side of the heart leading to large opening of aorta, small pulmonary artery opening, missing ventricular septum with straddling of aorta over malaligned VSD.

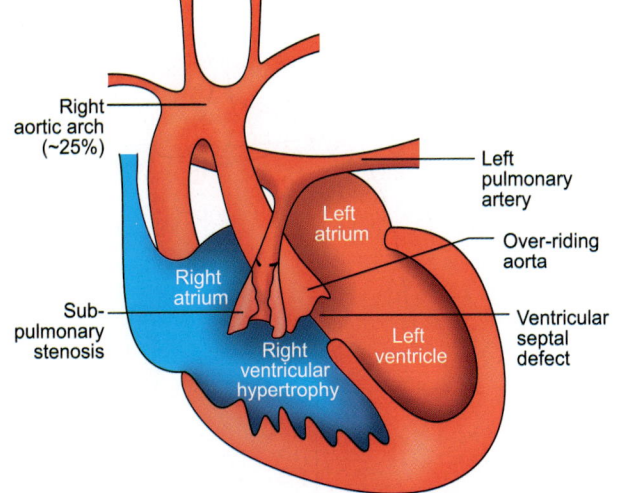

Fig. 12.2 Components of TOF: Infundibular stenosis, large VSD, overriding of aorta, right ventricular hypertrophy.

8. Why does cyanosis in TOF manifest beyond 6 months of age?
   - Fetal hemoglobin prevents the cyanosis at birth. It has a high affinity for oxygen.
   - Activity of the child increases beyond 6 months of age and this increases the oxygen demand. This aggravates the cyanosis.
   - The child also develops negativism by 6–7 months of age. These emotions cause spasm of smooth muscles.
   - Ductus arteriosus may be patent and this compensates for the decreased pulmonary blood flow.
   - Pulmonary infundibular muscular development occurs with the growth of the child. This leads to increased obstruction to the pulmonary blood flow.
9. Enumerate the characteristics of murmur in TOF.
   Fig. 12.3 shows the character of murmur in TOF according to severity.
10. *Define cyanosis. Enumerate the differences between central and peripheral cyanosis.
   Bluish discoloration of the skin and mucous membrane because of an increased quantity of reduced hemoglobin of >5 g/dL or 30% of total Hb PaO₂ less than 85% or because of abnormal hemoglobin pigments in the blood perfusing these areas as in Fig. 12.4

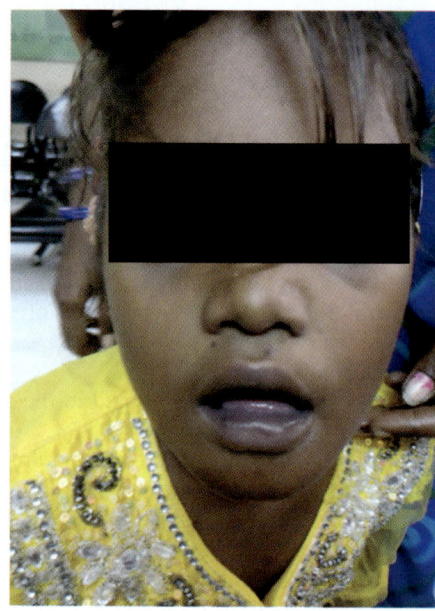

Fig. 12.4 (A) Bluish discoloration of tongue suggestive of central cyanosis. (B) Conjunctival congestion because of high Hb due hypoxic state.

Central Cyanosis	Peripheral Cyanosis
a) Reduced Hb is >5 g/dL	Sluggish blood flow to the affected parts
b) Sites: Soft palate, tongue, oral mucosa, nail bed, ear lobes, and soles	Sites: Tips of the fingers and toes, palms
c) Extremities will be warm	Extremities will be cold
d) Cyanosis may improve with oxygen	Does not improve with oxygen
e) PaO₂ is <85%	PaO₂ is 85%–100%
f) Warmth has no effect	Warmth improves cyanosis
g) Clubbing present	Clubbing absent
h) Polycythemia is present	Polycythemia is absent

Central Cyanosis	Peripheral Cyanosis
i) Causes: Right-to-left cardiac shunts – TOF, Transposition of Great Arteries (TGA), Truncus Arteriosus (TA), Total Anomalous Pulmonary Venous Connections (TAPVC); Eisenmenger complex; abnormal Hb – Methemoglobinemia	Causes: Decreased atmospheric oxygen, shock, hypothermia, high altitude, obstructive lung diseases such as asthma, ventilation–perfusion mismatch, foreign body obstruction, interstitial pneumonia

Cardiac Cyanosis	Respiratory Cyanosis
a) Symptom: Tachypnea	Symptom: Dyspnea
b) Age at onset: Early	Age at onset: Late
c) Intercostal retractions: Less	Intercostal retractions: More pronounced

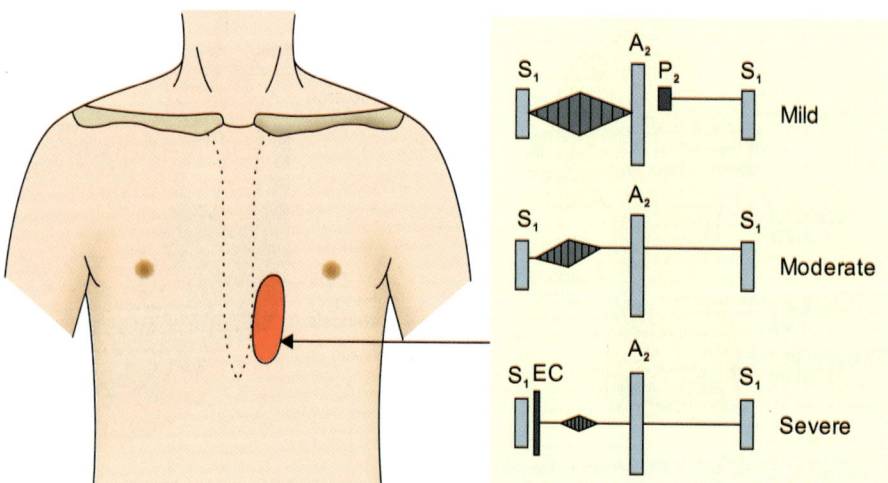

Fig. 12.3 Auscultation findings in TOF on the basis of severity.

Central Cyanosis	Peripheral Cyanosis
d) On crying, cyanosis aggravates	Crying improves the cyanosis
e) Hyperoxia test: No significant increase in pO_2	Hyperoxia test: Increases pO_2 to more than 150
f) pCO_2: Normal/low	pCO_2 may be increased

Differences Between Cardiac Cyanosis and Cyanosis in Methemoglobinemia

Cardiac Cyanosis	Methemoglobinemia
a) Associated symptoms present	Associated symptoms are absent
b) Clubbing may be present	Clubbing absent
c) Color of the blood improves on exposure to oxygen	Color of the blood does not improve on exposure to oxygen
d) No improvement with vitamin C/methylene blue	Clinical improvement seen with vitamin C/methylene blue
e) Predisposing factor: Exertion	Predisposing factor: Ingestion of dapsone

11. Discuss the types of cyanosis.
    Types of central cyanosis are as follows:
    a. *Intermittent cyanosis* – seen in Ebstein anomaly
    b. *Enterogenous cyanosis* – because of absorption of certain drugs from the intestine such as nitrites, nitrates, nitroglycerine, and sodium nitroprusside
    c. *Orthocyanosis* – cyanosis seen only in erect posture such as in pulmonary AV malformation
    d. *Circumoral cyanosis*
       - There occurs bluish discoloration around the lips because of the underlying veins being visible and diminished arterial supply.
       - Causes
         - Normal newborn
         - Occurs in some infants during feeding and resolves spontaneously following feeding
         - Drugs such as dapsone
       - Here other sites such as lips, tongue, and nail beds are pink.
    e. *Pseudocyanosis*
       There occurs bluish tinge of the skin and mucosa because of the ingestion of certain drugs such as amiodarone and clomipramine. There is no hypoxemia.
    f. *Mixed cyanosis*
       - It occurs because of both decreased oxygenation and diminished blood flow.
       - Causes
         - Cardiogenic shock
         - Acute pulmonary edema
         - CCF
         - Hypotension
    g. *Cyclical cyanosis* – bilateral choanal atresia
    h. *Ruddy cyanosis*
       In polycythemia vera, the mucosal congestion looks like cyanosis.
    i. *Differential cyanosis*

- The preductal (right upper extremity) saturation is more than the postductal saturation. The part of the body distal to the shunt is cyanosed.
  - Causes
    - PDA with reversal of shunt
    - PPHN
  - Reverse differential cyanosis
    - PDA reversal of shunt with TGV with severe pulmonary hypertension
    - PDA reversal of shunt with TGV with preductal COA
  - Cyanosis in left upper limb and lower limbs with right UL being pink
    - PDA with reversal of shunt with duct opening proximal to the left subclavian artery
12. Define clubbing.
    - Clubbing refers to selective bulbous enlargement of the distal portion of the distal phalanx because of proliferation of subungual connective tissue. It appears in the index finger first.
    - Time taken for the clubbing to develop in various conditions is as follows:
      - Lung abscess: 2 weeks
      - Infective endocarditis: 3 weeks
      - Cyanotic heart disease: 6 months
      - Bronchiectasis: 1 year
13. Enumerate the grading of clubbing.
    I. Softening and fluctuation of the nail bed
    II. Obliteration of the Lovibond angle (the normal angle is <165°) – Schamroth sign, as shown in Fig. 12.5A
    III. Parrot beak appearance due to increased convexity of the nail fold and drumstick appearance due to thickening of the whole distal finger as shown in Fig. 12.5B
    IV. Hypertrophic pulmonary osteoarthropathy (HPOA)
14. Discuss the types of clubbing.
    - *Unilateral clubbing:* AV malformation and aneurysm of any vessel
    - *Unidigital clubbing:* Gout, sarcoidosis, and trauma
    - *Bilateral*
      - Cardiac: Cyanotic congenital heart disease, infective endocarditis, and Eisenmenger syndrome
      - Respiratory: Bronchiectasis, lung abscess, and mesothelioma
      - GIT: Chronic liver disease and Inflammatory bowel disease (IBD)
    - *Pseudoclubbing:* It is seen in the following cases:
      - Hyperparathyroidism due to excessive reabsorption of the distal phalanx
      - Hansen disease due to excessive damage to the hands as a result of sensory neuropathy
      - Leukemia with secondary deposits in the bone causing destruction of bones
15. Discuss the theories in clubbing.
    Theories in clubbing are as follows:
    i. *PDGF mediated:* Normally megakaryocytes enter the pulmonary circulation where they are broken down and hence do not interact with the vascular endothelium. In case of reduced pulmonary circulation, megakaryocytes interact with the vascular endothelium, form plugs, and get activated to produce PDGF, which in turn leads to connective tissue proliferation and causes clubbing.

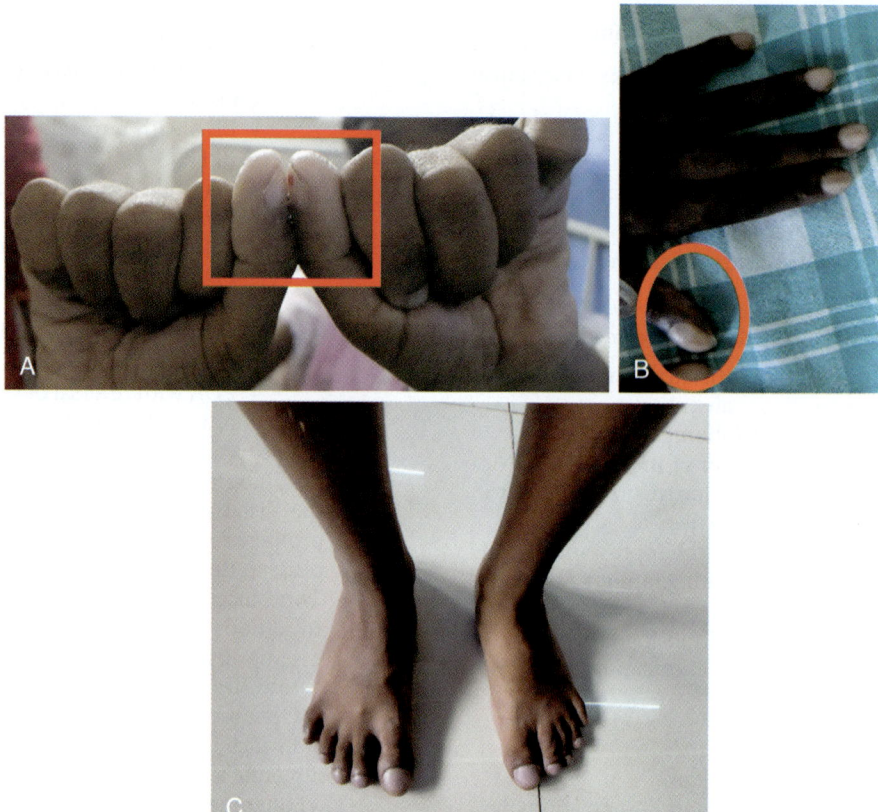

Fig. 12.5 (A) Obliteration of the Lovibond angle (normal angle is <165°) – Schamroth sign (red square). (B) Parrot beak appearance because of increased convexity of nail fold (red circle – parrot beak). (C) Clubbing grade 3, both legs (red circle).

ii. *Vagal stimulation:* Afferent nerves from the lungs to the brainstem cause reflex vasodilation. Vagotomy has helped to decrease symptoms in patients with lung carcinoma.

iii. *Hypoxic theory:* It explains clubbing in heart diseases that results in the formation of arteriovenous fistula, which in turn causes shunting of blood.

iv. *Tumor necrosis factor (TNF) and hepatocyte growth factor* cause connective tissue proliferation.

v. *Hormonal theory:* Certain lung diseases elaborate hormones, which causes vasodilation in the distal limb, e.g., growth hormone, parathormone, estrogen, prostaglandin, and bradykinin.

vi. *Ferritin:* Ferritin gets oxidized during pulmonary circulation. In conditions with reduced pulmonary blood flow, reduced ferritin is increased, which causes AV anastomosis. The ferritin enters the systemic circulation and causes vasodilation because it escapes degradation.

16. What are the conditions associated with TOF?
    - Chromosomal anomalies – Down syndrome and trisomy 18
    - Other syndromes – Goldenhar syndrome, Poland syndrome, Fetal hydantoin syndrome, Fetal alcohol syndrome, Alagille syndrome, VACTERL association (V-Vertebral abnormalities, A-Anal atresia, C-Cardiac anomalies, TE-Tracheoesophageal fistula, R-Renal anomalies, L-Limb anomalies), CHARGE syndrome (Coloboma Iris, heart defects, chonal atresia, growth retardation, genital abnormalities and ear abnormalities), Di-George syndrome, Down syndrome, and TAR syndrome (Thrombocytopenia -absent radius)
    - Maternal conditions such as phenylketonuria
    - Drugs such as thalidomide, trimethadione, and carbamazepine.

17. *Explain conotruncal facies and name some conditions associated with it.
    Conotruncal facies
    - Hypertelorism
    - Bloated eyelids
    - Small palpebral fissure
    - Small, deformed ears
    - Fish mouth
    Conditions with conotruncal facies are the following:
    - TOF, TGA, truncus arteriosus, and double aortic arch

18. What are the compensatory mechanisms in TOF?
    - Polycythemia: It relieves hypoxemia and aggravates cyanosis.
    - Collaterals: There are three types of collaterals – collaterals from the bronchial artery, from the branches of aorta (internal mammary, innominate, subclavian), and directly from the descending aorta. Usually in TOF, only collaterals from the bronchial artery will be present. But if TOF is associated with pulmonary atresia, all three types of collaterals can be seen.
    - PDA: There occurs delayed closure of ductus arteriosus.

19. *How does squatting help in cyanotic spell and what are the squatting equivalents?
    - Squatting causes kinking of great vessels in the inguinal region, so the venous return of more deoxygenated blood from the lower limbs is reduced.
    - It also increases the systemic vascular resistance (by kinking of femoral arteries).
20. Name some squatting equivalents.
    - Knee-chest position
    - Lying supine
    - Sitting with legs drawn underneath
    - Sitting on the mother's hips with legs flexed upon the abdomen
    - Crossing of legs while standing
      Name of these positions – **Taussig positions as in** Fig. 12.6
21. Why is cyanotic spell uncommon beyond 2 years?
    - The child develops adaptation to hypoxia.
    - The child knows to squat.
    - The smooth muscles of the infundibulum get fibrosed.
    - Collaterals develop.
    - Hyper-reactiveness of the respiratory system decreases with age.
22. Describe the various theories in cyanotic spell.
    - *Mechanoreceptor or Kothari theory*
      This is the widely accepted theory. Mechanoreceptors are found more in the right ventricle. When they get activated, there occurs intense right ventricular contraction and the blood is shunted to left ventricle.
    - *Young's theory or paroxysmal atrial tachycardia*
      Sudden tachycardia (because of the autonomic system) on waking up in the early morning increases the venous return and predisposes to cyanotic spell.
    - *Marfan's theory:* Hyper-responsiveness of the respiratory system
    - *Guntheroth theory:* Episodes of paroxysmal hyperpnea
    - *Wood's theory:* Infundibular spasm predisposing to cyanotic spell
    - *Catecholamine theory:* After prolonged sleep, the catecholamine sensitivity of the receptors increased
23. Explain the vicious cycle in a cyanotic spell.
    The vicious cycle in a cyanotic spell is depicted in Fig. 12.7.
24. How can one differentiate a cyanotic spell from a breath-holding spell?
    - Cyanotic spell: No trigger factor required
      The child remains hyperpneic.
    - Breath-holding spell: Trigger factor present
      The child remains apneic.
25. What are the other names of a cyanotic spell?
    Hypercyanotic spell, blue spell, tet spell, anoxic spell, paroxysmal hypercyanotic attacks, and hypoxic spell
    Full name of Fallot: **Etienne Louis Arthur Fallot**

26. Why do children with TOF not present with failure to thrive?
    - Decreased activity because of hypoxia
    - No CCF
27. Can tuberculosis occur in TOF? If "yes," why, and if "no," why?
    - "Yes" because of the extensive development of collaterals
    - "No" because of decreased pulmonary circulation and reduced oxygen tension
28. Mention few causes of cyanosis on day 1.
    - TGA with intact septum
    - TAPVC
    - Tricuspid atresia
    - Severe pulmonary stenosis
    - Pulmonary atresia
29. Mention some causes of nasal twang in TOF.
    Recurrent hypoxic episodes lead to improper approximation of the soft palate (velum) and pharyngeal muscles. This is called velopharyngeal insufficiency and is the reason for nasal twang.
30. Mention few causes of hemoptysis in TOF.
    - Pulmonary thrombi because of increased red cell mass causing sluggish blood flow and stasis
    - Pulmonary infarct
    - Disseminated intravascular coagulation
    - Bleeding tendencies
    - Rupture of collaterals
    - Rarely tuberculosis
31. Discuss the causes of stridor in TOF.
    - Pressure of an enlarged aorta over the trachea
    - Absence of pulmonary valve
    - Associated DiGeorge syndrome due to hypocalcemia
32. Enumerate the causes of wheezing in TOF.
    - Because of bronchopulmonary collaterals
    - Enlarged aorta compressing over bronchi
    - In absent pulmonary valve, compression of dilated main and branched pulmonary arteries over the bronchi
33. *Why is the second heart sound single and loud in TOF?
    - The second heart sound is loud and single; this is only the aortic component because the pulmonary component is soft and the aorta is anteriorly displaced.
34. Why is there no precordial bulge in TOF?
    The load in the right ventricle decompensates into a large dilated aorta and through the ventricular septal defect. Hence, there is no precordial bulge.
35. What are the causes of absence of ejection systolic murmur in TOF?
    - Cyanotic spell
    - Severe stenosis

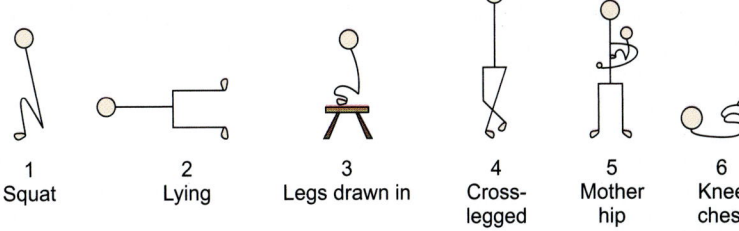

| 1 Squat | 2 Lying | 3 Legs drawn in | 4 Cross-legged | 5 Mother hip | 6 Knee chest |

Fig. 12.6 Squat postures and their equivalents.

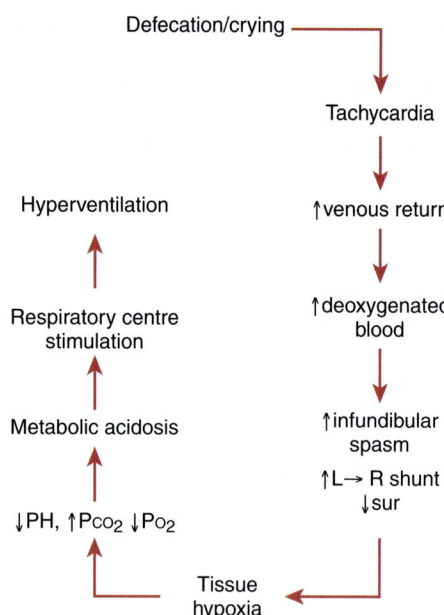

Fig. 12.7 Cycle of cyanotic spell.

The more severe the pulmonary stenosis, the shorter is the ejection systolic murmur and the more is the cyanosis.

36. What are the causes of wide pulse pressure in TOF?
    - TOF with PDA
    - TOF with collaterals
    - TOF with AR
37. What are the causes of TOF with an irregular pulse?
    - Abnormal coronaries
    - Pulmonary atresia
38. What are the causes of to-and-fro murmur in TOF?
    - TOF with AR
    - TOF with absent pulmonary valve
    - Because of collaterals
    - Post shunt
39. Where should one auscultate for collateral murmur?
    - Below the clavicles
    - On either sides of the sternum
    - At the back – interscapular space
40. What is the reason for ejection click in TOF?
    It is due to the blood flow through the large dilated aorta. It is otherwise called "Eddy sound" or "peacock's loud ringing second sound."
41. Where can one hear for ejection systolic murmur in TOF?
    It depends on the site of stenosis:
    - Valvular stenosis – left 2nd ICS
    - Infundibular stenosis – left 3rd ICS
    - Subinfundibular stenosis – left 4th ICS
    - Other murmurs in TOF – pansystolic murmur (pink TOF), to-and-fro murmur (absence of pulmonary valve, collaterals in pulmonary atresia), and early diastolic murmur (AR, PR)
42. What are the causes of LRI in TOF?
    - Associated asplenia/polysplenia
    - Compression of dilated aorta over the bronchus that causes stasis of the blood and infection
    - DiGeorge syndrome

43. What are the causes of raised JVP in TOF?
    - Tricuspid valve leaflet occluding VSD
    - Left jugular vein anomaly
    - Increased systemic vascular resistance
44. Explain the Hoffman variant of TOF.
    Right heart failure in TOF occurs because of tricuspid leaflet occluding VSD. It is called Hoffman variant.
45. Discuss the order of involvement of valve in IE in a child with TOF.
    - Pulmonary valve
    - Aortic valve
46. Discuss the associations of TOF with order of frequency.
    - Right-sided aortic arch (20%–25%)
    - Coronary artery anomaly (5%–10%)
    - Persistence of left superior vena cava (SVC) (10%)
    - Multiple Ventricular septal defects (more associated with postoperative complications)
    - TOF with complete AV canal defect (canal tet)
    - Pentalogy of Fallot – features in TOF with ASD
    - Trilogy of Fallot – Atrial septal defect (ASD) with right-to-left shunt + pulmonary stenosis + Right ventricular hypertrophy (RVH)
    - Congenital absence of pulmonary valve
    - Absence of a branch pulmonary artery
    - Can be associated with CATCH 22 (C-Cardiac defects, A-Abnormal facies, T-Thymic hypoplasia, C-Cleft palate, H-Hypocalcemia, deletion on chromosome 22)
    - Occasional defect in the atrial septum
47. Clinically how can one suspect right-sided aortic arch?
    Visible pulsations to the right of the sternum
48. Discuss the complications of TOF.
    1. Cyanotic spell
    2. Relative iron-deficiency anemia
    3. Infective endocarditis
    4. Thromboembolism
    5. Brain abscess
    6. Motor delay (because of chronic hypoxia)
    7. Polycythemia, hyperviscosity, and headache
    8. Subnormal intelligence
    9. Delayed sexual maturation
    10. Consumptive coagulopathy
    11. Bleeding
    12. Hyperuricemia, which leads to gouty arthritis
    13. Hypoxic arthropathy
    14. Gum disease (because of polycythemia, gingivitis and gum bleed can occur)
    15. Velopharyngeal insufficiency
    16. Stridor because of PA/aortic dilation
49. *What is the common age group for thromboembolism and brain abscess?
    - Thromboembolism is common in children younger than 2 years and the predisposing factors are dehydration and polycythemia.
    - Brain abscess is common in children older than 2 years. Causes are the following:
      - As the blood goes through pulmonary circulation, phagocytosis occurs. Phagocytosis is also bypassed and predisposes to infection because the pulmonary blood flow is reduced.
      - Dental abscess may lead to brain abscess.

- The common lobe is the right parietal lobe, at the junction of white and gray matter where the blood supply is rich.
- The four stages of abscess formation are early cerebritis (days 1–3), late cerebritis (days 4–9), early encapsulations (days 10–13), and late encapsulations (day 14 onwards). The abscess can rupture into the ventricles because the capsule is poorly formed on the medial aspect (ventricular side).
- Common organisms causing abscess are *Peptostreptococcus*, *Bacteroides*, and *Streptococcus*, which are commonly seen in the oral cavity.

50. What are the causes of failure in TOF?
- Anemia
- Infective endocarditis
- Systemic hypertension
- Myocarditis
- Presence of bronchopulmonary collaterals
- Patent ductus arteriosis (PDA)
- Atrial regurgitation (AR)
- Pink Fallot

51. *What are the differential diagnoses for TOF?
- TGA with pulmonary stenosis with VSD
- DORV with pulmonary stenosis with VSD
- Single ventricle with pulmonary stenosis
- VSD with pulmonary stenosis
- VSD with pulmonary atresia
- Type 4 truncus arteriosus
- Isolated pulmonic stenosis with intact aortic root with right-to-left shunt through the foramen ovale

52. Enumerate the differences between TOF and Double outlet right ventricle (DORV).

DORV	TOF
i. Early onset of cyanosis.	Onset of cyanosis only after 6 months of age
ii. CCF features can be present if pulmonary stenosis is not that severe.	Does not present with CCF
iii. Hyperactive precordium is present.	Precordial activities are not prominent
iv. A parasternal systolic ejection murmur is heard preceded by an ejection click. ESM is more prominent.	ESM is less prominent, usually grades 1–3 in left 2nd to 4th ICS
v. There is no fibrous continuity between mitral and aortic valves; instead, these valves are separated by a muscular conus.	The fibrous continuity between mitral and aortic valves is still maintained
vi. The overriding of aorta is >50%.	The overriding of aorta is <50%

53. What are the causes of DIVC in TOF?
- Polycythemia
- Reduced factors 5 and 7 leads to coagulopathy
- Thrombosis (increased RBC mass → anatomical alteration → thinning of medial wall of blood vessel and elastic tissue → thrombosis)

54. Why is fundus examination important in TOF?
- Congestion
- Papilledema due to raised ICP
- Roth spots due to IE

55. Discuss the investigations in TOF.
A. Complete blood count
- Anemia: Target Hb in TOF is 14–16 g/dL. If Hb is <14 g/dL, iron and folic acid should be started. On follow-up, iron should not be stopped once the Hb is normalized. Other parameters such as Mean Corpuscular Hemoglobin (MCH) and Mean Corpuscular Hemoglobin Concentration (MCHC) should also be checked. If the child is not hypochromic, then iron can be stopped.
- Polycythemia (Hct): The optimal value is 55%.
- Peripheral smear: It is performed to rule out anemia and Howell–Jolly bodies (associated splenic abnormalities).
- ESR: Elevated ESR in TOF can be due to abscess.
- Leukocytosis: Think of TOF.
- Thrombocytopenia: Disseminated Intravascular Coagulation (DIVC) is present.
B. Chest X-ray
- Normal-sized heart
- Clear lung fields because of pulmonary oligemia
- Coeur en sabot (wooden shoe with upturned toe/sheep nose shape) as in Fig. 12.8
  - The apex is upturned because of RVH. The hypertrophied right ventricle displaces the left ventricle to left and upwards (concave left heart border).
- Lazy reticular pattern if associated with pulmonary atresia
- Right-sided aortic arch seen in 25% of cases
C. ECG
- Monophasic pattern of R wave in V1
- Sudden transition of r waves to s waves in right chest leads V2
- Right-axis deviation
- Presence of Q wave in aVR
- Tall P waves
- BVH in case of pink Fallot
D. Echocardiography
- Demonstration of the malalignment
  - Large subaortic VSD
  - Pulmonary stenosis
  - Overriding of aorta
  - Right ventricular hypertrophy
E. Selective right ventriculography is performed to demonstrate the flow from the right ventricle to the aorta directly, which can be seen as simultaneous opacification of the pulmonary artery and aorta. It also enables to see the right-sided aortic arch and right ventricular hypertrophy.
F. Coronary arteriography is performed because in 5%–10% of the cases, an aberrant coronary artery crosses over the right ventricular outflow tract and this has to be ruled out before surgery.
G. Cardiac catheterization: Right heart catheterization is useful to differentiate TOF from pulmonary stenosis with a normal aortic arch.
H. Pressure studies: The pressure in the right ventricle is very high and approximates that in the left ventricle.

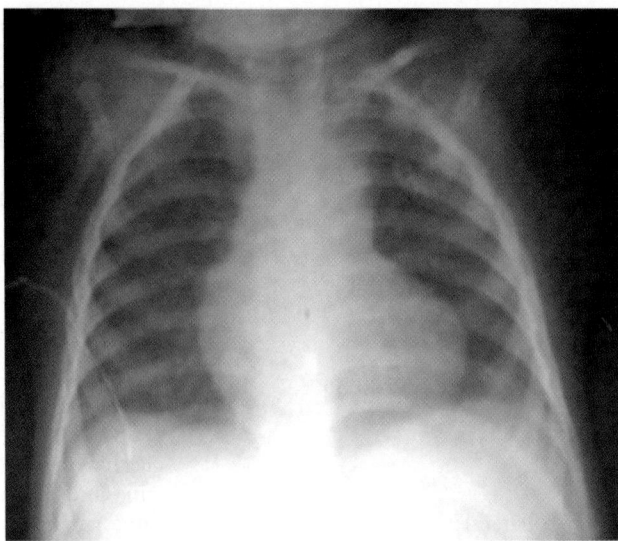

Fig. 12.8 Chest X-ray shows- Boot-shaped heart and pulmonary oligemia. (Source: Reproduced from Amy Kaji, Ryan A. Pedigo. *Emergency Medicine Board Review*, Congenital heart disease, eFIG. 13.1, Philadelphia, Elsevier Inc, 2022. (Credit line - From Kumar, V., Agrawal, V., Jain, D., & Shankar, O. (2012). Tetralogy of Fallot with Holt-Oram syndrome. *Indian Heart Journal* 64(1), 95–98.))

But the pressure in the pulmonary artery is low and is about (5–10 mm Hg).

I. CT brain: It is performed to rule out abscess and infarction.

56. *Discuss the medical management in TOF.
Medical management in TOF includes the following:
A. Management of cyanotic spell
B. Correction of anemia
C. IE prophylaxis
D. I.v. prostaglandin infusion at birth in case of pulmonary atresia

Management of cyanotic spell is performed as follows:
- Put the child in the knee-chest position.
- Oxygen administration: 8–10 L/min of oxygen through NRM will deliver 90%–95% FiO_2.
- Morphine 0.1–0.2 mg/kg s.c./i.v.
  ○ Mechanism: Anxiolytic
    - Depresses the respiratory center
    - Relieves infundibular spasm
    - Dilator of venous capacitance, so reduces venous return
  ○ Propranolol 0.05–0.25 mg/kg slow i.v.
    To reduce the tachycardia
    To reduce the infundibular spasm and improve the pulmonary circulation to some extent
  ○ Phenylephrine 0.02 mg/kg i.v.
    - To increase the systemic vascular resistance
  ○ Sodium bicarbonate 1 mEq/kg i.v.
    - To treat the metabolic acidosis, and the dose can be repeated in 10–15 minutes
  ○ Ketamine 1–3 mg/kg i.v.
    - To increase the systemic vascular resistance and sedate the child
  ○ Other drugs used in TOF
    - Trihydroxyaminomethane (THAM) in place of sodium bicarbonate
    - Methoxamine
    - Amyl nitrate

At the end of the management, always end up saying that I would then plan for surgery.

Management of hypercyanotic spells: Stepwise management is given as follows:
  ○ *Step 1: Immediate steps*
    - Check the airway; deliver oxygen by a face mask or nasal cannula.
    - Place the patient in the knee-chest position.
    - Sedate with morphine (0.2 mg/kg subcutaneously or ketamine 3–5 mg/kg/dose intramuscular).
    - Administer sodium bicarbonate at 1–2 mL/kg (diluted 1:1 or in 10 mL/kg N/5 in 5% dextrose).
    - Correct hypovolemia (10 mL/kg of dextrose normal saline).
    - Keep the child warm.
    - Transfuse packed red cell if the child is anemic (hemoglobin <12 g/dL).
    - Use beta-blockers unless contraindicated by bronchial asthma or ventricular dysfunction; metoprolol is given at 0.1 mg/kg i.v. slowly over 5 minutes and repeated every 5 minutes for maximum three doses; it may be followed by infusion at 1–2 microgram/ kg/ minute.
    - Monitor saturation, heart rates, and blood pressure; keep the heart rate less than 100/min.
  ○ *Step 2: Persistent desaturation and no significant improvement*
    - Consider vasopressor infusion – methoxamine 0.1–0.2 mg/kg/dose i.v. or 0.1–0.4 mg/kg/dose i.m., or
    - Phenylephrine 5 mic/kg as i.v. bolus and 1–4 mic/kg/min as infusion
  ○ *Step 3: If cyanotic spell persist*
    - Paralyze the patient.
    - Electively intubate and ventilate.
    - Plan for palliative or corrective surgery.
    - Seizures are managed with diazepam at 0.2 mg/ kg i.v. or midazolam at 0.1–0.2 mg/kg/dose i.v.

Step 4: Following a cyanotic spell
- Conduct a careful neurological examination; perform CNS imaging if focal deficits are present.
- Initiate therapy with beta-blockers at the maximally tolerated dose (propranolol 0.5–1.5 mg/kg continuous infusion 6–8 hours); it helps improve resting saturation and decreases the frequency of cyanotic spells.
- Ensure detailed echocardiography for disease morphology.
- Plan early corrective or palliative surgery.
- Administer iron in therapeutic (if anemic) or prophylactic dose.

Step 5: Prevention
- Counsel parents regarding the possibility of recurrence of cyanotic spells and precipitating factors (dehydration, fever, pain) and measures to avoid them (e.g., use of local anesthetic patches and/or sedation with i.m. ketamine to avoid pain during venesection).
- Encourage early surgical repair.

- *Prophylaxis in TOF*
  - Oral propranolol at a dose of 1 mg/kg q6h to prevent the cyanotic spell
  - Iron tablets (3 mg/kg) to treat the relative iron-deficiency anemia
  - Prophylaxis against infective endocarditis during any surgery/dental procedure along with good maintenance of oral hygiene
  - Advice to maintain good hydration
- *Prostaglandin infusion*
  If the TOF is associated with pulmonary atresia, prostaglandin E1 infusion at a dose of 0.05–0.2 mg/kg should be given to keep the ductus arteriosus patent.
- *Polycythemia*
  - Optimal hematocrit in TOF is 55%.
  - If Hct goes beyond 55%, then partial exchange transfusion should be planned.

57. Describe the indications and complications of shunt procedures.
    - *Indications*
      Shunt is preferred in the following conditions:
      - Infants weighing <2.5 kg
      - Hypoxic spell within 3–4 months of age
      - Pulmonary atresia
      - Hypoplastic pulmonary annulus
      - Hypoplastic pulmonary artery
      - Abnormal coronary artery anatomy
      - Nakata index <200
    - *Palliative shunt procedures*
      A. *Classic Blalock–Taussig shunt*
         - For a right-sided aortic arch, shunt is created between the left pulmonary artery and the left subclavian artery; for a left-sided aortic arch, shunt is created between the right subclavian artery and the right pulmonary artery.
         - It is performed only after 3 months of age because of risk of thrombosis before 3 months.
      B. *Modified Blalock–Taussig shunt*
         Shunt between the subclavian artery and the ipsilateral pulmonary artery is created using

Gore-Tex (polytetrafluoroethylene) interposition. It is left sided for the left aortic arch and right sided for the right aortic arch. The advantage of this procedure is that it can be performed even before 3 months of age. Mortality is <1%.

C. *Waterston shunt*
   Shunt is created between the ascending aorta and the right pulmonary artery. But it is no longer being performed.
   Complications include CCF, pulmonary hypertension, and narrowing/kinking of the right pulmonary artery.

D. *Potts–Smith shunt*
   Shunt is created between the descending aorta and the left pulmonary artery.
   Complications are CCF and pulmonary hypertension. Fig. 12.9 shows the palliative shunts.

E. *Glenn shunt*
   The superior vena cava is anastomosed to the right pulmonary artery as in Fig. 12.10.

F. *Barrett's procedure*
   Pleurae on both the sides are stripped, which leads to the formation of granulation tissue and predisposes to the development of collaterals.

- *Complications of a shunt*
  Junctional ectopic tachycardia, which is the most common complication
  Chylothorax
  Diaphragmatic hernia/paralysis
  Horner syndrome
  Arm length discrepancy

58. Describe the surgical management in TOF – timing, indications, and complications.
    - *Indications*
      - SpO$_2$ <75%–80%
      - Favorable pulmonary artery and RVOT anatomy

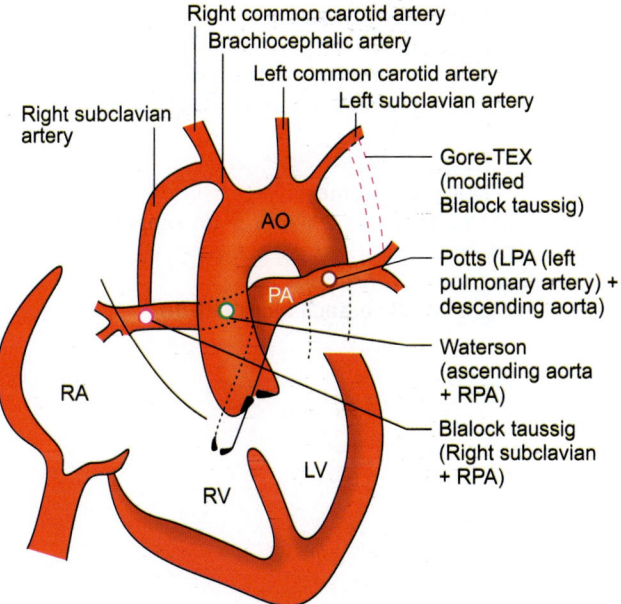

Fig. 12.9 Palliative shunt.

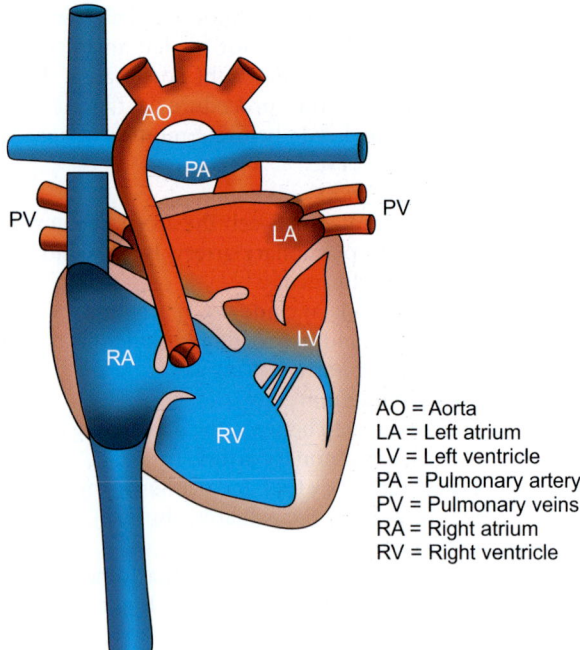

Fig. 12.10 Glenn shunt.

AO = Aorta
LA = Left atrium
LV = Left ventricle
PA = Pulmonary artery
PV = Pulmonary veins
RA = Right atrium
RV = Right ventricle

- One to 2 years following the shunt
- *Timing of surgery*
  - Three to 4 months of age
  - Elective primary repair by 1–2 years of age in case of pink Fallot/acyanotic CHD
- *Advantages of early correction*
  - Decreases the hypertrophy and fibrosis of RV
  - Normal growth of pulmonary artery
  - Decreased incidence of postoperative arrhythmias and death
- *Definitive procedure*
  - *Brock's procedure* – transventricular valvotomy or infundibulectomy
    Infundibulum resected
    Patch closure of VSD
    Pulmonary valvotomy
  - *Risk factors*
    - Younger than 3 months/older than 4 years
    - Severe pulmonary annulus hypoplasia
    - Multiple VSDs
    - Large MAPCAs
    - Down syndrome
  - *Mortality rate* is 2%–3% if uncomplicated TOF is present.
- *Complications of surgery*
  - Right bundle branch block (RBBB)

- Complete heart block
- Arrhythmias
- Pulmonary regurgitation
- Bleeding problems if polycythemic
- Anomalous coronary artery, which is a contraindication for primary repair because it needs placement of a conduit between RV and PA that is performed after 1 year of age.

59. How can one clinically detect a shunt block?
    The most common risk factor for shunt block is dehydration.
    Signs
    - Dyspneic
    - Disappearance of the continuous murmur and it should be auscultated in the infraclavicular and suprascapular regions
    - Reappearance of cyanosis
    - Decreasing saturation

60. Enumerate the signs of a good functioning shunt.
    - Symptoms improve.
    - Saturation increases by at least 10%–15%.
    - Continuous murmur is heard in the infraclavicular and suprascapular regions.
    - Cyanosis disappears.

61. Mention few ratios to identify the severity of pulmonary stenosis/atresia in TOF (two indices).
    1.
    $$\text{McGoon ratio} = \frac{\text{Diameter of right and left pulmonary arteries before branching}}{\text{Diameter of aorta above diaphragm}}$$
    Normal: 2–2.5
    >1.8: Candidate for Fontana procedure

    2.
    $$\text{Nakata index} = \frac{\text{Cross-sectional area of right and left pulmonary arteries}}{\text{Body surface area}}$$

    Body surface area
    Normal: 300 m^2
    >200: Rastelli operation
    >250: Fontan's procedure
    <200: Shunt procedure

62. What is central shunt?
    - Previously performed, not done nowadays
    - Davidson and Melbourne shunts
      - Steps
        - Ascending aorta to main pulmonary artery
        - Unifocalization of pulmonary artery
        - Connect right ventricle to pulmonary artery
        - Closure of VSD
          (There should be good pulmonary artery anatomy, i.e., it should supply 75% of the lung.)

Quick Bites

- Fallot's physiology: Ventricular septal defect with pulmonary stenosis
- Pink Fallot: Mild/moderate RVOT obstruction such as in acyanotic or pink TOF
- Extreme Fallot: Severe pulmonary stenosis and pulmonary atresia
- Compensatory mechanisms in TOF: Polycythemia, PDA, and collaterals
- Cyanotic spell: No trigger factor required (the child remains hyperpneic)
- Breath-holding spell: Trigger factor present (the child remains apneic)
- Common age group for thromboembolism, younger than 2 years; predisposing factors, dehydration and polycythemia
- Common age group for brain abscess, older than 2 years; predisposing factor, dental caries/abscess
- Hoffman variant of TOF: Right heart failure in TOF because of tricuspid leaflet occluding VSD
- Other names of cyanotic spell: hypercyanotic spell, blue spell, tet spell, anoxic spell, paroxysmal hypercyanotic attacks, and hypoxic spell

13

Rheumatic Fever

Following introduction, seek permission from the caregiver and introduce yourself to the patient before history elicitation, and identify the case.

Name____Age____Sex____Consanguinity____Order of birth____Place____Informant____

Presenting Complaints and Duration

- Breathlessness – duration, grading, progressive or nonprogressive, aggravating/relieving factor, and whether associated with paroxysmal nocturnal dyspnea (PND)/orthopnea
- Chest pain – duration, site, nature, aggravating/relieving factors, and radiation
- Palpitation
- Syncope
- Swelling of legs, puffiness of the face, abdominal distension, and reduced urine output

ETIOLOGY HISTORY

(If acquired heart disease is suspected)
- Fever with joint pain – localized to one joint, migratory or nonmigratory, and associated with swelling, redness, and warmth; restricted movements with difficulty in walking; response to oral medications; and with/without deformities
- Any skin rashes – site, origin, progression, and associated itch
- Any involuntary movements – proximal or distal, disappears during sleep, associated with emotional lability, and any clumsiness of activities with absence of school days

History to Rule Out Congenital Heart Disease

- Bluish discoloration of the tongue and nails
- Inadequate weight gain
- Recurrent respiratory tract infection

COMPLICATIONS HISTORY

- Hemoptysis
- Cough and breathlessness
- Fever, joint pain, rashes, skin changes, fatiguability, blood-stained urine, and painful fingertips

Past History

- Sore throat
- Similar illness in the past

Antenatal/Natal/Postnatal History

If significant

Developmental History

Attained age-appropriate milestones

Dietetic History

According to 24-hour recall method

Immunization History

According to National Immunization or IAP schedule

Family History

Any significant illness

Socioeconomic History

- Type of house
- Number of rooms, number of people, number of windows, type of ventilation, and drinking water facility

Summary

Acute onset of fever with migratory polyarthritis of flitting and fleeting type with complete resolution without any deformity ± evidence of carditis ± involuntary movements involving proximal muscles along with emotional lability – probably acute rheumatic fever

General Examination

- Conscious and oriented
- Comfortable at rest
- Any pallor/cyanosis/clubbing/pedal edema/lymphadenopathy
- Any external markers of heart disease
- Any external markers of infective endocarditis (IE)
- Mention whether the child is on oxygen support and i.v. line

Head-to-Foot Examination

- Dysmorphic facies
- Hair changes
- Eyes: Look for the following:
  Signs of aortic regurgitation
  Fundus for Roth spots in infective endocarditis
- Oral cavity: Look for oral hygiene and dental caries
- Chest wall deformities
- Kyphosis/scoliosis
- Extremities: Look for any anomalies, rashes, and skin nodule (signs of Infective endocarditis (IE))
- Skeletal deformities

- Joint swellings
- Involuntary movements
- Signs of infective endocarditis

Vital Signs

- Temperature (must be checked)
- PR: Rate, rhythm, volume, character, whether felt in all peripheries, and RR/RF delay
- RR: Rate, rhythm, and pattern of breathing
- BP: Both Upper limb (UL) and Lower limb (LL)
- SpO_2
- Jugular venous pressure (JVP)

Anthropometry

- Height, weight, and body mass index (BMI) – with interpretation

Cardiovascular System Examination

INSPECTION

- Trachea appearing in the midline
- Apical impulse in intercostal space (ICS) with respect to nipples
- Chest wall – any asymmetry
- Precordial prominence
- Visible pulsations
- Any scars and sinuses
- Any dilated veins
- Suprasternal/supraclavicular pulsations
- Back – any visible pulsations

PALPATION

- Tracheal position confirmed by palpation
- Apical impulse – left ICS at/medial/lateral to mid clavicular line (MCL), and any specific character
- Any thrill
- Parasternal heave
- Any palpable heart sounds
- Any thrill at the back

PERCUSSION

- The left heart border corresponds to the apex, and the right heart border corresponds to the right sternal margin.

AUSCULTATION

Mitral

- Soft S1
- S2 normal
- Holosystolic soft-blowing pansystolic murmur (PSM) of Grade___/6 best heard with diaphragm with breath held in expiration in the left lateral position conducted to the axilla
- Added sounds

Tricuspid, Pulmonary, Aortic

- Soft S1
- S2 normal
- Same murmur of less intensity heard
- Added sounds
- Carotid bruit
- Precordial rub

Other System Examination

RESPIRATORY SYSTEM

- Bilateral air entry +, any retractions, and no added sounds

ABDOMEN

- No organomegaly

CENTRAL NERVOUS SYSTEM EXAMINATION

- Tone
- Any focal deficits
- Any involuntary movements

Diagnosis

Acquired heart disease, probably rheumatic, with mild/moderate/severe mitral regurgitation (MR) with congestive cardiac failure ±, pulmonary hypertension ±, and features of infective endocarditis (IE) ± in sinus rhythm

Frequently Asked Questions

1. Define overcrowding.
   Age >9 years, two people of opposite sexes but not husband and wife sharing a living space of 1 × 10 square feet is called overcrowding.
2. What is the significance of overcrowding in rheumatic fever?
   Colonization of *Streptococcus* is common in overcrowding, which causes group A beta-hemolytic *Streptococcus* pharyngitis.
3. What is the significance of age in rheumatic fever?
   Rheumatic fever is common in the age group of 5–15 years because of the following:
   * Lack of immunity
   * Frequent contact with other children at home and in the school
4. Why is family history important in rheumatic fever?
   There is genetic predisposition in rheumatic fever:
   * DR3, DR4, DR2, DR1, DR7, DW10, and DRW53 associated with rheumatic fever
   * B-cell alloantigen (99% of patients with rheumatic fever have B-cell alloantigen)
5. Mention the significance of past history in rheumatic fever.
   * Sore throat 10–12 days prior to the onset of illness – a clue for streptococcal pharyngitis
   * Similar illness in the past – to know whether it is recurrence/relapse/rebound
6. Mention the importance of certain vaccines in rheumatic fever.
   a. Flu shot
      Inactivated influenza vaccine (IIV): Two doses are given 1 month apart to patients younger than 9 years, and single dose is given to patients older than 9 years.
      Annual reactivation with single dose is necessary.
   b. Varicella vaccine
7. How to differentiate streptococcal and nonstreptococcal pharyngitis?
   Differences between streptococcal and non-streptococcal pharyngitis are given as follows:
   * Age 5-15 years in streptococcal pharyngitis and non-streptococcal attacks all age group.
   * Streptococcal pharyngitis has sudden mode of onset while non-streptococcal is gradual in onset.
   * Initial symptoms include severe sore throat and high fever (>38°C) with anterior cervical nodes, erosions on edges of nose, hyperemic palate and petechiae on soft palate, in streptococcal pharyngitis but symptoms are mild in non-streptococcal pharyngitis.
8. Enumerate the clinical findings in throat examination in Group A Beta Hemolytic Streptococcus (GAS) pharyngitis.
   * The pharynx appears red.
   * Tonsils appear enlarged and are covered by white/gray/yellow exudates.
   * The soft palate may have petechiae or doughnut lesions in the soft palate.
   * The surface of the tongue may resemble a strawberry when the papillae are inflamed and prominent (strawberry tongue); initially it will be coated white with swollen papillae called "white strawberry tongue."
   * Tender anterior cervical lymph nodes will be present.

9. *What are modified McIsaac criteria?
   One point should be added for each of the following criteria:
   * Temperature of ≥38°C: 1
   * Absence of cough: 1
   * Tender anterior cervical lymphadenopathy: 1
   * Tonsillar exudates: 1
   * Age
   3–14 years: 1
      14–44 years: 0
      ≥45 years: −1
   * Otherwise called Centor criteria
   * At best, a score of ≥4 associated with a positive streptococcal pharyngitis in <70% of the children with pharyngitis
10. What are Canadian criteria?
    For the diagnosis of acute streptococcal sore throat:
    * Temperature more than 101°F
    * Sore throat
    * Painful deglutition
    * Erythema of the tonsillopharyngeal region with/without exudates
    * Cervical lymphadenopathy
11. *Discuss the treatment of streptococcal pharyngitis.
    Drugs used in treatment of streptococcal pharyngitis are given as follows:
    * Penicillin V - 250 mg qid for 10 days
    * Benzathine penicillin - 1.2 million units for weight more than 27 kg and 0.6 million units for below 27 kg single dose IM
    * Cephalexin - 15 mg/kg/day bd for 10 days
    * Clarithromycin – 15 mg/kg/day bd for 10 days
    * Clindamycin - 20 mg/kg/day tds for 10 days
    * Azithromycin 12.5 mg/kg/day od 5 days
12. Mention the antibiotics not useful in GAS pharyngitis.
    The following drugs are not useful in GAS pharyngitis:
    * Chloramphenicol (because of high toxicity and unpredictable efficacy)
    * Tetracycline (Resistant strains are prevalent)
    * Sulfonamides does not eradicate Group A streptococcus microbe in pharynx.
13. Enumerate the characteristics of polyarthritis in acute rheumatic fever.
    A. Clinical presentation
       a. Big joints are affected (order of involvement: knees > ankle > wrist > elbow > hip > shoulders).
       b. Joints are usually warm, swollen, red, and painful.
       c. Synovial joint fluid is sterile but has inflammatory cells (10,000–100,000 white blood cells/μL with a predominance of neutrophils, protein level of approximately 4 g/dL, normal glucose level, and formation of a good mucin clot).
       d. Pain is out of proportion to joint involvement.
    B. Character
       a. It is fleeting/migratory.
       b. Inflammation in the first joint recedes before the involvement of the next joint.

*Important question asked in the examination.

C. Course
a. Occurs in the first 2–4 weeks
b. Dramatic response to aspirin
14. *What are the variants of rheumatic arthritis?
- Additive arthritis (involvement of many joints at a time)
- Jaccoud arthritis: Progressing deforming arthropathy of the hands and feet in young adults following recurrent rheumatic fever/systemic lupus erythematosus
15. *Enumerate the differences between rheumatic arthritis and poststreptococcal reactive arthritis.
Differentiating features between rheumatic and poststreptococcal arthritis are given in Table 13.1.
16. Mention the differentiating features of rheumatic arthritis and rheumatoid arthritis.
Differences between rheumatic and rheumatoid arthritis are given in Table 13.2.
17. Name some differentials for fever with joint pain and CCF.
- Acute rheumatic fever
- Infective endocarditis
- Leukemias
- Systemic lupus erythematosus
- Viral myocarditis
- Lyme disease
- Kawasaki disease
18. *Mention some differentials for migratory polyarthritis.
- Rheumatic fever
- Gonococcal arthritis
- Meningococcal infection
- Lyme disease
- Whipple disease
19. Describe the clinical features of rheumatic carditis.
Clinical features of pancarditis are enumerated in Table 13.3.

20. Mention the indicators of recurrence of rheumatic fever in established heart disease.
- New murmur
- Change in preexisting murmur
- Unexplained CCF
- Enlargement of heart size clinically and on X-ray
- Pericardial rub
21. What are the named murmurs in acute rheumatic fever?
a. Seagull murmur is the pansystolic murmur heard at the apex because of mitral regurgitation.
b. Carey Coombs murmur is the mid-diastolic murmur heard at the apex because the thickened mitral valve leaflets cause mechanical obstruction to the blood flow through the valve as a result of edema.
c. Austin Flint murmur seen in severe aortic regurgitation – it is a jet flow vibrating the anterior mitral valve leaflet, which collides with the inflow of mitral valve during diastole, along with increased mitral inflow velocity from the narrowed mitral valve orifice that leads to the jet impinging on the myocardial wall.

TABLE 13.1	Differences Between Rheumatic and Poststreptococcal Arthritis	
Rheumatic Arthritis	Poststreptococcal Reactive Arthritis
Migratory	Nonmigratory
Latent period of 2–4 weeks	Short latent period of 1 week
Dramatic response to NSAID is present	No dramatic response to NSAID
Involves large joint	Involves small joints
	Axial involvement
Fulfills Jones criteria	Does not fulfill Jones criteria

TABLE 13.2	Differences Between Rheumatic and Rheumatoid Arthritis	
Features	Rheumatic Arthritis	Rheumatoid Arthritis
Age	5–15 years	Can occur in children younger than 3 years also
Onset	Acute	Chronic
Duration	Short	Long
Joints affected	Large joints	Smaller joints
Temporomandibular and interphalangeal joints, and spine	Not affected usually	Affected commonly
Symmetry	Asymmetrical in nature	Symmetrical usually
Character of pain	Migratory in nature	Nonmigratory
Diurnal variation	Not present	Stiffness present more in the morning
Fever	High grade commonly seen	Low grade
Muscle spasm	Absent	Present (jellying phenomenon)
Carditis	50%–70%	<10%
ASO	Positive	Negative
RA factor	Negative	Positive
Course	Acute Resolves with treatment Can recur	Chronic course
Residual defects	Not present Mild deformities seen in Jaccoud arthritis	Present Swan neck, boutonniere
Response to NSAIDs	Rapid (12–24 h) and dramatic	Slow and less
X-ray	Normal	Narrowing of space

Source: http://www.cardioiap.org/

TABLE 13.3	Clinical Features of Carditis	
Valvulitis	**Myocarditis**	**Pericarditis**
Apical pansystolic murmur	Tachycardia CCF	Pain pericardial
Apical mid-diastolic murmur	Unexplained cardiomeg-aly	rub pericardial
Basal early diastolic murmur	Soft S1 S3 gallop	effusion

22. What is the frequency of involvement of valves in ARF?
    • Mitral valve: 100%
    • Aortic valve: 20%–25%
    • Tricuspid valve: 5%
    • Pulmonary valve: Almost never involved
23. Mention some differentials for pansystolic murmur in a child with suspected heart disease.
    • Mitral regurgitation
    • Mitral valve prolapse syndrome
    • Ventricular septal defect
    • Postmyocarditis (high left ventricular load causes cardiomegaly and leads to annular dilatation, and hence mitral regurgitation)
    • Infective endocarditis
    • Collagen vascular disorders
24. Mention the differentiating features of mid-diastolic murmur in acute rheumatic fever and mitral stenosis.
    Mid-diastolic murmur because of mitral stenosis will have the following features:
    • Opening snap
    • Presystolic accentuation
    • Loud S1
    In contrast, these features are absent in a case of acute rheumatic fever.
25. How can one differentiate rheumatic fever from infective endocarditis?
    Differences between rheumatic fever and infective endocarditis are given in Table 13.4.
26. Mention some differentiating features of rheumatic carditis and infective endocarditis.
    Table 13.5 shows the differences between rheumatic carditis and infective endocarditis.

TABLE 13.4	Differences Between Rheumatic Fever and Infective Endocarditis	
Infective Endocarditis	**Rheumatic Fever**	
Any age	5–15 years	
Arthritis will be low grade	Arthritis will be high grade	
Fever will be prolonged	Not prolonged	
Clinical features such as hematuria, rashes, painful fingertips	Rashes are more of truncal distribution	
Rashes are more of peripheral distribution	Painless subcutaneous nodules	
Bivalvular involvement is uncommon	Bivalvular involvement is common	
Aortic valve more commonly involved than mitral valve	Mitral valve involvement is more common than aortic valve involvement	
Culture will be positive	Culture will be negative	
Vegetations will be present	Vegetations are absent	

TABLE 13.5	Distinguishing Features of Rheumatic Carditis and Infective Endocarditis	
	Infective Endocarditis	**Rheumatic Carditis**
Site	Ventricular wall	Valves
Appearance	Pedunculated	Sessile
Friability	Friable	Not friable
Prognosis	Wall defects, aneurysms	Valvular stenosis

TABLE 13.6	Classification of Carditis on the Basis of Severity		
Features	**Mild**	**Moderate**	**Severe**
Cardiomegaly	Absent	Present	Present
Complications	No CCF	No CCF	CCF, pericardial effusion
Treatment	Aspirin	Aspirin + steroids	Aspirin + steroids
Bed rest	4 weeks	6 weeks	Until CCF is controlled

27. Describe the features of mild, moderate, and severe carditis.
    Table 13.6 shows the classification of carditis.
28. Mention some salient features of subclinical and indolent carditis.
    • Subclinical carditis
      ◦ It is when the clinical examination is normal but echocardiogram is abnormal.
        Around 30% of the patients having chorea will present as subclinical carditis.
    • Indolent carditis
      Clinically the patient presents with CCF, murmur, and cardiomegaly but with no or very few features of carditis.
29. What is called the poor man's ECG and why is it called so?
    i. Subcutaneous nodules
    ii. More than 95% of the cases with subcutaneous nodule associated with carditis
30. Describe the features of subcutaneous nodules. How are they demonstrated?
    • Subcutaneous nodules are the firm, freely movable, painless, nontender nodules that occur in crops along the extensor aspect of bony prominences such as elbow, wrists, knees, ankles, shin of the tibia, Achilles tendon, and spinal process.
    • They are better felt than seen.
    • Hence, when the examiner asks to demonstrate the subcutaneous nodules, run your finger over the occiput, back of the neck, spine, extensor aspect of the elbow, forearm, tibial shin, and ankles, which is called the blessing sign.
31. Enumerate the features of erythema marginatum.
    • Erythema marginatum occurs in only 1% of the patients with acute rheumatic fever.
    • It is an erythematous, serpiginous, macular lesion with pale centers that are not pruritic.
    • It occurs primarily in the trunk and extremities (bathing suit appearance) and spares the face.
32. Mention some differentials for erythema marginatum.
    • Lyme disease – erythema chronicum migrans; here the lesions are much larger than those in erythema marginatum

- Acute glomerulonephritis
- Sepsis

33. What is the triad of Sydenham chorea?

Hypotonia, involuntary movements, and emotional lability (remember it as HIE)

34. Mention some history to be elicited in a child with chorea.

Poor school performance, clumsiness in activities, dropping things, emotional lability in the form of excessive crying or laughing, and worsening of handwriting (so always document the handwriting of the child in the case sheet in a case of rheumatic fever)

35. Describe the onset of chorea.

- The onset is 1–7 months from acute GAS infection.
- It is insidious in nature.
- It occurs in around 10%–15% of the patients with acute rheumatic fever.

36. Enumerate the clinical maneuvers to elicit the features of Sydenham chorea.

- Demonstration of milkmaid grip – irregular contractions and relaxations of the muscles of the fingers while squeezing the examiner's fingers (Fig. 13.1)
- Spooning and pronation of the hands when the patient's arms are extended (Fig. 13.2)
- Wormian darting movements of the tongue on protrusion
- St. Vitus dance – When asked to lift the arms up with palms facing each other, the forearm will pronate (Fig. 13.3)

37. What are the laboratory findings seen in acute rheumatic fever?

- Total count: Elevated
- Differential count: Polymorphonuclear leukocytosis
- Hemoglobin: Anemia
- ESR: Usually raised in rheumatic fever and anemia
  But ESR is reduced in the following conditions:
  - Congestive cardiac failure
  - Mild carditis
  - Chorea
  - Use of anti-inflammatory drugs
- C-reactive protein
  - It is a β-globulin that is increased in acute rheumatic fever.

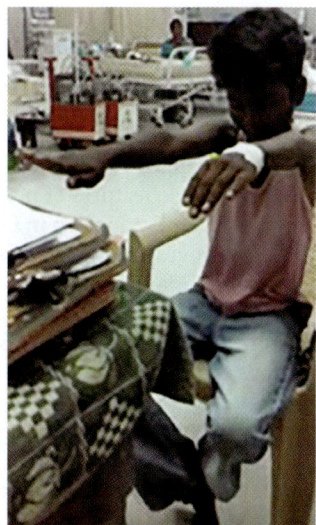

Fig. 13.2 Demonstration of spooning and pronation of the hands when the patient's arms are extended.

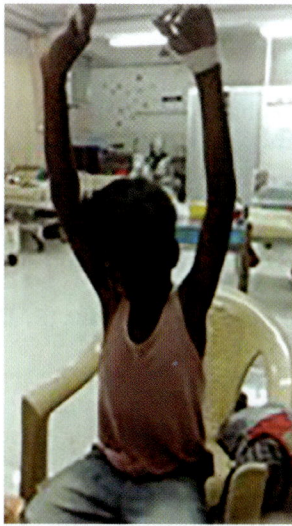

Fig. 13.3 Demonstration of pronator sign.

- It is the one first identified in the serum by its ability to react with C-polysaccharide of pneumococcus.
- It is a sensitive indicator running parallel to ESR but is not affected by anemia or CCF.
- *Evidence of preceding streptococcal infection*
  - *ASO titer*
    ASO is negative in the following conditions in rheumatic fever:
    - Twenty per cent of the cases negative
    - Seven days before and 5 weeks after the onset of rheumatic fever
    - In rheumatic chorea because it occurs 6 months after the onset of rheumatic fever
    - Early treated cases
    - Mild carditis
    - Technical errors
  - *Other streptococcal antibodies*
    Antihyaluronidase, antistreptokinase, antistreptozyme, anti-DNAse B, and anti-NADase

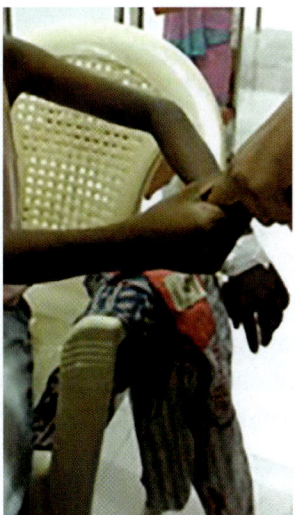

Fig. 13.1 Demonstration of milkmaid grip.

Positive throat culture
Rapid streptococcal antigen detection test
Evidence of carditis

 a. Chest X-ray: Cardiomegaly and pulmonary congestion
 b. ECG: Prolonged PR interval, varying degrees of heart block, features of pericarditis, T-wave inversion, and reduction in QRS voltages
 c. Echocardiography: Cardiac dilation, valve abnormalities, and rheumatic vegetations on mitral leaflets

38. What is the gold standard to diagnose GAS pharyngitis?
Throat culture is the gold standard for the detection of GAS pharyngitis.
Only 10%–20% of the cases grow *Streptococcus* at the time of sore throat.

39. Mention the steps to obtain a throat swab for culture.
 • The tongue should be depressed.
 • The throat should be clearly visualized and well lit.
 • The swab must be rubbed vigorously over the tonsillar fossa without touching the tongue and lips.

40. Mention the causes of false-positive and false-negative throat cultures.
False negative
 • Sampling errors
 • Prior antibiotic treatment
False positive
 • Misidentification of other bacteria as GAS
 • A case of streptococcal carrier now with acute pharyngitis caused by virus showing culture positivity

41. What are the other tests available for diagnosing GAS pharyngitis?
 a. **Rapid antigen detection tests (RADTs)**
 It has a high specificity of >95%. Hence, a positive RADT is considered accurate and a throat culture is unnecessary.
 But sensitivity is less and hence a negative RADT has to be confirmed with a culture.
 b. **ASO titer**
 Blood titers of antistreptolysin O start appearing in the blood in 10–15 days, reach a peak in 3–4 weeks after the acute infection, and remain in plateau for 2–3 months before declining; 20% of the cases remain positive for up to 6 months.
 Isolated rise in ASO titer in the absence of any major criterion can be a past or present streptococcal infection and not the acute rheumatic activity. Hence, it is not included in the minor criteria.
 There is no need to treat a single high ASO titer with secondary prophylaxis. Hence, in case of high clinical suspicion of acute rheumatic fever, rising titers should be demonstrated at an interval of 1 week.
 It is raised in 80% of children with acute rheumatic fever and 20% of normal children.
 c. **Streptozyme test**
 It tests the antibodies against DNAse, streptokinase, streptolysin O, and hyaluronidase.
 It is more sensitive but less specific.
 It is not recommended as a routine test.
 d. **Antideoxyribonuclease B (anti-DNAse B)**
 It will peak after 6–8 weeks of the infection.

 e. **Normal values of ASO titer and anti-DNAse B**
 • **ASO titer**
 Table 13.7 shows the normal values of ASO titer age-wise.
 • **Anti-DNAse B titer**
 Reference values of anti-DNAse B age-wise are given in Table 13.8.
 f. **Clinical correlation:**
 Clinical correlation of ASO and anti-DNAse B is given in Table 13.9.

42. What are the key points in the management of rheumatic fever?
 • General measures – supportive management
 • Control of inflammation
 • Follow-up
 • Primary and secondary prophylaxis

43. What are the supportive measures in the management of rheumatic fever?
General Measures
 a. Indications for hospitalisation:
 ° Diagnosis not clear
 ° Acute rheumatic fever with carditis, chorea, uncontrolled CCF and severe arthritis
 ° Patient with prolonged fever, not doing well on treatment illiterate patient or anxious parents
 b. Congestive heart failure is treated, if present
 c. Pain and constitutional symptoms: Paracetamol and codeine can be used till diagnosis is established. Aspirin is started only after establishing the diagnosis. Fever, myalgia, loss of appetite and anemia are treated to improve the management of rheumatic fever
 d. Rest:
 Indications for rest:

TABLE 13.7	ASO Titer Age-Wise	
Age Group		**Levels (Todd Units)**
Children (5–15 years)		>333
Adults		>250

TABLE 13.8	Age-Wise Anti-DNAse B	
Age		**Normal Levels (units)**
Preschool children		1:60
School children		1:480
Adults		1:340

DNAse B, deoxyribonuclease B.

TABLE 13.9	Clinical Correlation of ASO and Anti-DNAse B		
	Polyarthritis (%)	**Carditis (%)**	**Chorea (%)**
ASO	80	80	30
ASO + anti-DNAse	95	95	80

DNAse B, deoxyribonuclease B.

- Arthritis, carditis and chorea needs bed rest. Absolute bed rest needed only if carditis is severe, and rest is taken till the control of CCF (congestive cardiac failure).
- In the absence of carditis and chorea, rest taken for 15- 20 days. Carditis with no CCF rest is taken for 4-6 weeks.
- Sedatives are used in chorea and carditis with CCF to ensure rest.
- In the absence of carditis and chorea, once arthritis has subsided ambulatory restrictions are relaxed.

e. Diet: Salt restriction and adequate nutrition for growing child.

44. *How is inflammation in rheumatic fever treated?

A. *Arthritis only or with mild carditis -*
- Aspirin - start with 100 mg/kg/day for 2-3 weeks taper to 60-70 mg/kg/day until ESR is normal or symptoms are resolved
- Duration 6 weeks in case of arthritis and 8 weeks in mild carditis
- Naproxen is used if aspirin is not tolerated at dose of 10-20 mg/kg/day
- No response to aspirin in 4 days - rule out myeloproliferative disorder or chronic inflammatory disorders before starting steroids

B. *Moderate to severe carditis*
- Prednisolone 2 mg/kg/day (maximum 80 mg/kg/day) for 2 weeks thereby taper 2.5-5 mg every 3rd day for next 2-4 weeks then start aspirin at 50-70 mg/kg/day concurrently upto 12 weeks (*Aspirin cross over therapy*)
- Alternatively, the same dose of prednisolone can be given for 3-4 weeks and then tapered at 5 mg/week to cover a total period of 10-12 weeks. This is called *"no crossover therapy"*

C. *Non-responders*
- Methylprednisolone is used intravenously at 30 mg/kg/day
- **Precautions**
  - Consider giving antacids while the patient is on aspirin.
  - Avoid giving gastric irritants.
  - Allow frequent feeding.
  - Medicines must not be taken on an empty stomach.

45. How is a child on aspirin monitored?
- Earliest symptom of toxicity is tinnitus
- Later, epigastric pain, black stools or frank blood
- Others: reactivation of dormant comorbid conditions such as tuberculosis Ideal serum salicylate level: 20-25 mg/dl

46. *What are the types of prevention in rheumatic fever? Table 13.10 gives types of prevention in rheumatic fever.

47. What are the indications of secondary prophylaxis in rheumatic fever?
Indications of secondary prophylaxis are as follows:
a. Acute rheumatic fever confirmed by Jones criteria
b. Rheumatic heart disease by echocardiogram
c. Sydenham chorea
Remember
- Secondary prophylaxis mandatory after cardiac catheterization or surgical intervention.
- Isolated ASO titre is not a criterion to start secondary prophylaxis.
- Children who had previous drug allergies are treated cautiously (fatal allergic reaction to benzathine penicillin are rare).

48. What are the drugs used in secondary prophylaxis?
Drugs used for secondary prophylaxis in rheumatic fever are as follow:
- Inj. Benzathine penicillin G is given as 0.6 million units for weight less than 27 kg every 15 days and >27 kg, a dose of 1.2 million units every 21 days
- Oral drugs
  a. Penicillin V 250 mg bd daily
  b. Sulfadiazine or sulfisoxazole 0.5g for <27 kg and 1g if >27 kg once a day daily
- In children with penicillin allergy, erythromycin is used at 40 mg/kg/day as bd daily

49. What is the duration of secondary prophylaxis?
The duration of secondary prophylaxis in rheumatic fever are given below:
A. *Acute rheumatic fever (ARF) without carditis -* minimum for 5 years or until 18 years whichever is longer.
B. *ARF with carditis and no residual heart disease -* for 10 years or till 25 years of age whichever is longer.
C. *ARF with residual heart disease* lifelong secondary prophylaxis or till 40 years.

TABLE 13.10	Types of Prevention in Rheumatic Fever
Types of Prevention	**Salient Features**
Primordial prevention	Streptococcal sore throat prevention by proper hygiene, health education, and high-risk group vaccination
Primary prevention	Early recognition and treatment of streptococcal tonsillopharyngitis by appropriate antibiotic therapy, initiated on or before the 9th day of onset of symptoms
Secondary prevention	Continuous administration of specific antibiotics to children with a previous attack of rheumatic fever or well-documented rheumatic heart disease, to prevent colonization or infection of the upper respiratory tract with group A beta-hemolytic. *Streptococcus* and the development of recurrent attack of rheumatic fever. Significance: Prevents recurrence of GAS infection, which leads to recurrent ARF, reduces severity of RHD (can result in the cure of RHD after many years), prevent death from severe RHD
Tertiary prevention	To prevent the development of infective endocarditis in children with rheumatic valvular lesions; Prophylactic antibiotics are given prior to procedures such as dental extraction. Surgical correction of deformities of the cardiac valves or replacement of the valves with rehabilitation to prevent damage.

50. What are the precautions followed before administration of penicillin in rheumatic fever?
    - **Penicillin sensitivity testing:** It is an intradermal test using Benzylpenicillin 10,000 units/ml not benzathine penicillin with normal saline used as control (approximately 0.02 ml at the volar aspect of the forearm or lateral surface of the arm).
    - Test reading time is 15-30 minutes
    - A wheal of >2 mm than the control or >4 mm than the initial edema is taken as positive test.
    - Patient should not have taken antihistamines such as chlorpheniramine or terfenadine <24 hours, diphenhydramine hydrochloride or hydroxyzine in the past 4 days and astemizole in the preceeding 3 weeks.

51. What is the significance of performing penicillin sensitivity testing every time?
    - Each time penicillin predicts only the presence of IgE antibodies for the major or minor penicillin determinants at the time of application, does not predict the future development of IgE mediated reactions during subsequent course of penicillin. Also, it does not predict non IgE mediated reactions caused by other immune mechanisms such as cytotoxic antibody mediated reactions, antigen antibody immune complex mediated reactions and delayed type cell mediated reactions.

52. What are the indications of surgery in rheumatic fever?
    - Rupture of chordae tendineae
    - Valve rupture
    - Intractable CCF

DISCUSSION ON RHEUMATIC FEVER

53. Define rheumatic fever.
    It is an immunological, noninfectious, nonsuppurative sequela of infection of the pharynx by group A beta-hemolytic *Streptococcus*, which affects the heart, joints, CNS, skin, and subcutaneous tissue. It occurs 10 days to several weeks following the appearance of sore throat.

54. What is the prevalence of RHD in India?
    - The prevalence of RHD in India is 0.9 per 1000 population.
    - Risk of RF following streptococcal pharyngitis is 0.3%–3%.
    - Of all the cases of sore throats, 30% are caused by group A beta-hemolytic *Streptococcus* in the age group of 5–15 years.
    - Around 50%–90% of the patients with RF will end up with cardiac complications.
    - Only 30% (one-third) of the patients with RF will give the history of sore throat.

55. Describe the types of streptococcal strains causing pharyngitis and skin infections.
    - On the basis of hemolysis in 5% horse blood agar
      Alpha or partial hemolysis
      Beta or complete hemolysis
      Gamma or nonhemolytic type
      1. Alpha hemolysis: Greenish discoloration
      2. Beta or complete hemolysis
         - Colorless zone
         - Classified into 20 Lancefield groups (A–V except I and J) on the basis of carbohydrate Ag of the middle layer of the cell wall, of which most

pathogenic hemolytic *Streptococcus* is group A (*Streptococcus pyogenes*)
         - On the basis of M protein Ag of the outer layer of the cell wall of group A, 80 Griffith types present
      3. Gamma hemolysis
         Enterococcus group

56. Name the strains of *Streptococcus* causing pharyngitis and pyoderma.
    - Stains causing pharyngitis
      3, 5, 6, 12, 18, 19, 24, and 29
    - Strains causing pyoderma
      49, 55, 57, 60, and 63

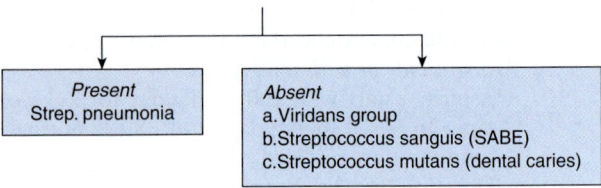

Present	Absent
Strep. pneumonia	a.Viridans group b.Streptococcus sanguis (SABE) c.Streptococcus mutans (dental caries)

57. Describe the structure of a streptococcal capsule.
    Structure of a streptococcal capsule (Fig. 13.4):
    - Capsule containing the hyaluronic acid affects the joints.
    - Peptidoglycan is responsible for the skin lesions.
    - Carbohydrate layer affects the cardiac valves.
    - M protein affects the myocardium.
    - Antibodies against the "N-acetyl-β-d-glucosamine" of the *Streptococcus* are directed against the intracellular β tubulins and extracellular lysoganglioside GM1 of the caudate putamen complex, which activates the calcium–calmodulin-dependent protein kinase 2 that increases dopamine release in the synapse and is responsible for Sydenham chorea.

58. Why does streptococcal skin infection not lead to rheumatic fever?
    - Less intense antibody response to GAS infection of the skin
    - Neutralization of streptococcal toxins by skin lipids

59. Mention the risk factors of rheumatic fever.
    - Overcrowding
    - Specific closed population
    - Socially and economically disadvantaged

60. *Enumerate the theories in rheumatic fever.
    - Cytotoxic theory
      GAS produces a number of enzymes such as streptolysin O that have a direct cytotoxic effect in mammalian cells.
      But the pitfall in this theory is its inability to explain the substantial latent period (2–4 weeks) between GAS pharyngitis and the onset of acute rheumatic fever.
    - Immunological theory
      The antigenicity of GAS cellular and extracellular epitopes and its immunological cross-reactivity with the cardiac antigenic epitopes support the hypothesis of molecular mimicry.
    - Superantigen theory
      The pyrogenic exotoxins of GAS are involved in the pathogenesis of acute rheumatic fever.
    - Recently proposed theory
      This theory states the binding of an M protein N-terminus domain (GAS) to a region of collagen type 4 (heart) that leads to an antibody response to the

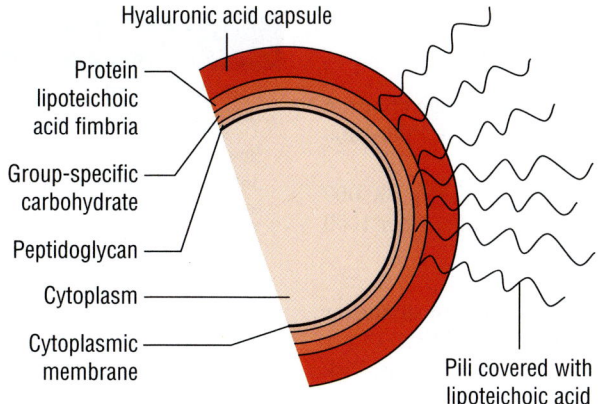

Fig. 13.4 Structure of the capsule of *Streptococcus*. (Source: Reproduced from S. C. Parija. *Textbook of Microbiology and Immunology*, Third Edition, Streptococcus and Enterococcus, Fig. 24-2, New Delhi, Elsevier India, 2016.)

collagen results in ground substance inflammation, especially in the cardiac valves and myocardium.

61. Who are considered as streptococcal carriers?

Patients who continue to harbor GAS in the pharynx despite appropriate antibiotic therapy are called carriers. They do not need treatment.

62. *Mention the indications for treatment in the carrier state.

Eradication might be attempted in selected circumstances:
  * When there is community outbreak of Acute rheumatic fever (ARF) or Post streptococcal glomerulonephritis (PSGN)
  * In an outbreak of GAS pharyngitis
  * In a closed community/nursing home/healthcare facility
  * When there are repeated episodes of symptomatic pharyngitis in a family with ping-pong spread among the family members despite adequate therapy
  * Where tonsillectomy is considered because of chronic carriage or recurrent streptococcal pharyngitis
  * Extreme anxiety called streptophobia

Source: Nelson, 21st edition, Chapter 409, p. 2196

63. How is a carrier state treated?
  * Clindamycin 20 mg/kg/day in three divided doses for 10 days
  * Amoxyclav 40 mg/kg/day in three divided doses for 10 days
  * Oral rifampin for 4 days + either i.m. benzathine penicillin one dose or 10 days of oral penicillin

64. What are the causes of recurrent pharyngitis?
  * Infection caused by a new M type
  * Infection with the same M type because of inadequate antibody response
  * Poor compliance of oral drug therapy
  * Resistance to macrolide if it was used

65. What is prolonged pharyngitis? Mention the possible causes.

Pharyngitis for more than 1 week is called prolonged pharyngitis.

Possible causes are the following:
  * Infectious mononucleosis
  * Lemierre syndrome
  * Neutropenia
  * Systemic lupus erythematosus
  * Inflammatory bowel disease

66. Mention the suppurative and nonsuppurative complications of GAS.

Suppurative
  * Parapharyngeal abscess
  * Mastoiditis

Nonsuppurative
  * Acute rheumatic fever
  * Poststreptococcal glomerulonephritis
  * Pediatric autoimmune neuropsychiatric disorder associated with *Streptococcus pyogenes* (PANDAS)
  * Childhood acute neuropsychiatric symptoms (CANS)

67. *What are modified Jones criteria?

Jones criteria were revised in 2015 as per the American Heart Association:
  * *Major criteria*
    ○ Carditis
    ○ Polyarthritis
    ○ Erythema marginatum
    ○ Subcutaneous nodules
    ○ Chorea
  * *Minor criteria*
    Clinical features
      - Fever
      - Arthralgia
    Lab features
      - Elevated acute phase reactants (ESR, CRP)
      - ECG (showing prolonged PR interval)*
  * *Supporting evidence of antecedent group A streptococcal infection*
    ○ Positive throat culture or rapid antigen detection test
    ○ Elevated or increasing ASO titer
  * *Diagnosis*

    The diagnosis of the first attack or recurrent attacks of acute rheumatic fever can be established only when a patient fulfills two major or one major and two minor criteria .

    *The PR interval is prolonged: >0.16 second in 3–12 years, >0.18 second in 12–14 years, and >0.20 second in >17 years

68. What are the modifications in the revised criteria?
  * There are two modifications in the major criteria and three modifications in the minor criteria.

- Before knowing the modifications, we must know what high-risk and low-risk groups are.
  - High-risk group
    - Incidence ≥2 per 100,000 in school-age children and prevalence of RHD in all ages of ≥1 per 1000
  - Low-risk group
    - Incidence in school-age children ≤2 per 100,000 and prevalence of RHD in all ages of ≤1 per 1000
- Modifications
  - Major
    - Carditis, which is now defined as clinical and/or subclinical (echocardiographic valvulitis)
    - Arthritis, which refers to polyarthritis in low-risk group of children and to polyarthralgia in high-risk group of children
  - Minor
    - Arthralgia in the low-risk group refers only to polyarthralgia but refers to even monoarthralgia in the high-risk group.
    - Fever refers to temperature of >38°C for the high-risk group and 38.5°C for the low-risk group.
    - ESR is >30 mm/h for the high-risk group and >60 mm/h for the low-risk group.

Source: Nelson, 21st edition, Chapter 210, p. 1445

Table 13.11 shows the echo findings in rheumatic valvulitis.

69. *What are the exceptions to Jones criteria?

There are three conditions in which the diagnosis of acute rheumatic fever may be made without strict adherence to Jones criteria; these are as follows:
  i. When chorea is seen as the only major manifestation of acute rheumatic fever
  ii. With indolent carditis
  iii. Recurrences of acute rheumatic fever, especially seen in high-risk groups

70. What is Caveat syndrome?
  - Arthralgia is not taken as a minor criterion in the presence of arthritis.
  - Prolonged PR interval is not taken as a minor criterion in the presence of carditis.

71. *Describe recurrence of rheumatic fever according to Jones criteria.
  - Recurrence of ARF without established heart disease: Two major or one major and two minor criteria with supportive evidence of streptococcal infection
  - Recurrence of ARF with established heart disease
    - Two minor criteria with supportive evidence of streptococcal infection (IAP consensus on acute rheumatic fever RHD, 2007)
    - Three minor criteria with supporting evidence of streptococcal infection (to diagnose recurrence of rheumatic fever in moderate- or high-risk population as given in *Nelson Textbook of Paediatrics*, 20th edition).

72. Describe the terms relapse, rebound, and recurrence in rheumatic fever.
  - Relapse
    Worsening of rheumatic fever while under treatment and often with carditis
  - Rebound
    Manifestations of rheumatic fever within 4–6 weeks of stopping the treatment or while tapering the drugs
  - Recurrence

TABLE 13.11	Echo Findings in Rheumatic Valvulitis	
Pathological MR (All Four Met)	**Pathological AR (All Four Met)**
Seen in at least two views	Seen in at least two views
Jet length of more than 2 cm in at least one view	Jet length of more than 1 cm in at least one view
Peak velocity of more than 3 m/s	Peak velocity of more than 3 m/s
Pansystolic jet in at least one envelope	Pandiastolic jet in at least one envelope

A new episode of RF following another GAS infection, occurring >8 weeks of stopping the treatment

73. What are Vijaya Lakshmi's echo criteria?

Vijaya Lakshmi's Echo criteria are as follows:
  - Echo findings in acute carditis
    i. Nodule: Focal, present at the body and the tip with no independent chaotic movement, and disappearing on follow-up
    ii. Prolapse of the tip of the valve because of minor chordal rupture
    iii. Pericardial inflammation/effusion
  - Echo findings in established Rheumatic heart disease
    i. Valve thickening
    ii. Restriction of leaflet movements
    iii. Valvular prolapse and annular dilatation
    iv. Thickening of subvalvular mitral apparatus
    v. Elongation of chordae
    vi. Ventricular dilatation secondary to valvular lesion
    vii. Mitral stenosis, mitral regurgitation, and aortic valve disease
    viii. Annular/commissural calcification
    ix. Simultaneous involvement of the tricuspid valve

74. Elaborate the reason behind the following statement: rheumatic fever licks the joint and bites the heart.
  - In arthritis, it is an exudative process and only the synovium is involved rather than the cartilage. Hence, there is no deformity.
  - In contrast, in the heart, it is a proliferative process.
  - There are three phases in rheumatic fever, namely, exudative, proliferative, and fibrotic.
  - The exudative phase responds only to anti-inflammatory therapy, whereas the proliferative and fibrotic phases do not respond to anti-inflammatory therapy.

75. *What is the pathological hallmark of rheumatic fever?

The Aschoff granuloma is the pathological hallmark of rheumatic fever. It consists of the central area of necrosis surrounded by cells of histiocytic multinucleated giant cells (Anitschkow cells) – macrophagic origin that showed a typical owl eye–shaped nucleus found mainly in the endocardium, and also found in the myocardium and pericardium.

76. What is the association of arthritis with other features of rheumatic fever?

The association of carditis with joint involvement is given in Table 13.12.

TABLE 13.12	Association of Carditis With Joint Involvement	
Arthritis	10%	
Arthralgia	33%	
No joint involvement	50%	

TABLE 13.13	Association of Carditis With Extracardiac Manifestations	
Arthritis	60%–75%	
Chorea	60%–75%	
Subcutaneous nodules	>95%	

The association of carditis with extracardiac manifestations is shown in Table 13.13.

DISCUSSION ON CHOREA

77. Define chorea.

Chorea is defined as a semipurposive, rapid, chaotic, continuous, nonrhythmic involuntary movement involving proximal muscles that increases during stress and disappears during sleep because of lesion in the caudate nucleus.

78. What are the causes of chorea?
- **Genetic causes**
  - Huntington disease
  - Neuroacanthocytosis
  - Leigh syndrome
  - Ataxia telangiectasia
  - Wilson disease
  - Structural basal ganglia lesion
  - Vascular chorea in stroke, vasculitis, and moyamoya disease
  - Mass lesions in the brain
  - Joubert syndrome
  - **Other causes**
    - Trauma
    - Parainfectious and autoimmune disorders
    - Sydenham chorea
    - Systemic lupus erythematosus
    - Chorea gravidarum
    - Antiphospholipid antibody syndrome
    - Infectious chorea
    - HIV encephalopathy
    - Toxoplasmosis
    - Cysticercosis
    - Diphtheria
    - Neurosyphilis
    - Acute intermittent porphyria
- **Metabolic causes**
  - Hyponatremia/hypernatremia
  - Hypocalcemia
  - Hyperthyroidism
  - Hypoparathyroidism
79. Name some drugs causing chorea.
- **Dopamine receptor blocking agents**
  - Phenothiazines
  - Butyrophenones
  - Benzamides
- **Antiparkinsonian drugs**
  - L-DOPA
  - Valproic acid
  - Psychostimulants
  - Amphetamines
  - Dopamine agonists
  - Anticholinergics
  - Antiepileptic drugs
  - Phenytoin
  - Carbamazepine
  - Methylphenidate
  - Cocaine
  - Flunarizine
  - Verapamil
  - Calcium channel blockers
  - Cinnarizine

80. Is penicillin prophylaxis needed in chorea and if so why?

Yes, penicillin prophylaxis should be started in a child with chorea. But anti-inflammatory therapy is not needed because 10%–20% of the cases with chorea develop an established heart disease.

81. Can chorea coexist with any other major manifestation?

Association with carditis is high but arthritis almost never coexists.

82. What are the variants of Sydenham chorea?
- Hemichorea: Chorea occasionally can be unilateral.
- Chorea gravidarum: Chorea occurs in pregnancy.
- Chorea mollis: There occurs extreme hypotonia with chorea. It is otherwise called paralytic chorea.

83. Describe the management in chorea.

Table 13.14 shows the management of rheumatic chorea.

84. What is the duration of the treatment in chorea?

Treatment of chorea should be continued for at least 2 weeks after the clinical subsidence of the signs of chorea.

85. What is the course of chorea?
- It is usually self-limiting – lasts for 2–6 weeks.
- Spontaneous recovery occurs within a few months.
- Although acute illness is distressing, chorea very rarely leads to permanent neurological sequelae.
- Recurrences are common.

86. *What are the atypical manifestations of rheumatic fever?
- Anemia
- Epistaxis in about 5%–10% of patients
- Acute abdominal pain attributed to mesenteric adenitis
- Rheumatic pneumonia seen in long-standing severe carditis and carries a grave prognosis

87. Mention the indications of surgery in mitral regurgitation.

Algorithm for the management of mitral regurgitation in rheumatic heart disease is shown in Table 13.15.

88. Mention the interventions performed in an established valvular heart disease.

Table 13.16 shows the interventions performed in established valvular heart diseases.

TABLE 13.14	**Management of Rheumatic Chorea**		
Mild Chorea		**Severe (Lifestyle-Limiting Chorea)**	**Resistant Chorea**
• Reassurance • Quiet environment • Drugs such as phenobarbitone, diazepam, and chlorpromazine are useful		• Haloperidol: 0.5–2.5 mg t.d.s. • Valproate: 15 mg/kg/day • Carbamazepine: 7–20 mg/kg/day	• Pimozide • Plasmapheresis

TABLE 13.15	**Management of Mitral Regurgitation in Rheumatic Heart Disease**	

Mild MR
• Child should be started on enalapril
• Periodic monitoring for the following:
  a. Progression of MR
  b. Chamber dilatation (Left atrium (LA), left ventricle (LV)
  c. Pulmonary hypertension
	Moderate or progressive MR
	• Monitor the LA and LV dimensions and left ventricular ejection fraction (LVEF) (%) periodically
	• If the LA and LV dimensions are <40 mm and LVEF is >60%, we can wait
	• If there are progressive dilations of the chambers along with left ventricular dysfunctioning, then surgery has to be planned
		Severe MR
		• It can be classified as symptomatic and asymptomatic
		• Symptomatic MR needs intervention surgically
		• If asymptomatic, plan the management according to the LA and LV dilation and LVEF as mentioned in "Moderate or progressive MR"

89. Enumerate the grading of mitral regurgitation.
   - **Mild MR**
     - History: Asymptomatic
       - Examination
       - Apical impulse: Normal
       - No cardiomegaly
       - Pansystolic murmur of grade <3/6
       - No pulmonary hypertension
       - Regurgitant volume <25%
   - **Moderate MR**
     - History: Fatigue and exertional dyspnea (New York Heart Association (NYHA) 1 and 2)
     - Examination
       - Apical impulse: Hyperdynamic
       - Cardiomegaly present
       - Pansystolic murmur of grade ≥3/6
       - Occurrence of pulmonary hypertension later because the left atrium is enlarged
   - **Severe MR**
     - History: Severe dyspnea (NYHA grade 3 and 4)
     - Examination
       - Apical impulse: Hyperdynamic
       - Parasternal heave present

- Pulmonary hypertension present
- Thrill present
- Wide split of second heart sound except in severe pulmonary hypertension
- S3 gallop
- Mid-diastolic murmur (the louder and longer the murmur, severe is MR)

90. What are the indications and contraindications of balloon mitral valvotomy in mitral stenosis?
   Table 13.17 gives the indications and contraindications for valvotomy in mitral stenosis.

91. What are the types of valves used in valve replacement surgery?
   Table 13.18 gives the comparison between prosthetic and bioprosthetic valves.

92. What are the complications of valvular surgery?
   - Paravalvular leakage
   - Thromboembolism
   - Bleeding manifestations
   - Hemolytic anemias (because of the mechanical force, RBC gets damaged when the valves close)

TABLE 13.16	**Interventions in Valvular Heart Diseases**
Conditions	**Interventions**
Mitral stenosis	Balloon mitral valvuloplasty
Mitral regurgitation	Valve repair or replacement
Aortic stenosis	Surgery in symptomatic cases
Aortic regurgitation	Prosthetic valve replacement

TABLE 13.17	**Indications and Contraindications of Valvotomy in Mitral Stenosis**		
	Indications	**Mechanism**	**Contraindications**
	a. Isolated MS without associated MR b. Mobile and non-calcified valve c. Severe mitral stenosis with a valve area of <1.5 cm² d. No thrombus e. Valve morphology should be suitable for valvuloplasty	a. Splitting of the fused commissure toward the mitral annulus b. Similar to the surgical mitral commissurotomy c. Balloon increases mitral valve flexibility by fracturing the calcified deposits in mitral valve leaflets	a. LA clot b. Calcified valve c. Associated lesions of other valves d. Commissural severe fibrosis e. MR grade 3 or more

TABLE 13.18	Comparison Between Prosthetic and Bioprosthetic Valves

Prosthetic Valves	Bioprosthetic Valves

A. Types
  • Björk–Shiley (tilting disk type – preferred one for young patients)
  • Starr–Edward valve (caged ball and socket type)
  • St. Jude's (tilting disk, bileaflet)
B. Disadvantage
  Needs prophylaxis for IE and anticoagulants lifelong
	A. Types
	  • Heterograft valve
	  • Porcine valve
	B. Disadvantage
	  It is not preferred for young patients because it deteriorates rapidly
	C. Advantage
	  It does not require anticoagulants because the incidence of thromboembolism is very low

Quick Bites

- Subcutaneous nodules are called poor man's ECG because they are usually associated with carditis.
- The clinical demonstration of subcutaneous nodules is called "blessing sign."
- The sites involved by erythema marginatum are described as "bathing suit appearance."
- ESR in acute rheumatic fever is increased in anemia, and reduced in CCF, carditis, chorea, and steroids.

- 10% to 20% of patients with chorea can develop RHD; hence, secondary prophylaxis is needed but anti-inflammatory therapy is not necessary.
- The high attack rate warrants 5 year prophylaxis in rheumatic fever. The attack rate is 50% in first year, reduces to 10% after 10 years. It falls to 1:10 probability in 15 years from initial attack and 1:20 in 20 years.

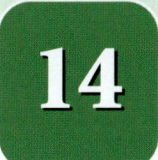

14 Ventricular Septal Defect

Following introduction, seek permission from the caregiver and introduce yourself to the patient before history elicitation, and identify the case.

Name____Age____Sex____Consanguinity____Order of birth____Place____Informant____

Presenting Complaints and Duration

Breathing difficulty

History of Presenting Illness

- Breathlessness – onset, duration, aggravating/relieving factors, improving or deterioration over a period of time, and postural variation
- Cough – onset, productive/nonproductive, aggravating/ relieving factors, diurnal variation, and seasonal variation
- Recurrent respiratory tract infections, three episodes in 1 year requiring i.v. antibiotics for 5–7 days
- Bluish discoloration of the nails and tongue
- Feeding difficulty, suck–rest–suck cycle, forehead sweating, decreased urine output, and presacral edema
- Orthopnea and paroxysmal nocturnal dyspnea (older children)
- Easy fatiguability/breathlessness on exertion
- Palpitations
- Chest pain/syncope (if older children)
- Inadequate weight gain
- Fever with rashes in the extremities

COURSE DURING HOSPITALIZATION

Required oxygenation, fluids, medications, and improvement or worsening of the condition

Past History

- Similar episodes with cough, fever, and breathlessness; child hospitalized and improved with i.v. antibiotics and other medications
- Detailed medical history at the time of discharge on previous admission
- Advised any surgery or drugs and follow-up

Antenatal History

Important points not to be missed are the following:
- Mother's age at conception
- Any drug ingestion (carbamazepine, trimethadione, thalidomide, sex hormones, alcohol, hydantoin, retinoic acid)
- Any maternal illness (fever, rash)
- Irradiation
- Immunization in pregnancy
- Any ultrasound or fetal echocardiography suggestive of heart disease

- Remember five I's not to be missed in AN: history of ingestion, illness, irradiation, immunization, and infections

Natal and Postnatal History

- Term/preterm
- Whether cried at birth
- Detailed feeding history
- Breathing pattern
- Any history of lethargy and poor feeding/frequent aspiration/vomiting
- Whether bluish discoloration noted at birth
- History of convulsions (DiGeorge syndrome because of hypocalcemia)
- Whether advised for surgery at that time
- History of prolonged jaundice (Alagille syndrome)

Developmental History

Developmental delay in case of chromosomal syndromes (Down syndrome, trisomy 18 syndrome)

Dietetic History

To rule out failure to thrive (as suggested earlier)

Immunization History

- It is important to know whether the child is receiving only selective vaccines (killed), e.g., in DiGeorge syndrome, because of T-cell dysfunction, live vaccines are contraindicated.
- In addition, in conditions such as polysplenia/asplenia, vaccine for capsulated organisms should be given.

Family History

History of similar illness in the family

Socioeconomic Status

Contact history of tuberculosis and measles

Summary

A…-year-old male/female child with a history suggestive of recurrent lower respiratory tract infection (LRI) with no symptoms suggestive of congestive cardiac failure (CCF), a child with acyanotic congenital heart disease – probably ventricular septal defect

General Examination

- Awake, active, and comfortable on the mother's lap
- On oxygen support

- Conjunctiva – pallor ±
- Clubbing of grade
- Central cyanosis ±
- Lymphadenopathy
- Edema
- External markers of heart disease/infective endocarditis

Head-to-Foot Examination

- Head size
- Dysmorphic facies: Any conotruncal facies (hypertelorism, bloated eyelids, small palpebral fissure, fish mouth, deformed ears) and Down facies
- Eyes: Congested conjunctiva (polycythemia), Ruth spots (Infective Endocarditis), cataract (Down syndrome), coloboma iris (CHARGE), posterior embryotoxon (Alagille syndrome), retinitis pigmentosa (Laurence–Moon–Biedl syndrome), and hypertelorism
- Ears deformities: Goldenhar syndrome and CHARGE syndrome
- Oral cavity: Dental caries, especially in children older than 2 years
- Chest deformities such as absence of pectoralis major in Poland syndrome
- Any joint abnormalities: TAR syndrome
- Nail changes
- Syndactyly and brachydactyly
- External genitalia: Normal (CHARGE syndrome)

Vital Signs

- Temperature: Fever in case of infective endocarditis
- Pulse rate: For example, in an order such as rate, rhythm, volume of pulse, condition of the vessel wall, and whether felt in all peripheries; pulsus alternans with CCF in large VSD
- Respiratory rate
- Blood pressure: Upper and lower limbs
- Saturation in all four limbs
- JVP: Increased in large VSD

Anthropometry

Height, weight, and BMI

Cardiovascular System Examination

INSPECTION

- Trachea
- Chest wall symmetry/any chest anomalies
- Apical impulse seen in usually normal position according to age
- Precordial bulge – yes or no
- Increased precordial activity – yes or no
- Visible pulsations – yes or no
- Any scars/sinuses
- Inspection of the back – pulsation, scars

(Moderate VSD, parasternal lift; large VSD, hyperdynamic precordium)

PALPATION

- Tracheal position confirmed
- Apical impulse position confirmed (expected to be normal)
- Any thrill (along the left sternal border)
- Parasternal heave in moderate VSD
- Palpable heart sounds P2 in moderate VSD
- Palpation at the back

PERCUSSION

- The left heart border corresponds to the apex, and the right heart border corresponds to the right sternal margin.

AUSCULTATION

Apex

a. S1 is loud at the apex (increased end-diastolic volume in LV).
b. S2 is widely split. As peripheral vascular resistance increases, split decreases.
c. S3 is flow related and can be heard (increased flow in ventricles).
d. Loud, harsh holosystolic murmur, associated with thrill beat, is heard in the left sternal border as in Fig. 14.1.
e. Mid-diastolic murmur can be heard because of increased flow through the mitral valve.

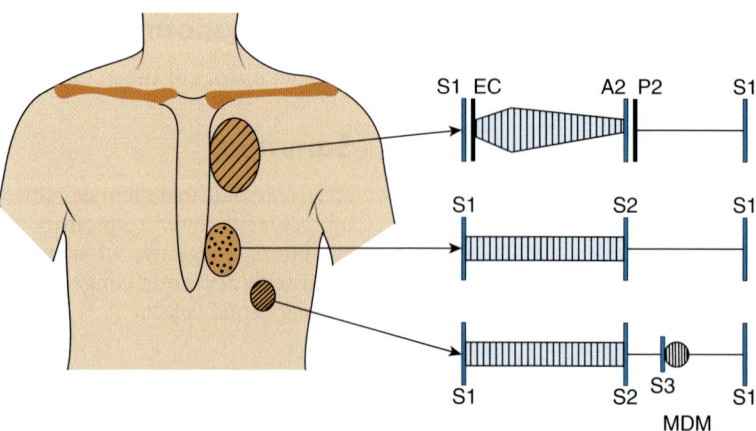

Fig. 14.1 Auscultatory findings in large VSD.

Pulmonary Area
a. P2 loud because of increased pulmonary flow
b. Soft, short systolic murmur in the pulmonary area
c. Early diastolic murmur in pulmonary hypertension (Graham Steell murmur)

Other System Examination

CENTRAL NERVOUS SYSTEM

Give importance to the central nervous system to rule out focal deficits (hemiparesis) and features of raised ICP.

RESPIRATORY SYSTEM

Signs of lower respiratory infection/pulmonary congestion

ABDOMEN

Hepatomegaly for CCF

Diagnosis

A child with congenital acyanotic heart disease with increased pulmonary flow, probably ventricular septal defect of size small/moderate/large with/without IE/CCF/focal deficits in sinus rhythm

Frequently Asked Questions

1. Discuss the embryology of ventricular septum.
   - The interventricular septum has two parts as in Fig. 14.2:
     - Muscular: It develops as an outgrowth from the floor of the primitive ventricle and grows toward the endocardial cushions. Growth of the septum ceases when it reaches the endocardial cushions and leaves an aperture called interventricular foramen.
     - Membranous: The interventricular foramen is closed by outgrowth of endocardial ridges and endocardial bar.
   - Closure of interventricular septum depends on the following:
     a. Continued growth of connective tissue situated on the crest of the muscular septum
     b. Downward growth of the ridges dividing conus and truncus arteriosus
     c. Projections from the arterioventricular canal from right-sided cushions
   - Points to remember
     - The membranous part extends from the tricuspid valve to the aorta and not up to the pulmonary component.
     - The membranous septum is more close to the aorta rather than to the pulmonary valve.
     - Hence, perimembranous VSD is also called the sub-aortic VSD.
     - Outlet (muscular part) VSD is subpulmonic VSD.
     - Crista ventricularis is a muscular ridge in the outlet muscular septum and it divides the outlet part into supracristal and infracristal VSD.
     - The supracristal VSD, because of the Venturi effect, causes prolapse of the right coronary cusp and hence produces AR murmur.

2. Classify VSD.
   I. **Classification on the basis of location of defect**
      Classification on the basis of anatomical location of defect is shown in Flowchart 14.1. The bundle

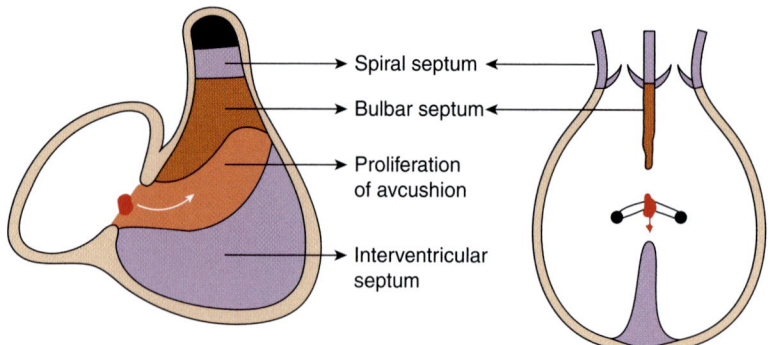

Fig. 14.2   Development of ventricular septum.

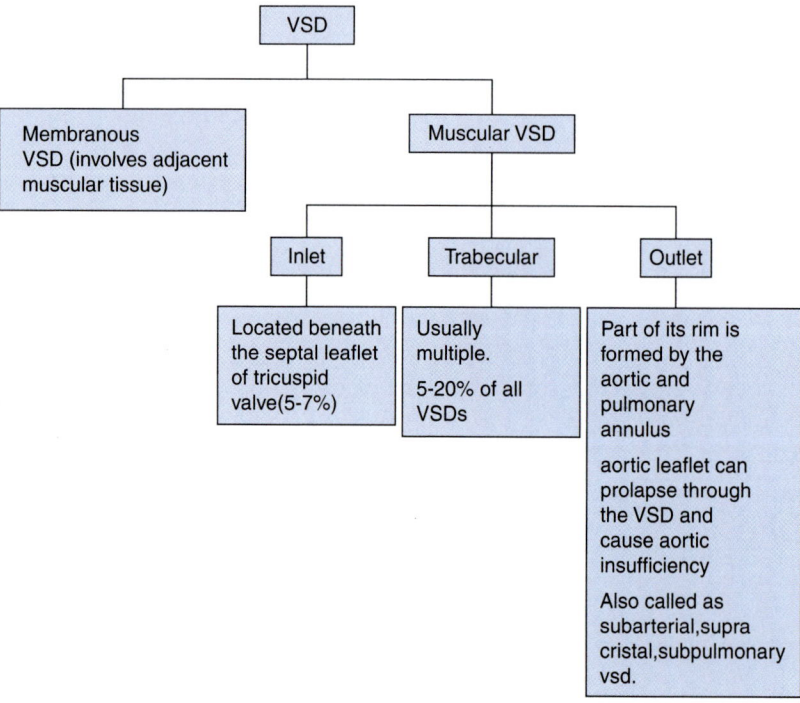

Flowchart 14.1   Anatomical classification of VSD.

of His is related to the posteroinferior quadrant of perimembranous defects and the superoanterior quadrant of inlet muscular defects. Fig. 14.3 shows anatomical classification of ventricular septal defect(VSD).

II. **Classification on the basis of size**
Small: <0.5 cm²/BSA, also called **maladie de Roger**
Moderate: 0.5–1 cm²/Body surface area (BSA)
Large: >1 cm²/BSA

III. **Classification on the basis of number**
  • **Single**
  • **Multiple:** Usually seen in trabecular VSD (Swiss cheese type)

IV. **On the basis of flow**
  • **Restrictive:** Small-sized defect. The defect limits the magnitude of the shunt.
  • **Nonrestrictive:** Large-sized defect. Here, the magnitude of the shunt is determined by pulmonary vascular resistance.

3. Discuss the conditions associated with VSD.
  • Conditions associated with VSD are as follows:
    1. Trisomies 13, 18, and 21
    2. CHARGE syndrome (C: Coloboma Iris, H: Heart Defects, A: Atresia Choanae, R: Growth Retardation, G: Genital Abnormalities, E: Ear Abnormalities), VAC-TERL association (V: Vertebral Abnormalities, A: Anal Atresia, C: Cardiac Defects, TE: Tracheoesophageal Fistula, R: Renal Anomalies, L: Limb Anomalies), Treacher Collins syndrome, fetal hydantoin syndrome, fetal alcohol syndrome, and DiGeorge syndrome
    3. Maternal diabetes and phenylketonuria
    4. Drugs: Amphetamines, estrogens, progesterones, and ACE inhibitors
  • The following are the associated defects with VSD:
    1. Pulmonary stenosis – most common
    2. Double Outlet Right Ventricle (DORV)
    3. Tetralogy of Fallot (TOF)
    4. Tricuspid atresia
    5. Transposition of Great Arteries (TGA)
    6. Truncus arteriosus

4. How can one differentiate ventricular septal defect on the basis of severity?
Differentiation of various sizes of VSD on the basis of severity is shown in Table 14.1.

5. Explain the hemodynamics in VSD.
  • Blood flows through interventricular defect from left to right throughout the systole, masking the first sound – pansystolic murmur as in Fig. 14.4.
  • The increased blood through the pulmonary artery causes delayed closure of the pulmonary valve, whereas

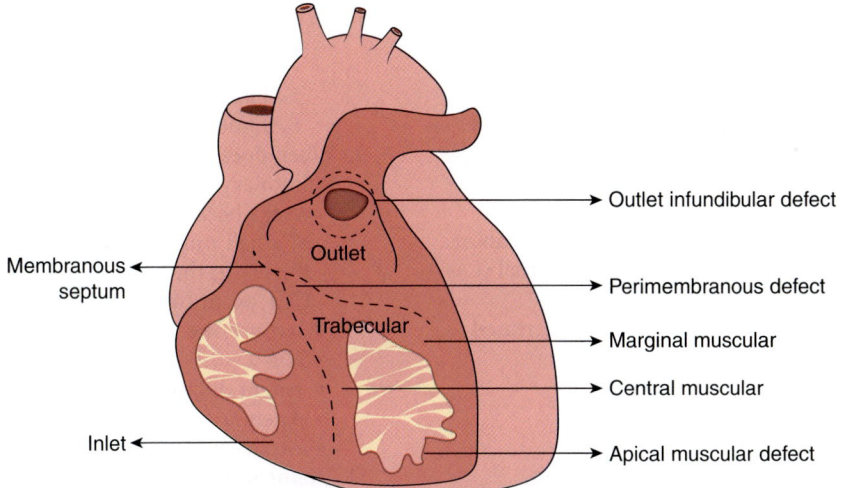

Fig. 14.3 Anatomical locations of VSD.

TABLE 14.1	Differentiation of Various Sizes of VSD on the Basis of Severity		
Feature	Small VSD	Moderate VSD	Large VSD
History	Asymptomatic usually; no failure to thrive (FTT)	Presents with CCF in initial 6 months of life	Presents with CCF in 6–8 weeks; cyanosis, clubbing if Eisenmenger develops
Pulse	Normal	Large volume	Large; normal volume once Eisenmenger develops
Inspection	Normal precordium	Precordial bulge Hyperdynamic precordium	Precordial bulge Hyperdynamic precordium
Palpation	Normal apical impulse; no thrill	Hyperdynamic apical impulse Systolic thrill+	Hyperdynamic apical impulse; systolic thrill + palpable P2 if pulmonary hypertension (HT)
Auscultation	S1, S2 normal; early systolic murmur	Loud S1 Holosystolic murmur	Loud S1, loud P2 if pulmonary HT Early systolic murmur; ejection systolic murmur (ESM) in pulmonary area
ECG	Normal	LVH (Left Ventricular Hypertrophy) LAD (Left Atrial Dilatation)	Biventricular hypertrophy
X-ray	Normal	Cardiomegaly Increased pulmonary vascularity	Normal heart size once Eisenmenger develops

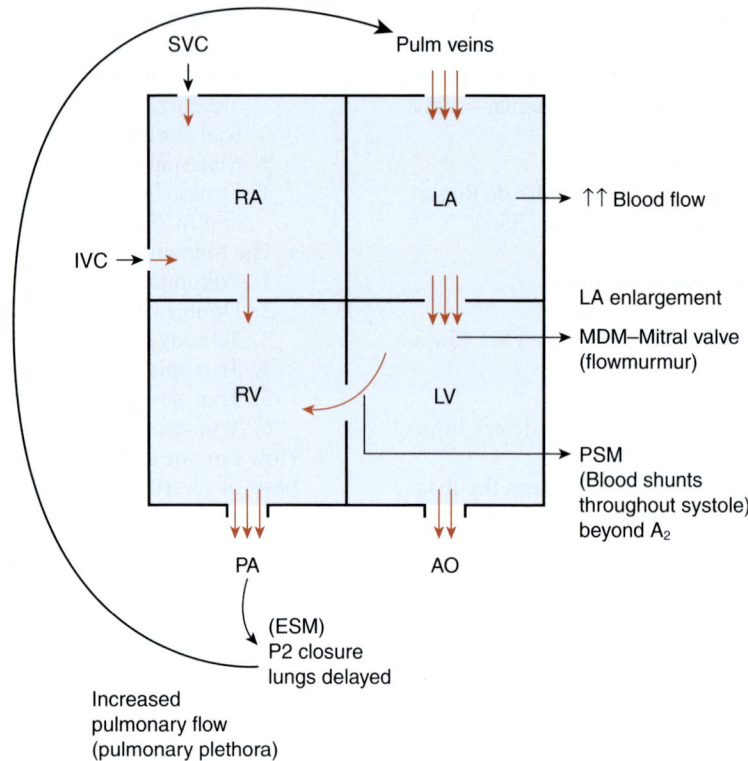

Fig. 14.4 Hemodynamics of VSD.

blood through the aortic valve is reduced, closing it earlier, and thus murmur persists beyond A2, masking it.
- S2 is widely split but varies with respiration.
- Increased blood flow occurs through the pulmonary valve – ejection systolic murmur.
- Blood flow to the lungs is increased – pulmonary plethora.
- Blood flow to the left atrium is increased – left atrial (LA) enlargement.
- Blood flow through the mitral valve is increased – mid-diastolic murmur (MDM).

6. Mention few differentials of VSD.
   A. Mitral regurgitation
   B. Tricuspid regurgitation
   C. Truncus arteriosus with increased blood flow
   D. c-TGA with VSD
   E. Moderate subaortic stenosis
   F. Common ventricle without PS

7. Enumerate some complications of VSD.
   a. Congestive cardiac failure (more in moderate VSD)
   b. Infective endocarditis (more in small VSD, low risk in trabecular VSD)
   c. Eisenmenger complex
   d. Recurrent respiratory infection
   e. Pulmonary hypertension (more in large VSD)
   f. Paradoxical embolism
   g. Failure to grow
   h. Hemoptysis (risk increases with age)

8. Mention few mechanisms of spontaneous closure of VSD.
   The mechanisms of closure of VSD are as follows:
   1. Approximation of the edges of VSD
   2. Hypertrophy of the septal muscles around the defect
   3. Closure of ventricular septal aneurysm
   4. Prolapse of the aortic and tricuspid valve leaflets

   5. Fibrous tissue proliferation
   6. Endocardial proliferation

9. When does CCF occur in VSD?
   Pulmonary vascular resistance decreases in the first few weeks because of the normal involution of the media of small pulmonary arterioles; hence, the shunt from the left to the right ventricle increases and the signs of CCF occur by 6–8 weeks of age.

10. What are the causes of CCF within 6 weeks of age in VSD?
    - patent ductus arteriosus (PDA)
    - Anemia
    - Atrial septal defect (ASD)

11. Name some maternal conditions associated with VSD.
    - Phenylketonuria
    - Infant of diabetic mother

12. Name some maternal drugs causing VSD.
    - Alcohol
    - Hydantoin
    - Valproate
    - Trimethadione

13. Describe the features of a small VSD.
    - Symptoms: Generally asymptomatic, and normal growth and development
    - Signs: Normal pulse volume and loud pansystolic murmur along the lower left sternal border usually not associated with thrill

14. Describe the clinical features of a large VSD.
    - Features of CCF at early infancy (6–8 weeks of age)
    - Failure to thrive
    - Pulse volume: Moderate to large VSD – normal/brisk
      - Large VSD with CCF – pulsus alternans
    - Apical impulse pushed down and out

- Parasternal heave present
- Loud P2
- Soft, more blowing holosystolic murmur associated with thrill heard in 3rd and 4th intercostal spaces along the left sternal border
- Mid-diastolic rumble heard in the apical area
- Ejection systolic murmur heard in the pulmonary area as a result of mild pulmonary insufficiency

15. What are the murmurs heard in VSD?
    a. VSD murmur
       Small: Harsh holosystolic murmur along the lower left sternal border; usually left 3rd and 4th intercostal spaces close to the sternum with/without thrill (this is called Roger's area; the murmur heard here is called Roger murmur)
       Large: Soft but more blowing holosystolic murmur
    (Size of VSD is inversely proportional to the intensity of murmur.)
    b. Mid-diastolic, low-pitched rumble heard at the apex because of increased flow across the mitral valve (when Qp:Qs is >2:1)
    c. Early diastolic decrescendo murmur of grades 1–3/6 because of aortic regurgitation in supracristal VSD
    d. Early decrescendo murmur in the pulmonary area because of pulmonary hypertension.

16. Differentiate VSD from mitral regurgitation.
    Differences between VSD and MR murmur are given in Table 14.2.

17. How can one differentiate VSD from tricuspid regurgitation?
    - Carvallo sign is a clinical sign seen in tricuspid regurgitation in which the pansystolic murmur increases in intensity during inspiration. This helps in differentiating from mitral regurgitation.
    - Hepatomegaly is common if tricuspid regurgitation is severe, whereas it is absent in VSD.

18. How is a child with VSD investigated?
    a. Chest X-ray
       Small VSD: Normal
       Moderate to large VSD: Cardiomegaly as in Fig. 14.5 (A and B)
       Increased pulmonary vascular markings
       Pulmonary edema
    b. ECG
       - Small: Normal
       - Moderate: left ventricular hypertrophy
       - Large: Biventricular hypertrophy with/without left atrial hypertrophy

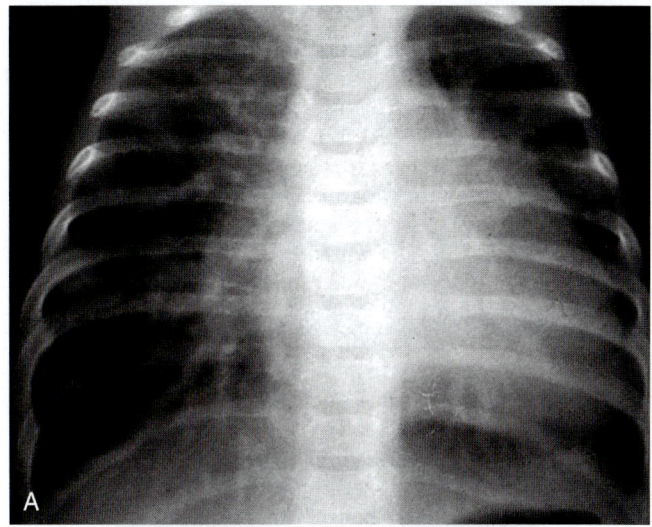

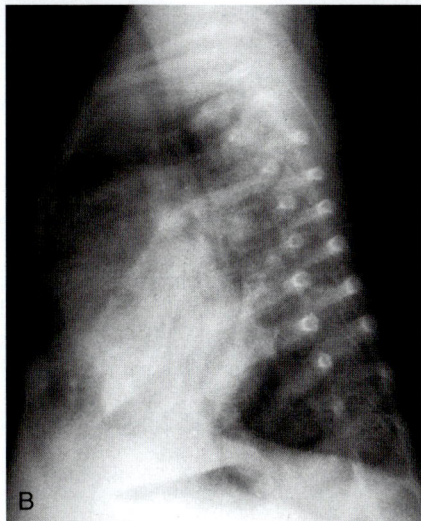

Fig. 14.5 X-ray chest in VSD. Posteroanterior (A) and lateral (B) radiograph. The flattened hemidiaphragms seen on the lateral view, a finding suggestive of associated pulmonary hypertension. *(Source:* Reproduced from Basil Zitelli, Sara McIntire, Andrew Nowalk et al. *Zitelli and Davis' Atlas of Pediatric Physical Diagnosis,* Eighth Edition, Cardiology, Fig. 5.25, Philadelphia, Elsevier Inc., 2023.)

  - Katz–Wachtel phenomenon: Tall, biphasic QRS complexes (>50 mm in height in the mid-precordial leads V2, V3, V4; typically seen in biventricular hypertrophy)
  - If associated with pulmonary vascular obstructive disease, predominantly right ventricular hypertrophy (RVH)
    c. Echo
    d. Cardiac catheterization

19. What is the medical management in VSD?
    - Congestive cardiac failure is treated.
    - The underlying anemia is corrected because it delays the spontaneous closure of VSD and delays surgery.
    - In case of small VSD, in the absence of pulmonary hypertension, no activity restriction is needed
    - Small VSDs with no CCF/pulmonary hypertension till 6 months of age and Qp:Qs <1.5:1 generally do not require surgery but are at an increased risk of infective endocarditis.

TABLE 14.2	Differences between Mitral Regurgitation (MR) and Ventricular Septal Defect (VSD)	
	Mitral Regurgitation	**VSD**
Murmur site	Apex	Lower left sternal border
Spread	Radiated to axilla	Conducted to axilla
ECG	Left ventricular hypertrophy	Biventricular hypertrophy if large
Pulmonary hypertension	Unlikely	More common

20. What is the incidence of VSD?
    - VSD is the most common congenital acyanotic heart disease which accounts for about 20%–25% of all congenital heart diseases.
    - Membranous VSD is more common than muscular VSD.
21. Comment on the prognosis in VSD.
    a. Small VSD: Closes spontaneously
    b. Moderate VSD: Spontaneous closure/CCF
    c. Large VSD: Pulmonary hypertension and CCF
    If the child improves clinically without treatment, consider restrictive VSD, acquired pulmonary stenosis, and pulmonary hypertension.
    - Important points
      - Eighty per cent of muscular VSDs close spontaneously but are uncommon beyond 8 years of age.
      - Thirty-five per cent of membranous VSDs close spontaneously but are uncommon beyond 5 years of age.
      - Only 8% of moderate to large VSDs close spontaneously.
      - Subpulmonic inlet VSDs are unlikely to close spontaneously.
22. What is Harrison groove due to?
    Harrison groove is due to chronic dyspnea.
23. Why does the left side of the heart enlarge earlier than the right side in VSD?
    During left-to-right shunt in VSD, the right ventricle is also in a contracted state. Hence, the blood flow is directed mainly toward the pulmonary artery that ultimately drains into the left atrium and left ventricle.
24. What is called Gerbode VSD?
    It is a type of defect in which blood shunts from the left ventricle to the right atrium.
25. What is called Gasul phenomenon?
    Acquired pulmonary infundibular stenosis in a case of ventricular septal defect is called Gasul phenomenon.
26. What are the indications of surgery in VSD?
    - Congestive cardiac failure and failure to thrive not responding to medical management (surgery can be planned by 3–4 months of age)
    - Pulmonary artery pressure more than 50% of systemic pressures (surgery can be planned by 6–12 months of age)
    - Patient older than 1 year if Qp:Qs >2:1
    - Subpulmonic VSD
27. What are the contraindications of surgery in VSD?
    Pulmonary:systemic vascular resistance >0.5 in the presence of right-to-left shunt
28. Discuss the type of incisions used in VSD surgery.
    a. Transatrial approach for perimembranous and inlet VSD
    b. Incision over the pulmonary artery for outlet VSD
    c. Right ventriculotomy for apical VSDs
29. What are the complications of VSD surgery?
    - Possibility of right bundle branch block because of the disruption of Purkinje fibers in right ventriculotomy
    - Complete heart block
    - Residual defects
    - Neurological complications
    - Mortality rate in surgery <1%

Quick Bites

- VSD is the most common congenital acyanotic heart disease that accounts for about 20%–25% of all congenital heart diseases.
- VSD murmur is otherwise called Roger murmur.
- Small VSD, <0.5 cm^2/BSA, is also called **maladie de Roger**.
- Gerbode VSD is a type of defect in which blood shunts from the left ventricle to the right atrium.
- Acquired pulmonary infundibular stenosis in a case of ventricular septal defect is called Gasul phenomenon.
- Katz–Wachtel phenomenon: Tall, biphasic QRS complexes are present (>50 mm in height in the mid-precordial leads V2, V3, V4; typically seen in biventricular hypertrophy).
- Prognosis: Small VSD closes spontaneously. Only 8% of moderate to large VSDs close spontaneously. Subpulmonic inlet VSD is unlikely to close spontaneously.

Atrial Septal Defect

Following introduction, seek permission from the caregiver and introduce yourself to the patient before history elicitation, and identify the case.

Name____Age____Sex____Consanguinity____Order of birth____Place____Informant____

Presenting Complaints and Duration

- Breathlessness
- Orthopnea and paroxysmal nocturnal dyspnea
- Platypnea
- Easy fatiguability/breathlessness on exertion
- Palpitations
- Chest pain/syncope
- Bluish discoloration of the skin and nails
- Recurrent respiratory tract infections
- Inadequate weight gain
- Fever, joint pain, swellings, and rashes in the peripheries

Past History

- Similar illness in the past
- Any previous hospitalization
- Medical history if any

Antenatal History

(Five I's to be remembered)
- Immunization
- Ingestion
- Infection (TORCH)
- Illness (maternal hypertension/gestational diabetes)
- Irradiation

Natal/Postnatal History

If significant

Developmental History

Age-appropriate milestones obtained or not

Dietetic History

According to 24-hour recall method

Immunization History

According to National Immunization or IAP schedule

Family History

Any history of similar illness in the family members

Socioeconomic History

According to the modified Kuppuswamy scale

Summary

Congenital acyanotic heart disease with/without CCF, with/without features of pulmonary hypertension, with/without features of infective endocarditis

General Examination

- Conscious and oriented
- Moderately nourished
- Pallor/icterus/cyanosis/clubbing/lymphadenopathy/edema
- External markers of congenital heart disease/infective endocarditis
- I.v. line/oxygen support to be mentioned, if any

Head-to-Foot Examination

- Dysmorphic facies
- Oral hygiene
- Abnormalities of the chest wall
  - Limb anomalies – thumb, radius, and phalanges
  - External markers of infective endocarditis, if any

Vital Signs

- Temperature
- PR – rate, rhythm, character, volume, felt in all peripheries, and RR/RF delay
- RR – rate, pattern, and work of breathing
- BP – in both the upper limb and the lower limb
- SpO_2 – in standing and supine positions
- JVP

Anthropometry

Height/weight/BMI – with interpretation

Cardiovascular System Examination

INSPECTION

- Position of the trachea
- Shape and symmetry of the chest wall
- Position of apical impulse in the ... space with respect to the nipples
- Precordial bulge
- Dilated veins over the chest
- Visible pulsations
- Any surgical scars

PALPATION

- Tracheal position confirmed by palpation
- Apical impulse felt in the left…ICS at/medial/lateral to MCL and character
- Thrill
- Parasternal heave with grading

PERCUSSION

- The left heart border corresponds to apical impulse.
- The right heart border corresponds to the sternal border.

AUSCULTATION

Pulmonary Area

- S1: Normal
- S2: Wide and fixed split +
- Soft and medium-pitched systolic ejection murmur of grade 2–3/6 heard in the left 2nd intercostal space with no radiation
- No added sounds

Tricuspid Area

- S1: Normal
- S2: Wide and fixed split +
- Short, rumbling mid-diastolic murmur of grade 2–3/6 heard along the left lower sternal border with no radiation
- No added sounds

Mitral and Aortic Areas

- S1: Normal
- S2: Wide and fixed split +
- No added sounds

Other System Examination

RESPIRATORY SYSTEM

BAE+/WOB/pattern of breathing

ABDOMEN

Soft/no tenderness/no organomegaly

CENTRAL NERVOUS SYSTEM EXAMINATION

Any focal deficits

Diagnosis

Congenital acyanotic heart disease, probably atrial septal defect with no CCF, with/without features of pulmonary hypertension, with/without features of infective endocarditis in sinus rhythm

Frequently Asked Questions

1. What is the significance of gender in ASD?
   - Female:male ratio is 2:1 in ostium secundum ASD.
   - ASD is equally distributed in sinus venosus type and ostium primum type.
2. *Why is ASD asymptomatic in infants?
   Paucity of symptoms in infants is because of the thick and compliant structure of the muscular tricuspid valve of the right ventricle in the early life and thus the left-to-right shunt is restricted.
3. What are the causes of early symptoms in ASD?
   - Scimitar syndrome
   - AV canal defects (Down syndrome)
4. Enumerate the symptoms of right and left heart failure.
   - Symptoms of right heart failure
     - Breathlessness on exertion
     - Cough
     - Easy fatiguability
   - Symptoms of left heart failure
     - Dependent edema
     - Abdominal distension
     - Orthopnea
     - Paroxysmal nocturnal dyspnea
     - Oliguria
5. Explain the significance of antenatal history in ASD.
   - Maternal drugs
     - Hydantoin
     - Alcohol
     - Amphetamines
     - Thalidomide
   - History for TORCH because ASD is associated with congenital rubella syndrome
6. Why is developmental history important in ASD?
   Down syndrome with endocardial cushion defects can have developmental delay.
7. Why family history is important in ASD?
   - ASD is usually sporadic.
   - But conditions such as Holt–Oram syndrome are inherited as autosomal dominant.
   - Familial ASD (ostium secundum type) is because of mutation in transcription factor Nkx2.5 and GATA4.
8. *Discuss the causes of cyanosis in ASD.
   - Large Eustachian valve selectively channeling inferior vena cava blood into the left atrium through secundum type of ASD or through IVC type of sinus venosus type
   - Coronary sinus type
   - Associated with PAPVC or TAPVC
9. What is orthodeoxia?
   Desaturation on standing that relieves with supine position
10. What is the cause of visible pulsation in ASD?
    Visible pulsation in the left 2nd intercostal space is because of the dilated and pulsatile pulmonary trunk in ASD.

11. *Enumerate the significance of head-to-foot examination in ASD.
    - Dysmorphic facies: Down syndrome with endocardial cushion defects (ostium primum type)
    - Polydactyly, short distal limbs, bell-shaped chest, and neonatal teeth: Ellis–Van Creveld syndrome
    - Absent radii with normal thumb: TAR syndrome
    - Hypoplastic or absent thumb, radii, triphalangism, and first-degree heart block with ASD: Holt–Oram syndrome
    - Microcephaly, downslanting eyes, cat cry, and ASD: Cri du chat syndrome
    - External features of trisomies 13 and 18
12. *What causes precordial bulge in ASD?
    The precordial prominence in ASD is because of the hyperdynamic right ventricle.
13. Describe the second heart sound in ASD.
    - The aortic and pulmonary components of the second heart sound are widely split and the split is fixed throughout the respiration.
    - Wide split
      The right ventricular volume is increased because of the extra flow from the left atrium. This leads to increased blood flow into the pulmonary artery. Hence, the pulmonary valve closure is delayed. At the same time, the left ventricular volume is decreased because of the same shunt and this causes early closure of the aortic valve. Hence, there is a wide split in the second heart sound.
    - Fixed split
      Normally the degree of split is more during inspiration, whereas it is decreased or heard as a single sound during expiration. During inspiration, the systemic venous return into the right atrium is more because of negative intrathoracic pressure, which causes delayed closure of the pulmonary valve and hence a wide split. The reverse of this happens in expiration – A2 is delayed and P2 is early. But in ASD, these differences are not present because there is a communication between the two atria and hence the split is fixed in all phases of respiration.
14. *Explain the causes of ASD with a variable split.
    - The split may become variable with the development of atrial fibrillation.
    - The split may get narrowed down with the development of pulmonary hypertension.
15. Enumerate the different types of ASD and their incidence.
    a. Ostium secundum: Most common type (50%–70%), at the site of fossa ovalis
       Anomalous pulmonary venous return is present in about 10% of the cases.
    b. Ostium primum defect: As both a part of complete endocardial cushion defect (30%) and isolated form (15%)
    c. Sinus venosus: 10%; located at the entry of SVC into RA (SVC type) – associated with anomalous drainage of the right upper pulmonary vein

---

*Important question asked in the examination.

In addition, rarely IVC type – anomalous drainage of right lung into IVC (Scimitar syndrome)

d. Coronary sinus type: Defect in the roof of the coronary sinus

16. What other valvular abnormalities can be associated with ostium secundum and primum types of ASD?
    - Ostium secundum ASD usually occurs in isolation but rarely can be associated with mitral valve prolapse syndrome or with mitral stenosis.
    - Ostium primum type of ASD may occur in isolation or in association with endocardial cushion defects, cleft mitral valve, mitral regurgitation, and tricuspid regurgitation.
    - Endocardial cushion defects can be either complete or incomplete:
      - Complete: ASD with MR with VSD
      - Incomplete: ASD with MR

17. *Explain the embryology of ASD.
    - The atrium develops from a common atrial canal.
    - It is divided into right and left atria by the downward growth of a septum called septum primum.
    - As the septum grows downwards toward the atrioventricular cushion, there is a communication between the septum primum and the atrioventricular cushion. This is called foramen primum (ostium primum).
    - As the septum fuses with the atrioventricular cushion, the foramen primum closes.
    - However, before the closure is complete, a defect occurs high above in the septum primum. This is called foramen secundum (ostium secundum).

- At this stage, another crescent-shaped fold grows down from the roof to the right of the septum primum. This is called septum secundum.
- The septum secundum grows downwards until it overlaps the foramen secundum. The opening left by the septum secundum is called foramen ovale.
- After birth, the pressure in the left atrium increases and the foramen ovale gets obliterated.
- The fossa ovalis represents the septum primum.
- The annulus ovalis or limbus fossa ovalis represents the lower free end of the septum secundum.
  Fig. 15.1 shows the embryology of ASD.

18. *What is Koch's triangle?
    - It indicates the landmark of AV node that is present in the lower end of the posterior surface of the right atrium.
    - It is bounded by the tricuspid valve, tendon of Todaro, and coronary sinus orifice.
      Fig. 15.2 shows the Koch's triangle.

19. *What are the syndromes associated with ASD?
    - Chromosomal disorders
      - Down syndrome
      - Edward syndrome
      - Patau syndrome
      - Klinefelter syndrome
    - Syndromes
      - Holt–Oram syndrome
      - Ellis–Van Creveld syndrome
      - Thrombocytopenia with Absent Radius (TAR) syndrome

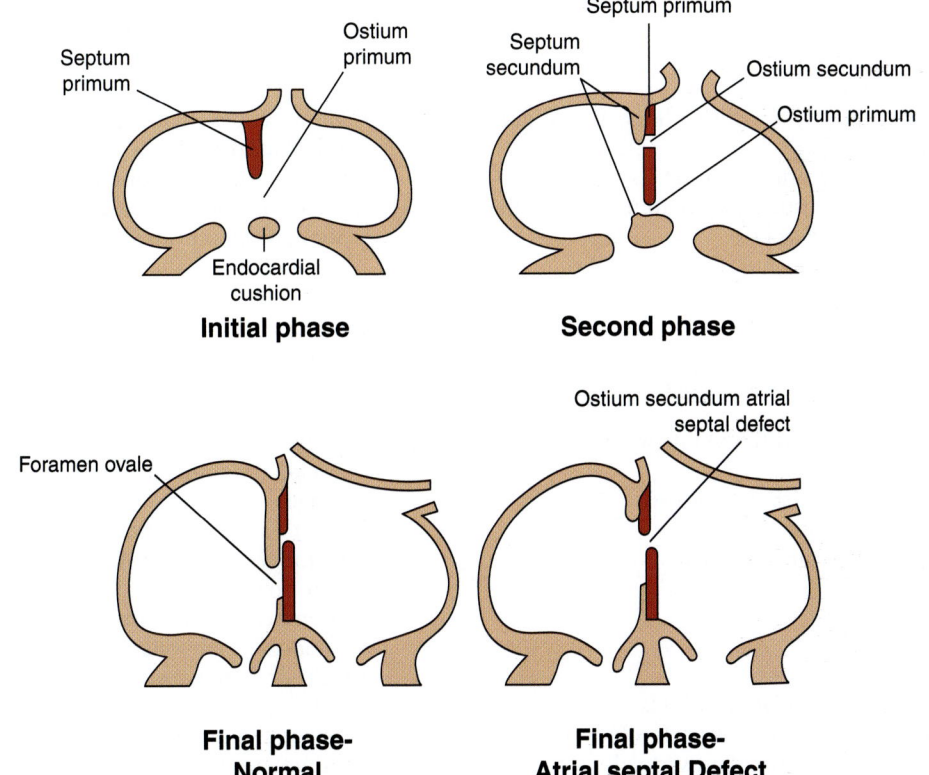

Fig. 15.1 Embryology of ASD. (*Source:* Reproduced from Kumar et al. Basic Pathology, 7th edition.)

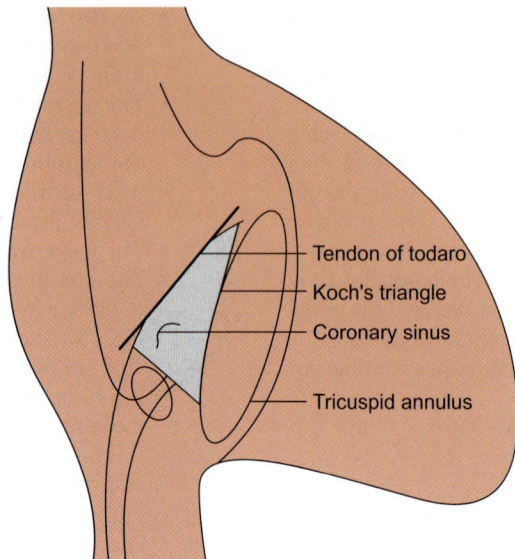

Fig. 15.2   Koch's triangle.

- Congenital rubella syndrome
- CHARGE syndrome
- VATER syndrome
- Fetal hydantoin syndrome
- Fetal alcohol syndrome
- Lutembacher syndrome (ASD + MS)
- Maternal conditions
  - Phenylketonuria
  - Rubella infection
- Familial recurrence
  - Scimitar syndrome
  - Holt–Oram syndrome
  - Ostium secundum type with/without AV conduction defect

20. Enumerate the clinical features in ASD.
    - A child with ASD is usually asymptomatic until the second or third decade of life.
    - The common symptoms in ASD are the following:
      - Palpitation on exertion
      - Fatigue
      - Dyspnea on exertion
      - Varying degrees of exercise intolerance in older children
    - Rarely ASD can present with the following:
      - Growth failure
      - Recurrent respiratory tract infections
      - Congestive heart failure

21. How is a child with ASD investigated?
    - ECG
      Ostium secundum type
      Right-axis deviation
      Mild RVH
      rsR′ pattern in precordial chest leads
      Incomplete Right Bundle Branch Block (RBBB) because of right ventricular overload
      Crochetage sign: ASD – notch in the apex of R wave in leads 2 and 3 and aVF
      Ostium primum type
      Left-axis deviation

Incomplete RBBB
Heart blocks
- Chest X-ray
  Cardiomegaly because of right atrial and right ventricular enlargement
  Ostium secundum type
  Jug handle appearance
  Sinus venosus when associated with PAPVC – figure of 8 appearance
  Pulmonary plethora
  Enlarged right pulmonary artery and dilated pulmonary trunk
- **Fluoroscopy:** Hilar dance of pulmonary arteries
- Echocardiography
- Cardiac catheterization (generally not catheterized)

22. *Discuss the natural course of ASD.
    - Spontaneous closure of the secundum defect occurs in about 40% of patients in the first 4 years of life.
    - If ASD is of size <3 mm, closure occurs by 1.5 years in 100% of patients.
    - If ASD is of size 3–8 mm, closure occurs by 1.5 years in 80% of patients.
    - If ASD is of size >8 mm, spontaneous closure is unlikely.
    - Overall spontaneous closure is unlikely beyond 4 years of age.

23. Explain the complications of ASD.
    - Pulmonary hypertension because of increased pulmonary flow
    - Eisenmenger syndrome
    - Paradoxical embolism
    - CCF and infective endocarditis, which are rare in ASD

24. * Explain the causes of CCF in ASD.
    - Ostium primum type associated with other lesions such as mitral regurgitation and tricuspid regurgitation
    - Large defect
    - Atrial arrhythmia
    - Anomalous pulmonary venous drainage with ASD

- Severe pulmonary hypertension
- Lutembacher syndrome
- Infective endocarditis (very rarely)

25. Enumerate the prerequisites for nonsurgical closure of ASD.
    - Amplatzer Septal Occluder and Helex Septal Occluder are approved for the secundum ASD closure.
    - Prerequisites are the following:
      - Secundum ASD measuring 5 mm or more in diameter
      - Hemodynamically significant left-to-right shunt with Qp:Qs ratio of 1.5:1 or more
      - Enough rim of at least 4 mm of septal tissue around the defect

26. *What is the timing for device closure?
    ASD closure devices can be implanted successfully in children younger than 2 years. Postdevice closure follow-up – aspirin 80 mg/day has to be prescribed for 6 months.

27. List the complications associated with device closure.
    - Complications are extremely rare. The overall risk of the procedure is 7.2%.
    - Complications include the following:
      - Device embolism
      - ECG abnormalities within 24 hours
      - Early or late erosion of the device into the aortic root
      - Release of nickel from the device with peak at 1 month after the implant
      - Rarely thrombus formation in the right and left atria

28. Explain the advantages of nonsurgical closure.
    - Complete avoidance of cardiopulmonary bypass
    - Avoidance of pain
    - Residual thoracotomy scars
    - Less than 24-hour hospital stay
    - Rapid recovery
    - Small residual leak

29. * Enumerate the indications and contraindications of surgical closure in ASD.
    - Indications
      - Ostium primum defect
      - If the device closure is not considered appropriate
      - Pulmonary artery pressure more than 50% of systemic pressure
      - CCF not responding to medical management
    - Contraindication
      - High pulmonary vascular resistance of >10 units/m^2 and that of 7 units/m^2 with vasodilators is a contraindication for surgery.

30. List the complications associated with surgical closure.
    - Atrial fibrillations/flutter, atrial tachycardia, and nodal rhythm are seen in the immediate postoperative period.
    - Sick sinus syndrome occurs after repair of the sinus venosus type.
    - Mortality rate is <0.5%.
    - Postoperative follow-up: Cardiomegaly on chest radiographs and enlarged RV dimensions on echo as well as the wide splitting of S2 may persist for 1 or 2 years after surgery.

Quick Bites

- Female:male ratio is 2:1 in ostium secundum ASD.
- Koch's triangle: Bounded by the tricuspid valve, tendon of Todaro, and coronary sinus orifice, it indicates the landmark of AV node.
- The most common association of ostium primum type of ASD is with endocardial cushion defects.
- The different types of ASD are ostium secundum (most common type, 50%–70%), ostium primum defect (complete [30%] and isolated [15%] forms), sinus venosus (10%), and coronary sinus (rare).
- Size of ASD
  - If ASD is of size <3 mm, closure occurs by 1.5 years in 100% of patients.
  - If ASD is of size 3–8 mm, closure occurs by 1.5 years in 80% of patients.
  - If ASD is of size >8 mm, spontaneous closure is unlikely.
  - Overall spontaneous closure is unlikely beyond 4 years of age.

16 Patent Ductus Arteriosus

Following introduction, seek permission from the caregiver and introduce yourself to the patient before history elicitation, and identify the case.

Name____Age____Sex____Consanguinity____Order of birth____Place____Informant____

Presenting Complaints and Duration

- Difficulty in breathing
- Fever

History of Presenting Illness

- Breathlessness
  - Duration
  - Classification according to NYHA/Ross classification if infant
  - Initially in grade … and now progressed to grade …
  - Changes with respect to position/respiration
  - Aggravating and relieving factors
- Other features of CCF
- Feeding difficulties
- Suck–rest–suck cycle
- Forehead sweating
- Presacral edema in case of infants; effort intolerance, swelling of legs, chest pain, and palpitation in case of older children
- History of fever and cough (to rule out respiratory cause of breathing difficulty)
- History of cyanosis, squatting episode, and spell (to rule out cyanotic heart disease)

COMPLICATIONS HISTORY

- Recurrent respiratory tract infections
- Inadequate weight gain (FTT)
- Fever with joint pain, skin rashes, and painful fingertips (infective endocarditis)
- History suggestive of pulmonary hypertension such as palpitation in case of older children or asking the mother whether she perceives increased precordial activity in case of infants; edema, breathlessness, and bluish discoloration of the nails and tongue (course – an asymptomatic period of the heart disease followed by onset of all these symptoms)

Past History

Detailed medical history if any – CCF, endocarditis, and reversal of shunt

Antenatal History

- Age of the mother at conception
- Any drug ingestion (alcohol, phenytoin, amphetamine)
- History of fever with rash, tender swelling in the neck (post-auricular, suboccipital adenopathy), and joint pain (TORCH infection – specifically congenital rubella syndrome)
- Maternal illness such as gestational diabetic mother and hypertension

Birth History

- Term/preterm
- Birth weight (low Birth weight, IUGR – a clue for TORCH)
- Any prolonged need for ventilation at birth
- Feeding/sucking history
- Any cyanosis
- Whether started on any drugs for CCF

Developmental History

Can think of syndrome in case of delay (congenital rubella syndrome [CRS])

Dietetic History

To rule out failure to thrive

Immunization History

Special vaccine – history of pnuemococcal and flu vaccines

Family History

Incidence of heart diseases in child is increased by 1–5% if siblings are known to have heart disease and by 3% if parents has.

Socioeconomic History

Children living at a high altitude have an increased chance of PDA (6% more chance).

General Examination

- Awake
- Comfortable at rest/tachypneic/dyspneic
- Need of oxygen
- Any NG tube in situ
- Pallor/icterus/clubbing/cyanosis/lymphadenopathy/edema
- Poorly nourished

Head-to-Foot Examination

- Head: Microcephaly (congenital rubella syndrome)
- Any dysmorphic facies
- Features of CCF: Facial, pedal, or presacral edema (in infants)

- Eyes: Pallor, cataract, fundus (Roth spots for IE), retina (cataract), microphthalmia, and pigmentary retinopathy (congenital rubella syndrome)
- Abnormalities in the chest such as Harrison groove and pigeon chest
- Extremities: Rashes and edema
- Nail changes
- Skeletal anomalies and craniofacial or limb anomalies
- Oral hygiene: Good
- Any external cardiac surgical scars

Vital Signs

- Temperature
- Pulse rate (PR) High volume pulse is felt in all peripheral pulses and capillaries of nails (mention the descriptive points of pulse – rate, rhythm, volume, character, condition of vessel walls, whether felt in all peripheries); Duroziez murmur – diastolic murmur felt in the femoral artery (bell of the stethoscope) and radiofemoral delay (coarctation of aorta)
- Respiratory rate
- Blood pressure: To look for wide pulse pressure
- Saturation in all four limbs
- Elevated JVP

Anthropometry

Height, weight, and BMI with interpretation

Cardiovascular System Examination

INSPECTION

- Trachea
- Chest wall symmetry/any chest anomalies
  - Apical impulse seen in the 6th ICS 0.5 cm lateral to the midclavicular line
  - Any precordial bulge
- Increased precordial activity: Hyperactive precordium
- Visible pulsations: Precordial pulsation over the left 2nd space (infraclavicular area)
- Inspection of the back: Any scars (surgical scar – shunt at the back)
- Look for Harrison sulcus
- Pigeon chest
- Engorged neck veins

PALPATION

- Confirm the tracheal position
- Confirm the apical impulse position – 6th ICS/0.5 cm lateral to the midclavicular line (PDA-BVH)
- Any thrill: Left 2nd space radiating toward the clavicle
- Continuous/systolic thrill in the left 2nd ICS: PDA (diastolic component disappears with the development of pulmonary hypertension/shunt reversal)
- Parasternal heave

- Palpable heart sounds: Over the left 2nd space
- Palpation at the back

PERCUSSION

- The left heart border corresponds to the apex.
- The right border corresponds to the sternum.

AUSCULTATION

- A grade 4 continuous murmur best heard in the left 2nd space in both systole and diastole, no variation with respiration, high pitch, and engulfing S2 (no radiation/no transmission)
- Disappearance of the diastolic component of the murmur as pulmonary hypertension develops
- MDM flow murmur ±
- Loud P2 in pulmonary area ±
- Other features of machinery murmur: Punctuated with Eddy sounds, randomly distributed in the second half of diastole, and obscuring S2
- Holosystolic murmur seen in PDA when pulmonary vascular resistance increases
- Spilt in PDA
  - Paradoxical split of S2 (larger shunt)
  - Single or closely split second heart sound with short pulmonary ESM and loud P2: Pulmonary hypertension
- To-and-fro murmur over the cranium of an infant in PDA: High flow and rapid diastolic runoff

Other Areas

- Tricuspid area: S1 and S2 heard
- Mitral area and aortic area: S1 and S2 heard
- Apical MDM: Larger shunt (these murmurs cannot be heard unless diastolic portion of the continuous murmur attenuated – increased PVR)

Other System Examination

RESPIRATORY SYSTEM

- Features of CCF (bilateral crepitations, tachypnea)

ABDOMEN

- Hepatomegaly and epigastric pulsations – right ventricular hypertrophy (seen in thin individuals)

CENTRAL NERVOUS SYSTEM EXAMINATION

- Any neurological deficit

Diagnosis

A child with acyanotic congenital heart disease and left-to-right shunt lesion, probably patent ductus arteriosus, and no syndromic features – with/without CCF, no signs of IE, with/without pulmonary hypertension in sinus rhythm, and poorly nourished (nutritional status)

Frequently Asked Questions

1. *Mention the significance of a child's age and sex in PDA.
   - Age and sex (female incidence is high): Female:male ratio is 2:1.
   - Place (high altitude): PDA is six times more common at 10,000 feet.
2. Mention some statistics in PDA.
   - PDA accounts for 5%–10% of all CHDs.
   - PDA is 1%–5% more common among siblings.
   - PDA is seen in 45% of infants with birth weight of <1.75 kg and 80% of infants with birth weight of <1.2 kg.
3. Describe the embryology of PDA.
   - It is a remnant of the left 6th aortic arch.
   - Ductus arteriosus is conical in shape with an apex/narrow area in the pulmonary artery side extending from the pulmonary artery to the descending aorta just (5–10 mm) distal to the origin of the left subclavian artery.
   - Bilateral PDA, which is because of the double aortic arch, is very rare.
4. *Mention few theories in PDA.
   - Oxygen theory
     - Oxygen → inhibits potassium channel → influx of calcium → vasoconstriction
   - Anatomical remodeling
     - Movement of cells from smooth muscle to intima
     - Intimal proliferation
     - Endothelial proliferation
   - Prostaglandin theory: After delivery, the placenta is cut off, so there are no more prostaglandins.
   - Prostaglandin receptor ineffectivity: The prostaglandin receptors also become ineffective (EP2 and EP4).
5. Describe genetics in PDA.
   - MYH1 gene
   - SNP gene mutation
   - TRAF1 and TRAF2B gene mutations
6. What are functional and anatomical closure of PDA?
   Functional closure
     - It occurs at 12–14 hours of life.
     - It occurs because of the constriction of the muscularis media layer of the ductus.
     - Factors responsible for the functional closure are rise in PaO_2 and reduced prostaglandin E synthesis.
     - Chances of spontaneous closure are as follows:
       - 50% by 24 hours
       - 25% by 48 hours
       - 15% by 72 hours
   Anatomical closure
     - Occurs by the 2nd to 3rd week
     - Three layer closure by the following:
       - Endothelium – infolding of the ductal epithelium by proliferation of the intima and fibrosis
       - Internal elastic lamina/intima – fragmentation and disruption
       - Smooth muscle – migration and contraction
       - Muscle fibers – fibrosis
       - Subendothelial layer – persisting ligamentum arteriosum

7. *When does a PDA reopen?
   PDA reopens due to vasodilation caused by prostaglandin E2 released by infections such as pneumonia.
8. What is the cause for PDA in term and preterm?
   - Term: Because of the lack of mucoid endothelium and muscularis mucosa
   - Preterm
     - Because of the insensitivity of smooth muscles to oxygen
     - Because of defect in elastic tissue in the walls of the ductus
     - Because of defective pulmonary circulation of PGE not metabolized and hence there is increased level of circulating PGE
9. What are the factors maintaining the ductus arteriosus in the fetal period?
   - Hypoxia
   - Prostaglandin production by the placenta
10. When do functional and anatomical closure of PDA occur?
    a. The normal process of functional closure occurs within 10–15 hours of birth and virtually completes by the 2nd week of birth.
    b. The ductus is anatomically closed by the ligamentum arteriosum by 2–3 weeks after birth.
11. Discuss the differentiating features of PDA in a term baby and a preterm baby.
    a. Functional closure of the ductus in term neonates occurs by 12–24 hours and in preterm neonates by 3–5 days.
    b. The ductus remains patent after 3 months in a term baby and beyond 1 year in a preterm baby and is unlikely to close.
    c. Indomethacin does not have much effect in term babies.
12. Discuss the mechanism of duct closure.
    - Spasm of muscular coil because of vasoactive amine
    - Intimal and subintimal proliferation
    - Endothelium ingrowth and infolding
    - Subendothelial edema
    - Connective tissue proliferation
    - Emboli of the ductus
    - Migration of the undifferentiated smooth muscle cells
13. *Classify PDA.
    - On the basis of size
      - Small: <0.5 cm
      - Moderate: 0.5–1 cm
      - Large: >1 cm
    - On the basis of Qp:Qs
      - Small: <1.5 cm
      - Moderate: 1.5–2.5 cm
      - Large: >2.5 cm
    - Size of PDA compared with that of the pulmonary artery
      - Small: <30% of the left pulmonary artery
      - Moderate: 30%–60% of the left pulmonary artery
      - Large: >60% of the left pulmonary artery

14. Mention few predisposing conditions in PDA.
    - Maternal factors
      - Drugs: Amphetamine, hydantoin, and alcohol
      - Congenital rubella
    - Neonatal factors
      - Preterm
      - Birth weight <1.5 kg
      - Fluid overload
      - Artificial ventilation
      - Intensive phototherapy
      - Exchange transfusion
        Drugs: Prostaglandins
    - Miscellaneous
      - High altitude (at 10,000 feet altitude, PDA is more common)
      - Anemia, CCF, infections, and acidosis

15. *Mention few causes of in utero closure of the ductus.
    - Right ventricular failure
    - Mother on NSAIDs

16. Name some syndromes associated with PDA.
    - Trisomies 13 and 18
    - CHARGE
    - Carpenter
    - Congenital rubella
    - VATER
    - Fragile X
    - Cri du chat
    - Klinefelter
    - Rubinstein–Taybi
    - Smith–Lemli–Opitz
    - Treacher Collins

17. Mention few maternal conditions associated with PDA.
    - Infant of diabetic mother
    - Phenylketonuria
    - Rubella

18. Classify PDA.
    The Krichenko angiographic classification of PDA is as follows:
    - Conical
    - Window
    - Tubular
    - Complex
    - Bead-like
    - Important points are the following:
      - Usually PDA is wider at the aortic end and narrower at the pulmonary end (conical).
      - Anatomical closure occurs first at the pulmonary end because the pulmonary artery responds more to oxygen.
      - Aneurysms are common at the aortic end.

19. What do restrictive and nonrestrictive PDA mean?
    a. When the ductus is restrictive, the PVR is normal, RV afterload is normal, and the hemodynamic consequences are negligible.
    b. When the ductus is nonrestrictive, systolic pressure at the aorta and pulmonary trunk equalizes at the systemic level. The direction of blood flow depends on the relative resistance in the systemic and coronary vascular beds. If pulmonary resistance lowers, left-to-right shunt is established. When it gets higher, reversal of shunt occurs.

20. *What is the cause of PDA in rubella?
    - Two-third of mothers with rubella will have a baby with congenital heart disease of whom one-third will have PDA.
    - Eighty per cent of cases are because of the first trimester infection.
    - Pathology: It includes mitotic arrest and differential retardation of tissue growth.

21. What does suck–rest cycle indicate?
    Suck–rest–suck cycle is adult equivalent of exertional dyspnea because of increased oxygen demand that cannot be met by a failing heart.

22. What are the clinical findings in PDA?
    - Silent PDA: No symptoms
    - Small PDA: Minimal symptoms and no CCF/PHT
      - Normal peripheral pulses
      - Normal pulse pressure
      - Systolic thrill in the left 2nd space
      - Machinery murmur
      - Cardiomegaly
    - Large PDA
      - Failure to thrive
      - Recurrent pneumonia
      - Pulmonary hypertension
      - CCF
      - Bounding peripheral pulses
      - Wide pulse pressure because of runoff of blood into the pulmonary artery during diastole
      - Moderately or grossly enlarged heart size
      - Thrill in the left 2nd intercostal space and radiating to the left clavicle
      - Increased precordial activity
      - S3
      - Apical diastolic rumble

23. Comment on split in PDA.
    - Spilt in PDA
      - Paradoxical split of S2: Larger shunt – LV ejection prolonged than RV ejection
      - Single or closely split second heart sound with short pulmonary ESM and loud P2: Pulmonary hypertension (Graham Steell murmur/PR murmur)

24. How can one differentiate between VSD and PDA?
    - History: Onset of failure in VSD is around 6–8 weeks, whereas in PDA it can occur in newborn also.
    - Examination
      a. VSD: Here bounding pulses are felt only in the radial artery but not in the posterior tibial and dorsalis pedis arteries.
         PDA: Bounding pulses are felt in the radial, posterior tibial, and dorsalis pedis arteries.
      b. VSD murmur is a holosystolic murmur heard best in the lower left sternal border, whereas PDA murmur is a continuous murmur that is best heard in the left sternal border away from the sternum.

25. When should one suspect PDA in preterm?
    - Difficulty in weaning
    - Apnea
    - Bounding pulses
    - Increased precordial activity
    - Wide pulse pressure

26. Discuss the murmur seen in PDA.

    The characteristic features of a continuous murmur are the following:
    - Murmur begins soon after S1, reaches maximal intensity during late systole, and wanes at the end of diastole.
    - It is heard in Gibson area.
    - Other names of the murmur are as follows:
      - Machinery murmur
      - Train in tunnel murmur
      - Gibson murmur
      - Crescendo–decrescendo murmur
    - DD of continuous murmur in the left 2nd space is the following:
      - Aorticopulmonary window
      - Coronary AV fistula
      - Ruptured sinus of Valsalva
      - Aberrant left coronary artery with major collaterals

27. Why is there a continuous murmur in PDA?

    Systolic pressure is 120 mm Hg and pulmonary pressure is 25 mm Hg. Blood flows from the aorta to the pulmonary artery during both systole and diastole and hence there is a continuous murmur.

28. What are the other murmurs in PDA?
    - Mid-diastolic flow in the mitral area because of increased blood flow through the valve – apical murmur
    - Aortic ejection click
    - Aortic ejection systolic murmur
    - Pulmonary Graham Steell murmur
    - Austin Flint murmur of pulmonary regurgitation
    - Pulmonary valve incompetence (dilated pulmonary trunk)

29. Describe the evolution of murmur in PDA.

    ESM → PSM → continuous → ESM

30. *Name some causes for absent murmur in PDA.
    - Infants with nonrestrictive PDA
    - CCF
    - Short large ductus
    - Shunt reversal with PHT
    - Thrombus and vegetations (infective endarteritis)

31. Mention the features of PDA with pulmonary hypertension.
    - Differential cyanosis
    - Disappearance of diastolic component of the murmur
    - Parasternal heave because of RVH
    - ECG: RVH
    - CXR: Cardiomegaly

32. How is the severity of PDA assessed?
    1. Wider the pulse pressure, larger the shunt
    2. Presence of S3
    3. Delayed diastolic murmur
    4. Cardiomegaly

33. *Name few causes of spontaneous appearance and disappearance of PDA murmur.
    - PDA with pulmonary hypertension
    - Acute angulation of ductus – positional change
    - Valve or wheel-like structure

34. Mention the differential diagnoses of PDA.
    1. Coronary/systemic/pulmonary AV fistula
    2. Truncus arteriosus
    3. Venous hum
    4. Collaterals in coarctation
    5. Persistent pulmonary artery stenosis
    6. Aortopulmonary window
    7. TAPVC
    8. Rupture of sinus of Valsalva
    9. MR with AR
    10. VSD with AR

35. What is the average age of Eisenmengerization in shunt lesions?
    - PDA: End of second decade
    - VSD: Third decade
    - ASD: Fourth decade

36. What is Bohn sign?

    Diastolic blood pressure falls during exercise. This is called Bohn sign.

    The greater the shunt, lower will be the diastolic pressure.

37. What is Gerhard's dullness?

    Dullness in the left 2nd intercostal space because of the presence of the ductus is called Gerhard's murmur.

38. Mention few complications in PDA.
    - Congestive cardiac failure
    - Failure to thrive
    - Infective endarteritis
    - Aneurysmal dilation of the pulmonary artery
    - Calcification of the ductus
    - Noninfective thrombus in the ductus with embolization
    - Paradoxical emboli

39. Mention few complications of PDA in preterm.
    - Laurens hypothesis: The myocardial dysfunction and ductal steal phenomenon cause poor systemic perfusion in preterm and it is called Laurens hypothesis.
    - IVH: Germinal matrix ischemia because of diastolic steal-off leads to abnormal cerebral blood flow.
    - NEC (Necrotising Enterocolitis): In addition, the reduced blood flow in the abdominal aorta and superior mesenteric artery, that is, "diastolic steal," in preterm infants with PDA causes NEC.

40. Discuss the ECG and chest X-ray features in PDA.
    - ECG
      - Small PDA: Normal
      - Moderate PDA: LVH
      - Large PDA: BVH (Biventricular Hypertrophy), left ventricular strain, and deep Q wave in left chest leads and tall T
      - PVOD (Pulmonary Veno-Occlusive Disease) (Eisenmenger syndrome): RVH
    - CXR
      - Small PDA: Normal
      - Large/moderate PDA: Cardiomegaly
        - Aortic knob seen
        - Enlarged left atrium and left ventricle
        - Increased pulmonary vascular markings
        - Prominent pulmonary artery
        - The space between pulmonary artery and aortic knuckle obliterated by PDA
        - Hilar dance on fluoroscopy
    - Cardiac catheterization
      - Either normal or increased pressure in the RV and PA
      - Presence of oxygenated blood shunting into the pulmonary artery – confirms the diagnosis of left-to-right shunt

- Oxygen studies
- Pressure studies: Pulmonary vascular obstructive disease – normal-sized heart and marked prominence of the PA segment and hilar vessels
- Echocardiography
  - 2D echocardiography in high parasternal view or suprasternal notch view
  - Larger the shunt, greater the dilatations of LA and LV

41. *Mention the echo criteria in a hemodynamically significant PDA.
    - Transductal diameter (mm): >3
    - Ductal velocity V_{max} (cm/s): <1.5
    - Antegrade PA diastolic flow (cm/s): >50

42. What is silent PDA?
    - Clinically there is no murmur.
    - Echo shows evidence of PDA.
    - It is usually not associated with pulmonary hypertension.
    - There is no need of any intervention.

43. What is obligatory PDA/desirable ductus?
    - Patent ductus is essential for the following conditions for the existence of life:
      - When duct is the only means of pulmonary blood flow
        - Tricuspid atresia with intact septum
        - Pulmonary atresia with intact septum
      - When duct is the only means of systemic blood flow
        - Hypoplastic left heart syndrome
        - Coarctation of aorta (preductal)
        - Aortic atresia
      - Bidirectional flow: TGA with intact septum
        - Maintenance of PDA
          - PGE1 is infused at the dose of 0.01–0.1 Microgram/kg/min (preparation: 30 Microgram added to 50 mL of normal saline at 1 mL/h). Ensure that the baby is mechanically ventilated before infusion because of risk of apnea and hypotension. PGE1 is usually given for 2–3 days till a maximum of 7 days; surgery should be planned in the meantime.
          - Adverse reactions include apnea, fever, cutaneous flushing, bradycardia, seizures, tachycardia, cardiac arrest, and edema.

44. Describe the medical management of PDA.
    - Fluid is restricted to 120 mL/kg/day with furosemide 1 mg/kg/day.
    - Drugs
      - Indomethacin
        - Loading dose: 0.2 mg/kg/dose
        - Subsequent dose: Intravenously (as per postnatal age)
          - Younger than 2 days: 0.1 mg/kg/dose every 12 hours – two doses
          - 2–7 days old: 0.2 mg/kg/dose every 12 hours – two doses
          - Older than 7 days: 0.25 mg/kg/dose every 12 hours – two doses
        - Administered as infusion over 30 minutes or as continuous infusion over 36 hours
        - Can prolong the first course by giving two more doses of 0.1 mg/kg q24 hourly (maximum two courses can be considered)

- Ibuprofen is administered as 10 mg/kg i.v. loading dose followed by two doses of 5 mg/kg every 24 hours for 2 days. It has got a low incidence of oliguria and cerebral complications. It is administered as an infusion over 30 minutes.
- Trial: Oral paracetamol 10 mg/kg is administered for 5 days; the same dose is repeated, with a maximum of two doses.
  - Indications: CCF, prolonged respiratory support, unexplained oxygen requirement (FiO_2 >30%), and recurrent apnea
  - Precautions: Urine output, RFT, and platelet count monitored
  - Contraindications
    - Urea >25 mg/dL
    - Creatinine >1.8 mg/dL
    - Platelets <80,000 cells/mm^3
    - Intracranial hemorrhage
    - NEC
    - Hyperbilirubinemia
  - Side effects: Renal impairment, Necrotising enterocolitis, GI hemorrhage, and impaired cerebral blood flow (paracetamol – no known renal impairment)
  - Drugs not effective in term babies

45. Discuss other modes of management.
    - Indication for closure
      a) Hemodynamically significant PDA causing failure to thrive, CCF, pulmonary overcirculation, and enlarged LA and LV
      b) Small PDA with murmur heard by standard auscultation techniques
    - Timing of surgery: Small, spontaneous; moderate, 2 years; and with symptoms, early closure
    - Nonsurgical closure of PDA
      a. Coils (Gianturco) can be used for small PDA (<3 mm).
        - For large PDA (3–12 mm), Amplatzer device should be used.
      b. Advantages
        - No need for general anesthesia
        - Short hospital stay
        - Elimination of thoracotomy scar
      c. Disadvantages
        - Residual leak
        - Hemolysis
        - Embolization of coil
        - Left pulmonary artery stenosis
        - Aortic occlusion for Amplatzer
        - Femoral vessel occlusion
    - Other procedures
      - Video-assisted thoracoscopic surgery (VATS)
      - Ligation + division
    - Surgical closure
      a. It is performed when the nonsurgical closure is not applicable.
      b. Methods
        - Ligation and division
        - Left posterolateral thoracotomy incision
        - Performed without cardiopulmonary bypass
      c. Complications
        - Injury to the recurrent laryngeal nerve
        - Vocal cord paralysis

- Chylothorax/pneumothorax
- Preterm: BPD
- Injury to the left phrenic nerve
- Injury to the thoracic duct
- Recanalization (reopening)
- Infection

d. Case fatality rate is <1%.

e. After surgery
  - CCF abates.
  - Failure to thrive improves immediately.
  - Pulse pressure is wide and machinery murmur normalizes.
  - But functional systolic murmur may be present in the left 2nd ICS because of turbulent flow into the dilated pulmonary artery.

f. Recurrence after surgery is 10%–15%.

46. *Mention few causes of death in PDA.
  - CCF, infective endarteritis, and dissecting aneurysm

Quick Bites

- High altitude: PDA is six times more common at 10,000 feet.
- Functional closure occurs at 12–14 hours of life; anatomical closure occurs by the 2nd to 3rd week.
- Drugs used for closure of PDA are ibuprofen, indomethacin, and paracetamol (under trial).
- Indomethacin does not have much effect in term babies.
- Drugs used for maintaining ductal patency are PGE3 and PGE1.
- The ideal age for PDA closure is 3 months for term and 1 year for preterm (as early as possible, when spontaneous closure is unlikely to occur).

Respiratory System

17

Examination of Respiratory System

General Examination

1. Sensorium
   - Altered sensorium in respiratory failure, lung abscess metastasizing to the brain, and TB meningitis
2. Posture
   - Mention in which position the patient prefers to lie.
   - A child with acute epiglottitis sits in a tripod position (sitting upright and leaning forward with the chin up and the mouth open while bracing on the arms).
   - Pleural effusion: Lying on the affected side relieves chest pain and lying on the normal side compresses the lung and compromises the lung volume, causing pain.
   - In unilateral bronchiectasis and lung abscess, the child prefers to lie on the affected side and sputum production is more when he or she lies on the healthy side.
3. Pallor
   - Hemoptysis
   - Infective seen in *Mycoplasma pneumoniae*
   - Hematological – acute chest syndrome because of sickle cell anemia
   - Large pulmonary embolism resulting in obstructive shock
   - Connective tissue disorders
   - Malignancies
4. Icterus
   - Secondary to hemolytic anemia in *M. pneumoniae* and SLE (Systemic Lupus Erythematosus)
   - Pulmonary infarct
   - Drug-induced (antituberculous drugs)
5. Cyanosis
   - Respiratory failure and hepatopulmonary syndrome
6. Clubbing
   - Empyema, lung abscess, bronchiectasis, cystic fibrosis, interstitial lung disease, long-standing tuberculosis, and pulmonary AV (Ateriovenous) malformations
   - Causes of unilateral clubbing: Local trauma, median nerve injury, subluxation of the shoulders, and subclavian artery aneurysm
7. Generalized lymphadenopathy
   TB, HIV, connective tissue disorders, and hematological malignancies
8. Pedal edema
   - Cor pulmonale and generalized lymphangiectasia (pleural effusion is the pulmonary manifestation)

Head-to-Foot Examination

1. Abnormal facies and respiratory system
   - Down syndrome: Recurrent respiratory tract infection, obstructive sleep apnea, hypoplastic lungs, diaphragmatic hernia, and TEF
   - Treacher Collins syndrome: Retrognathia and glossoptosis resulting in airway obstruction
   - DiGeorge syndrome: Immunodeficiency resulting in recurrent respiratory tract infections
   - Turner syndrome: Sternal malformations and scoliosis
   - Noonan syndrome: Generalized lymphangiectasia
2. Eyes
   - Pallor, icterus, phlycten, conjunctival congestion, and retinitis pigmentosa (primary ciliary dyskinesia)
3. Face
   - Malar rash and discoid rash (SLE)
4. Ears
   - Look for otitis media.
5. Nose and nasopharynx
   - Congestion, polyp, foreign body, adenoid hypertrophy, and deviation of the nasal septum
6. Paranasal sinus
   - Tenderness over the paranasal sinus region
7. Oral cavity and oropharynx
   - Macroglossia: Relative macroglossia – Down syndrome
   - Absolute macroglossia: Congenital hypothyroidism, glycogen storage disorders, MPS (Mucopolysaccharidosis) and histiocytosis
   - Dental caries
   - Odor of breath: Foul smelling (anaerobic lung infections) and acetone breath (DKA -Diabetic Ketoacidosis)
   - Cleft palate: Can result in aspiration
   - Tonsillar enlargement
   - Asymmetric enlargement of tonsils with the uvula pushed to the opposite side suggestive of peritonsillar abscess
   - Bulge in the lateral pharyngeal wall with medial displacement of tonsils: Lateral pharyngeal wall abscess
   - Bulge in the posterior pharyngeal wall: Retropharyngeal abscess
   - Trismus: Parapharyngeal abscess and Ludwig angina
8. Neck
   - Swellings causing airway obstruction – lymphadenopathy, Ludwig angina, and abscess
   - Engorged veins (cor pulmonale)
9. Extremities
   - Cyanosis, clubbing, palmar erythema, edema, and BCG (Bacille Calmette Guerin) scar
10. Chest
    - Chest wall symmetry, cutaneous swellings, bony deformities, visible pulsations, scars/sinuses, and intercostal drainage tube
11. Skin
    - Skin infections and exanthematous rash (SLE)
    - Scab, petechiae, and purpurae (*M. pneumoniae*, malignancies)
12. External markers of tuberculosis
    - Lupus vulgaris, scrofuloderma, erythema nodosum, and lichen scrofulosorum
13. Joints
    - Arthritis (*M. pneumoniae*, TB, SLE, malignancies, secondary to gout caused by pyrazinamide)

Vital Signs

1. Pulse
   - Low volume (obstructive shock because of massive pulmonary embolism)
   - Bounding pulse (CO_2 retention)
   - Pulsus paradoxus – severe airway obstruction
2. Blood pressure
   - Hypotension (obstructive shock because of massive pulmonary embolism)
   - Wide pulse pressure in CO_2 retention
3. Respiration
   Rate
   - Count the respiratory rate for 1 minute when the child is quiet and comfortable.
   - The normal range of respiratory rates is shown in Table 17.1.
   Types of respiration
   - Types of respiration according to the age are shown in Table 17.2.

Patterns of Respiration

   - Patterns of respiration and the corresponding level of lesions in the brain are shown in Table 17.3 and Fig. 17.1.
4. Temperature
   - Hyperthermia can cause tachypnea.
   - Fever can be suggestive of infections/connective tissue disorder/malignancy.
5. JVP (Jugular Venous Pressure)
   - Elevated in cor pulmonale

Examination of Respiratory System

UNIQUE FEATURES OF THE PEDIATRIC RESPIRATORY SYSTEM

- The tongue is relatively large in proportion to the oral cavity of the child.

TABLE 17.1	Normal Range of Respiratory Rates According to the Age
Age	**Respiratory Rate/Min**
0–3 months	30–60
3–6 months	30–45
6–12 months	25–40
1–3 years	20–30
3–6 years	20–25
6–12 years	14–22
Older than 12 years	12–18

TABLE 17.2	Types of Respiration According to the Age
Age	**Type of Respirations**
Infants	Abdominal
Young children	Abdominothoracic
Older than 7 years	Thoracic

- Infants younger than 2 months are obligate nose breathers and nasal obstruction can result in severe respiratory distress.
- The larynx is highly placed opposite C3–C4 vertebra as opposed to C4–C5 in adults.
- The cricoid ring is the narrowest portion of the respiratory tract.
- The chest wall is highly compliant resulting in reduced FRC (Functional Residual Capacity).
- The lungs are smaller with fewer alveoli and absent collateral channels of ventilation.
- The closing volume is higher than FRC leading to greater tendency for atelectasis and collapse.
- Infants and young children are at a high risk of respiratory failure because their diaphragms are flatter and more prone to fatigue.
- Poor immune response can result in frequent respiratory tract infections.

UPPER RESPIRATORY TRACT

- From anterior nares to larynx
- Nose and nasopharynx: Nasal flaring/rhinitis/deviated nasal septum/foreign body/polyp/adenoid hypertrophy/bleeding from the nose (can cause spurious hemoptysis) looked for
- Paranasal sinus: Tenderness
- Oral cavity and oropharynx: As mentioned in the section "General Examination"
- Ears: Otitis externa/otitis media

LOWER RESPIRATORY TRACT

- From larynx to alveoli
- Can divide the respiratory tract as a whole into conducting zone and respiratory zone as shown in Fig. 17.2
  - Conducting zone: Initial 16 generations of the airway (from nose to terminal bronchiole)
  - Respiratory zone: Final generations of the airway (from respiratory bronchiole to alveoli)

INSPECTION

Tracheal Position

- Trachea midline in loculated effusion, bilateral effusion, consolidation, and bronchiectasis
- Deviated to the opposite side in pleural effusion, pneumothorax, hydropneumothorax, and diaphragmatic hernia
- Pulled to the same side in collapse and fibrosis

Apical Impulse

If both trachea and apical impulse are shifted to the opposite side, it is suggestive of mediastinal shift. In contrast, if apical impulse alone is shifted, it is suggestive of dextrocardia.

Chest Wall

A. Shape and symmetry
   - Pectus excavatum: It is the most common of all chest wall defects. There occurs exaggeration of the normal hollowness of the lower end of the sternum. The apical impulse is deviated to the left. Pectus excavatum is associated with Marfan and Ehlers–Danlos syndromes,

Pattern		Level of lesions
1. Cheyne-stokes	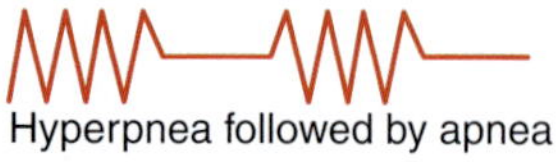 Hyperpnea followed by apnea	1. Cerebral hemisphere to 2. Pons-upper pearl 3. CCF, uremia
2. Kussmal's	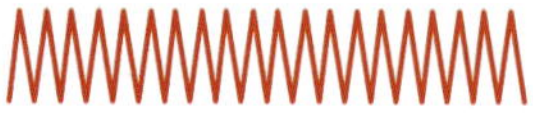 Hyperpnea & tachypnea	Metabolic, upper pons
3. Central hyperventilation	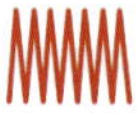 Rapid breathing	Mid brain, upper pons
4. Apneustic breathing	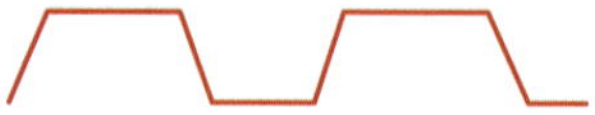 Inspiration followed by apnea exp followed by apnea	Pons
5. Blustes or blots breathing	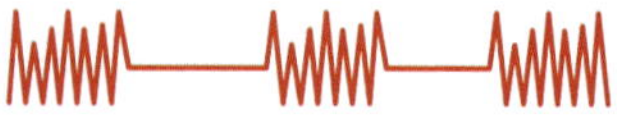 Blusts & breathing followed by apnea	Pons & upper medulla
6. Ataxic breathing	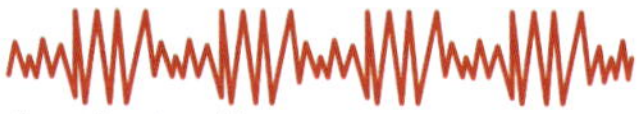 Inguinal pattern	Medulla

Fig. 17.1 Patterns of respiration and the corresponding level of lesions in the brain.

TABLE 17.3   Patterns of Respiration and the Corresponding Level of Lesions in the Brain

Breathing	Pattern	Level of Lesion
Cheyne–Stokes breathing	Hyperpnea followed by apnea	Diencephalus
Kussmaul breathing	Tachypnea with hyperpnea	Uremia, left ventricular failure, DKA
Central neurogenic hyperventilation	Regular rapid and deep respirations	Mid-brain
Apneustic breathing	Inspiration followed by apnea and expiration followed by apnea	Pons
Cluster or Biot's breathings	Clusters of breathing followed by apnea	Pons and upper medulla
Ataxic breathing	Chaotic pattern of breathing	Medulla

osteogenesis imperfecta, and progressive neuromuscular defects.
- Pectus carinatum: There occurs forward protrusion of the sternum and costal cartilages. Pectus carinatum is associated with Marfan syndrome, Noonan syndrome, and osteogenesis imperfecta.
- Haller index: The severity of pectus deformity can be determined by Haller index or pectus severity index (as shown in Fig. 17.3). In pectus excavatum, the value >2.5 is considered severe. In pectus carinatum, the value <2.0 is considered severe.
- Kyphosis: There occurs forward bending of the spine.
- Scoliosis: There occurs lateral deviation of the spine.
- Gibbus occurs.
- Other chest wall deformities include flail chest, fused ribs, and hemivertebra.
B. Chest wall movements
C. Suprasternal/sternal/intercostal/subcostal retractions
D. Intercostal fullness (empyema)
E. Empyema thoracis
F. Scars
- ICD (Intercostal Drain) scar is usually seen in the triangle of safety.
- VAT (Video Assisted Thoracoscopy) scar is seen in the axilla or posteriorly.
- Scar above the sternal notch is indicative of thoracotomy.

PALPATION

Tracheal Position

- Keeping the head in midline, looking straight, rest the second and fourth fingers of the examining hand at each sternoclavicular joint and use the third finger to assess the tracheal position by passing it in the midline and on either side deeply and inferiorly as well as shown in Fig. 17.4A–C.

Apical Impulse

Assess for the apical impulse by first placing both palms on either side of the chest at the level of the nipple (this helps to pick up dextrocardia). Once you are sure of the side, place the ulnar

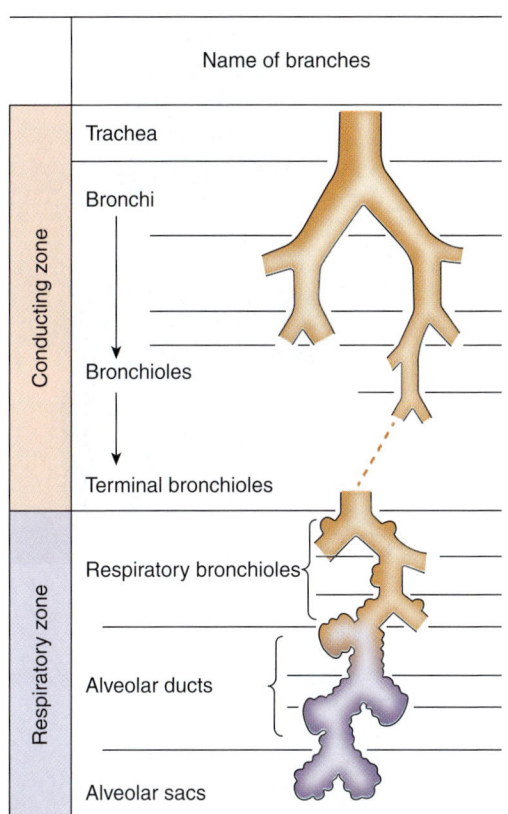

Fig. 17.2 Conducting zones and the respiratory zones of the airway. (*Source: Reproduced from Ganong Textbook of Physiology, 25th edition, Chapter 34.*)

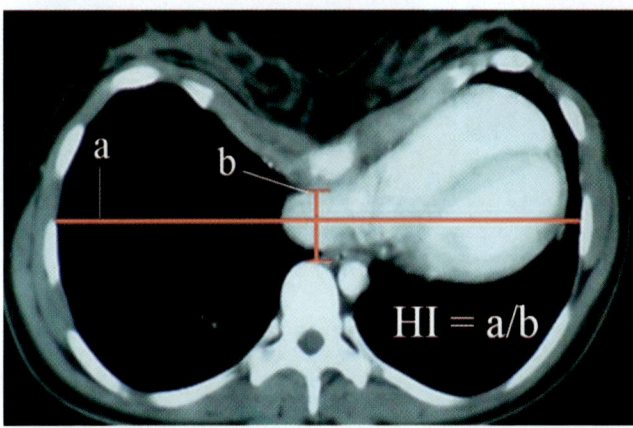

Fig. 17.3 Haller index (HI) = maximum transverse diameter (a)/minimum anteroposterior diameter (b). (Source: Reproduced from Ferdynand Hebal, Elissa Port, Catherine J. Hunter et al. and A novel technique to measure severity of pediatric pectus excavatum using white light scanning, *Journal of Pediatric Surgery*, 54:656-662.)

border of the hand; use the index to pinpoint the location of the apical impulse.

Chest Wall Movements

- Apical expansion: Stand behind the patient and place hands on both supraclavicular fossa (Fig. 17.5A).
- Anterior expansion in the upper chest: Stand in front of the patient and keep both palms over either side of the upper chest.

- Anterior expansion in the lower chest: Stand in front of the patient, and encircle both hands around the chest below the nipple so the two thumbs meet in the midline. Ensure that all fingers, not just thumbs and index fingers, are in contact with the body (Fig. 17.5B).
- Posterior chest expansion: The above-mentioned method is performed from the posterior aspect (Fig. 17.5C).

Chest Measurements

- Although not much used in pediatrics, it is important to know how to measure the chest. Important measurements are chest circumference (Fig. 17.6A), transverse diameter (Fig. 17.6B), hemithoracic diameter, and anteroposterior diameter (Fig. 17.6C).

Other Findings in Palpation

- Tenderness
- Chest crepitus – because of subcutaneous emphysema in pneumothorax and trauma to the chest wall
- Vocal fremitus

PERCUSSION

Technique

- It was discovered by Dr Leopold Auenbrugger.
- The middle finger of the left hand (pleximeter) is placed over the intercostal space (ICS)/area to be percussed with slight extension of the distal interphalangeal joint.
- The middle finger of the examiner's right hand (plexor) is used to strike the middle phalanx of the pleximeter.
- Movement of the plexor is at the wrist joint and not at the elbow.
- Always compare both sides.
- The movement should be sudden and the plexor should be withdrawn suddenly on striking the pleximeter.
- Fig. 17.7A–E shows the technique of percussion.

Areas of Percussion

1. Right and left supraclavicular
2. Right and left clavicular (direct percussion)
3. Right and left mammary
4. Right and left inframammary
5. Right and left axillary
6. Right and left infra-axillary
7. Right and left suprascapular
8. Upper and lower interscapular
9. Right and left infrascapular

Types of Percussion Note

- Percussion note and its various types are mentioned in Table 17.4.

Areas of Chest and the Corresponding Lobes of Lungs

The areas of chest and the corresponding lobes of lungs are shown in Table 17.5 and Fig. 17.8.

Shifting Dullness

- Percuss the chest with the child sitting and note for dullness.
- When dullness is noted, ask the patient to lie down on the opposite side and percuss after a few seconds.
- If the area becomes resonant, shifting dullness is present. It is seen in hydropneumothorax.

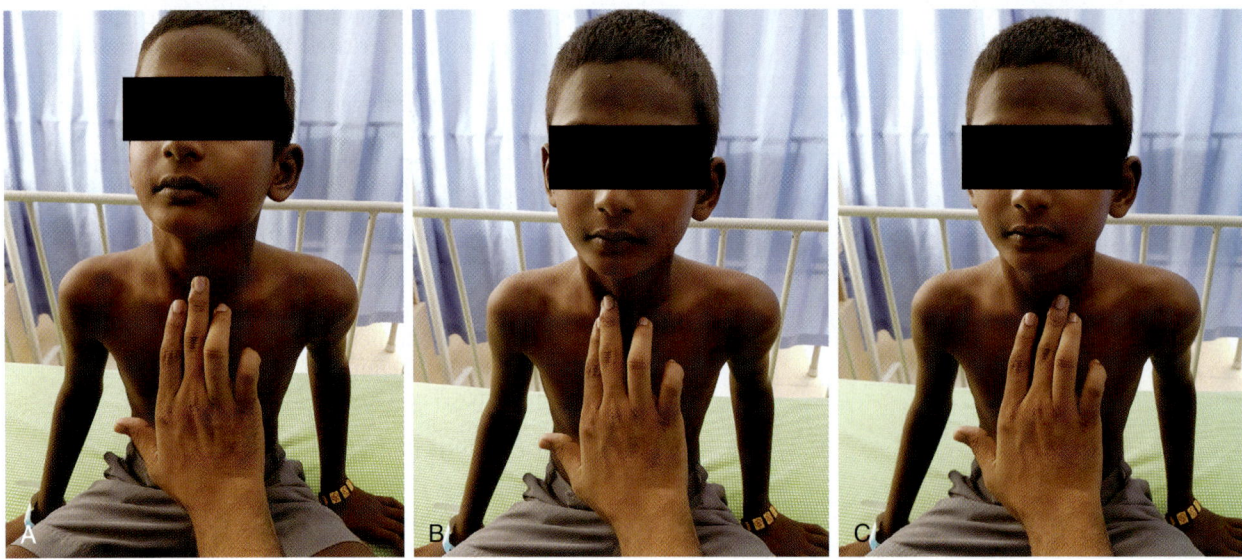

Fig. 17.4 (A–C) Palpation of tracheal position.

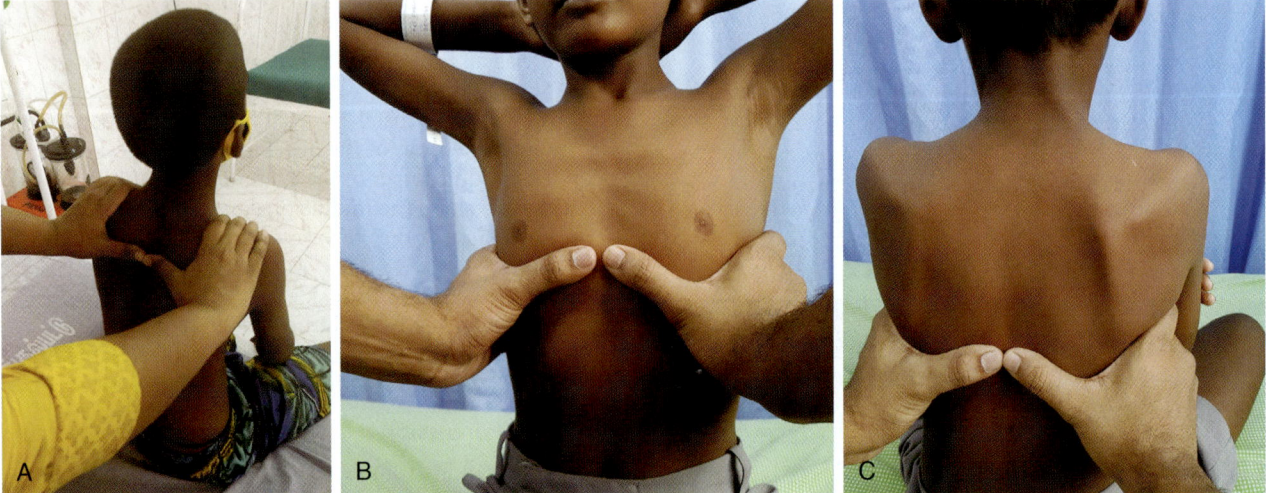

Fig. 17.5 (A) Assessment of upper lobe expansion. (B) Assessment of anterior chest wall expansion. (C) Posterior aspect of posterior expansion.

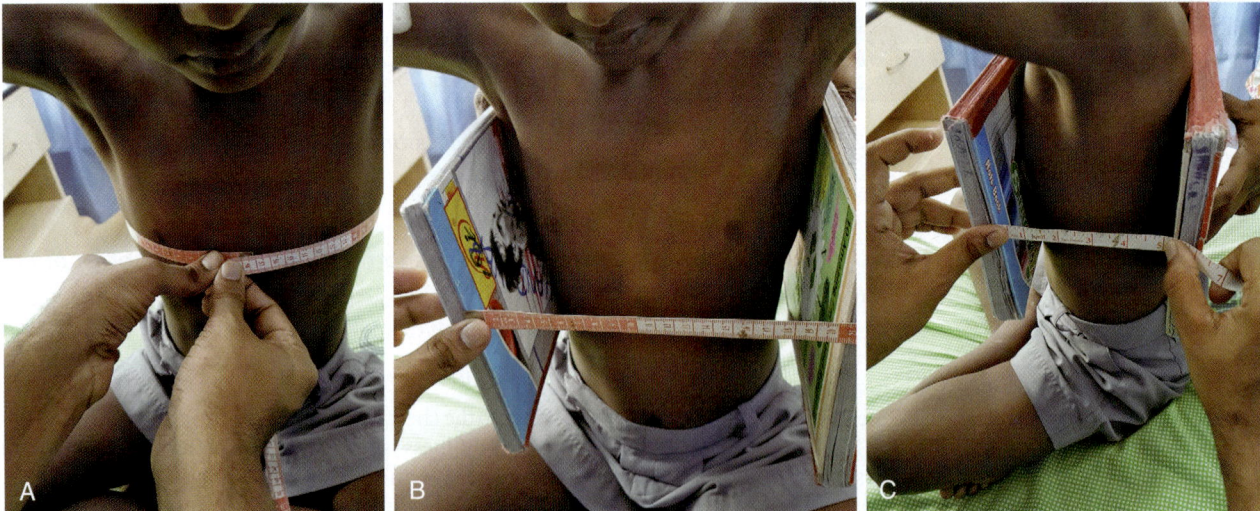

Fig. 17.6 (A) Measurement of chest circumference. (B) Measurement of transverse diameter. (C) Measurement of anteroposterior diameter.

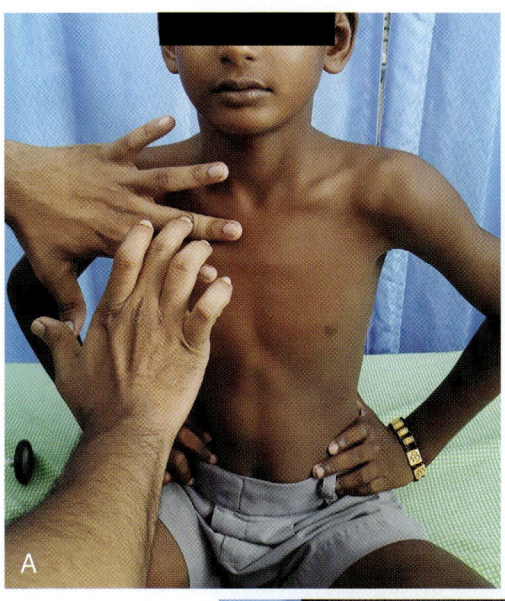
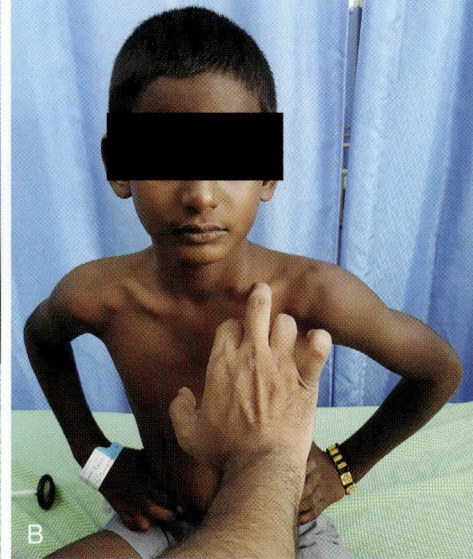
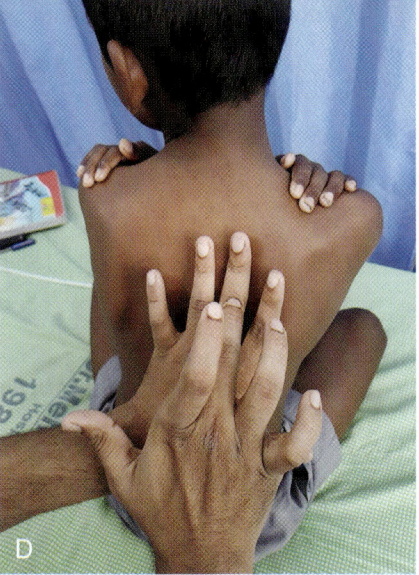
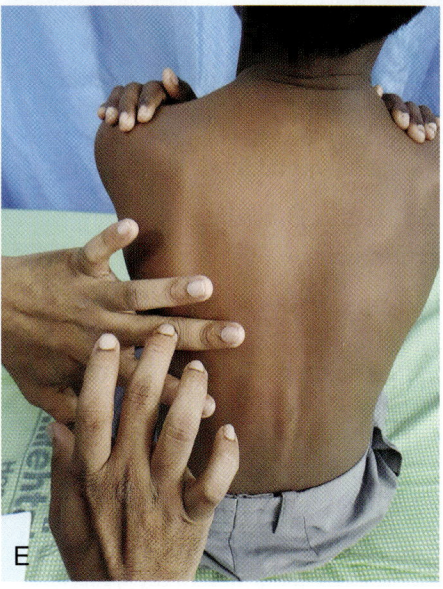

Fig. 17.7 (A) Percussion technique shown over the infraclavicular region. (B) Direct percussion over the clavicle. (C) Percussion over the infra-axillary region. (D) Percussion of the interscapular region. (E) Percussion of the infrascapular region.

TABLE 17.4	Types of Percussion Note	
Percussion Note	**Conditions**	
Resonant	Normal	
Hyper-resonant	Pneumothorax	
Dull	Consolidation, collapse, abscess, sequestration	
Stony dull	Pleural effusion	

TABLE 17.5	Areas of Chest and the Corresponding Lobes of Lungs	
Area of Chest	**Right Lung**	**Left Lung**
Supraclavicular, clavicular, infraclavicular	Upper lobe	Upper lobe
Mammary	Middle lobe	Upper lobe
Inframammary	Lower lobe	Lower lobe
Axillary	Upper lobe	Upper lobe
Infra-axillary	Lower lobe	Lower lobe
Suprascapular	Upper lobe	Upper lobe
Infrascapular	Lower lobe	Lower lobe

Tidal Percussion

- The anterior wall of the chest is percussed from the right 2nd intercostal space along the midclavicular line. Once the dullness is noted in the inferior part with the percussing finger in position, the patient is asked to take a deep breath.
- Again the same spot is percussed.

- If the dullness is because of pleural effusion, it will persist.
- If the dullness is because of the liver, the area becomes resonant (because the liver will be pushed down by the expanding lung)

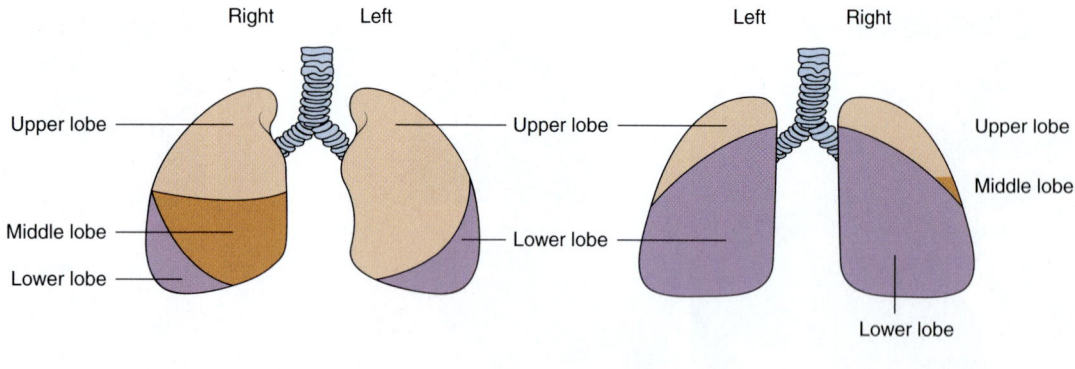

Fig. 17.8 Anterior and posterior aspects of lungs. *(Source: Reproduced from Michael Glynn, William M Drake. Hutchison's Clinical Methods, 24th Edition, Fig 12.2, Edinburgh, Elsevier Ltd, 2018)*

Traube's Space

The surface anatomy of Traube's space is shown in Fig. 17.9.

Surface Anatomy of Traube's Space
- Two parallel vertical lines drawn, first at the 6th costochondral junction and second at the 9th rib in the midaxillary line
- Two horizontal lines drawn, first at the level of the 6th costochondral junction and second at the left costal margin (as shown in Fig. 17.5)
- Boundaries
  - Right: Left lobe of the liver
  - Left: Spleen
  - Above: Lower border of the left lung
  - Below: Left costal margin
- Contents: Fundus of the stomach
- Traube's space obliterated in liver enlargement of the left lobe, splenomegaly, left pleural effusion, and massive pericardial effusion

"S"-Shaped Curve of Ellis
- In moderate-sized pleural effusion, the uppermost level of dullness is highest in the axilla and lowest in the spine, and tends to assume the shape of the letter "S." It is thought to be because of capillary suction between two layers of pleura resulting in the highest level of fluid at the axilla.

AUSCULTATION

Breath Sound
- Breath sounds originate from turbulent airflow in the larger airways.
- They are of two types: bronchial and vesicular.
- Differences between bronchial and vesicular breath sounds are listed in Table 17.6 and Fig 17.10.

Bronchial Breathing
Types of bronchial breathing are listed in Table 17.7.

Added Sounds
- Rales and crepitations are older terms and should be avoided.
- Differences between wheeze and crepitations are listed in Table 17.8.

Pleural Rub
- It is a superficial, localized squeaking or grating sound best heard with a firm pressure of the stethoscope. It is associated with pain.

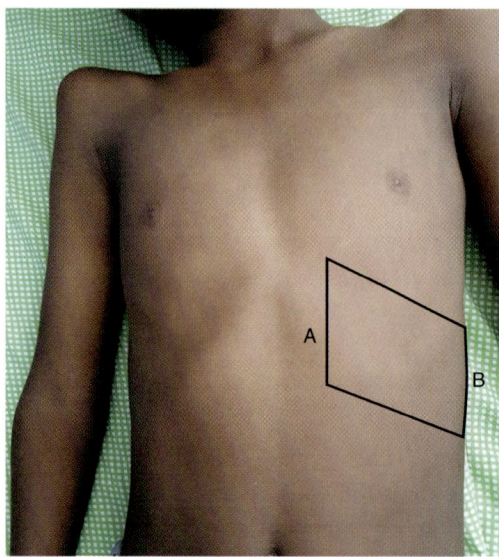

Fig. 17.9 Surface anatomy of Traube's space.

TABLE 17.6	Bronchial and Vesicular Breath Sounds	
Vesicular		**Bronchial**
They are low pitched and quieter		They are high pitched and louder
Normal lung tissue makes the sound quieter and filters some frequencies		They are produced when underlying lung tissue is consolidated and transmits the sound generated in large airways to the chest
Inspiration:expiration = 3:1 with no pause in between		Expiratory sound lasts longer than inspiratory with a pause in between

Note: Broncho-vesicular-Intermediate pitch, where inspiratory and expiratory sound are almost equal, often heard in 1st and 2nd intercostal space anteriorly and between the scapula posteriorly.

Breath sounds

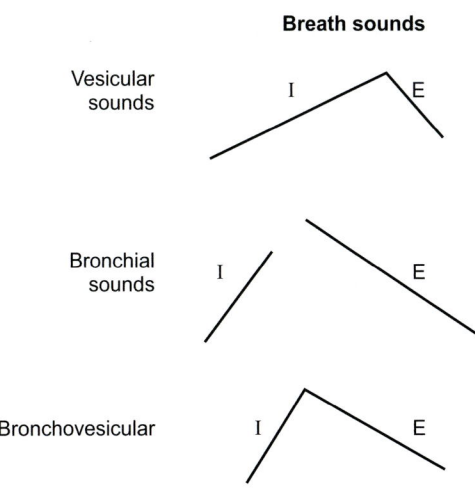

Fig.s 17.10 Types of breath sounds.

TABLE 17.7	Types of Bronchial Breathing	
Bronchial Sound	**Quality**	**Condition**
Tubular	High pitched	Seen in consolidation, above the level of pleural effusion
Cavernous	Low pitched	Seen in the presence of a cavity communicating with a bronchus
Amphoric	Low pitched with a metallic quality	Seen in bronchopleural fistula, tension pneumothorax

Succussion Splash

- It is a splashing sound heard over the chest when the patient is shaken suddenly by the examiner.
- Ask the patient to lie down on the healthy side.
- Determine the air–fluid level in the paraspinal region and place the stethoscope there.
- Grasp the nondependent shoulder and shake it suddenly.

TABLE 17.8	Differences Between Wheeze and Crepitations	
Wheeze	**Crackles**	
Musical sounds produced by passage of air through narrowed airways	Short explosive sounds; produced by sudden changes in pressure related to opening of airways	
Monophonic – localized narrowing (FB-Foreign body)	Coarse crackles – bronchiectasis	
Polyphonic – asthma	Fine crackles – ILD (Interstitial Lung Disease)	

- Sound like a splash of water can be heard.
- It is seen in hydropneumothorax and diaphragmatic hernia.

d'Espine Sign

- It is the presence of high-pitched tubular breathing and whispering pectoriloquy over the thoracic spine below T4 in children and infants.
- It is because of transmission of bronchial breath sound through a mass or central pneumonia in the middle or posterior mediastinum.

Voice Sounds

1. Bronchophony: Voice sounds appear to be heard near the earpiece of the stethoscope and words are unclear, e.g., consolidation.
2. Egophony: On saying "E," it will be heard as "A," e.g., consolidation.
3. Whispering pectoriloquy: The patient is asked to whisper words at the end of expiration, and this whispered voice is transmitted without distortion so that the individual syllables are recognized clearly, e.g., consolidation.

Various Diseases of Respiratory System

- A summary of findings of various pathologies in the respiratory system is listed in Table 17.9.

TABLE 17.9	Summary of Findings of Various Pathologies in the Respiratory System						
Pathology	**Tracheal Position**	**Chest Movements on the Affected Side**	**Vocal Fremitus**	**Percussion**	**Breath Sounds**	**Vocal Resonance**	**Added Sounds**
Consolidation	Midline	Reduced	Increased	Dull	Tubular	Increased	Indux, fine crackles; redux, coarse crackles
Pleural effusion	Shifted to the opposite side	Reduced	Decreased	Stony dull	Tubular above the level of effusion	Decreased	Pleural rub may be heard above the level of effusion
Collapse	Pulled to the same side	Reduced	Decreased	Dull	Diminished or absent	Decreased	None
Bronchiectasis	Midline	Reduced	Normal or increased (if there is consolidation)	Normal or dull (if there is consolidation)	Cavernous if there is a large cavity Tubular if there is consolidation	Normal or increased (if there is consolidation)	Coarse crackles
Pneumothorax	Shifted to the opposite side	Reduced	Decreased	Hyper-resonant	Amphoric	Decreased	None

Pleural Effusion

Following introduction, seek permission from the caregiver and introduce yourself to the patient before history elicitation, and identify the case.

Name____Age____Sex____Consanguinity____Order of birth____Place____Informant____

Presenting Complaints and Duration

Cough/fever/breathlessness/chest pain

History of Presenting Illness

- Cough
  - Duration
  - Whether associated with sputum? If yes
    - Quantity
    - Color
  - Diurnal variation
  - Postural variation
  - Aggravating/relieving factors
- Fever
  - Duration
  - Associated with chills/rigors and whether resolving with medications
- Breathlessness
  - Duration/grade
  - Associated with chest – indrawing
  - Feeding difficulty
  - Whether associated with pedal edema/facial puffiness/abdominal distension
- Chest pain
  - Duration
  - Site
  - Nature of the pain
  - Aggravating and relieving factors
  - Radiation
  - Whether associated with sweating and palpitations

COMPLICATIONS HISTORY

- Cyanosis
- Altered sensorium

ETIOLOGICAL HISTORY

- Exanthematous rash and skin infections
- Throat infections
- Aspiration
- Weight loss/failure to gain weight
- Trauma to the chest
- Easy fatigability/skin rashes with joint swelling and joint pain

COURSE DURING HOSPITAL

Mention whether any medications given (antibiotics, ATT-Anti-tuberculosis therapy), and investigations and surgical procedures performed

Past History

- Similar illness in the past
- Prior viral respiratory tract illness
- Head injury
- Comorbidities

Antenatal History/Natal History/ Postnatal History

- Any significant history

Development History

- Attained age-appropriate milestones

Nutrition History

- According to 24-hour recall method

Immunization History

- Mention whether any additional vaccines were given apart from those in the National Immunization Schedule.

Allergy History

- Any history of allergic rhinitis

Contact History

- History of contact with TB

Family History

- History of acute respiratory tract illness in family members

Socioeconomic History

- Overcrowding and hygiene/passive smoking/poor ventilation

Summary

A _____-year-old child, aged _____, presented with acute onset of cough and fever followed by breathlessness and _____-sided pleuritic type of chest pain, with/without complications, and with/without contact history of TB, probably a case of _____-sided pleural effusion with/without consolidation.

General Examination

- Patient's sensorium
- Posture: Supine/semirecumbent/lying on the affected side
- Any oxygen support
- Pallor
- Cyanosis
- Clubbing
- Any icterus
- Generalized lymphadenopathy
- Pedal edema

Head-to-Foot Examination

- Eyes: Pallor, icterus, phlycten, conjunctival congestion, and iridocyclitis
- Face: Malar rash and discoid rash
- External markers of tuberculosis
- BCG (Bacille Calmette Guerin) scar
- Signs of malnutrition
- Skin lesions: Infections – impetigo and scab
- Petechiae and purpura
- Markers of CO_2 retention
- Malodorous breath

Vitals Signs

- Pulse
- BP
- Respiration: Rate, rhythm, and type of respiration
- Temperature
- JVP (Jugular Venous Pressure)

Anthropometry

- Wasting
- Stunting

Respiratory System Examination

- Upper respiratory tract
- Lower respiratory tract

INSPECTION

- Tracheal position
- Apical impulse
- Chest shape and symmetry
- Kyphosis
- Scoliosis
- Gibbus
- Scars
- Chest movements
- Intercostal fullness
- Empyema thoracis

PALPATION

- Tracheal position
- Apical impulse
- Tenderness

TABLE 18.1	Areas to be Examined for Vocal Fremitus	
Areas	**Right**	**Left**
Supraclavicular		
Infraclavicular		
Mammary		
Inframammary		
Axillary		
Infra-axillary		
Suprascapular		
Upper interscapular		
Lower interscapular		
Infrascapular		

- Vocal fremitus: Look for reduced vocal fremitus in the areas given in Table 18.1. Vocal fremitus may be increased in the presence of consolidation.
- Chest movements
- Chest measurements

PERCUSSION

- Look for stony dullness in the areas mentioned in Table 18.1
- Tidal percussion
- Traube's space percussion
- Percussion for shifting dullness
- "S"-shaped curve of Ellis

AUSCULTATION

- Vesicular breath sounds
- Bronchial breath sounds±
- Air entry in both the lungs
- Vocal resonance: Look for reduced vocal resonance in the areas mentioned in Table 18.1 (vocal resonance may be increased in the presence of a consolidation)
- Added sounds
- Pleural rub
- Succussion splash

Other System Examination

CARDIOVASCULAR SYSTEM

S3 gallop and murmurs

ABDOMEN

Signs of DCLD (Decompensated Chronic Liver Disease) and HSM

CENTRAL NERVOUS SYSTEM

Altered sensorium, meningeal signs, signs of raised ICT (Intracranial Tension), and focal neurological deficit

Diagnosis

A case of _____-sided pleural effusion with/without consolidation
  With/without complications
  Probable etiology

Frequently Asked Questions

1. What is the significance of age in a patient with pleural effusion?
   - Age can give a clue to the etiology.
   - Parapneumonic effusions are the most common cause in children.
   - Tuberculous effusion is rare in children younger than 2 years.
2. What is the significance of gender in a patient with pleural effusion?
   Effusions secondary to connective tissue disorders (Systemic lupus erythematosus) are common in females.
3. Explain the physiology of cough
   - Cough receptors are present in the upper and lower airways (up to terminal bronchioles), external auditory meatus, pleura, pericardium, and esophagus.
   - The intrathoracic pressure generated during cough is 50–300 cm H_2O.
   - The air is expelled rate of 300 m/s.
   - Children can expectorate only by 7 years of age.
*4. What is the duration of acute and chronic cough?
   - Acute cough: <3 weeks
   - Chronic cough: >8 weeks (Hutchison) and >4 weeks (Nelson's symptomatology)
5. Enumerate the etiologies of cough.
   The etiologies of cough have been enumerated in Table 18.2.

---

*Important question asked in the examination.

TABLE 18.2	Various Etiologies of Cough
Acute	**Chronic**
Infections	Asthma
Foreign body	Cystic fibrosis
Aspiration	Airway anomalies
	Passive smoking
	GERD (Gastroesophageal Reflux Disease)

TABLE 18.3	Characteristics of Cough in Different Conditions
Characteristics	**Etiology**
Abrupt	Pulmonary embolism, FB (Foreign Body)
Followed by whoop	Pertussis
Brassy, barking	Croup, epiglottitis
Nocturnal	Asthma, sinusitis
Following exercise	Asthma
Seasonal	Allergic sinusitis, asthma
Following feed	TEF (Tracheoesophageal Fistula)
All day but absent during sleep	Habit cough
Staccato	Pertussis, foreign body
Hacking	Postnasal drip

6. What are the different characteristics of cough?
   The various characteristics of cough have been enumerated in Table 18.3.
7. Enumerate the causes of chronic cough with normal chest X-ray.
   - Asthma
   - GERD
   - Postnasal drip
   - Passive smoking
   - Postviral URTI (Upper Respiratory Tract Infection)
8. What are the histories to be elicited when a child presents with cough?
   - Duration
   - Whether associated with sputum; if yes
     - Quantity
     - Color
     - Diurnal variation
     - Postural variation
     - Aggravating/relieving factors
     (For discussion on sputum and hemoptysis, kindly refer chapter 19 -Chronic Suppurative Lung Disease.)
*9. Define breathlessness.
   - Dyspnea is defined as a subjective sensation of breathing discomfort and is inappropriate to the level of physical activity. Everyone has breathlessness on strenuous exertion.
   - Eupnea is defined as normal unlabored breathing.
10. Explain the correlation between the severity of breathlessness and the site of pathology.
    The severity of breathlessness and the site of pathology are described in Table 18.4.
    - Effortless tachypnea is seen in the following:
      - Exercise
      - Hyperthermia
      - Anemia
      - Metabolic acidosis
      - Abdominal distension
      - CNS lesions (neurogenic hyperventilation)
      - Psychogenic
11. Enumerate the various causes of acute breathlessness.
    Various causes of acute breathlessness are described in Table 18.5.
12. Enumerate the drugs causing breathlessness.
    - Anticancer: Azathioprine, bleomycin, busulfan, cyclophosphamide, and methotrexate
    - Antibiotics: Penicillins, sulfonamides, erythromycin, nitrofurantoin, and isoniazid
    - Antiepileptics: Phenytoin and carbamazepine
    - Others: Hydralazine, penicillamine, imipramine, and cocaine
*13. What is the Medical Research Council grading of dyspnea (for older children and adults)?
    - **Grade 1:** Breathlessness on strenuous exercise
    - **Grade 2:** Breathlessness when hurrying on a level ground or walking up a hill
    - **Grade 3:** Walks slower than people of the same age on the level because of breathlessness, or breathlessness when walking at own pace
    - **Grade 4:** Stops for breath after about 100 m or after a few minutes on the level

TABLE 18.4	Severity of Breathlessness According to the Site of Pathology			
Symptom/Sign	Extrathoracic Airway Obstruction	Intrathoracic Extrapulmonary Airway Obstruction	Intrapulmonary Airway Obstruction	Parenchymal Disease
Breathlessness	+	+	++	++++
Retractions	++++	++	++	+++

TABLE 18.5	Etiologies of Acute Breathlessness	
Cardiac	Respiratory	Others
• Acute rheumatic fever • Infective endocarditis • Myocarditis • Pericardial effusion • Acute mitral regurgitation/aortic regurgitation	• Airway: Bronchiolitis, asthma, foreign body, bronchiectasis • Parenchymal: Pneumonia, lung abscess • Interstitial: Pulmonary edema • Pleural: Pleural effusion, pneumothorax • Vascular: Pulmonary embolism	• Anemia • Metabolic acidosis • Anaphylaxis • Abdominal distension • CNS lesions (neurogenic hyperventilation) • Hyperthermia • Drugs (usually in adolescents) • Psychogenic

TABLE 18.6	Differences Between Pleuritic and Pericardial Pain	
Pleuritic Pain	Pericardial Pain
Lateral location	Central in location
Stabbing character	Sharp pain
Aggravated by deep inspiration	Aggravated by deep inspiration and cough, lying supine
Relieved by lying on the affected side	Relieved by sitting and leaning forward

- **Grade 5:** Too breathless to leave the house, or breathless on doing day-to-day activities such as bathing and going to the toilet
- For infants, it is graded on the basis of the ability to feed, retractions, nasal flaring, grunting, and cyanosis.
  Source: The MRC dyspnoea scale by telephone interview to monitor health status in elderly COPD patients. | Semantic Scholar

14. What does fever in a patient with pleural effusion suggestive of?
    - Infection and connective tissue disorders (SLE)
    - Malignancy
    - Failure of the fever to resolve with appropriate antibiotics suggestive of complications (empyema), TB effusion, connective tissue disorders, and malignancy
15. What is the significance of stridor in a patient with pleural effusion?
    Neurogenic stridor resulting in aspiration and secondary bacterial infection
*16. Enumerate the causes of chest pain in children.
    - Ask about the onset, nature of pain, site, radiation, aggravating and relieving factors, and associated symptoms when a child gives a history of chest pain.
    - Causes
      ○ Idiopathic: Most common cause
      ○ Musculoskeletal: Second most common cause
      ○ Respiratory
      ○ Others: Gastrointestinal (GERD, peptic ulcer, hiatal hernia, acute pancreatitis), cellulitis, and herpes zoster
      ○ Cardiac cause: <5% in children
17. Differentiate between pleuritic type of chest pain and pericardial pain.
    Differences between pleuritic and pericardial pain are listed in Table 18.6.
*18. What does altered sensorium in a child with effusion signify?
    - Hypoxia

- Metastatic abscess (complication of empyema)
- TB meningitis
- Altered sensorium, which can cause aspiration
19. Enumerate the etiological histories to be asked in a child with pleural effusion.
    - *Staphylococcus aureus* pneumonia secondary to measles: History of exanthematous rash
    - Foci of infection: History of skin infections/throat infection
    - Aspiration pneumonia: History of recurrent aspiration
    - TB: History of recent weight loss
    - Malnutrition: History of failure to gain weight
    - Hemothorax: History of trauma to the chest
    - *Mycoplasma* infection/connective tissue disorders/malignancy: History of easy fatigability/skin rashes with joint swelling and joint pain
20. What is the significance of past history in pleural effusion?
    - Similar episodes in past (recurrent pneumonia)
    - Prior viral exanthematous illness
    - Head injury/seizures (result in aspiration)
    - Comorbid illness (CCF -Congestive Cardiac Failure, liver, renal disorders, hematological malignancy, connective tissue disorders)
21. What is the significance of perinatal history?
    Delayed umbilical cord fall – primary immunodeficiency disorder (LAD Leucocyte Adhesion Deficiency)
22. What are a contact and history of contact?
    - History of contact: In a symptomatic child, contact with any form of active TB within 2 years is considered as a positive contact history. In an asymptomatic child, contact with smear-positive TB is considered as a positive contact history.
    - Contact: It refers to any person who has been exposed to the index case. It is of two types:
      ○ Household contact: Any person who has shared the same enclosed living space as the index case during the 3 months before the beginning of the current treatment episode
      ○ Close contact: Any person who has shared the same enclosed space such as social gathering and workplace as the index case during the 3 months before the beginning of the current treatment episode

23. What is the significance of family history?
    - Any acute respiratory tract illness in the family members
    - Immunodeficiency disorders in family members
24. List the significant general examination findings to be looked for in a patient with pleural effusion.
    The significance of general examination findings is listed in Table 18.7.
*25. List the significant head-to-foot findings to be looked for in a patient with pleural effusion.
    - Eyes: Pallor, icterus, phlycten (TB), conjunctival congestion (viral exanthematous fever), and iridocyclitis (connective tissue disorders)
    - Face: Malar rash and discoid rash seen in SLE
    - Markers of tuberculosis: Phlycten, lupus vulgaris, scrofuloderma, erythema nodosum, erythema induratum, tuberculosis chancre, warty tuberculosis, and granuloma annulare
    - BCG scar
    - Signs of malnutrition
    - Skin lesions: Infections – impetigo and scab
    - Skin bleed: Petechiae and purpura (*Mycoplasma* infection, connective tissue disorders, malignancy)
    - Markers of CO_2 retention
    - Malodorous breath: suggestive of anaerobic infection
26. What are the markers of CO_2 retention?
    - Headache
    - Drowsiness
    - Head bobbing
    - Diminished vision
    - Cyanosis
    - Palmar erythema
    - Twitching
    - Asterixis
    - Bounding pulse
    - Wide pulse pressure

*27. What is the significance of vital signs in a patient with pleural effusion?
    - Pulse
        - Bounding pulse because of anemia, CO_2 retention, and DCLD
        - Low-volume pulse because of CCF
    - BP
        - Wide pulse pressure in anemia, CO_2 retention, and DCLD
        - Hypotension because of CCF
    - Respiration: Tachypnea
    - Temperature: Suggestive of infection/connective tissue disorders/malignancy
    - JVP: Elevated in right heart failure
28. List the findings to be looked for in inspection.
    - Upper respiratory tract: Otitis/sinusitis/pharyngitis/tonsillitis
    - Lower respiratory tract
    - Chest shape and symmetry
        - Tracheal position and apical impulse: Trachea midline in loculated effusion and bilateral effusion
        - Trail's sign: Prominence of the clavicular head of the sternomastoid on the side of deviation of the trachea; this is because of relaxation of the pretracheal fascia covering the clavicular head of the sternomastoid, thus making it prominent on the side of deviation
    - Examination of the back
        - Kyphosis
        - Scoliosis
        - Gibbus (TB spine)
    - Scars
        - ICD (Intercostal Drain) scar is usually seen in the 5th ICS in the midaxillary line.
        - VAT (Video Assisted Thoracoscopy) scar is seen in the axilla or posteriorly.
        - Scar above the sternal notch is indicative of thoracotomy.
    - Chest movements: Diminished on the affected side
    - Intercostal fullness: Empyema
    - Empyema thoracis
29. What are the findings to be looked for in palpation?
    - Tracheal position and apical impulse: Trachea midline in loculated effusion and bilateral effusion
    - Tenderness: Empyema
    - Vocal fremitus: Reduced on the affected side
    - Chest movements: Diminished on the affected side
    - Chest measurements
*30. What are the causes of tenderness in chest?
    - Trauma
    - Costochondritis
    - Intercostal muscle pain
    - Herpes zoster infection
    - Inflammatory conditions
    - Empyema
    - Abscess
*31. Explain Grocco's and Garland's triangles.
    - Grocco's triangle: It is a triangular area of dullness – the posterior region of the chest opposite to the side of effusion.
    - Garland's triangle: It is an area of resonance on the posterior region of the chest on the same side of effusion (as shown Fig. 18.1).

TABLE 18.7	Significance of General Examination Findings in a Patient With Pleural Effusion	
Clinical Finding	**Significance**
Patient's sensorium	Altered sensorium in hypoxia, metastatic abscess, TB meningitis
Posture	In pleural effusion, the patient prefers to lie on the affected side
Oxygen support	Need for oxygen support can signify hypoxia
Pallor	Malnutrition, infection (*Mycoplasma* presenting as hemolytic anemia), CCF, hypothyroidism, connective tissue disorders, hematological malignancy
Cyanosis	Respiratory failure
Icterus	Secondary to hemolytic anemia in *Mycoplasma* and SLE, DCLD presenting with ascites
Clubbing	Empyema, lung abscess
Generalized lymphadenopathy	TB, HIV, connective tissue disorders, hematological malignancies
Pedal edema	Malnutrition, CCF, DCLD, nephrotic syndrome

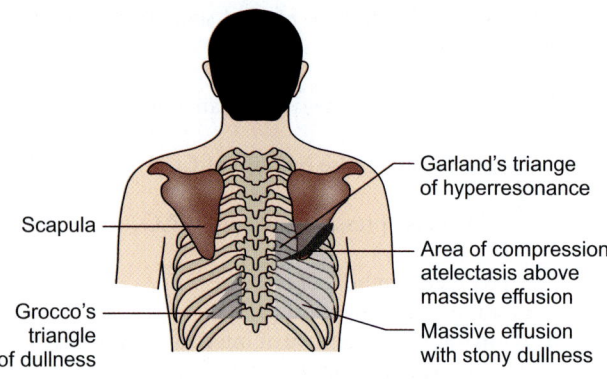

Scapula

Grocco's triangle of dullness

Garland's triange of hyperresonance

Area of compression atelectasis above massive effusion

Massive effusion with stony dullness

Fig. 18.1   Grocco's and Garland's triangles.

TABLE 18.9	Stages of Empyema	
Stage	Duration (Days)	Feature
Exudative stage	0–3	An outpouring of fluid from lung interstitium and also because of increased capillary permeability. Pleural fluid is sterile (simple parapneumonic effusion).
Fibrinopuru-lent stage	3–14	Bacteria invade the pleural cavity. Pus accumulates (complicated parapneumonic effusion).
Organization stage	>14	Fibroblast proliferation from parietal and visceral pleural results in the formation of a thick peel, which prevents expansion of lung.

- Both of these are seen in a patient with U/L and moderate-to-large effusion.
32. Explain the differences between vesicular and bronchial breath sounds.
    Differences between vesicular and bronchial breath sounds are listed in Table 18.8.
33. List the findings to be looked for in other systems in pleural effusion.
    - CVS: S3 and murmurs (CCF)
    - Abdomen: Signs of DCLD and HSM (Hepatospleno-megaly) (because of TB, malignancy)
    - CNS: Altered sensorium, meningeal signs (TB meningitis), signs of raised ICT, and focal neurological deficit (TB meningitis, metastatic abscess)
*34. Enumerate the complications of pleural effusion.
    - Empyema
    - Lung abscess
    - Subdiaphragmatic abscess
    - Pericardial abscess
    - Intracranial abscess
    - Collapse
35. What are the stages in the evolution of empyema?
    Stages of empyema are listed in Table 18.9.
36. List the investigations to be performed in pleural effusion.
    1. CBC (Complete Blood Count)
        a. Neutrophilia: s/o parapneumonic effusion
        b. Lymphocytosis: TB effusion and hematological malignancies
        c. Anemia: s/o *Mycoplasma* infection/malnutrition/malignancy/connective tissue disorders
    2. LFT (Liver Function Test) and RFT (Renal Function Test): To rule out hepatic and renal causes, respectively

3. CRP and ESR (Erythrocyte Sedimentation Rate): Serial measurements that can help in guiding prognosis of parapneumonic effusion
4. TB and retroviral workup
5. Chest X-ray
6. Chest USG (Ultrasonogram)
7. CT chest
8. Thoracocentesis and pleural fluid analysis
37. List the findings to be looked for in chest X-ray in pleural effusion.
    - Look for the tracheal shift, hilar lymphadenopathy, consolidation, cavity, pneumatocele, pleural effusion, and cardiomegaly (as shown in Fig. 18.2).
    - Findings specific for pleural effusion are the following (AAP, *Pediatric Pulmonology*, 2011):
        - The earliest finding is the blunting of costophrenic angles, which is evident only on an erect film.
        - Homogenous opacity is seen with obliteration of the costophrenic and cardiophrenic angles and a curved upper border.
        - Lateral decubitus film can identify minimal pleural effusion as little as 50 mL. If there is no shift of fluid with lateral view, then it is a loculated effusion.

TABLE 18.8	Bronchial and Vesicular Breath Sounds	
Vesicular Breath Sounds	**Bronchial Breath Sounds**	
They are low pitched and quieter	They are high pitched and louder	
Normal lung tissue makes the sound quieter and filters some frequencies	They are produced when the underlying lung tissue is consolidated and transmits the sound generated in large airways to the chest	
Inspiration:expiration = 3:1 with no pause in between	Inspiration = expiration with a pause in between	

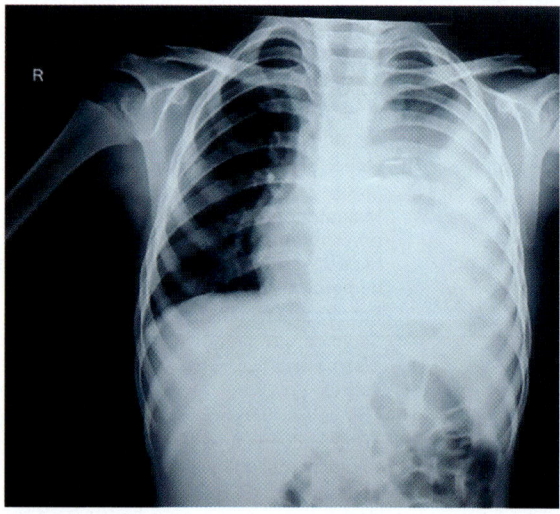

Fig. 18.2   Left lower lobe consolidation with left-sided pleural effusion.

- Presence of air–fluid level is suggestive of hydropneumothorax.

*38. What is the role of chest USG in pleural effusion?

According to AAP, *Pediatric Pulmonology*, 2011:
- Can detect effusions much earlier than they are detected in a chest X-ray
- Can differentiate free from loculated pleural fluid
- On the basis of the USG, effusions classified into simple (transudative) and complex (exudative)
- TB effusion – diffuse small nodules on the pleural surface
- Used for thoracocentesis and also for the diagnosis of loculated pleural effusion

39. What is the role of CT chest in pleural effusion?

It is rarely indicated. It may be used in complicated cases where routine management fails, prior to the surgery for delineating the exact anatomy of defect, to look for intrapulmonary abscess.

40. Discuss the management of pleural effusion/empyema.
- Bed rest
- Oxygen support
- Dehydration and electrolyte imbalance corrected
- I.v. antibiotics – third-generation cephalosporin + vancomycin – being the initial empirical treatment for uncomplicated parapneumonic effusion
- Closed chest tube drainage with/without fibrinolytics
- Video-assisted thoracoscopic adhesiolysis and pleural debridement
- Open drainage and decortication

41. List the indications for closed chest tube drainage with fibrinolytics.

Indications are as follows:
- Complicated parapneumonic effusion
- Empyema
- Moderate effusions (opacifies less than one-half of hemithorax on chest X-ray) causing respiratory compromise
- Large effusions (opacifies more than one-half of hemithorax on chest X-ray)
- Repeat chest X-ray to be taken after 12 hours to look for lung expansion (chest tube should be placed for at least 1 week; the tube can be removed if the fluid is <30 mL/day or <1 mL/kg/h)
- No response to the above-stated treatment discussed in the following flowchart.

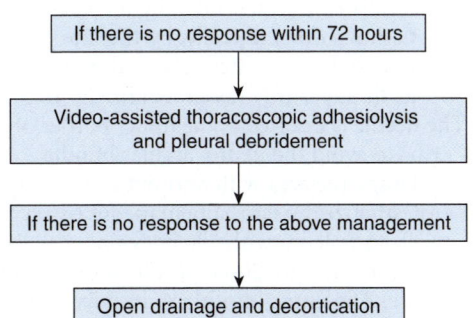

42. What is the dose of fibrinolytics?
- Streptokinase is given as 15,000 units/kg in 50 mL of 0.9% normal saline daily for 3–5 days.

- Urokinase is given as 40,000 units in 40 mL normal saline every 12 hours for six doses.
- Complications include anaphylaxis and hemorrhage.

43. What is the prognosis of empyema?

Clinical response in empyema is slow; even with optimal treatment, there may be little improvement for as long as 2 weeks. With staphylococcal infections, systemic antibiotic therapy is required for 3–4 weeks. The overall prognosis for adequately treated empyema is excellent.

44. What is the etiopathogenesis of pleural effusion?
- Pleural fluid physiology
  - The pleural space normally contains 0.3 mL/kg of fluid.
  - Fluid enters the pleural space from the following:
    - Capillaries of parietal pleura
    - Interstitial spaces of the lung
    - Peritoneal cavity from pores in the diaphragm
- The fluid is absorbed by the lymphatics of parietal pleura.
- Pleural effusion results when there is an imbalance between production and absorption.

*45. Differentiate between transudative and exudative pleural effusion.

Differences between transudative and exudative pleural effusion are listed in Table 18.10.

*46. What are Light's criteria and Roth's criteria for pleural effusion?

A. Light's criteria
- Ratio of pleural fluid protein to serum protein >0.5
- Ratio of pleural fluid Lactate dehydrogenase (LDH) to serum LDH >0.6
- Pleural fluid LDH >2/3rd normal upper limit of serum LDH

At least one criterion to be met by exudative pleural effusion and no criterion to be met by transudative pleural effusion (these criteria can misidentify 25 percent of transudates as exudates)

Source: https://www.google.co.in/url?sa5i&url5 https%3A%2F%2Fwww.pinterest.com%2Fp-in%2F302163456246684253%2F&psig5AOvVaw 3zkActXr7Py1C5X-tlnPEQ&ust51613482519436 000&source5images&cd5vfe&ved50CAIQjRxqF woTCLCc0YCB7O4CFQAAAAAdAAAAABAD.

B. Roth's criteria: If the patient meets one or more of the above-mentioned criteria for exudative effusion but has features s/o of transudate, then measure serum-pleural albumin gradient. If this is greater than 1.2 g/dL, then it is transudative pleural effusion, and if this is less than 1.2 g/dL, then it is exudative pleural effusion.

47. What are the causes of various types of effusion?

Etiologies of pleural effusion are listed in Table 18.11.

48. What are the salient features of tuberculous effusion? (RNTCP (Revised National TB Control Programme), 2019)
- It is caused by the discharge of tubercle bacilli into the pleural cavity from either subpleural pulmonary focus or a caseated lymph node.
- It is rare in children younger than 2 years.
- Children present with low-grade fever, chest pain, anorexia, and weight loss. The child is usually nontoxic; rarely the patient may present with high-grade fever.

TABLE 18.10	Differences Between Transudative and Exudative Pleural Effusion	
Feature	**Transudative Pleural Effusion**	**Exudative Pleural Effusion**
Causes	CCF Nephrotic syndrome DCLD Malnutrition Hypothyroidism Peritoneal dialysis	• Infections: Viral, bacterial, TB, fungal, parasitic • Connective tissue disorders • Malignancies • Pulmonary embolism • GI: Acute pancreatitis, esophageal perforation, intra-abdominal abscess • Chylothorax • Hemothorax • Postradiation • Drugs: Nitrofurantoin, dantrolene, bromocriptine, amiodarone
Pathogenesis	Increased hydrostatic pressure/decreased oncotic pressure	Pleural inflammation/infiltration
Appearance	Clear/straw colored	Turbid, purulent/blood/stained/milky
pH	>7.2	<7.2
Specific gravity	<1.020	>1.020
Glucose	>40 mg/dL	<40 mg/dL
LDH	<200 IU/L	>200 IU/L
Cells	WBC <1000/mm^3	WBC >1000/mm^3
Amylase	Absent	Present in pancreatitis/esophageal perforation
Gram stain/culture	Absent	Present in parapneumonic effusion
Interferon gamma/ADA	Absent	Present in TB effusion

TABLE 18.11	Etiologies of Pleural Effusion			
Bilateral Pleural Effusion	**Recurrent Pleural Effusion**	**Left-Sided Pleural Effusion**	**Chylous Effusion**	**Pseudochylous Effusion**
CCF Hypoalbuminemia Malignancy Connective tissue disorders	CCF Malignancy TB effusion Connective tissue disorders	Acute pancreatitis Esophageal perforation	TB Trauma to the thoracic duct Tumor – mediastinal lymphadenopathy	TB Rheumatoid arthritis Lung fluke infection

- It is usually unilateral.
- It never occurs in miliary TB.
- Pleural fluid analysis reveals the following:
  - Cells: >1000/mm^3 initially; polymorphs followed by lymphocyte predominance
  - Protein: 2–4 g/dL
  - Glucose: <40 mg/dL
  - AFB (Acid-Fast Bacillus): Rarely positive
  - Culture: Positive only in 30% of patients
  - ADA (Adenosine Deaminase) and interferon gamma: Elevated (ADA has limited utility in children)
  - Pleural biopsy: Diagnostic (it is performed with Cope's or Abraham's pleural biopsy needle; the yield of pleural biopsy is 80%)
  - TST (Tuberculin Skin Test): Positive in 70%–80% of patients with TB effusion
- The prognosis is excellent.

49. Describe the procedure of pleural fluid aspiration.
    The British Thoracic Society guidelines (2010) are as follows:
    - Obtain an informed consent from the patient.
    - A recent chest radiograph should be available prior to performing a pleural aspiration.
    - Thoracic ultrasound guidance is strongly recommended for pleural fluid aspiration. The complications and failure rates are less compared with those with clinically localized aspiration. USG-guided aspiration is also needed for loculated effusions.
    - Position: The patient may either sit upright, leaning forward with hands positioned above the head, or lie supine with hands positioned over the head.
    - Site of aspiration: The procedure is performed in the triangle of safety.
      This triangle is bordered by the lateral edge of pectoralis major anteriorly, by the lateral edge of latissimus dorsi laterally, by the line of the 5th intercostal space inferiorly, and by the base of the axilla superiorly (as shown in Fig. 18.3).
    The needle is inserted at the upper border of the lower rib (to avoid the neurovascular bundle).
    - Drape the area with antiseptics.
    - Anesthetize the skin, subcutaneous tissue, ribs, chest wall, and pleura with 1% lidocaine.
    - Advance 18- to 20-G needle into the intercostal space. The entry into pleural cavity is indicated by loss of resistance or appearance of fluid.
    - Gently aspirate the fluid and send the samples for analysis. For therapeutic aspiration, the volume of fluid should not exceed 20 mL/kg.
    - Cover the site of aspiration with dressing.

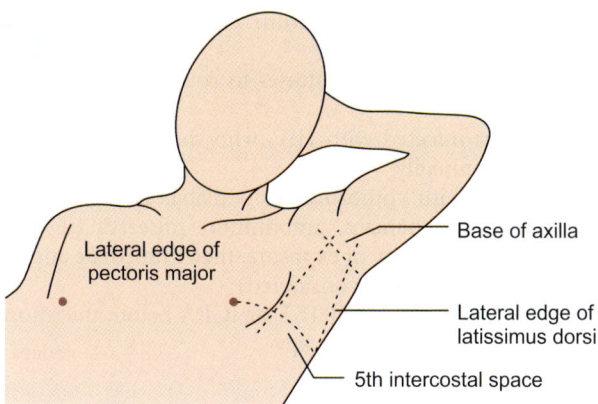

Fig. 18.3 Site for thoracocentesis.

- Routine postprocedure chest X-ray is needed for all procedures. Chest X-ray should be taken if the patient becomes symptomatic, if air is withdrawn, or multiple attempts have been made.

DISCUSSION ON TUBERCULOSIS

Epidemiological Triad in Tuberculosis

AGENT

- The causative agent is *Mycobacterium tuberculosis* complex that belongs to the family Mycobacteriaceae and order Actinomycetales.
- *M. tuberculosis* complex consists of the following subspecies:
  - *M. africanum*
  - *M. bovis*
  - *M. canetti*
  - *M. microti*
  - *M. pinnipedii*
  - *M. tuberculosis*

HOST FACTORS

- Age: All ages are equally susceptible. However, the age group of 5–14 years is called the favored age. An infected child younger than 1 year has a 40% chance of developing disease within 9 months.
- Gender: Males are at a slightly higher risk of acquiring TB infection.
- Malnutrition and immunodeficiency are the risk factors for acquiring TB.
- Patients with the following are highly contagious:
  - Cavity
  - Laryngeal TB
  - Extensive pulmonary infection
  - Sputum containing 10^5–10^7 bacilli/mL
  - Neonate with congenital TB
- Infection with atypical mycobacteria offers cross-immunity.

ENVIRONMENTAL FACTORS

Overcrowding, poor hygiene, and low socioeconomic status are the risk factors.

Pathogenesis

- The manifestations of tuberculosis depend on the host immune response.
- Macrophage-activating cell-mediated immunity is the major mechanism of host immunity. This is responsible for granuloma formation.
- Tissue-damaging delayed-type hypersensitivity is a less common mechanism. It is characterized by bacterial death along with tissue destruction.
- The pathological reaction depends on the balance between the mycobacterial antigen load and the host's tissue sensitivity as given in Table 18.12.

Terminologies

- Exposure: The child has a contact with an adult patient with TB but lacks evidence of infection. Skin test/IGRA is positive or negative.
- Infection: There are no signs or symptoms, physical examination is normal, TST or IGRA (Interferon-Ƴ Release Assay) result is positive, and CXR reveals only granuloma or calcifications in the lung parenchyma.
- Disease: Features of infection and clinical signs or symptoms are present.
- TB calendar (Wallgren calendar): The time interval between the infection and the clinical manifestations is variable and is given in Table 18.13.
- TB in children: It should be suspected in case of the following:
  - Persistent fever and/or cough for more than 2 weeks
  - Loss of weight (>5% highest recorded body weight in the last 3 months)/no weight gain
  - History of contact with infectious TB cases
- Presumptive extrapulmonary TB: It refers to the presence of organ-specific symptoms and signs (headache, neck stiffness, joint pain, constitutional symptoms such as fever and night sweats).
- History of contact and a positive contact
  - History of contact: In a symptomatic child, contact with any form of active TB within 2 years is considered as a positive contact history. In an asymptomatic child, contact with smear-positive TB is considered as a positive contact history.

TABLE 18.12	Relationship Between Antigen Load and Host's Tissue Sensitivity	
Antigen Load	Tissue Sensitivity	Reaction
Low	High	Localized granuloma
High	High	Caseous necrosis
High	Low	Caseous necrosis with dissemination

TABLE 18.13	Wallgren Calendar
Clinical Manifestation	Time Interval to Manifest After Acquisition of Infection
Miliary/meningeal	2–6 months
Nodal/endobronchial	3–9 months
Bone and joints	Many years

- Contact: It refers to any person who has been exposed to the index case. It is of two types:
  - Household contact: Any person who has shared the same enclosed living space as the index case during the 3 months before the beginning of the current treatment episode
  - Close contact: Any person who has shared the same enclosed space such as social gathering and workplace as the index case during the 3 months before the beginning of the current treatment episode

Investigations for TB in Children

Chest radiograph

Highly suggestive chest X-ray findings for TB are as follows:
- Miliary shadows
- Lymphadenopathy (hilar or mediastinal)
- Chronic fibrocavitary shadows
- Consolidations, inhomogenous shadows, or bronchopneumonia – nonspecific findings

Tuberculin skin test/mantoux/pirquet test

- A total of 2 TU (Tuberculin Units) of PPD is used.
- A total of 0.1 mL of 2 TU PPD (Purified Protein Derivative) is injected in the flexor aspect of the left forearm such that it produces a wheal of 6–10 mm.
- Sensitized T cells are recruited to the site of injection and produce erythema and induration.
- The test is read after 48–72 hours. However, it can be read as late as 7 days. If the patient reports after 7 days, the test is repeated in the opposite forearm.
  <6 mm: Negative
  6–9 mm: Doubtful
  ≥10 mm: Positive
  ≥20 mm: Strong positive
- Strong positives are at a higher risk of having active disease than positives. Similarly, patients with TST <6 mm are at a higher risk of having active disease than those with TST 6–9 mm.
- False negative: It occurs in case of measles, being immunocompromised, and malnutrition.
- False positive: It occurs in case of BCG vaccination and atypical mycobacterial infection.
- A patient can test positive during the beginning of the steroid treatment.
- 10% of immunocompetent children can have a negative result.
- Fifty per cent of patients with TB meningitis and those with disseminated TB have negative TST.
- Fifty per cent of infants who receive BCG vaccine never develop TST and reactivity usually wanes in 2–3 years.
- In older children and adults vaccinated with BCG, the reactivity is lost after 5–10 years.

Indications for TST (American Academy of Pediatrics (AAP), 2018)

- Can be performed as early as 3 months
- Contacts of people with confirmed or suspected contagious tuberculosis
- Children with radiographic or clinical findings suggesting tuberculosis disease
- Children immigrating from countries with endemic infection
- Children with travel histories to countries with endemic infection
- Children infected with HIV, who should have TST performed annually
- Children with comorbidities – diabetes, nephrotic syndrome, malignancies, autoimmune diseases (if history suggests possibility of exposure, then immediate and periodic TST should be considered)
- Should perform initial TST or IGRA before initiation of immunosuppressive therapy

Definition of a Positive TST

≥5 mm
- Children in close contact with known or suspected contagious people with tuberculosis disease
- Children with findings on chest radiograph consistent with active or previous tuberculosis disease
- Clinical evidence of tuberculosis disease
- Children receiving immunosuppressive therapy or with immunosuppressive conditions, including HIV infection

≥10 mm
- Children younger than 4 years
- Children with other medical conditions, including Hodgkin disease, lymphoma, diabetes mellitus, chronic renal failure, or malnutrition
- Children born in high-prevalence regions of the world
- Children often exposed to adults who are HIV infected, homeless, users of illicit drugs, residents of nursing homes, incarcerated or institutionalized, or migrant farm workers
- Children who travel to high-prevalence regions of the world

≥15 mm
Children ≥4 years of age without any risk factors
Fig. 18.4 shows a positive Mantoux test.

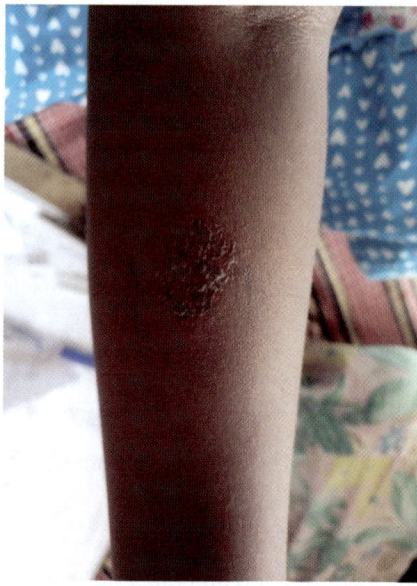

Fig. 18.4 Positive Mantoux test.

MICROBIOLOGICAL TESTS

Specimens for Pulmonary TB

Gastric Aspirate

It is the preferred specimen.

It needs overnight fasting, and requires hospitalization and skilled staff.

It should be collected after a minimum of 4–6 hours of fasting.

Induced Sputum

- The patient should be fasting for 2–3 hours prior to the collection procedure.
- Priming with salbutamol can be performed through either a metered dose inhaler (i.e., MDI) or nebulization with 5 mL of 3% sterile hypertonic saline.
- While the child is being nebulized, give a container to the child to collect any expectorated sputum.
- If the child is still unable to expectorate, sputum can be collected by suction through the nasopharynx or oropharynx.

Specimens for Extrapulmonary TB

The specimens include the following;
- Serous cavity fluids
- Tissue specimens
- CSF (Cerebrospinal Fluid)
- Synovial fluid

Smear Microscopy

- Needs 5000–10,000 bacilli/mL of sputum
- Ziehl−Neelsen method: Cost-effective
- Fluorescence microscopy: Lowers work effort
- LED (Light-Emitting Diode) microscopy

Culture

- Can detect as few as 10–100 viable AFB per milliliter of sputum

Solid Medium

- Löwenstein–Jensen is an egg-based medium. It contains egg albumin and malachite green.
- Middlebrook 7H10 medium is an agar-based medium. It contains bovine serum albumin and an antibiotic combination of polymyxin B, amphotericin B, nalidixic acid, trimethoprim, and azlocillin (PANTA) or polymyxin B, amphotericin B, carbenicillin, and trimethoprim (PACT). It takes 4–8 weeks to get visual colonies. It is used for primary isolation, antibiotic susceptibility studies, and differentiation of mycobacterial species.

Liquid Medium

- Contains 10% calf serum and an antibiotic combination (PACT)

BACTEC 460 System

- ^{14}C-labeled palmitic acid in 7H12 media is used.
- Mycobacteria metabolize the palmitic acid and $^{14}CO_2$ is released.
- The presence of free $^{14}CO_2$ in the vial is measured by the BACTEC system and is reported in terms of growth index.
- The use of radiolabeled carbon has led to its withdrawal by the manufacturers.

BACTEC MGIT 960 System

- It is the gold standard for the primary isolation as well as for the drug susceptibility testing.
- It is a fully automated, nonradiometric, and noninvasive system.
- A fluorescent compound embedded in silicon is at the bottom of each MGIT tube that is sensitive to oxygen. Mycobacteria consume oxygen and allow the compound to fluoresce. This change in fluorescence is detected by the system and is reported in terms of growth units.
- The BACTEC system can detect growth as early as in 1–3 weeks.

Thin Layer Agar (TLA) Method. The solid agar–based method allows the detection of mycobacteria within 9–14 days on the basis of its colony morphology. It is used for the detection of multi-drug-resistant TB (MDR-TB) directly from the specimens.

Genotypic Methods

Line Probe Assay (LPA). It allows the molecular identification of the *M. tuberculosis* complex and its associated genotypic susceptibilities to rifampicin and isoniazid.

GeneXpert

- It is a real-time PCR Xpert MTB assay (Xpert® MTB/RIF) for the detection of rifampicin-resistant *M. tuberculosis* exceptionally sensitive for the detection of *M. tuberculosis* even in smear-negative specimens.
- The result is made available in 2 hours.
- It can be used for both pulmonary and extrapulmonary specimens.
- The sensitivity of GeneXpert for extrapulmonary specimen is lymph node and CSF > pericardial, ascitic, and synovial fluid > pleural fluid.
- Negative GeneXpert does not rule out TB.

Interferon-Gamma Release Assays. These tests detect IFN-γ generation by the patient's T cells in response to specific *M. tuberculosis* antigens (ESAT-6, CFP-10, and TB7.7).

QuantiFERON-TB Test

- Measures whole blood concentrations of IFN-γ

T-SPOT.TB Test

- It measures the number of lymphocytes/monocytes producing IFN-γ. It is highly specific for *M. tuberculosis* because the antigens are not present on *M. bovis* and atypical mycobacteria. However, the test does not differentiate between infection and disease. Indeterminate results are obtained in children younger than 5 years and in those with immunosuppression.

Age of the Child and Test Preferred

- TST preferred in children younger than 5 years
- IGRA preferred in the following:
  - Children older than 5 years who have received the BCG vaccine
  - Children older than 5 years who are unlikely to return for TST reading

OTHER TESTS

USG

- Assesses pleural fluid collection

- Detects ascitis
- Differentiates between thymus and anterior mediastinal node
- USG-guided aspiration/biopsy

CT Scan

- CT patterns highly suggestive of TB: Mediastinal lymph-adenopathy and centrilobular nodules with tree-in-bud pattern and cavities with surrounding consolidations
- May also help in CT-guided biopsy

Case Definitions of TB

Case definitions are shown in Flowchart 18.1.
- Microbiologically confirmed TB: A patient in whom TB has been diagnosed by microbiological methods, such as smear and culture, or genotypic methods
- Clinically confirmed TB: A patient in whom microbiological methods were negative but TB has been diagnosed by clinical/radiological features or histopathology
- Anatomic classification – pulmonary and extrapulmonary (includes pleura also): A patient with both pulmonary and extrapulmonary TB classified as having pulmonary TB
- Classification on the basis of history of treatment
  Category 1: New case – a patient with confirmed TB who has not taken treatment or taken treatment for not more than 4 weeks
  Category 2: Any previously treated patient
   a. Relapse: A patient who has been treated for TB, declared cured, and now found to be a microbiologically confirmed TB
   b. Treatment after failure: A patient who has been previously treated for TB and whose treatment has failed at the end of most recent course of treatment
   c. Treatment after loss to follow-up: A patient who has been previously treated for TB for 1 month or more and declared lost to follow-up at the end of most recent course of treatment and now found to be microbiologically confirmed TB

Treatment of TB

ANTITUBERCULOUS DRUGS

Antituberculous drugs are given in Table 18.14.

NEWER ANTITUBERCULOUS DRUGS

Bedaquiline

- Is a diarylquinoline, and acts by inhibiting ATP (Adenosine Triphosphate) synthase
- Indication: For age >18 years
- Adverse effects: QT prolongation and hepatotoxicity
- Contraindications: Pregnancy and heart disease

Delamanid

- Is a nitroimidazole, and acts by inhibiting mycolic acid synthesis
- Indications: For MDR (Multiple Drug Resistance)-TB in age >6 years
- Dose: 50 mg b.i.d. (6–11 years) and 100 mg b.i.d. (12–17 years)
- Contraindications
  - Children younger than 6 years
  - Pregnancy and lactation
  - Prolonged QT interval

IAP RNTCP (2019) GUIDELINES FOR ATT

RNTCP (2019) guidelines for ATT are given in Table 18.15.

DOSE OF ANTITUBERCULOUS DRUGS

Dose of ATT is given in Table 18.16.

ROLE OF STEROIDS IN TB

The following are the indications for steroids in a patient with TB (TBM):
- Pericarditis

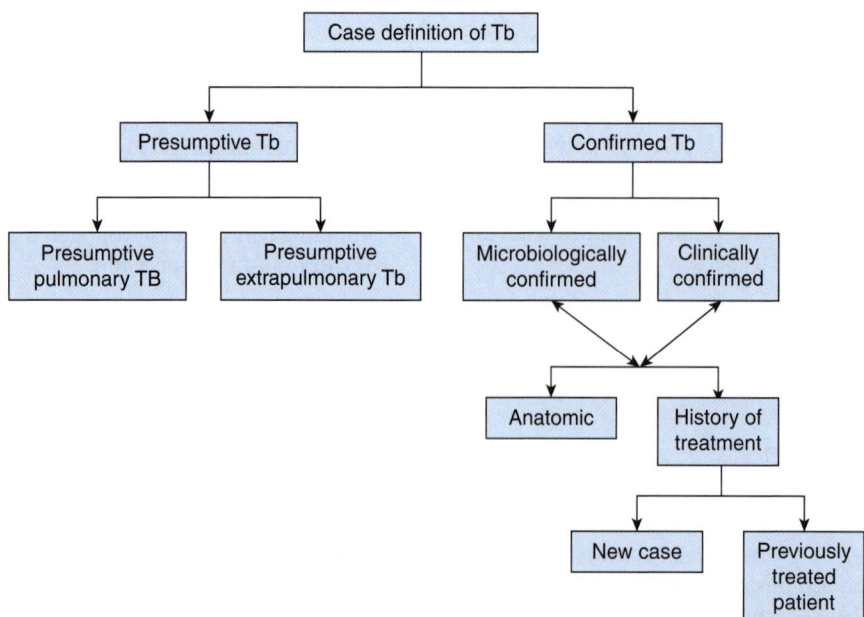

Flowchart 18.1   Case definitions of TB.

TABLE 18.14	Antituberculous Drugs	
Group	**Drugs**	
1. First-line oral drugs	INH (Isoniazid), rifampicin, ethambutol, pyrazinamide, rifampicin	
2. Injectable agents	Kanamycin, amikacin, capreomycin, streptomycin	
3. Fluoroquinolones	Moxifloxacin, levofloxacin, ofloxacin	
4. Oral bacteriostatic second-line agents	Ethionamide, prothionamide, cycloserine, PAS (Para-aminosalicylic Acid)	
5. Agents with unclear efficacy	Clofazimine, linezolid, amoxicillin/clavulanate, high-dose INH, clarithromycin	

TABLE 18.15	IAP RNTCP (2019) Guidelines for ATT	
Type of Patient		**Drug Regimen**
• New microbiologically confirmed pulmonary TB		2HRZE + 4HRE
• New clinically diagnosed pulmonary TB		
• New microbiologically confirmed extrapulmonary TB		
• New clinically diagnosed, rifampicin-sensitive extrapulmonary TB		
• ᵃDrug-sensitive, previously treated TB (recurrence, treatment after loss to follow-up, treatment after failure)		

ᵃThese children shall be evaluated as DR (Drug Resistant)-TB suspects. In case they are found to be drug sensitive, they shall be started on the above-mentioned regimen as for a new case. This group was earlier treated with CAT (Category) II regimen according to the older guidelines that are now withdrawn from RNTCP. For neuro and spinal TB, the continuation phase is extended to 8 months.

- Addison disease
- Miliary TB
- Endobronchial TB
- TB uveitis
- Abdominal TB (AAP, *Red Book*, 2018)
- Dose: Prednisolone 1–2 mg/kg/day or dexamethasone 0.6 mg/kg/day for 4 weeks and then tapered over next 4 weeks

MONITORING DURING TREATMENT

- All patients started on INH should be supplemented with 10 mg/day of pyridoxine to prevent peripheral neuropathy.
- Clinical monitoring: Follow-up should be performed every month during treatment and every 6 months up to 2 years after completion of treatment.
- During each follow-up, look for the following:
  - Improvement in clinical symptoms

TABLE 18.16	Dose of Antituberculous Drugs	
Drug		**Dose (mg/kg/day)**
Isoniazid (INH or H)		10
Rifampicin (R)		15
Pyrazinamide (Z)		20
Ethambutol (E)		20
Streptomycin (S)		35

- Physical examination
- Adverse effects of medications
- Treatment of comorbid conditions
- Laboratory monitoring
  - Microbiological: Tested at end of IP and end of treatment
  - MGIT (Mycobacteria Growth Indicator Tube) culture: Should be performed if the child is not responding even after 4 weeks of therapy
  - Follow-up chest radiographs: Should be performed only at the end of therapy or earlier if there is no response to therapy or if there is any deterioration

ADVERSE DRUG REACTIONS TO TB DRUGS

ATT-Induced Liver Injury

- Criteria: Defined by any one of the following.
  - In an asymptomatic patient, rise of ALT (Aanine Tansaminase)/AST (Aspartate Aminotransferase) >5 times the upper limit of normal levels
  - Rise of ALT/AST >3 times when the patient has nausea, vomiting, and diarrhea
  - Rise in level of serum total bilirubin above 1.5 mg/dL
  - **Risk factors for ATT-induced liver injury**
    - Malnutrition
    - Hypoalbuminemia
    - Infections – HIV, and hepatitis B and hepatitis C infections
    - Extensive TB disease
    - Slow acetylators of INH
  - **Management of ATT-induced liver injury**
    - Continue ATT in symptomatic patients with monitoring of symptoms and repeat enzymes after a week.
    - Stop ATT in all symptomatic patients.
    - Critically ill patients can be started on ethambutol, streptomycin, and levofloxacin.
    - Introduce primary drugs once the liver enzymes are <2 times ULN (Upper Limit of Normal).
    - Start with full dose of rifampicin and other drugs should be added every 3 days, with regular LFT monitoring.

Drug-Resistant TB

Terminologies used in drug-resistant TB are given in Table 18.17.

PRESUMPTIVE MDR-TB

Presumptive case of MDR-TB in children include the following:
- Children who are contacts of adults with MDR-TB/drug-resistant TB
- Those who are lost to follow-up after initiating treatment
- Those who present with recurrence of disease after previous treatment
- Those who do not respond to therapy with first-line drugs
- Those living with individuals with HIV

All patients with presumptive drug-resistant TB should undergo microbiological confirmation and drug susceptibility testing. If there is no microbiological confirmation, bacteriologically negative clinically diagnosed DR-TB can be considered after ruling out an alternative diagnosis.

TABLE 18.17	Terminologies in Drug-Resistant TB				
Monoresistant (MR) TB	**Polydrug-Resistant (PDR) TB**	**[a]Rifampicin Resistance (RR)**	**Multidrug-Resistant (MDR) TB**		**Extensive Drug Resistance**
Resistant to H/R/Z/E/S	Resistant to Z/E/S, except H and R	Resistant to R with/without resistance to H/Z/E/S	Resistant to both H and R with/without resistance to other first-line drugs Patients may also have additional resistance to any/all FQ (Fluoroquinolone) or any/all second-line injectable anti-TB drugs		MDR-TB + Resistance to all second-line injectable ATT + Any of the fluoroquinolones

[a]Isolated R resistance is very rare. Patients who are R resistant are also found to be H resistant. Therefore, R-resistant patients are treated as MDR-TB.

METHODS FOR DRUG SUSCEPTIBILITY TESTING

Molecular Methods

These are the first-choice method of testing:
CBNAAT (Cartridge- Based Nucleic Acid Amplification Test): Detects TB and resistance to R
Line probe assay (LPA): Detects MTB complex, resistance to first-line drugs R and H, fluoroquinolones, and injectable drugs

Growth-Based Phenotypic Drug Susceptibility Testing

- Includes liquid and solid media.
- Mycobacteria growth indicator tube (MGIT) – the commonest system used
- Requires 2–8 weeks to yield results
- Will be used for long-term follow-up of patients on DR-TB treatment and better yield in tuberculous meningitis.
- Additionally detects resistance to linezolid, clofazimine, bedaquiline, and delamanid

TREATMENT REGIMENS FOR DRUG-RESISTANT TB

Table 18.18 gives regimens for drug-resistant TB.
Total period of treatment for Multi-Drug Resistant TB is 18 months. Some examiners can ask about TB drug groups which is as follows:
- Group 1: First line oral anti-tuberculosis agents (H- Isoniazid, R- Rifampicin, E- Ethambutol, Z- Pyrazinamide, Rfb-Rifabutin)
- Group 2: Injectable agents (Km-kanamycin, Am-Amikacin, Cm-Capreomycin, S-Streptomycin)
- Group 3: Fluoroquinolones (Lfx-Levofloxacin, Mfx-Moxifloxacin, Ofx-Ofloxacin)
- Group 4: Oral bacteriostatic second line agents (PAS-Para aminosalicylic acid, Cs-Cycloserine, Eto-Ethionamide, Cfz-Clofazimine)
- Group 5: Agent with unclear role in drug-resistant TB (Lzd-Linezolid, Amx/clv-Amoxyclavulanate, Clr-Clarithromycin, High dose Isoniazid, Imp/Cls Imepinem/Cilastin).

PRETREATMENT EVALUATION FOR PATIENTS WITH DR-TB

- Detailed history including screening for mental illness, seizure disorder, and drugs/alcohol abuse
- Weight
- Height

TABLE 18.18	Regimens for Drug-Resistant TB	
Type of Drug Resistance		**Regimen**
Monodrug-resistant TB (H resistance with/without resistance to other first-line drugs apart from R)		6Lfx REZ uniphasic regimen
R resistance/MDR-TB (conventional shorter regimen)		Intensive phase: 4–6 Mfx Km Eto Cfz Z H E Continuation phase: 5Mfx Cfz Z E
MDR-TB		6–9 Km Lfx EtoCs Z E 12–18 Lfx Eto Cs E
[a]XDR-TB		6–8 dlm(bdq) 6 Lf(Mfx) Lzd Cfz Cs 12 Lf(Mfx) Lzd Cfz Cs

Lfx- Levofloxacin, H- Isoniazid, R- Rifampicin, E- Ethionamide, Z- Pyrazinamide, Mfx- Moxifloxacin, Km- kanamycin, Eto- Ethionamide, Cs- Cycloserine, Cfz- Clofazimine, DLM-Delamanid, BDQ- Bedaquiline, LZD-Linezolid
MDR, multidrug resistant.
[a]Not for children younger than 6 years. Bdq should be replaced by Dlm between 6 and 12 years. This is not for EPTB (Extra-pulmonary Tuberculosis) other than lymph node or pleural effusion.

- CBC with platelets counts
- Blood sugar to screen for Diabetes mellitus
- LFT
- RFT (blood urea, serum creatinine)
- TSH and other thyroid functioning tests
- Urine examination: Routine and microscopic
- Chest X-ray
- ECG (Electrocardiogram)
- Serum electrolytes

TB With HIV Coinfection

SPECIAL CONSIDERATIONS

- The clinical symptoms of HIV and TB can overlap, making early identification difficult.
- Sputum has poor sensitivity in detecting TB in patients with HIV because the organism count in sputum is low.
- Patients with TB–HIV coinfection can have a normal chest radiograph.
- The sensitivity of IGRA and TST is low.
- TST of >5 mm is considered positive and patients need annual TST.
- The likelihood of having extrapulmonary TB is higher.
- Severity and rate of progression of TB is high.

TABLE 18.19	Management of TB–HIV Coinfections
Patient Category	**Timing of ATT and ART**
TB–HIV coinfection with CD4 count >50/mm³	• Start ATT first • Initiate ART after 2–12 weeks if ATT is tolerated
TB–HIV coinfection with CD4 count <50/mm³	• Start ATT first and initiate ART within 2 weeks with clinical monitoring

- The rate of drug resistance is higher in patients with HIV.
- Mortality from TB is high among patients with HIV.
- CBNAAT is the frontline test for the diagnosis of TB in children with HIV.
- Management of TB–HIV coinfections is given in Table 18.19:

  Rifampicin is a potent enzyme inducer and thus reduces the therapeutic levels of protease inhibitors, so children younger than 3 years can be superboosted with lopinavir/ritonavir and those older than 3 years can be started on efavirenz.

MONITORING DURING TREATMENT

- HIV-infected children on ATT: LFTs are administered at baseline, day 15, month 1, and month 3. After 3 months, a symptom-directed approach is useful.
- If symptoms of drug toxicity develop, a physical examination and liver enzyme measurement should be repeated.
- Guidelines for ATT-induced liver disease remain the same.

IMMUNE RECONSTITUTION INFLAMMATORY SYNDROME (IRIS)

IRIS and Its Types

IRIS is of two types as given in Table 18.20.

Diagnostic Criteria for IRIS

The onset of TB-associated IRIS should be within 3 months of starting ART (Anti-retroviral Therapy).
Diagnosis is made with one major and two minor criteria. Table 18.21 gives the diagnostic criteria for IRIS.

Treatment for IRIS

- Mild IRIS: Symptomatic treatment

TABLE 18.20	Immune Reconstitution Inflammatory Syndrome (IRIS)
Paradoxical IRIS	**Unmasking IRIS**
A diagnosis of TB is already made ATT is started A good initial response to TB therapy is observed before the patient started on ART	Diagnosis of TB was not made After ART is initiated, a good initial response is seen Then the TB manifestations become manifest

TABLE 18.21	Diagnostic Criteria for IRIS
Major Criteria	**Minor Criteria**
• New/enlarging lymph nodes or other focal tissue enlargement • New/worsening radiological features • New/worsening CNS tuberculosis • New/worsening serositis	• New/worsening constitutional symptoms such as fever • New/worsening respiratory symptoms such as cough • New/worsening abdominal pain

- Moderate to severe IRIS: Oral prednisolone 1–2 mg/kg for 1–2 weeks followed by gradual taper

INH Preventive Therapy

DOSE OF INH PROPHYLAXIS

- 10 mg/kg/day for 6 months Pyridoxine at a dose of 10-50mg/day for 6 months to prevent drug-induced neuritis.

INDICATIONS FOR INH PREVENTIVE THERAPY

- All asymptomatic contacts (younger than 6 years) of a smear-positive case after ruling out active TB disease and irrespective of BCG vaccination
- All HIV-infected children who had a known exposure to an infectious TB case or are tuberculin skin test (TST) positive (≥5 mm induration) but have no active TB disease
- All TST-positive children who are receiving immunosuppressive therapy
- A child born to mother who was diagnosed to have TB in pregnancy should receive prophylaxis for 6 months, provided congenital TB has been ruled out; BCG vaccination can be given at birth even if INH preventive therapy is planned

MANAGEMENT OF INTERRUPTION OF INH PROPHYLAXIS

Management of interruption of INH prophylaxis is given in Table 18.22.

Management of a Neonate Exposed to Tuberculosis (AAP, *Red Book*, 2018)

Table 18.23 gives the management of a neonate exposed to tuberculosis.

TABLE 18.22	Management of Interruption of INH Prophylaxis		
Duration of Treatment (months)	**Duration of Discontinuation (months)**	**Management**	
<1	<1	Restart the regimen	
>1	<1	Continue the regimen	
>1	1–3	Restart the regimen	
>1	>3	Do not reinitiate the prophylaxis	

TABLE 18.23	Management of a Neonate Exposed to Tuberculosis		
Management	**Mother (or Household Contact) Has Evidence of TB Infection and a Normal Chest Radiograph**	**Mother (or Household Contact) Has a Positive TST or IGRA and Abnormal Findings on Chest Radiography But No Evidence of TB Disease**	**Mother (or Household Contact) Has Clinical Signs and Symptoms and/or Abnormal Findings on Chest Radiograph Consistent With TB Disease**
Separation of the newborn from the mother	Not needed	Not needed	Infant should be separated: • Until the mother and the infant are started on appropriate anti-TB therapy • If the mother is having poor adherence to therapy • If the mother is found to have MDR-TB
Management of the infant	No therapy for infant	No therapy Regular follow-up	Evaluate the infant for congenital TB If there is no evidence of congenital TB, the infant should be started on INH prophylaxis
Management for the mother	Mother to be treated for TB infection Household members should have TST or IGRA	Mother to be treated for TB infection Household members should have TST or IGRA	TB workup HIV screening Start anti-TB therapy Screen the household members

MDR, multidrug resistant.

Quick Bites

- TB effusions are rare in a child younger than 2 years.
- The child is nontoxic in TB effusion and high-grade fever is rare.
- In children younger than 1 year, empyema is common; and in children older than 1 year, effusion secondary to bacterial infection is common.
- Most parapneumonic effusions are preceded by viral respiratory tract illness.
- Ascites + pedal edema + pleural effusion: CCF, DCLD, nephrotic syndrome, and malnutrition.
- The trachea can be in the midline in a child with loculated effusion and bilateral pleural effusion.
- The role of USG chest in a patient with pleural effusion is diagnosing loculated effusion and thoracocentesis.
- CT has a very limited role in effusion. It may be used in complicated cases where routine management fails, prior to the surgery for delineating the exact anatomy of defect, and to look for intrapulmonary abscess.
- All cases of empyema need intercostal tube drainage.
- Multiloculated effusions need open drainage and decortication.

Chronic Suppurative Lung Disease

Following introduction, seek permission from the caregiver and introduce yourself to the patient before history elicitation, and identify the case.

Name____Age____Sex____Consanguinity____Order of birth____Place____Informant____

Presenting Complaints and Duration

- Recurrent episodes of fever/cough/sputum/hemoptysis/breathlessness

History of Presenting Illness

- Age of onset of the initial episode mentioned
- How the initial episode started
- Severity of the initial episode (associated with altered sensorium, inability to feed)
- Any treatment given
- Oxygen requirement, nebulization, i.v. antibiotics, ATT (Anti-tuberculosis Therapy), and any bronchoscopy procedures performed
- Number of episodes per year
- Interval between each episode
- Whether the subsequent episodes are of increasing severity/occurring at frequent intervals
- Whether the child is responding to the same line of treatment for each episode/requiring longer duration of treatment
- Then the current episode mentioned

COMPLICATIONS HISTORY

- Apneic episodes during sleep/frequent awakenings from sleep
- Breathlessness/abdominal distension/pedal edema
- Fever with chills/cough with sputum

ETIOLOGICAL HISTORY

- Aspiration after feeding
- Noisy breathing
- Recurrent ENT infections
- Passing oily stools
- Failure to gain weight
- Exposure to passive smoking
- Pedal edema/abdominal distension

ANTENATAL HISTORY

- HIV/TB in mother

POSTNATAL HISTORY

- Delayed passage of meconium
- Neonatal jaundice
- Delayed umbilical cord fall
- Neonatal respiratory distress
- Neonatal rhinitis

DEVELOPMENT HISTORY

Age-appropriate milestones

DIETETIC HISTORY

According to 24-hour recall method and any caloric deficit (suggestive of malnourishment)

IMMUNIZATION HISTORY

- Mention whether any additional vaccines were given apart from those in the National Immunization Schedule.

CONTACT HISTORY

Any history of contact with TB

ALLERGY HISTORY

If significant

FAMILY HISTORY

Similar illness in family members

SOCIOECONOMIC HISTORY

Overcrowding and hygiene/passive smoking/poor ventilation

Summary

A _____-year-old child presented with recurrent respiratory tract infections with/without sputum, with/without hemoptysis since_____ years of age, with/without complications, and with/without history of contact with TB, probably a case of chronic suppurative lung disease.

General Examination

- Patient's sensorium/posture
- Any oxygen support
- Pallor
- Icterus
- Cyanosis
- Clubbing
- Pedal edema
- Generalized lymphadenopathy

Head-to-Foot Examination

- Alopecia
- Ocular telangiectasia
- Oculocutaneous albinism
- Nasal polyps
- Vitiligo

- Oral cavity: Oral ulcers, presence of tonsils, oral candidiasis, and cleft palate
- Skin: Eczema, abscess, and cutaneous granulomas
- Yellow nails and lymphedema
- Markers of TB
- Signs of malnutrition

Vital Signs

- Temperature
- Pulse rate
- Respiration: Rate, rhythm, and type of respiration
- BP
- JVP

Anthropometry

Wasting
Stunting
Macrocephaly

Respiratory System Examination

- Upper respiratory tract
- Lower respiratory tract

INSPECTION

- Tracheal position
- Apical impulse
- Chest shape and symmetry
- Kyphosis
- Scoliosis
- Gibbus
- Scars
- Chest movements
- Intercostal fullness
- Empyema thoracis

PALPATION

- Tracheal position
- Apical impulse
- Tenderness
- Vocal fremitus (vocal fremitus may be normal or increased in the areas shown in Table 19.1)
- Chest movements
- Chest measurements

PERCUSSION

- May note resonance or dullness in the areas discussed in Table 19.1

TABLE 19.1	Areas to Be Examined for Vocal Fremitus	
Areas	**Right**	**Left**
Supraclavicular		
Clavicular		
Infraclavicular		
Mammary		
Inframammary		
Axillary		
Infra-axillary		
Suprascapular		
Upper interscapular		
Lower interscapular		
Infrascapular		

- Tidal percussion
- Traube's space percussion

AUSCULTATION

- Normal vesicular breath sounds
- Bronchial breath sounds
- Air entry in both the lungs
- Vocal resonance (vocal resonance may be normal or increased in the areas discussed in Table 19.1)
- Added sounds: Coarse crackles

Other System Examination

CARDIOVASCULAR SYSTEM

Dextrocardia, S1, S2, and murmurs

ABDOMEN

Features of DCLD (Decompensated Chronic Liver Disease) and hepatosplenomegaly

CENTRAL NERVOUS SYSTEM

- Features of hydrocephalus and neuromuscular disorders

Diagnosis

- A case of chronic suppurative lung disease
- Bronchiectasis of _____ lung
- Probable etiology
- With/without complications

Frequently Asked Questions

1. What is the significance of age in a patient with chronic suppurative lung disease?
   A. Conditions presenting in the neonatal period: Primary ciliary dyskinesia and primary immunodeficiency disorders (except B-cell deficiency)
   B. Presentation of B-cell deficiency after 6 months (because maternal antibodies are protective in the first 6 months)
   C. Cystic fibrosis: Has a varied presentation
   D. In infancy: Infections
   E. In childhood: Allergic bronchopulmonary aspergillosis (ABPA), sinusitis, and nasal polyps
   F. Adulthood: ABPA, sinusitis, nasal polyps, and respiratory failure
2. What is the significance of gender?
   X-linked agammaglobulinemia and IPEX (Immune Dysregulation, Polyendocrinopathy, Enteropathy, X-linked) – males
3. List the histories to be elicited when a child presents with sputum.
   - Duration – for how many days
   - Quantity – massive sputum production seen in bronchiectasis, lung abscess, empyema rupturing into the bronchus, and necrotizing pneumonia
   - Color
     - Green: Acute bacterial infections
     - Rusty sputum: Pneumococcal pneumonia
     - Red currant jelly: *Klebsiella pneumoniae*
     - Pink frothy sputum: pulmonary edema
   - Diurnal variation (in chronic bronchitis, sputum production is more in the early morning)
   - Postural variation (in bronchiectasis and lung abscess, sputum production is more when the patient lies on the healthy side)
   - Aggravating/relieving factors
*4. Define hemoptysis and enumerate the causes of hemoptysis in children.
   - It is defined as coughing out of blood, or bloody sputum.
   - Spurious hemoptysis occurs because of bleeding from the upper respiratory tract.
   - Massive hemoptysis is defined as hemoptysis of quantity >250 mL in 24-hour period (Nelson) and >300 ml in 24 hour period-AAP, *Pediatric Pulmonology*, 2011).
   The causes of hemoptysis are listed in Table 19.2.
5. Differentiate between hemoptysis and hematemesis.
   The differences between hemoptysis and hematemesis are listed in Table 19.3.
6. Enumerate the histories for complications to be elicited in chronic suppurative lung disease.
   - Sleep-disordered breathing: History of apneic episodes during sleep/frequent awakenings from sleep
   - Right heart failure: History of breathlessness/abdominal distension/pedal edema
   - Lung abscess: History of fever with chills/cough with sputum

---

*Important question asked in the examination.

TABLE 19.2	Causes of Hemoptysis	
Focal Lesions		**Diffuse Lesions**
Infections		Acute idiopathic pulmonary hemorrhage of infancy
Bronchiectasis		
Trauma		Congenital heart diseases (resulting in pulmonary hypertension)
Foreign body		
Pulmonary AV (Arteriovenous) malformations		Connective tissue disorders
		Coagulopathy
Pulmonary embolism		Celiac disease
Hemangiomas		Neoplasms

TABLE 19.3	Differences Between Hemoptysis and Hematemesis	
Hemoptysis		**Hematemesis**
• Bright red in color		• Dark red/coffee-colored
• Followed by cough		• Followed by nausea and vomiting
• Frothy, may contain sputum		
• Alkaline		• May contain food particles
• Melena absent		• Acidic
		• Melena present

7. Enumerate the etiological histories in chronic suppurative lung disease.
   - Tracheoesophageal fistula: Aspiration after feeding
   - Airway anomalies, neurogenic stridor, and foreign body: Noisy breathing
   - Neuromuscular incoordination and GERD (Gastroesophageal Reflux Disease): Recurrent aspiration
   - Immunodeficiency disorders: Recurrent ENT infections (otitis media, sinusitis, rhinitis) and skin infections/recurrent diarrhea
   - Cystic fibrosis: Passing oily stools
   - Malnutrition: Failure to gain weight
   - Airway injury: Exposure to passive smoking
   - To rule out cardiac cause of recurrent respiratory tract infections: Any pedal edema/abdominal distension
8. What is the significance of postnatal history?
   Cystic fibrosis: Delayed passage of meconium/neonatal jaundice
   Leukocyte adhesion deficiency: Delayed umbilical cord fall
   Primary ciliary dyskinesia: Neonatal respiratory distress/neonatal rhinitis
9. What is the significance of immunization history?
   - BCG (Bacille Calmette Guerin) is contraindicated in T-cell deficiency and HIV.
   - All live vaccines are contraindicated in B-cell and T-cell defects.
   - In agammaglobulinemia, pertussis and influenza vaccine can be given.
   - In phagocytic defects, all live bacterial vaccines are contraindicated, and all live viral vaccines can be given.
   - In complement defects, all live vaccines can be given.
10. What is the significance of family history?
    Similar illness in family members: Primary immunodeficiency disorders and cystic fibrosis

11. List the findings to be looked for in general examination and head-to-foot examination.
    General examination
       The significance of general examination findings is shown in Table 19.4.
    Findings in head-to-foot examination
    - Markers of TB (phlycten, tinea versicolor, lupus vulgaris, scrofuloderma, scrofula, erythema nodosum, tuberculosis verrucosa cutis, lichen scrofulosorum, papulonecrotic tuberculid)
    - Signs of malnutrition
    - Retinitis pigmentosa: Primary ciliary dyskinesia
    - Nasal polyps: CF
    - Yellow nails and lymphedema: Yellow nail syndrome
    - Signs of primary immunodeficiency disorders
    - Vitiligo and alopecia: B-cell defects and chronic mucocutaneous candidiasis
    - Ocular telangiectasia: Ataxia telangiectasia
    - Oculocutaneous albinism: Chédiak–Higashi syndrome
    - Oral ulcers: HIV and chronic granulomatous disease
    - Presence of tonsils (rules out X-linked agammaglobulinemia)
    - Oral candidiasis
    - Cleft palate (DiGeorge syndrome)
    - Eczema: Wiskott–Aldrich syndrome
    - Skin abscess: Chronic granulomatous disease, leukocyte adhesion deficiency, and hyper-IgE syndrome
    - Cutaneous granulomas: Chronic granulomatous disease and severe combined immunodeficiency disorder

12. What is the significance of vital signs?
    - Pulse: Bounding pulse because of anemia, CO_2 retention, and DCLD
    - BP: Wide pulse pressure in anemia, CO_2 retention, and DCLD
    - Respiration: Occurrence of tachypnea in acute exacerbation of bronchiectasis

    - Fever: Suggestive of infection
    - JVP: Elevated in right heart failure

13. List the findings in the upper respiratory tract.
    Upper respiratory tract: Look for otitis, sinusitis, rhinitis, nasal septal deviation, and polyps.

14. List the findings in the respiratory system specific for bronchiectasis.
    - Trachea: Midline
    - Chest wall movements: Reduced
    - Vocal fremitus: Normal or increased (if there is consolidation)
    - Percussion: Resonant or dull (if there is consolidation)
    - Air entry: Equal
    - Bronchial sounds: Tubular (if there is consolidation)
    - Vocal resonance: Normal or increased (if there is consolidation)
    - Added sounds: Coarse crackles

15. What is the significance of cardiovascular system examination in chronic suppurative lung disease?
    Congenital heart disease in TOF, truncus arteriosus in Di George syndrome, dextrocardia in Kartagener syndrome, and cor pulmonale

16. What is the significance of examination of the gastrointestinal system in chronic suppurative lung disease?
    - Ascites (cor pulmonale, DCLD secondary to CF) and HSM (immunodeficiency disorders)
    - Situs inversus (Kartagener syndrome)

17. What is the significance of CNS examination in chronic suppurative lung disease?
    Hydrocephalus (primary ciliary dyskinesia) and neuromuscular disorders (cause recurrent aspiration)

18. Define bronchiectasis (Robbins).
    Bronchiectasis is the permanent dilatation of bronchi and bronchioles caused by the destruction of smooth muscles and the supporting elastic tissue. It typically results from or is associated with chronic necrotizing infections. The two important predisposing factors needed for the bronchiectasis to develop are obstruction of airway and infection.

19. Classify bronchiectasis.
    The classification of bronchiectasis is shown in Table 19.5.

TABLE 19.4	Significance of General Examination Findings in a Patient With Bronchiectasis
Clinical Finding	**Significance**
Patient's sensorium	Altered sensorium in hypoxia, metastatic abscess, TB meningitis
Posture	In unilateral bronchiectasis, the patient prefers to lie on the affected side
Oxygen support	Need for oxygen support can signify hypoxia
Pallor	Can be because of hemoptysis/malnutrition/hemolytic anemia in T-cell and B-cell defects, ALPS – autoimmune lymphoproliferative disorders
Cyanosis	Respiratory failure
Icterus	Secondary to hemolytic anemia in *Mycoplasma* and SLE (Systemic Lupus Erythematosus), DCLD presenting with ascites
Clubbing	Bronchiectasis, CF (Cystic Fibrosis)
Generalized lymphadenopathy	TB, HIV, lymphomas occurring in CVID (Common Variable Immunodeficiency), ALPS (Autoimmune Lymphoproliferative Syndrome)
Pedal edema	Cor pulmonale, DCLD (secondary to cystic fibrosis)

TABLE 19.5	Classification of Bronchiectasis		
On the Basis of the Extent of Lung Involved	**On the Basis of the Pathology**	**Clinical Classification**	
a. Focal: Because of localized obstruction (FB, lymph node, tumor) b. Diffuse: Cystic fibrosis, primary ciliary dyskinesia, immunodeficiency, autoimmune diseases	a. Cylindrical b. Saccular – most severe form c. Varicose	**Prebronchiectasis:** Recurrent endobronchial infection, nonspecific HRCT (High Resolution Computed Tomography) changes, reversible **HRCT bronchiectasis:** Clinical symptoms with HRCT evidence of bronchiectasis, may resolve, progress **Established bronchiectasis:** Irreversible	

*20. What are the syndromes associated with bronchiectasis?
The syndromes associated with bronchiectasis are shown in Table 19.6.

21. List the investigations to be performed in a child with bronchiectasis.
   • CBC
      a. Raised TLC (Total Leucocyte Count): Suggestive of infection
      b. Neutrophilia in the range of 30,000–100,000: Suggestive of leukocyte adhesion deficiency
      c. Lymphopenia: T-cell deficiency
      d. Lymphocytosis: TB
      e. Anemia: Can be because of hemoptysis/malnutrition/hemolytic anemia in T-cell and B-cell defects, and ALPS – autoimmune lymphoproliferative disorders
      f. Thrombocytopenia: Wiskott–Aldrich syndrome
   • LFT (Liver Function Test) – features of DCLD (because of cystic fibrosis)
   • Chest X-ray
   • HRCT
   • Flexible bronchoscopy
   • Etiological workup

22. List the findings that are seen in a chest X-ray and HRCT in a patient with bronchiectasis.
The radiological findings in bronchiectasis are listed in Table 19.7.

23. What is the etiological workup to be performed in a patient with bronchiectasis?

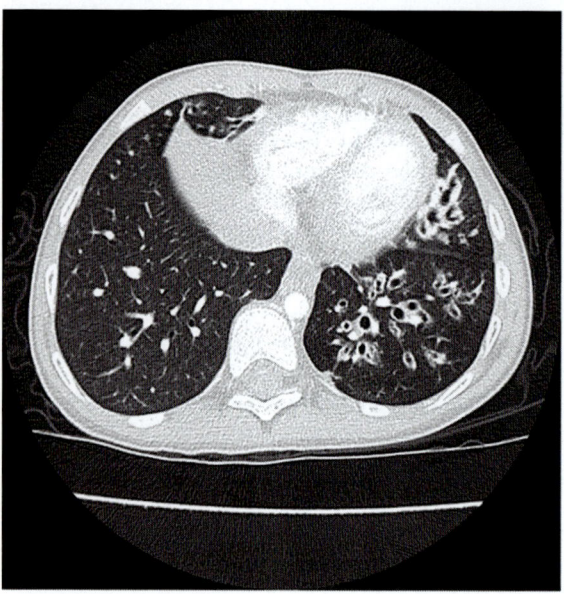

Fig. 19.1 CT chest showing signet ring sign. (Source: Reproduced from Sam Janes. *Encyclopedia of Respiratory Medicine*, Second Edition, Bronchiectasis in Childhood (Including PBB), Fig. 3, Oxford, Academic Press, 2022.)

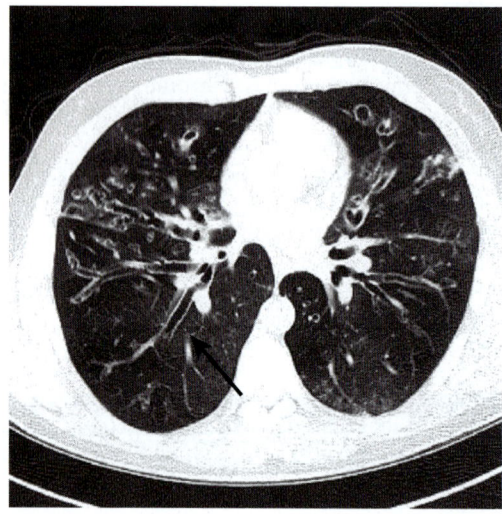

Fig. 19.2 CT chest showing tram-track sign. (*Source: https://www.researchgate.net/figure/Tram-track-sign-seen-in-cylindrical-bronchiectasis-on-the-chest-CT-scan-in-a-patient_fig13_313820333.*)

   a. TB workup
   b. Retroviral workup
   c. Investigations for primary immunodeficiency disorders
   d. Sweat chloride test and DNA analysis for cystic fibrosis
   e. Ciliary biopsy and DNA analysis for primary ciliary dyskinesia
   f. Flexible bronchoscopy – to rule out foreign body obstruction and airway abnormalities (bronchoscopy also allows collection of bronchoalveolar lavage [BAL] fluid, which can be subject to microbiological analysis)

24. What are the diagnostic criteria for acute exacerbations of bronchiectasis?
Defined by two major or one major + two minor or one major + one laboratory diagnostic criteria for bronchiectasis, as shown in Table 19.8

TABLE 19.6   Syndromes Associated With Bronchiectasis

Syndrome	Manifestations
Mounier-Kuhn syndrome	Tracheobronchomegaly
Williams–Campbell syndrome	Esophagobronchomalacia
Yellow nail syndrome	Yellow nail, pleural effusion, lymphedema
Right middle lobe syndrome	Extrinsic compression of right middle lobe bronchus by lymph nodes
Kartagener syndrome	Situs inversus, chronic sinusitis, bronchiectasis, azoospermia

TABLE 19.7   Radiological Findings in Bronchiectasis

Chest X-Ray	HRCT
Increased interstitial markings	Airway lumen greater than adjacent blood vessel ("signet ring sign") as shown in Fig. 19.1
Thickened airway walls	Tram-track markings as shown in Fig. 19.2
Dilated airway lumen	Extension of airway markings to the periphery
Hyperinflation	Lack of tapering of airways toward the periphery
Consolidation	Mucus plugging and centrilobular opacities ("tree in bud") as shown in Fig 19.3.
Lung abscess	The mosaic pattern of perfusion
	Beaded contour (String of pearls) appearance depicting alternating areas of dilatation and constriction.

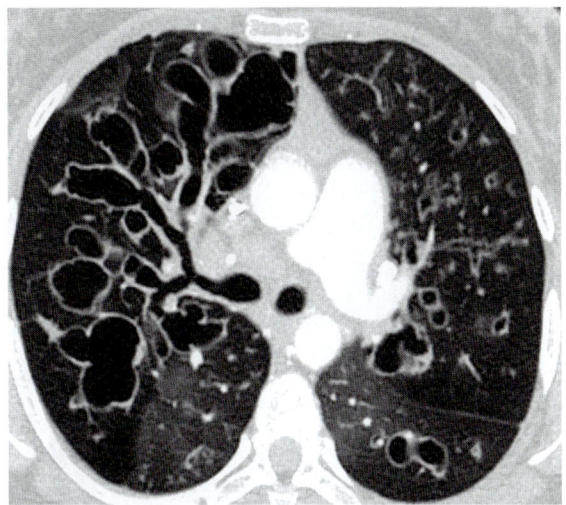

Fig. 19.3 CT chest showing tree in bud appearance (centrilobular nodules, peripheral airway mucus plugging and bronchial wall thickening). (*Source: Reproduced from Lane Donnelly.* Fundamentals of Pediatric Imaging, *Third Edition, Chest, Figure 3-37, Chennai, Academic Press, 2022.*)

TABLE 19.9 Stages of Pneumonia		
Stages	**Clinical Findings**	**Pathological Findings**
1. Stage of congestion	Fine/scattered crackles (indux crackles), decreased breath sounds	Heavy, red, boggy because of increased vascularity
2. Stage of red hepatization	Tubular type of bronchial breath sound	Liver-like consistency
3. Stage of gray hepatization	Tubular type of bronchial breath sound	Lung: Dry/gray RBC (Red Blood Cells) lysis (fibrinosuppurative exudates)
4. Stage of resolution	Coarse crackles (redux crackles)	Exudates in alveoli (thickening/adhesions)

TABLE 19.8 Diagnostic Criteria for Bronchiectasis		
Major Criteria	**Minor Criteria**	**Laboratory Criteria**
Wet cough >72 h or cough worsening over 72-h period	Change in sputum color, chest pain, breathlessness, crackles, wheeze	CRP (C-reactive Protein) >3 mg/dL IL-6 (Interleukin-6) >2 ng/L SAAP (Serum Amyloid A Protein) >5 mg/L Elevated neutrophil count

25. What is the treatment for bronchiectasis?
    - General management
        - Diet: High-calorie diet, with supplementation of fat-soluble vitamins, MCT (Medium Chain Triglyceride) oil, and adequate oral hydration (for patients with cystic fibrosis)
        - Vaccination
    - Specific management
        - Treatment of acute exacerbations with i.v. antibiotics
        - Mucolytics: Human recombinant DNAse 2.5 mg daily, *N*-acetylcysteine, and hypertonic saline
        - Chest physiotherapy
        - Bronchodilators
        - Treatment of underlying disorders
        - Surgery: Segmental or lobar resection for cases refractory to above-mentioned therapy
        Lung transplantation
26. Define pneumonia.
    - Inflammation of the lung parenchyma is called pneumonitis.
    - Pneumonia is the inflammation secondary to an infection.
27. What are the stages of pneumonia?
    The stages of pneumonia are listed in Table 19.9.

*28. What are the various classifications of pneumonia?
    A. Anatomical
        - The anatomical classification of pneumonia is listed in Table 19.10.
    B. On the basis of the duration of symptoms
        - The classification of pneumonia on the basis of the duration of symptoms is listed in Table 19.11.
    C. On the basis of the site of acquisition of infection
        - The classification of pneumonia on the basis of the site of acquisition of infection is listed in Table 19.12.
    D. **On the basis of the etiology**
        - The classification of pneumonia on the basis of the etiology is listed in Table 19.13.
    E. **Clinical classification**
        - The clinical classification of pneumonia is listed in Table 19.14.
29. Enumerate the antimicrobial treatment in pneumonia.
    - Antimicrobial treatment in pneumonia – WHO (World Health Organisation) (Table 19.15)
    - Updates in antimicrobial therapy for pneumonia (Nelson) as shown in Table 19.16
        Source: Nelson's textbook of pediatric antimicrobial therapy, 2019
30. What segments are commonly involved in a child with aspiration?
    - In recumbent position: Both the upper lobes and the apical segment of the right lower lobe
    - In erect position: Posterior segment of both the upper lobes

TABLE 19.10 Anatomical Classification of Pneumonia		
Lobar Pneumonia	**Bronchopneumonia**	**Interstitial Pneumonia**
Replacement of alveoli with exudates as shown in Fig. 19.4	Spreading inflammation along bronchial walls as shown in Fig. 19.5	Proliferation and desquamation of alveolar cells and thickening of alveolar walls as shown in Fig. 19.6

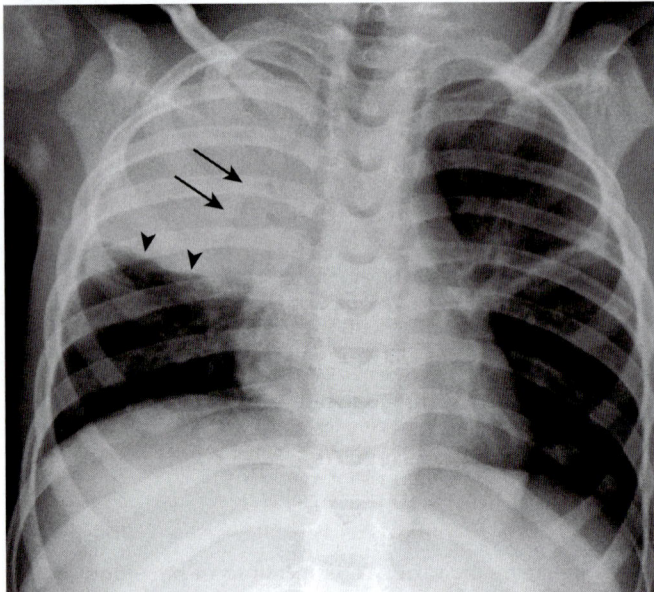

Fig. 19.4 Right upper lobe pneumonia with inferior bulging of the minor fissure (arrowheads) and air bronchograms (arrows). *(Source: Reproduced from Keith Kleinman, Lauren McDaniel, Matthew Molloy. The Harriet Lane Handbook, Twenty Second Edition, Radiology, FIGURE EC 26.F, Philadelphia, Elsevier Inc., 2021.)*

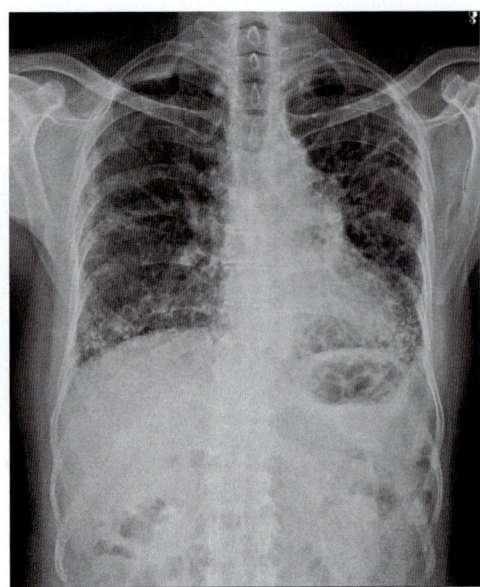

Fig. 19.6 Interstitial pneumonia – reticular and linear pulmonary opacification seen in peripheral subpleural region predominantly in the basal region suggestive of interstitial pneumonia. *(Source: https://radiopaedia.org/cases/usual-interstitial-pneumonia-7?lang=gb.)*

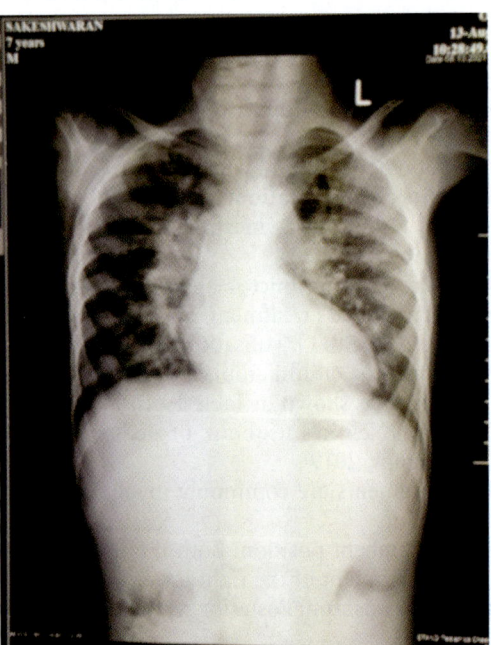

Fig. 19.5 Bronchopneumonia.

TABLE 19.11	Classification of Pneumonia on the Basis of Duration of Symptoms
Recurrent Pneumonia	**Persistent Pneumonia**
Two or more episodes in 12-month duration or three or more in a lifetime with radiological clearance in between	Defined as persistence of symptoms and radiographic abnormalities in a child with LRTI (Lower Respiratory Tract Infection) for >1 month despite antibiotic therapy for at least 10 days (*Indian Journal of Paediatrics*, 2009) (some authors use 3-month duration)

TABLE 19.12	Classification of Pneumonia on the Basis of the Site of Acquisition of Infection
Community Acquired	**Hospital Acquired**
Defined as pneumonia acquired by an immunocompetent child outside healthcare setting	Defined as pneumonia occurring in a child after 48–72 h after admission to hospital that was not present at the time of admission

TABLE 19.13	Etiological Classification of Pneumonia	
Infective Pneumonia		**Noninfective Pneumonia**
Bacteria: Pneumococci, Hib, group A *Streptococcus*, *Staphylococcus aureus*, *E. coli*, *Klebsiella*, *Legionella*, *Mycoplasma*, *Chlamydia*, TB Viral: RSV (Respiratory Syncytial Virus), influenza, parainfluenza, adenovirus, human metapneumovirus Fungal: *Histoplasma*, coccidioidomycosis, *Cryptococcus*, mucormycosis, pneumocystosis Parasites: *Strongyloides*, ascariasis		Aspiration Radiation Hypersensitivity

31. Differentiate between bacterial and viral pneumonia.
    The differences between bacterial and viral pneumonia are listed in Table 19.17.
32. List the indications for blood culture in a child with pneumonia.
    - No improvement or deterioration
    - Severe pneumonia
    - Pneumonia requiring hospitalization
    - Abscess and cellulitis in the presence of an infective focus

TABLE 19.14	Clinical Classification of Pneumonia	
WHO Classification	**IMNCI (Integrated Management of Neonatal and Childhood Illness) Classification**	

WHO Classification:
- Pneumonia with fast breathing and/or chest indrawing Treatment: Amoxicillin 80 mg/kg/day b.d. – 5 days
- Severe pneumonia: Pneumonia with any general danger sign Treatment: Ampicillin (50 mg/kg/6 hourly + gentamicin (7.5 mg/kg i.m. or i.v. o.d.) Or Ceftriaxone 75 mg/kg/day b.d. – 5 days
- Empirical *Pneumocystis jiroveci* treatment for HIV-infected or exposed infants younger than 1 year

IMNCI Classification:
1. In young infants (younger than 2 months)
   - Very severe disease: Fever or hypothermia, wheezing or stridor in a calm child, abnormally sleepy, stopped feeding well, convulsions
   - Severe pneumonia: Fast breathing or chest indrawing
   - No pneumonia: Cough, no fast breathing and chest indrawing
2. Children aged 2 months to 5 years
   - Very severe disease: Pneumonia with general danger signs
   - Severe pneumonia: Fast breathing with chest indrawing
   - Pneumonia: Fast breathing
   - No pneumonia: Cough, no fast breathing

TABLE 19.15	WHO Treatment in Pneumonia	
WHO Classification	**Treatment**	
• Pneumonia with fast breathing and/or chest indrawing • Severe pneumonia: Pneumonia with any general danger sign	Treatment: Amoxicillin 80 mg/kg/day b.d. – 5 days Treatment Ampicillin (50 mg/kg/6 hourly + gentamicin (7.5 mg/kg i.m. or i.v. o.d.) Or Ceftriaxone 75 mg/kg/day b.d. – 5 days Empirical *Pneumocystis jiroveci* treatment for HIV-infected or exposed infants younger than 1 year	

TABLE 19.16	Recent Updates in Antimicrobial Therapy for Pneumonia	
Clinical Diagnosis	**Treatment**	
Mild to moderate illness Moderate to severe illness	• No antibiotic therapy (majority of the infections are viral, especially in preschool children) • For regions with low pneumococcal resistance to penicillin: Ampicillin 150–200 mg/kg/day in four divided doses • For regions with high pneumococcal resistance to penicillin: Ceftriaxone 50–75 mg/kg/day q24h • Empirical oral outpatient therapy for less severe illness: High-dosage amoxicillin 80–100 mg/kg/day p.o. div. t.i.d.	
For suspected *Mycoplasma*/atypical pneumonia	Add azithromycin 10 mg/kg i.v., p.o. on day 1, and then 5 mg/kg o.d. for days 2–5 of treatment	

TABLE 19.17	Differences Between Bacterial and Viral Pneumonia	
Bacterial Pneumonia	**Viral Pneumonia**	
Occurs at any age	Most common between 1 month and 5 years	
Toxic appearance, **rapid progression**, child nontoxic in *Mycoplasma* infection	Nontoxic, playful child, associated with upper respiratory tract infection	
Crackles+	Wheeze+	
Raised TLC, CRP, procalcitonin	Normal	
CXR – consolidation, bronchopneumonia, pleural effusion	Chest X-Ray – Bilateral Hyperinflated lungs, interstitial pneumonia	
The definitive diagnosis of a bacterial infection requires isolation of an organism from the blood, pleural fluid, or lung; **blood cultures positive only in 10% of patients**	The definitive diagnosis of a viral infection rests on the isolation of a virus or detection of the viral genome or antigen in respiratory tract secretions	

- Malnutrition
- Suspected sepsis
- Pneumonia in an immunocompromised child

33. List the indications for chest X-ray in a child with pneumonia.
- Indications for chest X-ray
  - Persistent pneumonia
  - Severe pneumonia
  - Pneumonia in a child with ambiguous clinical findings
  - Complications: Pleural effusion, empyema, abscess, necrotizing pneumonia, and bronchopleural fistula
  - Pneumonia in SAM (Severe Acute Malnutrition)/immunocompromised
- Indication for repeat CXR
  - First CXR collapse or collapse consolidation (to rule out congenital lung disease, lung mass)
  - No improvement or worsening of symptoms within 48–72 hours after appropriate therapy

34. Explain the role of USG chest in pneumonia.
- Performed if no improvement or worsening of symptoms within 48–72 hours after appropriate antibiotic therapy
- To identify complications such as empyema or a loculated effusion

*35. When should *Staphylococcus aureus* pneumonia be suspected?
- Cavitary pneumonia
- Pneumatocele as shown in Fig. 19.7.
- Necrotizing pneumonia as shown in Fig. 19.8
- Pneumonia in a child with SAM
- Following influenza epidemic
- Not responding to regular antibiotics
- Complications (pleural effusion, empyema, lung abscess)

36. What is the usual response to therapy in pneumonia? The response to therapy in pneumonia is listed in Table 19.18.

37. Enumerate the factors to be considered while selecting antibiotic therapy for pneumonia.
- Age – gives a clue to etiology

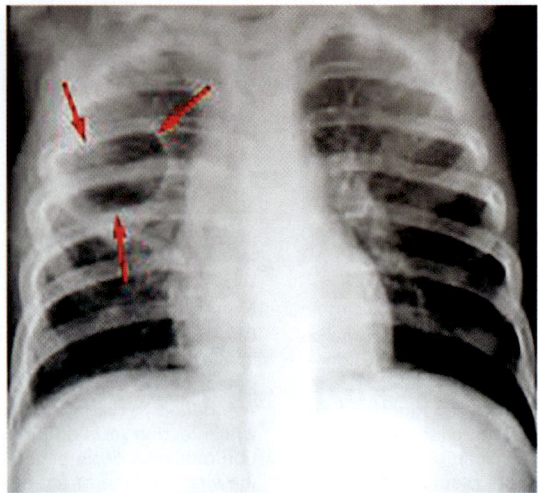

Fig. 19.7 Pneumatocele. *(Source: https://br.pinterest.com/pin/64394444 6690764128/.)*

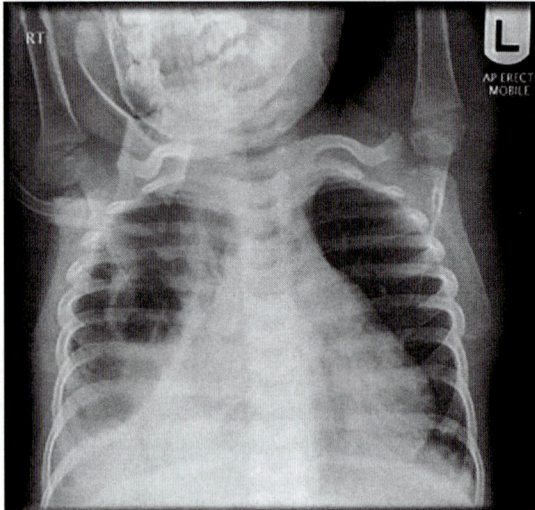

Fig. 19.8 Necrotizing pneumonia with cavity. *(Source: Reproduced from David A Spencer, Matthew F Thomas. Necrotising pneumonia in children, Paediatric Respiratory Reviews 15(3):240-245.)*

TABLE 19.18	Response to Therapy in Pneumonia	
Feature	**Duration**	
Fever	Within 4 days	
Abnormal physical findings	Can persist up to 7 days	
Raised TLC	Resolves within 4 days	
Radiological findings	Resolve within 6 weeks	

- Site of acquisition – community-acquired, most commonly caused by pneumococci
- Hospital-acquired – Most common cause is S.aureus followed by Pseudomonas.
- Nutrition – malnutrition (Gram-negative and *S. aureus*)
- Underlying disease – CF (Cystic Fibrosis) (*Pseudomonas, S. aureus*), sickle cell, nephrotic syndrome (*S. pneumo-*

cocci), HIV (Gram-negative), and neutropenia (Gram-negative, *S. aureus*)
- Previous antibiotic therapy – results in change of microbial flora to Gram negative
- Duration of illness – prolonged duration (TB)

38. What are the criteria for admission in hospital in a child with pneumonia?
- Age <6 months
- Multiple lobe involvement
- Toxic appearance
- Moderate to severe respiratory distress
- Dehydration
- No improvement on oral antibiotics
- Severe acute malnutrition
- General danger signs
- With coinfections
- Social factors (cannot come for follow-up; mother not confident in managing at home, far away from a health facility)

39. If a child with pneumonia does not improve within 48–72 hours of appropriate therapy, what are the possibilities?
1. Complications: Pleural effusion, empyema, and lung abscess
2. Drug factors: Inadequate dose, poor compliance, and bacterial resistance
3. Nonbacterial etiology
4. Comorbid conditions: Immunodeficiency and cystic fibrosis
5. Bronchial obstruction: Foreign body and mucous plug
6. Other noninfectious agents: Bronchiolitis obliterans, hypersensitivity, or eosinophilic pneumonitis

40. Define cystic fibrosis.
- It is also called mucoviscidosis (Robbins).
- It is an inherited disorder of ion transport that affects fluid secretion in exocrine glands and the epithelial lining of respiratory, gastrointestinal, and genitourinary tracts.
- It is characterized by hypertonic sweat and dehydrated mucus in epithelial-lined tracts.

41. What is the pathogenesis of CF (Robbins)?
- Caused by mutations in genes encoding CFTR (Cystic Fibrosis Transmembrane Conductance Regulator) protein in chromosome 7
- Most common mutation being the one causing deletion of phenylalanine at position 508
- CF type with normal sweat chloride test: class 5 CF 3849+10kbC → T
- Classes of mutations: Six (Robbins) and five (Nelson)
  - Class 1: Defective protein synthesis
  - Class 2: Defective packaging
  - Class 3: Defective regulation
  - Class 4: Decreased conductance
  - Class 5: Reduced abundance
  - Class 6: Altered function in regulation of ion channel
    - CFTR protein is a chloride channel located in sweat ducts and respiratory, GIT (Gastrointestinal Tract), and genitourinary tracts.
    - CFTR also regulates ENaC (Epithelial Sodium Channels), K, and HCO_3 channels.
    - In the sweat duct (as shown in Fig. 19.9), CFTR stimulates ENaC. Hence, when CFTR is mutated,

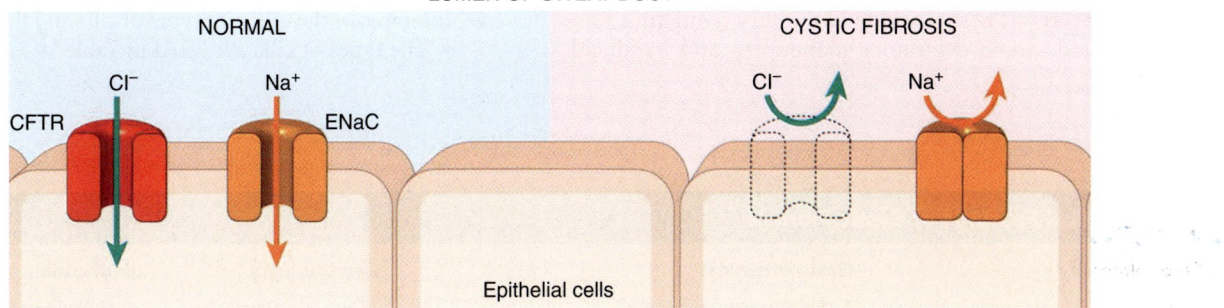

Fig. 19.9 CFTR protein in the lumen of sweat duct. (*Source:* Modified from Vinay Kumar, Abul Abbas, Jon Aster. *Robbins Basic Pathology, International Edition*, 9th Edition, Genetic and Pediatric Diseases, Fig 6.4, Philadelphia, Saunders, 2013.)

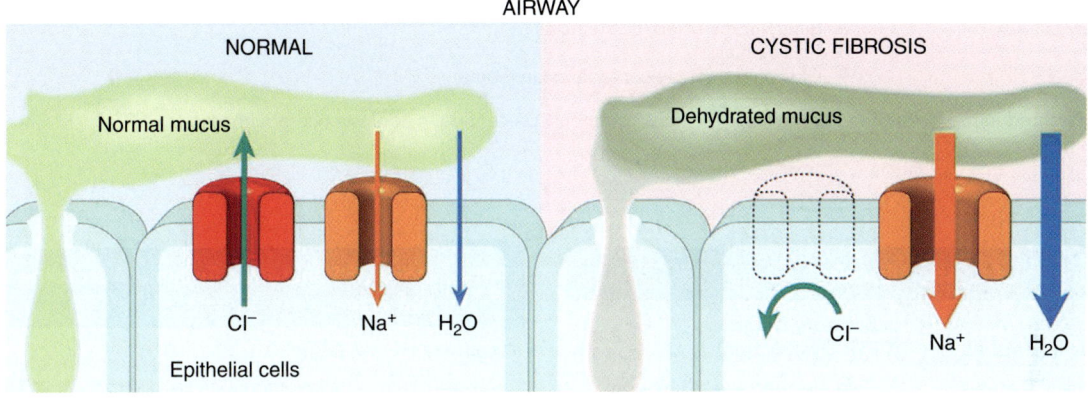

Fig. 19.10 CFTR protein in the airway lumen. (*Source:* Modified from Vinay Kumar, Abul Abbas, Jon Aster. *Robbins Basic Pathology, International Edition*, 9th Edition, Genetic and Pediatric Diseases, Fig 6.4, Philadelphia, Saunders, 2013.)

ENaC is also inhibited leading to accumulation of sodium and chloride in the lumen of the sweat duct.

- In respiratory, GIT, and genitourinary tracts (as shown in Fig. 19.10), normal CFTR protein inhibits ENaC. Hence, when CFTR is mutated, the ENaC is activated. This results in passive water reabsorption from the lumen resulting in dehydrated mucus.

- CFTR mutation in the above epithelial-lined tracts results in diminished HCO_3 secretion that results in acidity of luminal fluids, which causes increased mucin precipitation and ductal plugging and adherence of bacteria to mucin plugs.

42. What are the factors favoring infection of the respiratory tract in a patient with CF?
- Defective clearance of secretions is present.
- Abnormal CFTR creates a proinflammatory state.
- CF epithelia provide a favorable environment for *S. aureus*, *Pseudomonas*, and *Burkholderia*.
- *Pseudomonas* undergoes mucoid transformation in CF airways and this results in the formation of a biofilm.
- Antimicrobial activity is diminished in CF airways because of an acidic environment.
- Fatty acid deficiency is also postulated to be a predisposing factor.

43. What are the clinical features of cystic fibrosis?
The clinical features of cystic fibrosis are listed in Table 19.19.

*44. What are the diagnostic criteria for cystic fibrosis?
The diagnostic criteria for cystic fibrosis are listed in Table 19.20.

45. What are the newer therapies in CF?
- Lumacaftor, ivacaftor, and tezacaftor: FDA (Food and Drug Administration)-approved drugs for patients with class 3 mutations

46. Name some noninjectable antipseudomonal agents used in patients with cystic fibrosis.
- Oral: Ciprofloxacin (the only oral antibiotic that is effective against *Pseudomonas*)
- Aerosol: Aztreonam, colistin, gentamicin, and tobramycin

47. What is the dose of pancreatic enzymes in patients with cystic fibrosis?
- Enzymes should be given before and during meals.
- They should not be crushed, powdered, or chewed because this will allow gastric acid to penetrate the enteric coating and destroy the enzymes.
- The North American Cystic Fibrosis Foundation guidelines for the dosing of enzymes are shown in Table 19.21.

*48. Describe the method of chest physiotherapy.
- Chest PT (Physiotherapy) is recommended one to four times a day.

- Cough, huffing, or forced expirations are encouraged after each lung segment is drained.
- Methods: These include voluntary coughing, repeated forced expiratory maneuvers, and handheld oscillatory devices. The methods of chest physiotherapy are shown in Figs. 19.11 and 19.12.
49. Enumserate the different types of cilia and their functions.
    - The types of cilia are listed in Table 19.22.

TABLE 19.19	Clinical Features of Cystic Fibrosis		
Sinopulmonary	**Gastrointestinal**	**Genitourinary**	**Endocrine**
1. Sinusitis	1. Fetal echogenic bowel	1. Pseudo Bartter syndrome	1. Delayed puberty
2. Polyposis	2. Meconium ileus	2. Renal calculi	2. Cystic fibrosis–related diabetes mellitus
3. Allergic bronchopulmonary aspergillosis	3. Pancreatic insufficiency (most common)	3. Osteoporosis	
4. Bronchiectasis (hemoptysis)	4. Distal intestinal obstructive syndrome	4. Renal failure	
5. Pneumothorax	5. Rectal prolapse		
6. Respiratory failure	6. Intussusception		
	7. Biliary fibrosis/hepatic steatosis		
	8. Cholelithiasis		
	9. Digestive tract cancer (adenocarcinoma)		

Note: Text highlighted in red color refers to the features more commonly presenting in adolescence/adulthood.

TABLE 19.20	Diagnosis of Cystic Fibrosis	
History/Clinical Features	**Laboratory Diagnosis (CFTR Dysfunction)**
1. Typical clinical features (GIT, pulmonary, gut) Or	1. Two elevated sweat chloride test on separate days Or
2. History of cystic fibrosis in sibling Or	2. Identification of two CF mutations Or
3. Positive newborn screening	3. Abnormal nasal potential difference measurement

TABLE 19.21	Dose of Pancreatic Enzyme According to the Age	
Age	**Dose**
Infants	2000–4000 units lipase/120 mL of breast milk or formula
1–4 years	1000 units lipase/kg/meal initially, and then titrate per response
Older than 4 years	500 units lipase/kg/meal initially, up to maximum of 2500 units lipase/kg/meal or 10,000 units lipase/kg/day or 4000 units lipase/g fat ingested per day

Note: Complications of pancreatic enzyme replacement include kidney stones and fibrosing colonopathy.

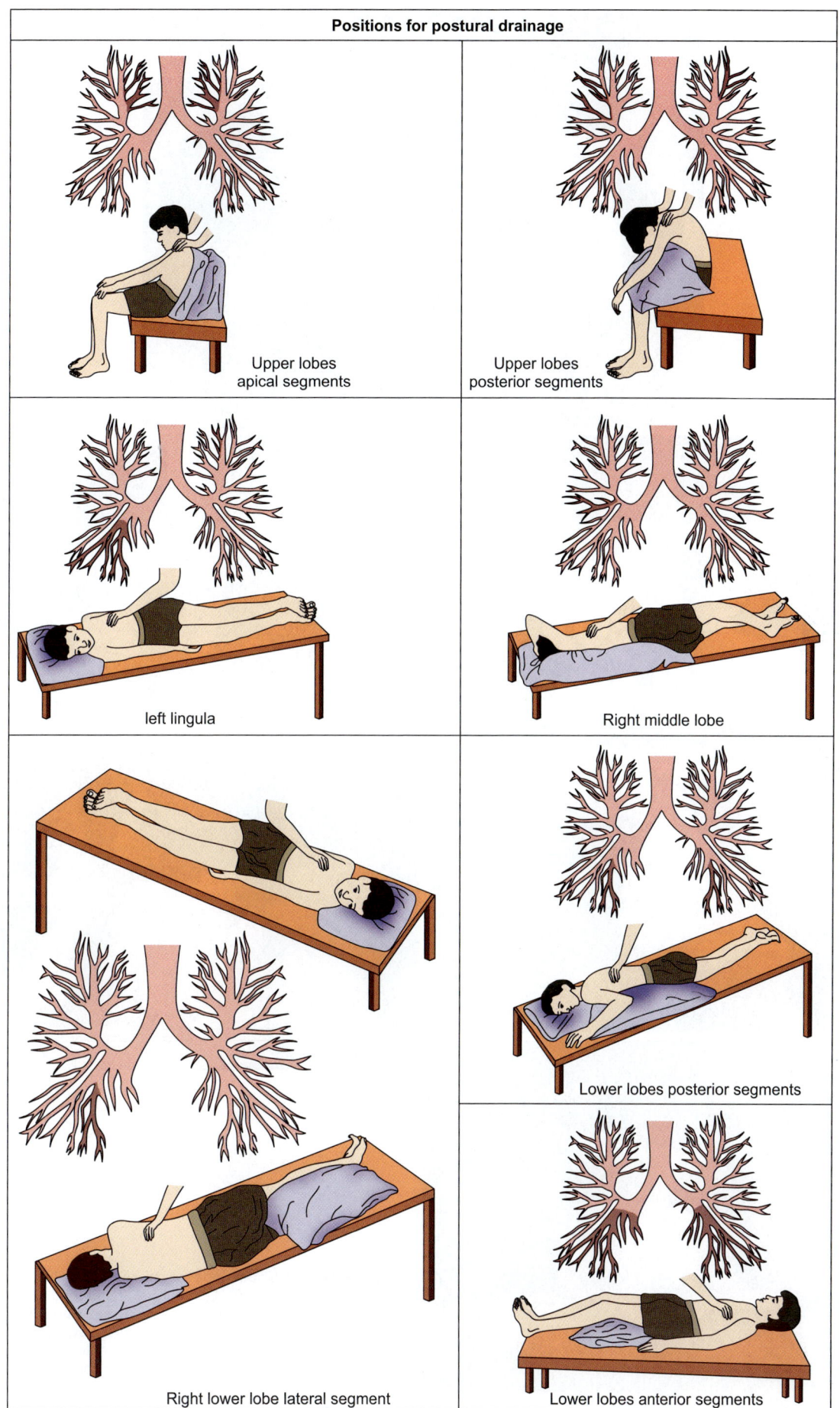

Fig. 19.11   Schematic presentation of methods of chest physiotherapy.

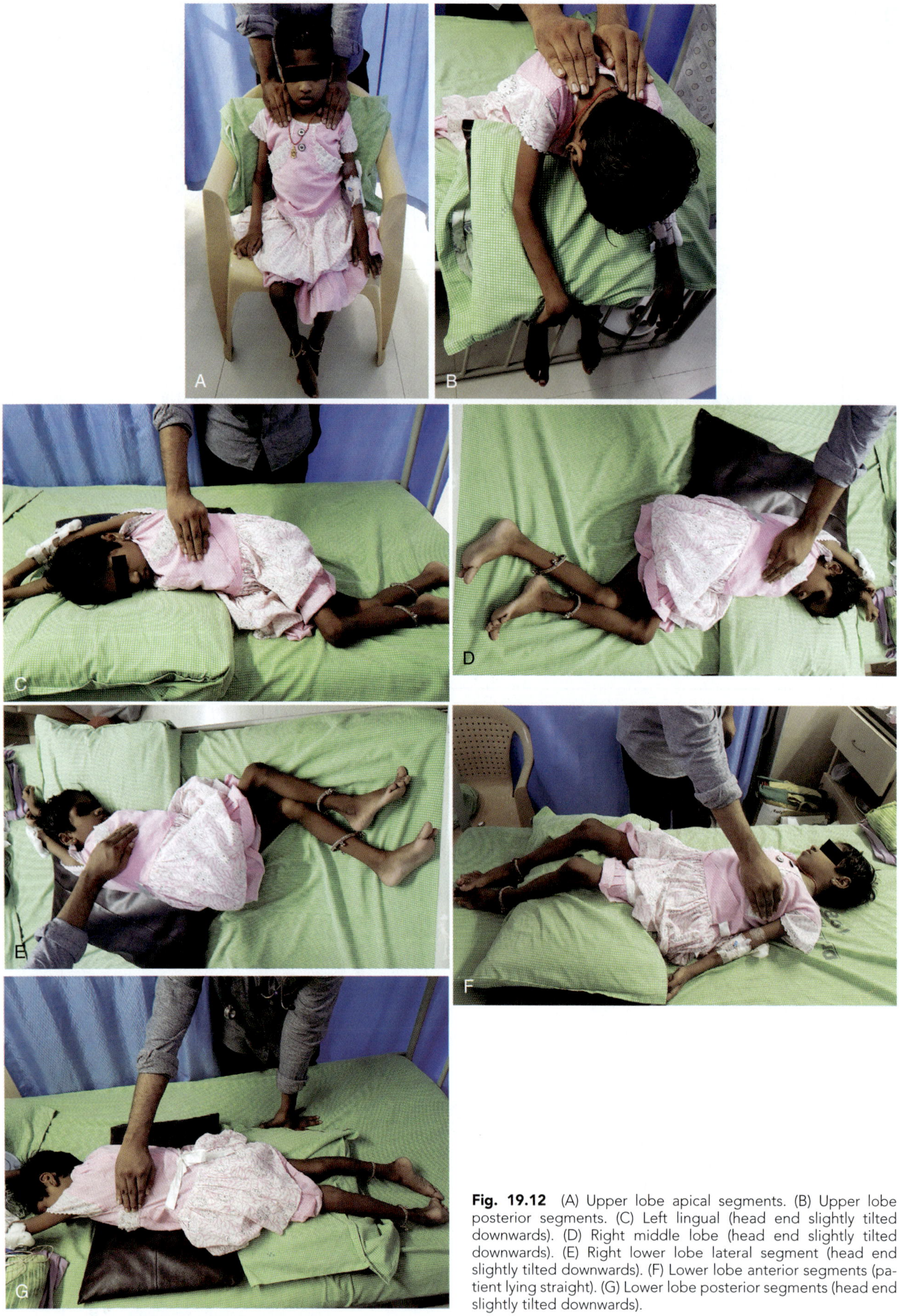

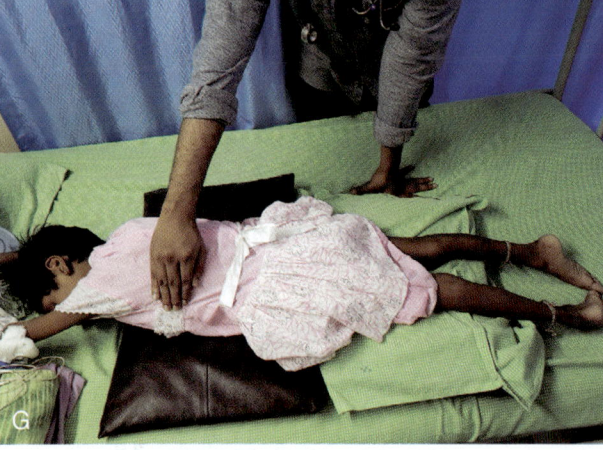

Fig. 19.12 (A) Upper lobe apical segments. (B) Upper lobe posterior segments. (C) Left lingual (head end slightly tilted downwards). (D) Right middle lobe (head end slightly tilted downwards). (E) Right lower lobe lateral segment (head end slightly tilted downwards). (F) Lower lobe anterior segments (patient lying straight). (G) Lower lobe posterior segments (head end slightly tilted downwards).

TABLE 19.22	Types of Cilia	
Cilia	**Location**	**Function**
Motile cilia	Eustachian tube, paranasal sinuses, conducting airways	Movement of fluids, mucus, and inhaled particles
Primary (sensory) cilia	Renal nephron, bile ductules, chondrocytes, astrocytes, and cells in sensory organs	They are mechanoreceptors, chemosensors, osmosensors
Nodal cilia	Present during the embryonic period	Establish body sidedness by regulating extracellular fluid movement

Quick Bites

- A history of recurrent episodes of cough with sputum is a pointer toward bronchiectasis.
- Cystic fibrosis is the most common cause of bronchiectasis in children.
- Primary ciliary dyskinesia should be ruled out in a patient with chronic suppurative lung disease having a history of neonatal rhinitis.
- HRCT is the investigation of choice for the diagnosis of bronchiectasis.
- Lumacaftor, ivacaftor, and tezacaftor are the latest FDA-approved drugs for cystic fibrosis.
- Ciprofloxacin is the only oral antimicrobial agent that is effective against *Pseudomonas*.
- The diagnosis of community-acquired pneumonia is clinical.
- The etiology of community-acquired pneumonia varies according to the age.

SECTION D

Abdomen System

Gastrointestinal System Examination

General Examination

SENSORIUM

Altered sensorium in hepatic encephalopathy, acute pancreatitis, and gastrointestinal (GI) bleed

POSTURE

- Mention the position in which the patient prefers to lie.
- In massive ascites, the patient prefers an upright or semirecumbent posture.
- In GERD (Gastroesophageal Reflux Disease), there occurs arching and turning of the head.

PALLOR

- Because of blood loss: GI bleed, worm infestations, and GI tract malignancy
- Hypoproliferative anemia: Nutritional (secondary to malabsorption), HBV infections (aplastic anemia), anemia of chronic disease (because of inflammatory bowel disease, chronic liver disease,), and *H. pylori* infection
- Anemia because of increased destruction: Autoimmune hepatitis, hypersplenism, and IBD (Inflammatory Bowel Disease)

ICTERUS

Prehepatic, hepatic, and posthepatic causes

CYANOSIS

Hepatopulmonary syndrome

CLUBBING

DCLD (Decompensated Chronic Liver Disease), IBD, polyposis coli, severe gastrointestinal hemorrhage, and small bowel lymphoma

GENERALIZED LYMPHADENOPATHY

TB and GI lymphomas

EDEMA

DCLD, protein-losing enteropathy, and Aagenaes syndrome

Head-to-Foot Examination

SYNDROMIC FACIES AND GI SYSTEM

- Down syndrome (refer to chapter 39 on Down syndrome)
- Treacher Collins syndrome: Retrognathia and glossoptosis resulting in airway obstruction

- Turner syndrome: IBD and celiac disease
- Syndromic diarrhea: Facial dysmorphism with prominent forehead, broad nose, and hypertelorism; secretory diarrhea; chronic liver disease; trichorrhexis nodosa; and pili torti
- Aagenaes syndrome, Zellweger syndrome, and Alagille syndrome: Neonatal cholestasis

EYES

- Pallor, icterus, and phlycten
- Bitot spots and subconjunctival hemorrhage (vitamin deficiency secondary to malabsorption)
- Posterior embryotoxon and microcornea – Alagille syndrome
- Cataract, chorioretinitis, and salt and pepper fundus – TORCH infections

ORAL CAVITY AND OROPHARYNX

- Macroglossia: Relative macroglossia, Down syndrome; absolute macroglossia, congenital hypothyroidism, glycogen storage disorders, MPS (mucopolysaccharidosis), and histiocytosis
- Dental caries
- Dental erosions: GERD
- Odor of breath: Fetor hepaticus
- Cleft palate
- Oral ulcers: Peutz–Jeghers syndrome

EXTREMITIES

- Cyanosis
- Clubbing
- Palmar erythema
- Asterixis
- Dupuytren's contracture
- Nail changes in liver failure
- Edema
- BCG scar

CHEST

- Gynecomastia
- Spider angioma
- Subcutaneous emphysema: Boerhaave syndrome

SKIN

- Skin changes in cirrhosis (refer to chapter 21 on chronic liver disease)
- Petechiae and purpura (secondary to hyperspelnism)
- Gianotti–Crosti syndrome and polyarteritis nodosa: HBV infections
- Grey Turner and Cullen signs: Acute pancreatitis

- Blueberry muffin lesions: Neonatal cholestasis
- Telangiectasia (GI bleed)
- Enterocutaneous fistulas: Crohn disease

Skin Manifestations in Inflammatory Bowel Disease

- Erythema nodosum
- Pyoderma gangrenosum
- Sweet syndrome
- Metastatic Crohn disease
- Psoriasis
- Epidermolysis bullosa acquisita
- Perianal skin tags
- Polyarteritis nodosa

EXTERNAL MARKERS OF TUBERCULOSIS

- Lupus vulgaris, scrofuloderma, tinea versicolor, and scrofula

JOINTS

Arthritis (HBV infection, IBD, Alagille syndrome)

GENITALS

Testicular atrophy (liver failure)

Vital Signs

TEMPERATURE

Elevated in infections, autoimmune disorders, and malignancy

PULSE RATE

- Low volume (GI bleed, acute pancreatitis)
- Bounding pulse (DCLD)

RESPIRATORY RATE

Tachypnea in hepatopulmonary syndrome, massive abdominal distension, and GI infection

BLOOD PRESSURE

- Hypotension (GI bleed, acute pancreatitis)
- Wide pulse pressure and DCLD

JVP

Hepatojugular reflex absent in Budd–Chiari syndrome

Anthropometry

- Acute/chronic malnutrition: Seen in malabsorption, IBD, chronic liver disease, and GERD
- Short stature: Malabsorption disorders and Crohn disease
- Obesity: Associated with GERD, fatty liver disease, gallstones, and recurrent pancreatitis

Abdomen Examination

ORAL CAVITY

As described earlier

SEGMENTS OF ABDOMEN

The abdomen can be divided into nine segments by drawing two imaginary vertical lines at the midclavicle on either side and two imaginary horizontal lines – one midway between xiphisternum and umbilicus, and the other midway between umbilicus and pubic symphysis as in Fig. 20.1 (kindly avoid using the term "quadrant" because quadrant means four).

Note: Some examiners refer:

- External genitalia as the 10th segment
- Renal angle as the 11th segment
- Per rectal examination as the 12th segment
- Supraclavicular fossa as the 13th segment

Inspection

- Shape: Normal shape scaphoid; pear-shaped abdomen seen in obesity
- Distension: Uniform distension in ascites and localized in organomegaly
- Umbilicus
  - Normal: Retracted and inverted
  - Everted: Umbilical hernia
  - Horizontal slit: Ascites
  - Pushed down: In upper abdominal mass
  - Pushed up: In pelvic mass
- Flanks: Full flanks in ascites
- Hernia orifices: Obliterated in inguinal hernia
- Movements of segments of the abdomen
- Skin
- Purple striae in Cushing syndrome
  - Stretched and shiny skin in massive ascites
  - Doughy skin: Severe dehydration
- Veins over the abdomen (refer the chapter 22 on UGI bleed)
- Scars: Laparotomy, right subcostal scar, inguinal scar, right iliac fossa scar, and peritoneocentesis scar looked for
- Sinuses: Gastrointestinal TB and Crohn disease
- Fistula: Crohn disease and persistent vitellointestinal fistula
- Colostomy opening

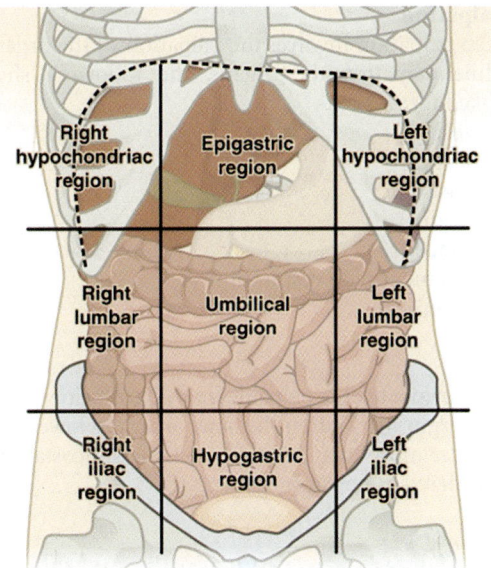

Fig. 20.1 Segments of abdomen. *(Source: Abdominal Quadrant Regions – Quadrants and Regions of Abdomen, Wikipedia.)*

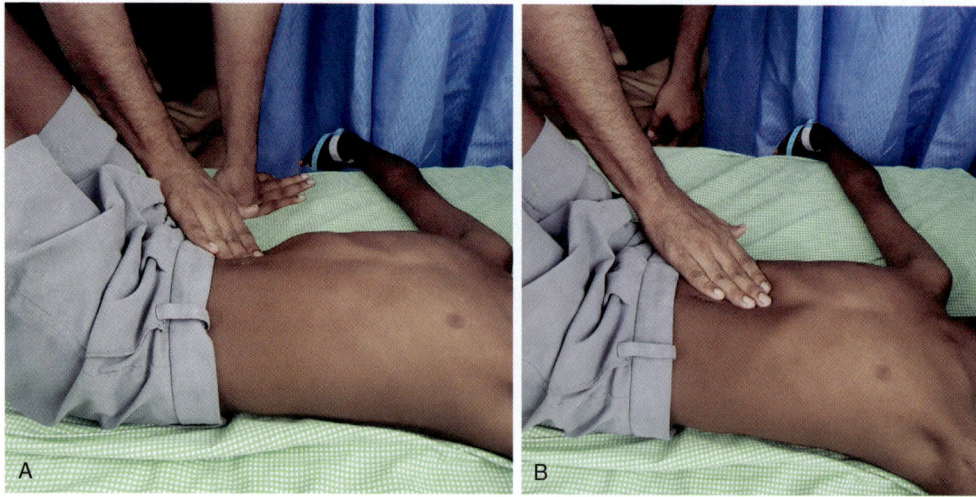

Fig. 20.2   (A and B) (Left to right) Examination of liver – with hands parallel to right costal margin palpating from RIF using radial border of index finger.

- Visible gastric peristalsis: Pyloric stenosis and intestinal obstruction
- External genitalia

Palpation
- Before starting the palpation of the abdomen, remember the following:
  - Check the patient's position (supine/lateral/sitting).
  - Check the examiner's position to the patient (right/left).
  - Explain the procedure to the patient.
  - The examiner's hands should be clean and warm (cold hands can cause reflex contraction of abdominal muscles).
  - Ensure that the patient is relaxed.
  - Always remember that the palpation should start in the left lower segment.

Superficial Palpation
- It includes warmth and tenderness in each of the nine segments of the abdomen.

Deep Palpation
- Deep palpation involves the palpation of the organs.
- While palpating the organs, the following should be looked for:
  - Size
  - Location
  - Consistency
  - Margins
  - Surface
  - Movement with respiration
  - Tenderness

Liver
- The normal liver is palpable up to 2 cm below the subcostal margin in children. In newborns, the lower border of the liver more than 3.5 cm below the subcostal margin is considered as hepatomegaly.

Palpation of Liver
- Two methods are used for palpation of the liver:
  1. Place both the hands side by side flat on the abdomen lateral to the rectus and below the right subcostal margin with fingers pointing toward the right subcostal margin (Hutchinson). Some textbooks mention using one hand. As the patient takes a deep breath, the index and middle fingers are used to palpate the liver edge as shown in Fig. 20.2A and B.
  2. Place the right hand below and parallel to the right subcostal margin. Start palpating from RIF. As the patient takes a deep breath, the radial border of the index finger is used to palpate the liver edge.

Spleen
- Soft and thin spleen is palpable in 15% of neonates, 10% of children, and 5% of adolescents.
- It has to be enlarged to two or three times its usual size before it becomes palpable.
- Enlargement takes place in a superior and posterior direction before it becomes palpable subcostally.
- Palpate for the splenic notch along the anterior border.

Clinical Features of Splenic Mass. Table 20.1 gives the features of splenic mass.

Enlarged Liver, Enlarged Spleen, and Enlarged Kidney, and Their Differences. Table 20.2 gives the differences between enlarged liver, enlarged spleen, and enlarged kidney.

Renal Mass and Splenic Mass and Their Differences. Table 20.3 gives the differences between renal mass and splenic mass.

Palpation of Spleen. Methods of palpation of spleen are discussed in Table 20.4.

TABLE 20.1	**Clinical Features of Splenic Mass**

Firm swelling
Sharp margins
Rounded anterior border
Moves downwards on inspiration
Upper border cannot be felt (i.e., cannot get above the swelling)
Dull to percussion
Not bimanually palpable/not ballotable
Cannot insinuate into the space between left costal margin and spleen (hook sign – hooking the left costal margin is not possible)
Enlarges downward and medially
No bowel sound over the spleen

TABLE 20.2	Differences Between Enlarged Liver, Enlarged Spleen, and Enlarged Kidney		
Features	Enlarged Liver	Enlarged Spleen	Enlarged Kidney
Site	Right hypochondrium and epigastrium	Left hypochondrium	Loin
Extent	Cannot get above the mass	Cannot get above the mass	Hand can get between mass and costal margin
Mobility	Moves with respiration	Moves with respiration	Moves with respiration but not markedly
Shape	Sharp lower border	Rounded, notched lower border	Smooth, round lower pole
Percussion	Dullness to percussion up to 5th rib in the midaxillary line	Dullness to percussion extend across the costal margin	Resonant to percussion anteriorly
Bimanually palpable/ballotable	Not unless very large	Not unless very large – separate from the erector spinae	Yes and fills the flank

TABLE 20.3	Differences Between Splenic Mass and Left Kidney	
Spleen	Left Kidney
Sharp edge	Round edge
Notch – medial border	No notch
Crosses midline	Does not cross midline
Moves with respiration	Does not move with respiration
Cannot get above it	Can get above it
Neither bimanually palpable nor ballotable	Bimanually palpable and ballotable
Finger insinuation not possible	Fingers can be insinuated
Band of colonic resonance absent	Band of colonic resonance present

Percussion

Liver Span
- Mark the upper border of the liver by percussing in the midclavicular line from the 2nd ICS.
- The lower border is palpated by any of the above-mentioned two methods.

- The distance between the two borders gives the liver span.
- The liver span remains normal in conditions causing pushed-down liver (asthma, bronchiolitis).

Spleen
- Percussion is performed to confirm the findings of the palpation. Dullness extends from the left lower ribs into the left hypochondrium and left lumbar region. Three methods to identify splenic enlargement by percussion method are given in Table 20.5.

Shifting Dullness
- With the patient in supine position, percuss laterally from the midline keeping the fingers in the longitudinal axis until dullness is detected.
- In normal individuals, the flanks are resonant.
- In patients with moderate ascites, the flanks are dull.
- Maneuver: Ask the patient to lie on the other side in lateral decubitus position, and after 30–60 seconds (to allow for the fluid to shift), the previous dull area over the flank becomes resonant as illustrated in Fig. 20.10.

TABLE 20.4	Palpation of Spleen	
Position	Clinical Method
1. Supine position a. Classical method	• Place the left hand over the lowermost rib cage posterolaterally. Then start palpation from RIF with right hand, slowly advancing toward left costal margin and spleen is palpated using the tip of fingers as in Fig. 20.3.
b. Bimanual method (support with left hand, palpate with right hand)	• Place left hand on left lower ribs. • Right hand placed beneath the costal margin well out to left. • Press in deeply with fingers of right hand beneath the costal margin (medial–lateral) as shown in Fig. 20.4.
2. Right lateral position (left leg flexed at hip and knee)	Bimanual palpation – support with left hand palpate with right hand as shown in Fig. 20.5.

3. Stand on the left side of patient (examiner standing left side facing toward the foot end)
  a. Hooking method (supine position)
  b. Middleton maneuver (right lateral position)
	a. Hooking method (supine position)
	  • Examiner standing on left side facing toward the foot end. From above, spleen may be continently palpable with two hands arching below the left costal margin while the patient takes in a deep breath as shown in Fig. 20.6.
	b. Middleton maneuver (right lateral position)
	  • Patient in right lateral position. Examiner standing on left side facing toward the foot end. Left-hand fingers hooked under left costal margin. Now exert pressure over the postero-lateral aspect of lower thorax using right hand. Spleen felt at the end of deep inspiration as shown in Fig. 20.7.

4. The patient lies in supine position and the examiner stands on the right side of the patient	Dipping method – Usually done in the presence of ascites (as shown in fig. 20.8).

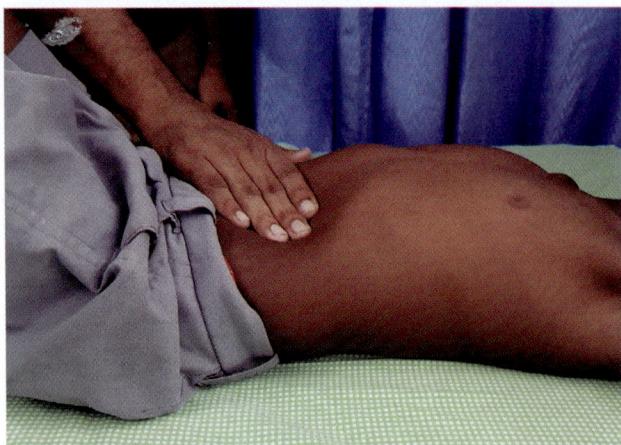

Fig. 20.3   Conventional method of spleen palpation.

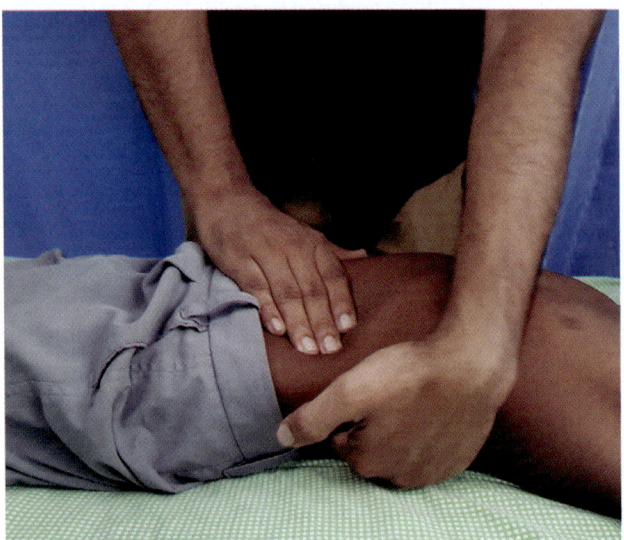

Fig. 20.4   Bimanual palpation of spleen.

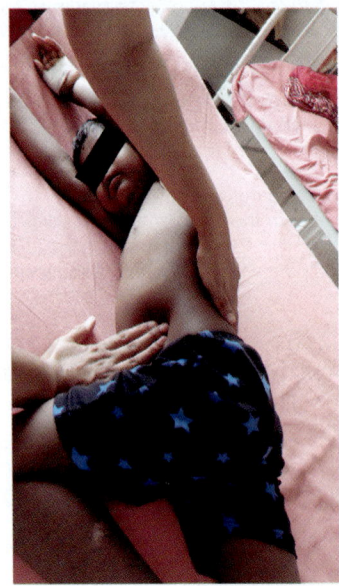

Fig. 20.5   Patient in right lateral position – bimanual palpation.

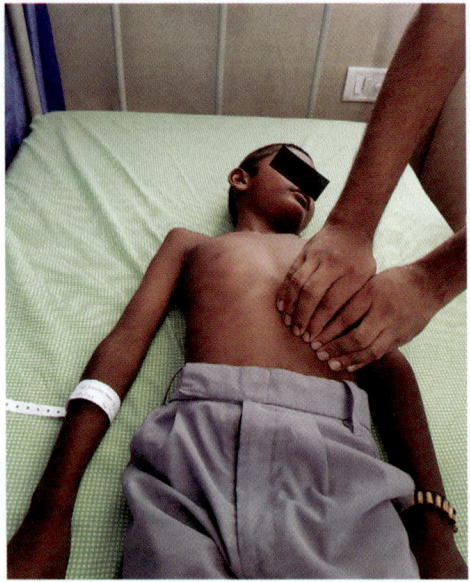

Fig. 20.6   Hooking method: Examiner standing on the left side of patient. Using hooked fingers of both hands placed under LCM for palpation of mildly enlarged spleen.

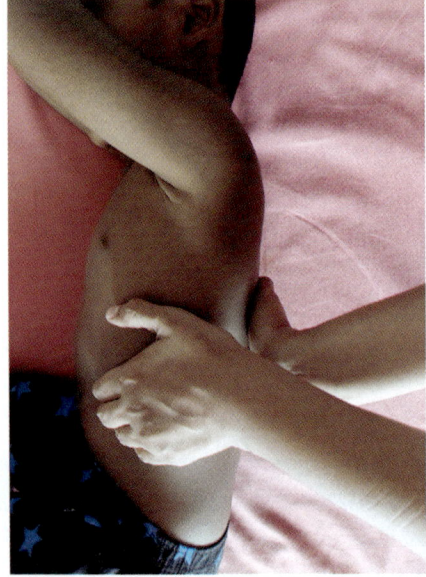

Fig. 20.7   Middleton maneuver: Patient in right lateral position, examiner on left side of the patient, hooked fingers of one hand placed over LCM and other hand on posterolateral aspect of thorax, and pressure is exerted.

Fig. 20.11A–D demonstrates shifting dullness and shift of fluid in a patient with moderate ascites when placed in lateral position.

- This is because of the shift of fluid in the peritoneal cavity. To elicit this sign, at least 1000 mL of fluid should be present in the peritoneal cavity.
- This sign is negative in loculated ascites.

Fluid Thrill

- The patient lies on his or her back. Place one hand over the lumbar region of one side; ask an assistant or the patient himself or herself to put the side of his or her hand firmly

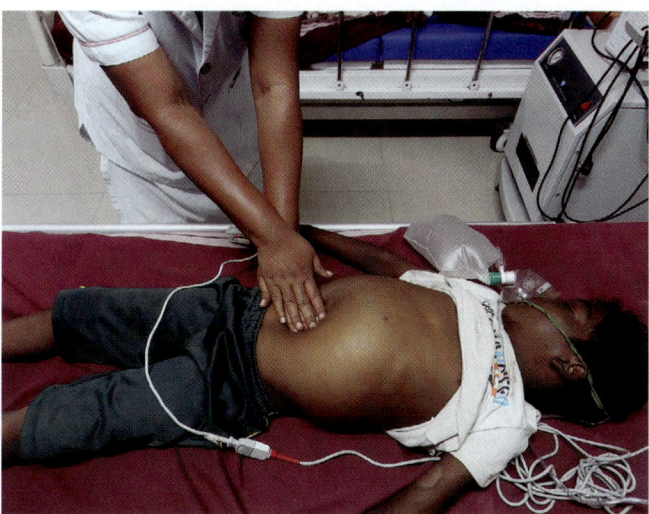

Fig. 20.8 Dipping method: Usually done in ascites one hand is placed upon other and gentle pressure is given outward and inward. Any enlarged viscera is felt by the palpating finger. In Dipping method, pressure given by one hand will displace the ascitic fluid and the other hand will feel the enlarged viscera.

TABLE 20.5	Methods to Identify Splenic Enlargement by Percussion Method
Method	**Demonstration**
Nixon method	• Position: Right lateral decubitus • Percussion started from the midpoint of left costal margin and continued upward for 8 cm perpendicular to left costal margin • Normally, the level of dullness does not extend more than 8 cm above the costal margin; if the dullness extends beyond 8 cm, splenomegaly is diagnosed as shown in Fig. 20.9
Castell method	Position: Supine Castell spot located at the junction of lowest intercostal space and the left anterior axillary line; in full inspiration, dullness felt if spleen is enlarged
Traube sign	Position: Supine Superiorly: 6th rib Inferiorly: Costal margin Laterally: Left anterior axillary line Splenomegaly: Dullness

in the midline of the abdomen (to dampen any impulse that may be transmitted through the fat of the abdominal wall) and then flick or tap gently the lumbar region as shown in Fig. 20.11.
• A fluid thrill or wave is felt as a definite impulse by the detecting hand held flat in the opposite lumbar region.
• To elicit this sign, >2000 mL of fluid should be present in the peritoneal cavity.

Puddle Sign
• Ask the patient to lie in the arm–knee position so that the middle portion of the abdomen is dependent.
• On percussion around the umbilicus, the previously resonant area becomes dull because of collection of fluid in the dependent region as shown in Fig. 20.12A. Fig. 20.12B

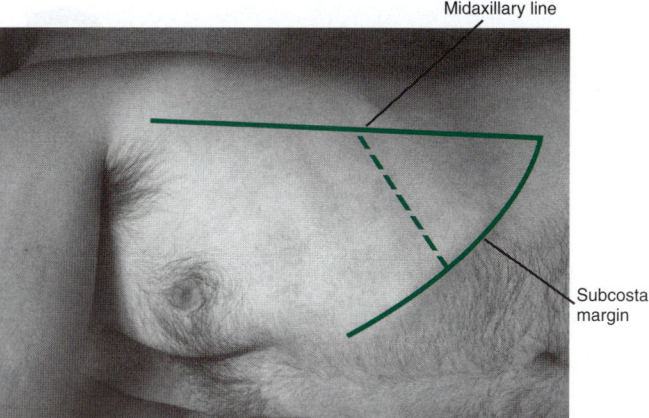

Fig. 20.9 Nixon method: Patient in right lateral position. Percussion started at midpoint C of left costal margin (AB) and proceeds perpendicularly (CD). Splenomegaly is diagnosed if the upper limit of dullness extends more than 8 cm above the costal margin (above D). (Source: Reproduced from Katrina Hurley, Peter Green, Rose Mengual. *OSCE and Clinical Skills Handbook*, Second Edition, Gastrointestinal system, Figure 3-6, St. Louis, Saunders Canada, 2012.)

shows demonstration of puddle sign to identify minimal fluid collection.
• This method can elicit as little as 120–150 mL of fluid.

Auscultopercussion
• With the patient in the similar position as mentioned previously, place a stethoscope over the umbilical region and scratch the abdominal wall from periphery toward the umbilicus as shown in Fig. 20.13.
• A change in the quality of sound is perceived while crossing the fluid column.
• This sign is false positive in massive splenomegaly and distended bladder.

Grading of Ascites
Grading of ascites is as follows:
    • +: Detectable only by careful examination
    • ++: Easily detectable but of relatively small volume
    • +++: Obvious ascites but not tense
    • ++++: Tense ascites

Auscultation

Bowel Sounds
• Increased in malabsorption, GI bleed, and carcinoid syndrome
• Absent in intestinal obstruction

Succussion Splash
• It is heard in a normal stomach within 2 hours after a meal, and is pathological in pyloric stenosis.

Bruit
• Bruit heard in aortic aneurysm and renal artery stenosis
• Bruit over the liver – hemangioma, hepatic artery aneurysm, and hepatocellular carcinoma

Venous Hum
• It is heard between xiphisternum and umbilicus because of turbulent blood flow in collaterals as a result of portal hypertension (Cruveilhier–Baumgarten murmur).

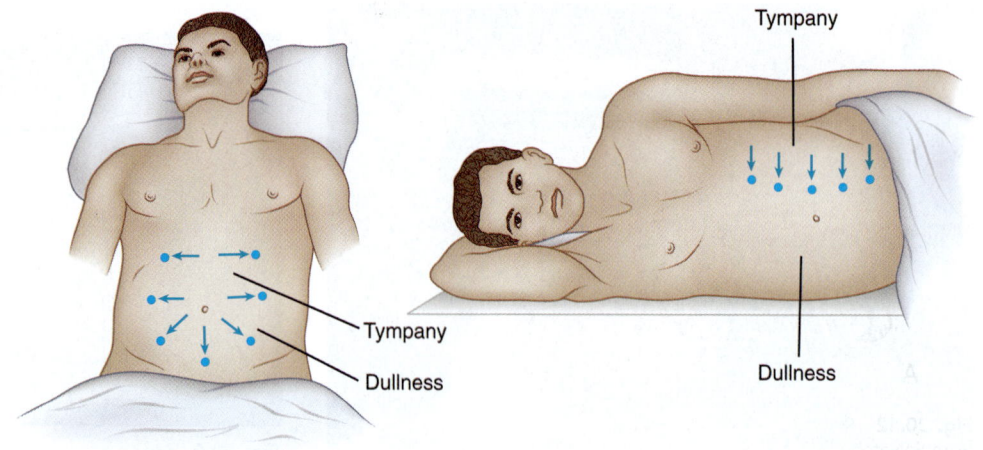

Fig. 20.10 Illustration of fluid shift. (*Source:* Reproduced from Jane Ball, Joyce Dains, John Flynn. *Seidel's Guide to Physical Examination: An Interprofessional Approach,* Tenth Edition, Abdomen, Fig. 18.23, St. Louis, Elsevier Inc, 2023.)

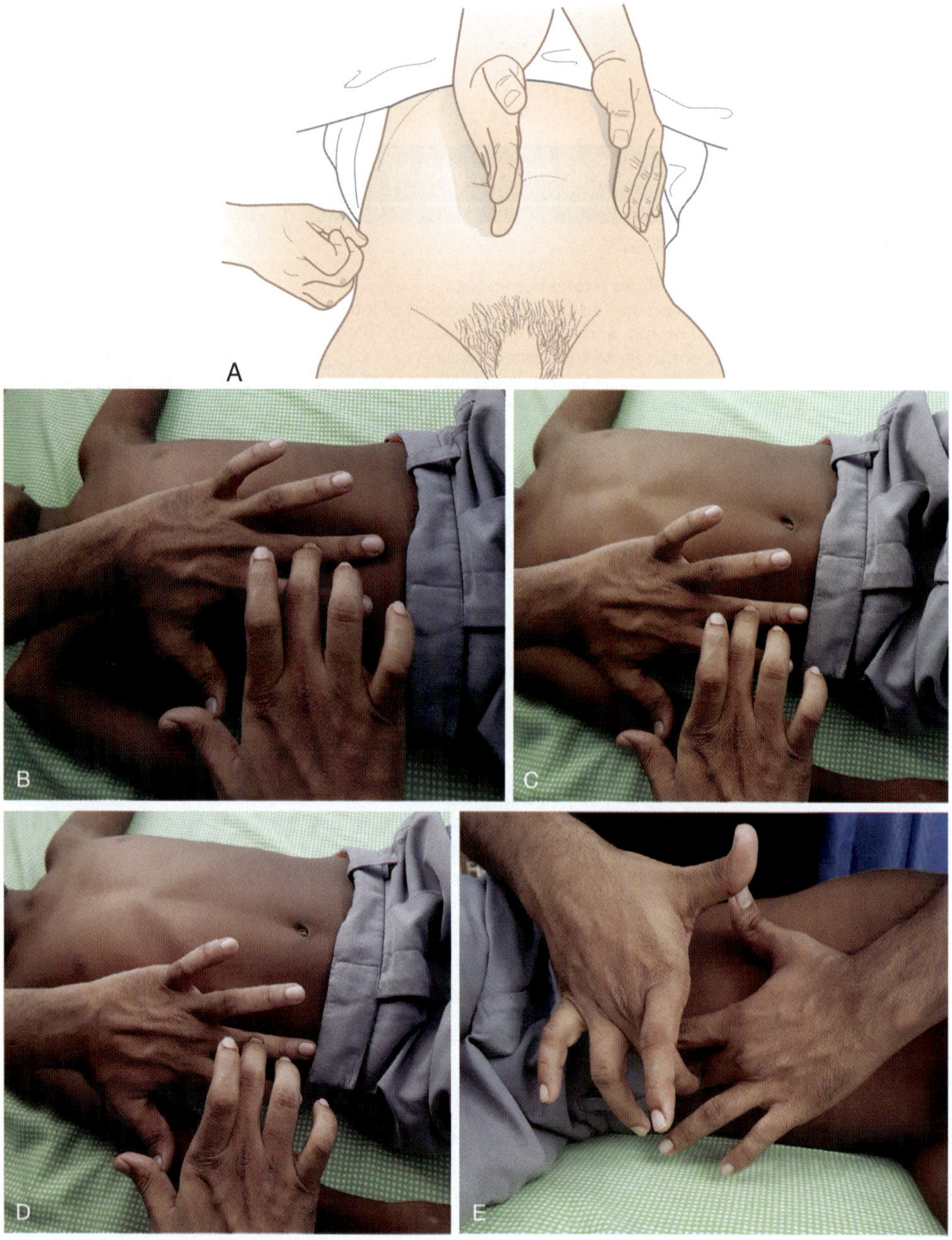

Fig. 20.11 (A) Demonstration of fluid thrill. (B) Percuss from epigastric to umbilicus in midline. (C) Percuss from umbilicus laterally to area of dullness. (D) Percussion in flanks at maximum point of dullness. (E) Percussion after lateral decubitus. (Source A: Reproduced from Michael Glynn, William M Drake. *Hutchison's Clinical Methods: An Integrated Approach to Clinical Practice,* Twenty-Fourth Edition, Gastrointestinal system, Figure 14.25, Edinburgh, Elsevier Ltd, 2018.)

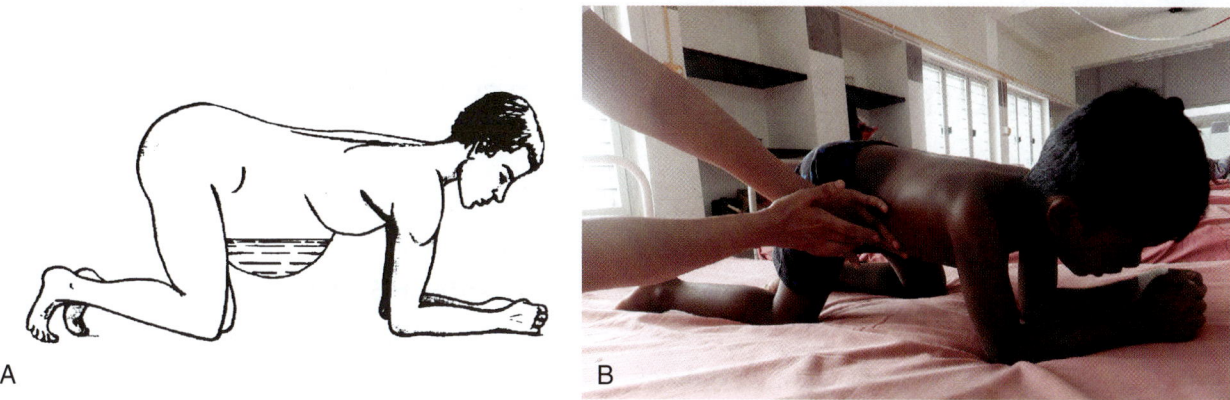

Fig. 20.12 (A) Patient in arm-knee position and collection of fluid around the umbilicus. (B) Demonstration of Puddle sign. (Source: Reproduced from Salvatore Mangione, Peter Sullivan, MIchael Wagner. *Physical Diagnosis Secrets*, Third Edition, The Abdomen, Fig. 13.18, Philadelphia, Elsevier Inc., 2022. (Credit line- From Dioguardi, N. & Sanna, G. P. (1975). Moderni Aspetti di Semeiotica Medica. Milan: Societa Editrice Universo.)

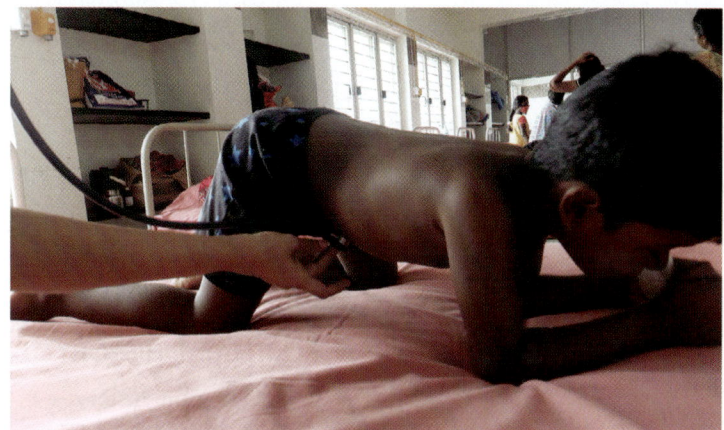

Fig. 20.13 Auscultopercussion method.

Chronic Liver Disease (CLD)

Following introductions, seek permission from the caregiver and introduce yourself to the patient before history elicitation, and identify the case.

Name____Age____Sex____Consanguinity____Order of birth____Place____Informant____

Presenting Complaints and Duration

- Yellowish discoloration of eyes/skin/urine
- Abdominal distension

History of Presenting Illness

- Jaundice
  - Onset, duration of jaundice
  - Whether associated with clay-colored stools
  - Whether associated with generalized itching
- Abdominal distension
  - Duration
  - Uniform/localized
  - Whether associated with swelling of legs/puffiness of face/breathlessness/oliguria, (abdominal distension without oliguria/puffiness of face or breathlessness more in favor of organomegaly)
- Other associated symptoms — abdominal pain/vomiting/anorexia

COMPLICATIONS HISTORY

- Hematemesis/melena
- Oily stools/foul-smelling stools
- Altered sleep pattern/abnormal behavior/seizures
- Fever/abdominal pain/vomiting
- Night blindness/bony deformities/bleeding manifestations
- Failure to gain weight

ETIOLOGY HISTORY

- Fever/recurrent blood transfusions/needle injury
- Breathlessness/palpitations/pedal edema
- Sudden onset of abdominal pain/jaundice/abdominal distension
- Recurrent seizures/failure to gain weight
- Long-term drug intake/native medications
- Recurrent respiratory tract infections/oily stools

COURSE DURING HOSPITAL

Mention about biopsy/Upper GI endoscopy/medications/transfusions given.

ANTENATAL HISTORY

- TORCH infections
- Hypothyroidism
- Acute fatty liver of pregnancy
- Recurrent fetal loss (neonatal iron storage disease)
- Drug intake by mother — sulfonamides, nitrofurantoin, antimalarials; any regular i.v. infusions
- Scan abnormalities such as oligo-/polyhydramnios
- History s/o any sepsis near term/timing of ROM (Rupture Of Membranes) and timing of delivery

NATAL HISTORY

- Term or preterm
- Birth weight (to know whether preterm/IUGR (Intra Uterine Growth Restriction))
- Birth asphyxia
- Any intolerance to feed
- Breathing efforts

POSTNATAL HISTORY

- Meconium history
- Sepsis
- TPN (Total Parenteral Nutrition)
- Any seizures
- Jaundice

PAST HISTORY

Any drug intake/native medication/previous hospitalization/blood transfusion

DEVELOPMENTAL HISTORY

Any development delay

DIETETIC HISTORY

Any calorie deficit, malnutrition

IMMUNIZATION HISTORY

According to national or IAP (Indian Academy of Paediatrics) schedule

FAMILY HISTORY

- Metabolic disorders
- Previous sibling death (metabolic diseases)
- Jaundice in family members

SOCIOECONOMIC HISTORY

According to modified Kuppuswamy scale

Summary

A _____-year-old _____ child, presented with yellowish discoloration of eyes/skin and urine for ___ months (usually >6 months), with/without clay-colored stools, with/without complications, a case of chronic liver disease, probable due to...

General Examination

- Sensorium
- Pallor
- Icterus
- Clubbing
- Cyanosis
- Pedal edema
- Generalized lymphadenopathy

Head-to-Foot Examination

- Head
  - Microcephaly
  - Any bulging AF
  - Wide-open fontanelles
- Dysmorphic facies
- Eyes: Pallor, icterus, epicanthic folds, bitot spots, Kayser–Fleischer (KF) ring, posterior embryotoxon, Brushfield spots in the iris, cataract, chorioretinitis, cherry red spot, papilledema.
- Parotid enlargement
- Macroglossia
- Gynecomastia
- Fetor hepaticus
- Spider angiomas
- Palmar erythema, petechiae, ecchymosis
- Xanthomas
- Dupuytren contracture
- Nails — leukonychia, Muehrcke nails/Terry nails/blue lunulae
- Bony deformities
- Dilated veins in abdominal wall
- Umbilical hernia
- Scratch marks of anklets in lower limbs
- Midline defects, micropenis
- Testicular atrophy
- Blueberry muffins

Vitals Signs

- Temperature
- Pulse rate
- Respiration — rate, rhythm, type of respiration
- Blood pressure

Anthropometry

Failure to thrive, Microcephaly

Abdominal Examination

INSPECTION

- Distended in upper part/uniform distension
- Skin — stretched and shiny
- Scars
- Dilated veins
- Umbilicus — transverse slit, umbilical hernia
- Flanks — full or free
- Hernia orifices
- All quadrants move equally with respiration
- External genitalia – micropenis, testicular atrophy, scrotal edema/vulval edema

PALPATION

- Warmth
- Tenderness
- Any organomegaly
- Fluid thrill

PERCUSSION

- Shifting dullness
- Liver span

AUSCULTATION

- Bowel sounds
- Bruit

Other System Examination

CARDIOVASCULAR SYSTEM

- Features of CCF (Congestive Cardiac Failure)

RESPIRATORY SYSTEM

- Look for signs of bronchiectasis and pleural effusion

CENTRAL NERVOUS SYSTEM

- Look for hypotonia
- Look for the signs of hepatic encephalopathy and raised ICT (Intracranial Tension)

Diagnosis

A case of decompensated chronic liver disease (DCLD), with/without complications
Probable etiology

Frequently Asked Questions

1. Enumerate the causes of chronic liver disease.
   Flowchart 21.1 explains the causes of chronic liver disease.

*2. List the features suggestive of chronic liver disease.
   - History — duration >6 months
   - Examination — signs of liver failure (seen in DCLD (Decompensated Chronic Liver Disease)), firm/nodular liver
   - Signs of portal hypertension
   - Investigations — A:G reversal, USG abdomen showing coarse echotexture of liver/portal hypertension

3. Describe the characteristic pathological features of cirrhosis (Robbins).
   - Parenchymal injury resulting in fibrosis
   - Regeneration resulting in nodules
   - Disruption of hepatic vascular architecture

4. Describe the morphological classification of cirrhosis.
   - Macronodular >3 mm — HBV/HCV, Wilson disease, galactosemia, alpha-1 antitrypsin
   - Micronodular <3 mm — EHBA (Extrahepatic Biliary Atresia), hemochromatosis

5. List the manifestations of compensated (latent) cirrhosis.
   - Essentially asymptomatic
   - Liver may shrink
   - Left lobe enlarges to compensate for right lobe destruction
   - Liver function tests – normal
   - Mild elevation of enzymes and GGT
   - Liver biopsy confirms the diagnosis

*6. mention the skin changes in cirrhosis.
   - Spider angiomas: These consist of a central arteriole from which numerous fine blood vessels radiate. They are found on the vascular territory of the superior vena cava (necklace area, face, forearm, and dorsum hands). These disappear following hypotension due to hemorrhage or shock. If these are more than five in number, these are considered significant. Skin is warm and patient looks flushed despite being afebrile. This reflects decreased peripheral vascular resistance and increased blood volume, complicating cirrhosis. Fig. 21.1 shows spider angioma.

   Palmar erythema (Dawson sign):
   - Paper money skin (American dollar sign)
   - Scratch marks
   - Hyperpigmentation
   - Xanthomas around eyes, flexural areas, and scar tissues
   - Dupuytren contracture

7. Mention the nail changes in cirrhosis.

Nail Changes	Disease
Clubbing	• More common in biliary cirrhosis; because of hypoxia, there is development of AV fistulas in lungs, steatorrhea, and platelet-derived growth factors (PDGF) → dilate peripheral vessels • Fig. 21.2 shows clubbing of nails
Blue lunulae	• Wilson disease • Fig. 21.3 shows blue nails
Leukonychia (white nail)	Causes: • Mainly due to hypoalbuminemia • Liver cell failure • Nephrotic syndrome • Protein losing enteropathies Fig. 21.4 shows leukonychia (white nail)
Muehrcke lines: White bands seen in hypoalbuminemia of any cause	White bands seen in hypoalbuminemia of any cause Fig. 21.5 shows Muehrcke lines
Terry nail	Approximately 80% of the proximal part of the nail become opaque (usually thumb and index fingers) and the remaining 20% retain the normal pink color (80 and 20 nail) Fig. 21.6 shows Terry nail

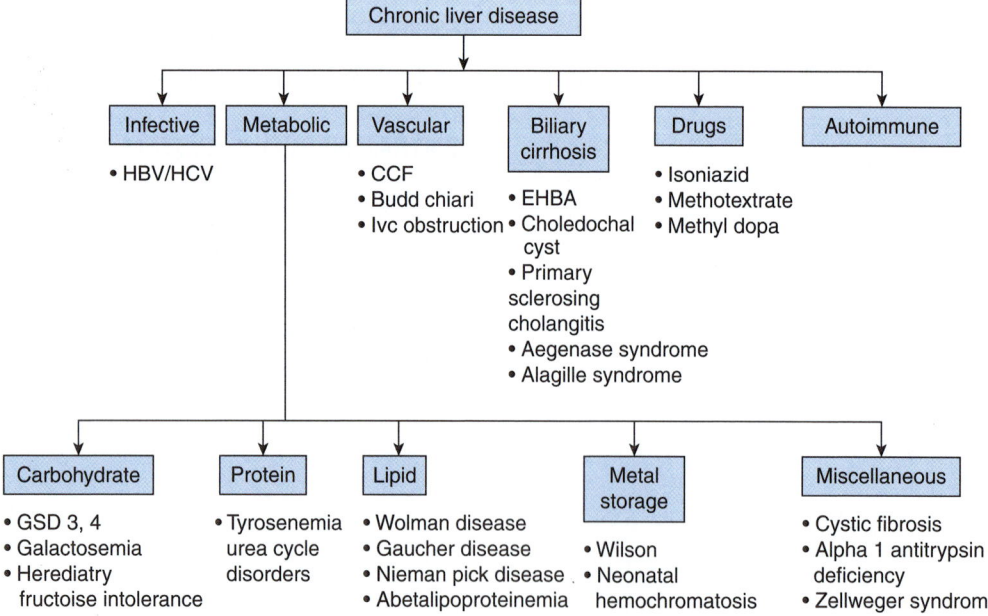

Flowchart 21.1 Causes of chronic liver disease.

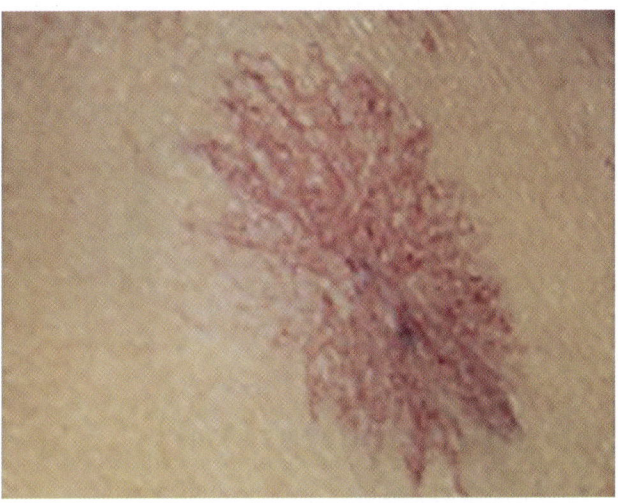

Fig. 21.1 Spider angioma. (*Source: Spider angioma - Wikipedia*)

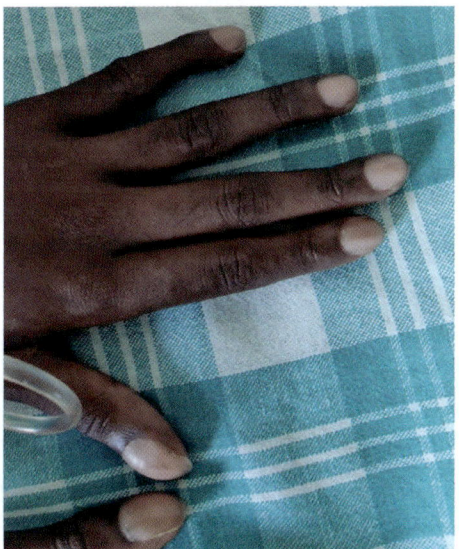

Fig. 21.2 Clubbing of nails.

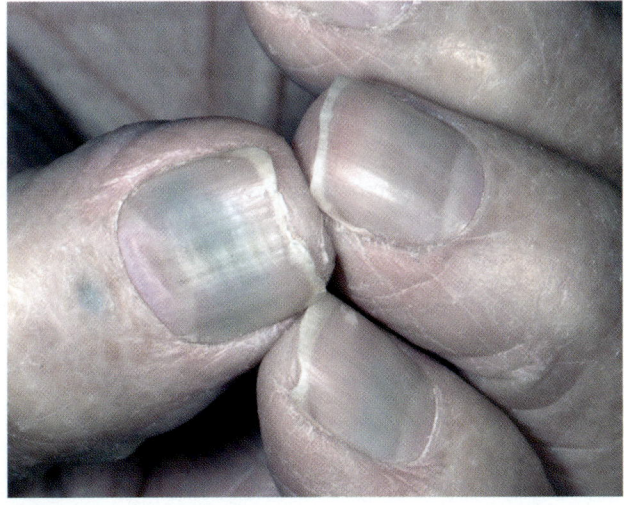

Fig. 21.3 Blue nails. (*Source: Reproduced from James Dinulos. Habif's Clinical Dermatology: A Color Guide to Diagnosis and Therapy, Seventh Edition, Acne, Rosacea, and Related Disorders, FIG 7.35, London, Elsevier Inc., 2021.*)

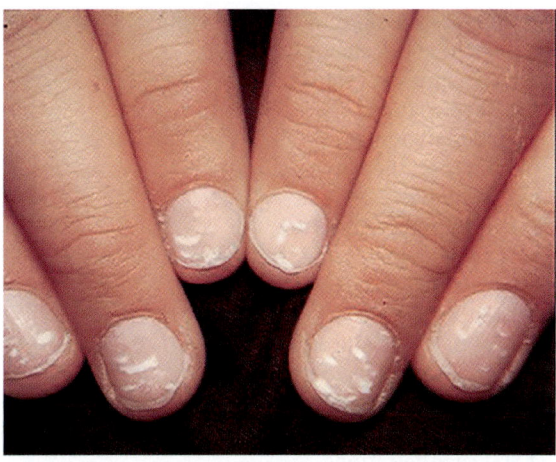

Fig. 21.4 Leukonychia. (*Source: https://www.google.co.in/url?sa=i&url= https%3A%2F%2Fwww.medicinenet.com%2Fimage-collection% 2Fleukonychia_striata_picture%2Fpicture.htm&psig=AOvVaw0coHzKthTO HEhMtdrJXZeu&ust=1613025357221000&source=images&cd=vfe&ved= 0CAIQjRxqFwoTCND26u_Z3u4CFQAAAAAdAAAAABAP)*)

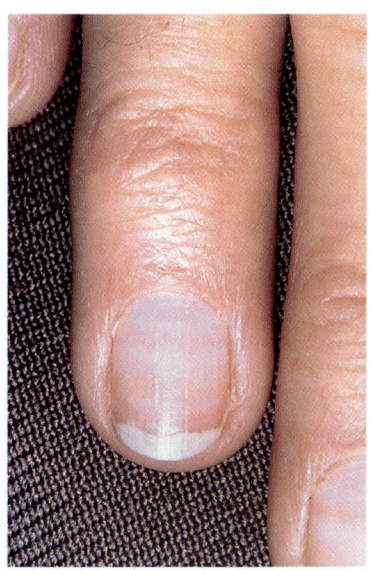

Fig. 21.5 Muehrcke lines. (*Source: Reproduced from William D. James, Dirk Elston, James R. Treat. Andrews' Diseases of the Skin: Clinical Dermatology, Thirteenth Edition, Diseases of the Skin Appendages, Fig. 33.48, London, Elsevier Inc., 2020.*)

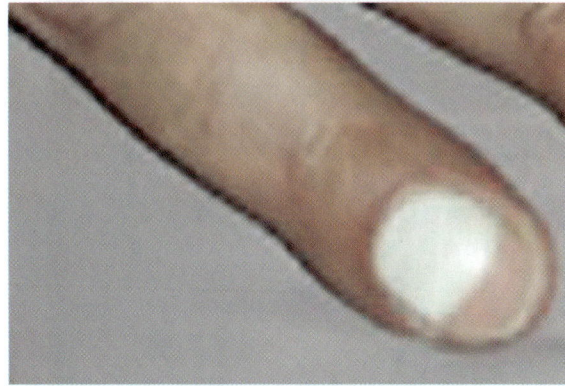

Fig. 21.6 Terry nail. (*Source: https://www.google.co.in/url?sa=i&url= https%3A%2F%2Fonlinelibrary.wiley.com%2Fdoi%2Ffull%2F10.1111% 2Fj.1440-1746.2012.07184.x&psig=AOvVaw2vEUxmcYFQjlgyXXfDp7j0& ust=1613025451003000&source=images&cd=vfe&ved=0CAIQjRxqFwo TCPiyiJ_a3u4CFQAAAAAdAAAAABAD)*)

*8. enumerate the signs of liver cell failure.
- Parotid enlargement
- Gynecomastia (Fig. 21.7)
- Fetor hepaticus
- Spider angiomas
- Palmar erythema
- Xanthomas
- Dupuytren contracture
- Nails − leukonychia, Muehrcke nails/Terry nails/blue lunulae
- Ascites
- Loss of pubic and axillary hair
- Signs of portal hypertension
- Signs of hepatic encephalopathy

9. Enumerate the extrahepatic manifestations of cirrhosis.
  a. GI manifestations
    - Upper GI bleeding
    - Gastroesophageal reflux
    - Pigment gallstones are common in cirrhosis because of:
      - Hemolysis secondary to hypersplenism
      - Decreased bile acid pool and bile stasis
      - Diarrhea due to bile acid deficiency, malabsorption, and malnutrition
      - Acute pancreatitis due to hypertriglyceridemia
      - Spontaneous bacterial peritonitis
  b. Hematologic manifestations
    Anemia in cirrhosis is caused by:
      - Nutritional anemia
      - Anemia of blood loss − GI bleeding
      - Hemolytic anemia − secondary to hypersplenism
      - Pancytopenia − due to hypersplenism
      - Coagulopathy
  c. Cardiovascular manifestations
    - Large volume pulse (due to AV (Aterio-venous) fistulas, vasodilators such as GABA (Gamma Amino Butyric Acid), prostaglandins, VIP (Vasoactive Intestinal Polypeptide), substance P, and nitric oxide)
    - High output cardiac failure .

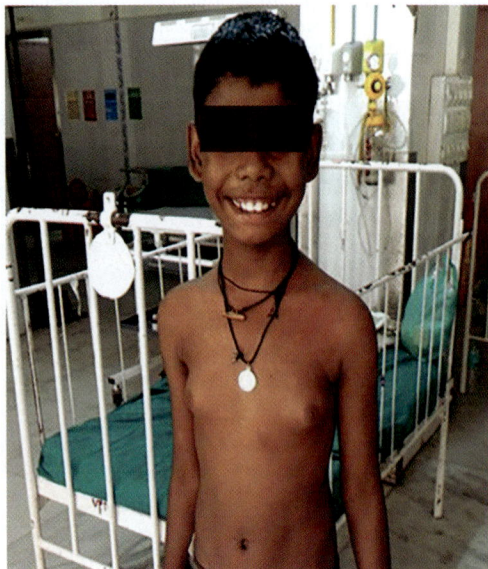

Fig. 21.7 Gynecomastia.

  d. Dermatologic manifestations (as mentioned in Q. 5 and 6)
  e. Endocrinologic manifestations
    - Gynecomastia and decreased pubic and axillary hair
    - Delayed puberty
    - Diabetes mellitus
    - Decreased libido, decreased facial hair and impotence in the adolescent
  f. Nutritional manifestations
    - Anorexia
    - Malabsorption
    - Steatorrhea
    - Hypoalbuminemia
    - Deficiency of fat-soluble vitamins
    - PEM is common in decompensated cirrhosis and is caused by all the above-mentioned factors
  g. Neurological manifestations
    - Intracranial bleeding
    - Hepatic encephalopathy
    - Seizures
    - Extrapyramidal signs (in cirrhosis secondary to Wilson disease)
    - Psychiatric manifestations
  h. Pulmonary manifestations
    - Hepatopulmonary syndrome
    - Portopulmonary hypertension
    - Pleural effusion
  i. Renal manifestations
    - Hepatorenal syndrome
    - Hematuria − secondary to coagulopathy

10. What are the causes of hypogonadism in cirrhosis?
    Hypserestrogenism (males) and suppression of HPA axis

*11. What is the mechanism of portal hypertension in cirrhosis?
    - Sinusoidal obstruction.
    - Splanchnic vasodilatation due to increased nitric oxide. This is also responsible for hyperdynamic circulation.

12. Describe the mechanism of ascites in cirrhosis.
    - Hypoalbuminemia.
    - Splanchnic vasodilatation resulting in reduced systemic perfusion and activation of renin−angiotensin system. This results in water and sodium retention.
    - Percolation of hepatic lymph into peritoneal cavity.

13. What is the cause for A:G reversal in DCLD?
    - Hypoalbuminemia due to reduced hepatic synthetic function
    - Hypergammaglobulinemia − due to reduced Kupffer cell activity, microorganisms from gut reach the systemic circulation where they activate the B lymphocytes leading to increased immunoglobulin production

14. List the complications of cirrhosis.
    - Portal hypertension
    - Coagulopathy
    - Ascites
    - Hepatorenal syndrome
    - Hepatic encephalopathy
    - Hepatopulmonary syndrome
    - Portopulmonary hypertension
    - Osteopenia
    - Malnutrition
    - Fat malabsorption
    - Hypogonadism

*15. Enumerate the causes of bleeding in a patient with DCLD.
- Reduced clotting factor synthesis
- Reduced clearance of anticoagulants
- Vitamin K deficiency
- Thrombocytopenia due to hypersplenism

16. List the investigations to be carried out in DCLD.
A. Liver function tests
- Serum bilirubin
- Transaminases
- A low serum albumin with a normal or elevated globulin is common in cirrhosis
- Alkaline phosphatase, gamma-glutamyl transpeptidase, 5-nucleotidase, and cholesterol are elevated in biliary cirrhosis
B. Investigations for complications
- CBC (Complete Blood Count) – elevated TLC (Total Leucocyte Count) in spontaneous bacterial peritonitis
- Pancytopenia
- RFT (Renal Function Test) – may be abnormal in hepatorenal syndrome
- Coagulation profile
- USG abdomen
- Upper GI endoscopy – look for varices, congestive gastro-pathy
C. Investigations for etiology
Tests for infections
- HBV, HCV
Tests for metabolic liver diseases
Wilson disease:
- Alpha-1 antitrypsin deficiency: Serum alpha-1 antitrypsin level and serum protein electrophoresis
- Glycogen storage disease: Fasting blood sugar level, lactic acid, uric acid, lipid profile, and liver and muscle tissue enzyme levels
- Hereditary tyrosinemia type 1: Serum amino acids and urine succinylacetone
- Galactosemia: Fasting blood sugar level, urine reducing sugar and RBC galactose-1-phosphate uridyl transferase
- Hemochromatosis: Serum iron, ferritin, and total iron-binding capacity
Cystic fibrosis:
- Elevated sweat chloride level abnormal nasal potential difference/identification of two CF mutations
Autoimmune cause:
- ANA (Anti-Nuclear Antibody), anti–smooth-muscle antibody, antibodies to LKM (Liver-Kidney-Microsome)
USG Doppler:
- To rule out Budd–Chiari syndrome and IVC (Inferior Vena Cava) obstruction

17. Define hepatic encephalopathy (HE).
It is defined as the presence of neuropsychiatric manifestations in a patient with acute/chronic liver disease.

18. Describe the etiological classification of hepatic encephalopathy.
Etiological classification of hepatic encephalopathy (2015) – American Association for the Study of Liver Disease

A: Associated with acute liver failure
B: Associated with portosystemic bypass in the absence of structural liver disease
C: Associated with cirrhosis

*19. Explain the West Haven grading of hepatic encephalopathy.
West Haven grading of hepatic encephalopathy is given in Table 21.1

20. What is the newer classification of hepatic encephalopathy?
Table 21.2 gives newer – International Society for Hepatic Encephalopathy and Nitrogen Metabolism (ISHEN) – classification of hepatic encephalopathy.

21. Enumerate the factors precipitating hepatic encephalopathy.
- Infection – most common in children
- Hypokalemia
- Metabolic alkalosis
- High protein diet
- Constipation
- UGI bleeding
- Dehydration
- Benzodiazepines

22. Enumerate the management of hepatic encephalopathy.
Management of hepatic encephalopathy is enumerated in Table 21.3.

23. What is critical flicker frequency threshold?
- It is used to identify low-grade HE.
- It is based on the ability to identify the point of switch over from steady red light to flickering light.
- A normal human eye can identify flicker at a frequency of 60 Hz, whereas patients with hepatic encephalopathy can identify flicker only at a rate of 39 Hz.
- This test can be used only in children older than 8 years.

24. List the false neurotransmitters in HE.
- Tyramine
- Octopamine
- Beta-phenylethanolamine

*25. Explain the Child–Pugh score.
Child–Pugh score is given as follows.
For parameters, remember A, B, C, D, E:
A: Albumin ->3.5 (score 1), 3.5-3 (score 2), and <3 (score 3)
B: Bilirubin -<2 (score 1), 2-3 (score 2), and >3 (score 3)
C: Coagulopathy (PT seconds prolonged) -<4 (score 1), 4-6 (score 2), and >6 (score 3)
D: Distension - None (score 1), easily controlled (score 2), and Poorly controlled (score 3)
E: Encephalopathy stage - None (score 1), stages 1 and 2 (score 2) and stages 3 and 4 (score 3)

TABLE 21.1	West Haven Grading of Hepatic Encephalopathy		
Stage	**Symptoms**	**Signs**	**EEG**
1	Periods of lethargy, euphoria, altered sleep pattern	Trouble drawing figures and performing mental tasks	Normal
2	Disorientation, agitation, mood swings	Asterixis, incontinence and fetor hepaticus	Generalized slowing, q wave
3	Stupor but arousable, incoherent speech	Asterixis, hyper-reflexia, rigidity	Abnormal triphasic waves
4	a Pain responsive b Unresponsive	Areflexia, flaccidity	Markedly abnormal slowing, d waves

TABLE 21.2	**ISHEN Classification of Hepatic Encephalopathy**	

Old Classification	Symptoms and Signs	ISHEN (International Society for Hepatic Encephalopathy and Nitrogen Metabolism) Classification
Unimpaired		No present or previous HE
Minimal HE	Psychometric or neuropsychological alterations without clinical evidence of mental change	Covert HE
Grade 1	Trivial lack of awareness Shortened attention span Euphoria or anxiety Impaired performance of addition	
Grade 2	Lethargy or apathy Minimal disorientation for time or place Subtle personality change Inappropriate behavior Impaired performance of subtraction	Stage 2 overt HE
Grade 3	Somnolence to semistupor, but responsive to verbal stimuli Confusion Gross disorientation	Stage 3 overt HE
Grade 4	Coma (unresponsive to verbal or noxious stimuli)	Stage 4 overt HE

Source: Modified from Vilstrup H, Amodio P, Bajaj J, et al.: Hepatic encephalopathy in chronic liver disease: 2014 Practice Guideline by the American Association for the Study of Liver Diseases and the European Association for the Study of the Liver. Hepatology. 2014; 60(2): 715–35.

TABLE 21.3	**Management of Hepatic Encephalopathy**	

Investigations	Treatment
• Sepsis work-up	• Manage Airway, Breathing, Circulation and Disability — grade 3/4 requires mechanical ventilation and treatment of raised ICT
• Serum electrolytes/blood sugar	• Low-protein diet
• Serum ammonia	• To reduce ammonia production — ampicillin, lactulose, and bowel wash
• Coagulation profile	• To increase ammonia metabolism — sodium benzoate, zinc (increases urea production)
• CT brain — to rule out intracranial hemorrhage and cerebral edema	• Treat the precipitating factors

- Class A: Score up to 6
- Class B: 7−9
- Class C: 10 or more

The Child−Pugh scoring is a reliable scoring system to determine
  - The prognosis
  - The likelihood of complications (bleeding from cirrhosis, spontaneous bacterial peritonitis)
  - The need for transplantation (classes B and C)

26. What is PELD score?
- **P**ediatric **E**nd-stage **L**iver **D**isease
- Parameters − age, albumin, bilirubin, INR, and nutritional status
- Used for children younger than 12 years

27. Define fulminant hepatic failure.
- Biochemical evidence of liver injury in <8 weeks duration
- No pre-existing liver disease
- Coagulopathy not corrected by vitamin K
- INR: 1.5−1.9 or PT 15–19 seconds in the presence of encephalopathy or
- INR: >1.9 or PT >19 seconds irrespective of encephalopathy

28. List the indications for liver transplantation.
- EHBA − the most common indication
- Cholestatic and metabolic liver disease
- Fulminant hepatic failure
- Autoimmune liver disease
- Chronic hepatitis with cirrhosis: hepatitis B or C
- Graft versus host disease
- Tumors

29. Enumerate the various types of liver transplantation.
A. Orthotopic liver transplantation: In this procedure, the recipient's liver is removed.

   Whole orthotopic liver transplantation involves excision of the diseased liver, by the division of the common bile duct, hepatic artery, portal vein, and IVC above and below the liver. Orthotopic liver replacement is accomplished by anastomosis of the corresponding structures with the donor liver and achieving hemostasis.

   Partial orthotopic transplantation: Left lateral segment of the donor is transplanted.

   Living donor liver transplantation: A portion of liver from a parent or a sibling is removed and placed in the diseased person.

B. Auxiliary liver transplantation: In this procedure, the recipient's liver is not removed completely. It is particularly useful in children with acute liver failure and inborn errors of metabolism.

DISCUSSION ON WILSON DISEASE

30. Describe the normal metabolism of copper in the body.
    - Approximately 40%–60% of ingested copper is absorbed, the rest is passed in stools.
    - Flowchart 21.2 gives metabolism of copper in the body.
31. Enumerate the clinical features of Wilson disease (ESPGHAN (European Society of Paediatric Gastroenterology Hepatology and Nutrition) and NSPGHAN (North American Society of Paediatric Gastroenterology Hepatology and Nutrition), 2018) enumerates clinical features of Wilson disease in Table 21.4.
32. Explain the significance of Kayser−Fleischer ring. Fig. 21.8 shows KF ring.
    - It is a greenish yellow ring, 1–3 mm in diameter seen in the periphery of the cornea. It starts at the inferior pole, then involves the superior pole and other parts of cornea.
    - It is an incomplete ring. There is a gap between the limbus and KF ring.
    - It is due to deposition of copper−sulfur complex in the Descemet's membrane.

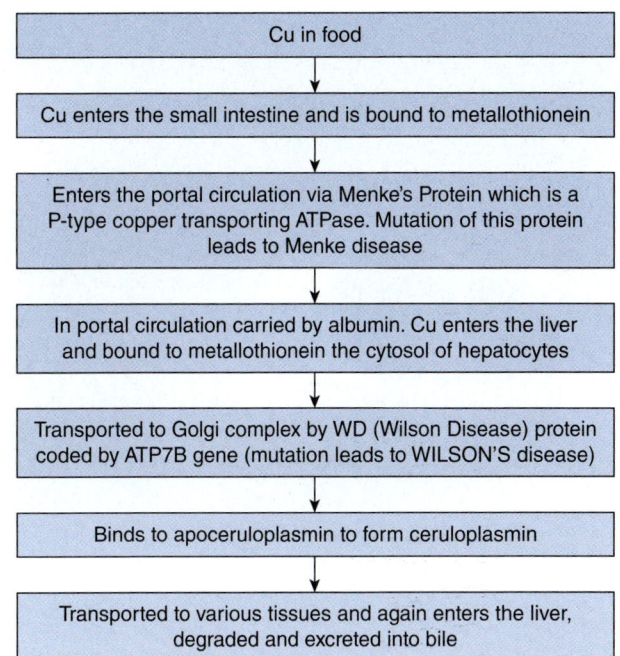

Flowchart 21.2 Metabolism of copper in the body.

TABLE 21.4	Clinical Features of Wilson Disease
Age at Onset of Symptoms	**Clinical Features**
2 years	Hepatic • Incidental finding of increased serum transaminases • Hepatomegaly • Fatty liver • Acute hepatitis • Acute liver failure with hemolysis • Portal hypertension: Esophageal varices, splenomegaly, and low platelet count • Decompensated cirrhosis with ascites
Older than 10 years	• Ophthalmic 　• KF ring 　• Sunflower cataract
Usually older than 15 years	• Neurological and psychiatric 　• Mood/behavior changes including depression and irritability 　• Declining performance at school 　• Incoordination (e.g., handwriting deterioration) 　• Resting and intention tremors 　• Stroke-like symptoms 　• Gait disturbance, dystonia, rigidity 　• Mask-like face, risus sardonicus 　• Dysarthria
Older than 17 years	• Hematological 　• Coombs negative − hemolytic anemia • Renal 　• Renal tubular dysfunction (Fanconi syndrome, tubular acidosis, aminoaciduria) 　• Nephrolithiasis 　• Nephrocalcinosis • Cardiac 　• Cardiomyopathy, subclinical dysfunction 　• Arrhythmia • Bone and joints 　• Bone fractures 　• Osteomalacia 　• Osteochondritis 　• Arthralgia • Others 　• Skin hyperpigmentation 　• Hypoparathyroidism 　• pancreatitis

The flowchart (21.2) contents:
- Cu in food
- Cu enters the small intestine and is bound to metallothionein
- Enters the portal circulation via Menke's Protein which is a P-type copper transporting ATPase. Mutation of this protein leads to Menke disease
- In portal circulation carried by albumin. Cu enters the liver and bound to metallothionein the cytosol of hepatocytes
- Transported to Golgi complex by WD (Wilson Disease) protein coded by ATP7B gene (mutation leads to WILSON'S disease)
- Binds to apoceruloplasmin to form ceruloplasmin
- Transported to various tissues and again enters the liver, degraded and excreted into bile

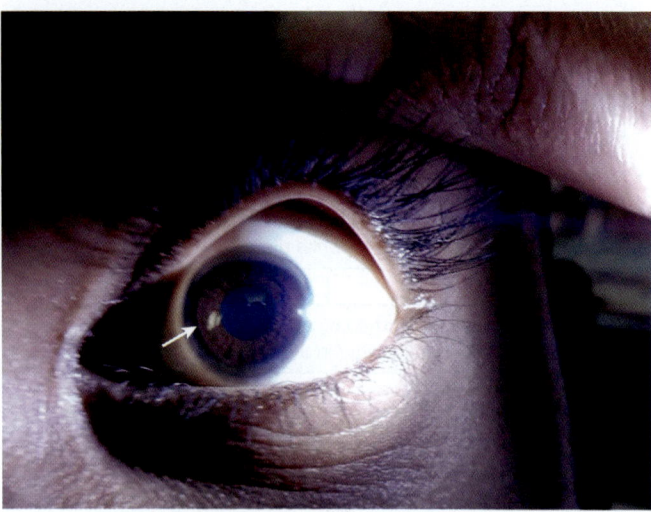

Fig. 21.8 Kayser–Fleischer (KF) ring.

TABLE 21.5	False-Positive and False-Negative Ceruloplasmin Conditions	
False-Positive Conditions		**False-Negative Conditions**
• Liver failure • Malabsorption • Glycosylation disorders • Menkes disease • Protein–energy malnutrition • Nephrotic syndrome • Protein-losing enteropathy • Acquired copper deficiency • Hereditary aceruloplasminemia		• Hyperestrogenic states • Acute inflammatory conditions

- It signifies the amount of copper load and duration of exposure to copper.
- It is present in 50% of patients with hepatic Wilson disease and 90% of patients with neuro Wilson disease.
- In early stages, it can be seen only with slit lamp examination. In late stages, it can be seen with +40D lens and also with naked eye.
- It does not affect the vision.
- It resolves completely with the treatment.

33. When to suspect Wilson disease?

   Wilson disease should be suspected in any children older than 1 year presenting with any of the following:
   - Asymptomatically increased serum transaminase level
   - Asymptomatic HSM
   - Cirrhosis
   - ALF
   - Any teenager with unexplained cognitive, psychiatric, or movement disorder

34. List the investigations to be performed in a patient with suspected Wilson disease.

   Liver function test:
   - Increased total bilirubin, increased ALT, AST, and ALP; Berman's ratio – ALP:total bilirubin < 2
   - If serum ceruloplasmin level is <20 mg/dL, suspect Wilson disease

   Table 21.5 gives conditions causing false-positive and false-negative ceruloplasmin.

   24-hour urine copper
   - Normal value < 40 µg
   - Wilson disease > 100 µg
   - Following D-penicillamine challenge (500 mg 12 hours apart), 24-hour urine copper level can be as high as >1600 µg

   Mutation analysis

   Liver biopsy
   - The size of specimen should be at least 1 cm to improve the accuracy
   - Normal: <50 µg/g of liver
   - Wilson disease: >250 µg/g of liver

- Disadvantages of liver copper:
  ○ Copper is not uniformly distributed in the liver giving rise to false-negative results
  ○ In acute fulminant hepatitis, copper may be released from necrosed hepatocytes giving rise to false-positive values
- Increased liver copper level is also seen in
  ○ Healthy children up to 14 months of life
  ○ Biliary atresia
  ○ Congenital disorders of glycosylation

Other liver biopsy findings:
- Early: Glycogen deposition and microvesicular steatosis
- Late: Mallory hyaline, macronodular cirrhosis, periportal fibrosis, and bridging necrosis

Radio-labelled copper assay

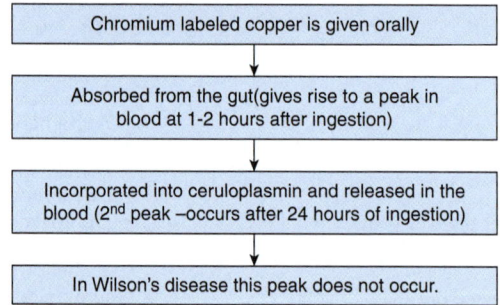

Chromium labeled copper is given orally

↓

Absorbed from the gut(gives rise to a peak in blood at 1-2 hours after ingestion)

↓

Incorporated into ceruloplasmin and released in the blood (2nd peak –occurs after 24 hours of ingestion)

↓

In Wilson's disease this peak does not occur.

35. Enumerate the stepwise approach to the diagnosis of Wilson disease.

   Stepwise approach to the diagnosis of Wilson disease is as follows (ESPGHAN and NASPGHAN, 2018):

   Step 1
   ○ Clinical evaluation – hepatosplenomegaly, ascites, and KF ring
   ○ Liver tests – bilirubin total/direct, INR, ALP, ALT/AST
   ○ Biochemical tests of copper metabolism – serum ceruloplasmin, 24-hour urinary copper excretion

   Step 2
   ○ Molecular testing evaluation for common mutations and whole gene sequencing

   Step 3
   ○ Liver copper (if molecular testing inconclusive or not available)
   ○ Ferenci score calculated at each step
   ○ 4 points or more confirm diagnosis – once diagnosis is confirmed, further testing is not required; start therapy directly

TABLE 21.6	**Ferenci Scoring System**				
Score	**−1**	**0**	**1**	**2**	**4**
Kayser−Fleischer rings		Absent		Present	
Neuropsychiatric symptoms suggestive of Wilson disease (or typical brain MRI)		Absent		Present	
Coombs negative − hemolytic anemia, high serum copper		Absent	Present		
Urinary copper (in the absence of acute hepatitis)		Normal	1–2 times ULN ((Upper Limit of Normal)	>2 times ULN or >5 times ULN 1 day after, challenge test with two doses of 0.5 g D-penicillamine	
Liver copper quantitative	Normal		<250 mg/g	>250 mg/g	
Rhodanine-positive hepatocytes (only if quantitative copper measurement is not available)		Absent	Present		
Serum ceruloplasmin (nephelometric assay	>0.2 g/L	0.1–0.2 g/L	<0.1 g/L		
Disease-causing mutations detected		None	1		4

Note: 0–1, unlikely; 2–3, probable; 4 or more, highly likely.
Source: Psychiatric manifestations in Wilson's disease: possibilities and difficulties for treatment. March 2018. Therapeutic Advances in Psychopharmacology 8(7).DOI:10.1177/2045125318759461

*36. What is the Ferenci scoring system for the diagnosis of Wilson disease?
   Table: 21.6 gives Ferenci scoring system.

37. Describe the importance of family screening for Wilson disease.
   - All siblings of the patient with Wilson disease should be screened
   - Assessment should include:
     - Physical examination
     - Serum ceruloplasmin
     - Liver function tests
     - Molecular testing for ATP7B mutations
   - Considering the possibility of late-onset Wilson disease, ESPGHAN and NASPGHAN (2018) guidelines recommend the screening of the parents of the affected child.

38. What is the management of Wilson disease?
   Dietary management
     - Avoid cooking in copper vessels
     - Avoid copper-containing foods − nuts, chocolate, fish, and mushrooms
   Drugs:
     D-PENICILLAMINE
     - It does not decrease copper levels, but detoxifies copper
       - Dose: 20 mg/kg/day in three divided doses to be taken 1 hour or 2 hours after food
       Adverse effects
         - Agranulocytosis
         - SLE
         - Elastosis perforans serpiginosa
         - Cutis laxa
         - Pemphigus
         - Lichen planus aphthous
         - Stomatitis
       Response to treatment
         - Response is assessed by decrease in the urine copper
   Trientine
     - Same action as that of D-penicillamine
     - Same dose as that of D-penicillamine
   Zinc
     - It increases hepatocyte metallothionein and hence has a copper-detoxifying effect

   - It can be used for the maintenance therapy after initiating chelators and also as a monotherapy in asymptomatic patients
   Dose
     - For children younger than 6 years: 25 mg b.d.
     - For children older than 6 years: 25 mg t.d.s.
   BAL
     - It forms inert complex with copper in the blood, and hence reduces the toxic effect of copper
   Ammonium tetrathiomolybdate
     - Useful for neuro Wilson disease
     - Treatment of complications − ascites and portal hypertension
   Liver transplantation
     - Indications − decompensated liver disease and acute liver failure

39. List the patterns of drug-induced liver injury.
   Drug-induced liver injury and its pattern are given in Table 21.7.

TABLE 21.7	**Drug-Induced Liver Injury and Its Pattern**
Disease	**Drug**
Centrilobular necrosis	Acetaminophen Halothane
Microvesicular steatosis	Valproic acid
General hypersensitivity	Sulfonamides Phenytoin
Acute hepatitis	Isoniazid
Cholestasis	Chlorpromazine Erythromycin Estrogens
Fibrosis	Methotrexate
Portal and hepatic vein thrombosis	Estrogens Androgens
Veno-occlusive disease	Irradiation plus busulfan Cyclophosphamide
Hepatic adenoma or hepatocellular carcinoma	Oral contraceptives Anabolic steroids
Biliary sludge	Ceftriaxone

Quick Bites

- Chronic liver disease presents clinically by symptoms persisting for more than 6 months, firm/nodular liver, and signs of portal hypertension.
- Fibrosis, nodules, and distortion of hepatic vasculature are the three characteristic pathological features of cirrhosis.
- Infection is the most common precipitating factor of hepatic encephalopathy in children.
- The differentiation between covert hepatic encephalopathy and stage 2 covert hepatic encephalopathy is difficult in children because it requires their cooperation to perform psychometric tests.
- EHBA is the most common indication for liver transplantation in children.
- Wilson disease can present at any age between 3 and 74 years.
- Hepatic Wilson disease can present as asymptomatic HSM, acute hepatitis, ALF, and DCLD.
- Kayser−Fleischer does not affect the vision and resolves completely with treatment.
- Ferenci scoring system and mutational analysis aid in the diagnosis of Wilson disease in children. Liver biopsy should be considered in equivocal cases.
- Screening should be offered for siblings as well as the first-degree relatives of the patient.

22 EHPVO – Upper GI Bleeding

Following introduction, seek permission from the caregiver and introduce yourself to the patient before history elicitation, and identify the case.

Name____Age____Sex____Consanguinity____Order of birth____Place____Informant____

Presenting Complaints and Duration

- Vomiting of blood
- Brought for routine endoscopic procedure

History of Presenting Illness

- Blood vomiting – number of episodes, quantity, color, associated with clots, cool peripheries/altered sensorium, whether required hospitalization and blood transfusion
- Abdominal pain/retching
- Melena
- Jaundice
- Abdominal distension/pedal edema/breathlessness
- Routine endoscopic procedure:
  - Describe the initial event which resulted in the child undergoing this procedure
  - How often the child is undergoing the procedure
  - Medications given
  - Surgical procedures performed
  - Any blood transfusions given

COMPLICATIONS HISTORY

- Altered sensorium
- Oliguria
- Easy fatigability/breathlessness
- Dysphagia and vomiting
- Failure to gain weight/height

ETIOLOGY HISTORY

- Fever
- Drug intake
- Bleeding from other sites
- Erythematous rash/joint pain
- Diarrhea/dysentery
- Abdominal distension/jaundice

PAST HISTORY

- Trauma to the abdomen
- Similar episodes
- Whether the child was normal between the episodes
- Blood transfusion
- Drug intake
- Comorbidities – cardiac, renal, and bleeding disorders

PERINATAL HISTORY

- Neonatal sepsis (umbilical sepsis)
- Umbilical vein catheterization can result in EHPVO (Extrahepatic Portal Vein Obstruction)

DEVELOPMENT HISTORY

Age-appropriate milestone attained

DIETETIC HISTORY

By 24 hours recall method

IMMUNIZATION HISTORY

According to national immunization or IAP schedule

FAMILY HISTORY

Bleeding disorders and liver disorder in the family

SOCIOECONOMIC HISTORY

According to modified Kuppuswamy scale

Summary

A _____-year-old _____ child, presented with major/minor upper gastrointestinal (UGI) bleeding, with/without complications, probably variceal/nonvariceal bleeding

General Examination

- Patient's sensorium
- Pallor
- Icterus
- Clubbing
- Cyanosis
- Pedal edema
- Generalized lymphadenopathy

Head-to-Foot Examination

- Signs of liver cell failure
- Signs of Turner syndrome
- Petechiae/purpura
- Hyperpigmented lesions in oral cavity
- Hemangiomas
- Oral ulcers/perianal skin tags/pyoderma gangrenosum/erythema nodosum

Vital Signs

- Pulse
- BP

- Respiration — rate, rhythm, and type of respiration
- Temperature
- JVP

Anthropometry

- Short stature in Turner syndrome
- Failure to thrive in DCLD

Abdominal Examination

INSPECTION

- Distended in upper part/uniform distension
- Skin — stretched and shiny
- Scars
- Dilated veins
- Umbilicus — transverse slit, umbilical hernia
- Flanks — full or free
- Hernia orifices
- All quadrants move equally with respiration
- External genitalia – scrotal edema/vulval edema

PALPATION

- Warmth
- Tenderness
- Organomegaly
- Fluid thrill

PERCUSSION

- Shifting dullness
- Liver span

AUSCULTATION

- Bowel sounds
- Bruit

Other System Examination

CARDIOVASCULAR SYSTEM

Ejection systolic murmur due to anemia

RESPIRATORY SYSTEM

Features of pleural effusion

CENTRAL NERVOUS SYSTEM

Signs of hepatic encephalopathy

Diagnosis

A case of major/minor UGI bleeding
- Nonvariceal/variceal
- With or without signs of liver cell failure
- With/without complications
- Probable etiology

Frequently Asked Questions

1. Classify gastrointestinal bleeding.
   Flowchart 22.1 shows classification of UGI (Upper Gastrointestinal) bleeding.
2. What is the significance of age in UGI bleeding?
   - Classic hemorrhagic disease of newborn − most commonly presents as UGI bleeding at 2–7 days of life.
   - In newborns, UGI bleeding can also be due to swallowed maternal blood.
   - Extrahepatic portal hypertension most commonly presents at the age of 6 years.
3. What is the significance of gender in UGI bleeding?
   Turner syndrome can also present with telangiectasia causing UGI bleeding.
4. What are the presentations of UGI bleeding?
   - Hematemesis: It has a coffee ground color (due to conversion of Hb (Haemoglobin) to hematin in the presence of HCl (Hydrochloric Acid)). It can be bright red if there is an active bleeding.
   - Melena: It is defined as a passage of black, tarry foul-smelling stools which stick to the pan because of bleeding proximal to the ileocecal valve including an UGI bleeding.
   Approximately 15%–20% of UGI bleeding presents as melena without hematemesis.
     - Blood should be present in the GI tract for at least 12 hours and a minimum of 60 mL of blood is needed to cause melena.
     - Single episode of UGI bleeding can cause melena up to 6–7 days (easy to remember: Rule of 6 – blood should be present for at least minimum 6 hours in GI tract, 60 mL in quantity, can cause melena up to 6 days)
     - Black color results from bacterial breakdown of Hb in the gut.

*5. Differentiate major and minor UGI bleeding.
   Table 22.1 gives differences between major and minor UGI bleeding.
*6. Differentiate between variceal and nonvariceal bleeding.
   - Variceal bleeding is a painless bleeding, with sudden onset, not associated with retching/abdominal pain. It is usually a major bleeding.
   - Nonvariceal bleeding is usually associated with abdominal pain and retching. It is usually a minor bleeding.
7. Differentiate between variceal bleeding due to extrahepatic and intrahepatic portal hypertension.
   - Extrahepatic portal hypertension: UGI bleeding is the most common manifestation. Child is normal between the episodes of bleeding.
   - Intrahepatic portal hypertension: Child has other features of liver disease apart from UGI bleeding.
*8. Can anemia occur immediately after an episode of massive bleeding?
   Immediately following a massive bleeding, there is a significant reduction of plasma as well as the blood cells. Hence, there is no reduction in Hb. After this, there is a shift of fluid from extravascular space to compensate for volume loss, and hence anemia manifests usually at 72 hours following a major bleeding. Hence, it is important to give whole blood transfusion following such bleeding episode.
9. What are the causes of jaundice in a patient with EHPVO?
   - Hemolytic − due to hypersplenism
   - Hepatocellular − transfusion-related hepatitis
   - Obstructive − due to hypertensive portal biliopathy

---

*indicates important question asked in examination

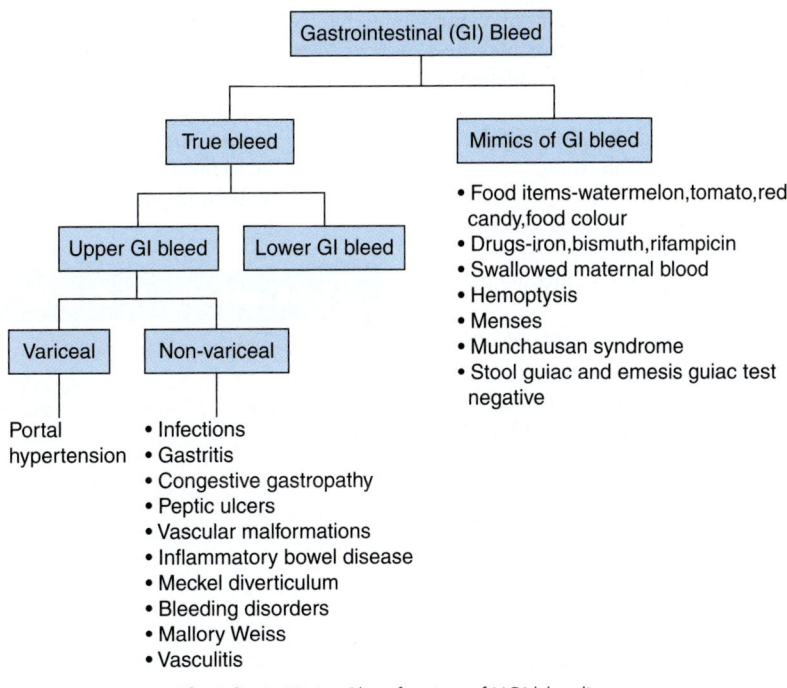

Flowchart 22.1 Classification of UGI bleeding.

TABLE 22.1	Differences Between Major and Minor UGI Bleeding	
Major Bleeding	**Minor Bleeding**	

Major Bleeding	**Minor Bleeding**
• Quantity: Handful, bright red in color, associated with clots, features of hypovolemic shock, requiring resuscitation, requiring blood transfusion	Quantity: Less, no features of shock, blood transfusion history not required, no need for resuscitation
• Variceal bleeding: Sudden onset, unprovoked painless, and massive bleeding	Nonvariceal bleed, associated with vomiting, retching, and heartburn
• Nonvariceal bleed: Associated with abdominal pain, retching, and retrosternal burn	
Signs of liver cell failure may be present	Signs of liver cell failure usually absent
Etiology: Portal hypertension, peptic ulcer, coagulopathy, polyp, and vascular malformation	Etiology: Inflammatory bowel disease, sepsis, trauma, erosive gastritis, drug-induced gastritis, GERD, Mallory–Weiss syndrome, and vasculitis

10. Mention some causes of breathlessness in UGI bleeding.
   • Major bleeding: Hypovolemia causing ischemia → lactic acidosis → breathlessness
   • Chronic anemia
   • DCLD (Decompensated Chronic Liver Disease) presenting with ascites
   • Patient with CCF (Congestive Cardiac Failure) presenting with congestive gastropathy, portopulmonary hypertension, and hepatopulmonary syndrome
*11. Enumerate causes of altered sensorium in UGI bleeding.
   • Major UGI bleeding — leading to hypovolemia
   • Hepatic encephalopathy
   • Cushing ulcer (due to head injury)
   • Sepsis
12. Mention some causes of abdominal pain in UGI bleeding.
   • Gastritis
   • Peptic ulcer
   • Barret ulcer
   • Congestive gastropathy
   • Budd–Chiari syndrome
   • HSP
13. List some complications in UGI bleeding.
   • Hypovolemic shock — history of altered sensorium
   • Prerenal AKI (Acute Kidney Injury) — history of oliguria
   • Anemia — history of easy fatiguability/breathlessness
   • Strictures secondary to sclerotherapy — history of dysphagia and vomiting
   • Chronic anemia — failure to gain weight/height
14. List the etiological histories in UGI bleeding.
   • Infection — history of fever
   • Drug-induced gastritis — history of drug intake
   • Coagulopathy — history of bleeding from sites
   • Henoch Schonlein Purpura (HSP) — history of erythematous rash/joint pain
   • Hemoconcentration → thrombosis → Budd–Chiari syndrome — history of diarrhea/dysentery
   • DCLD — history of abdominal distension/jaundice
15. What is the significance of past history in UGI bleeding?
   • Similar episodes — 30% of patients usually rebleed within 1 year of diagnosis
   • If the patient is symptom-free between the episodes, it is more likely to be EHPVO
   • Any history of drug intake — drug-induced gastritis
   • Bleeding from other sites/FFP (Fresh Frozen Plasma) transfusion — s/o coagulopathy
   • Renal failure — UGI bleeding due to uremic platelet dysfunction

16. What is the significance of neonatal history in UGI bleeding. Any umbilical vein catheterization and umbilical sepsis can result in EHPVO.
17. What is the significance of family history in UGI bleeding.
   • Bleeding disorders in the family
   • Liver disorders
   • Syndromic causes — Peutz–Jeghers syndrome/Ehlers–Danlos syndrome
18. List the examination findings in UGI bleeding.
   Table 22.2 gives examination findings in UGI bleeding.
19. List the significance of head-to-foot examination.
   • Signs of liver cell failure
   • Signs of Turner syndrome (GI vascular malformations)
   • Petechiae/purpura (HSP-Henoch Schonlein Purpura)
   • Hyperpigmented lesions in oral cavity — Peutz–Jeghers syndrome
   • Hemangiomas — GI vascular malformations
   • Oral ulcers/perianal skin tags/pyoderma gangrenosum/erythema nodosum — IBD (Inflammatory Bowel Disease)
   • Hyperextensible joints/lax skin — Ehlers–Danlos syndrome
20. What is the significance of vital signs?
   • Tachycardia/hypotension — may be found immediately following a major bleeding.
   • Bounding pulse and wide pulse pressure — may be suggestive of cirrhosis/anemia
   • Hypertension — due to COA (Coarctation of Aorta) seen in Turner syndrome
   • Tachypnea — due to shock/anemia/hepatopulmonary syndrome/portopulmonary hypertension

TABLE 22.2	Examination Findings in UGI Bleeding	
Clinical Finding	**Significance**	

Clinical Finding	**Significance**
• Patient's sensorium	Altered sensorium in hepatic encephalopathy/hypovolemic shock
• Pallor	Anemia secondary to bleeding, hypersplenism secondary to portal hypertension, inflammatory bowel disease
• Cyanosis	Hepatopulmonary syndrome
• Icterus	• Hemolytic — due to hypersplenism
	• Hepatocellular — transfusion-related hepatitis, DCLD
	• Obstructive — due to hypertensive portal biliopathy
• Clubbing	DCLD, inflammatory bowel disease
• Pedal edema	DCLD

- Fever − suggestive of infective causes of UGI bleeding
- JVP − negative hepatojugular reflex in Budd−Chiari syndrome

21 What is head-tilt test?

After tilting the head up to 45°, if the pulse rate increases by >20/min or diastolic pressure falls by >10 mm Hg, it is suggestive of volume loss of 25%. It is also seen in patients with autonomic dysfunction.

22. What is the significance of anthropometry in UGI bleeding?
- Short stature in Turner syndrome
- Failure to thrive – DCLD, anemia

23. List the findings in systemic examination.

Abdomen
- Distension – uniform distension is suggestive of ascites; upper abdominal distension is suggestive of organomegaly
- Flanks full – ascites
- Umbilicus – transverse slit – ascites
- Dilated veins – portal hypertension
- Tenderness – gastritis, peptic ulcer
- Organomegaly
- Cruveilhier−Baumgarten murmur

Cardiovascular system
- ESM due to anemia

Respiratory system
- Features of pleural effusion

Central nervous system
- Altered sensorium/signs of hepatic encephalopathy

24. List the investigations in UGI bleeding.
a. CBC (Complete Blood Count)
  - Hb: <8 g/dL – transfuse and maintain hemoglobin
  - Elevated TLC (Total Leucocyte Count) – infective cause
  - Pancytopenia – due to hypersplenism
b. RFT – elevated plasma urea:creatinine ratio following a massive bleeding (prerenal AKI)
c. LFT – deranged in DCLD/ischemic hepatitis following a massive bleeding

   A/G reversal – seen in cirrhotic liver, A:G ratio normal in noncirrhotic liver disease
d. USG abdomen findings in portal hypertension
  - Portal vein diameter >17 mm
  - Absence of increase in diameter during inspiration
  - Portal diameter:surface area >12
  - Collaterals greater than 1.7 times the aorta caliber
  - Thickening of lesser omentum/omentum congested
  - Splenomegaly
  - Ascites
  - Lesser omentum and aorta diameter ratio
e. Upper GI scopy
  - Diagnostic and therapeutic
  - To locate the site of bleeding and cause of bleeding
  - To grade the varices
  - Therapeutic – sclerotherapy and banding
f. Doppler study
  - Flow velocity, omentum:aorta ratio, pulsatility of varices
  - To determine the pressure gradient (mm Hg) between portal vein and IVC: 6–10, preclinical portal hypertension; 10–12, varices; >12, bleeding and ascites

g. Etiology work-up − to rule out infections, HSP, inflammatory bowel disease

*25. Enumerate the USG findings in a cirrhotic and a noncirrhotic liver.

Table 22.3 gives USG findings in a cirrhotic and a noncirrhotic liver.

26. List the etiologies of UGI bleeding (ISPGHAN, 2017).

Table 22.4 gives etiologies of UGI bleeding.

27. Mention few causes of lower GI bleeding (ISPGHAN (Indian Society of Paediatric Gastroenterology Hepatology and Nutrition), 2017).

Table 22.5 gives etiologies of lower GI bleeding.

*28. Define obscure gastrointestinal bleeding.

It is defined as bleeding of unknown origin with negative findings on bidirectional endoscopy. It can be classified as overt or occult on the basis of presence or absence of clinically evident bleeding. Obscure-occult bleeding is generally determined by a positive fecal occult blood test result and/or iron-deficiency anemia.

29. Enumerate the causes of obscure gastrointestinal bleeding.
- Small intestinal polyps
- Meckel diverticulum
- Vascular malformations
- Crohn disease
- Anastomotic ulcers
- Intestinal duplications

30. Give some hematological causes of EHPVO.

Thalassemia, hereditary spherocytosis, and splenic cyst

31. What is Smith−Howard syndrome?

In a patient with portal hypertension, following an episode of UGI bleeding, the spleen size reduces because of decrease in congestion.

32. Enumerate some causes of painful spleen.
- Sickle cell crisis
- Rheumatological vasculitis
- Paroxysmal nocturnal hemoglobinuria
- Splenic infarct

33. Mention few causes of bruit in spleen.
- Systemic mastocytosis
- Splenic hemangioma
- AV fistula

*34. Differentiate between portal vein obstruction and IVC obstruction.

Table 22.6 gives difference between portal vein and IVC obstruction.

TABLE 22.3	USG Findings in a Cirrhotic and a Noncirrhotic Liver	
Cirrhotic Liver	**Noncirrhotic Liver**
Altered liver echoes	Normal liver echoes
Portal vein – dilated and well seen	Portal vein malformations – cavernoma, portal vein obstruction, venae comitans
Collaterals – splenorenal, renorenal	Gastrosplenic collaterals common
Omental thickening	Absence of omental thickening

TABLE 22.4	Etiologies of UGI Bleeding		
Site	**<1 year**	**1–5 Years**	**>5 Years**
Esophagus		Esophagitis Esophageal varices Mallory–Weiss syndrome	Esophagitis Esophageal varices Mallory–Weiss syndrome
Stomach	Gastritis	Gastritis Gastric ulcer Gastric varices Vascular malformations Coagulopathy Infections	Gastritis Gastric ulcer Gastric varices Vascular malformations Coagulopathy Infections Dieulafoy lesion Congestive gastropathy Hemobilia
Duodenum		Duodenitis Duodenal ulcers	Duodenitis Duodenal ulcers
Variable location	Vitamin K deficiency Sepsis Trauma (from NG tube) Cow's milk protein allergy Coagulopathy	Caustic ingestion Foreign body Drugs	Caustic ingestion Foreign body Drugs Polyps Crohn disease Telangiectasia Aortoenteric fistula

Source: https://www.espghan.org/dam/jcr:d958c7e2-614e-47ec-9f41-0f929515b3ad/European_Society_for_Paediatric_Gastroenterology__Hepatology_ and_Nutrition_Position_on_Training_in_Paediatric_Endoscopy.pdf

TABLE 22.5	Etiologies of Lower GI Bleeding		
<1 Year	**1–5 Years**	**>5 Years**	
Nonspecific colitis	Polyps	Polyps	
Anal fissure	Anal fissure	Anal fissure	
Milk allergy	Infectious entero-colitis	Infectious entero-colitis	
Duplication of bowel	Intussusception	Intussusception	
Volvulus	Meckel diverticulum	Meckel diverticulum	
Hirschsprung disease	Henoch–Schönlein purpura	Henoch–Schönlein purpura	
Necrotizing enterocolitis	Hemolytic-uremic syndrome	Hemolytic-uremic syndrome	
Bleeding diathesis	Lymphonodular hyperplasia	Lymphonodular hyperplasia	
	Angiodysplasia	Angiodysplasia	
	Bleeding diathesis	Inflammatory bowel disease	
		Bleeding diathesis	

Source: https://www.espghan.org/dam/jcr:d958c7e2-614e-47ec-9f41-0f929515b3ad/European_Society_for_Paediatric_Gastroenterology__Hepatology_and_Nutrition_Position_on_Training_in_Paediatric_Endoscopy.pdf

35. Differentiate between extrahepatic and intrahepatic portal hypertension.

Table 22.7 gives differences between extrahepatic and intrahepatic portal hypertension.

*36. Describe various grading of varices.

Modified Paquet classification

    I. Varices extending just above mucosal surface

    II. Varices projecting up to one-third of lumen

    III. Varices projecting up to >50% of lumen

SARIN classification

    Gastroesophageal varices

        I. Along lesser curvature

        II. Along greater curvature

    Isolated gastric varices

        I. In fundus

        II. Anywhere in stomach

Fig. 22.1 shows Sarin classification of esophageal and gastric varices.

Grading of varices by UGI scopy

    I. Not visible on routine UGI scopy but visible on performing Valsalva maneuver

TABLE 22.6	Differences Between Portal Vein and IVC Obstruction
Portal Vein Obstruction	**IVC Obstruction**
Dilated veins in anterior abdominal wall	Dilated veins in flanks
Caput medusae +	Caput medusae absent
The direction of flow is away from umbilicus	The direction of blood flow is upward and toward umbilicus
Cruveilhier–Baumgarten murmur +	Cruveilhier–Baumgarten murmur absent

TABLE 22.7	Differences Between Extrahepatic and Intrahepatic Portal Hypertension	
Extrahepatic Portal Hypertension	**Intra-/Posthepatic Portal Hypertension**	
1. UGI bleeding/splenomegaly	UGI bleeding + splenomegaly + *DCLD* features	
2. Hepatic venous wedged pressure is normal	Hepatic venous wedge pressure is normal in presinusoidal and increased in postsinusoidal and posthepatic portal hypertension	
3. Hepatic encephalopathy uncommon	Common if there is *DCLD*	

Gastro-esophageal varices (GOV)

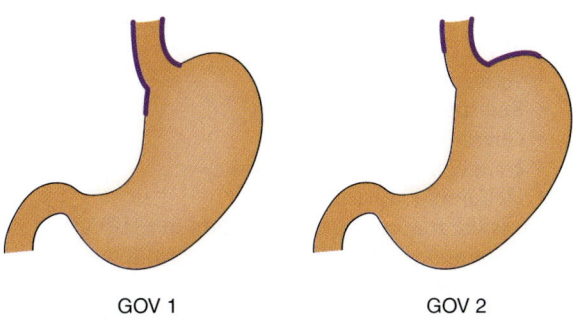

GOV 1   GOV 2

Isolated gastric varices (IGV)

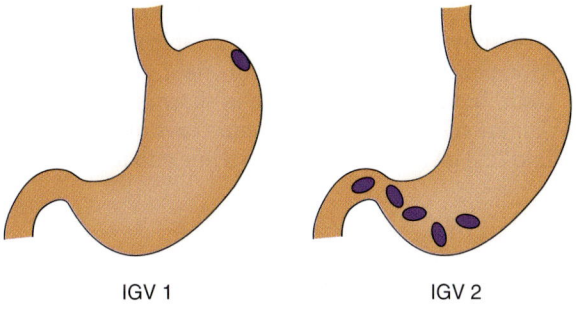

IGV 1   IGV 2

Fig. 22.1 Sarin classification of esophageal and gastric varices. (*Source: https://www.tigejournal.org/article/S1096-2883(04)00102-0/fulltext*)

II. Visible on routine UGI scopy
III. Visible and occludes half the lumen
IV. Visible and occludes more than two-third of lumen

37. List the findings in UGI scopy other than varices.
    - Gastric submucosal vascular ectasia — Dieulafoy disease
    - Watermelon stomach — angiomatous malformation of antrum of stomach
    - Barret ulcer/peptic ulcer
    - Polyps
    - Mallory—Weiss tear

38. Discuss the management of UGI bleeding.
    Flowchart 22.2 shows overall management of UGI bleeding.

*39. Mention dose and mechanism of action (MOA) of vasopressin/octreotide and other drugs used in UGI bleeding.
    Vasopressin (terlipressin)
    - MOA — splanchnic vasoconstriction, constricts lower esophageal sphincter, inhibits the release of vasodilatory peptides and glucagon
    - Dose — 0.3 U/kg infusion over 20 minutes followed by 0.3 U/kg/h
    - Adverse effects — myocardial infarction, bowel ischemia, and limb ischemia
    - Better tolerated — terlipressin because of less cardiac toxicity, and it acts by itself
    - If bleeding not controlled in 4–6 hours — stop the infusion
    Octreotide
    - It is a somatostatin analogue

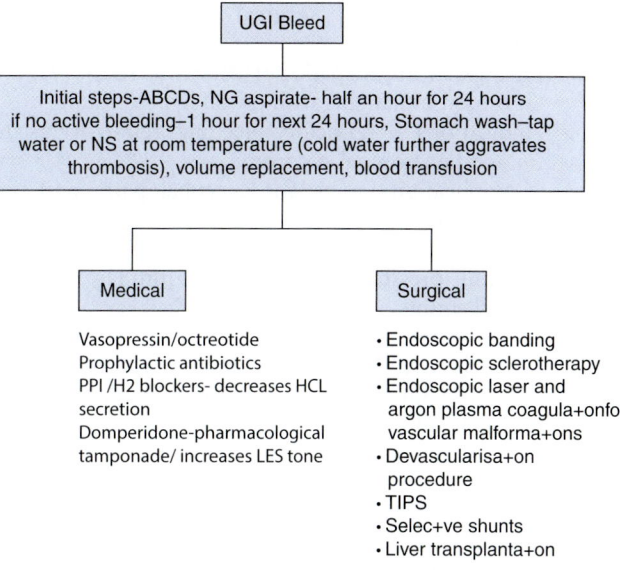

Flowchart 22.2 Management of UGI bleeding.

- MOA — splanchnic vasoconstriction/suppresses GI motility, and has a long half-life
- Dose — 1 microgram/kg bolus followed by 2–5 micrograms/kg/h infusion
- If there is no bleeding for 48 hours — taper and stop the infusion
- Adverse effects — flatulence/malabsorption
Other drugs in the management of UGI bleeding
- Nitrates, clonidine, ketanserine — decreases intrahepatic flow, thereby causing vasodilation

*42. What is the role of antibiotics and H2 blockers in UGI bleeding?
- Role of antibiotics: During UGI bleeding, bacterial translocation of the gut occurs and can lead to infection. Hence, i.v. ceftriaxone can be given.
- H2 blocker: They inhibit pepsin secretion which lyses the clot.

*44. Name some commonly used sclerosants.
    Ethanolamine oleate, sodium tetradecyl sulfate, polidocanol, ethoxy scleral, 50% dextrose, 5% sodium morrhuate: They are injected either intervariceal, paravariceal, or combined. Complications: Necrosis, hemorrhage, ischemia, bowel necrosis, respiratory arrest, pneumonitis, and retrosternal pain.

45. Name the drug used for prophylaxis of portal hypertension.
- Propranolol – reduces portal blood flow
- Therapeutic effect is thought to result when heart rate reduces by >25%

46. Enumerate the schedule of sclerotherapy.
    Surveillance UGI scopy should be performed once in 8 weeks, and depending on the grading, sclerotherapy can be performed once in 6–12 months. Endoscopy is therapeutic as well as diagnostic.

47. Mention few indications for surgery in EHPVO.
- Failure of EST
- Hypersplenism
- Child living in remote areas or with rare blood groups
- Growth retardation

48. Enumerate various surgical procedures for UGI bleeding.

    Transjugular intrahepatic portosystemic shunt (TIPSS)

    It is used in patients with portal hypertension

    Indications − refractory bleeding, refractory ascites, and hepatorenal syndrome

    Complications − hepatic encephalopathy and stent stenosis

    A successful TIPSS results in reduction of portosystemic pressure gradient to 8–12 mm Hg

    Surgical shunts

    Nonselective portosystemic shunts

    - These shunts decompress the portal venous pressure but result in hepatic encephalopathy

    Selective shunts

    - Warren shunt (distal splenorenal shunt) − most commonly used shunt
    - Rex shunt (mesenterico-left portal bypass)

    Devascularization surgery

    - Sugiura operation

    Esophageal transaction + splenectomy + esophagogastric devascularization + truncal vagotomy + pyeloplasty

49. Mention the predictors of bleed in a child with esophageal varices.

    The following are the predictors of bleeding in esophageal varices:

    - Grade 3/4 varices
    - Red spots – red whale sign
    - Cherry red spot
    - Daughter varices (varices on a varix)
    - Hemocystic varices

50. What is the role of blood transfusion in EHPVO?

    - Maintain the target Hb of 8 g/dL to avoid overtransfusion because it causes increase in pressure → increases the collateral flow → increases the chance of bleeding.

51. Describe the anatomy of portal vein.

    - Anatomy: It is 8 cm long and 12 mm in diameter. It is formed by the union of superior mesenteric vein and splenic behind the neck of pancreas at the level of L2 vertebra. Normal portal venous pressure is 7–10 mm Hg.
    - Tributaries: Superior mesenteric, splenic vein, superior pancreaticoduodenal vein, right and left gastric vein, and para umbilical vein as shown in Fig. 22.2.

52. What are the sites of portosystemic anastomosis?

    Table 22.8 gives sites of portosystemic anastomosis.

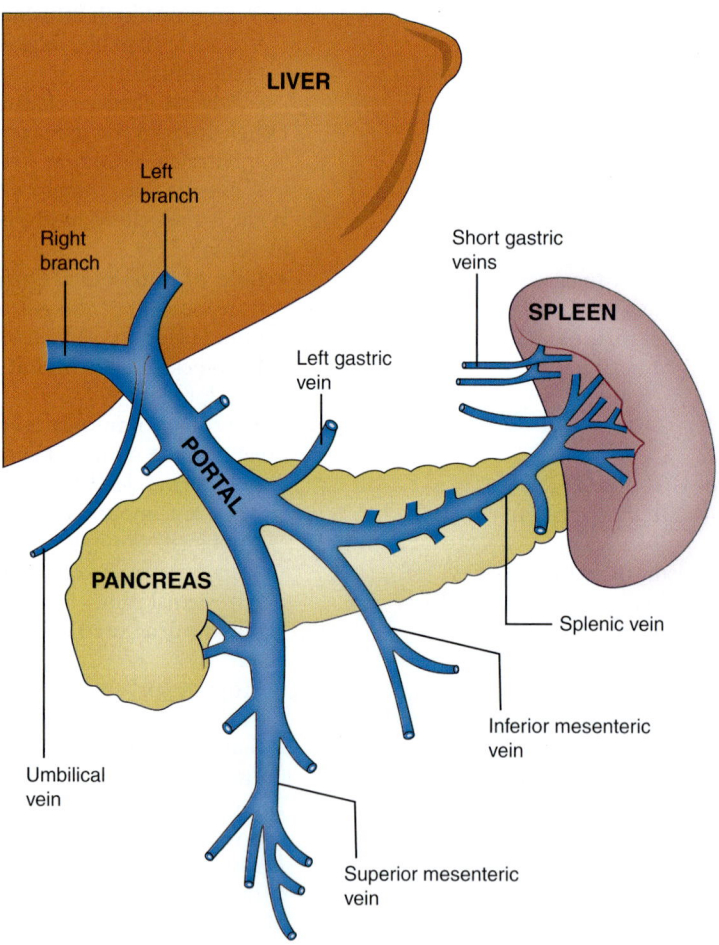

Fig. 22.2 Anatomy of portal vein and its tributaries. (*Source: https://www.google.com/imgres?imgurl=https%3A%2F%2Fi.pinimg.com%2F736x%2F4d%2Fb2%2F38%2F4db238b104c5fbc33555df655f95981e.jpg&imgrefurl=https%3A%2F%2Fza.pinterest.com%2Fpin%2F709528116268914850%2F&tbnid=4DiMieGJsos-M&vet=10CAMQxiAoAGoXChMI2Ne6hcvu7gIVAAAAAB0AAAAAEBQ..i&docid=XJbxt-peAQ0TM&w=638&h=479&itg=1&q=anatomy%20of%20portal%20vein%20and%20tributaries&ved=0CAMQxiAoAGoXChMI2Ne6hcvu7gIVAAAAAB0AAAAAEBQ)*

TABLE 22.8	Sites of Portosystemic Anastomosis	
Site	Portal	Systemic
Anterior abdominal wall	Left branch of portal vein	Umbilical vein
Lower end of esophagus	Left gastric	Azygous and hemiazygous vein
Lower end of rectum	Superior rectal vein	Middle and inferior rectal vein
Posterior abdominal wall	Veins of retroperitoneal organs	Veins of posterior abdominal wall
Liver	Hepatic venules	Phrenic and intercostal veins

Quick Bites

- The most common cause of UGI bleeding in children is variceal bleeding secondary to portal hypertension.
- Approximately 15%–20% of UGI bleeding can present as melena without hematemesis.
- Vomiting of bright red blood is indicative of ongoing UGI bleeding.
- A patient presenting with recurrent episodes of painless major UGI bleeding and normal between the episodes is more likely to have EHPVO.
- A patient with EHPVO can also present with jaundice.
- UGI scopy is both diagnostic and therapeutic.
- Endoscopic banding and variceal ligation are the treatment of choice for bleeding varices.

Neonatal Cholestasis Syndrome

Following introduction, seek permission from the caregiver and introduce yourself to the patient before history elicitation, and identify the case.

Name____Age____Sex____Consanguinity____Order of birth____Place____Informant____

Presenting Complaints and Duration

Yellowish discoloration of the eyes/skin and urine

History of Presenting Illness

- Describe the onset and duration of jaundice
- Whether associated with clay-colored stools
- Abdominal distension — upper abdomen or uniform distension
- Associated with swelling of legs/puffiness of face/ breathlessness incessant cry, skin rashes/scratch marks

COMPLICATIONS HISTORY

- Hematemesis
- Melena
- Altered sensorium/seizures in the absence of fever
- Skin swellings
- Oily stools
- Bony deformities

ETIOLOGY HISTORY

- Fever
- Early-morning seizures/repeated vomiting/failure to thrive
- Abnormal facies/swelling in the umbilicus
- Delayed passage of meconium

COURSE DURING HOSPITALIZATION

Any blood transfusion/drugs

ANTENATAL HISTORY

- History suggestive of TORCH infections
- Hypothyroidism
- Acute fatty liver of pregnancy/recurrent fetal loss
- Drug intake by mother – sulfonamides, nitrofurantoin, and antimalarials
- Regular i.v. infusions
- Scan abnormalities such as oligo-/polyhydramnios
- Any sepsis near term/timing of ROM (Rupture of Membranes) and timing of delivery

NATAL HISTORY

- Term or preterm

- Birth weight
- Birth asphyxia

POSTNATAL HISTORY

- Meconium history
- Sepsis
- Total parental nutrition
- Any seizures
- Volume of cry
- Jaundice, need for exchange transfusion
- Intolerance to feed

PAST HISTORY

Any history of drug intake, native medications, and blood transfusion

DEVELOPMENT HISTORY

Any developmental delay

DIETETIC HISTORY

Exclusive breastfeeding, any calorie deficit

IMMUNIZATION HISTORY

According to national or IAP (Indian Academy of Paediatrics) immunization schedule

FAMILY HISTORY

- Metabolic disorders
- Previous sibling death (metabolic diseases)
- Hemolytic diseases

Summary

A _____ -month-old child, aged _____, presented with yellowish discoloration of eyes/skin and urine ___days, with/without clay-colored stools, with/without complica-tions, probably a case of neonatal cholestasis (intrahepatic/extrahepatic)

General Examination

- Whether sick looking
- Sensorium
- Pallor
- Icterus
- Cyanosis
- Clubbing
- Edema
- Generalized lymphadenopathy

Head-to-Foot Examination

- Head
  - Microcephaly
  - Bulging AF (Anterior Fontanelle)
  - Wide-open fontanelles
- Dysmorphic facies
- Eyes:
  Pallor, icterus, epicanthic folds, bitot spots, posterior embryotoxon, Brushfield spots in the iris, cataract, chorioretinitis, cherry red spot, and papilledema
- Macroglossia
- Spider angiomas
- Palmar erythema, petechiae, ecchymosis
- Xanthomas
- Bony deformities
- Dilated veins in the abdominal wall
- Umbilical hernia
- Scratch marks of anklets in lower limbs
- Midline defects, micropenis
- Blueberry muffins

Vitals Signs

- Temperature
- Pulse rate
- Respiration – rate, rhythm, type of respiration
- Blood pressure
- JVP (Jugular Venous Pressure)

Anthropometry

- Failure to thrive
- Microcephaly

Abdominal Examination

INSPECTION

- Distended in upper part/uniform distension
- Skin – stretched and shiny
- Scars
- Dilated veins
- Umbilicus – transverse slit, umbilical hernia

- Flanks – full or free
- Hernia orifices
- All quadrants move equally with respiration
- External genitalia – micropenis, scrotal edema/vulval edema

PALPATION

- Warmth
- Tenderness
- Organomegaly
- Fluid thrill

PERCUSSION

- Shifting dullness
- Liver span

AUSCULTATION

- Bowel sounds
- Bruit

Other System Examination

CARDIOVASCULAR SYSTEM

Any ejection systolic murmur (ESM)

RESPIRATORY SYSTEM

Look for signs of bronchiectasis and pleural effusion.

CENTRAL NERVOUS SYSTEM

Hypotonia; look for the signs of hepatic encephalopathy and raised ICT (Intracranial Tension).

Diagnosis

- A case of neonatal cholestasis
- Probably intrahepatic/extrahepatic
- With/without complications
- Probable etiology

Frequently Asked Questions

*1. Define neonatal cholestasis.
- Cholestasis is the obstruction of bile flow anywhere from the hepatocyte canalicular membrane to the duodenum. It is defined:
- Clinically as yellowish discoloration of eyes and urine with/without clay-colored stools.
- Pathologically as histological presence of bile in hepatocyte and bile duct with secondary cell injury.
- Biochemically as persistent elevation of serum conjugated bilirubin beyond first 14 days of life.

2. What is the significance of age in neonatal cholestasis?
Age is a predictor of outcome in a child with EHBA (Extrahepatic Biliary Atresia). Kasai procedure has an outcome of 90% when performed before 8 weeks.

3. Enumerate the histories to be elicited when the mother reports yellowish discoloration of the eyes in a child.
- Urine is high colored/staining of diapers seen in hepatocellular jaundice
- Stools are pigmented/clay-colored (persistently pigmented stools rules out EHBA; however, persistent clay-colored stools does not always suggest EHBA because it can be seen in late stages of intrahepatic cholestasis also).
  Fig. 23.1 shows clay-colored stools. (The mother is asked to collect 3 consecutive day early-morning stool sample in an empty glass tube.)

4. What are the other features of cholestasis?
Pruritus and abdominal distension

5. What does fever in a patient with neonatal cholestasis syndrome (NCS) signify?
- Sepsis
- Cholangitis
- Recurrent respiratory tract infection (due to cystic fibrosis)

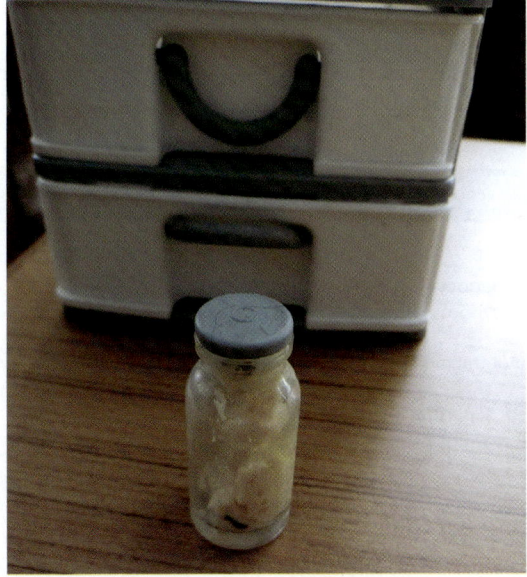

Fig. 23.1 Clay-colored stools.

6. What are the types of jaundice?
- Hemolytic
- Hepatocellular
- Obstructive
- Mixed (gallstones seen in patients with hemolytic anemia)

*7. What are the complications of cholestasis?
- Secondary biliary cirrhosis
- Portal hypertension
- Coagulopathy
- Fat malabsorption
- Deficiency of fat-soluble vitamins
- Failure to thrive

8. Enumerate the causes of altered sensorium in NCS.
- Hepatic encephalopathy
- Raised ICT secondary to intracranial bleeding
- Sepsis
- Metabolic liver disease

9. List the causes of seizures in NCS.
- Metabolic liver disease
- Hepatic encephalopathy
- Raised ICT
- Sepsis

10. What history is suggestive of pruritus in an infant?
History of incessant cry (<6 months) and frequent rubbing of legs (results in increased noise of anklets — the mother usually perceive this as a happy and playful child).

*11. Enumerate the etiological histories in neonatal cholestasis.
- Sepsis — fever
- Metabolic liver disease — early-morning seizures/repeated vomiting/failure to thrive
- Congenital hypothyroidism — history of abnormal facies/swelling in the umbilicus/delayed passage of meconium
- Cystic fibrosis — delayed passage of meconium

12. What are the significant antenatal histories in NCS.
- TORCH infections (maternal fever, rash)
- Hypothyroidism
- Acute fatty liver of pregnancy
- Recurrent fetal loss (neonatal iron storage disease)
- Drug intake by mother – sulfonamides, nitrofurantoin, and antimalarials; any regular i.v. infusions (IVIG (Intravenous Immunoglobulin) once in a week in case of a previous child with neonatal hemochromatosis)
- Abnormal antenatal scan such as oligo-/polyhydramnios
- Sepsis near term/timing of ROM and timing of delivery (early-onset neonatal sepsis)

13. What does acute fatty liver of pregnancy in antenatal mother signify?
Medium-chain acyl-CoA dehydrogenase deficiency and carnitine palmitoyl transferase-1 deficiency in the fetus

14. Explain the significance of natal history in neonatal cholestasis.
- Low birth weight/IUGR — suggestive of TORCH
- Birth asphyxia — leads to ischemic hepatitis

*15. What is diving reflex?
In birth asphyxia, blood flow is diverted to vital organs such as brain, heart, and adrenal glands. This impairs the blood flow to the liver resulting in ischemic hepatitis.

16. Explain the significance of dietetic history in neonatal cholestasis.
    - Bottle feeding/prelacteal feed may lead to sepsis.
    - If a child is on a milk-free diet, it may be indicative of galactosemia.
    - Prolonged TPN can lead to cholestasis.
17. How should a child with NCS having bleeding manifestations be immunized?
    - Vaccinations can be given after correction of coagulopathy with FFP (Fresh Frozen Plasma).
    - Use 23 G or smaller needles. Apply firm pressure at the injection site for 5–10 minutes. Some vaccines such as Hib and PCV (Packed Cell Volume) can be given subcutaneously also.
18. Explain the significance of a positive family history in neonatal cholestasis.
    - Idiopathic neonatal hepatitis
    - Metabolic liver disease
    - Syndromic causes
    - PFIC (Progressive Familial Intrahepatic Cholestasis)
    - Hypothyroidism
*19. List the findings in general examination in NCS.
    Table 23.1 gives examination findings in a patient with neonatal cholestasis.
20. Enumerate the differential diagnosis of yellowish discoloration of the skin.
    - Jaundice
    - Carotenemia (seen in palms and soles, sclera is spared)
    - Uremia
    - Drugs – quinacrine
*21. List the findings in head-to-foot examination in NCS.
    1. Head
       - Microcephaly – TORCH infections
       - Bulging AF – intracranial bleeding
       - Wide-open fontanelles – hypothyroidism
    2. Dysmorphic facies
       - Down syndrome
       - Edward syndrome
       - Alagille syndrome
       - Zellweger syndrome
       - Hypothyroidism
    3. Eyes
       - Pallor
       - Icterus

- Epicanthic folds – Down syndrome, Zellweger syndrome
- Bitot spots – vitamin A deficiency
- Posterior embryotoxon – Alagille syndrome
- Brushfield spots in iris (Down syndrome)
- Cataract – Down syndrome, TORCH infection, and galactosemia
- Chorioretinitis – TORCH infection
- Cherry red spot – Niemann–Pick disease
- Papilledema – due to raised ICT
4. Spider angiomas: They are 5 mm in size. They consist of central dilated arterioles with radiating blood vessels. They are seen in thorax and back. More than five are considered significant. They occur secondary to hyperestrogenism.
5. Palmar erythema
6. Petechiae, ecchymosis
7. Xanthomas
8. Bony deformities secondary to vitamin D malabsorption
9. Dilated veins in the abdominal wall
10. Umbilical hernia – hypothyroidism
11. Scratch marks of anklets in lower limbs
12. Midline defects, micropenis – hypopituitarism
13. Blueberry muffins skin lesions – centrally raised greenish-blue nodule with surrounding skin discoloration (D/D – congenital rubella and neuroblastoma) – it is a sign of extramedullary hematopoiesis
22. What is the significance of vital signs in NCS?
    1. Pulse
       - Large volume (hyperdynamic circulation)
       - Sinus bradycardia can occur because of depression of SA node caused by bile salts
    2. Blood pressure
       - Wide pulse pressure (hyperdynamic circulation)
       - Hypotension (bleeding manifestation)
       - Hypertension (due to raised ICT)
    3. Temperature
       Fever suggestive of sepsis/cholangitis/recurrent respiratory tract infections due to cystic fibrosis
    4. Respiratory rate
       Tachypnea in sepsis/respiratory tract infection due to cystic fibrosis

TABLE 23.1	Examination Findings in Neonatal Cholestasis
Clinical Finding	**Significance**
Sick child	Sepsis, metabolic disorders, and HLH (Hemophagocytic Lymphohistiocytosis)
Nonsick child	EHBA, choledochal cyst, inspissated bile duct syndrome/hypothyroidism/Alagille syndrome, Down syndrome
• Patient's sensorium	Altered sensorium in hepatic encephalopathy/intracranial bleeding/metabolic disorders presenting with encephalopathy/sepsis
• Pallor	Anemia secondary to bleeding, hypersplenism secondary to portal hypertension, TORCH infection (syphilis), hypothyroidism
• Cyanosis	Hepatopulmonary syndrome
• Icterus	• Lemon yellow – hemolytic jaundice • Greenish yellow – hepatocellular jaundice • Dark yellow/orange tint – obstructive jaundice
• Clubbing	DCLD, Alagille syndrome (due to TOF – Tetralogy of Fallot), cystic fibrosis
• Generalized lymphadenopathy	Congenital syphilis, HLH
Pedal edema	DCLD, (Decompensated Chronic Liver Disease) Aagenaes syndrome

23. Explain the significance of anthropometry in cholestasis.
    1. Failure to thrive
       * TORCH
       * Metabolic — galactosemia, hereditary fructose intolerance, Gaucher disease, Niemann—Pick disease, tyrosinemia, NISD (Neonatal Iron Storage Disease), Wolman disease, cystic fibrosis, and Zellweger syndrome
       * Cystic fibrosis
    2. Microcephaly
       * TORCH, metabolic disorders
24. List the findings in systemic examination.
    A. Abdomen
       * Distension — uniform distension is suggestive of ascites; upper abdominal distension is suggestive of organomegaly
       * Flanks full — ascites
       * Umbilicus — transverse slit — ascites
       * Umbilical hernia — hypothyroidism
       * Dilated veins — portal hypertension
       * Early splenomegaly is seen in TORCH infection and metabolic disorders
       * Splenomegaly occurs late in the course of extrahepatic cholestasis
       * Liver becomes firm early in the course of EHBA
       * Micropenis – in hypopituitarism
    B. Cardiovascular system
       ESM (Alagille syndrome)
    C. Respiratory system
       * Interstitial lung disease (Gaucher disease and Niemann—Pick disease)
       * Pleural effusion (secondary to ascites)
       * Recurrent respiratory tract infections (cystic fibrosis, alpha-1 antitrypsin deficiency, and polycystic kidney disease)
    D. Central nervous system
       * Hypotonia (Down syndrome, hypothyroidism, Zellweger syndrome, and metabolic liver disease)
       * Signs of hepatic encephalopathy
       * Raised ICT
*25. Enumerate the etiologies of neonatal cholestasis.
    Table 23.2 gives etiologies in neonatal cholestasis.

*26. Classify biliary atresia.
    1. NASPGHAN (North American Society of Paediatric Gastroenterology Hepatology and Nutrition) (2017)
       * There are three types of biliary atresia.
         a. Nonsyndromic form — most common type
         b. Syndromic form without situs inversus
         c. Syndromic form with situs inversus
       * The syndromic form is usually associated with anomalies of cardiovascular and gastrointestinal systems.
    2. Kasai classification
       * It is based on the extent of biliary tract involved:
         a. Type I: Obliteration of common bile duct (patent cystic and common hepatic duct)
         b. Type II
            IIa: Obliteration of common hepatic duct (patent cystic and common bile duct), sometimes with a cyst at hilum, hence termed cystic biliary atresia
            IIb: Obliteration of common hepatic duct, cystic, and common bile duct
         c. Type III: It is the most common type (90%); obliteration of left and right main hepatic ducts at or above the level of porta hepatis
       Fig. 23.2 shows Kasai classification of biliary atresia.
*27. List the investigations in neonatal cholestasis.
    * CBC (Complete Blood Count)
    * LFT (Liver Function Test) and RFT (Renal Function Test)
    * USG abdomen
    * Upper GI endoscopy
    * Hepatobiliary iminodiacetic acid (HIDA) scan
    * Liver biopsy
    * Etiological work-up — sepsis work-up, viral markers, TORCH screening, thyroid function tests, metabolic work-up, sweat chloride test, alpha-1 antitrypsin levels, and serum bile acids
    * X-ray, MRI brain – depending on clinical scenario
*28. Explain the significance of CBC in neonatal cholestasis.
    * Elevated total leukocyte count — sepsis
    * Anemia — TORCH infections, bleeding manifestations, hypersplenism, and hypothyroidism
    * Polycythemia — Alagille syndrome (due to TOF)
    * Pancytopenia — hypersplenism
    * Thrombocytopenia – sepsis and TORCH

TABLE 23.2	**Etiologies of Neonatal Cholestasis**
Intrahepatic	**Extrahepatic (in the Decreasing Order of Frequency)**

• Idiopathic neonatal hepatitis
• Sepsis
• TORCH infections
• Endocrine: Congenital hypothyroidism, panhypopituitarism
• Syndromic: Down syndrome, Zellweger syndrome, Alagille syndrome, Aagenaes syndrome
• Metabolic:
  a. Carbohydrate metabolism — galactosemia
  b. Lipid metabolism — Niemann—Pick type C, Wolman disease
  c. Protein metabolism — urea cycle disorders, tyrosinemia
• Others:
• Neonatal iron storage disease
• Alpha-1 antitrypsin deficiency
• Cystic fibrosis
• Progressive familial intrahepatic cholestasis
• Disorders of bile acid metabolism
	• Biliary atresia
	• Total parenteral nutrition
	• Choledochal cyst
	• Inspissated bile duct syndrome
	• Spontaneous perforation of bile duct
	• Biliary strictures
	• Choledocholithiasis

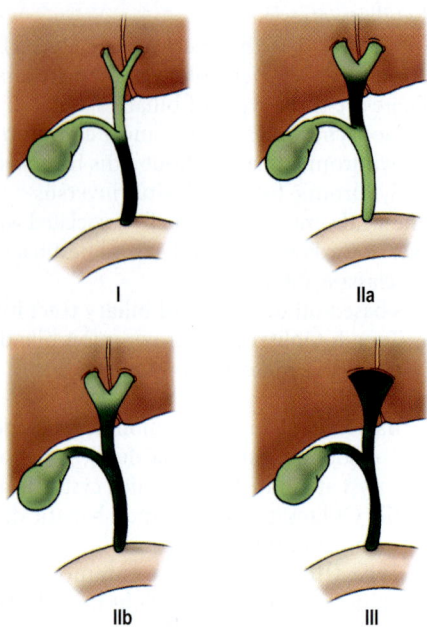

Fig. 23.2 Kasai classification of biliary atresia. (*Source: Reproduced from George Holcomb, J. Patrick Murphy, Shawn St Peter. Holcomb and Ashcraft's Pediatric Surgery, Seventh Edition, Biliary Atresia, Fig. 43.1, London, Elsevier Inc., 2020. (Credit line - From Lefkowitch JH. Biliary atresia. Mayo Clin Proc 1998;73:90–95).*

29. What is the relevance of clinical jaundice and bilirubin levels?
    - Neonates: >5 mg/dL
    - Children and adults: >2–3 mg/dL
*30. What is delta bilirubin?
    - It is also called biliprotein.
    - It is seen because of impaired excretion of conjugated bilirubin in patients with obstructive jaundice. It represents the fraction of conjugated bilirubin bound to serum albumin.
    - Hence, the clearance rate of delta bilirubin from serum approximates the half-life of albumin (12–14 days) as compared to half-life of bilirubin (4 hours) and there is delayed fall in bilirubin levels during recovery phase of obstructive jaundice.
31. Explain the significance of bilirubin in cholestasis.
    - The predominance of conjugated bilirubin occurs in extrahepatic cholestasis.
    - Total bilirubin is usually <40 mg/dL in extrahepatic cholestasis because the bile salt excretion in the gut is impaired and it is excreted in the kidneys. Bile salts also increase the renal excretion of bilirubin; hence, the total bilirubin does not raise higher than 40. Opposite of this occurs in intrahepatic cholestasis.
32. Explain bilirubin formation from RBCs.
    Approximately 90% is formed from Hb. Remaining 10% from heme-containing proteins such as cytochrome c and myoglobin. One gram of Hb gives rise to 35 mg of bilirubin and 1.34 mg of iron.
33. What is the ratio of binding of unconjugated bilirubin to albumin?
    3:1.

*34. Explain the significance of urinary examination in cholestasis.
    Urine bile salt, bile pigment, and urobilinogen findings are given in Table 23.3
    A. Urine screening for metabolic disorders
    B. Urine routine examination, culture, and sensitivity for sepsis work-up
35. Enumerate the types of liver enzymes.
    A. Transaminases
        - AST (Aspartate Transaminase) is a mitochondrial and cytosolic enzyme (remember MSC); also seen in heart, skeletal muscle, brain, and pancreas.
        - ALT (Alanine Transaminase) is cytosolic. It is specific for liver (remember "L" for liver).
        - Transaminases are the first laboratory abnormality to be detected in viral hepatitis.
          The level of transaminases does not correlate with the degree of liver damage. Sudden fall in transaminase level may indicate fulminant hepatic failure and is a poor prognostic sign. Transaminase levels are elevated: >10 times in hepatocellular jaundice and <5 times in cholestatic jaundice.
          Table 23.4 gives levels of transaminases in various liver disorders.
    B. Alkaline phosphatase
        - It is the enzyme secreted by canalicular membrane of hepatocytes.
        - It is also produced by bone, leukocytes, kidney, placenta, and small intestine.
        - It is elevated up to 5 times in cholestatic liver disease.
        - It does not differentiate between intrahepatic and extrahepatic cholestasis.
        - Zinc is a co-factor for ALP, so reduced ALP is seen in zinc deficiency.
    C. Gamma-glutamyl transferase (GGT)
        - It is synthesized by bile duct and hepatocytes.
        - It is elevated more in extrahepatic cholestasis than intrahepatic cholestasis.
        - Normal GGT levels in a patient with cholestasis are seen in PFIC-1, PFIC-2, and benign recurrent intrahepatic cholestasis (Summerskill syndrome).

TABLE 23.3	Urinary Examination in Cholestasis		
Urine	Hemolytic	Hepatocellular	Obstructive
Bile salts/bilirubin	Nil	Positive	Positive
Urobilinogen	Positive	Positive	Nil

TABLE 23.4	Levels of Transaminases in Various Liver Disorders		
2–3 Times the normal	3–20 Times the normal	>20 Times the normal
Infections — nonhepatotropic virus, bacterial sepsis, liver abscess	Wilson	Dengue
NASH (Non-Alcoholic Steato Hepatitis)	Autoimmune hepatitis	Toxin/drug-induced

36. Explain the role of ultrasound abdomen in cholestasis.
    - USG abdomen after 4–5 hours of milk-free diet shows absent gallbladder (ghost sign)
    - Triangular cord sign seen as echogenic foci 4 mm in size, seen anterior to right branch of portal vein is highly suggestive EHBA.
    - Other findings in USG:
      - Choledochal cyst
      - Choledocholithiasis
      - Liver echoes
      - Portal hypertension
      - Renal cysts in Zellweger syndrome
      - Polysplenia, malrotation in EHBA
      - Splenomegaly

*37. What is HIDA scan?
    - HIDA scan, also known as cholangioscintigraphy, is performed in patients with "pale-pigmented stools" in which radioactive tracer is injected into a vein. (HIDA has highest hepatic extraction rate and shortest transit time.) Pretreatment with phenobarbital (5 mg/kg/day) for 5 days to increase the biliary secretion by stimulating the hepatic enzymes is helpful to minimize the possibility of false-positive study in a child with patent biliary system with poor excretion.
    - Intrahepatic cholestasis – uptake is impaired, excretion normal.
    - Extrahepatic cholestasis – uptake is normal, excretion impaired.
    - No tracer activity in the small intestine after 24 hours is suggestive of EHBA.

*38. What is the definitive diagnosis of NCS?
    The definitive diagnosis is established by laparotomy and peroperative cholangiogram. This should be followed by liver biopsy.

39. What are the liver biopsy findings in neonatal hepatitis and EHBA?
    - Giant cell transformation can be seen in 20%−50% of patients with BA (Biliary Atresia). But it is not as prominent as that seen in idiopathic neonatal hepatitis.
    - Parenteral nutrition−associated cholestasis, CF (Cystic Fibrosis), and alpha-1 antitrypsin deficiency have histological features similar to biliary atresia.
    Table 23.5 shows liver biopsy findings in neonatal hepatitis and EHBA.

40. What are the bile duct paucity/ductopenic syndromes?
    - Ductopenia is defined as the ratio of bile duct to portal tract <0.5.

- Ductopenia = number of portal tracts without bile ducts/total number of portal tracts examined. A minimum of 10 portal tracts have to be examined.
- Seen in
  - Alagille syndrome
  - Alpha-1 antitrypsin deficiency
  - HSV (Herpes Simplex Virus) and CMV (Cytomegalo Virus)
  - Gaucher type 4
  - GVHD (Graft Versus Host Disease)

41. List the radiological investigations in NCS.
    - X-ray DL (Dorso-Lumbar) spine AP and lateral views to look for butterfly-shaped vertebra.
      X-ray DL spine showing the butterfly-shaped vertebra is shown in Fig. 23.3.
    - X-ray long bones to look for Wimberger sign in congenital syphilis, celery stalk appearance of metaphysis in congenital rubella syndrome
    - X-ray knees for stippled calcifications in Zellweger syndrome
    - X-ray chest − signs of bronchiectasis and pleural effusion
    - X-ray chest with abdomen for signs of sepsis (narrow pedicle, hyperinflated lungs, tented diaphragm, and dilated bowel loops)
    - X-ray abdomen showing ground-glass appearance suggestive of meconium peritonitis (seen in cystic fibrosis), duodenal atresia (Down syndrome), signs of necrotizing enterocolitis in preterm infants (prone to cholestasis due to prolonged TPN)
    - CT brain − look for calcifications, periventricular calcifications seen in Cytomegalovirus (CMV) infection (Clue: Both CMV and Periventricular have an alphabet ''V'' in common) as shown in Fig. 23.4). Diffuse calcifications- toxoplasmosis as shown in Fig. 23.5.

42. Mention the conditions with high serum bile acids.
    PFIC (Progressive Familial Intrahepatic Cholestasis)-1 and PFIC-2 diseases with high serum bile acids

43. What are the causes of delayed passage of meconium in a child with NCS?
    Hypothyroidism, cystic fibrosis, and Down syndrome

*44. Explain the dietary management of NCS.
    - Calories – according to RDA (Recommended Dietary Allowance)
    - Proteins – avoid animal protein in patients with DCLD.
    - FAT – MCT (Medium Chain Triglyceride) oil
    - Vitamin A – 10,000–15,000 IU/day
    - Vitamin D – 5000–8000 IU/day
    - Vitamin E – 50–400 IU/day
    - Vitamin K – 5 mg/kg for 3 days followed by 5 mg every 4 weeks (5 mg every week according to IAP)
    - Calcium – 25–100 mg/kg/day
    - Phosphorous – 25–50 mg/kg/day
    - Zinc – 1 mg/kg/day
    - Iron – 5–6 mg/kg/day
    - Magnesium – 1–2 mEq/kg/day
    - Water-soluble vitamins – twice the RDA

45. What is the treatment and prognosis of biliary atresia?
    - Definitive treatment is Kasai procedure
    - Survival depends on the day of operation of Kasai procedure

TABLE 23.5	Liver Biopsy Findings in Neonatal Hepatitis and EHBA	
Neonatal Hepatitis	**EHBA**
Giant cell hepatitis	Periportal fibrous cord expansion
Kupffer cell hyperplasia	Bile duct epithelial proliferation
Distortion of intralobular bile ducts	Hepatic lobule intact
Panlobular involvement	Bile lakes
No bile duct epithelial proliferation	

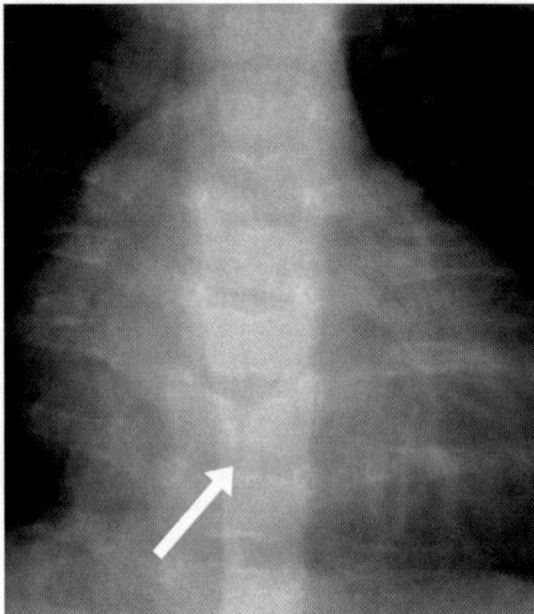

Fig. 23.3   X-ray DL spine — butterfly-shaped vertebra. *(Source: Reproduced from Hyun-Hae Cho, Woo Sun Kim, Young Hun Choi et al. and Ultrasonography evaluation of infants with Alagille syndrome: In comparison with biliary atresia and neonatal hepatitis, European Journal of Radiology, 85(6):1045-1052.)*

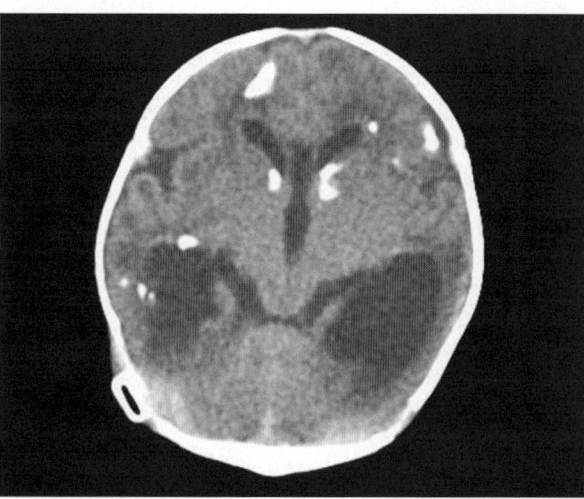

Fig. 23.5   CT brain — multiple calcified lesion seen in cerebral toxoplasmosis. *(Source: Reproduced from Andrej Spec, Gerome Escota, Courtney Chrisler et al. Comprehensive Review of Infectious Diseases, Infections of Pregnancy, Fig. 20.3, Oxford, Elsevier Inc., 2020. (Credit line - From Montoya JG, Boothroyd JC, Kovacs JA et al. Imaging studies of central nervous system toxoplasmosis in Toxoplasma gondii. In: Bennett JE, Dolin R, Blaser MJ, eds. Mandell, Douglas, and Bennett's Principles and Practice of Infectious Diseases. Updated 8th ed. Elsevier; 2015).*

- Hundred per cent mortality by 18 months, if untreated
- Eighty per cent bile flow restoration, if <60 days
- Sixty per cent restoration if 60–90 days
- Ten per cent restoration if >90 days
- Successful Kasai fall in bilirubin to less than 2 mg/dL in 6 months after surgery

*46. What are the effects of ursodeoxycholic acid (UDCA) in cholestasis?
- Choleretic
- Cytoprotective
- Antiapoptotic
- Anti-inflammatory
- Immunomodulatory

47. Describe the grading of pruritis.
- Grade 1: No pruritus
- Grade 2: Mild scratching, but can be distracted
- Grade 3: Active scratching without abrasion
- Grade 4: Active scratching with abrasions
- Grade 5: Cutaneous mutilation with bleeding/scarring

48. Enumerate the various treatment options available for pruritis.
- UDCA
- Antihistaminic
- Phenobarbitone
- Steroids
- Rifampicin
- Carbamazepine
- Opioid antagonist
- ondansetron
- UV rays
- Biliary diversion
- Plasmapheresis

49. What are the causes of rickets in NCS?
    Vitamin D malabsorption and tyrosinemia (presents as Fanconi syndrome)

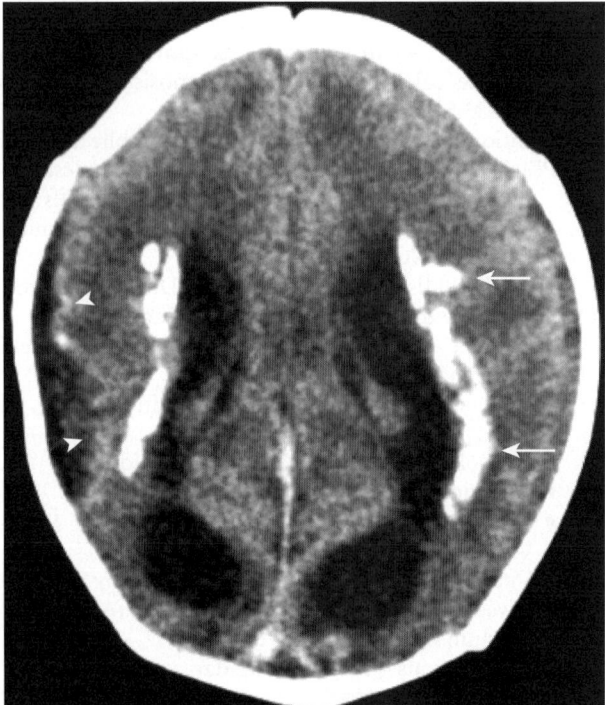

Fig. 23.4   Radiocontrast CT brain — CMV encephalitis. *(Source: Reproduced from Brian Coley. Caffey's Pediatric Diagnostic Imaging, Thirteenth Edition, Infection and Inflammation, Figure 34.31, Philadelphia, Elsevier Inc., 2019.)*

50. What is the method of estimation of serum bilirubin in the laboratory?
    - It is called Van den Bergh reaction.
    - In this, bilirubin reacts with Ehrlich's diazotized sulfanilic acid to produce chromogenic molecules which can be detected colorimetrically.
    - It is of two types: Direct and indirect.
    - Direct Van den Bergh reaction detects conjugated bilirubin because it is done in an aqueous medium.
    - Indirect Van den Bergh detects total bilirubin and this test is carried out in methanol.
51. What are the common sites for xanthomas?
    Lower eyelids, hands, and feet
52. What is the cause of butterfly vertebra in Alagille syndrome?
    Incomplete fusion of anterior arch of the vertebra

*53. List the poor prognostic factors in NCS.
    - Hard liver
    - Increased periosteal fibrosis
    - Elevated GGT
    - Alpha-1 antitrypsin deficiency
    - PFIC-3
54. What are the theories behind cholestasis?
    a. Reflux of pancreatic juice into biliary system
    b. Occlusion of arterial system to biliary tree
    c. Reovirus infection (can cause both intrahepatic and extrahepatic cholestasis)
*55. Enumerate the differences between neonatal hepatitis and EHBA.
    Table 23.6 gives differences between neonatal hepatitis and EHBA.

TABLE 23.6	Differences Between Neonatal Hepatitis and EHBA	
Features	**Intrahepatic Cholestasis**	**Extrahepatic Cholestasis**
HISTORY		
Onset	Anytime in neonatal period	End of 1st week
Gestational age	Preterm/IUGR/SGA	Term/normal birth weight
Sex	Males	Females
Family history	15% – metabolic cause	–
History of high-colored urine	Yes	Yes
History of pale stools	No; can be present in late-stage	Yes
Seizures	+	–
Failure to thrive	+	–
EXAMINATION		
General condition	Sick	Initially normal
Dysmorphic facies	+	–
Liver size	Small	Large
Liver consistency	Soft initially, firm in later stages	Firm
Spleen	Early	Late finding (seen after portal hypertension develops)
Polysplenia, accessory spleen	–	+
INVESTIGATIONS		
Liver enzymes	High	Very high
Alkaline phosphatase		
Transaminases	Very high	High
TORCH	Positive	Negative
Alpha-fetoprotein	High	Normal
USG	Gallbladder visualized	Gallbladder not visualized
UGI scopy	Bile visualized	Not visualized
Scintigraphy	Radioactivity + in small intestine	Radioactivity absent in small intestine
Liver biopsy (refer Q. No. 39)		
Cholangiogram	Normal	Block visualized
Prognosis	Poor	Better

Quick Bites

- Biliary atresia is the most common cause of neonatal cholestasis.
- Cholestasis in a well-thriving, nonsick child is more likely to be due to extrahepatic causes.
- Persistent pigmented stools in a child with cholestasis rules out EHBA. However, persistent pale stools are not always suggestive of EHBA because it can occur in end stages of intrahepatic cholestasis also.
- Normal GGT levels and elevated serum bile acids levels are seen in PFIC-1 and PFIC-2.

- Peroperative cholangiogram followed by liver biopsy is the investigation of choice.
- Parenteral nutrition−associated cholestasis, CF, and alpha-1 antitrypsin deficiency have histological features similar to biliary atresia.
- HIDA scan has limited specificity and can be used in patients with "pale-pigmented stools."
- There is no role for ERCP (Endoscopic Retrograde Cholangiopancreatography) and MRCP (Magnetic Resonance Cholangiopancreatography).
- Kasai procedure is the treatment of choice for EHBA and has an excellent prognosis when performed before 8 weeks of age.

Short Cases

Hydrocephalus

Following introduction, seek permission from the caregiver and introduce yourself to the patient before history elicitation, and identify the case.

Name____Age____Sex____Consanguinity____Order of birth____Place____Informant____

Presenting Complaints and Duration

- Abnormal increase in size of the head or large head since birth
- Delayed motor milestones (head control)

History of Presenting Illness

- Abnormal increase in size of the head noticed since when?
- Progressive/static
- Involving predominantly which part of the skull – occipital or frontal
- Flailness of lower limbs
- Gait disturbance – frequent fall
- Irritability, vomiting, and poor feeding (if more than 2 years)

CENTRAL NERVOUS SYSTEM HISTORY

Higher Function

- Seizures, early handedness, speech abnormality, scholastic backwardness, altered sensorium

Cranial Nerve History

- Ability to perceive light
- Ability to move eyeballs in all four directions
- Abnormal eye movements (sunset sign/roving eye movements), diplopia, abnormal eye position (not able to move eye in the upward direction)
- Ability to chew food
- Facial asymmetry, ability to close both eyes while sleeping, drooling of saliva, deviation of angle of mouth
- Ability to hear and respond to sound
- Nasal twang of voice, nasal regurgitation
- Ability to move the head side to side
- Deviation of tongue on protrusion

Motor System

- Thinness noticed by the mother on all four limbs
- Stiffness/scissoring of lower limbs
- Ability to move legs along the cot or above the cot or only flicker of movements
- Gait abnormalities with frequent falls

Cerebellar Features

- Swaying of body
- Abnormal eyeball or head movement or tremors

Bladder/Bowel Disturbance

- Bladder/bowel involvement (dribbling of urine, leaky stools)

Sensory Features

- History of perception of pain or crying while giving vaccination or any intramuscular injection; any history of loss of sensation in an older child

Autonomic Features

- Flushing, sweating, palpitation episodes

Spine and Cranium

- Any abnormality in head size noted by the mother compared with sibling or peers
- Any swelling, tuft of hair, sinus, discharge, abnormal curvature − any shunt or tube placement – when was it placed; whether it is functioning

COMPLICATION HISTORY

- Head banging (infant), headache, blurring of vision, altered sensorium
- If VP shunt in situ − any redness, swelling over the shunt tube, recent altered sensorium, sudden increase in size of head (shunt block, added infection)
- Stridor (especially seen in coning)

ETIOLOGICAL HISTORY

- Poor feeding, failure to thrive, stridor
- Suck−rest cycle, breathing difficulty, sacral edema
- Protuberant/flat occiput
- Recurrent ear infection, obesity, prominent forehead, unusual facies

PAST HISTORY

- Fever with seizures; hospitalized followed by regression of milestone and progressive increase in head size (meningitis),
- Head trauma

ANTENATAL HISTORY

- First trimester – intrauterine infection, drug intake, irradiation exposure
- Second trimester – antenatal ultrasound, increased liquor, any fetal surgery (in utero shunt – ventriculo-amniotic shunt)

NATAL HISTORY

- Prematurity/malpresentation (dystocia)/PROM/traumatic delivery/instrumentation/birth asphyxia

POSTNATAL HISTORY

- Preterm, seizures − NICU admission, any lumbar puncture (CNS − infection, meningitis), hypopigmented macule (neurocutaneous marker), swelling at the back, and limb weakness (myelomeningocele)

DEVELOPMENTAL HISTORY

- Delay (predominant motor delay – delay in head control because of large head), or neuroregression

DIETETIC HISTORY

- Exclusive breastfeeding or started any complementary feed

IMMUNIZATION HISTORY

- Any feeding difficulty, immunization − as per universal immunization or IAP Indian Academy of Pediatrics

FAMILY HISTORY

- Large head
- Similar illness in the family members

TREATMENT HISTORY

- Any surgery (shunt, meningomyelocele surgery)/medication

Summary

A …-month/year-old child with history of progressive increase in size of the head/abnormal enlargement of the head noticed since ……, with or without higher function involvement (seizures/speech), with or without cranial nerve involvement, with or without complications, with or without developmental delay (global or predominant motor), surgery done − Ventriculoperitoneal shunt in situ or not

General Examination

- Posture of the child
- Head appears – big
- Any shunt tube placed
- Check for the functioning of the tube

Head-to-Foot Examination

Head
a) Head circumference and shape of the skull in terms of AP diameter, biparietal diameter, any evidence of frontal bossing and occipital prominence
b) Presence of dilated veins over the scalp
c) Skin stretched and shiny
d) Anterior and posterior fontanelles (note their size, shape, borders, pulsation, tension in sitting and supine positions) − always look for the AF tension at 45°
e) Any sutural separation
f) Transillumination
g) Prominent/flat occiput
h) Craniotabes − pingpong feeling of the occipital skull due to thinning of skull.
i) Macewen sign – only seen when the AF is closed; tap over the parietal bone on one side, keep the examiner ear on the temporal side of the same side – seen when there is sutural separation
j) Cranial bruit – heard all over the skull

Eyes
- Sunset sign, chorioretinitis, cherry red spot, papill-edema, cataract, optic atrophy

Neurocutaneous markers
- Hypopigmented macule, café au lait spots, port-wine stain

Facies
- Dysmorphic features/coarse facies

Extremities
- Short limb, normal trunk
- Rash/lymphadenopathy

Spine
- Look for tuft of hair/skin tag/any hemangioma

Vital Signs

- Temperature
- Pulse rate − bradycardia (raised Intracranial Pressure (ICP)), tachycardia and bounding pulse (Congestive Cardiac Failure − vein of Galen malformation), bounding carotid (vein of Galen malformation)
- Respiratory rate − shallow respiration
- Blood pressure − hypertension – raised ICP, hypotension – congestive cardiac failure seen in vein of Galen malformation

Anthropometry

- Weight, height, weight for height with interpretation
- Head circumference – percentile

Central Nervous System Examination

HIGHER FUNCTIONS

- Sensorium, speech, progressive loss of scholastic performance

CRANIAL NERVES

- Cranial nerve II – bilateral optic atrophy (3rd ventricular dilatation)
- Cranial nerve VI – raised intracranial pressure
- Cranial nerve VIII – TORCH – sensory neural deafness
- Cranial nerves IX, X, XI, XII – shallow breathing/apnea (Arnold−Chiari and Dandy−Walker malformation)

MOTOR SYSTEM EXAMINATION

Signs of Pyramidal Tract Involvement

- Bulk − any wasting of limbs
- Tone – hypertonia (features suggestive of pyramidal involvement), lower limbs > upper limbs
- Power − decreased in all four limbs
- Reflexes – brisk or exaggerated, plantar – extensor
- Mention about anal reflex (normal anal wink present or absent)
- Gait – truncal ataxia is seen in Dandy–Walker malformation, magnetic gait

CEREBELLAR SYSTEM

Any titubation, nystagmus, dysdiadochokinesia, tremors

SENSORY SYSTEM

- Ask about cry or any response while giving immunization

EXAMINATION OF SPINE AND CRANIUM

- Mention about anterior fontanelle — size, pulsatile, bruit (any pulsation in the fontanelle, sutural separation, posterior fontanelle)
- Spina bifida — any spinal swelling, tuft of hair, sacral dimple >25 mm from anal verge, >5 mm depth – significant for occult spina bifida
- Shunt — side, site, patency, whether reservoir present or absent; any redness or swelling over the shunt – suggestive of shunt infection

Other System Examination

CARDIOVASCULAR SYSTEM

- Hyperdynamic precordium, continuous murmur — congestive heart failure (vein of Galen malformation), infective endocarditis (VP shunt)

ABDOMEN

- Any surgical scar, any signs of peritonitis

RESPIRATORY SYSTEM

- Abnormal pattern of breathing (impending coning)

Diagnosis

A child with hydrocephalus most probably due to ……, with or without raised intracranial pressure, with developmental delay (global or predominant motor), with/without focal neurological deficits, nutritional status, other comorbidities – anemia, vitamin deficiency if any

Frequently Asked Questions

1. What is sunset sign?

   Impingement of the dilated suprapineal recess on the brainstem tectum produces setting sun sign (normal during infancy) as shown in Fig. 24.1.

2. What is the significance of etiological history in hydrocephalus?

   Etiological history and its significance are given in Table 24.1.

3. What is the significance of antenatal and birth history in a child with hydrocephalus?

   Table 24.2 gives clues in antenatal and natal history.

4. What is the significance of postnatal history in a hydrocephalus child?

   a. Preterm – intracranial bleeding (intraventricular/subarachnoid hemorrhage – posthemorrhagic hydrocephalus)

   b. Traumatic delivery – intracranial bleeding

   c. Postnatal – fever seizures – infection (meningitis)

   d. Neurocutaneous marker – hypopigmented macule (tuberous sclerosis); port-wine stain in the face – Sturge–Weber syndrome; swelling at the back; and limb weakness (myelomeningocele)

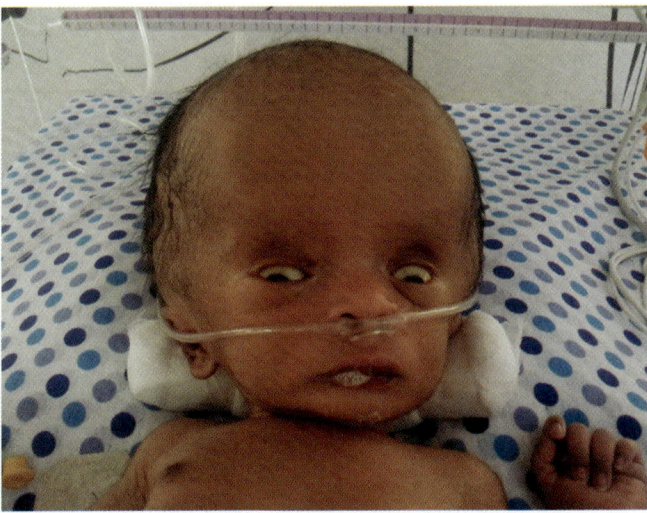

Fig. 24.1 Sunset sign.

TABLE 24.1	Etiological History	
Clinical Clues	**Etiology**
Poor feeding, failure to thrive, stridor	Nasal encephalocele
Suck–rest cycle, breathing difficulty	Vein of Galen malformation presenting with CCF
Protuberant occiput	Dandy–Walker malformation
Flat occiput	Arnold–Chiari malformation
Fever with seizures/focal deficit (acquired cause)	Neurocysticercosis, toxoplasmosis, mumps
Recurrent ear infection, obesity, prominent forehead, unusual facies	Achondroplasia

TABLE 24.2	Clues in Antenatal and Natal History	
Clues	**Significance**
Intrauterine infection	Toxoplasma, mumps, congenital aqueductal stenosis
Drug intake	Vitamin A toxicity – pseudotumor
Polyhydramnios	Myelomeningocele (Arnold–Chiari malformation)
Fetal surgery	In utero shunt – ventriculo-amniotic shunt
Birth history	Prematurity/dystocia/Premature Rupture of Membranes (PROM)/traumatic delivery/instrumentation/birth asphyxia

   e. Feeding difficulty, breathing difficulty – congestive cardiac failure – vein of Galen malformation

5. What are the causes of congenital aqueductal stenosis?

   Intrauterine infection – mumps, L1CAM gene mutation causing L1 syndrome, developmental errors causing abnormal folding of the neural plate, Bickers–Adams–Edwards syndrome or X-linked hydrocephalus

6. *What is the size of aqueduct of Sylvius?

   The cross-sectional size of aqueduct of Sylvius is 3×2 mm.

7. What are the neurodegenerative syndromes associated with large head?

   Neurodegenerative syndrome associated with large head – CATS (Canavan disease, Alexander disease, Tay–Sachs disease, Sandhoff disease)

8. What is the significance of family history in a child with hydrocephalus?

   - Familial – history of large head in family (mother and father with large head)

   - Congenital or hereditary – X-linked (aqueduct stenosis), autosomal form of hydrocephalus, malformations of brain in family

9. How to identify Ventriculo-Peritoneal (VP) shunt tube functioning?

   Fig. 24.2 shows flushing test.

   - Flushing test gives three different possible test results to identify the shunt patency

   - Step 1 – normal: Compress the dome with moderate force – check for complete emptying. If it empties completely and reinflates in less than or equal to 1 second, then test is negative – tube function is normal.

   - Step 2 – shunt proximally occluded: If the dome empties completely, but there is no or slow refilling (reinflation time >1 second), then shunt is occluded proximally – either complete or partial obstruction.

   - Step 3 – shunt distally occluded: If the dome is not compressible or only hard to press, then shunt is occluded distally (partial or full occlusion).

10. What are the common causes of cerebrospinal fluid (CSF) shunt dysfunction in children?

    Table 24.3 gives common causes of CSF shunt dysfunction in children.

11. What is the significance of head-to-foot examination in a child with hydrocephalus?

    Table 24.4 gives the significance of head-to-foot examination in a child with hydrocephalus.

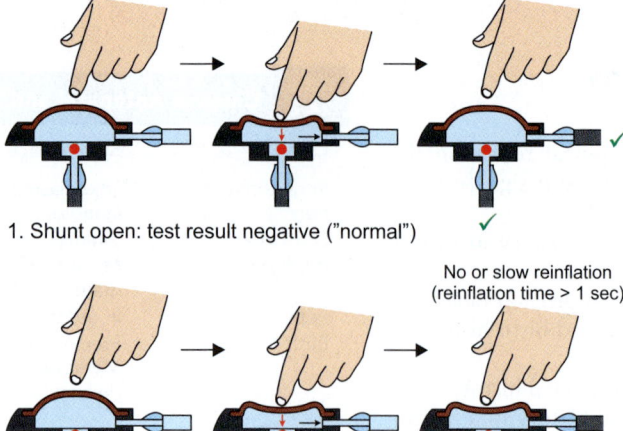

1. Shunt open: test result negative ("normal")

No or slow reinflation
(reinflation time > 1 sec)

2. Shunt proximally occluded: test result positive ("not-normal")

Not compressible
(or hard to compress)

3. Shunt distally occluded: test result positive ("not-normal")

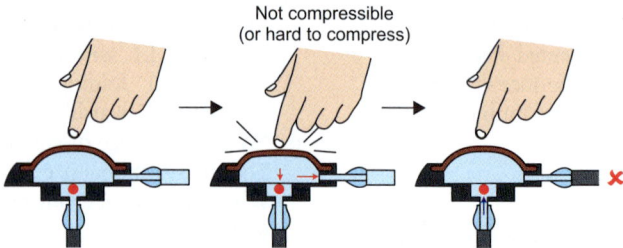

Fig. 24.2 Flushing test.

TABLE 24.3	Common Cause of CSF Shunt Dysfunction in Children	
Time From Shunt Placement or Revision	**Common Cause of Shunt Dysfunction**
0–6 months	Infection, abdominal dislocation
6 months to 4 years	Overdrainage, underdrainage, shunt occlusion
4 years or more	Disconnection, kinking, lacerations, and shunt occlusion

12. What are the endocrine problems associated with hydrocephalus?

Precocious puberty/delayed puberty, short stature, hypothyroidism, and hypopituitarism are the endocrine abnormality associated with long-standing/chronic hydrocephalus.

13. Why there is features of pyramidal signs in a child with hydrocephalus?

Pyramidal signs (hypertonia, brisk reflex, extensor plantar) are due to stretching and disruption of corticospinal fibers which lie along the ventricles.

14. Why lower limb is more affected than upper limb in a child with hydrocephalus?

The lower limbs are affected first in hydrocephalus because the tracts supplying the lower limb run closer to the ventricles.

15. What are the features of raised Intra Cranial Pressure (ICP)?

Raised ICP can present as headache, irritability, worsening in flexion of neck, coughing, sneezing, increase in symptoms when the child wakes up from sleep (early morning), associated with photophobia. It should be differentiated from migraine (unilateral, often frontal, relieved after sleeping). Clinical signs include upward gaze palsy.

16. What are the types of intracranial pressure?

There are two types of ICP:
- Primary – idiopathic
- Secondary – to a specific condition (trauma, brain tumor, meningitis, vasculitis, toxin and drug, head and neck infection)

17. What are the clinical features of shunt infection?

Redness and tenderness along the line of the shunt, high fever, headache, vomiting, neck stiffness, abdominal distension (peritonitis), irritability/sleeplessness (Fig. 24.4)

18. What are the organisms that cause shunt infection?
- *Staphylococcus epidermidis* is the most common cause of shunt infection. Other causative organisms are *Staphylococcus aureus*, streptococci, Gram-negative bacteria, *Pneumococcus*, *Haemophilus influenzae*, and meningococcus.
- Treatment:
  - Tapping the reservoir for CSF analysis and treatment with intravenous and intraventricular antibiotics (if ventriculitis present or refractory to systemic antimicrobial therapy)
  - Surgical removal of the infected shunt, instillation of external ventricular drain, placement of

TABLE 24.4	Head-to-Foot Examination in Hydrocephalus
Head	a. Frontal bossing or flat occiput – achondroplasia, Arnold–Chiari malformation b. Occipital prominence – Dandy–Walker, posterior fossa tumor/arachnoid cyst c. Transillumination positive – Dandy–Walker malformation d. Bruit over skull – vein of Galen malformation
Transillumination	• Transillumination – more than 2 cm in frontal and more than 1 cm in occipital region (it is positive only if the cerebral mantle is less than 1 cm) Fig. 24.3A shows transillumination test in a child with hydrocephalus Fig. 24.3B shows transillumination test positive in a child with encephalocele
Eyes	a) Sunset sign b) Chorioretinitis (TORCH infection) c) Cherry red spot – storage disorder d) Papilledema e) Optic atrophy – raised ICP
Short limb, normal trunk	Achondroplasia
Coarse features	Storage disorder, achondroplasia
Neurocutaneous markers	• Hypopigmented patches in tuberous sclerosis • Café au lait, port-wine stain – Sturge–Weber syndrome
Spine	• Tuft of hair/skin tag/any hemangioma • Neural tube defects – myelomeningocele with Arnold–Chiari type 2
Rash/lymphadenopathy/cataract/hepatosplenomegaly	Intrauterine infection

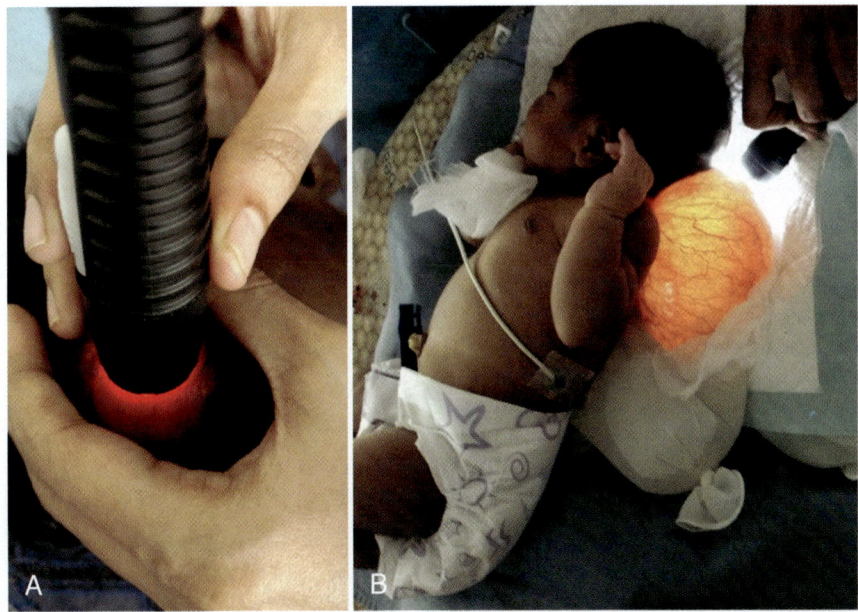

Fig. 24.3 (A) Transillumination positive in hydrocephalus. (B) Transillumination positive in encephalocele.

new shunt after three consecutive CSF sample are sterile
• Empirical antibiotics – inj. vancomycin for shunt infection

19. When to suspect overdrainage of CSF?
When there is overriding of sutures, depressed AF, altered level of consciousness, subdural effusion, hematoma, distal infection – peritonitis

DISCUSSION ON HYDROCEPHALUS

20. Define hydrocephalus.
Hydrocephalus is a disorder in which the cerebral ventricular system contains an excessive amount of CSF and is dilated either with or without raised intracranial pressure.

21. What is the incidence of hydrocephalus in children?
Approximately 0.3–2.5 per 1000 live births

22. *What are the salient features of Arnold–Chiari and Dandy–Walker syndrome?
Table 24.5 gives salient features of Arnold–Chiari and Dandy–Walker malformation.

23. Enumerate the causes of hydrocephalus.
Table 24.6 gives differentiating features of communicating and noncommunicating hydrocephalus.

24. What are the differential diagnoses of hydrocephalus?
Table 24.7 gives differential diagnoses of hydrocephalus.

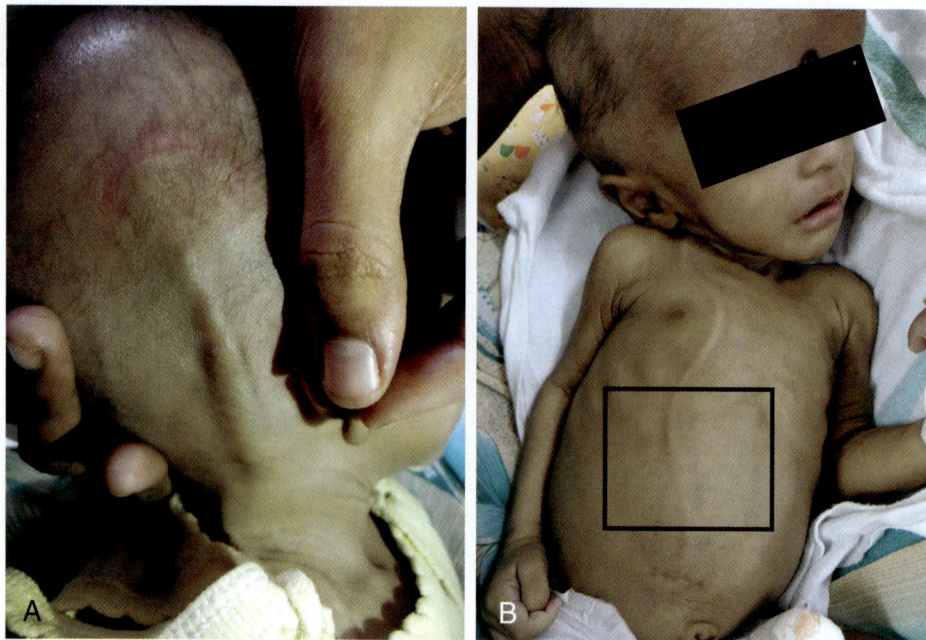

Fig. 24.4   (A) VP shunt with infection in the proximal catheter. (B) Redness along the line of the shunt suggestive of infection.

TABLE 24.5	Salient Features of Arnold–Chiari and Dandy–Walker Malformations

Arnold–Chiari Malformation	Dandy–Walker Malformation
Four types	• Most common posterior fossa malformation
• Type 1 to type 4	• Dilatation of posterior part of 4th ventricle because of defective formation of roof of 4th ventricle as shown in Fig. 24.6
Type 1	• Associated malformations
• Most common	• Cranial
• Herniation of cerebellar tonsil	1. Agenesis of corpus callosum
• Absent myelomeningocele, absent hydrocephalus	2. Cerebral atrophy
• Present in adults (headache, vomiting, neck stiffness, gait disturbance, spasticity, frequent urination)	3. Holoprosencephaly, schizencephaly
• Less severe form	4. Vermis hypoplasia
• MRI – only syrinx (syringomyelia)	• Extracranial
Type 2	1. Hypertelorism
• Most common in children	2. Low set ears
• More severe	3. Syndactyly/polydactyly
• Herniation of lower brainstem	
• Associated with myelomeningocele, hydrocephalus as shown in Fig. 24.5	
• Present in infancy as stridor and apnea	
Type 3	
• With occipital encephalocele +	
Type 4	
• Cerebellar agenesis	
CT/MRI brain	
• Lemon sign and banana sign	
• Platybasia (both are associated with invagination of base of skull)	
• Distance between the inferior margin of foramen magnum and inferior margin of tonsil measured	
<5 mm = Tonsillar ectopia	
>5 mm = Arnold–Chiari malformation	
Treatment = Surgical decompression up to C3 vertebra	
Fig. 24.5 shows Arnold–Chiari malformation type 2, hydrocephalus + myelomeningocele	

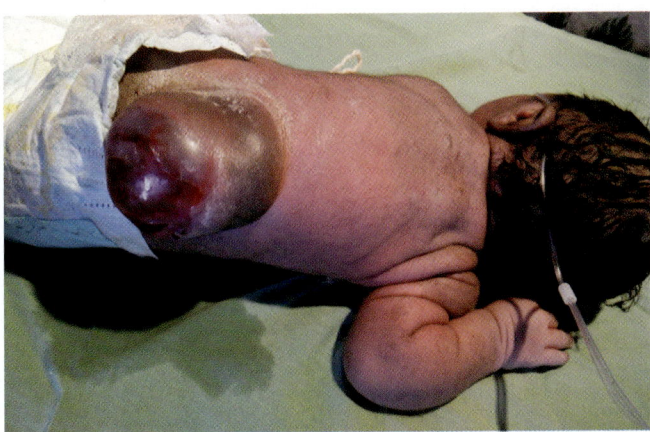

Fig. 24.5 Child with Arnold—Chiari malformation – hydrocephalus.

TABLE 24.6	Differentiating Features of Communicating and Noncommunicating Hydrocephalus	
Communicating/ Nonobstructive Hydrocephalus	**Noncommunicating/ Obstructive Hydrocephalus**	

• Most common
  a. Infection
  b. Pneumococci, tuberculous meningitis
 	
• Other causes
  a) Subarachnoid hemorrhage
  b) Malignancy
  c) Achondroplasia
  d) Benign enlargement of subarachnoid space
	• Most common
	  a. Aqueductal stenosis (X-linked, congenital)
	  b. Infection – toxoplasmosis, mumps, neurocysticercosis
	  c. Neurofibromatosis
	• Other causes
	  a. Malformation — vein of Galen
	  b. Arnold—Chiari malformation and Dandy—Walker malformation
	  c. Tumor
	  d. Hematoma
	  e. Abscess	

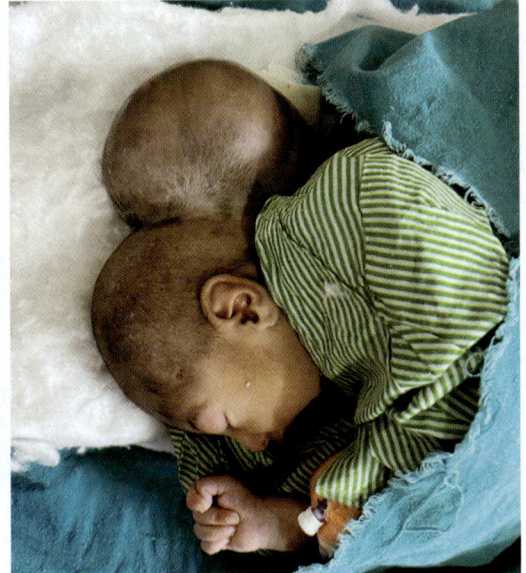

Fig. 24.6 Dandy—Walker – posterior fossa malformation.

25. How to differentiate between stiffness of tetanus spasm and meningitis neck stiffness clinically?

In tetanus spasm, there is trismus and child's sensorium is normal, whereas in meningitis, there are neck stiffness and altered sensorium.

26. What is bobble head?

Intermittent obstruction of arachnoid cyst causes bobbling of head in children.

27. What are the infections that cause hydrocephalus directly?
- TORCH – toxoplasmosis, cytomegalovirus
- Others – mumps, neurocysticercosis

28. What are Wormian bones?
- Wormian bones (intrasutural bones) — extra bone pieces that occur within a suture (joint) in the cranium.
- They are irregular isolated bones, in addition to the centers of ossification of the cranium.

TABLE 24.7	Differential Diagnosis in Hydrocephalus		
Macrocephaly (Increased Skull Size)	**Megalencephaly (Increased Brain Parenchyma)**	**Hydranencephaly (Absent Hemisphere; Only CSF)**	

• Anemia
• Rickets
• Osteogenesis imperfecta
Storage disorder – Mucopolysaccharidosis (MPS), Maple syrup urine disease (MSUD)
Leukodystrophy – CATS mnemonic
	Increased brain weight: Volume as shown in Fig. 24.7
	
	>2 SD above normal for age
	
	• Most common: Benign familial megalencephaly
	• Other
	  a. Sotos syndrome: Most common cause of syndromic hydrocephalus
	    Associated with 100% macrocephaly at the age of 1 year
	  b. Weaver syndrome
	  c. Fragile X syndrome
	  d. Gorlin syndrome: Macrocephaly with cutis marmorata telangiectasia
		Absent cerebral hemisphere with intact midbrain and brainstem as shown in Fig. 24.8
		
		Cause: Bilateral occlusion of internal carotid artery during fetal development
		
		Present as spastic quadriparesis	

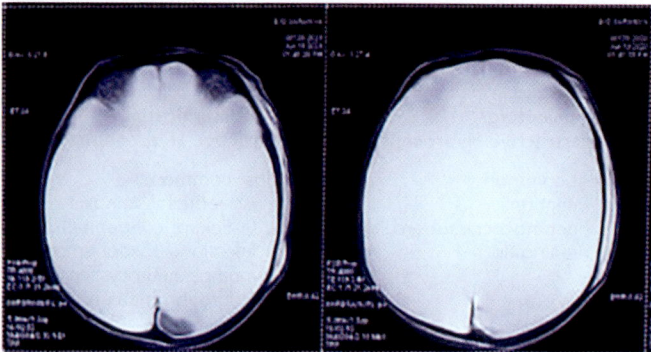

Fig. 24.7 Megalencephaly — CT brain.

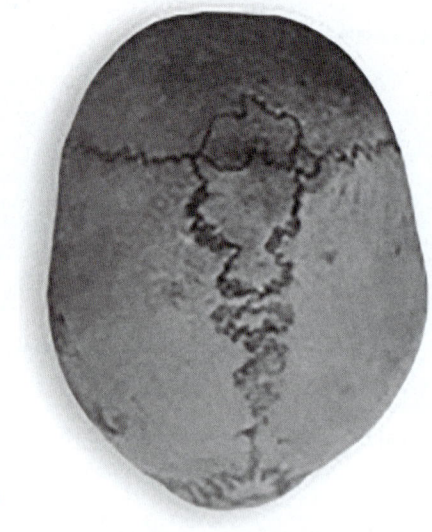

A

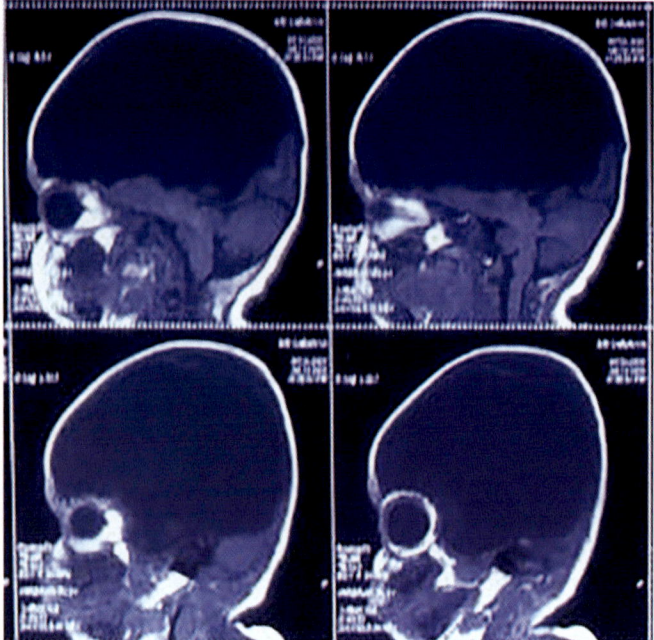

Fig. 24.8 Hydranencephaly.

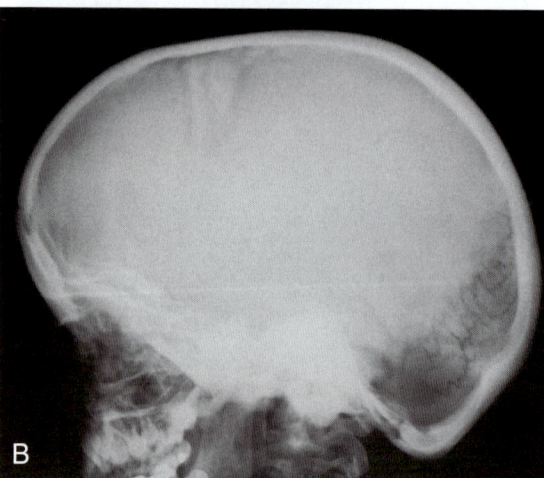

B

Fig. 24.9 (A) Diagrammatic representation of Wormian bones. (B) X-ray skull — Wormian bones seen in cleidocranial dysplasia. *(Source: (A) Wormian bones - Wikipedia; (B) Reproduced from Thomas Pope, Hans Bloem, Javier Beltran. Musculoskeletal Imaging, Second Edition, Dysplasias, eFIGURE 104-47, Philadelphia, Saunders, 2015.)*

- They occur most frequently in the course of the lambdoid suture, may also occur in sagittal or coronal sutures. Fig. 24.9A shows diagrammatic representation of Wormian bones and Fig. 24.9B shows X-ray of Wormian bone — seen in cleidocranial dysplasia.

29. What are the conditions associated with Wormian bones?
    - Pyknodysostosis
    - Osteogenesis imperfecta
    - Rickets
    - "Kinky-hair" Menkes syndrome
    - Cleidocranial dysostosis
    - Hypothyroidism and hypophosphatasia
    - Otopalatodigital syndrome
    - Primary acro-osteolysis
    - Down syndrome
      These causes can be remembered by the mnemonic "PORKCHOPS."

30. *What are the differentials for open Anterior Fontanelle (AF)?
    Open AF can occur because of delayed bone closure or rapidly enlarging brain or increased intracranial volume
    a) Rickets
    b) Hydrocephalus
    c) Hypothyroid
    d) Preterm
    e) All trisomy
    f) Achondroplasia

31. *Give examples of condition associated with bulging AF.
    a. Meningitis – early stage
    b. Hydrocephalus
    c. Increased intracranial hypertension
    d. Pseudotumor cerebri – vitamin A poisoning, nalidixic acid
    e. Intracranial tumors

32. What are the neurocutaneous syndromes associated with hydrocephalus?
    Neurofibromatosis, tuberous sclerosis, Sturge−Weber syndrome
33. What is HARDE syndrome?
    - H − hydrocephalus
    - A − agyria, various
    - RD − retinal dysplasia, corneal opacity, or microphthalmia
    - E − encephalocele
34. What are the stages of hydrocephalus?
    Table 24.8 gives various stages of hydrocephalus.
35. What is the cause of sudden death in a child with hydrocephalus?
    Herniation
36. What is unilateral hydrocephalus?
    Unilateral hydrocephalus is due to obstruction of foramen of Monro and is associated with corpus callosal anomalies. Acquired unilateral hydrocephalus is seen in obstruction at the foramen of Monro by thalamic or intraventricular neoplasm, colloid cyst, tuberculoma, and ventriculitis.
37. What is double compartment hydrocephalus?
    Double compartment is a rare shunt complication which produces independent supra- and infratentorial hydrocephalus because of occlusion of the aqueduct of Sylvius and 4th ventricle outlets, after shunting the lateral ventricles and causes dilation of 4th ventricle which in turn causes brainstem dysfunction and cerebellar signs.
38. What is huge hydrocephalus?
    Head circumference > height of the infant
39. What is external hydrocephalus?
    - CSF collection over the cerebral convexity, interhemispheric fissure, basal cisterns
    - Usually asymptomatic, occurs in infancy to distinguish from chronic Sub Dural Hematoma (SDH)
    - Usually resolves by 3 years of age; rarely requires surgery
40. What are the types of hydrocephalus depending on the onset of symptoms?
    - Acute hydrocephalus: In this, symptoms develop within hours as the intracranial pressure rises because of acute dilatation of the ventricular system proximal to the block. Death usually occurs rapidly unless treatment is immediate.
    - Chronic hydrocephalus: It occurs because of slow evolution or arrested pathological signs of injury to the central nervous system as a result of compensatory mechanisms that dissipate the pressure due to the hydrocephalus.
    - Arrested hydrocephalus: No evolution in symptoms occurs because CSF pressure has returned to normal and the pressure gradient between the cerebral ventricles and brain parenchyma has been dissipated.
41. *What is arrested hydrocephalus?
    - Arrested hydrocephalus or normal pressure hydrocephalus is defined as state of chronic hydrocephalus where CSF pressure has returned to normal.
    - The rate of CSF absorption is equal to the rate of CSF formation in "arrested" hydrocephalus and the size of the ventricles remains stable or decreases.
    - No new neurologic signs appear, and there is evidence of continuing psychomotor development with increasing age.
    - It occurs as a result of spontaneous arrest of hydrocephalus most likely when the CSF obstruction is incomplete and when the block is distal (subarachnoid space) rather than proximal (intraventricular).
42. What is vein of Galen?
    Great cerebral vein is otherwise called vein of Galen.
43. Where is vein of Galen malformation located?
    Seen in base of the brain
44. *What is vein of Galen malformation?
    Vein of Galen malformation are due to dilation of great cerebral vein of Galen secondary to as a result of force of arterial blood into the venous system instead of connecting to capillaries, cerebral arteries are connected directly to great cerebral vein through arteriovenous fistula or by a tributary vein as shown in Fig. 24.10, which results in high blood flow into the great cerebral vein causing steal phenomenon.
45. What are the clinical clues in vein of Galen malformation?
    Presents usually in neonatal and infancy as high output cardiac failure (right-sided heart failure − dilation of right side cardiac chamber and pulmonary arteries) and intracranial hemorrhage
46. What is the treatment of vein of Galen malformation?
    Arterial embolization or coiling of the feeding vessels
47. What is the name of the torch used for transillumination test?
    Shongran's torch
48. *Where to look for bruit in a child with hydrocephalus?
    Over the eyeball, temporal region, all over the skull (vein of Galen malformation)
49. What are the investigations done in a child with hydrocephalus?
    a. TORCH screening
    b. X-ray skull
    c. USG skull
    d. CT and MRI (to find the cause)
    e. Intracranial CSF pressure monitoring
    f. EEG (if associated with convulsions)
    g. Lumbar puncture – to rule out CNS infection/shunt infection, TB meningitis, CSF pressure monitoring, CSF opening pressure
    h. Angiography – to look for aneurysm of vein of Galen
    i. Others – to monitor for complications – hemoglobin, CBC, lumbar puncture to rule out shunt infection

TABLE 24.8	Stages of Hydrocephalus	
Stage	**Clinical Features**
Stage 1	Compensated stage
Stage 2	Raised ICP – headache, sunset sign, crackpot resonance
Stage 3	Worsening headache and cranial nerve involvement
Stage 4	Coma, decorticate, decerebrate posturing

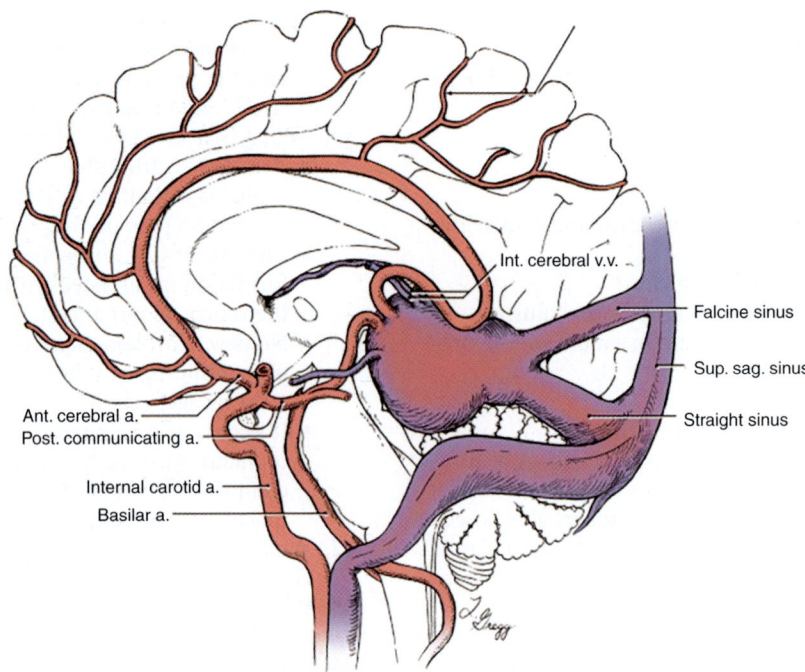

Fig. 24.10   Vein of Galen. *(Source: Reproduced from Monica Pearl, Lydia Gregg, Dheeraj Gandhi. Cerebral Venous Development in Relation to Developmental Venous Anomalies and Vein of Galen Aneurysmal Malformations, Seminars in Ultrasound CT and MRI 32(3):252-263.)*

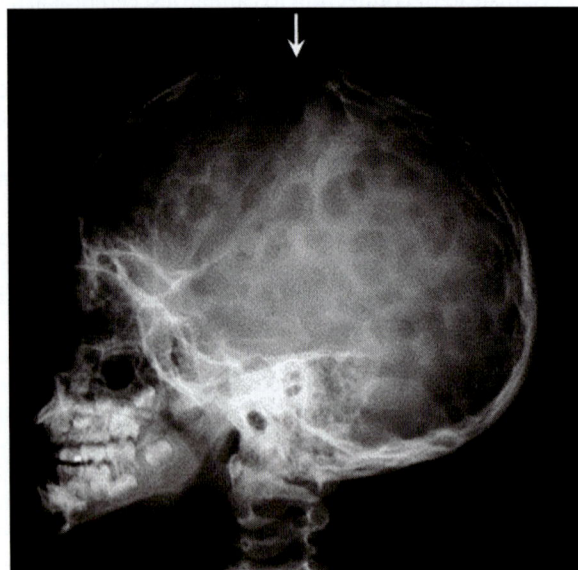

Fig. 24.11   Copper-beaten appearance – hydrocephalus. *(Source: Reproduced from Rajesh Thakker, Michael Whyte, John Eisman. Genetics of Bone Biology and Skeletal Disease, Second Edition, Hypophosphatasia and How Alkaline Phosphatase Promotes Mineralization, Figure 28.6, Chennai, Academic Press, 2018. (Credit line - Source: Reproduced with permission from Whyte MP. Hypophosphatasia, in "pediatric bone: biology & diseases" 3rd ed. In: Glorieux FH, Jueppner H, Pettifor J, editors. San Diego (CA): Elsevier (Academic Press); 2012. p. 777).*

50. What are the findings in X-ray skull in a child with hydrocephalus?
    1. X-ray skull: Islands of bone in sea of membrane
    2. Macrocrania
    3. Erosion of clinoid, sutural separation, increased convolution markings – silver-/copper-beaten appearance as shown in Fig. 24.11, thinning of skull bones

4. Calcification (toxoplasmosis – diffuse, CMV – periventricular, candle wax dripping sign – tuberous sclerosis)
    5. Lacunar skull (Arnold–Chiari malformation II)
51. What is the role of ultrasound in hydrocephalus?
    1. Intraventricular hemorrhage – preterm/newborn
    2. Follow-up ultrasound to measure the ventricular size
52. What are the CT and MRI findings in hydrocephalus?
    1. Evans ratio – maximal frontal horn width (biventricular diameter)/transverse inner diameter (biparietal diameter) >0.33 suggestive hydrocephalus
       Normal values
       * 14 weeks: 0.61
       * 27 weeks: 0.29
       * After birth: 0.26
       * Hydrocephalus: >0.33
    2. Acute hydrocephalus: Transependymal seepage of CSF around the frontal horns and less in occipital horn seen in acute and active hydrocephalus
    3. Mickey Mouse sign – ballooning of frontal horns and 3rd ventricle
       Fig. 24.12A shows schematic representation of Mickey Mouse sign. Fig. 24.12B shows CT brain showing Mickey Mouse sign – dilatation of lateral, 3rd and 4th ventricles
    4. Rule out any malformations of corpus callosum. MRI is preferred for posterior fossa and spinal cord.
53. *What is colpocephaly?
    Disproportionate prominence of occipital horns of lateral ventricle as shown in Fig. 24.13 due to congenital abnormality of corpus callosum. Example: Dysgenesis of corpus callosum (Aicardi syndrome), Lissencephaly type I. Diagnosis of colpocephaly is likely when ratio of posterior to anterior horn of lateral ventricle is more than or equal to 3.

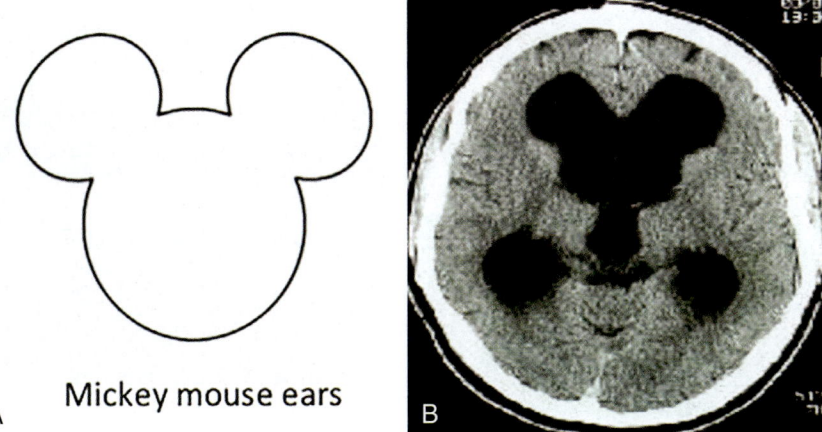

Fig. 24.12 (A) Schematic representation of Mickey Mouse sign. (B) CT brain showing Mickey Mouse sign – dilatation of lateral, 3rd and 4th ventricles.

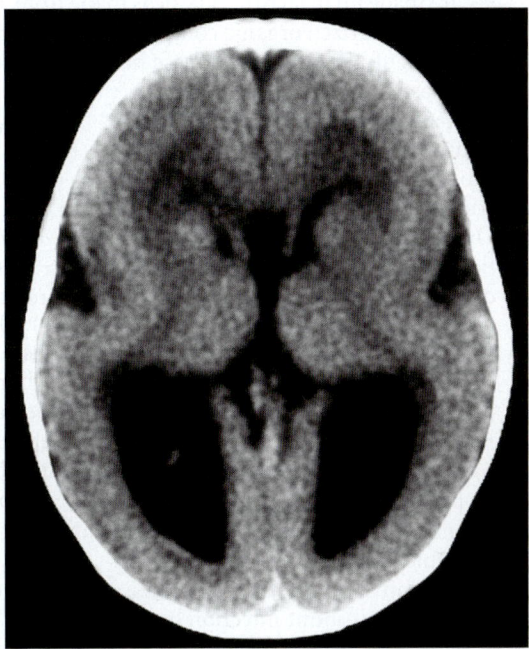

Fig. 24.13 Colpocephaly – prominent occipital horn of lateral ventricle. *(Source: Reproduced from Joseph Volpe, Terrie Inder, Basil Darras et al. Volpe's Neurology of the Newborn, Sixth Edition, Neuronal Migration, Figure 6.14, Philadelphia, Elsevier Inc., 2018. (Credit line - With permission from Dobyns WB. The neurogenetics of lissencephaly. Neurol Clin. 1989;7:89–105.).*

54. How to treat hydrocephalus?
    A. Medical treatment
       1. I.v. mannitol 0.25−0.5 g/kg/dose over 20 minutes
       2. Diuretics
          • Tab. acetazolamide – 25 mg/kg/day in three divided doses
          • Tab. frusemide – 1 mg/kg/day
    B. Surgical treatment
       • Emergency management – external ventricular drainage (EVD) – relieve acute hydrocephalus. Procedure: Under aseptic precaution, 23-gauge spinal needle is inserted on the right side 3 cm laterally in the anterior fontanelle in the midpupillary line and advance toward nasion. Around 30 mL of CSF can be drained to tide over impending respiratory arrest. Avoid repeating puncture not more than twice.
       • Surgical procedures
          1. Ventriculoperitoneal (most commonly used)
          2. Ventriculopleural
          3. Ventriculoatrial
          4. Lumboperitoneal
          5. Endoscopic third ventriculostomy – performed in obstructive hydrocephalus
          6. Shunt between lateral ventricle and cisterna magna – Torkildsen shunt
          7. Treatment for Arnold−Chiari malformation – ventriculolumbar shunt – Tuohy shunt needle (side effects – scoliosis)
          8. Dandy−Walker syndrome – two catheters are placed – Y-shaped one in ventricle and then in cyst connected to a common chamber which is connected to peritoneum

55. What are the complications of hydrocephalus?
    • Complications are mainly due to ischemia causing ependymal layer damage
    • Others include
       1. Raised intracranial pressure
       2. Cognitive impairment/speech disturbance
       3. Strabismus, visual field defect
       4. Hearing defect
       5. Weakness, gait disturbance
       6. Precocious puberty – due to increased gonadotropin secretion secondary to raised ICP
       7. Long-term complication – chronic hydrocephalus – headache, poor school performance, failure to thrive

56. What are the complications of shunt procedure?
    Table 24.9 gives complications of shunt procedure.

57. Comment on prognosis of hydrocephalus.
    Prognosis
       1. Depends on etiology − good with neural tube defects, poor with systemic infection
       2. Increased risk of developmental abnormality
       3. Visual evoked potential takes some time to resolve following shunt surgery

TABLE 24.9	**Complications of Shunt Procedure**	
Immediate Complications	**Late Complications**	
1. Infection	1. Abscess	
2. Malfunction – detected by Shunt- o- gram (injection of radioactive tracer)	2. Craniostenosis – most common is dolichocephaly	
3. Bowel perforation	3. Tube disconnection	
4. Hemiparesis	4. Blindness – posterior cerebral artery infarct	
5. Intracranial hemorrhage	5. Inguinal hernia, hydrocele	
6. Peritubal leak	6. Peritoneal pseudocyst/peritonitis/ascites	
7. Wound dehiscence	7. Length shortening/tip migration	
8. Seizures/SDH/Herniation of brainstem	8. Silicone allergy	

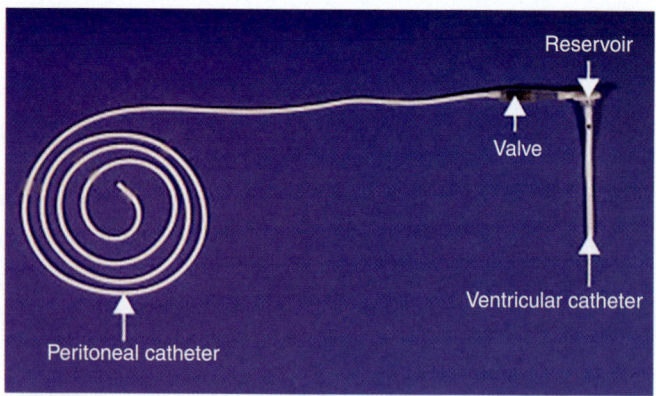

Fig. 24.14 Shunt catheter system. (*Source: References in Hydrocephalus - Surgery - Oxford International Edition (surgeryjournal.co.uk)*)

TABLE 24.10	**Three Types of Newer Shunt Valves**	
Pressure Regulated	**Flow Regulated**	**Programmable Valve**
Two types – differential pressure valve and adjustable pressure valve Differential pressure valve: Low – 5 cm, medium – 10 cm (most commonly used), high pressure – 15 cm	Used in infants Maintains constant flow irrespective of pressure They are used in large ventricles with thin cortical mantle to avoid overdrainage	Noninvasive Ball spring mechanism; uses magnet
Example: Chhabra shunt – low cost; used in developing countries; PS Medical, Hakim Microprecision	Examples: Delta and Orbis Sigma OSV 2	Examples: Sophy and Polaris

    4. Survival
       50%: Normal intelligence
       25%: Mild intellectual impairment
       25%: Severe MR

58. When to remove CSF shunt?
    Shunt placement in most of the cases is lifelong except for some conditions such as tumor. Revision surgery is required for twice in lifetime (because of normal growth of a child and CSF shunt tube becoming short compared to the size of the child): One in infancy and the other in adulthood.

59. What are the types of CSF shunt valves?
    Older name
    a) Upadhyaya shunt
    b) Chopra shunt
    c) Pudenz shunt
    d) Spitz−Holter shunt
    Newer shunt valves are as given in Table 24.10.

60. What are the parts of CSF shunt system?
    1. Proximal − ventricular catheter
    2. Reservoir − unidirectional valve (antireflux valve)
    3. Distal − peritoneal catheter
    Shunt catheter system consists of three parts as shown in Fig. 24.14.

61. Comment on the material used in shunt system.
    They are made up of silastic. Silastic is made from a family of polymerized organic compounds called silicone. No cases of autoimmune disease have been linked to the silastic used in shunts so far.

62. Comment on shunt infection.
- Shunt infection is common in newborns (5% to 10%). Most of them occur in the first 6 months of age. Ventriculitis may develop.
- Organisms causing shunt infections are own skin flora, such as *Staphylococcus epidermidis*, less frequently *S. aureus*, enteric bacteria, diphtheroids, and *Streptococcus* species.
- Infection must be considered when there is persistent and prolonged fever in a child with shunt.
- Antibiotics should be started, but antibiotics alone is not effective usually. An infected shunt must be removed and an external ventricular drain is temporarily placed.
- Shunt infections may contribute to impaired cognitive outcome and death.
- Perioperative antibiotic prophylaxis reduces the risk of subsequent shunt infection by 50%.

63. *What are the criteria for diagnosis of CSF shunt infection?
    Criteria for CSF shunt infection include both of the following:
    A. Positive CSF or CSF shunt tip culture in children with signs or symptoms of shunt malfunction or obstruction or clinical presentation of acute bacterial meningitis
    B. At least one of the following parameters of bacterial inflammation of the CSF
      a. CSF lactate concentration of >3.5 mmol/L
      b. Leukocyte count of >0.25 ×10^9/L with predominant polymorphonuclear cells
      c. Glucose ratio (CSF glucose/serum glucose): <0.4
      d. CSF glucose value of <2.5 mmol/L if no simultaneous blood glucose is observed

64. Comment on shunt failure.
    a) The failure rate (including infection) is approximately 40% in the first year and 5% in subsequent years.
    b) Most of the shunt failures result from obstruction at the ventricular catheter. This is due to overdrainage of shunt, which reduces the size of the ventricles and catheter that lie against the ependyma and choroid

plexus which block the holes at the end of the catheter.
c) Fractured tubing is the cause in around 15% of cases.
d) Other causes include migration of part or all of the shunt (7.5%) and problems with overdrainage (7%).
65. What is slit ventricle syndrome?
a. Usually seen 5−10 years postshunt because of intermittent transient shunt dysfunction; presents as headache for about 10−90 minutes
b. CT brain − small ventricles
c. Treatment – overdrainage treated with upregulation of valve pressure, shunt revision with a high-pressure valve with addition of antisiphon device

DISCUSSION ON CEREBROSPINAL FLUID

66. What is the normal CSF pathway?
Flowchart 24.1 and Fig. 24.15 show normal CSF pathway.
67. What is the normal secretion and absorption of CSF?
• Approximately 75% of CSF is secreted by choroid plexus and 25% by capillary endothelium of brain parenchyma
• Secretion of CSF is around 25 mL/h, total volume 50 mL (children), and 150 mL in adult
• Adrenergic receptors will inhibit and cholinergic will stimulate the CSF production

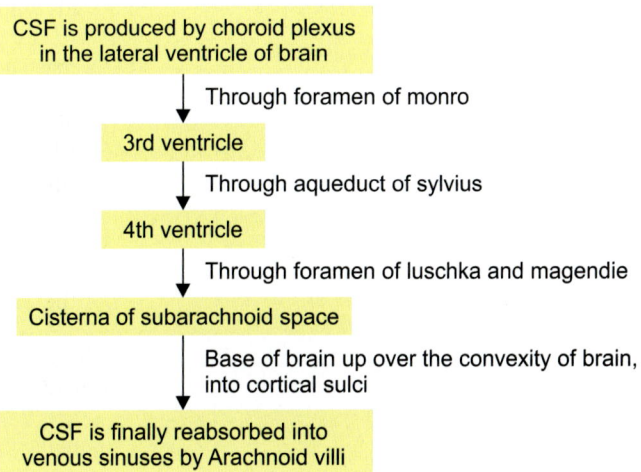

Flowchart 24.1 Normal CSF pathway.

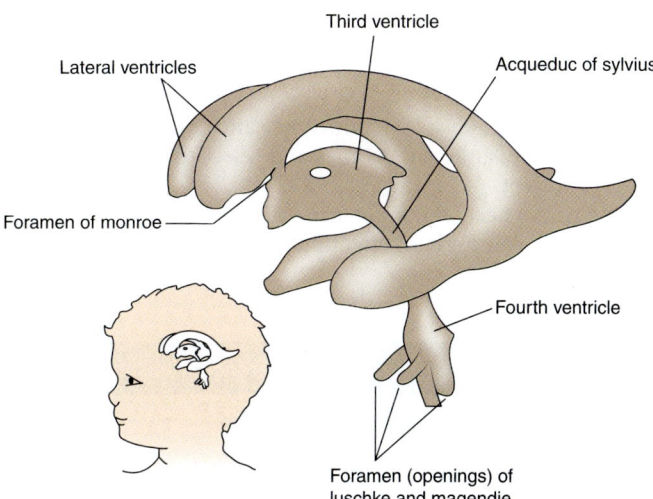

Fig. 24.15 Diagrammatic representation of normal CSF pathway.

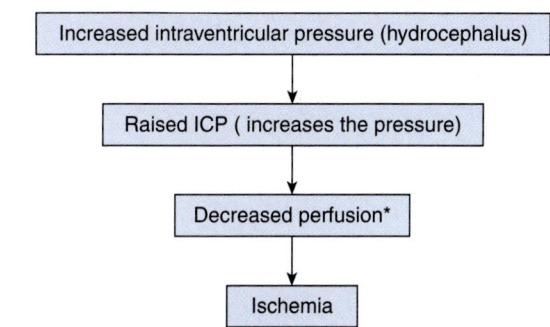

Fig. 24.16 Sequence of events occurring in brain because of hydrocephalus.

68. How does hydrocephalus affect cerebral perfusion?
Fig. 24.16 shows sequence of events due to hydrocephalus.
*Monro–Kellie hypothesis: The Monro–Kellie hypothesis states that the cranial compartment is incompressible and that the volume inside the cranium is fixed. The cranium and its constituents (blood, CSF, and brain tissue) create a state of volume equilibrium, such that any increase in volume of one of the cranial constituents must be compensated by a decrease in volume of another.

Quick Bites

- Measure the head circumference after 24 hours of birth.
- Take measurement 3 times and select the largest nearing to 0.1 cm.
- Normal head circumference – always use growth charts.
- Rough rule for head circumference is shown in Table 24.11.
- Dyne's formula: Head circumference measurement from length in first 400 days= length in cm/2 + (9.5 + or - 2.5 cm).
- Clinical clues are shown in Table 24.12.
- Cranial bruit is heard all over the skull for vein of Galen malformation.

TABLE 24.11	Rough Rule in Head Circumference Measurement
Age	**Head Circumference**
0–3 months	2 cm/month
3–6 months	1 cm/month
7–12 months	0.5 cm/month
1–3 years	1 cm/6 month
3–5 years	1 cm/year

TABLE 24.12	Clinical Clues	
Clinical Features		**Diagnosis**
Prominent occiput		Dandy−Walker malformation
Flat occiput		Arnold−Chiari malformation
Hydrocephalus + myelomeningocele		Arnold−Chiari malformation type 2
Diffuse calcification in brain		Toxoplasmosis
Periventricular calcification in brain		Cytomegalovirus infection

Meningomyelocele

Following introduction, seek permission from the caregiver and introduce yourself to the patient before history elicitation, and identify the case.

Name____Age____Sex____Consanguinity____Order of birth____Place____Informant____

Presenting Complaints and Duration

- Fluid-filled swelling in the back with/without leak
- Seizures/tonic spasms
- Flailness of both lower limbs

History of Presenting Illness

- Swelling in the back – noticed since birth, fluid filled, whether ruptured, operated
- Any leakage of fluid from the swelling
- Paucity of movement of lower limbs, bilateral, symmetrical
- Any worsening/improvement noted

CENTRAL NERVOUS SYSTEM HISTORY

Higher Functions

- Seizures, early handedness, speech and language, mental retardation, behavior abnormality

Cranial Nerve Involvement

- Usually cranial nerve (CN) findings are normal in myelomeningocele if associated with hydrocephalus, the following findings are seen: Abnormal eye position, lower CN involvement presents with difficulty feeding, choking, stridor, and pooling of secretions
- CN I – history could not be elicited
- CN II – ability to perceive light
- CN III, IV, and VI – abnormal position of eyeball
- CN V – ability to chew food
- CN VII – facial asymmetry, able to close both eyes while sleeping, drooling of saliva, deviation of angle of mouth
- CN VIII – ability to hear and respond to sound
- CN IX and X – nasal twang of voice, nasal regurgitation, choking, stridor, pooling of secretion
- CN XI – ability to move head side to side
- CN XII – any deviation of tongue on protrusion

Motor System

a. Thinness noted by the mother on both lower limbs
b. Floppiness noted by the mother on both legs
c. Ability to move limbs above the cot or whether it is only sideways or whether there are only just some flickers
d. Abnormal posturing of the lower limb
e. Involuntary movements/fasciculations
f. Ability to perceive pain sensation ask the mother whether child cries while giving injection
g. Leaky stools, dribbling of urine (retention/incontinence)
h. Big head size as compared with peers noticed by the mother

HISTORY OF COMPLICATIONS

- Rupture of sac during birth process
- Any fluid (cerebrospinal fluid) leak
- Vomiting/convulsions/increasing head size/altered sensorium
- Fever/convulsions/altered sensorium
- Fever, hematuria, dysuria, increased urgency, increased frequency
- Bedsores, ulcers, limb/foot deformity

ANTENATAL HISTORY

- Repeated abortions
- Previous fetal death
- X-ray/irradiation during pregnancy
- Fever/rash/lymphadenopathy during pregnancy (Intrauterine infection)
- Drug ingestion during pregnancy – thalidomide/valproate/phenytoin/carbamazepine
- Maternal malnutrition/folic acid deficiency
- Hair loss/skin lesions – s/o zinc deficiency
- Alcohol ingestion during pregnancy
- Polyhydramnios
- Any antenatal screening done
- Maternal diabetes mellitus

BIRTH HISTORY

- Delayed onset of labor/prolonged labor
- Cesarean section (malpresentation)
- Difficulty in delivery of head (large head)

NEONATAL HISTORY

Birth asphyxia, limpness or decreased spontaneous movement of lower limbs, swelling over the back – skin intact or ruptured, leaky CSF, large head, feeding difficulties, drooling or pooling of secretions, breathlessness/abnormal breathing pattern, decreased movement, weak cry, abnormal posture/contractures, convulsions in neonatal period, dribbling of urine/leaky stools

DEVELOPMENT HISTORY

Delayed motor milestone, other milestones – normal

DIETETIC HISTORY

Any feeding difficulty

IMMUNIZATION HISTORY

Immunization as per universal immunization schedule or IAP schedule

FAMILY HISTORY

- Other siblings affected with similar complaints
- Mental retardation or other congenital anomalies and delayed milestone

Summary

A......-month/year-old infant with fluid-filled sac in the back with or without seizures, with flailness/paucity of movements of both lower limbs, leaky stools/dribbling of urine with or without big size head, with or without polyhydramnios in the antenatal period, with or without significant birth history, with delayed motor milestone, with feeding difficulties with or without significant family history with or without VP shunt, most likely spinal dysraphism; proceed with examination.

General Examination and Head-to-Foot Examination

- Posture – lies in the cot/extended posture, knees along the side of the cot/paucity of movement of both lower limb
- Alert, recognizes the mother
- Neurocutaneous markers
- Bedsores/contractures/trophic ulcers/callosities
- Skull examination
  - Head circumference/transillumination/fontanelles/separation of sutures
  - Eyes – look for conjugate movements of eyes/sunset sign
  - Face – dysmorphic facies
  - Ventriculoperitoneal shunt – whether present
- Any operated scars noted
- BCG scar, gibbus and spinal deformity
- Examination of the back
  - Site
  - Size
  - Shape of the defect (globular)
  - Midline or not
  - Skin over the swelling
  - Pigmentation
  - Leakage from the sac
  - Cough impulse/crying (does the swelling increase in size)
  - Curvature of the spine gibbus underlying the defect

Vital Signs

- Temperature
- Pulse rate
- Respiratory rate – breathing pattern any evidence of respiratory distress
- Blood pressure

Anthropometry With Interpretation

- Head circumference – hydrocephalus

CNS Examination

HIGHER FUNCTIONS

- Sensorium – recognizes the mother, alert, speech, early handedness, mental retardation, behavior or sleep disturbance

CRANIAL NERVES

- CN I – could not be tested
- CN II – ability to perceive light, fundus – optic atrophy
- CN III, IV, VI – look for sunset sign, whether moves eyeball in all four cardinal directions, strabismus, no ptosis
- CN V – pain sensation over the face, able to chew food, jaw jerk
- CN VII – wrinkling of forehead present; look for any facial asymmetry
- CN VIII – normal
- CN IX, X – low voice volume, choking, stridor, apnea, vocal cord paralysis
- CN XI – able to lift head from supine position; whether turns head on both side
- CN XII – any deviation of tongue, fasciculation, or wasting

MOTOR SYSTEM EXAMINATION

Motor system examination is given in Table 25.1.

TABLE 25.1 Motor System Examination		
Motor System Examination	**Right**	**Left**
Bulk	Upper limb – normal Lower limb wasting	Upper limb – normal Lower limb wasting
Tone[a]	Upper limb – normal Lower limb – hypotonia	Upper limb – normal Lower limb – hypotonia
Power[a]	Shoulder joint: 5/5 Elbow: 5/5 Wrist: 5/5 Finger grip – normal Hip joint: 2/5 Knee joint: 2/5 Ankle joint: 2/5 Toe grip – weak	Shoulder joint: 5/5 Elbow: 5/5 Wrist: 5/5 Finger grip – normal Hip joint: 2/5 Knee joint: 2/5 ankle joint: 2/5 Toe grip – weak
Superficial reflexes	Anal reflex – absent anal wink Cremasteric reflex – absent	Anal reflex – absent anal wink Cremasteric reflex – absent
Plantar	No response	No response
Deep tendon reflexes	Biceps ++ Triceps ++ Supinator ++ Knee jerk absent Ankle jerk absent	Biceps ++ Triceps ++ Supinator ++ Knee jerk absent Ankle jerk absent

[a]Depends on the level of defect.

SENSORY SYSTEM

Response to sensory stimuli in all extremities (paresthesia)

MUSCULOSKELETAL SYSTEM

Look for congenital dysplasia of hip and CTEV

Other System Examination

CVS EXAMINATION

Rule out congenital heart disease

RS EXAMINATION

Pattern of breathing, respiratory distress

ABDOMEN

Rule out renal malformation, palpable bladder

Diagnosis

A child with open/closed neural tube defect (NTD) probably with or without hydrocephalus with or without signs of raised ICP with or without VP shunt

Frequently Asked Questions

1. Enumerate spinal cord lesion and its corresponding clinical features

   Table 25.2 gives level of spinal lesion and its corresponding clinical findings.

2. *What is spinal dysraphism?

   The term spinal dysraphism indicates Neural Tube Defect (NTD), due to of closure of posterior vertebral arch. It refers to a spectrum of disorders in which there is defective midline closure of neural, bony, or other mesenchymal tissues, whereas the term myelodysplasia indicates spinal cord malformation.

3. What are the causes of Neural Tube Defect (NTD)?

   Etiology of NTD is Multifactorial. It includes both environmental and Genetic causes.

   Genetic determinants include mutations in folate-responsive or folate-dependent pathways (polymorphism of the MTHF reductase gene), hyperhomocysteinemia which is seen in people of northern European or Hungarian origin.

4. What are the complications seen in hydrocephalus?
   - Rupture of sac during birth process
   - CSF leak
   - Meningitis
   - Raised intracranial pressure
   - Urinary tract infection
   - Bedsores, ulcers, limb/foot deformity, scoliosis, kyphosis

5. What are the risk factors in myelomeningocele?

   Table 25.3 gives risk factors associated with myelomeningocele.

6. *List the significance of clinical clues in myelomeningocele.

   Table 25.4 gives clinical clues in myelomeningocele.

_____

*Important question asked in the examination.

TABLE 25.2	Level of Lesion and Clinical Findings	
Spinal Cord Level	**Clinical Features**
Above L3	• Complete paraplegia noted • Dermatomal anesthesia • Bowel and bladder incontinence
L4 and below	• Same as for above L3, except for the hip function is preserved • Flexors of hip, adductors of hip and knee extensors are affected • The child is ambulatory with aids, bracing or surgery
S1 and below	• Same as for L4 and below, except for the following: Preservation of feet dorsiflexors and partial preservation of hip extensors and knee flexors • The child is ambulatory with minimal aids
S3 and below	• Lower extremity motor function normal • Saddle anesthesia • Variable bladder–rectal incontinence

TABLE 25.3	Risk Factors Associated With Myelomeningocele
Nutritional status of mother (folate deficiency)	
Folic acid supplementation during pregnancy	
Maternal obesity	
Hair loss/skin lesions suggestive of zinc deficiency	
Hyperthermia	
Family history of neural tube defects	
Maternal exposure to X-ray, hazardous waste sites, disinfection products found in drinking water and pesticides	
Drug intake – thalidomide/valproate/phenytoin/carbamazepine and drugs to induce ovulation	
Fever/rash/lymphadenopathy during pregnancy (intrauterine infection)	
Alcohol ingestion during pregnancy	
Trisomies 13 and 18, triploidy, Meckel syndrome	

TABLE 25.4	Clinical Clues in Myelomeningocele	
Arnold–Chiari (AC) malformation Fig. 25.1A–C gives clinical findings in Arnold–Chiari malformation type 2	• Frontal prominence • High-pitched cry • Stridor, apnea, and hoarseness of voice • Lower cranial nerve palsy • Flaccid paralysis of the lower extremities • Lack of response to touch and pain • Lower extremity deformities (clubfeet, ankle and/or knee contractures, and subluxation of the hips, spine kyphotic gibbus) • Constant urinary dribbling and a relaxed anal sphincter
Hydrocephalus	Prominent scalp veins, shiny skin, sunset sign, shunt scars, nystagmus, bulging anterior fontanelle

7. What is the significance of vital signs in myelomeningocele?
   - Increased respiratory rate – aspiration pneumonia
   - Blood pressure – hypertension seen in renal failure

8. What are the clues in anthropometry in myelomeningocele?
   - To compare head size with centile chart (hydrocephalus)
   - Height is decreased in kyphoscoliosis and shorter lower limbs are due to reduced growth and contracture

9. What is the importance in other systemic examination in myelomeningocele?
   - Abdomen – to look for scars (ventriculoperitoneal shunt), palpable bladder, renal malformation kidneys
   - Respiratory system – aspiration pneumonia

10. *How common is hydrocephalus in myelomeningocele?

    About 75% of patients with meningomyelocele have hydrocephalus, whereas patients with only meningocele rarely have hydrocephalus.

11. What are the causes of hydrocephalus in myelomeningocele?
    - Meningitis
    - Arnold–Chiari type 2 malformation
    - Aqueductal stenosis

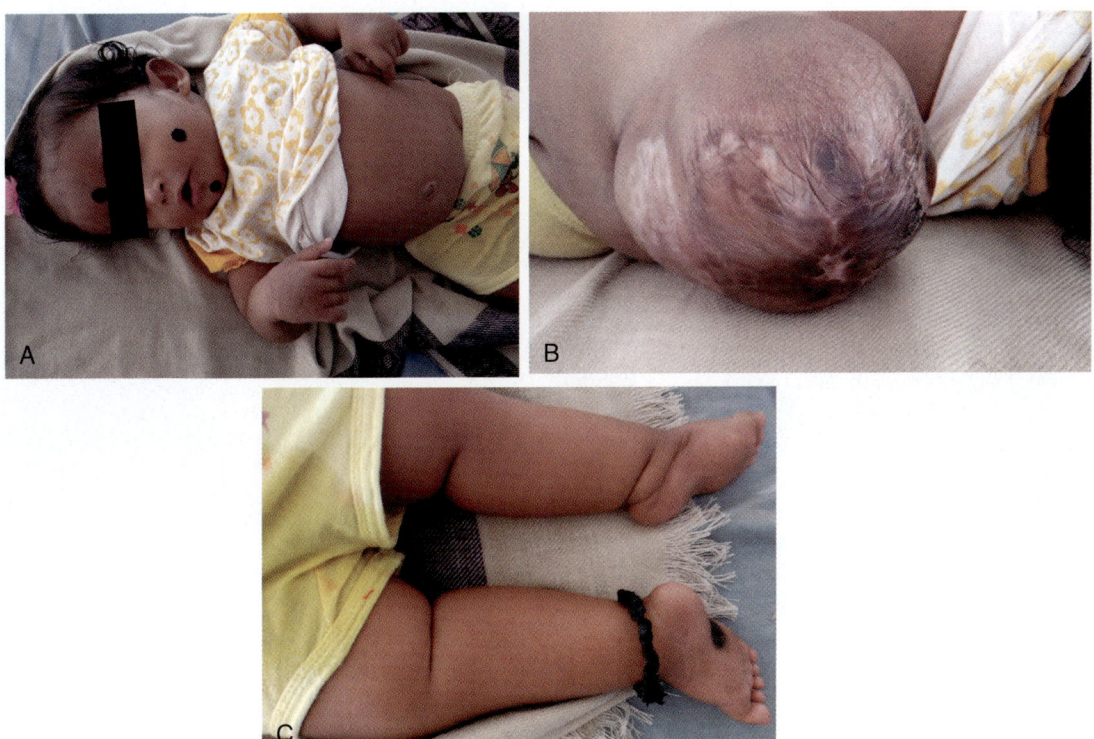

Fig. 25.1 (A) Arnold–Chiari malformation (hydrocephalus). (B) Arnold–Chiari malformation – myelomeningocele. (C) Arnold–Chiari malformation paraparesis.

12. What are the clinical clues in myelomeningocele according to age?
    a. Newborn – paucity of movement, flailness of lower limb, arthrogryposis or contractures, dribbling of urine, leaky stools
    b. Infancy stridor, weak cry, and apnea, childhood abnormalities of gait, spasticity, and increasing incoordination during childhood
13. What are the findings in motor system examination in myelomeningocele?
    • Flaccid paralysis of the lower extremities
    • An absent Deep tendon reflex (DTR)
    • A lack of response to touch and pain
    • Lower extremity deformities (clubfeet, ankle and/or knee contractures, and subluxation of the hips, kyphosis, gibbus)
    • Constant urinary dribbling and a relaxed anal sphincter
    Fig. 25.2A shows relaxed anal sphincter (absent anal wink), Fig. 25.2B shows absent deep tendon reflex (DTR), and Fig. 25.2C shows absent plantar reflex in a child with myelomeningocele.
14 What are the clinical clues in myelomeningocele? Remember as "4 P"
    • Palpable bladder
    • Paresthesia
    • Patulous anus
    • Paraparesis
15. What are the symptoms of Chiari crisis?
    Chiari crisis is due to downward herniation of the medulla and cerebellar tonsils through the foramen magnum. It is due to endogenous malformations in the cerebellum and brainstem.

16. What are the symptoms of hindbrain dysfunction?
    Symptoms include apnea, stridor, difficulty feeding, choking, vocal cord paralysis, pooling of secretions, and spasticity of the upper extremities. If left untreated, it can lead to death.
17. *What are the criteria for surgery in NTD?
    • Emergency surgery in open NTD
    • Elective surgery in closed NTD by 6 months of age
18. What are the immediate complications of myelomeningocele?
    1. Hydrocephalus
    2. Paralysis and deformities of legs
    3. Urinary problems – incontinence and difficulty emptying bladder
    4. Bowel – constipation
19. Comment on long-term prognosis of myelomeningocele.
    a. Survival can be up to 17 years in repaired meningocele
    b. Long-term outcome depends on
        ○ Neurosurgical issues
        ○ Raised ICP
        ○ Shunt infection
        ○ Seizures
    c. Motor outcomes depends on the level of paralysis
    d. Intellectual outcome: >75% have IQ >80
20. What are the long-term complications of hydrocephalus?
    • Urologic and renal complications
    • Urinary tract infections
    • Growth and nutrition
    • Endocrinopathies
    • Orthopedic complications
    • Rehabilitation
    • Latex allergy

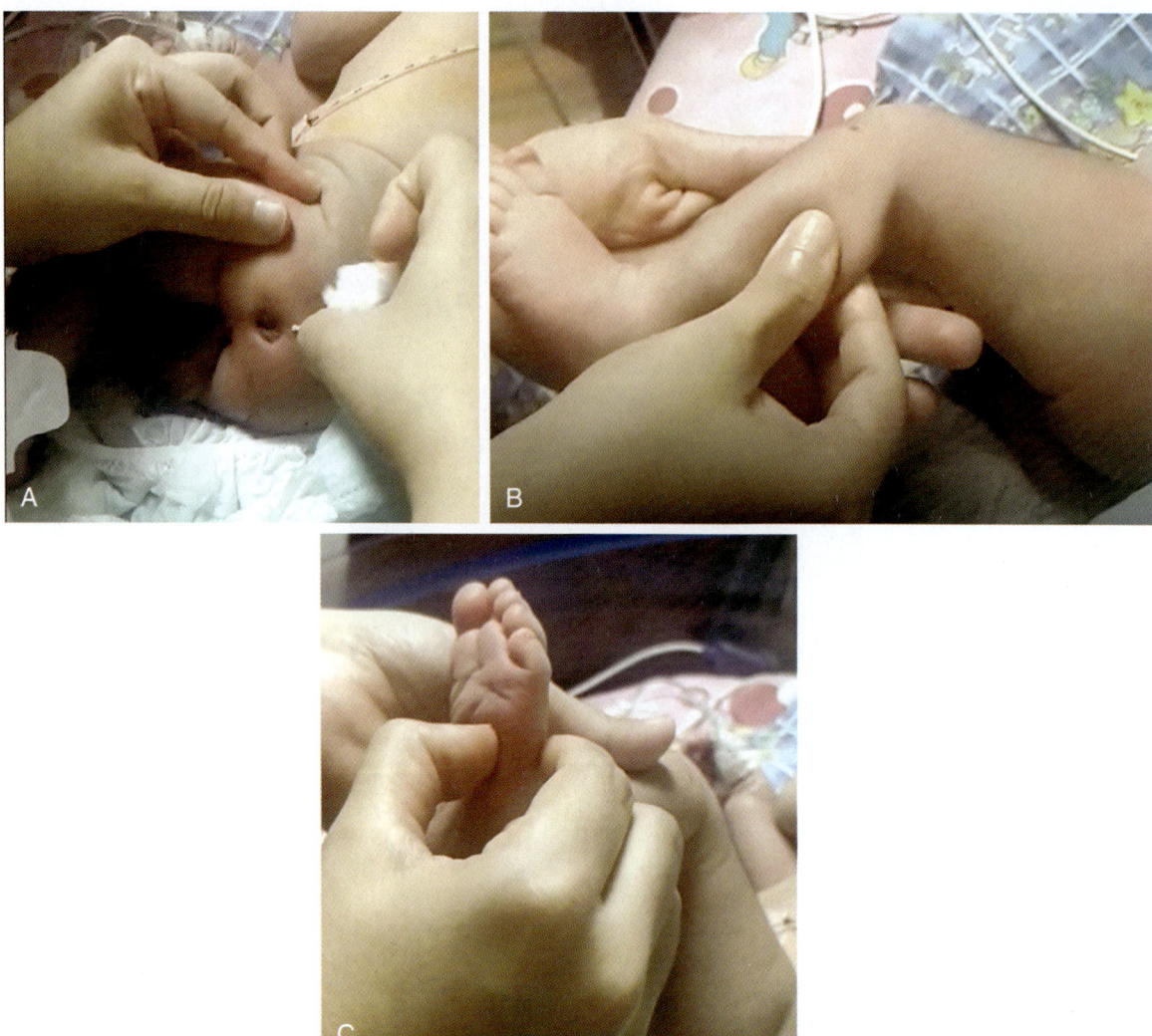

Fig. 25.2 (A) Relaxed anal sphincter – absent anal wink. (B) Absent deep tendon reflex (DTR). (C) Absent plantar reflex.

21. What are the investigations done in NTD?
    Investigations
    1) Routine investigations
    2) X-ray chest
       Spine
       Pelvic Joints
    3) CT brain
    4) MRI if suspecting posterior fossa tumor and syringomyelia
    5) Tests of renal functions
       ◦ Urodynamic studies
       ◦ IVP (Intravenous pyelogram)
       ◦ USG of urinary tract
       ◦ Micturating cystourethrogram
    6) Tests of vision and hearing
22. *What are the surgical procedures performed in myelomeningocele?
    The following procedures are performed in a child with myelomeningocele:
    a. Repair of a myelomeningocele
    b. Shunting procedure for hydrocephalus

    c. Clubfeet taping or casting
    d. Operation of dislocated hips
23. How to follow a child with myelomeningocele?
    • Multidisciplinary approach
    • Pediatrician – drugs, counseling
    • Neurosurgeon
    • Neurologist
    • Nephrologist
    • Ophthalmologist
    • Physiotherapist
    • Periodic monitoring of head circumference – every 3 months
24. *What is the cause of mortality in a child with myelomeningocele?
    Most common cause of mortality in a child with myelomeningocele is renal dysfunction.
25. What is the incidence of NTD?
    1 in 2000 live births
26. *How to differentiate between open and closed NTD?
    Table 25.5 gives differences between open and closed NTD.

TABLE 25.5	Differences Between Open and Closed Neural Tube Defects
Open Neural Tube Defect	**Closed Neural Tube Defect**
Also called primary neural tube defect	Also called secondary neural tube defect
More common	Less common
Because of primary failure of closure of neural tube or disruption of closure between 18 and 25 days of gestation	Abnormal closure of the lower sacral or coccygeal segments during secondary neurulation
Defect in cranial vault or vertebra	Defect in cranial vault or vertebra
Brain or spinal cord is exposed, not covered by skin	Brain or spinal cord is not exposed, covered by skin
Examples: Anencephalocele (Fig. 25.3A), encephalocele (Fig. 25.3B), spina bifida (occulta; Fig. 25.3C), myelocele, myelomeningocele (Fig. 25.3D)	Lipomyelomeningocele (Fig. 25.4), lipomeningocele, diastematomyelia, tethered cord (Fig. 25.5)

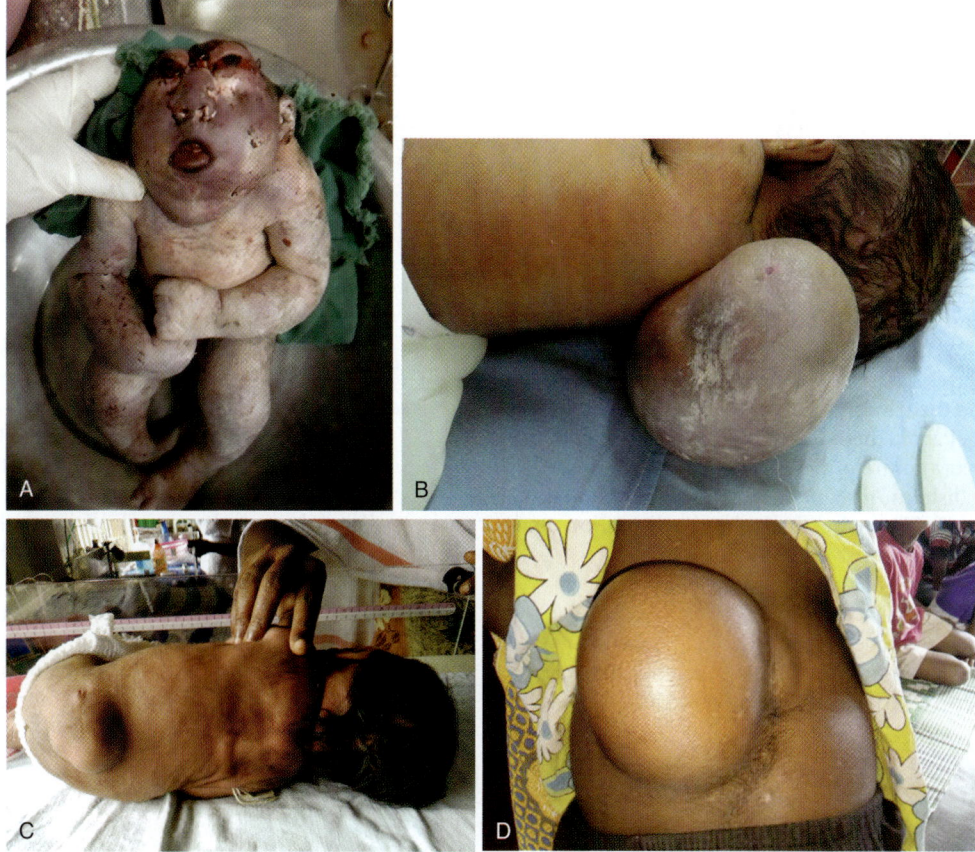

Fig. 25.3 (A) Anencephaly. (B) Encephalocele. (C) Spina bifida occulta. (D) Myelomeningocele.

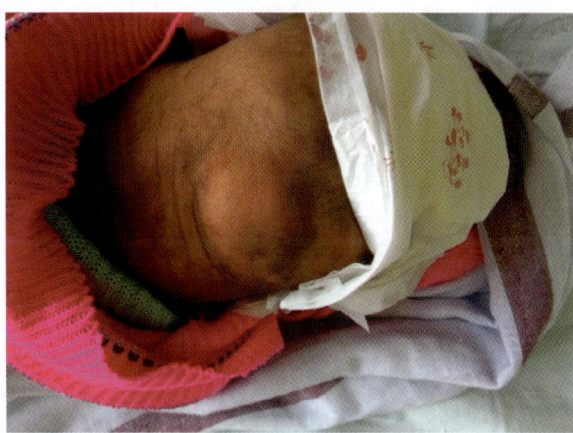

Fig. 25.4 Lipomyelomeningocele.

27. *What is spinal bifida and what are its types?
    - Spina bifida is an open NTD. it is of two types – spina bifida cystica and occulta.
    - Examples of spina bifida cystica are meningocele and myelomeningocele.
    - Spina bifida occulta is also called hidden spilt spine. It is due to defect in the parts of the bones of the spine, called the spinous process, and the neural arch that appears abnormal on a radiogram, without any involvement of the spinal cord and spinal nerves.
28. What are spina bifida occulta and spina bifida cystica?
    - Spina bifida occulta = spilt spine (deformity in spinous process and vertebral arches)
    - Spina bifida cystica = meningocele, myelomeningocele
    - Meningocele = herniation of meninges

Tethered **Normal**

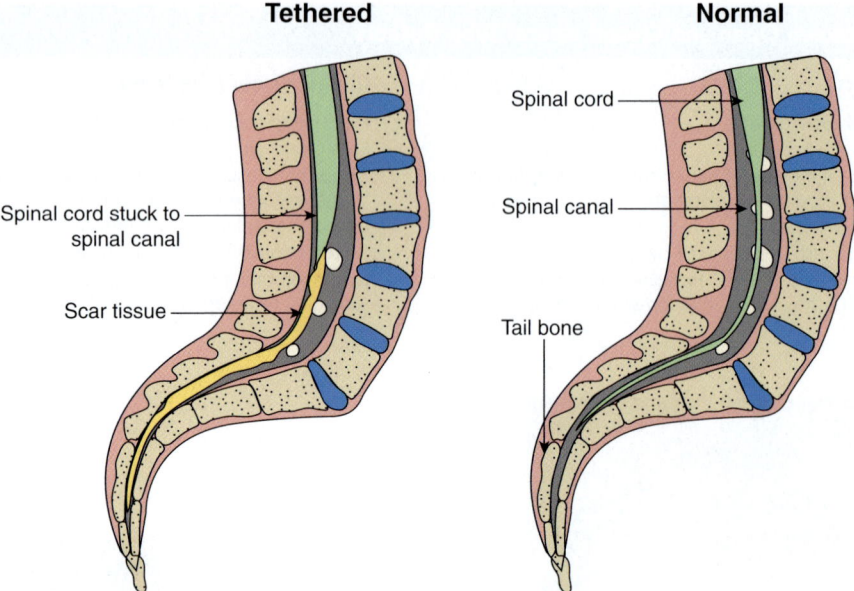

Spinal cord stuck to spinal canal

Scar tissue

Spinal cord

Spinal canal

Tail bone

Fig. 25.5 Tethered cord (schematic representation). *(Source: DOI:10.33762/BSURG.2018.160100. TETHERED SPINAL CORD: REVIEW OF LITERATURE)*

- Myelomeningocele = herniation of meninges + spinal cord
  Fig. 25.6 gives schematic representation of spina bifida.
29. What are the theories in the formation of NTD.
  - The "nonclosure theory" proposes that NTDs represent primary failure of neural tube closure.
  - The "overdistention theory," introduced by Morgagni, states that NTDs arise through overdistention and rupture of a previously closed neural tube.
30. What are the stages of spinal cord development?
  Three stages:
    - Gastrulation stage − conversion of bilaminar disk into a trilaminar disk (ectoderm, endoderm, and mesoderm) initiated by primitive streak = 23 weeks

- Primary neurulation = 34 weeks
- Secondary neurulation = 56 weeks
31. Describe neural tube formation and the stages of neural tube formation.
  - The neural tube is an embryonic structure. It forms the brain and spinal cord during the process called neurulation.
  - The edges of the neural plate are thickened and migrate toward the midline of the embryo and result in fusion in the midline and form the hollow neural tube.
  - Neurulation starts on day 20 and completely closed by day 29 in humans.
  - An initial anterior-posterior patterning is seen before the neural tube closure, with four distinct regions in

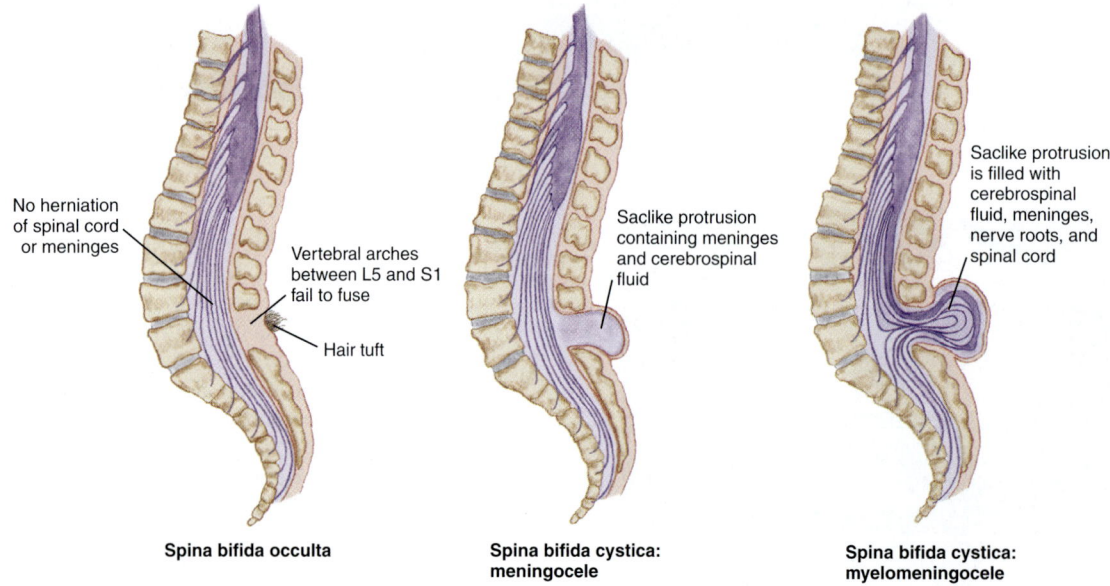

No herniation of spinal cord or meninges

Vertebral arches between L5 and S1 fail to fuse

Hair tuft

Saclike protrusion containing meninges and cerebrospinal fluid

Saclike protrusion is filled with cerebrospinal fluid, meninges, nerve roots, and spinal cord

Spina bifida occulta **Spina bifida cystica: meningocele** **Spina bifida cystica: myelomeningocele**

Fig. 25.6 Spina bifida (schematic representation). *(Source: Reproduced from Emily McKinney, Susan James, Sharon Murray. Maternal-Child Nursing, Sixth Edition, The Child With a Neurologic Alteration, FIG 52.2, St. Louis, Elsevier Inc., 2022.)*

the neural tube as follows: Prosencephalon (fore-brain), mesencephalon (midbrain), rhombencephalon (hindbrain), and the future spinal cord. The stages of neural tube formation are primary neurulation and secondary neurulation.
- Primary neurulation: Rostral spinal cord formation (brain + up to the level of S2)
- Secondary neurulation: Distal spinal cord formation (distal to S2 level)

32. How to classify spinal dysraphism on the basis of embryology?
    Flowchart 25.1 shows classification of spinal dysraphism on the basis of embryology.

33. Enumerate the salient features of each spinal dysraphism.
    Table 25.6 gives salient features of various spinal dysraphism.

34. *What are the clinical clues in tethered cord syndrome
    Clumsiness of gait, stunted growth, leg length discrepancy, thinness of limb, deformity of one foot or leg, and disturbances in bladder function are the clinical clues. Fig. 25.7A shows a child with tethered cord over the back. Fig. 25.7B shows neuropathic changes in left foot as a result of spinal cord tethering. Fig. 25.7C shows sagittal T1 MRI showing thickening and fatty infiltration of the filum terminale.

35. Enumerate the clinical features of myelomeningocele according to the vertebral body level.
    Table 25.7 gives clinical features of myelomeningocele according to the vertebral body level.

36. What are the biomarkers in identifying NTD antenatally?
    Failure of closure of the neural tube allows excretion of fetal substances (α-fetoprotein [AFP], acetylcholinesterase) into the amniotic fluid, which are the biochemical markers for an NTD. Most specific biochemical marker for an NTD is acetylcholine esterase.

37. What are the antenatal screening findings in NTD?
    - Maternal serum Alpha feto protein > 2.5 MoM (Multiples of Median) in the second trimester (Normal AFP <2.5 MoM before 14 weeks)
    - Ultrasound findings − direct visualization of spinal defect or through indirect signs such as lemon shaped head, banana cerebellum, ventriculomegaly

38. Mention some causes of decreased AFP.
    Trisomy 13, trisomy 18, and trisomy 21

39. *What is MoM in antenatal screening test of AFP?
    - Multiple of the median (MoM) is a measure of how far an individual test result deviates from the median. It is a medical screening test and the results are highly variable.
    - MoM is a method that normalizes the data from participating laboratory values of AFP, so that individual test results can be compared.

    $$\text{MoM (of the Patient)} = \frac{\text{Result (Patient)}}{\text{Median (patient population)}}$$

    - For example, alpha feto protein testing is used to screen for NTD. During the second trimester, if the median AFP at 16 weeks of gestation is 30 ng/mL and that of a pregnant woman's AFP at that same gestational age is 60 ng/mL, then her MoM is equal to 60/30 = 2.0. Otherwise, her AFP result is 2 times higher than the normal. Normal MoM is 0.7−2.5.

40. What is MOMS trial in NTD?
    MOMS trial (Management of Myelomeningocele Study) is a clinical trial for the treatment of myelomeningocele. It compared the prenatal (before birth)

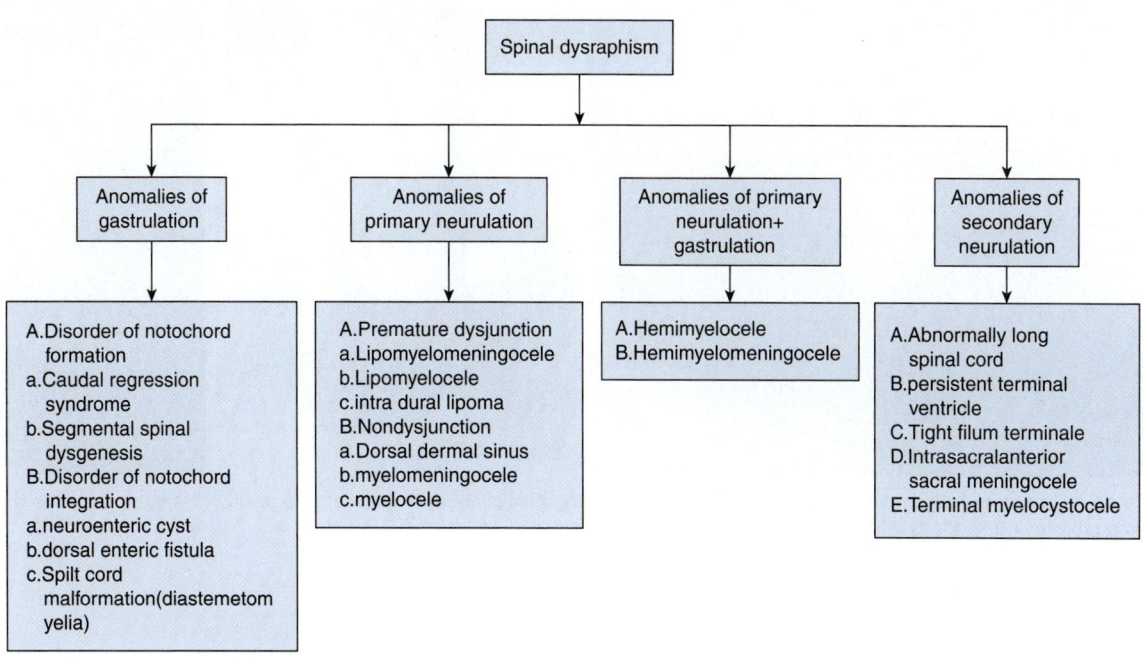

Flowchart 25.1 Classification of spinal dysraphism based on embryology

TABLE 25.6	Salient Features of Various Spinal Dysraphism

1. Anomalies of gastrulation
   A. Caudal regression syndrome
   - a. Lumbosacral vertebral body dysgenesis/hypogenesis
   - b. Truncated blunt spinal cord ends above the expected level

   B. Segmental spinal dysgenesis
   - a. Congenital thoracic or lumbar kyphosis
   - b. Bulky, thickened and low-lying cord below the dysgenetic segment

   C. Split cord malformations (Diastematomyelia [DSM])
   Splitting of the spinal cord into two hemicords:
   Type 1: The two hemicords are located within individual dural tubes separated by an osseous or cartilaginous septum
   Type 2: There is a single dural tube containing two hemicords, not separated by osseous or cartilaginous septum

2. Anomalies of primary neurulation
   A. Lipomyelomeningocele
   - Closed dysraphism with lumbosacral skin covered masses
   - The placode – lipoma interface lies outside of the spinal canal because of expansion of the subarachnoid space

   B. Lipomyelocele
   - Closed dysraphism with lumbosacral skin covered masses
   - The placode – lipoma interface lies within the spinal canal

   C. Intradural lipoma
   - Closed dysraphism
   - Lipoma located along the dorsal midline that is contained within the dural sac
   - Lumbosacral most common location

   D. Myelomeningocele
   - Open dysraphism
   - Neural placode protrudes above the skin surface
   - Almost always associated with Chiari type 2 malformation

   E. Myelocele
   - Open dysraphism
   - neural placode lies exposed on the surface of the back without any covering of the skin or the meninges

3. Anomalies of combined primary neurulation + gastrulation
   A. Hemimyelomeningocele
   - Diastematomyelia associated with myelomeningocele or myelocele of one of the hemicords

4. Anomalies of secondary neurulation and retrogressive differentiation
   A. Tight filum terminale
   Low-lying cord with thickened filum
   B. Terminal myelocystocele
   Herniation of large terminal syrinx (syringocele) into a posterior meningocele through a posterior spinal defect; usually do not communicate with each other
   C. Abnormally long spinal cord
   Persistent cord termination below L2−L3 after the first month of life in a full gestation infant

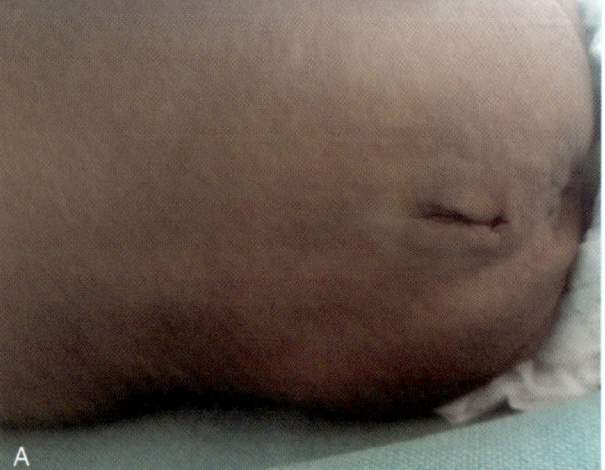
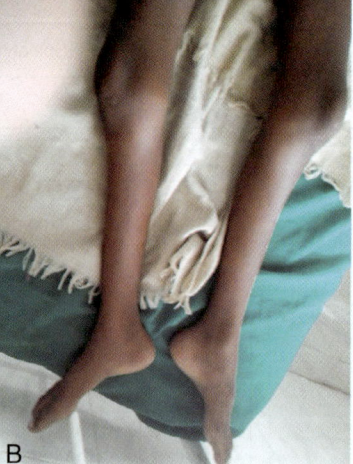
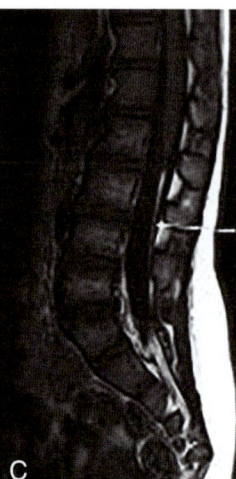

Fig. 25.7 (A) A child with tethered cord syndrome in the back. (B) Neuropathic changes in left foot as a result of tethered spinal cord. (C) Sagittal T1 MRI showing thickening and fatty infiltration of the filum terminale. (*Source: (C) Nelson 21st, Chapter 624, Fig. 624.1, page, 3239.*)

TABLE 25.7	Clinical Features of Myelomeningocele According to the Vertebral Body Level

Vertebral Level of Lesion	Clinical Features
Upper thoracic or cervical region	a. Very minimal neurologic deficit b. Do not have hydrocephalus c. Neurogenic bladder and bowel may be present
Thoracic lesion	a. Spastic paraplegia b. Spastic bladder c. Sensory loss d. Segmental withdrawal of reflexes below the level of lesion indicates the presence of intact but isolated spinal cord segment below the cyst
Conus medullaris lesion	a. Flaccid paraplegia b. Lumbosacral sensory loss c. Distended bladder with overflow incontinence d. Lack a withdrawal response in the legs, high incidence of lower extremity deformities (clubfeet, ankle and/or knee contractures), and subluxation of the hip

and postnatal (after birth) surgery to repair myelomeningocele defect. The study concluded that

- Among the babies who underwent fetal repair of spina bifida, only 50% were likely to require ventricular shunt after birth.
- Chiari malformations were less common in the fetal repair group.
- Standardized test scores for motor skills were superior in the fetal surgery group as many as twice the number of children were walking independently at 30 months as compared with the postnatal surgery group.

41. What is the role of folic acid in the prevention of NTDs?

Folic acid cannot be synthesized de novo by the body, and must be obtained either from diet or supplementation. Folic acid present in the diet is not active metabolite. It is converted into tetrahydrofolate (THF), which acts as a cofactor for the conversion of methionine to homocysteine which undergoes methylation and helps in the formation of DNA and acetylcholine (neurotransmitter).

42. What is the therapeutic and preventive dose of folic acid?

Folic acid at a dose of 0.4 mg/day decreases the incidence of NTD when taken 3 months before conception to 1 month after pregnancy. In case of previous sibling affected with NTD, 4 mg/day (10 times that of the therapeutic dose) is given.

43. What is the percentage of reduction of NTD with antenatal folic acid consumption?

Approximately 50%–70% decreased chance of NTDs

44. What is engagement pill?

Folic acid is called engagement pill because it helps in maturation of Graafian follicle in ovum.

45. What are the food rich in folate?

Green leafy vegetables, fruits, animal liver and kidney, legumes, egg yolk, and citrus fruits

46. What are the associated anomalies with NTD?

Arnold−Chiari type 2 malformation, Meckel syndrome, trisomy 13, trisomy 18, trisomy 21, triploidy

47. What are the drugs that inhibit folic acid metabolism?

Methotrexate, pyrimethamine, anticonvulsants such as phenobarbitone and phenytoin

48. What is the ideal threshold for RBC folate level?

Normal RBC folate levels are 150−600 ng/mL (serum folic acid level is 520 ng/mL).

Quick Bites

- Incidence of neural tube defect is 1:2000 live births.
- Antenatal folic acid consumption shows 50%−70% decreased chance of neural tube defects.
- Mode of inheritance in neural tube defects is multifactorial polygenic or oligogenic.
- Folic acid preventive dose of 0.4 mg/day decreases the incidence of neural tube defect, and the therapeutic dose is 4 mg/day.
- Spina bifida occulta = spilt spine (deformity in spinous process and vertebral arches)
- Spina bifida cystica = meningocele, myelomeningocele
- Meningocele = herniation of meninges
- Myelomeningocele = herniation of meninges + spinal cord
- Clinical clues in myelomeningocele: Remember as "4 P" − Palpable bladder, Paresthesia, Patulous anus, Paraparesis.
- Most common cause of mortality in a child with myelomeningocele is renal dysfunction.

26

Facial Palsy

Frequently Asked Questions

1. Trace facial nerve course.
   Three courses: (1) Intracranial course, (2) intratemporal course, and (3) extracranial course as shown in Fig. 26.1. Flowchart 26.1 gives the course of facial nerve.
2. How to locate the level of facial nerve palsy?
   Site of lesion and its corresponding level in facial palsy are given in Table 26.1.
3. How to examine facial nerve?
   Inspection
   a. Any asymmetry of face at resting position
   b. Movements during spontaneous facial expression (as child talks and smiles)
   c. Tone, atrophy, and fasciculations of facial muscles
   d. Pattern of spontaneous blinking for frequency and symmetry
   e. Widening of palpebral fissures and facial dystonia with knitting of brow (omega sign)

Examination of motor function
   To examine the muscles on voluntary and emotional responses. Palpate the tone of the muscle.
   a. Wrinkle forehead by looking upwards
   b. Close eyes as tight as possible
   c. Blow cheeks against closed mouth
   d. To blow whistle
   e. To show teeth, angle of mouth is deviated on healthy side
Examination of facial reflexes
   a. Orbicularis oculi reflex – pulling the skin lateral to outer canthus with thumb and index causes reflex closing of eyes
   b. Cochleopalpaberal reflex – closure of eyes to loud noise
   c. Visuopalpalpebral or menace reflex – closure of eyes to strong visual stimuli or light

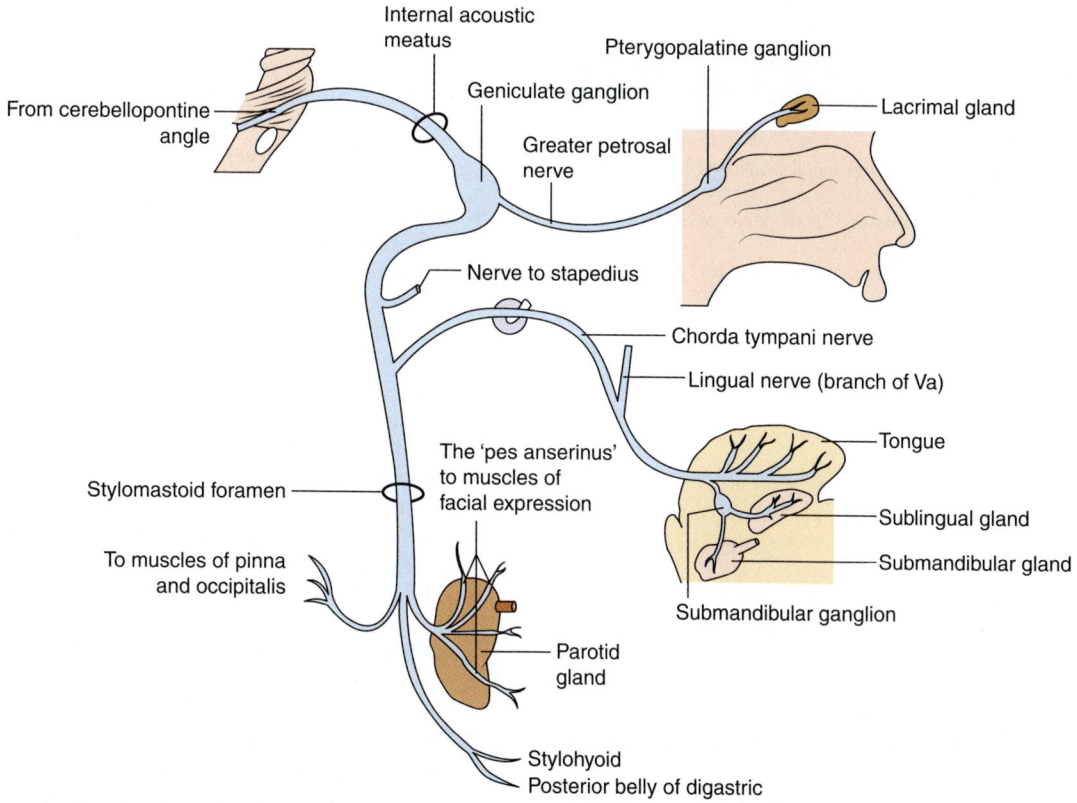

Fig. 26.1 Course of facial nerve. (Source: https://www.google.com/imgres?imgurl=https%3A%2F%2Fmedicine.uiowa.edu%2Fiowaprotocols%2Fsites%2Fmedicine.uiowa.edu.iowaprotocols%2Ffiles%2Fwysiwyg_uploads%2FCN%252520VII.png&imgrefurl=https%3A%2F%2Fmedicine.uiowa.edu%2Fiowaprotocols%2Ffacial-nerve-cranial-nerve-vii-general-information&tbnid5OWrg4JK6TScHFM&vet=12ahUKEwij1ojHgfHuAhVESisKHccuAswQMygBegUIARDHAQ..i&docid=nOSmJ81DZwqRiM&w=640&h=589&q=facial%20nerve%20course&ved=2ahUKEwij1ojHgfHuAhVESisKHccuAswQMygBegUIARDHAQ)

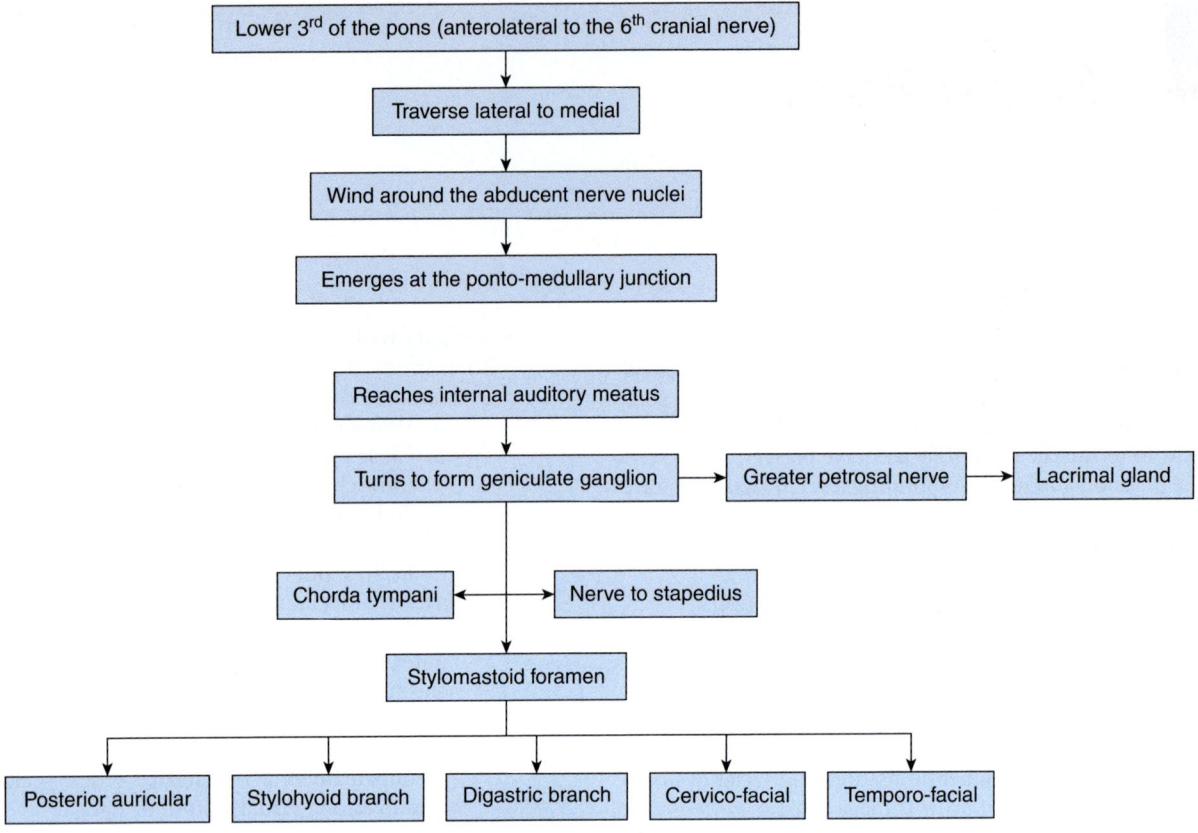

Flowchart 26.1 Facial nerve course.

TABLE 26.1	Site of Lesion in Facial Palsy
Site	**Clinical Clue**
Cortex (supranuclear)	Contralateral lower facial weakness with hemiparesis
Pons (nuclear)	LMN type ipsilateral facial nerve palsy with abducent nerve palsy
Facial canal (petrous bone)	LMN type ipsilateral weakness with loss of taste, salivation and lacrimation (lesion proximal to chorda tympani)
	Hyperacusis, if lesion is proximal to stapedius
Parotid gland	Weakness of facial muscles due to respective branch
Neuromuscular junction	External ophthalmoplegia, dysphagia, dysarthria
Muscles	Tenderness of muscles

  d. Orbicularis oris reflex – percussion over upper lip or side of nose causes contraction of muscles to elevate the angle of mouth
  e. Corneal reflex – brisk closure of eyes when cornea is touched by a wisp of cotton
  f. Stapedial reflex – hyperacusis of low tones in facial nerve lesion
  g. Chvostek sign – tetanic contraction of ipsilateral facial muscles on tapping the pes anserine anterior to ear
Examination of sensory function
  Taste sensation in anterior two-third of the tongue.

Examination of secretion function
  a. Lacrimation – Schirmer test, nasolacrimal reflex
  b. Salivation – on placing flavored substance on the tongue, salivary secretion seen in submandibular duct at floor of mouth
4. What is mimetic or emotional facial palsy?
  In mimetic facial palsy, only emotional fibers are affected but volitional fibers are intact. It is seen in frontal lobe white matter, thalamus, and hypothalamus lesions. For example, when the patient laughs, he or she will have facial palsy but when he or she is quiet or during any voluntary facial movement, he or she will be without facial palsy.
5. What is volitional facial palsy?
  It refers to the paresis of facial muscles during voluntary movements sparing activation on emotion. It is seen in motor cortex lesion and pyramidal tract lesion.
6. How to differentiate between upper motor neuron (UMN) and lower motor neuron (LMN) type of facial palsy?
  Differences between UMN and LMN type of facial palsy are given in Table 26.2.
  Fig. 26.2 shows LMN type of facial palsy.
7. What is Schirmer test?
  The greater petrosal branch of facial nerve that innervates lacrimal glands is paralyzed if the lesion is at geniculate ganglion. Schirmer test is performed to confirm the absence of tears on the affected side, by placing a blotting paper underneath the lower eyelid.

TABLE 26.2	Differences Between Upper Motor Neuron (UMN) and Lower Motor Neuron (LMN) Type of Facial Palsy	
Features	UMN	LMN
Lesion	Above facial nerve nucleus	At or below the facial nerve nucleus
Clinical features	Upper part of face affected Lower half is spared	One half of the face is affected including upper part of face
Bell phenomenon	Never occurs	Bell phenomenon – present
Taste sensation	Not affected	May be affected
Corneal reflex	preserved	lost

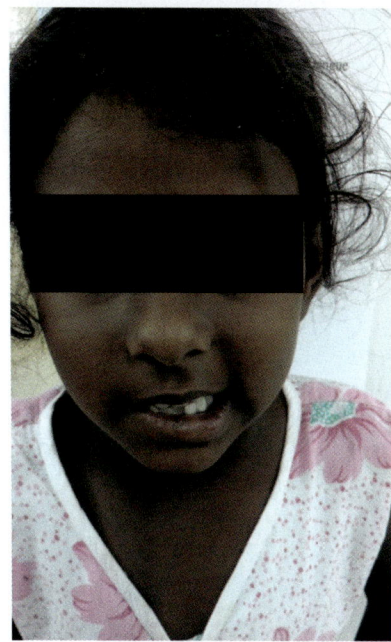

Fig. 26.2 Right LMN type of facial palsy – absent nasolabial fold on the right side.

8. What are the clinical clues to identify the UMN and LMN of lesion in facial palsy?
   The clinical clues to identify the UMN and LMN of lesion in facial palsy are given in Table 26.3.
9. What are the causes of unilateral and bilateral UMN facial palsy?
   The causes of UMN facial palsy are enumerated in Table 26.4.
10. What are the causes of unilateral and bilateral LMN facial palsy?
    The causes of LMN facial palsy are enumerated in Table 26.5.
11. What are the complications of facial palsy?
    Ophthalmological
    1. Exposure keratitis
    2. Corneal drying
    Hyperkinetic complication
    1. Synkinesis
    2. Hemifacial spasm
    3. Facial asymmetry
12. What is Bell phenomenon?
    The eyeball moves upward and inward on attempting to close the eyes normally. It is called Bell phenomenon seen in LMN type of facial nerve palsy. Fig. 26.3 shows Bell phenomenon.

TABLE 26.3	Site of Upper Motor Neuron (UMN) and Lower Motor Neuron (LMN) of Lesion in Facial Palsy	
Type of Cranial Nerve VII	Site of Lesion	Side of Lesion
UMN type of cranial nerve VII palsy	Above pons	Opposite side
LMN type of cranial nerve VII palsy	At the level of the pons	Crossed hemiplegia Same side of the lesion
No facial nerve involvement	Below pons	Incomplete hemiplegia

TABLE 26.4	Causes of Upper Motor Neuron (UMN) Facial Palsy	
Unilateral UMN Facial Palsy	Bilateral UMN Facial Palsy	
Bell palsy	Guillain–Barré syndrome	
Cerebellopontine lesion	Myasthenia gravis	
Parotid tumor	Myopathies	
Facial trauma	Leprosy	
	Tuberculosis	

TABLE 26.5	Causes of Lower Motor Neuron (LMN) Facial Palsy	
Unilateral LMN Facial Palsy	**Bilateral LMN Facial Palsy**	
Cerebrovascular accidents	Pseudobulbar palsy	
Demyelination	Emotional paralysis	

13. What is Melkersson syndrome?
    - It is a benign disease of idiopathic etiology characterized by
      a) Deep furrowed tongue
      b) Recurrent facial edema
      c) Recurrent unilateral or bilateral facial palsy.
14. What is Moebius syndrome?
    It refers to bilateral facial and abducent nerve palsy due to congenital absence or hypoplasia of bilateral facial and abducent nerve nuclei. It may present with delayed milestone.
15. What is House—Brackmann scale?
    This scale helps is grading the recovery of facial palsy.
    - Grade 1: Normal symmetrical function
    - Grade 2: Slight weakness only on close inspection
    - Grade 3: Obvious weakness
    - Grade 4: Obvious disfiguring weakness
    - Grade 5: Motion barely perceptible
    - Grade 6: No movement, loss of tone, no synkinesis, contracture or spasm

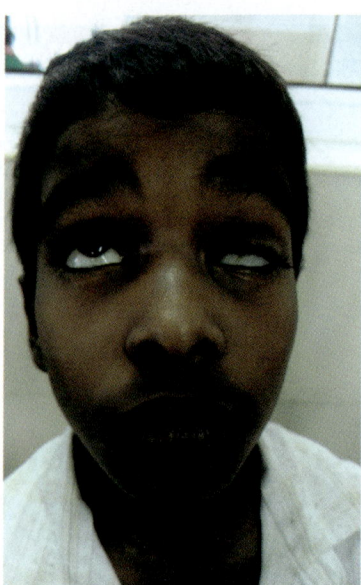

Fig. 26.3   Bell phenomenon.

27

Microcephaly

Frequently Asked Questions

1. Define microcephaly.
   - Microcephaly is defined as head circumference that measures more than below the mean for age and sex.
   - Borderline microcephaly – occipitofrontal length between 2 and 3 SD below the mean for age and sex.
   - Moderate microcephaly – occipitofrontal length between 3 and 5 SD below the mean for age and sex.
   - Severe microcephaly – occipitofrontal length between ≥5 SD below the mean for age and sex (Flowchart 27.1 shows Approach to microcephaly).

2. How is head circumference measured?
   - Use tape that cannot be stretched.
   - Place tape above the glabella – supraorbital ridges – maximum prominence of occiput as shown in Fig. 27.1.
   - Take measurement 3 times and select the largest nearing to 0.1 cm.

3. What is dyne formula?
   - Denotes the relation between length and head circumference
   - HC = length/2 + 9.5± 2.5
   - Accurate for 95% measurements in first 400 days

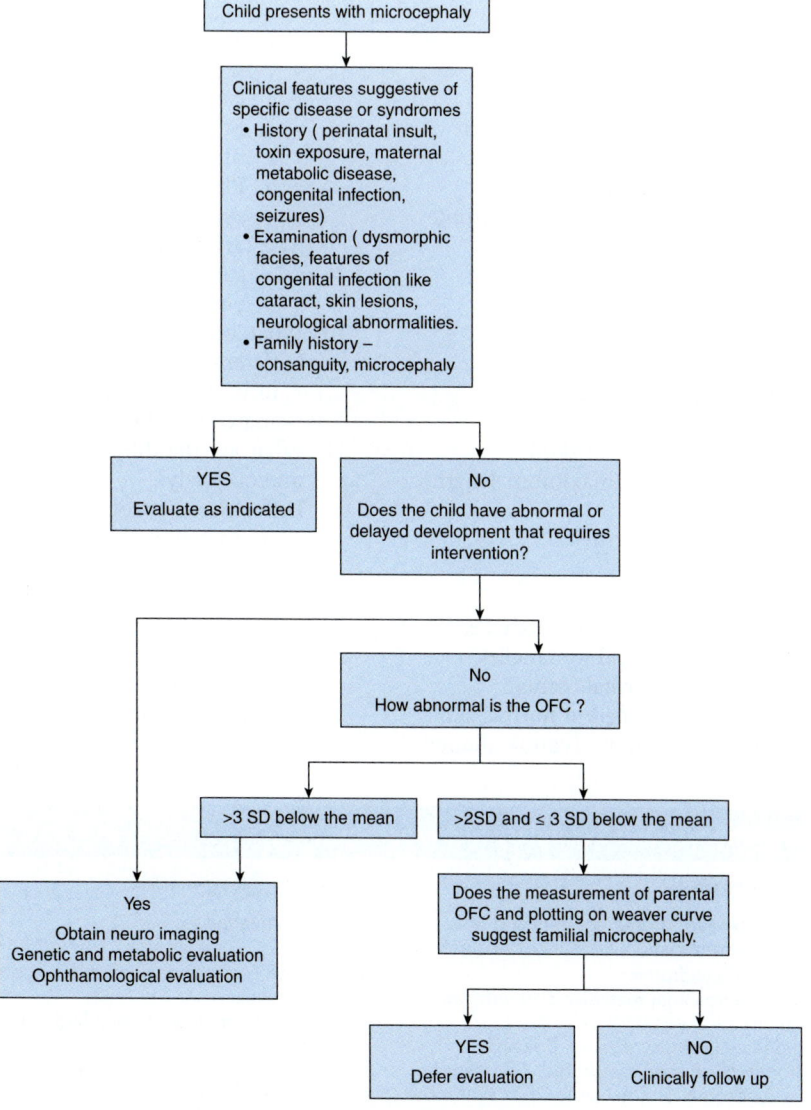

Flowchart 27.1 Approach to microcephaly.

353

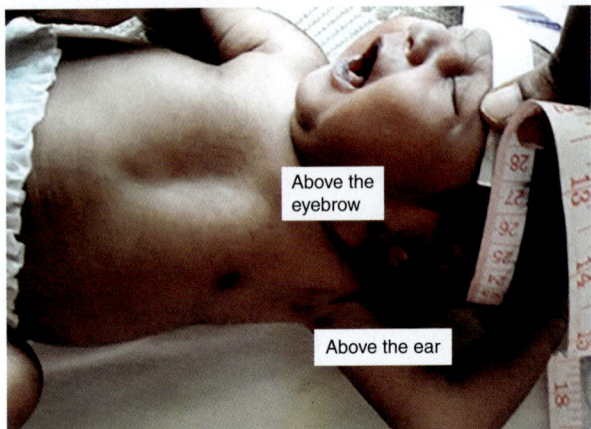

Fig. 27.1 Measuring head circumference.

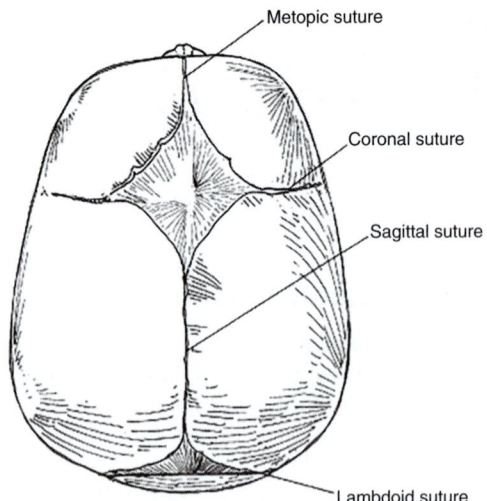

Fig. 27.2 Normal infant skull with sutures identified. *(Source: Reproduced from RE Bristol and SP Beals, and Craniosynostosis, Encyclopedia of the Neurological Sciences* 1(2): 894-895.)

4. How to classify microcephaly and differentiate between the two?
   A. Genetic/nongenetic
      - Primary (genetic) – present at birth or at 36 weeks of gestation
      - Secondary (nongenetic) microcephaly – failure of normal growth of brain that was of normal size at birth (Table 27.1)
   B. By etiology – genetic or environmental
   C. By growth parameters – symmetric or asymmetric
   D. Pure microcephaly or syndromic microcephaly
5. What are the causes of acquired microcephaly?
   Rett syndrome, Angelman syndrome, Seckel syndrome, GLUT1 transporter defect
6. What are the environmental causes of microcephaly?
   a. Maternal infection – TORCH
   b. In utero drug or toxin exposure
   c. Hypoxic-ischemic injury
   d. Intraventricular hemorrhage or stroke
   e. Severe malnutrition
7. Which index helps to determine shape of skull?
   Cephalic index = (maximum width/maximum length) × 100
8. What are the fontanelles present at birth?
   a. Anterior fontanelle
   b. Posterior fontanelle
   c. Two anterolateral – pair of sphenoidal fontanelles
   d. Two posterolateral – pair of mastoid fontanelles
9. What are the different types of abnormal crania?
   Fig. 27.2 shows cranial sutures identified in normal skull
      a. Dolichocephaly/scaphocephaly (canoe-shaped cranium) – AP length is more than width because of premature closure of sagittal suture as shown in Fig. 27.3A
      b. Turricephaly/oxycephaly/acrocephaly – high-peaked skull because of premature closure of coronal and lambdoid suture as shown in Fig. 27.3B
      c. Brachycephaly – premature closure of coronal suture as shown in Fig. 27.3C
      d. Plagiocephaly – irregular and abnormal closure of sutures as shown in Fig. 27.3D
      e. Trigonocephaly – premature closure of metopic suture, so the skull is narrow anteriorly and wide posteriorly as shown in Fig. 27.3E
10. What are the differential diagnoses for microcephaly?
    Differential diagnosis of microcephaly are craniosynostosis and plagiocephaly and their differences are shown in Table 27.2.
11. What are the differences between craniosynostosis and microcephaly?
    Differences between craniosynostosis and microcephaly are shown in Table 27.3.
12. Does congenital torticollis can cause plagiocephaly?
    Yes, congenital torticollis can cause plagiocephaly and vice versa.
13. What is Virchow's law?
    When premature closure of sutures occurs, skull growth is restricted perpendicular to fused suture and growth occurs parallel to it.

TABLE 27.1	Differences Between Primary and Secondary Microcephaly	
Features	**Primary (Genetic)**	**Secondary (Nongenetic)**
Clinical features	Receding forehead, prominent ears and nose, severe mental retardation, prominent seizures	Nondistinctive facies
Causes	• Familial and syndromic • Familial – autosomal recessive and autosomal dominant • Syndromic – Down syndrome, Edwards syndrome, cri-du-chat syndrome, Cornelia de Lange syndrome, Smith–Lemli–Opitz syndrome	a. Infection – congenital infection, acquired infection – meningitis/encephalitis b. Drugs – fetal alcohol, fetal hydantoin c. Radiation d. Metabolic – maternal diabetes, maternal hyperphenylalaninemia e. Significant fever – during first 4–6 weeks of gestational age can cause microcephaly f. HIE – hypoxic-ischemic encephalopathy

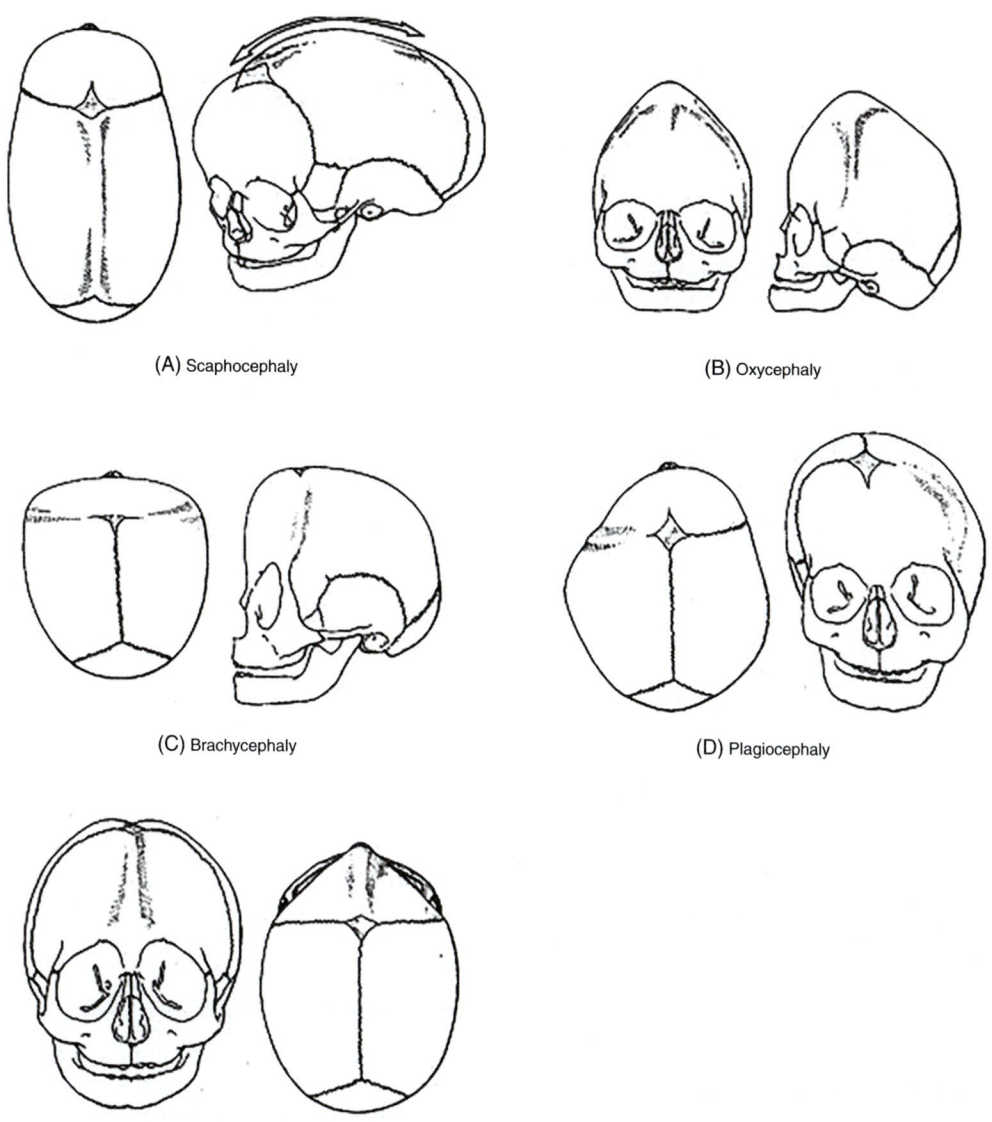

(A) Scaphocephaly

(B) Oxycephaly

(C) Brachycephaly

(D) Plagiocephaly

(E) Trigonocephaly

Fig. 27.3 Abnormal crania. (Source: Reproduced from RE Bristol and SP Beals, and Craniosynostosis, *Encyclopedia of the Neurological Sciences* 1(2): 894-895.)

TABLE 27.2	**Differences Between Craniosynostosis and Plagiocephaly**	
Clinical Features	**Craniosynostosis**	**Plagiocephaly**
Definition	Premature closure of cranial sutures	Cranial flattening/asymmetry due to extrinsic molding forces
Shape	Trapezoid	Parallelogram
Features	Mastoid prominence	Ipsilateral anteriorly placed ear/contralateral occipital prominence
Overriding of sutures	Yes	No
Ridges	Ridges palpable	No ridges palpable
Treatment	Surgery	Helmet/repositioning/physiotherapy

TABLE 27.3	**Differences Between Craniosynostosis and Microcephaly**	
Clinical Features	**Craniosynostosis**	**Microcephaly**
Shape	Abnormal	Normal
Sutural line	Ridges palpable	Normal
Overriding of bones	Present	Absent
Ipsilateral ear	Posteriorly placed	Anteriorly placed
Investigations	CT brain 3D reconstruction	CT brain/MRI brain

Duchenne Muscular Dystrophy

Following introduction, seek permission from the caregiver and introduce yourself to the patient before history elicitation, and identify the case.

Name____Age____Sex____Consanguinity____Order of birth____Place____Informant____

Presenting Complaints and Duration

- Delayed walking
- Difficulty in getting up from squatting position, climbing stairs, abnormal gait — waddling gait with lordotic posture
- History of toe walking
- Tripping while walking
- Clumsiness/frequent falls recently
- Swelling in the calf region

History of Presenting Illness

- Narrate as a story: Child was apparently normal till ———-years of age, then mother noticed child had difficulty in climbing stairs which was gradual in onset, progressive; noticed in school initially; subsequently child had difficulty in getting up from squatting/sitting position, difficulty in carrying school bags then needed assistance for toileting (Indian style); no diurnal variation of symptoms
- At present . . . . . . (what the child is able to do; explain the daily activities).

CENTRAL NERVOUS SYSTEM HISTORY

Higher Function History

- Cognitive delay, speech delay, seizures, preferential use of one hand (early handedness), intelligence, behavior or sleep disturbance

Cranial Nerve History

- Ability to perceive light
- Any history of drooping of eyelids, ability to move eyeballs in all four directions or restriction of eyeball movement, double vision
- Ability to chew food
- Able to close both eyes while sleeping, drooling of saliva, deviation of angle of the mouth, lack of facial expression
- Ability to hear and respond to sound
- History of nasal twang of voice, nasal regurgitation
- Ability to move head side to side
- Any deviation of the tongue on the protrusion

Motor System

- Swelling in the calf region noted by the mother on both sides
- Flailness noted by the mother in both legs
- Difficulty in reaching the things from top shelves
- Difficulty in buttoning clothes, mixing food

- Difficulty in getting up from squatting/sitting position
- Unable to hold the slippers or slipping, buckling of knees
- Any difficulty in daily routine activities
- Any history of involuntary movements

Cerebellar Features

- Abnormal eyeball or head movement or tremors

Bladder/Bowel Disturbance

- History of urinary incontinence or dribbling of urine, constipation

Sensory Features

- Perception of pain or crying while giving vaccination/injection

Autonomic Features

- Flushing, sweating, palpitation episodes

Spine and Cranium

- Any abnormality in head size compared with sibling or peers noted by the mother
- Any swelling, tuft of hair, sinus, discharge, abnormal curvature

HISTORY OF COMPLICATIONS

- Repeated lower respiratory infections/feeding difficulties, contractures, deformities, any assistant or devices for mobility, behavioral problem

ETIOLOGICAL HISTORY

- Constipation, lethargy, neck swelling, delayed milestones
- Thinning of limb muscles
- Drug ingestion
- Rash, photosensitivity, pain
- Cramps, exercise intolerance
- Pain and weakness
- Facial involvement — double vision, inability to close eyes tightly, easy fatiguability, diurnal variation
- Exercise intolerance, muscle cramps
- Breathlessness, palpitations, puffiness of eyelid, edema, features of congestive heart failure
- Breathing difficulty, chest retraction, nocturnal hypoventilation
- Dark brown urine

PAST HISTORY

- When was the disease diagnosed initially
- Any previous hospitalizations
- Any onset of deterioration, commencement of steroids, any surgical procedure for release of contractures

ANTENATAL HISTORY

- Decreased fetal movements, polyhydramnios

BIRTH HISTORY

Poor cry at birth, need for resuscitation or ventilation, weak cry, feeding difficulty, breech, hip deformity, contractures

DEVELOPMENT HISTORY

- Dissociated delay or selective motor delay – predominant motor delay – other milestones normal

DIETETIC HISTORY

- As per 24 hours recall method

IMMUNIZATION HISTORY

Hemophilus influenza b, – pnuemococcal, flu vaccine

FAMILY HISTORY

- Similar illness in family members, history of congestive heart failure, early childhood or adolescent death in sibling, spine deformity, wheelchair bound or any similar complaints in sibling or in maternal aunt's children
- Mother complains of weakness, calf pain, calf hypertrophy

Summary

A ...-year-old boy with weakness noticed after ——- years of age; proximal weakness, with prominent muscle bulk in calf, in the absence of higher function, or cranial nerve involvement or hand muscle involvement with or without a family history; would like to think in terms of muscular dystrophy and proceed further with examination

General Examination

- Attitude and posture
- Wheelchair bound, lying in bed or ambulant or lordotic posture
- Oxygen support
- Nasogastric tube feed

Head-to-Foot Examination

a. Head – normal in size and shape
b. Face – no dysmorphic facies
c. Eye – cataract, violaceous discoloration of eyelids, ophthalmoplegia, Gottron plaques
d. Chest – any deformity
e. Hypertrophy of muscle (deltoid, calf muscle)
f. Skeletal deformities – kyphosis, scoliosis, lumbar lordosis, pes cavus
g. Scar – biopsy scar, tenotomy scar, tendon release scar
h. Umbilical hernia, goiter
i. Ulceration over knuckles
j. Muscle pain or tenderness
k. Features of rickets

Vital Signs

- Temperature
- Pulse rate
- Respiratory rate
- Blood pressure
- SpO_2

Anthropometry

Weight, height, weight/height or BMI

Central Nervous System Examination

HIGHER FUNCTIONS

Mnemonic COSSHMIB:
- C – consciousness
- O – orientation
- S – Sleep
- S – Speech and Language
- H – handedness
- M – memory
- I – intelligent
- B – behavior

CRANIAL NERVES

- Perceive smell in both nostril
- Cranial nerve VI – six points
  Light perception, visual acuity, color vision, field of vision, direct and consensual light reflex, fundus
- Ptosis, moves eyeball in all four cardinal directions, strabismus
- Pain sensation over the face, able to chew food, jaw jerk
- Wrinkling of forehead present
- Ability to close eyes on both sides while sleeping, nasolabial fold
- Any deviation of the angle of mouth
- Any drooling of saliva
- Hearing – normal
- Palatal movement – normal, uvula in the midline, any pooling of secretions present
  palatal arches – normal; palatal and pharyngeal reflexes – normal
- Ability to lift head from supine position
- Fibrillation or wasting, myotonia, tongue fasciculations

MOTOR SYSTEM EXAMINATION

Attitude and Posture

- Wheelchair bound, lying in bed or ambulant
- Clinical findings in motor system examination are given in Table 28.1
- Gait – Gowers sign positive
- Involuntary movements – no involuntary movement seen

CEREBELLAR FUNCTIONS

Normal

SENSORY SYSTEM

Normal

TABLE 28.1 Motor System Examination		
Motor System Examination	**Right**	**Left**
Bulk	Increased on lower limb	Increased on lower limb
Tone	Hypotonia	Hypotonia
Power[a]	Lower limb < upper limb	Lower limb < upper limb
	Predominant proximal muscle weakness	Predominant proximal muscle weakness
Superficial reflexes	Norma	Normal
Plantar	Norma	Normal
Deep reflexes	Knee jerk – absent	Knee jerk – absent
	Ankle jerk – retained till late	Ankle jerk – retained till late

[a]Detailed muscle charting (refer Frequently Asked Questions).

SPINE AND CRANIUM

Normal

Other System Examination

CARDIOVASCULAR SYSTEM

Apical impulse, murmur, arrhythmia/heart block

RESPIRATORY SYSTEM

Respiratory distress, seesaw breathing

ABDOMEN

Features of constipation, undescended testes, hepatomegaly

Diagnosis

A child with gradual onset of progressive proximal weakness with calf muscle hypertrophy with or without cardiac, pulmonary involvement, with intellectual impairment, with or without a positive family history – suggestive of Duchenne muscular dystrophy (DMD)

Frequently Asked Questions

1. How to correlate age of onset and presentation of different types of dystrophies?
   Age of onset
   a. Neonatal: Transient myasthenia, congenital myopathy, congenital muscular dystrophy
   b. Infancy: Pompe disease, Duchenne Muscular Dystrophy (DMD)
   c. Childhood: DMD, inflammatory myopathies, dermatomyositis
   d. Older children: Limb-girdle muscular dystrophy (LGMD), facioscapulohumeral dystrophy (FSHD), Becker muscular dystrophy
   e. Adolescence or later: FSHD and LGMDs

2. How to elicit history for proximal weakness in children?
   Upper limb
   a. Trouble lifting objects over their head
   b. Combing and brushing hair
   c. Difficulty in reaching things to get from top shelves
   d. Brushing teeth, shaving (older children)
   e. Difficulty in carrying a school bag
   Lower limb
   a. Difficulty in getting up from a sitting/squatting position
   b. Difficulty in climbing stairs in school

3. How to elicit history for distal weakness in children?
   Upper limb distal symptoms:
   a. Difficulty opening jars or tap
   b. Buttoning clothes
   c. Turning a key in the ignition
   d. Mixing food
   e. Using keyboard
   f. Holding water before washing face
   Lower limb distal symptoms:
   a) Tripping over a curb
   b) Difficulty in walking on uneven ground
   c) Foot slapping
   d) Unable to hold the slippers or slipping, buckling of knees, stumbling over
   e) Tripping and falling, unable to hold chappals

4. Give an example for buckling and fall and triple and fall.
   - Buckle and fall – proximal weakness (myopathies)
   - Triple and fall – distal weakness (peripheral neuropathy)

5. How to elicit history of day-to-day activities in children?
   Getting up from the bed, brushing, bathing/toileting (western or Indian), walking, playing, sleeping, dressing, eating, ambulation, going to school – how far from home it is located, ground floor, first floor – difficulty in climbing stairs

6. What are the clinical ways of presentation in myopathies?
   Various clinical presentations of myopathies are described in Table 28.2.

7. *How to classify muscular disorder depending on the course of the disease?
   Course of muscular disorder is given in Table 28.3.

8. What are the differentials to be suspected in muscular disorder with hearing defect?
   DMD, mitochondrial disorder, myotonic dystrophy

9. What are the bladder/bowel disturbances seen in a child with myopathy?

TABLE 28.2	Various Clinical Presentation in Myopathies	
Clinical Presentation	**Examples**
Myopathies with constant weakness	Muscular dystrophies, inflammatory myopathies
Episodic periods of weakness with normal strength in between	Periodic paralysis, metabolic myopathies (due to certain glycolytic pathway disorders)
The fluctuating weakness that is provoked by fatigue	Neuromuscular junction disorder (myasthenia gravis)

TABLE 28.3	Course of Muscular Disorder	
Course	**Examples**
Progressive	Duchenne muscular dystrophy
Nonprogressive	Congenital myopathies, myotonic dystrophy, congenital myasthenia syndrome
Fluctuating weakness	Myotonic dystrophy, myasthenia gravis, juvenile dermatomyositis
The episodic weakness with complete recovery	Channelopathy (familial hypokalemic, periodic paralysis), metabolic (glycolytic enzyme defect)

Urinary incontinence and constipation seen in children with myopathy and hypothyroid

10. List the significance of etiological history in a child with muscular disorder.
    Etiological history and its significance are described in Table 28.4.

11. *What are the clinical clues in the examination in a child with muscular disorder?
    Clues in examination in muscular disorder are given in Table 28.5.

12. *What are the muscle hypertrophies in DMD?
    First calf muscle (gastrocnemius, soleus) as shown in Fig. 28.5, followed by deltoid, infra-spinatus, brachioradialis, and tongue. Calf muscle hypertrophy is better appreciated when seen from the side of the child.

13. Enumerate the importance of vital sign in myopathies.
    - Temperature instability – familial dysautonomia
    - Heart rate – bradycardia – heart block seen in myotonic muscular dystrophy
    - Respiratory pattern – seesaw breathing – respiratory muscle weakness – congenital myopathies, bulbar weakness – myasthenia syndrome
    - Blood pressure – hypotension or hypertension – familial dysautonomia

14. What are the possible differentials if higher functions are affected in a child with myopathy?
    a. Intelligent Quotient (IQ) – DMD, myotonic muscular dystrophy, congenital muscular dystrophy, mitochondrial disease
    b. Stroke-like episodes, myoclonus, epilepsy, deafness, ataxia, and encephalopathy – mitochondrial disorder

TABLE 28.4	Etiological History and Its Significance
History	**Etiology**
Constipation, lethargy, neck swelling, delayed milestones Thinning of limb muscles	Hypothyroidism • Drug-induced myopathy – anabolic steroids; toxic – alcohol, cocaine, glucocorticoids; lipid-lowering drugs, statin, antimalarials colchicine • Zidovudine intake (mitochondrial myopathy)
Rash, photosensitivity, pain Cramps, exercise intolerance Pain and weakness	Polymyositis McArdle disease and other metabolic myopathies 1. Infection – viral myositis, leptospirosis, trichinella 2. Inflammation – Guillaine Barre Syndrome 3. Drug-induced myopathies 4. Thyroid myopathy 5. Inherited metabolic myopathies 6. Dermatomyositis
Facial involvement	Myasthenia gravis – double vision, ptosis, inability to close eyes tightly, easy fatiguability, diurnal variation
Exercise intolerance, muscle cramps	Glycogen Storage Disorder, McArdle disease, carnitine palmitoyl transferase deficiency
Congestive heart failure	Congenital myotonic dystrophy, rarely mitochondrial
Respiratory – breathing difficulty, chest retractions, nocturnal hypoventilation, respiratory infection, reduced vital capacity, scoliosis	Congenital muscular dystrophy, Duchenne muscular dystrophy
Dark brownish urine	McArdle disease, malignant hypothermia, rhabdomyolysis, muscle injury, Diabetic Ketoacidosis

TABLE 28.5	Examination Clues in Muscular Disorder
Clinical Features	**Muscular Disorder**
Cataract	Myotonic muscular dystrophy
Ptosis, ophthalmoplegia	Myasthenia gravis – ptosis as shown in Fig. 28.1
Dolichocephaly, hanging jaw, open mouth, expressionless facies	Congenital myopathy (nemaline rod myopathy)
Inverted V-shaped upper lip, loss of muscle mass in the temporal fossa	Myotonic muscular dystrophy
Cleft lip/high-arched palate	Congenital myopathy
Male – baldness	Myotonic dystrophy
Cherubic facies	• Glycogen storage disorder • Cherubic facies as seen in glycogen storage disorder as shown in Fig. 28.2
Heliotrope rash, Gottron papules	Dermatomyositis – Fig. 28.3A and B shows heliotrope rash and Gottron papules
Herculean appearance – generalized muscle hypertrophy (resembling bodybuilder)	Fig. 28.4 shows herculean appearance in Thomsen disease
Umbilical hernia, goiter	Hypothyroid

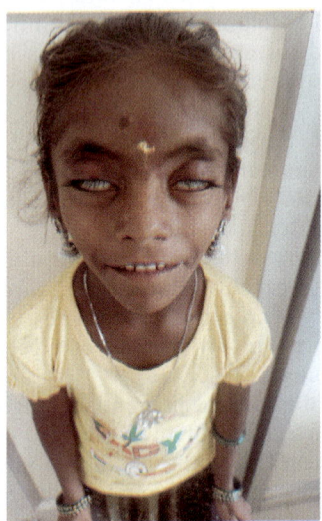

Fig. 28.1 Ptosis.

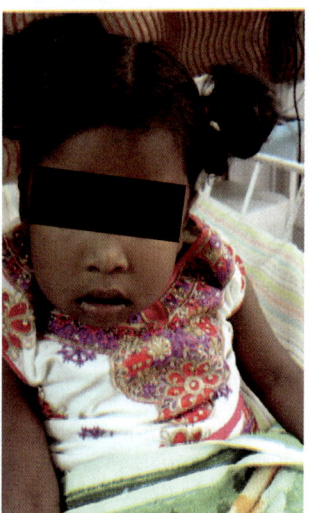

Fig. 28.2 Cherubic facies

TABLE 28.13	Examples of Inherited and Acquired Causes of Muscle Disorder
Inherited	**Acquired**
1. Congenital myopathies (central core disease, nemaline rod myopathy, centronuclear [myotubular] myopathy) 2. Muscular dystrophy (DMD, Becker dystrophy, FSHD, LGMD) 3. Myasthenic syndromes 4. Channelopathies (Channelopathies- Myotonia congenita (two types -Autosomal dominant-Thomsen disease, Autosomal recessive - Becker disease) 5. Metabolic (Pompe disease, GSD types 3, 5, and 7 and mitochondrial)	1. Inflammatory myopathies (dermatomyositis, polymyositis) 2. Endocrine – thyroid 3. Toxic 4. Systemic disease

TABLE 28.14	Various Causes of Muscle Weakness on the Basis of Their Level of Weakness			
Proximal Muscle Weakness	**Distal Muscle Weakness – Wrist and Small Muscles of Hand (C7–T1)**	**Peripheral Muscle Weakness (in All Four Limbs)**	**Non-neuronal Cause**
1. DMD 2. Facioscapulohumeral dystrophy 3. Proximal limb girdle dystrophy 4. Dystrophia myotonica (face, skeletal muscles, quadriceps) 5. Rickets 6. Metabolic myopathy (thyroid) 7. Polymyositis – difficulty running, jumping, and walking up steps, waddling gait	1. Cervical spondylosis 2. Cervical cord tumor 3. Motor neuron disease 4. Syringomyelia 5. Hereditary Motor Sensory Neuropathy (HMSN)	1. Peroneal muscular atrophy (Charcot–Marie tooth disease) 2. HMSN (Hereditary Motor Sensory Neuropathy)	1. Chronic illness 2. Chronic renal failure 3. Tuberculosis 4. Cachexia 5. Undiagnosed illness

3. In the absence of radiculopathy, central nervous system, and spinal involvement
4. Muscle biopsy showing evidence of degeneration + regeneration

71. Enumerate the causes of muscle weakness on the basis of their level of weakness.
    Table 28.14 gives the various causes of muscle weakness on the basis of their level of weakness.
72. How to differentiate between the neurological and non-neurological causes of muscle weakness?
    The features of non-neurological causes of muscle weakness are as follows:

1. Complain of weakness, not objectively weak when muscle strength is formally tested
2. Functionally limited
3. Inability to perform a specific task such as climbing stairs or combing hair

In non-neuronal causes:
1. Features of underlying cause predominate
2. Despite advanced generalized muscle atrophy, muscle strength is relatively preserved in patients with underlying chronic illness

Quick Bites

a. Features of DMD: Remember as 4 Ps — Progressive weakness, Proximal > Distal, Preserved reflex, Pseudohypertrophy.

b. Severe childhood autosomal recessive muscular dystrophy (SCARMD) — severe DMD-like phenotype is seen in female. Mental subnormality is very uncommon.

c. Incidence of DMD is 1:3600 live male birth.

d. First reflex to be lost in DMD is knee jerk reflex. Ankle jerk is retained till last.

e. Most common cause of death in DMD – respiratory failure; second common cause is cardiac failure due to dilated cardiomyopathy.

Approach to Hepatosplenomegaly

- The following case sheet format is an example of history taking and examination of a child with fever + hepatosplenomegaly (HSM) + jaundice. When given a case with HSM, the case sheet format will be of the same pattern, except for few history elicitations depending on the etiology.

  Name____Age____Sex____Consanguinity____Order of birth____Place____Informant____

Presenting Complaints and Duration

- Age –
  - EBV (Epstein-Barr Virus) common among older children and adolescents
  - Chronicity of HBV (Hepatitis B Virus) is more common in infants
- Gender – autoimmune, connective tissue disorders common in females

History of Presenting Illness

- Ask for duration of symptoms – acute/acute on chronic/chronic
- Fever – continuous/intermittent
- Chills (leptospirosis, brucella, infective endocarditis, malaria)
- Sweating (malaria)
- Jaundice – whether associated with high-colored urine, associated with pruritus
- Abdominal distension – whether localized/uniform; associated with pedal edema, breathlessness, facial puffiness, oliguria (to rule out other causes of distension)
- Abdominal pain/vomiting

COMMON PRESENTATION OF LIVER DISEASES

Remember A to P for symptoms:
- Anorexia
- Bowel symptoms
- Vomiting, constipation
- Coma
- Distension of abdomen
- Ecchymoses
- Fever and fetor hepaticus
- GI bleeding
- Hair loss
- Infections
- Jaundice
- Kidney failure
- Lassitude
- Menarche delay

- Neurological signs and night blindness
- Edema
- Pruritus and pale stools and pain abdomen

COMPLICATION HISTORY

- Bleeding manifestations/generalized edema/altered sensorium/seizures (liver cell failure)
- Oily bulky stools/night blindness/bony deformities (malabsorption)

ETIOLOGICAL HISTORY

a. Skin rash (enteric fever, leptospirosis, rickettsia, EBV, SOJIA (Systemic-Onset Juvenile Idiopathic Arthritis)
b. Breathlessness/palpitations/cyanosis (infective endocarditis)
c. Joint pain/joint swelling – infective causes, SOJIA, histiocytosis
d. Blood transfusions/needle stick injuries – HBV/HCV
e. Failure to gain weight/loss of weight – TB, HIV, malignancy

PAST HISTORY

- Similar episodes – acute on chronic
- Previous blood transfusion
- Heart disease
- Drug intake – ATT (Anti-Tuberculosis Treatment), ART (Antiretroviral Therapy), anti-inflammatory drugs (connective tissue disorders), chemotherapeutic drugs (hemophagocytic lymphohistiocytosis and Langerhans cell histiocytosis)

PERINATAL HISTORY

HBV, HCV (Hepatitis C Virus), and HIV (Human Immunodeficiency Virus) in mother

IMMUNIZATION HISTORY

BCG (Bacille Calmette-Guerin), typhoid, HBV, HAV

CONTACT HISTORY

History of contact with TB

FAMILY HISTORY

Autoimmune hepatitis, familial hemophagocytic lymphohistiocytosis

DIETETIC HISTORY

As per 24 hours recall method

SOCIOECONOMIC HISTORYS

Infective causes

General Examination

- Sensorium is altered in acute liver failure, cerebral malaria, Langerhans cell histiocytosis
- Anemia present in EBV, enteric fever, leptospirosis, malaria, kala-azar, infective endocarditis, SOJIA, tuberculosis, hemophagocytic lymphohistiocytosis, Langerhans cell histiocytosis
- Clubbing – infective endocarditis (IE), cirrhosis
- Cyanosis seen in infective endocarditis (if associated with cyanotic heart disease) portopulmonary hypertension due to cirrhosis
- Pedal edema
- Generalized lymphadenopathy seen in EBV, tuberculosis, HIV, SOJIA, hemophagocytic lymphohistiocytosis, Langerhans cell histiocytosis

Head-to-Foot Examination

- Eyes – pallor, icterus, proptosis (Langerhans cell histiocytosis)
- Oral cavity – tonsillitis – EBV
- Face – rose spots – enteric fever
- Petechiae/purpura – bleeding manifestations/leptospirosis/ hemophagocytic lymphohistiocytosis, Langerhans cell histiocytosis
- Exanthematous rash seen in SOJIA
- Seborrheic dermatitis seen in Langerhans cell histiocytosis
- Features of liver cell failure
- Markers of TB
- Markers of infective endocarditis
- Arthritis – SOJIA
- Scratch marks
- BCG scar

Vital Signs

- Temperature
- Pulse rate
- Respiratory rate
- BP – wide pulse pressure in IE and cirrhosis, hypotension in bacterial sepsis
- SpO$_2$

Abdominal Examination

INSPECTION

Look for shape, skin, veins over abdomen, flanks, umbilicus, hernial orifices, and external genitalia.

PALPATION

- Start in the left lower quadrant. All the organs in the upper abdomen move downward with inspiration and hence ask the patient to take a deep breath in.

- During this time, the examiner's hands should be still so that the organ in question comes on to the examining hand or slips by underneath it.
- Before starting the palpation of the abdomen, remember the following:
  1. Patient's position (supine/lateral/sitting)
  2. Examiner's position to the patient (right/left)
  3. Explain the procedure to the patient
  4. Examiner's hands should be clean and warm (cold hands can cause reflex contraction of abdominal muscles)
  5. Ensure that the patient is relaxed
- Palpation of liver – as discussed in Chapter 20 – examination of abdomen
- Palpation of spleen – discussed in Chapter 20 – examination of abdomen
  - Remember the following points for organomegaly:
    - Size: Mild, moderate, and massive
    - Edge: Sharp, thick, rounded, even/uneven
    - Surface: Smooth, granular, irregular
    - Consistency: Soft, firm (grades I and II) and hard, cystic, pleomorphic
    - Tenderness: Present/absent
    - Upward enlargement
    - Palpable rub
    - Vertical span of liver
    - Bruit, HJ (Hepato-Jugular) reflux

Other System Examination

CARDIOVASCULAR SYSTEM

- Gallop rhythm, regurgitant murmurs

CENTRAL NERVOUS SYSTEM

- Sings of hepatic encephalopathy

Diagnosis

A case of HSM with fever with jaundice with/without complications; probable etiology.

Investigations

For a child with fever +HSM+ jaundice
  1. CBC
     - Raised total leukocyte count – infection
     - Differential count – lymphocytosis in EBV, pancytopenia – hemophagocytic lymphohistiocytosis and Langerhans cell histiocytosis
  2. Peripheral smear – normocytic normochromic anemia in SOJIA, infective endocarditis; look for malarial parasite
  3. Liver function test – raise in bilirubin (total, direct, and indirect)
  4. Renal function test – can be deranged in leptospirosis, CCF (Congestive Cardiac Failure) due to IE
  5. Urine – RBCs – leptospirosis and infective endocarditis
  6. Chest X-Ray – cardiomegaly, pleural effusion in CCF due to IE
  7. USG (Ultrasonogram) abdomen – liver echoes, suggestive of portal hypertension

8. Etiology:
- Blood cultures/serology/viral markers
- Tuberculosis/retroviral screening
- (Echocardiography)
- ANA (Anti-Nuclear Antibody), anti–smooth muscle antibodies, ANCA (Anti-Neutrophilic Cytoplasmic Antibody) (autoimmune hepatitis)
- Bone marrow biopsy – hemophagocytic lymphohistiocytosis/Langerhans cell histiocytosis

Treatment (Fever + HSM + Jaundice)

1. Supportive management
2. Management of liver cell failure
3. Treat the specific cause

Overall Approach to HSM on the Basis of Following Methodology

- History + clinical examination
- Provisional diagnosis
- Differential diagnosis in order of priority
- Laboratory test
  1. Preliminary tests: Urgent tests and less urgent tests (Box 29.1)
  2. Selective tests: Rapid diagnosis and routine diagnosis (Box 29.2)
  3. Specific test (Box 29.3)

BOX 29.1   PRELIMINARY TEST

1. Complete blood count Anemia, leukemia, hypersplenism, RBC morphology, infection
2. Reticulocyte count: Hemolytic anemia
3. Mantoux test
   X-ray chest and abdomen: Koch septicemia, congestive heart failure, anemia, space-occupying lesion – mediastinal widening in lymphomas
4. Liver function test: Liver dysfunction
5. Total protein and A:G ratio: Severity of liver disease
6. Post–vitamin K prothrombin time: Severity of liver dysfunction
7. Serum preprothrombin time: Alpha -1 antitrypsin (AAT) deficiency, severity in Chronic Liver Disease (CLD)
8. Blood group and typing: Blood transfusion
9. Blood glucose: Reye syndrome, fulminant hepatic failure and glycogen storage disorder
10. Blood Venereal Disease Research Laboratory (VDRL) test: Congenital syphilis (mother and baby)

BOX 29.2   SELECTIVE TESTS (ANY ONE OR TWO)

1. HSM + anemia: Bone marrow smear, reticulocyte count, endoscopy, barium swallow liver biopsy, protein electrophoresis, work up for hemolysis
2. HSM + fever: Preliminary lab tests, Microscopic Agglutination Text (MAT) leptospirosis, TORCH screening
3. HSM + lymphadenopathy: Bone marrow liver and lymph node biopsy
4. HSM + bleeding: Endoscopy
5. HSM + jaundice: Depends on type
6. HSM + neurological signs: Work up for underlying clinical condition

---

BOX 29.3   SCREENING FOR SPECIFIC DISEASE

For metabolic disease and hematological disease:
1. Ultrasound, endoscopy, barium swallow
2. Liver biopsy, laparoscopy, venous phase angiography
3. Hepatography – IVC graphy, minilaparotomy – FNAC
4. CT/HIDA Hepatobiliary Iminodiacetic Acid (HIDA)

Further Discussion

The rest of the discussion is on grading, surface marking of liver and spleen, and various causes of HSM.

HEPATOMEGALY

Liver Span

Normal liver span:
- Birth: 5.5–5.9 cm
- 2 months to 1 year: 5 cm
- 1 year to 12 years: 6–7 cm
- 12 years: 7–8 cm in boys/6–6.5 cm in girls

Any liver span >10 cm of any age – hepatomegaly

Grades of Hepatomegaly

On the basis of extension of liver edge below right costal margin as shown in Fig. 29.1:
- Mild: <4 cm
- Moderate: 4–7 cm
- Severe: >7 cm

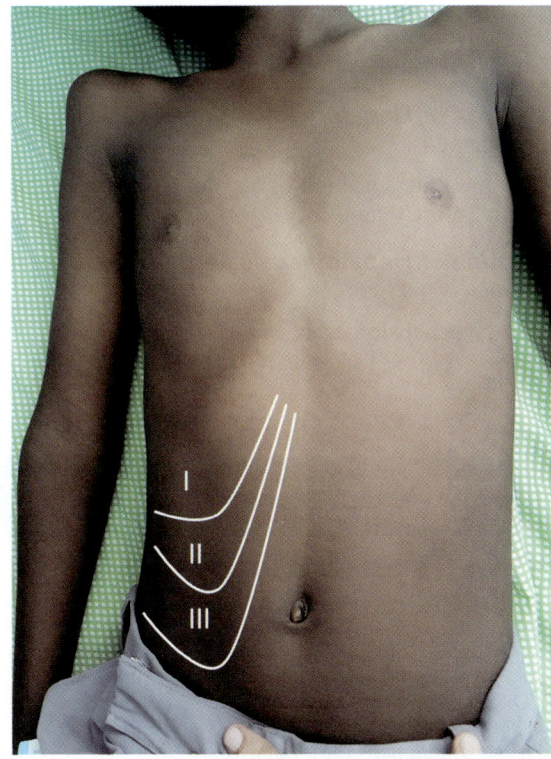

Fig. 29.1   Grades of hepatomegaly.

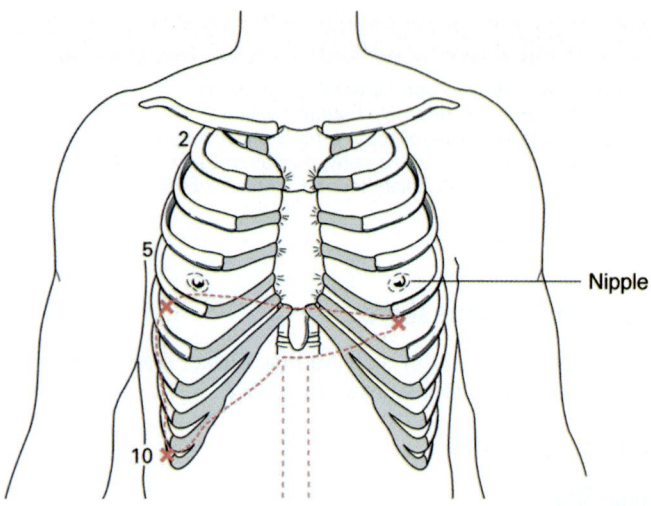

Fig. 29.2 "*" marks the outline of liver, which reaches from the right 5th intercostal space in the midaxillary line to the left 5th intercostal space in the midclavicular line and from the latter to the lower margin of the right 10th rib. (*Source: https://basicmedicalkey.com/2-the-abdomen-and-pelvis/*)

TABLE 29.2	Hepatomegaly and Its Consistency	
Soft	**Firm**	**Hard**
Acute and sub-acute conditions	Cirrhosis	Congestive cardiac failure
Anemia	Koch infection	Liver metastasis (primary and secondary)
Fatty liver	Metabolic conditions, e.g., Wilson galactosemia	
Leukemia	Tyrosinemia – long-standing	Postnecrotic macronodular cirrhosis
Septicemia	Neonatal hepatitis	Chronic abscess
Push down liver		

BOX 29.4   CAUSES OF TENDER HEPATOMEGALY

Infections: Liver abscess, hepatitis, infectious mononucleosis, leptospirosis, pyogenic liver abscess, CCF
Postinvasive procedure (liver biopsy, Percutaneous transhepatic cholangiography (PTC)
Trauma: Hematoma, Hematobilia
Hydatid cyst: Infected
Any condition: Perihepatitis
Acute Budd–Chiari syndrome
Primary malignancy

Surface Marking of Liver

Surface marking of liver is shown in Fig. 29.2.
   Conditions in which hepatomegaly considered as insignificant:
- Newborn (<2 cm, soft).
- Older children (1 cm and soft) Hepatosplenomegaly.
- In diverse conditions such as iron-deficiency anemia, rickets, septicemia, recurrent respiratory infection, UTI, and parasitic infestation.
- Push down organomegaly such as in asthmatic wheeze.
- Emphysema and pleural effusion.

Classification of Hepatomegaly on the Basis of Liver Surface

Table 29.1 gives classification of hepatomegaly on the basis of liver surface (more than 8 cm).

Classification of Hepatomegaly on the Basis of Consistency

Table 29.2 gives hepatomegaly and its consistency.

Causes of Tender Hepatomegaly

Box 29.4 shows causes of tender hepatomegaly.

SPLEEN

Features of Spleen

Soft, thin spleen is palpable in 15% of neonates, 10% of normal children, and 5% of adolescents.

Splenomegaly Grades

Hackett's Semiquantitative Assessment. Hackett's semiquantitative assessment is shown in Fig. 29.3.
   Mild:
      Class 0: Not palpable even on deep inspiration
      Class 1: Palpable on deep inspiration
      Class 2: Palpable but not beyond an imaginary horizontal line half way between the costal margin and umbilicus (measured along vertical line from L nipple)
   Moderate:
      Class 3: Palpable more than half way to umbilicus, but not below the line running through it.
      Class 4: Palpable below umbilicus but not below horizontal line half way between umbilicus and pubic symphysis
   Severe:
      Class 5: Palpable below class 4

Grading on the Basis of Extension From Left Costal Margin
- Mild: <3 cm
- Moderate: 4–7 cm
- Severe: >7 cm

Surface Marking of Spleen

The spleen lies in the left hypochondrium and the surface marking of spleen is given as follows:
- Long axis: corresponds to posterior part of 10th rib

TABLE 29.1	Classification of Hepatomegaly Based on Liver Surface	
Smooth	**Uneven Surface**	
Glycogen storage disorder (GSD)	Congestive cardiac failure with polycystic disease	
Indian Childhood Cirrhosis (ICC)	Metastatic malignancy	
EHPVO (Extra Hepatic Portal Vein Obstruction)	Multiple hydatids	
Budd chiari syndrome/ Inferior vena caval obstruction	Hamartoma	
Hepatic amebiasis	Inborn error of metabolism with sequelae (cirrhosis)	

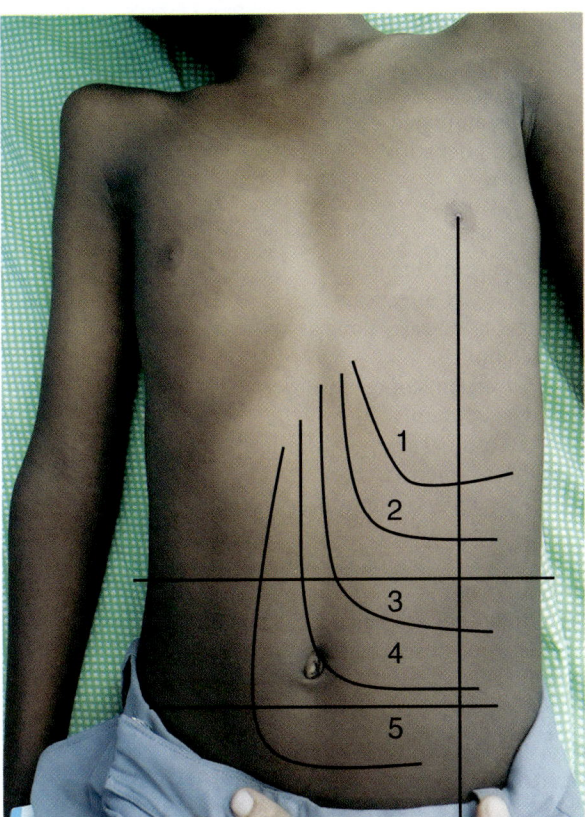

Fig. 29.3 Hackett method of grading splenomegaly.

- Upper border: corresponds to the upper border of 9th rib
- Lower border: corresponds to the lower border of the eleventh rib
- Medial end: 1.5 inches lateral to 10th thoracic spine
- Lateral end: reaches the mid-axillary line

Discussion on Various Causes of Splenomegaly

Table 29.3 gives causes of splenomegaly.

Further Discussion on Etiology of Hepatosplenomegaly

The etiology of HSM in children can be grouped either by
 a. Associated symptoms such as fever, anemia, jaundice, lymphadenopathy, and developmental delay or
 b. The age of presentation

TABLE 29.3	Causes of Splenomegaly	
Mild (<4 cm)	**Moderate (4–7 cm)**	**Massive (>8 cm)**
• Acute and subacute infections	• Chronic infections	• Chronic myeloid leukemia
• Acquired hemolytic anemia	• Portal hypertension	• Storage disorders
• Acute leukemia	• Congenital hemolytic anemia	• Gaucher disease
• Iron-deficiency anemia	• Polycythemia vera	• Kala-azar
		• Hypersplenism
		• Chronic malaria
		• Myeloid leukemia
		• Banti spleen
		• Tumors/cysts

ETIOLOGY OF HEPATOSPLENOMEGALY ON THE BASIS OF ASSOCIATED SYMPTOMS

Hepatosplenomegaly With Fever

A. Infections
- Enteric fever
- Leptospirosis
- Disseminated TB
- Syphilis
- Viral hepatitis
- EBV
- CMV
- Dengue
- HIV
- Chronic malaria
- Kala-azar

B. Rheumatological
- SLE
- Systemic onset JIA

C. Malignancy
- Leukemia
- Lymphoma
- Histiocytosis

D. Others
- Autoimmune hepatitis

Hepatosplenomegaly With Jaundice

A. Infections – same as above

B. Metabolic disorders
- Glycogen storage disorder
- Galactosemia
- Tyrosinemia
- Neonatal hemochromatosis
- Wilson disease
- Wolman disease

C. Hematological
- Hemolytic anemia

D. Rheumatological
- SLE

E. Malignancy
- Leukemia
- Lymphoma
- Histiocytosis

F. Others
- Cardiac cirrhosis
- Autoimmune hepatitis

Hepatosplenomegaly With Anemia

A. Infections – same as above

B. Rheumatological
- SLE
- Systemic onset JIA
- Sarcoidosis

C. Hematological
- Hemolytic anemia

D. Metabolic
- Gaucher type 1
- Nieman–Pick type B
- Wilson disease

E. Malignancy
- Leukemia
- Lymphoma
- Histiocytosis

F. Others
- Osteopetrosis
- Congestive cardiac failure
- Autoimmune hepatitis

Hepatosplenomegaly With Lymphadenopathy

A. Infections
- Disseminated TB
- Congenital syphilis
- HIV
- EBV
- CMV
- Congenital rubella syndrome
- Histoplasmosis
- Kala-azar

B. Rheumatological
- Sarcoidosis
- Systemic onset JIA

C. Malignancy
- Leukemia
- Lymphoma
- Histiocytosis
- Secondaries

D. Others
- Castleman disease

Hepatosplenomegaly With Developmental Delay

- Glycogen storage disorder
- Galactosemia
- Lysosomal storage disorders except Fabry disease
- Mucolipidosis
- Mucopolysaccharidosis
- Tyrosinemia
- Neonatal hemochromatosis
- Wilson disease

Classification of HSM according to the associated symptoms is depicted in Fig. 29.4.

(Note: Jaundice and anemia have similar causes to remember.)

CLASSIFICATION OF HEPATOSPLENOMEGALY ACCORDING TO THE AGE OF PRESENTATION

<1 Month

a. Infective
- TORCH infections
- Bacterial sepsis
- Congenital TB
- Nonpolio enterovirus
- Congenital malaria

b. Hematological
- Alloimmune hemolytic anemia
- Hereditary spherocytosis and hereditary elliptocytosis
- Alpha-thalassemia
- G6PD deficiency

c. Metabolic
- Galactosemia
- Tyrosinemia
- Neonatal hemochromatosis

d. Others
- Congestive cirrhosis
- Osteopetrosis

1 Month to 6 Months

a. Infective
- Enteric fever
- Disseminated TB
- Viral hepatitis
- EBV
- CMV
- Dengue
- Congenital malaria
- TORCH infections

b. Hematological – same as above

c. Metabolic
- Glycogen storage disorder
- Galactosemia
- Lysosomal storage disorders except Fabry disease
- Mucolipidosis
- Mucopolysaccharidosis
- Tyrosinemia
- Neonatal hemochromatosis

d. Malignancy
- Infantile leukemia
- Histiocytosis

e. Others
- Congestive cirrhosis
- Osteopetrosis

6 Months to 5 Years

a. Infective
- Enteric fever
- Leptospirosis
- Disseminated TB
- Syphilis
- Viral hepatitis
- EBV
- CMV
- Dengue
- HIV
- Chronic malaria
- Kala-azar

b. Hematological – same as above plus
- Thalassemia
- Sickle cell anemia
- PNH
- Autoimmune hemolytic anemia

c. Metabolic
- Glycogen storage disorder
- Lysosomal storage disorders except Fabry disease
- Mucolipidosis
- Mucopolysaccharidosis
- Wilson disease

d. Malignancy
- Leukemia
- Lymphoma
- Histiocytosis
- Secondaries

e. Others
- Congestive cirrhosis

>5 Years

a. Infective
- Enteric fever

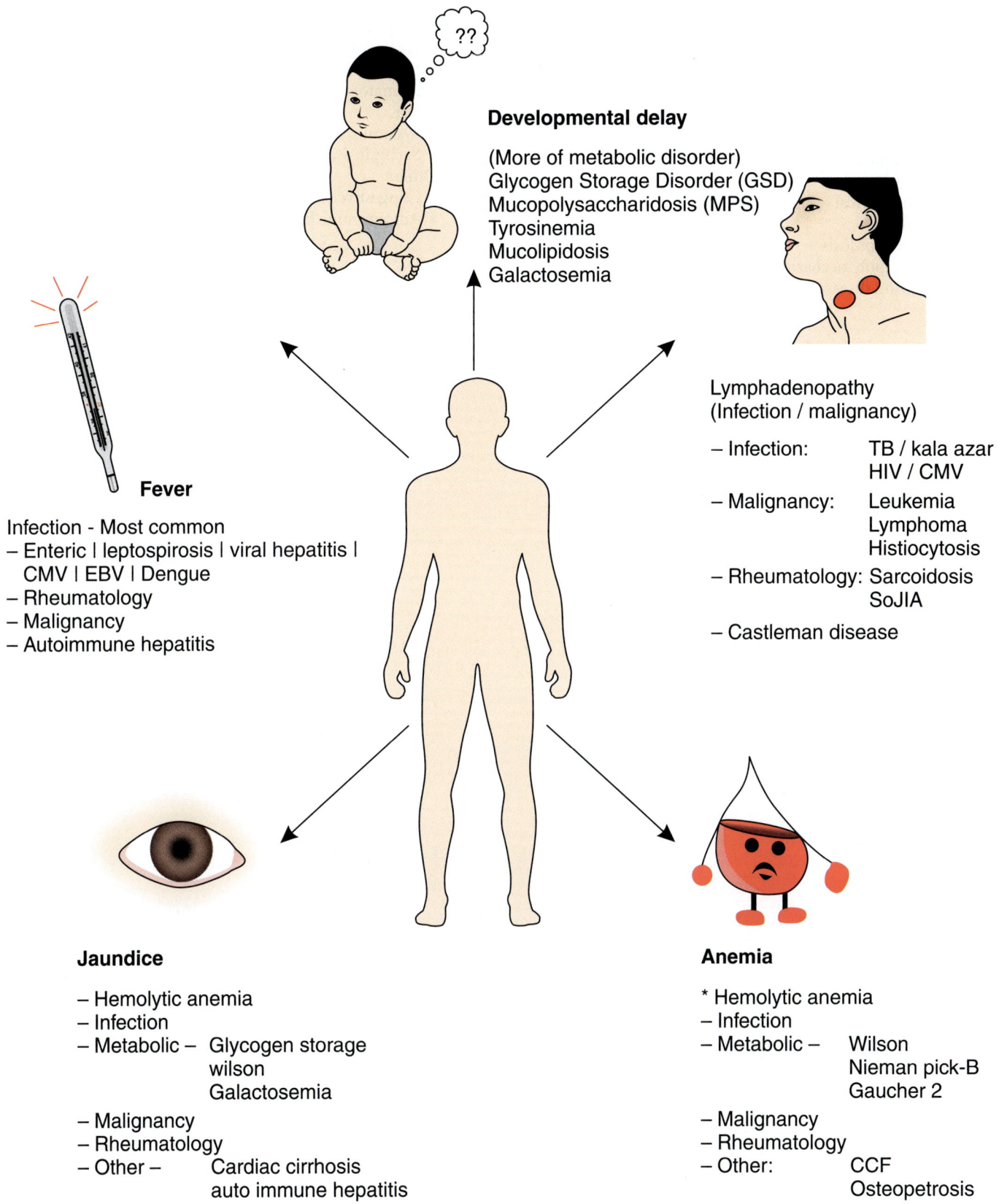

Developmental delay

(More of metabolic disorder)
Glycogen Storage Disorder (GSD)
Mucopolysaccharidosis (MPS)
Tyrosinemia
Mucolipidosis
Galactosemia

Fever

Infection - Most common
– Enteric | leptospirosis | viral hepatitis |
CMV | EBV | Dengue
– Rheumatology
– Malignancy
– Autoimmune hepatitis

Lymphadenopathy
(Infection / malignancy)

– Infection: TB / kala azar
                  HIV / CMV
– Malignancy: Leukemia
                  Lymphoma
                  Histiocytosis
– Rheumatology: Sarcoidosis
                  SoJIA
– Castleman disease

Jaundice

– Hemolytic anemia
– Infection
– Metabolic – Glycogen storage
               wilson
               Galactosemia
– Malignancy
– Rheumatology
– Other –   Cardiac cirrhosis
               auto immune hepatitis

Anemia

* Hemolytic anemia
– Infection
– Metabolic –   Wilson
                Nieman pick-B
                Gaucher 2
– Malignancy
– Rheumatology
– Other: CCF
                Osteopetrosis

Fig. 29.4 Classification of HSM on the basis of associated factors.

- Leptospirosis
- Disseminated TB
- Syphilis
- Viral hepatitis
- EBV
- CMV
- Dengue
- HIV
- Chronic malaria
- Kala-azar

b. Hematological – same as above

c. Metabolic
- Mucolipidosis
- Mucopolysaccharidosis
- Wilson disease

d. Malignancy
- Leukemia
- Lymphoma
- Histiocytosis
- Secondaries

e. Rheumatological
- SLE
- Systemic onset JIA
- Sarcoidosis

f. Others
- Congestive cirrhosis
- Autoimmune hepatitis

Ascites

Following introduction, seek permission from the caregiver and introduce yourself to the patient before history elicitation, and identify the case.

Name____Age____Sex____Consanguinity____Order of birth____Place____Informant____

Presenting Complaints and Duration

- Abdominal distension and its duration

History of Presenting Illness

- Abdominal distension: Localized or uniform/whether associated with pedal edema/facial puffiness/oliguria
- Explain the sequence of symptoms: Duration, associated symptoms – pain, early satiety, nausea, pedal edema

COMPLICATION HISTORY

- Breathlessness
- Fever
- Abdominal pain
- Oliguria

ETIOLOGICAL HISTORY

- Breathlessness
- Palpitations
- Oliguria
- Facial puffiness
- Jaundice
- UGI bleeding
- Fever
- Abdominal pain
- Recurrent diarrhea
- Failure to gain weight/weight loss
- Rash/joint pain/joint swelling
- Trauma

PAST HISTORY

- Previous blood transfusions
- Surgeries − VP (Ventriculoperitoneal) shunt
- Comorbidities − cardiac, renal, hepatic, malignancies

ANTENATAL/NATAL/PERINATAL HISTORY

- TORCH infection
- Rh incompatibility
- Abnormal antenatal scan (cardiac anomalies, chromosomal anomalies, posterior urethral valve, congenital nephrotic syndrome presents with increased placental weight)
- Jaundice in newborn period − can be suggestive of hepatic cause of ascites/immune hemolytic anemia

DEVELOPMENTAL HISTORY

Development delay (hypothyroidism, chromosomal anomalies, malnutrition, TORCH infections)

IMMUNIZATION HISTORY

Immunized up to age according to IAP or National Immunization Schedule

DIETETIC HISTORY

- History of protein intake
- High-fat diet – acute pancreatitis

CONTACT HISTORY

Any history of contact with TB

FAMILY HISTORY

- Chromosomal anomalies
- Metabolic liver disease
- Socioeconomic history

Summary

A _____-year-old _____ child, presented with abdominal distension of____ days, associated with_____, with/without complications, probably due to___

General Examination

- Sensorium − altered in hepatic encephalopathy, acute pancreatitis
- Anemia − malnutrition, cirrhosis, TORCH infections, hypothyroidism, lymphatic malignancies
- Jaundice − cirrhosis, CCF (Congestive Cardiac Failure), Budd−Chiari syndrome
- Clubbing − cirrhosis, CCF secondary to cyanotic congenital heart disease
- Cyanosis − cirrhosis (hepatopulmonary syndrome), CCF secondary to cyanotic congenital heart disease
- Generalized lymphadenopathy − TB, lymphatic malignancies
- Pedal edema

Head-to-Foot Examination

- Head
  Size − microcephaly
  Hair − hypopigmentation, easily pluckable hair, flag sign
  AF (Anterior Fontanelle) bulge − due to raised ICT (Intracranial Tension)
- Eyes − pallor, icterus, phlycten, periorbital puffiness

- BCG scar
- Prominent neck veins/pulsations in the neck
- Cullen sign/Grey Turner syndrome sign
- Dilated veins in abdomen/peritoneocentesis scar
- VP shunt
- Petechiae/purpura
- Arthritis
- Features of liver cell failure
- Features of chromosomal anomalies
- Features of hypothyroidism

Vital Signs

- Fever – peritonitis, connective tissue disorders, malignancies
- Pulse rate – bradycardia in hypothyroidism, low volume pulse in CCF, wide pulse pressure in cirrhosis
- Blood pressure – hypotension in CCF, wide pulse pressure in cirrhosis
- JVP (Jugular Venous Pressure) – raised in CCF, absent hepatojugular reflex in Budd—Chiari syndrome

System Examination

ABDOMEN

Inspection

- Distended in upper part/uniform distension
- Skin — stretched and shiny
- Scars
- Dilated veins
- Umbilicus — transverse slit, umbilical hernia
- Flanks — full or free
- Hernial orifices
- All quadrants move equally with respiration
- External genitalia – scrotal edema/vulval edema

Palpation

- Warmth
- Tenderness
- Guarding/rigidity
- Organomegaly
- Fluid thrill

Percussion

- Shifting dullness
- Liver span

Auscultation

Bowel sounds, hepatic or renal bruit

CARDIOVASCULAR SYSTEM

Gallop rhythm, murmurs

RESPIRATORY SYSTEM

Pulmonary edema – due to acute left ventricular failure, signs of pleural effusion

CENTRAL NERVOUS SYSTEM

Features of hepatic encephalopathy

Diagnosis

A case of mild/moderate/massive ascites, with or without complication; probably etiology

Frequently Asked Questions

1. Enumerate the causes of ascites.
   Flowchart 30.1 shows various causes of ascites.
2. Explain the significance of age in ascites.
   Etiology of ascites varies according to age:
   Neonatal period:
   > Infections − TORCH
   > CVS − congenital heart block and HLHS (Hypoplastic Left Heart Syndrome)
   > Neonatal hemochromatosis
   Infancy:
   > Tumors − Wilms tumor and neuroblastoma
   > Renal/urogenital − congenital nephrotic syndrome, PUV (Posterior Urethral Valve)
   > Chromosomal anomalies
   > Iso-/alloimmune hemolytic anemia
3. Explain the significance of gender in ascites.
   Females − Turner syndrome, Meigs syndrome, and struma ovarii; males − PUV
4. Explain the significance of appearance of symptoms in ascites.
   Pedal edema → ascites = cardiac cause
   Ascites → pedal edema = hepatic cause
   Facial puffiness → ascites → pedal edema = renal cause
*5. Describe the grading of ascites (also refer the chapter 20 on examination of gastrointestinal system).
   Mild: Puddle sign +
   Moderate: Shifting dullness +
   Severe: Fluid thrill +, respiratory embarrassment
6. Enumerate the complication histories to be elicited in ascites.
   Massive ascites − breathlessness
   Spontaneous bacterial peritonitis − fever and abdominal pain
   Secondary to intravascular volume depletion − oliguria
*6. Enumerate the etiological history in ascites.
   CCF − history of breathlessness and palpitations
   Renal cause − history of oliguria and facial puffiness
   Cirrhosis − history of jaundice and UGI bleeding
   Peritonitis − history of fever and abdominal pain
   Protein-losing enteropathy secondary to malabsorption − history of recurrent diarrhea
   Malnutrition − history of failure to gain weight/weight loss
   Connective tissue disorders (SLE (Systemic Lupus Erythematosus) and JIA) (Juvenile Idiopathic Arthritis) − history of rash/joint pain/joint swelling
   Acute pancreatitis − history of trauma
7. Explain the significance of perinatal history in ascites.
   Antenatal history
   > TORCH infection
   > Rh incompatibility
   > Abnormal AN (Antenatal) scan (cardiac anomalies, chromosomal anomalies, PUV; congenital nephrotic syndrome presents with increased placental weight)
   Postnatal history
   > Respiratory distress in newborn period − CCF
   > Jaundice in newborn period − can be suggestive of hepatic cause of ascites/immune hemolytic anemia
8. List the examination findings in ascites and their significance.
   Table 30.1 gives examination findings and their significance in ascites.
*9. List the head-to-foot examination findings in ascites.
   • Head
     Size − microcephaly

Flowchart 30.1 Various causes of ascites.

ASCITES

Cardiac	G.I	Renal	Infective	Malignancies	Miscellaneous
• Congestive cardiac failure	• Cirrhosis • Acute pacreatitis • Budd-chiari syndrome	• Nephrotic syndrome • PUV (Posterior Urethral Valve)	• Peritonitis • Torch infections	• Lymphomas • Neuroblastoma • Wilms tumor • Meigs syndrome • Struma ovari	• Trisomies 13,18, 21 • Turner syndrome • Chylous ascites • Hypothyroidism • VP (Ventriculoperitoneal) shunt

TABLE 30.1	Examination Findings and Its Significance in Ascites	
Clinical Finding	**Significance**	
Patient's sensorium	Altered sensorium in hepatic encephalopathy, acute pancreatitis	
Posture	Upright posture in massive ascites, sitting and leaning forward in acute pancreatitis	
Oxygen support	CCF (Congestive cardiac failure), pleural effusion	
Pallor	Malnutrition, cirrhosis, TORCH infections, hypothyroidism, connective tissue disorders, lymphatic malignancies	
Cyanosis	Cirrhosis (hepatopulmonary syndrome), CCF secondary to cyanotic congenital heart disease	
Icterus (Fig 30.1)	Cirrhosis, Budd−Chiari syndrome	
Clubbing	Cirrhosis, CCF secondary to cyanotic congenital heart disease	
Generalized lymphadenopathy	Abdominal Tuberculosis connective tissue disorders, hematological malignancies	

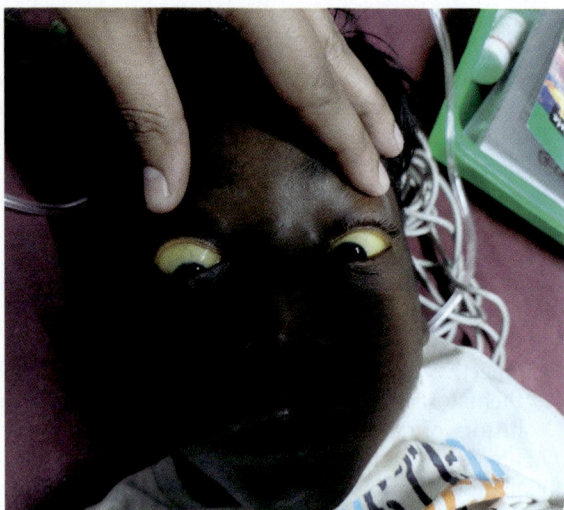

Fig. 30.1   Icterus noted in bulbar conjunctiva in a child with cirrhosis.

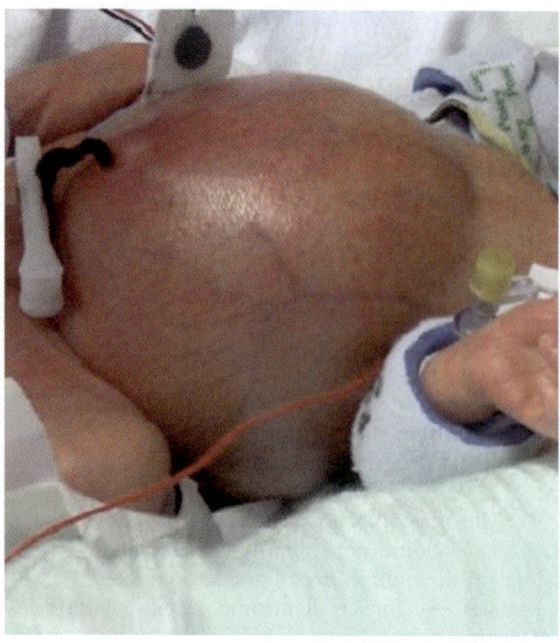

Fig. 30.2   Child with massive ascites with dilated veins over the abdomen. (*Source:* Reproduced from Suhail A. Khan, Manjiri Khare, Haitham Dagash et al. and Meconium pseudocyst presenting as massive ascites in a new-born, *Radiol Case Rep*, 14(2): 235–237.)

Hair − hypopigmentation, easily pluckable hair, flag sign
AF bulge − due to raised ICT
- Eyes − pallor, icterus, phlycten, periorbital puffiness
- BCG scar
- Prominent neck veins/pulsations in the neck
- Cullen sign/Grey Turner syndrome sign
- Dilated veins in abdomen/peritoniocentesis scar
- VP shunt
- Petechiae/purpura
- Arthritis
- Features of liver cell failure
- Features of chromosomal anomalies
- Features of hypothyroidism
Fig. 30.2 shows a child with massive ascites with dilated veins over the abdomen.

10. What is the significance of vital signs in ascites?
Pulse – bradycardia in hypothyroidism, low volume pulse in CCF, wide pulse pressure in cirrhosis
BP − hypotension in CCF, wide pulse pressure in cirrhosis
JVP − raised in CCF, absent hepatojugular reflex in Budd−Chiari syndrome
Fever − peritonitis, connective tissue disorders, malignancies
*11. Mention other systemic findings in ascites.
- CVS − gallop rhythm and murmurs
- RS − pulmonary edema – due to acute LVF (Left Ventricular Failure), features of pleural effusion
- CNS − features of hepatic encephalopathy
12. List the investigations to be performed in ascites.
a. CBC
Raised total leukocyte count − infective cause
Lymphocytosis − TB and lymphatic malignancies
Polycythemia − cyanotic congenital heart disease presenting as CCF; polycythemia is also a risk factor for Budd−Chiari syndrome
b. RFT, urine proteins − to rule out renal cause of ascites
c. LFT − abnormal in cirrhosis
d. Hypoalbuminemia − nephrotic syndrome, cirrhosis, and protein-losing enteropathy
e. Serum amylase, lipase − increased in acute pancreatitis
f. TB work up

g. Chest X-Ray − cardiomegaly, pulmonary edema, and pleural effusion
h. Abdominal Xray
Hellmer sign − lateral liver edge is displaced medially from abdominal wall
Mickey Mouse appearance − due to fluid in paravesical fossa
i. USG abdomen
Can detect as little as 100 mL fluid.
To look for loculated ascites
To detect the etiology − cirrhosis, Budd−Chiari syndrome, acute pancreatitis, malignancies (Wilms tumor and neuroblastoma)
j. Ascitic fluid analysis
*13. Describe the technique of ascitic fluid tapping.
- Explain the procedure and obtain an informed consent.
- Place the patient in supine position.
- Site: It is in midline half way between umbilicus and pubic symphysis, because linea alba is avascular. (The lower quadrants are the most frequent sites for paracentesis. The left lower quadrant is preferred because of the greater depth of ascites and the thinner abdominal wall [Harrison].)
- Drape the area with antiseptic.
- Anesthetize the skin over the insertion site with 1% lidocaine.
- Using 18- to 20-G needle, puncture the anesthetized skin. Keeping the needle perpendicular to the abdominal wall, advance the needle slowly until fluid flows freely into the syringe.
- While advancing the syringe, maintain constant, gentle suction. When there is a return of fluid, begin to aspirate.
- When enough fluid has been withdrawn, quickly withdraw the needle. Cover the insertion site with a sterile pressure dressing.

14. List the gross appearance of ascites in various conditions.
    Straw colored − cirrhosis, as shown in Fig. 30.3A
    Blood stained − traumatic, malignancies, and TB
    Dark brown − biliary
    Black − pancreatic etiology, as shown in Fig. 30.3B
    Milky − chylous ascites, as shown in Fig. 30.3C
*15. Differentiate between transudative and exudative ascites.
    Table 30.2 lists the differences between transudative and exudative ascites.
*16. Explain the significance of SAAG (Serum Ascites Albumin Gradient) in ascites.

SAAG: It does not differentiate between transudate and an exudate. It tells whether the ascites is due to portal hypertension or not.
SAAG > 1.1 g%: Ascites is due to portal hypertension
SAAG < 1.1 g%: Ascites is due to other mechanisms
Both sensitivity and specificity of SAAG in identifying portal hypertension are 97%.
Table 30.3 lists the conditions with high and low SAAG.
17. Differentiate between chylous and pseudochylous ascites.
Pseudochylous ascites contains phospholipid−protein complex which makes the fluid opalescent.
Table 30.4 shows the differences between chylous and pseudochylous ascites.

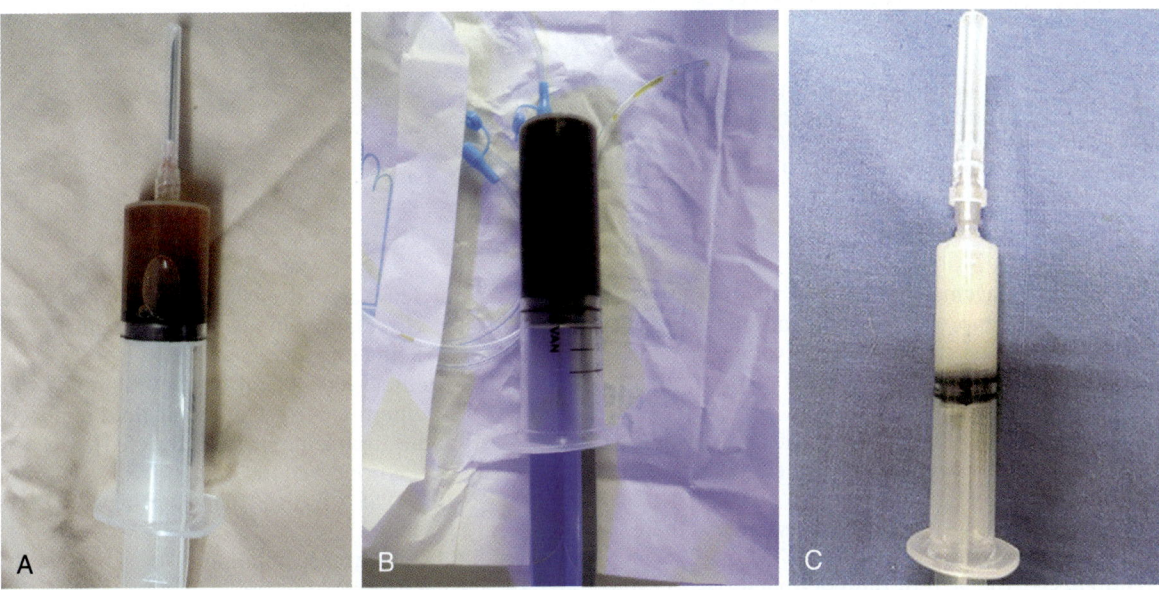

Fig. 30.3 (A) Straw-colored fluid aspirate − cirrhosis. (B) Black-colored fluid seen in pancreatitis. (C) Chylous ascites. (*Source: https://www.researchgate.net/figure/Milky-white-colour-of-the-aspirated-ascitic-fluid_fig3_273351923*)

TABLE 30.2	Differences Between Transudative and Exudative Ascites	
Feature	**Transudative**	**Exudative**
Cells	<250/mm³	>250 neutrophils s/o SBP (Spontaneous Bacterial Peritonitis)
Protein	<3 g%	>3 g%
Specific gravity	<1.015	>1.015
IDH	Low	High
Glucose	<50 mg%	>50 mg%
Triglycerides	Low	High (high in TB, chylous, and rheumatoid arthritis)
ADA (Adenosine Deaminase)	Low	High in TB
Amylase	Low	Increased in pancreatic ascites

TABLE 30.3	Conditions With High and Low SAAG		
High SAAG, High Ascitic Fluid Protein	**High SAAG, Low Ascitic Fluid Protein**	**Low SAAG, High Ascitic Fluid Protein**	**Low SAAG, Low Ascitic Fluid Protein**
Early Budd−Chiari syndrome	Cirrhosis	Peritonitis	Nephrotic syndrome
Constrictive pericarditis	Late Budd−Chiari syndrome	Malignancy	Malnutrition
CCF		Acute pancreatitis	
		Chylous ascites	

TABLE 30.4	Differences Between Chylous and Pseudochylous Ascites	
Feature	**Chylous Ascites**	**Pseudochylous Ascites**
Fat globules	Present	Absent
Ether test	Fat dissolves and top layer becomes clear	Remains turbid
Alkali test	No change in color	Alkali dissolves cellular proteins and fluid becomes clear

TABLE 30.5	Differences Between Primary and Secondary Bacterial Peritonitis
Primary (Spontaneous) Bacterial Peritonitis	**Secondary Bacterial Peritonitis**
• It is the bacterial infection of peritoneal cavity without an identifiable intraabdominal cause • Pneumococci is the most common cause followed by *Escherichia coli*, *Klebsiella*, *Staphylococcus aureus*, and *Mycoplasma pneumoniae* • Monomicrobial • Drug of choice is cefotaxime/ceftriaxone for 10–14 days • Culture-negative neutrocytic ascites is a variant of primary bacterial peritonitis and is characterized by ascitic fluid WBC > 500/mm^3, negative ascitic fluid culture; treatment is same as that of primary bacterial peritonitis	• It is the bacterial infection of peritoneal cavity secondary to an intra-abdominal cause, most common among which is the perforation of the appendix • *E. coli*, *Klebsiella*, and anaerobic organisms • Polymicrobial • Therapy should include both Gram-negative and anaerobic coverage

18. Describe the management of ascites.
    A. Bed rest — improves plasma volume and renal perfusion and hence prevents activation of renin–angiotensin system
    B. Dietary management
       Calorie — RDA (Recommended Dietary Allowances)
       Protein — RDA (avoid animal protein in cirrhosis)
       No added salt to diet
       Fluid restriction — not necessary unless there is hyponatremia
    C. Diuretics — the goal of diuretic therapy is to cause weight loss of 0.5 kg/day if there is no peripheral edema or 0.8–1 kg/day if there is peripheral edema
       Spironolactone is the preferred diuretic because it inhibits aldosterone
       If there is no response, furosemide/thiazide diuretic can be added
    D. Therapeutic paracentesis
       Indications:
       Tense ascites causing respiratory embarrassment
       No response to medical treatment
       Refractory ascites
       Volume: 200–400 mL/kg/day, followed by infusion of albumin 6–8 g/L of ascitic fluid removed
    E. Other treatments — usually reserved for refractory ascites
       1. Peritoneovenous shunts
       2. TIPSS (Transjugular Intrahepatic Portosystemic Shunt)
       3. Liver transplantation
*19. Define refractory ascites.
     Ascites not responding to salt restriction and maximal tolerable dose of two diuretics.
*20. Define recidivant ascites.
     Ascites recurs frequently (3 or more times in a year) in spite of salt restriction and diuretic usage.
21. Differentiate between primary and secondary bacterial peritonitis.
    Table 30.5 lists the differences between primary and secondary bacterial peritonitis.

Quick Bites

- Uniform abdominal distension, which is progressive and is associated with oliguria/pedal edema, is more likely to be due to ascites with an exception of localized ascites.
- The sequence of symptoms, i.e., abdominal distension, facial puffiness, and pedal edema, can give a clue to the cause of ascites.
- Sudden onset of ascites is seen in peritonitis, Budd–Chiari syndrome and acute pancreatitis.
- Patients with Budd–Chiari syndrome have negative hepatojugular reflex.
- Ascites with abdominal pain is also seen in the above-mentioned conditions.
- Gross appearance of ascitic fluid can give a clue to an underlying condition.
- SAAG does not differentiate between a transudative and an exudative ascites. It can only signify whether the underlying mechanism of ascites is due to portal hypertension or not.
- Primary bacterial peritonitis is most commonly caused by pneumococci and is usually monomicrobial, whereas secondary bacterial peritonitis occurs secondary to an intra-abdominal cause and is polymicrobial.
- Spironolactone is the initial diuretic of choice because it inhibits aldosterone.
- The treatment of refractory ascites is
  - Peritoneovenous shunts
  - TIPSS
  - Liver transplantation

Nephritic/Nephrotic Syndrome

Following introduction, seek permission from the caregiver and introduce yourself to the patient before history elicitation, and identify the case.

Name_____Age_____Sex_____Consanguinity_____Order of birth_____Place_____Informant_____

Presenting Complaints and Duration

- Facial puffiness/generalized swelling of the body
- Oliguria
- Cola-colored urine

History of Presenting Illness

FACIAL PUFFINESS

- Duration
- At what time of the day
- Whether associated with pedal edema, ascites, or generalized edema
- History of presacral edema in infants asked for
- If there is ascites or generalized edema, whether it is associated with breathlessness/palpitations/jaundice

OLIGURIA

- Quantity of urine output in the previous 24 hours enquired about
- In infants, ask about the diaper weight/number of times the diaper has been changed
- Cola-colored urine

ASSOCIATED SYMPTOMS

- Fever
- Nausea
- Vomiting
- Fatigue
- Dysuria

COMPLICATION HISTORY

- Headache/projectile vomiting/seizures
- Cough/breathlessness/palpitations
- Fever, abdominal pain, and vomiting
- Diarrhea
- Hematemesis/melena
- Recurrent infections
- Cushingoid features – short stature/increased weight gain/skin changes/defective vision//behavioral changes/headache

ETIOLOGICAL HISTORY

- Sore throat/skin infections
- Fever with exanthematous rash

- Jaundice/previous blood transfusions
- Fever with chills and sweating
- Insect bite/bee sting/food allergy/snake bite
- Drug intake
- Rash, joint pain, and joint swelling
- Easy fatigability/bleeding gums/bone pain/weight loss

TREATMENT HISTORY

- Drug dose/frequency/duration/compliance asked about
- Any intravenous medications given
- Transfusions given (FFP-Fresh Frozen Plasma)
- Biopsy performed

PAST HISTORY

- Similar complaints (if yes, describe in detail about the duration of symptoms, investigations performed, duration of the treatment)
- Medications – duration/compliance
- Blood/FFP transfusions
- Comorbidities

ANTENATAL HISTORY

Abnormal antenatal scan and oligohydramnios

NATAL HISTORY

- Term/preterm
- Respiratory distress
- Edema/oliguria

DEVELOPMENTAL HISTORY

Developmental milestones – normal

DIETETIC HISTORY

Mention about the following in the last 24-hour period:
- Calorie intake
- Protein intake
- Fluid intake
- Salt intake

Immunization History

Immunized according to IAP or Universal Immunization

CONTACT HISTORY

Any contact with TB-tuberculosis

ALLERGY HISTORY

Exposure to any known allergens

FAMILY HISTORY

- Sore throat in family members
- Similar illness in family members

SOCIOECONOMIC HISTORY

According to the modified Kuppuswamy scale

Summary

A _____-year-old _____ child presented with facial puffiness/generalized edema, with oliguria, with/without cola-colored urine, with/without complications, and with/without similar episodes in the past, probably because of a renal cause.

General Examination

- Sensorium
- Posture
- Pallor
- Cyanosis
- Icterus
- Generalized lymphadenopathy
- Edema

Head-to-Foot Examination

- Facial puffiness
- Facies: Cushingoid facies and hirsutism
- Eyes: Pallor, icterus, cataract, anterior lenticonus, retinitis pigmentosa, hypertensive retinopathy, and papilledema
- Oral cavity: Tonsillitis and ulcers
- Ear: Preauricular skin tag and SNHL (Sensory Neural Hearing Loss)
- Nails: Leukonychia
- Skeletal deformity/bone fractures
- Skin: Infections/scab/erythematous rash
- Arthritis
- Scrotal edema/vulval edema
- Peritoneal tap marks
- Signs of steroid toxicity: Cushingoid facies/buffalo hump/acanthosis nigricans/purple striae

Vitals Signs

- Pulse rate
- Blood pressure
- Respiration: Rate, rhythm, and type of respiration
- Temperature
- JVP (Jugular Venous Pressure)

System Examination

ABDOMEN

Inspection

- Uniformly distended
- Skin: Stretched and shiny, any scars, and purple striae
- Umbilicus: Transverse slit
- Flanks: Full or free
- Hernia orifices
- Equal movements of all quadrants with respiration
- External genitalia: Scrotal edema/vulval edema

Palpation

- Warmth
- Tenderness
- Guarding
- Abdominal wall edema
- Organomegaly
- Kidneys ballotable
- Fluid thrill

Percussion

- Puddle sign
- Shifting dullness

Auscultation

Any renal bruit (auscultate on either side of the umbilicus or below the xiphisternum)

CARDIOVASCULAR SYSTEM

Gallop rhythm/pericardial rub

RESPIRATORY SYSTEM

Look features suggestive of pleural effusion/basal crackles.

CENTRAL NERVOUS SYSTEM

Signs of ↑ ICT (Intracranial Tension)/focal neurological deficit

Diagnosis

- A case of nephritic or nephrotic syndrome
- Steroid-responsive/SDNS (Steroid Dependant Nephrotic Syndrome)/SRNS (Steroid Resistant Nephrotic Syndrome)
- With/without complications
- Probable etiology

Frequently Asked Questions

*1. What is the significance of age in a child with nephritic/nephrotic syndrome?
   - 0–3 months: Congenital nephrotic syndrome
   - 3 months to 1 year: Infantile nephrotic syndrome
   - 2–6 years: Minimal change disease
   - 5–15 years: MPGN (Membranoproliferative Glomerulonephritis)/secondary nephritic syndrome
   - 5–12 years: PIGN (PostInfectious Glomerulonephritis)

2. Explain the significance of gender in a child with nephritic/nephrotic syndrome.
   - Males: Minimal change disease, Alport syndrome, and nephrotic syndrome secondary to Fabry disease
   - Females: Nephrotic syndrome secondary to SLE (Systemic Lupus Erythematosus)

*3. Define oliguria and anuria.
   - Oliguria is defined as urine output <1 mL/kg/day in infants, <0.5 mL/kg/day in children, and <400 mL/day in adolescents and adults (Nammalvar and Harrison, 20th edition).
   - Anuria is defined as nil urine output for 12 hours in the absence of urinary tract obstruction.

4. Enumerate the complications in nephritic/nephrotic syndrome.
   Complications due to disease
   - Hypertensive encephalopathy, cortical vein thrombosis, and electrolyte imbalance: Headache/projectile vomiting/seizures
   - Pulmonary edema/acute left ventricular failure: Cough/breathlessness/palpitations
   - Spontaneous bacterial peritonitis: Fever, abdominal pain, and vomiting
   - Bowel wall edema and peritonitis in nephrotic syndrome: Diarrhea
   - Immunosuppression in nephrotic syndrome: Recurrent infections
   Complications due to drugs (steroids)
   - Abdominal pain and GI bleeding (gastritis)
   - Cushingoid features
   - Short stature
   - Increased weight gain
   - Skin changes (purple striae, acanthosis nigricans)
   - Defective vision (cataract)
   - Behavioral changes (psychosis)
   - Headache (pseudotumor cerebri)

5. Enumerate the significance of etiological histories in nephritic/nephrotic syndrome.

History	Etiology
• Sore throat/skin infections	• AGN (Acute Glomerulonephritis)
• Fever with exanthematous rash	• Mumps, chicken pox
• Jaundice/previous blood transfusions	• HBV (Hepatitis B Virus)/HCV (Hepatitis C Virus) infection
• Fever with chills and sweating	• Malaria, infective endocarditis
• Allergic reactions	• Insect bite/bee sting/food allergy

History	Etiology
• Drug intake	• Minimal change nephrotic syndrome: Penicillamine, captopril, NSAIDs (Non-Steroidal Anti-Inflammatory Drugs), probenecid, ethosuximide, methimazole
	• Proliferative glomerulonephritis: Procainamide, chlorpropamide, phenytoin, trimethadione, paramethadione
• Rash, joint pain, joint swelling	• Systemic lupus erythematosus
• Easy fatigability/bleeding gums/bone pain/weight loss	• Leukemia/lymphoma

*6. What is the significance of past history in nephritic/nephrotic syndrome?
   - Relapse/steroid-dependent nephrotic syndrome: Similar complaints in the past
   - Medications: Duration/compliance
   - HBV and HCV: Blood/FFP transfusions
   - Comorbidities: Congenital heart disease and infective endocarditis that predisposes to nephrotic syndrome

7. Mention the significance of perinatal history.
   - Antenatal period
     - Abnormal AN (Antenatal) scan: Placental weight >25% in Finnish type of congenital nephrotic syndrome and oligohydramnios
   - Natal period
     - Preterm birth: Finnish type of congenital nephrotic syndrome
     - Respiratory distress in the newborn period (pulmonary hypoplasia associated with Potter syndrome)
     - Edema/oliguria in the newborn period: Congenital nephrotic syndrome

8. Explain the significance of developmental history.
   - Delayed development of language secondary to hearing loss in Alport syndrome
   - Mental retardation in Laurence–Moon–Biedl syndrome

9. What is the significance of family and socioeconomic history?
   - Family history: Sore throat in family members (AGN-Acute Glomerulonephritis)
   - Socioeconomic history: Poor hygiene/overcrowding (AGN)
   - Disease impact on the child (number of school days and playtime missed) and impact on family (financial constraints)
   - Familial causes of nephrotic syndrome

*10. List the findings in general examination.
    Table 31.1 gives the general examination findings in nephritic/nephrotic syndrome.

*11. List the findings in head-to-foot examination.
    - Facial puffiness
    - Facies: Cushingoid facies and hirsutism
    - Eyes
      - Pallor

TABLE 31.1	General Examination Findings in Nephritic/Nephrotic Syndrome
Clinical Finding	**Significance**
Patient's sensorium	Altered in cerebral venous thrombosis, hypertensive encephalopathy, uremic encephalopathy/electrolyte imbalance
Posture	The patient might prefer an upright posture in case of massive ascites
Pallor	Malaria, kala-azar, sickle cell anemia, infective endocarditis, connective tissue disorders, loss of transferrin in nephritic syndrome, leukemia/lymphoma
Cyanosis	Respiratory failure because of pulmonary edema/pleural effusion
Icterus	HBV, HCV
Generalized lymphadenopathy	Connective tissue disorders, hematological malignancies
Pedal edema	Fast edema (pitting lasting for <20 s)

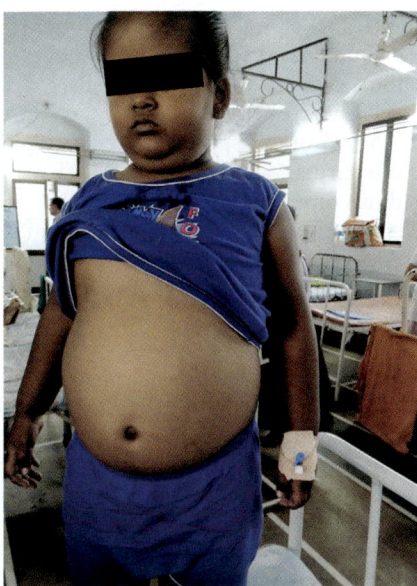

Fig. 31.1 Ascites in a child with nephrotic syndrome.

- Icterus
- Cataract (steroid-induced)
- Anterior lenticonus (Alport syndrome)
- Retinitis pigmentosa (Laurence–Moon–Biedl syndrome)
- Roth spots: Infective endocarditis
- Hypertensive retinopathy
- Papilledema (because of raised ICT)
- Oral cavity
  - Tonsillitis: Streptococcal infection
  - Ulcers: SLE
- Ears: Preauricular tag and (Sensorineural Hearing Loss) (Alport syndrome)
- Nails: White nails – hypoalbuminemia and chronic kidney disease
- Skeletal deformity: Renal/nutritional rickets
- Skin: Infections/scab/erythematous rash
- Bone
  - Arthritis: SLE
  - Bone fractures: Steroid-induced osteoporosis
- Scrotal edema/vulval edema
- Peritoneal tap marks
- Signs of steroid toxicity: Cushingoid facies/buffalo hump/acanthosis nigricans/purple striae
- Signs of dehydration

12. What is the significance of vital signs in nephritic/nephrotic syndrome?
    - Pulse: Low-volume pulse suggestive of intravascular volume depletion/secondary to acute LVF (Left Ventricular Failure) (AGN)
    - BP: High in AGN
    - RR: Increased because of pleural effusion/pulmonary edema
    - Temperature: suggestive of infection/spontaneous bacterial peritonitis/connective tissue disorder/malignancy
    - JVP: Elevated in pericardial effusion
13. Enumerate the findings in system examination.
    Abdomen
    - Inspection: Uniformly distended; skin – stretched, shiny, and purple striae; umbilicus – transverse slit; flanks – full; and external genitalia – scrotal edema/

vulval edema Fig. 31.1 shows ascites in a child with nephrotic syndrome.
    - Palpation: Tenderness, guarding, abdominal wall edema, organomegaly (infection, connective tissue disorders/malignancy), and deep – kidneys ballotable (nephromegaly)
    - Percussion: Puddle sign, shifting dullness, and fluid thrill
    - Auscultation: Any renal bruit (auscultate on either side of the umbilicus or below the xiphisternum)
    Cardiovascular system
    - Gallop rhythm because of (Congestive Cardiac Failure)
    - Pericardial rub – uremic pericarditis
    Respiratory system
    - Look for features of pleural effusion
    - Basal crackles in pulmonary edema
    Central nervous system
    - Signs of raised intracranial tension and focal neurological deficit

DISCUSSION ON ACUTE GLOMERULONEPHRITIS

14. Enumerate the clinical course of Post Streptococcal Glomerulonephritis (PSGN).
    - Recovery rate is usually 95%–97%. Mortality is 0.5%.
    - Hypertension resolves in 1 week usually but can take up to 4–6 weeks.
    - Albuminuria takes 4–6 weeks to resolve.
    - Gross hematuria resolves in 3–5 days but microscopic hematuria can persist for up to 1 year.
15. Name few organisms causing acute glomerulonephritis.
    - Coagulase-positive and coagulase-negative *Staphylococcus aureus*
    - *Streptococcus pneumoniae*
    - Gram-negative bacteria
    - *Mycoplasma pneumoniae*
    - Rickettsia

- Fungi
- Viral: Influenza, hepatitis B and C, parvovirus, CMV (Cytomegalovirus), EBV (Epstein-Barr Virus), mumps, varicella, and rubella

16. When should one suspect non−poststreptococcal glomerulonephritis?
    - Insidious onset and protracted course
    - Systemic features: Fever, rash, joint pain, and heart disease
    - Absence of serological evidence of streptococcal infection and normal levels of C3 in acute illness
    - Mixed picture of glomerulonephritis and significant proteinuria
    - Uremia requiring dialysis

17. Mention few complications of acute glomerulonephritis.
    a) Hypertension: Seen in 60% of patients but hypertensive encephalopathy seen in only 10% of patients
    b) Acute left ventricular failure and pulmonary edema
    c) Acute renal failure requiring dialysis
    d) Metabolic: Hyponatremia, hyperkalemia, hypocalcemia, and hyperphosphatemia

18. Name some diseases under nephritic syndrome spectrum.
    - Postinfectious glomerulonephritis
    - IgA nephropathy
    - MPGN
    - Membranous nephropathy
    - RPGN (Rapidly Progressive Glomerulonephritis)
    - HSP (Henoch-Schönlein Purpura) nephritis
    - SLE
    - Sickle cell disease
    - Wegener granulomatosis
    - Alport syndrome
    - Goodpasture syndrome
    - Shunt nephritis
    - Endocarditis

19. List the investigations performed in AGN.
    1. Urine examination
       a. Macroscopic: Color of the urine
       b. Microscopic: To look for RBCs, RBC (Red Blood Cells) casts, WBCs, (White Blood Cells) granular casts, and epithelial cells
          ○ *Hematuria in AGN*
            - It is gross in 30% of patients.
            - It is microscopic in 100% of patients.
            - Gross hematuria resolves in 3–5 days.
            - Microscopic hematuria resolves in 1 month to 1 year.
            - *Hematuria*: There are >5 RBCs/HPF (High Power Field) in centrifuged urine.
          ○ Cast in urine
            - The major component of casts is Tamm–Horsfall protein.
            - RBC casts are present.
          ○ It is the hallmark of glomerulonephritis. It is also seen after strenuous exercise.
          ○ Spin 12 mL of urine at 1500–2000 rpm for 5 minutes. The sediment is mixed with a drop of urine and examined under a microscope. Look at the edge of coverslip for casts:
            - WBC casts: Pyelonephritis
            - Hyaline casts: Nephrotic syndrome
       c. Urine for spot PCR (Protein Creatinine Ratio)

       d. Urine albumin/24-hour urine protein
       e. Urine culture and sensitivity: To rule out urinary tract infection
    2. *CBC*
       - Anemia because of hemodilution
       - Leukocytosis because of glomerular inflammation
    3. ESR: Increased
    4. RFT
       - Renal failure common in AGN than in nephrotic syndrome
       - Hyponatremia because of volume overload and hyperkalemia because of impaired renal function
    5. Serum electrolytes: Hyponatremia (dilutional)
    6. USG abdomen
       USG in nephritic syndrome
         ○ Kidneys enlarged with increased echoes in 25% of patients
         ○ To look for ascites
         ○ To rule out other causes of hematuria
    7. Chest X-ray (cardiomegaly and pulmonary edema)
    8. Antibody titer
       ASO (Antistreptolysin O) titer
         ○ Normal: 170–330 Todd units/mL
         ○ Abnormal: >200 IU (International Units) (or >330 Todd units)
         ○ Appears in 7–10 days following streptococcal infection
         ○ Peaks at 3–6 weeks
         ○ At 3 months, positive in 75% of patients
         ○ At 6 months, positive in 20% of patients
       Anti-DNase B
         ○ Normal: ≤170 Todd units/mL
         ○ Peaks at 6–8 weeks
         ○ Remains positive for longer than ASO (110 days compared with 90 days with ASO)
       Streptozyme test
         ○ Against four antigens – streptolysin O, DNase B, hyaluronidase, and streptokinase
         ○ Normal: <1 in 100 (antizymogen assay is superior to ASO and anti-DNase B)
    9. Throat swab
    10. Complements C3 and C4
        Persistently low complement
         ○ SLE
         ○ MPGN
         ○ RPGN
         ○ Shunt nephritis
         ○ Bacterial endocarditis
         ○ Visceral abscess
         ○ Nonstreptococcal PIGN
         ○ Essential mixed cryoglobulinemia

20. Enumerate the management in AGN.
    Treatment
    - Daily monitoring of weight and abdominal girth
    - Bed rest, which increases renal blood flow
    - Strict intake–output chart
    - No added salt
    - Fluid restriction on the basis of the urine output and hydration status
    - Cautious use of loop diuretics if needed for the management of edema and hypertension – furosemide at 1–2 mg/kg/dose

- Antibiotics: Penicillin oral for 10 days to prevent possibility of transmission of nephritogenic strains to the community and to reduce the antigenic load in the index child
- Management of complications such as hypertension, pulmonary edema, and renal failure

21. Mention the role of furosemide in PIGN.
    - Should be used only in case of severe pulmonary edema
    - Should not be used routinely

22. Why is routine antibiotic prophylaxis not indicated after PIGN?
    - Second attacks are extremely rare.
    - In addition, there is no permanent damage to the kidneys following an attack of PIGN.

23. Mention few drugs used to treat hypertension in postinfectious glomerulonephritis.
    - Nifedipine: 0.25–0.5 mg/kg/dose b.d. or t.d.s. (maximum of 1 mg/kg t.d.s.) orally
    - ACE (Angiotensin-Converting Enzyme) inhibitors can be used if there is no impaired renal function/renal vein thrombosis/renal artery stenosis after ruling out hyperkalemia
      - Enalapril 0.1 mg/kg/day (maximum of 0.5 mg/kg/dose b.d.) orally
      - Hydralazine 0.2–0.6 mg/kg/dose i.v. or 0.25 mg/kg/dose t.d.s.–q.i.d. (maximum of 7.5 mg/kg/day)

DISCUSSION ON NEPHROTIC SYNDROME

24. Classify nephrotic syndrome.
    Flowchart 31.1 shows the classification of nephrotic syndrome.

25. List the investigations in nephrotic syndrome.
    1. Investigations to confirm diagnosis
       - Urine albumin: Greater than or equal to 3+
       - Urine PCR: >2.0
       - 24-Hour urine proteins: >3.5 g/day or >40 mg/m²/h
       - Serum cholesterol >200 mg/dL
       - Serum albumin: <2.5 g/dL
    2. Investigations to look for complications
       - RFT (Renal Function Tests): To rule out renal failure
       - Electrolytes: Hyponatremia, hypokalemia (secondary to diuretics), and hyperkalemia (renal failure)
       - Chest X-Ray: Cardiomegaly/pericardial effusion, pleural effusion, and pulmonary edema
       - Ultrasonogram abdomen: To look for ascites, renomegaly in early stages, and RPD (Renal Pelvic Dilation) grading (compare with liver texture)
       - Grade 1: Equal to liver texture
       - Grade 2: More echogenic than the liver texture but corticomedullary differentiation maintained
       - Grade 3: More echogenic than the liver texture and corticomedullary differentiation lost
       - Grade 4: Reversal of corticomedullary differentiation, more than the papillary sinuses
    3. Investigations prior to starting steroids
       - Sepsis work-up: CBC, CRP (C-Reactive Protein), urine WBCs, urine culture, and blood culture
       - TB work-up
    4. Investigations to look for etiology (depending on the clinical condition)
       - Peripheral smear: Malaria
       - HBsAg and anti-HCV
       - ANA (Anti-Nuclear Antibodies) and anti-dsDNA
       - C3 and C4 (C3 decreased in AGN, both C3 and C4 reduced in lupus nephritis)

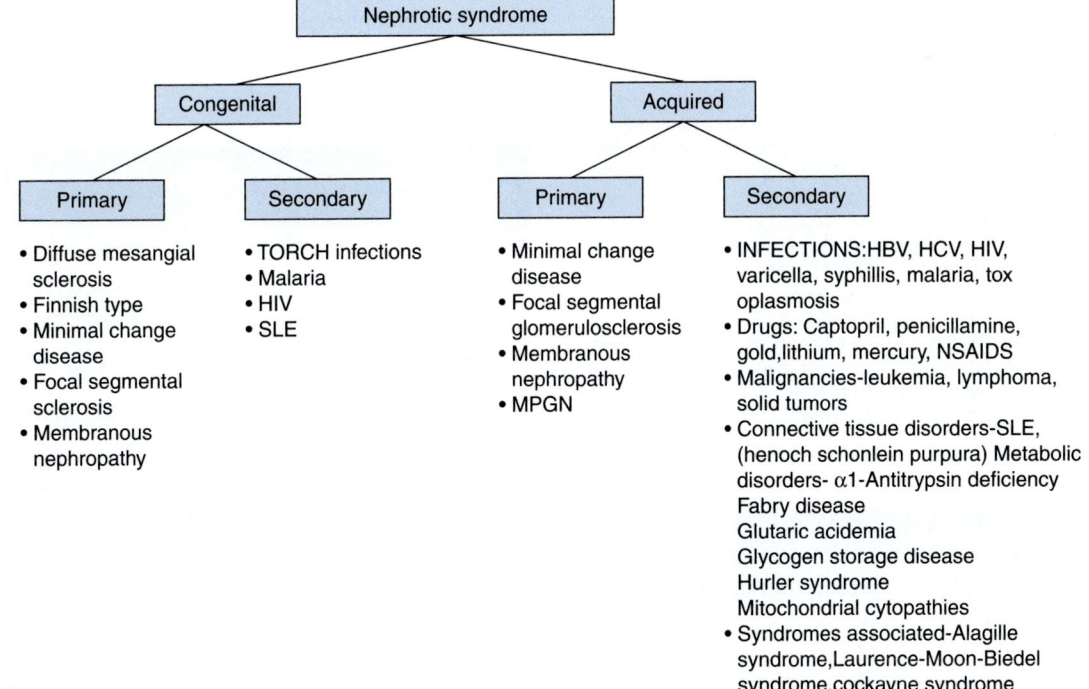

Flowchart 31.1 Classification of nephrotic syndrome.

5. Renal biopsy
   Table 31.2 shows the indications for renal biopsy in nephritic/nephrotic syndrome.
*26. What is the management of nephrotic syndrome?
   • Hospitalize if it is the first episode with severe edema and nephrotic syndrome with complications
   A. Diet
      • Calories: RDA (Recommended Dietary Allowances)
      • Protein: 1.5–2 g/kg/day
      • Salt: No added salt to the diet; this diet allows the following:
         - 1–1.5 g/day for children younger than 5 years
         - 2 g/day for schoolchildren
         - 3–4 g/day for adolescents
         - To avoid pickles, chips, and fried items
      • Fluid intake
         - Mild: No extra water
         - Moderate: Previous-day urine output + insensible water loss
         - Massive edema (anasarca and/or edema causing respiratory embarrassment): Insensible water loss
         - On the basis of body surface area, insensible water loss = 400 mL/m^2/day (for calculating body surface area, use Mosteller formula, BSA (Body Surface Area) = $\sqrt{\text{weight [kg]} \times \text{height [cm]}/3600}$)
         Table 31.3 lists the insensible water loss according to various ages.

B. Medications
   1. Diuretics
      Furosemide is the first choice; potassium-sparing diuretics can be added to prevent hypokalemia. Thiazide can be added as second line in cases refractory to furosemide.
   2. Albumin infusion
      - It improves intravascular volume and renal perfusion, and also prevents edema.
      - Indications: These include massive ascites causing respiratory embarrassment, pleural effusion, and severe peripheral edema with skin breakdown.
      - Dose: The dose is 0.5–1 g/kg of 25% human albumin (maximum of 25 g). It is given as slow infusion over 6–8 hours followed by furosemide injection. The dose can be repeated every 12 hours.
      - If urine output does not improve in a child with oliguria/anuria after two doses of albumin, evaluate for acute renal failure.
      - Albumin infusion in the presence of sepsis can further aggravate it because bacteria use plasma proteins as a nutrient.
   3. Steroids
   4. Steroid-sparing agents
   5. Rituximab
   6. ACE inhibitors
*27. Enumerate the various steroid regimens for the treatment of nephrotic syndrome.
   Table 31.4 lists the various steroid regimens for the treatment of nephrotic syndrome.
28. Name some steroid-sparing agents.
   • Cyclophosphamide
   • Chlorambucil
   • Calcineurin inhibitors
   • Levamisole
   • Mycophenolate mofetil

TABLE 31.2	Indications for Renal Biopsy in Nephritic/Nephrotic Syndrome
Renal biopsy in nephrotic syndrome	1. Age <1 or >12 years 2. Gross hematuria, persistent microscopic hematuria 3. Low serum C3 > 3 months 4. Sustained hypertension 5. Renal failure not attributed to hypovolemia 6. Presence of systemic features such as arthritis, skin rashes, HSM (Hepatosplenomegaly), abdominal pain, serositis 7. Steroid-resistant nephrotic syndrome 8. Before starting calcineurin inhibitors 9. Nephritic-onset nephrotic syndrome
Indications for renal biopsy in PIGN	1. Presence of nephrotic syndrome 2. Acute renal failure 3. Absence of evidence of glomerulonephritis 4. Normal complement levels or persistent hypocomplementemia >2 months 5. Persistent hematuria >2 months

TABLE 31.3	Insensible Water Loss According to Various Ages	
Age		**Volume (mL/kg/day)**
Younger than 1 month		30
1 month to 1 year		25
1–5 years		20
Older than 5 years		15

TABLE 31.4	Various Steroid Regimens for the Treatment of Nephrotic Syndrome	
Regimen	**Duration of Therapy of Prednisolone**	
APN (Arbeitsgemeinschaft für Pädiatrische Nephrologie)	2 mg/kg daily for 6 weeks 1.5 mg/kg/day EOD (Every other day) for 6 weeks	
ISPN (Indian Society of Pediatric Nephrology)	2 mg/kg/day – single or divided doses – for 6 weeks 1.5 mg/kg – single morning dose EOD – for 6 weeks	
ISKDC	2 mg/kg daily for 4 weeks 1.5 mg/kg/day for 3 consecutive days in 1–4 weeks	
Modified ISKDC (International Study of Kidney Disease in Children)	Same as above except that 1.5–mg/kg dose is given on alternate days	
KDIGO (Kidney Disease Improving Global Outcomes)	2 mg/kg/day – single dose – daily for 6 weeks 1.5 mg/kg EOD for 6 weeks followed by tapering over 2–5 months	

- Rituximab
- ACE inhibitors/ARB (Angiotensin Receptor Blockers)
29. Mention the dose and adverse effects of steroid-sparing agents.

    Table 31.5 lists the dose and adverse effects of steroid-sparing agents.
30. Enumerate the treatment options for steroid-resistant nephrotic syndrome.
    A. Mendoza regimen as given in Flowchart 31.2
    B. Calcineurin inhibitors: Tacrolimus 0.12–0.15 mg/kg/day; if there is no remission after 3–6 months, tacrolimus resistant; triple therapy started
    C. Triple therapy: Oral prednisolone + mycophenolate mofetil + tacrolimus – 1 year; if remission does not occur in 6 months, then triple therapy resistant
    D. If triple therapy resistant, rituximab started

TABLE 31.5	Dose and Adverse Effects of Steroid-Sparing Agents	
Drug	**Adverse Effects**
Cyclophosphamide (i.v. monthly for 6 months – 500 mg/m²/month), cumulative dose not more than 168 mg/dL	BM suppression, gonadal toxicity, hemorrhagic cystitis, withhold when WBCs <4000/mm³
Levamisole	Leukopenia, GI upset
Cyclosporine (4–5 mg/kg/day daily – 12–24 months)	Hirsutism, hyperglycemia, hyperkalemia, hypertension, hypomagnesemia, neurotoxicity, tubulointerstitial nephritis
Tacrolimus (0.1–0.2 mg/kg/day) – 12–24 months	Except for neurotoxicity and hyperglycemia, all the effects are less compared with those with cyclosporine
MMF (Mycophenolate Mofetil) (800–1200 mg/m²) – 12–24 months	Leukopenia, esophagitis, GI hemorrhage, lymphoma
Rituximab (375 mg/m²/week) – 2–4 weekly	Hypogammaglobulinemia

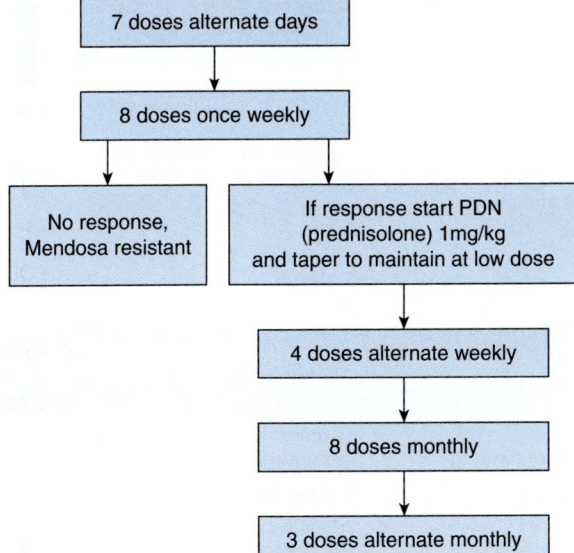

Flowchart 31.2 Mendoza regimen.

E. If no response to above-mentioned treatment, ACE/ARB inhibitors
31. What is West regimen?

    West regimen is given in Flowchart 31.3.
32. What is Ponticelli regimen?
    - Three doses of cyclophosphamide, three doses of methylprednisolone alternate monthly
    - First, 3rd, and 5th months: Pulse methylprednisolone 30 mg/kg alternate day; from day 6 prednisolone 1 mg/kg/day
    - Second, 4th, and 6th months: I.v. cyclophosphamide 500 mg/m²; from day 2 prednisolone 1 mg/kg for 6 months; prednisolone continued to delay renal failure
*33. Enumerate the management of complications.
    A. Refractory edema
    - Dietary management
    - Diuretics
    - Albumin infusion
    - ACE inhibitors
    - PG (Prostaglandins) inhibitors
    - Peritoneal dialysis
    - Head-out water immersion technique (not practiced these days)
    B. Hypertension: ACE inhibitors/ARB
    C. Hyperlipidemia: Dietary restriction of fat and statins (when cholesterol >500 mg/dL and in SRNS)
    D. Hypercoagulability
    - Indications for starting anticoagulants (KDIGO)
        - Serum albumin <2.0–2.5 g/dL + one or more of the following:
            - Body mass index (BMI (Body Mass Index)) >35 kg/m²
            - Proteinuria >10 g/day
            - Family history of thromboembolism with a documented genetic predisposition
            - Recent abdominal or orthopedic surgery, or prolonged immobilization
            - New York Heart Association class III or IV congestive heart failure
    - Heparin should be given in higher than usual dose because part of the action of heparin depends on antithrombin III, which may be lost in the urine.
    - Maintain INR (International Normalized Ratio) of 2–3.
        Source: ref-https://kdigo.org/wp-content/uploads/2017/02/KDIGO-GN-GL-Public-Review-Draft_1-June-2020.pdf.
    E. Infections: If repeated infections occur, serum immunoglobulins should be measured. If serum IgG <600 mg/day, the infection risk can be reduced by monthly administration of i.v. immunoglobulin 10–15 g to keep serum IgG >600 mg/dL. However, there is limited evidence to the above-mentioned therapy.

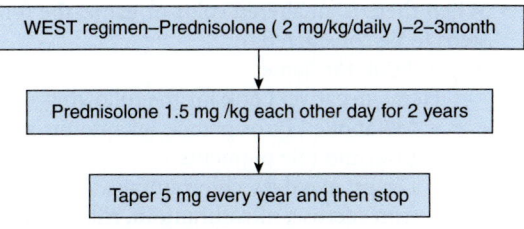

Flowchart 31.3 West regimen.

*34. Explain the principles behind immunization in nephrotic syndrome (KDIGO).
- Pneumococcal vaccination should be given to all the children.
- Influenza vaccination should be given annually to all the children and their household contacts.
- Avoid live vaccines until prednisone dose is either <20 mg/day or 2 mg/kg on alternate days (<40 mg on alternate days).
- Live vaccines are contraindicated in children who receive corticosteroid-sparing immunosuppressive agents.
- Immunize healthy household contacts with live vaccines to minimize the risk of transfer of infection to the immunosuppressed child. Avoid direct exposure of the child to gastrointestinal, urinary, or respiratory secretions of vaccinated contacts for 3–6 weeks after vaccination.
- Following close contact with varicella infection, for nonimmune children on immunosuppressive agents, vaccine is given against varicella zoster immune globulin, if available.
   Source: ref-https://kdigo.org/wp-content/uploads/2017/02/KDIGO-GN-GL-Public-Review-Draft_1-June-2020.pdf.

SPECIAL SITUATIONS IN NEPHROTIC SYNDROME

35. What is the management of nephrotic syndrome with varicella infection?
- If the child is on low-dose steroids <1 mg/kg/day or <2 mg/kg EOD, stop steroids. Restart steroids 4 weeks after scabbing.
- If the child is on steroids greater than above-mentioned dose, taper steroids by 0.5 mg/kg every 5 days and stop; restart steroids 4 weeks after scabbing.

36. What is the management of nephrotic syndrome with UTI (Urinary Tract Infection)?
   If the culture is positive, treat UTI. It is followed by chemoprophylaxis for 2 weeks. Restart steroids 4 weeks after completing chemoprophylaxis.

37. What is the management of Mantoux-positive children with nephrotic syndrome?
   Start INH prophylaxis after ruling out active TB. Start steroids 4 weeks after starting INH (Isoniazid) prophylaxis. If active TB is present, steroids should be started after completing the intensive phase.

DISCUSSION ON HEMATURIA

*38. Describe the approach to gross hematuria.
- Gross hematuria is defined as passing frank blood in the urine that is visible to the naked eye.
- Urine RBCs are >5/HPF.
- When there is an altered color of urine, the following steps to be considered.
   Step 1: Look for heme.
   - Heme negative: Look for the following:
      - Metabolic: Tyrosinemia, alkaptonuria, melanuria, and bile pigments
      - Drugs: Azo dyes, chloroquine, desferrioxamine, iron sucrose, nitrofurantoin, rifampin, and sulfasalazine

   - Red diaper syndrome: Red staining of diapers because of deposition of urate crystals
   - Heme positive: Go to the next step.
   Step 2: Look for RBCs.

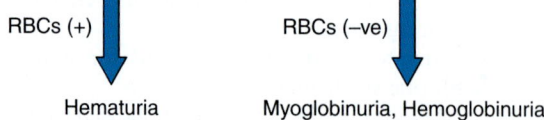

   Step 3: If heme (positive) and RBCs (positive), look for the origin of hematuria (refer Q. 28).
   Source: Own collection.

39. Enumerate the types of hematuria.
   Table 31.6 shows the various types of hematuria.

40. Differentiate between glomerular and nonglomerular hematuria.
   Table 31.7 lists the differences between glomerular and nonglomerular hematuria.

41. Enumerate the causes of asymptomatic, recurrent, and gross hematuria.
- Causes of asymptomatic hematuria
   - Benign familial hematuria
   - Idiopathic hypercalciuria
   - Cystic diseases of the kidney
   - Hemangioma of the urinary tract
- Causes of recurrent hematuria
   - IgA nephropathy
   - Alport syndrome
   - Benign familial hematuria

TABLE 31.6	Various Types of Hematuria
Macroscopic hematuria	• Dipstick (peroxidase test) positive for true hematuria or myoglobinuria or hemoglobinuria and negative for food and drugs • Detects 3–10 RBCs/microgram litre (100% sensitive and 99% specific) • False positive: pH >9, contamination with menstrual blood, oxidizing agent, fever, exercise • False negative: Formalin, ascorbic acid • Confirmatory test: Always microscopic examination of RBCs and RBC casts • Spectrophotometry: Hemoglobinuria, myoglobinuria
Microscopic hematuria	• Centrifugation: 10 mL urine + 2000 RPM + 5 minutes • Centrifuged sample: >5 RBCs/HPF
Transient hematuria	Fever, infection, trauma, exercise

TABLE 31.7	Differences Between Glomerular and Nonglomerular Hematuria	
Urinary Finding	**Glomerular Hematuria**	**Nonglomerular Hematuria**
1. Color	Cola or brown	Red
2. Casts/crystals	Absent	± Present
3. Proteinuria	2+ or more	<2+
4. RBC morphology	Dysmorphic	Eumorphic

- Nutcracker syndrome
- ADPKD (Autosomal Dominant Polycystic Kidney Disease) (50% present with gross hematuria)
- Nephrolithiasis (25%)
- Urinary tract infection (25%)
- HSP
- SLE
- Causes of recurrent gross hematuria
  - IgA nephropathy
  - Alport syndrome
  - Benign familial hypercalciuria
  - Thin basement membrane disease

42. Enumerate the causes of hematuria following an episode of URI (Upper Respiratory Tract Infection).
    - PIGN: It occurs 1–3 weeks after an episode of URI (streptococcal pharyngitis). Hematuria lasts for 4–5 weeks.
    - IgA nephropathy: It occurs 1–2 days after an episode of URI. Hematuria lasts for 5 days.

DISCUSSION ON PROTEINURIA

43. Mention the various tests for the estimation of proteinuria.
    Table 31.8 lists the tests for the estimation of proteinuria.

44. Explain the grading of edema in nephrotic syndrome.
    - Grade 1: Facial + pedal edema
    - Grade 2: Grade 1 + ascites
    - Grade 3: Grade 2 + anasarca

45. Enumerate the causes of abdominal pain in a child with renal disease.
    - Nephrotic syndrome: Spontaneous bacterial peritonitis
    - Nephrolithiasis: Loin to groin/colicky abdominal pain
    - Renal vein thrombosis: Abdominal pain + renal mass + hematuria
    - Urinary tract infection (cystitis/pyelonephritis)

46. What are the causes of palpable mass in a child with renal disease?
    1. Multicystic dysplastic kidney (most common cause of abdominal mass in newborn)
    2. Hydronephrosis
    3. Polycystic kidney disease
    4. Urinary bladder
    5. Renal vein thrombosis
    6. Wilms tumor

47. When do the clinical features resolve in AGN?
    Table 31.9 lists the time of resolution of clinical features in AGN.
    Monitoring/follow-up up to 1 year
    - Blood pressure – thrice daily until normal
    - Monthly urine albumin – 6 months
    - Annual blood pressure/serum creatinine for follow-up

48. List the terminologies in nephrotic syndrome.
    1. REMISSION - Urine albumin nil or trace (i.e., proteinuria, 4 mg/m2/h) for three consecutive early morning samples
    2. RELAPSE - Urine albumin 3+ or 4+ (proteinuria > 40 mg/m2/h) for three consecutive early morning samples who have been in remission previously
    3. INFREQUENT RELAPSE - < 2 in 6 months < 3 per year
    4. FREQUENT RELAPSE - ≥ 2 in 6 months, ≥ 3 in 1 year
    5. STEROID RESPONSIVE - Achievement of remission within 4 weeks of starting steroid therapy
    6. STEROID DEPENDENT - Two consecutive relapses on alternate steroid or within 14 days of stoppage of therapy
    7. STEROID RESISTANT - Absence of remission with steroid therapy for 4 weeks (*Indian Academy of Pediatrics*), 8 weeks (*Nelson's Textbook of Pediatrics*)

49. List the various mutations in congenital nephrotic syndrome.
    Table 31.10 lists the various mutations in congenital nephrotic syndrome.

50. Differentiate between Finnish type and diffuse mesangial sclerosis type of congenital nephrotic syndrome.
    Table 31.11 lists the differences between Finnish type and diffuse mesangial sclerosis type of congenital nephrotic syndrome.

TABLE 31.8	Tests for Proteinuria
Test	**Procedure**

1. Qualitative
  a. Heat coagulation test
  b. Sulfosalicylic acid
  c. Heller nitric acid test
	a. 10 mL urine + boil; turbidity + add six drops of 5% acetic acid; turbidity because of phosphates disappears, turbidity because of proteins persists
	b. 5 mL urine, 5–10 drops of 20% sulfosalicylic acid; watch for turbidity
	c. Heller nitric acid test: 5 mL concentrated nitric acid + urine (few drops) = white ring at the junction of two layers

2. Semiquantitative test Urine dipstick test – only albumin	• Negative • Trace: 10–29 mg/dL • 1+: 30–100 mg/dL • 2+: 100–300 mg/dL • 3+: 300–1000 mg/dL • 4+: >1000 mg/dL

3. Quantitative test
  a. Spot PCR
  b. 24-Hour urine protein
	a. Spot PCR
	  • Normal values
	    • <0.5 in children younger than 2 years
	    • <0.2 in children older than 2 years
	  • 0.2–2: Nephritic range of proteinuria
	  • 2: Nephrotic range of proteinuria
	b. 24-Hour urine protein
	  • <4 mg/m²/h or 100 mg/m²/day: Normal
	  • 4–40 mg/m²/h: Nephritic range
	  • >40 mg/m²/h: Nephrotic range
	  • <150 mg/day: Normal (Nelson)
	  • >3 g/1.73 m²/day: Nephrotic range (Nelson's symptomatic approach)

TABLE 31.9	Time of Resolution of Clinical Features in AGN
Feature	**Time of Resolution**
Gross hematuria	4–6 weeks
Proteinuria and hypertension	4 weeks
C3 returns to normal	6–8 weeks
Microscopic hematuria	1 year

TABLE 31.10	**Various Mutations in Congenital Nephrotic Syndrome**	
Type	**Protein Affected**	**Renal Disease**
NPHS 1 Autosomal Recessive	Nephrin	Finnish type of congenital nephrotic syndrome
NPHS 2 Autosomal Recessive	Podocin	FSGS
NPHS 3 Autosomal Recessive	PLCE1 mutation	Early onset nephrotic syndrome
WT1 Autosomal Dominant	Wilms tumor suppressor gene	• Denys–Drash syndrome, which causes diffuse mesangial sclerosis • Frasier syndrome – FSGS
LMX1B Autosomal Dominant	Homeodomain protein – LIM	Nail–patella syndrome
SMARCAL1 Autosomal Recessive	SWI/SNF2-related matrix-associated actin-dependent regulator of chromatin subfamily A like protein 1	Schimke immuno-osseous dysplasia with FSGS
LAMB2 Autosomal Recessive		• Pierson syndrome • Microcoria

TABLE 31.11	**Differences Between Finnish Type and Diffuse Mesangial Sclerosis Type of Congenital Nephrotic Syndrome**	
Feature	**Finnish Type**	**Diffuse Mesangial Sclerosis**
Genetics	Mutation in NEPHS1 gene	Mutation of WT1 gene
Amniotic fluid alpha-fetoprotein	Increased	Normal
Placental weight	>25% of birth weight	Normal
Natal history	Preterm	Term
Onset of proteinuria	Intrauterine	In the 1st year of life
Proteinuria	Severe, >20 g/L	Less severe
GFR (Glomerular Filtration Rate)	Normal in the initial 6–12 months of life	Presents with end-stage renal disease within few months of life
Renal biopsy findings	Radial dilatation of proximal tubules at 3–8 months of age	Mesangial sclerosis and interstitial fibrosis
Treatment	Bilateral nephrectomy followed by renal transplantation	Bilateral nephrectomy followed by renal transplantation

Quick Bites

- Age is one of the most important factors in a child with nephritic/nephrotic syndrome because it gives a clue to the etiology and prognosis and is also one of the indications for renal biopsy.
- The most common cause of acute glomerulonephritis in children is post–group A beta-hemolytic *Streptococcus* infection.
- IgA nephropathy is the most common chronic glomerular disease and the most common cause of recurrent gross hematuria in children.
- Minimal change disease is the most common cause of nephrotic syndrome in children.
- Ninety per cent of patients with minimal change disease are steroid responsive.
- Congenital nephrotic syndrome has a very poor prognosis and the treatment includes bilateral nephrectomy followed by renal transplantation.

Thalassemia

Following introduction, seek permission from the caregiver and introduce yourself to the patient before history elicitation, and identify the case.

Name_____Age_____Sex_____Birth order_____
Consanguinity_____Address_____Informant_____

Complaints and Duration

The history starts from ... years back, so start the presentation from the time of onset of symptoms:
- Progressive pallor
- Easy fatiguability and lethargy
- Abdominal distension
- Insidious in onset
- Gradually progressive till date
- Involving predominantly the upper abdomen
- Not associated with abdominal pain/facial puffiness/leg swelling/diminished urine output
- Associated with pallor – as noticed by the doctor

NEGATIVE HISTORY

- Abdominal pain/passing worms in the stools
- Pica
- Bleeding manifestations/hematuria
- Jaundice
- Fever
- Chronic diarrhea/altered bowel habits
- Leg ulcers
- Bone pain/loss of weight/loss of appetite
- Recurrent infections
- Skin hyperpigmentation
- Joint pain/skin rashes

BLOOD TRANSFUSIONS

- After evaluation, the child reported to have hematological illness, for which regular blood transfusions given
- Multiple blood transfusions
- Once in a month
- Getting transfused, around 16–18 transfusions per year (each transfusion probably of 10 mL/kg, thereby approximately 160–180 mL/kg/year)
- The child started on oral medication to prevent transfusion-related complications
- At around 3–4 weeks after each transfusion, development of progressive pallor and lethargy in the child that improves only with subsequent blood transfusions

AT PRESENT

- Stunted growth
- Breathlessness/palpitations/generalized swelling of body
- Jaundice/hematemesis/melena
- Fractures

- Skin hyperpigmentation
- Polyuria/polydipsia/polyphagia
- Hard of hearing and visual disturbances
- Constipation

Past History

- Other significant illness requiring admissions other than blood transfusions
- Any history of chronic drug intake/chronic comorbid illness

Antenatal History

- Abortions/miscarriages
- Booked and immunized
- Maternal fever with rash/joint pain/swelling over the neck
- Any drug intake/radiation exposure
- Any maternal diseases complicating pregnancy
- Antenatal scans

Natal History

- Mode of delivery
- Birth weight
- Cried immediately after birth

Postnatal History

- Any NICU admission, low birth weight, neonatal jaundice, and neonatal seizures
- Exclusively breastfed until ... months of age and then started on complementary feeds

Developmental History

- Attained age-appropriate developmental milestones
- Average scholastic performance

Dietetic History

- As per 24-hour recall method

Immunization History

- Immunization is up to age as per IAP (Indian Academy of Pediatrics) or National Immunization Schedule.
- Special vaccines such as pneumococcal/meningococcal vaccines have been advised.

Family History

- Similar illness/any blood disorders in the family
- Any regular blood transfusions in the family members
- Abdominal surgeries

Socioeconomic History

As per the modified Kuppuswamy scale

General and Head-to-Foot Examination

- Conscious and oriented
- Cooperative for examination
- Comfortable at rest and not dyspneic
- Facies, characterized by frontal bossing and malar prominence +
- Neck: Any goiter/midline swelling
- Severe pallor +
- Chest deformities
- Abdominal distension + (more in the upper abdomen)
- Limbs: Normal
- Icterus/cyanosis/clubbing
- Generalized lymphadenopathy/pedal edema
- Markers of bleeding
- Ulcers/pigmentary changes of the skin
- Bony deformities; spine normal

Anthropometry

- Weight
- Height
- BMI

Vital Signs

- Heart rate: Pulses – normal volume, regular rhythm, any specific character, felt in all peripheral vessels, any radioradial or radiofemoral delay, and any vessel wall thickening
- Respiratory rate
- Blood pressure (mm Hg; measured in the right arm in a sitting posture)

Systemic Examination

ABDOMEN

Inspection

- Abdomen distended – more in the upper half
- Flanks free
- Umbilicus in midline and inverted
- Equal movement of all quadrants with respiration
- Skin over the abdomen normal
- No dilated veins/no scars/no sinuses

- Hernial orifices free
- External genitalia normal

Palpation

Superficial

- Warm and not tender
- Mass palpable in the right hypochondrium and left hypochondrium

Deep

- Liver: Palpable ... cm from the right costal margin, firm, nontender, margins well defined, and moves with respiration
- Liver span: ... cm
- Spleen: Palpable ... cm along the long axis, firm, nontender, moves with respiration, and splenic notch felt in the anterior border

Percussion

- No free fluid

Auscultation

- Bowel sounds heard and no audible bruits

GENITALIA

- Examine the testis on both the sides.
- Testicular volume should be measured using an orchidometer.

CARDIOVASCULAR SYSTEM

- First heart sound and second heart sound heard – normal
- P2 normal
- A systolic murmur of grade 2/6 heard in the pulmonary area

RESPIRATORY SYSTEM

- Normal vesicular breath sounds heard
- Air entry equal on both sides

CENTRAL NERVOUS SYSTEM

- No focal neurological deficit

Diagnosis

A child with chronic hemolytic anemia, probably thalassemia major, with no signs of iron overload and chronic malnutrition

Frequently Asked Questions

1. Discuss the significance of age in hemolytic anemia.
   - Neonatal
     - ABO incompatibility
     - Rh incompatibility
     - Hereditary spherocytosis
     - Glucose-6-phosphate dehydrogenase deficiency
   - Six to 12 months
     - β-Thalassemia
     - Sickle cell anemia
   - Older than 2 years
     - Thalassemia intermedia

2. Why does thalassemia major manifest at the age of 6 months?
   - Until 6 months, there is no manifestation of thalassemia major because of the presence of fetal hemoglobin ($\alpha 2 \gamma 2$).
   - By 6 months of age, there is a gradual switch from fetal to adult hemoglobin and hence thalassemia major begins to manifest.

3. Enumerate the different types of hemoglobin according to different stages of life.
   - **Embryonic Hemoglobin (Hb)**
     - Prominent up to 4–8 weeks of gestational age and almost disappears by 12 weeks
     - Gower 1 ($\zeta 2 \varepsilon 2$)
     - Gower 2 ($\alpha 2 \varepsilon 2$)
     - Portland ($\zeta 2 \gamma 2$)
   - **Fetal Hb ($\alpha 2 \gamma 2$)**
     - It is prominent from 12 to 24 weeks of gestational age (almost 90%).
     - By the third trimester, fetal Hb declines to 70% and gradually adult Hb increases up to 30%.
   - **At term**
     - Adult Hb ($\alpha 2 \beta 2$) accounts for 30% of cases.
     - Fetal Hemoglobin (HbF) accounts for 70% of cases.
     - HbA2 ($\alpha 2 \delta 2$) accounts for <1% of cases.
   - **6 to 12 months of age**
     - Adult Hb ($\alpha 2 \beta 2$): 95%
     - HbA2 ($\alpha 2 \delta 2$): 2%–3.4%
     - Fetal Hb ($\alpha 2 \gamma 2$): <2.5%
     - Normal HbA:HbA2 pattern: 30:1

4. Classify hemolytic anemia on the basis of the mode of onset.
   Acute onset
     - Autoimmune hemolytic anemias
     - Glucose- 6- phosphate- dehydrogenase (G6PD) deficiency
     - Hemolytic uremic syndrome
     - Sickle cell crisis
   Chronic hemolysis
     - Hereditary spherocytosis
     - β-Thalassemia

5. What are the differential diagnosis for transfusion-dependent anemias?

With Organomegaly	Without Organomegaly
Thalassemia Major	
Hereditary spherocytosis	Transient eryhtroblastopenia of childhood
G6PD Deficiency	
Autoimmune hemolytic anemia	Diamond–Blackfan syndrome
Congenital dyserythropoietic anemia	Aplastic anemias
Sickle cell anemia	Pearson syndrome

   Anemia requiring transfusions at 6 months
     - Thalassemia major
     - Osteopetrosis
     - Gaucher disease
     - Congenital dyserythropoietic anemia
     - Pure red call aplasia
     - Anemia of prematurity in preterm
   Conditions requiring recurrent blood transfusions
     - Thalassemia major
     - Aplastic anemia
     - Myelodysplastic syndromes
     - Leukemia
     - Congenital dyserythropoietic anemia type 1
     - Extrahepatic portal venous obstruction (EHPVO)
   Conditions requiring occasional blood transfusions
     - Thalassemia intermedia
     - G6PD deficiency
     - Sickle cell anemia
   Neonatal conditions requiring blood transfusions
     - Hereditary spherocytosis
     - G6PD deficiency
     - α-Thalassemia severe

6. Discuss the points in favor of thalassemia major.
   - Age of presentation
   - Need of transfusions
   - No history of jaundice
   - Previous sibling's death

7. Discuss the points against sickle cell anemia in a child.
   No past admissions with pain crisis, dactylitis, acute chest symptoms, and leg ulcers
   Absence of jaundice in the newborn period

8. Discuss the pathophysiology in β-thalassemia.
   - Thalassemia refers to a group of genetic disorders of globin chain production in which there is an imbalance between the α- and β-globin chain productions.
   - In β-thalassemia syndromes, there is a decrease in the synthesis of β-globin chain synthesis and this results in a relative excess of α-globin chain and hence results in an abnormal adult hemoglobin.
   - It results in α-globin tetramers ($\alpha 4$) and appears as red cell inclusions.

9. Describe ineffective erythropoiesis in thalassemia.
   - As the α-globin tetramers ($\alpha 4$) precipitate in the red cells, they make the red blood cell unstable, damage the red blood cell membrane, and shorten the red cell survival that results in anemia.
   - This in turn causes increased erythropoiesis but with early erythroid precursor death in the bone marrow itself.
   - That is why it is called ineffective erythropoiesis and has a low reticulocyte count.

10. Why is jaundice uncommon in thalassemia?

As the abnormal hemoglobins are unstable (α tetramers), they are destroyed in the bone marrow level itself before they reach the circulation. That is why jaundice is uncommon in thalassemia.

11. Classify β-thalassemia.
    - **Thalassemia major ($\beta^0\beta^0$)**
      - It is also called Cooley anemia.
      - It is the most severe form of β-thalassemia.
      - It is transfusion dependent.
      - Hb electrophoresis shows HbF >90%, HbA2 2%, and HbA 5%–10% or even absent.
    - **Thalassemia intermedia ($\beta^0\beta^+/\beta^+\beta^+$)**
      - It presents with anemia of intermediate severity and Hb <8 g/dL.
      - It manifests at the age of 2 years only.
      - Hb electrophoresis shows HbF (10%–50%), HbA2 3%–3.5%, and HbA 30%.
    - **Thalassemia minor ($\beta\beta^+/\beta\beta^0$)**
      - It is otherwise called thalassemia minor or thalassemia trait.
      - It is the mildest form.
      - HbA2 more than 3.5% is the gold standard to diagnose thalassemia trait.
      - The red cell indices show mild anemia, with Mean Corpuscular Volume (MCV), Mean Corpuscular Hemoglobin (MCH) reduced, and Mean Corpuscular Hemoglobin Concentration (MCHC) being normal.

12. Name the closest differentials for thalassemia trait.

The closest differential diagnosis is iron-deficiency anemia.

The differentiating points are as follows:

Thalassemia Trait	Iron-Deficiency Anemia
Red cell distribution width is normal	Red cell distribution width is increased
Red blood cell count is normal or increased	Red blood cell count is low
Mentzer index is low	Mentzer index is high
HbA2 is high (>3.5%)	HbA2 is low

- The normal value of red cell distribution width is 11.5–14.5.
- Mentzer index = Mean Corpuscular Volume (MCV)/Red Blood Cell (RBC). It is more than 13 in iron-deficiency anemia.

13. What is Shine and Lal index?
    - It is $(MCV)^2 \times MCH \times 100$.
    - It is >1530 in iron-deficiency anemia and <1530 in thalassemia intermedia.

14. Name two conditions associated with raised MCHC.
    - Hereditary spherocytosis
    - Hereditary stomatocytosis (xerocytosis variety)

15. Discuss the peripheral smear findings in thalassemia.
    - Microcytic hypochromic anemia
    - Anisocytosis
    - Poikilocytosis
    - Target cells
    - Basophilic stippling
    - Teardrop cells

16. Draw a target cell and explain it.
    - Target cell is otherwise called a codocyte or a Mexican hat cell.
    - It gives the appearance of a shooting target with a bull's eye.
    - It has a dark center (a central, hemoglobinized area) surrounded by a white ring (an area of relative pallor), followed by a dark outer (peripheral) second ring containing a band of hemoglobin.
    - Target cells have an excess of cell membrane relative to cell volume (disproportionate increase in membrane area to volume) – relative membrane excess as in Fig. 32.1.

17. Name some conditions associated with raised HbF.
    - Thalassemia major
    - Sickle cell anemia
    - Aplastic anemia such as Fanconi, Diamond–Blackfan anemia, and Pearson syndrome
    - Treatment with erythropoietin

18. Name two conditions with high and low HbA2.
    - **HbA2 is increased in the following:**
      - Thalassemia minor
      - Megaloblastic anemia
    - **HbA2 is decreased in the following:**
      - Iron-deficiency anemia
      - α-Thalassemia

19. Name some macrocytic anemias with dysmorphic features.
    - Down syndrome
    - Hypothyroidism
    - Diamond–Blackfan anemia
    - Congenital dyserythropoietic anemia type 1
    - Fanconi anemia
    - Aplastic anemia

20. What is a reticulocyte?
    - Reticulocyte is an immature RBC that takes 48 hours to mature.
    - Reticulocyte count = No. of reticulocytes per 500 RBCs. Normally it is 2%–3% only.
    - Reticulocyte index or corrected reticulocyte count
    $$= \frac{\text{Reticulocyte count} \times \text{Patient Hematocrit (Hct)} \times 1}{\text{Observed Hematocrit (Hct)} * \text{Maturation factor } (\mu)}$$

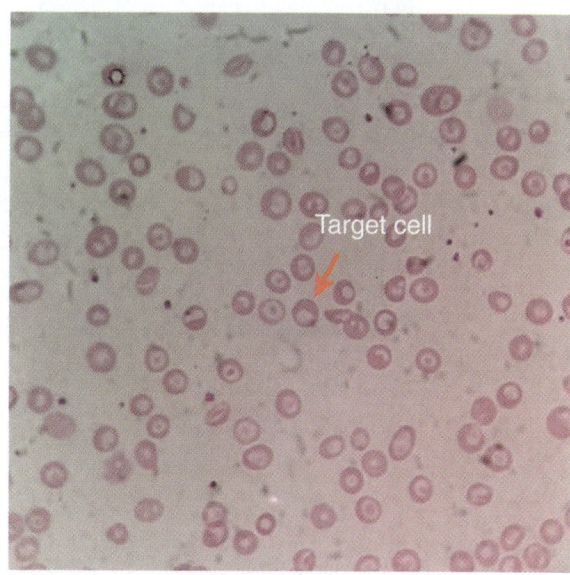

Fig. 32.1 Target cell.

- Absolute reticulocyte count $= \dfrac{\text{Reticulocyte count}(\%) \times 100}{\text{Total RBC count}}$
- The normal value is 25,000–75,000.
21. Name the stains to view iron and reticulocytes.
    - Iron: Prussian blue
    - Reticulocyte count
      Methylene blue
      Supravital stain
      Cresyl violet
      Brilliant cresyl blue
22. Which chromosome encodes for β-chain and α-chain?
    - β-Chain: Chromosome number 11
    - α-Chain: Chromosome number 16
23. Discuss the significance of antenatal history in hemolytic anemia.
    - Rh incompatibility
    - α-Thalassemia with four gene deletions
24. What is the cause for developmental delay in anemia?
    - In untreated or poorly transfused cases of hemolytic anemia, tissues are deprived of oxygen because of chronic anemia and hence this leads to motor delay.
    - In storage disorders, there will be a global delay.
25. Describe thalassemia facies.
    - It is called chipmunk facies or rodent facies.
    - The dysmorphic facies occurs because of marrow expansion as a result of ineffective erythropoiesis causing bony deformities.
    - Features are the following:
      - Maxillary hyperplasia
      - Flat nasal bridge
      - Frontal bossing
      - Widely spaced eyes

- Unequal development of upper and lower jaws, which causes malocclusion of teeth and hence projection of the upper incisor – like a chipmunk
26. What is the earliest radiological feature seen in thalassemia?
    The earliest change is seen in the hands as early as 4 months of age. It is seen as a reticular pattern of the metacarpals because of widening of the medulla and thinning of the cortex with a coarse trabecular pattern in the medulla as in Fig. 32.2.
27. What is the reason for hair-on-end appearance?
    The hair-on-end appearance is because of the widened diploic spaces in the skull as in Fig. 32.3.
28. Enumerate the causes for short stature in thalassemia.
    Stunting of child as in Fig. 32.4 is because of the following:
    - Chronic disease
    - Endocrine abnormalities
    - Chelation side effects (deferoxamine)
    - Nutritional
    - Psychological
29. Is conjugated hyperbilirubinemia possible in hemolytic anemia?
    Yes. Hemolytic anemia with concurrent gallstones can cause biliary obstruction, which results in conjugated hyperbilirubinemia.
30. What is the skin change seen in thalassemia?
    Repeated blood transfusions cause hemosiderosis, which results in bronze discoloration of the skin.
31. Discuss the cardiac findings in thalassemia.
    - Hemic murmur: Chronic anemia
    - Loud P2: Pulmonary hypertension in thalassemia intermedia

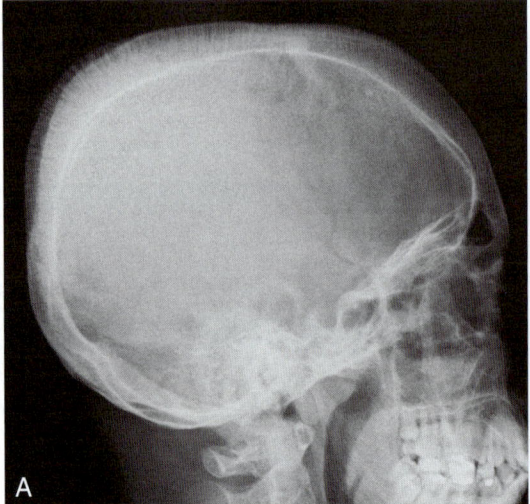
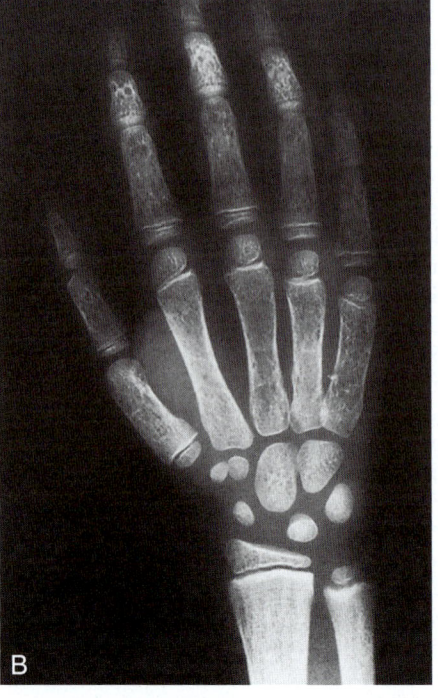

Fig. 32.2 X-ray – widening of medulla in metacarpals. (*Source: Reproduced from* Michele Walters, Richard Robertson. *Pediatric Radiology: The Requisites*, Fourth Pedition, Musculoskeletal Imaging, Figure 7.53, Philadelphia, Elsevier Inc., 2017.)

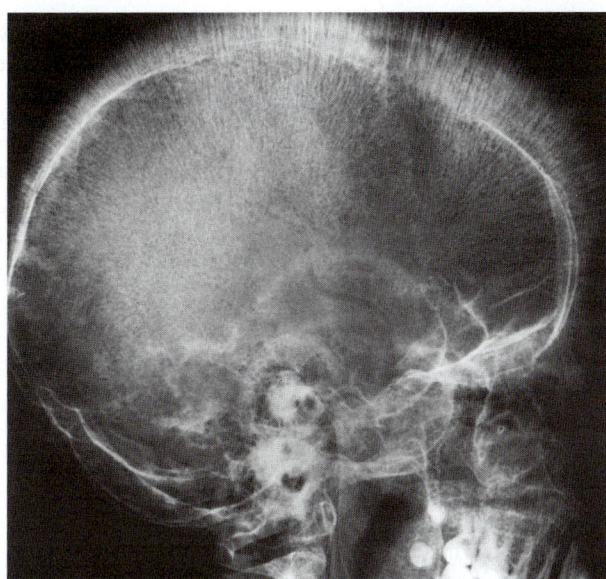

Fig. 32.3 Hair-on-end appearance. (*Source: Reproduced from* Ronald Eisenberg, Nancy Johnson. *Comprehensive Radiographic Pathology, Seventh Edition,* Hematopoietic System, Fig. 9.4, St. Louis, Mosby, 2021.

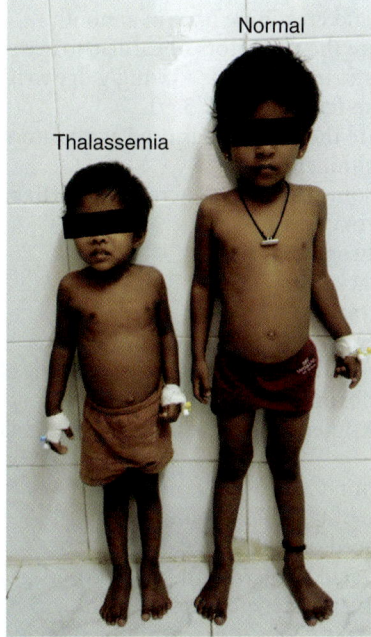

Fig. 32.4 Stunting of child with thalassemia compared with child of same age.

32. **Why does a child with thalassemia require blood transfusion?**
    - To improve oxygenation, growth, and development
    - To decrease hemolysis
    - To reduce hepatosplenomegaly
    - To reduce cardiomegaly
    - To reduce extramedullary hematopoiesis
    - To reduce the iron overload

33. **At what interval is a child with thalassemia transfused and why is it so?**

Patients are generally transfused once in 4 weeks because the life span of an in vitro RBC is 3 weeks, and it takes another 1 week for the patient to develop signs of anemia and get admitted for transfusion.

34. **Mention few factors that decide the need for regular transfusions.**
    - Severity of ineffective erythropoiesis
    - Disturbance of growth and development
    - Complications of extramedullary hematopoiesis

35. **How can one identify whether transfusions are inadequate in a child with thalassemia?**
    - Disturbance of growth and development
    - Steady-state hemoglobin of <7 g/dL for more than 2 weeks apart
    - Severe extramedullary hematopoiesis in the form of fractures

36. **Discuss the various transfusion regimens.**
    - Moderate transfusion regimen: It involves pretransfusion Hb of >9 g/dL and a mean Hb of 11 g/dL.
    - Hypertransfusion regimen: It involves pretransfusion Hb of >10 g/dL and a mean Hb of 12 g/dL.
    - Supertransfusion regimen: It involves pretransfusion Hb of >12 g/dL and a mean Hb of 14 g/dL.
    - Note: 3.5 mL/kg of blood will improve Hb by 1 g.

37. **Discuss the guidelines followed in regular blood transfusions.**
    - Pretransfusion Hb should be 9–9.5 g/dL (in cardiac patients 10–11 g/dL).
    - Transfuse every 2–4 weeks.
    - Post-transfusion Hb should be <14 g/dL.
    - Transfuse only fresh RBCs of <2 weeks old.
    - Blood should be group and type specific with an Hct of 65%–75% and Coombs matched.
    - Leukoreduction should be done by any of the following methods:
      - Centrifugation
      - Triple saline wash
      - Decentralized red cells
      - Third-grade leukocyte filters (target $<1 \times 10^6/\mu L$)
      - Irradiation

38. **Mention few points if the child does not improve with regular transfusion in thalassemia.**
    - Hypersplenism
    - Alloimmunization
    - Chronic viral infections by parvovirus
    - Folic acid and vitamin B12 deficiency

39. **Mention few causes of hepatomegaly in thalassemia.**
    - Extramedullary hematopoiesis
    - Secondary iron deposition
    - Transfusion-associated infections such as hepatitis B and C

40. **What are the causes for splenomegaly in thalassemia?**
    - Extramedullary hematopoiesis
    - Hypertrophy in response to extravascular hemolysis

41. **Name few causes of infections in thalassemia.**
    - Hypersplenism causing leukopenia
    - High basal metabolic rate causing increased nutritional demand but low intake
    - Blockage of monocytes and phagocytes
    - High free Fe
    - Transfusion-associated infections

42. Which infection is least common in thalassemia?
Malaria
43. Which infection can cause aplastic crisis in thalassemia?
Parvovirus infection
44. Discuss the complications of thalassemia.
Cardiac
   - Systolic and diastolic dysfunctioning
   - Arrhythmias

Liver
   - Iron overload
   - Extramedullary hematopoiesis
   - Hepatitis B and C
   - Drug toxicity
   - Biliary gallstone

Spleen
   - Enlargement of spleen

Endocrine
   - Hypopituitarism (34%)
   - Hypoparathyroidism (5%)
   - Hypothyroidism (10%)
   - Type 2 diabetes (20%)
   - Hypogonadism (35%–55%)

Skeletal system
   - Medullary enlargement
   - Osteopenia
   - Osteoporosis

Iron overload
   - Because of frequent transfusions

Drug-related complications (iron chelator therapy)
   - Transfusion-related complications
      - Liver affected first (within 1 year of transfusion)
      - Endocrine system affected after 3–5 years of transfusion
      - Cardiac system affected after about 7–10 years of transfusion

45. Define iron overload.
   - Ferritin level >1000 µg/L
   - Number of transfusions >15–20 per year
46. What are the indications for chelation therapy in a child receiving chronic transfusions?
   - Chelation is generally not advisable for children younger than 2 years.
   - Chelation is usually delayed until 3–4 years of age.
   - Indications for chelation are the following:
      - Cumulative transfusion load of 120 mL/kg or greater (around 10–12 times of Packed red blood cell (PRBC) transfusion)
      - Serum ferritin >1000 ng/mL

   - Liver iron concentration >2500 µg/g dry weight of the liver
47. Discuss the drugs used for iron chelation.
   - Parenteral: Deferoxamine; 20–60 mg/kg/day in three divided doses given as infusion for 8 hours subcutaneously or intravenously for 5 days a week; t½ less than 30 minutes; excreted via feces or urine
   - Oral
      - Deferiprone: 25 mg/kg/day three times a day; t½ 3 hours; excreted via urine
      - Deferasirox: 20–30 mg/kg/day once a day; t½ 16 hours; excreted via feces
48. Discuss the adverse effects of drugs used for chelation.
Table 32.1 **gives the adverse effects of drugs used for chelation.**
49. How is a child on iron chelator monitored?
   - Deferoxamine
      - Complete anthropometry once in 6 months
      - Hearing and vision screening annually
   - Deferiprone
      - Blood counts once in a month
      - Serum zinc once in 6 months
      - Clinical examination of joints in each visit
   - Deferasirox: Serum glutamic oxaloacetic transaminase (SGOT)/Serum glutamic pyruvic transaminase (SGPT), urea, and creatinine once in a month
50. What are the predictors of cardiac toxicity?
   - Hepatic iron load of >15 mg/g dry weight of the liver
   - Serum ferritin of >2.5 g/L
51. What are the other drugs used as chelators?
Desferrithiocin
52. Name some drugs that increase fetal Hb synthesis.
   - Hydroxyurea
   - Erythropoietin
   - 5-Azacytidine
   - Butyrates
   - Myleran
   - Histone deacetylase inhibitor (glutaric acid analog)
   - Pyridoxine hydrazine
53. Discuss other supportive therapies in a child with thalassemia.
   - Vitamin C
   - More of tea intake
   - Reduced oral iron intake
   - Folic acid to increase new RBC production
54. What is shuttle hypothesis?
   - This therapy includes a combination of deferoxamine and deferiprone.

TABLE 32.1	Adverse Effects of Drugs Used for Chelation	
Deferoxamine	**Deferasirox**	**Deferiprone**
• Ototoxicity • Retinal changes, cataract, reduction of visual field and visual acuity, night vision • Bone dysplasia, truncal shortening • Local reactions such as swelling, rashes (allergic reactions) • Pulmonary and neurological complications	• Gastrointestinal disturbances, GI bleeds • Transaminase elevation, hepatic failure • Rise in serum creatinine, proteinuria and rashes	• Gastrointestinal disturbances • Transaminase elevation • Agranulocytosis/neutropenia • Arthralgia • Zinc deficiency (Weekly blood count monitoring is essential)

- Deferiprone shifts the iron from intracellular to extracellular component and deferoxamine enhances the excretion of iron.
- Advantages include the following:
  - Dosage of both the drugs can be reduced.
  - Cost can be minimized.
  - Compliance will be good.

55. Discuss tests to identify iron overload.
- Noninvasive tests: These include urine iron, superconducting quantum interface device – biomagnetic liver susceptometry (SQUID-BLS), and T2 WT MRI for myocardial iron estimation.
- Invasive tests: These include serum iron, liver iron content, and plasma non-transferrin-bound iron (NTBI). Estimation of iron in gram per kilogram of the liver content **is the gold standard test for iron overload**.

56. What are the indications for splenectomy in thalassemia?
- Cumulative transfusion load of >250 mL/kg/day (>1.5 times the basal requirement for a patient maintaining pretransfusion Hb of 10 g/dL)
- Serum ferritin >1500 ng/mL
- Massive splenomegaly causing symptoms such as pain, early satiety because of compression over the stomach, and splenic rupture risk
- Evidence of leukopenia/thrombocytopenia (hypersplenism)

57. Name one hemolytic anemia in which splenectomy is contraindicated.
Hereditary stomatocytosis

58. Discuss the peripheral smear findings in a post-splenectomy case.
- Howell–Jolly bodies
- Thrombocytosis
- Heinz bodies

59. Mention few prerequisites for bone marrow transplant.
- Matching sibling donor
- A donor older than 2 years needed
- High cost
- Lucarelli risk stratification – liver >2 cm, liver fibrosis, irregularity in iron chelation
Class 1: No risk
Class 2: One or two risks

Class 3: All three risks (Lucarelli class 3 – hepatomegaly >5 cm and age >7 years [very high risk])

60. What is Pesaro risk stratification?
The following three parameters are monitored:
- Liver size by more than 2 cm below the costal margin
- Fibrosis in liver biopsy
- Inadequacy in transfusion and chelation
  - Low risk: No risk factors (96% thalassemia-free survival)
  - Intermediate risk: One risk factor (90% thalassemia-free survival)
  - High risk: Two or more risk factors (80% thalassemia-free survival)

61. Describe the follow-up of a child with thalassemia.
Table 32.2 gives the follow-up of a child with thalassemia.

62. What are the prenatal tests available to diagnose thalassemia?
- Fetal blood with $\beta:\alpha$ cell ratio of <0.025 indicates thalassemia major.
- Chorionic villous sampling can be done at 9–11 weeks.
- Amniocentesis can be done at 15–18 weeks.

63. Mention few points on prenatal counseling in thalassemia.
- Prevention of marriage between the traits
- Antenatal diagnosis
- Termination of pregnancy if it is found to be thalassemia major

64. Discuss few screening tests available to diagnose thalassemia.
- Naked eye single tube red cell osmotic fragility test (NESTROFT) is the test available to diagnose thalassemia.
- NESTROFT alone has a sensitivity of 95%; together with Mean corpuscular volume, it has 100% sensitivity.

65. How can one screen parents of a child with thalassemia for future pregnancy?
Flowchart 32.1 shows antenatal screening for a high-risk pregnancy (previous child with thalassemia).

66. Which is preferred – High-performance liquid chromatography (HPLC) or Hb electrophoresis?
- High-performance liquid chromatography is the preferred test.
- Hb electrophoresis can reveal whether Hb pattern is normal or abnormal.
- But HPLC can give the estimation (%) of the abnormal hemoglobins such as HbS and HbA2.

TABLE 32.2	Follow-Up in Thalassemia	
Investigation	**Timing**	**Frequency**
Serum ferritin	Pretransfusion	Once in 6–12 months
Liver biopsy	After 10–20 transfusions	Annually
Cardiac load	At 10 years	Annually
Liver enzymes and renal function tests	Pretransfusion	Once every 3 months
Short stature (anthropometry)	At diagnosis	Once in 6 months
Gonadal examination	At 10 years	Until puberty
Thyroid function test	At 12 years	Annually
Parathyroid assessment	At 12 years	Annually
Diabetes	Pretransfusion	Every 6 months once
Bones Dual-energy X-ray absorptiometry (DEXA)	At 10 years	Annually
Infections (hepatitis B and C, Human immunodeficiency viruses (HIV))	Pretransfusion	Once in 2–3 years

HIV, human immunodeficiency virus.

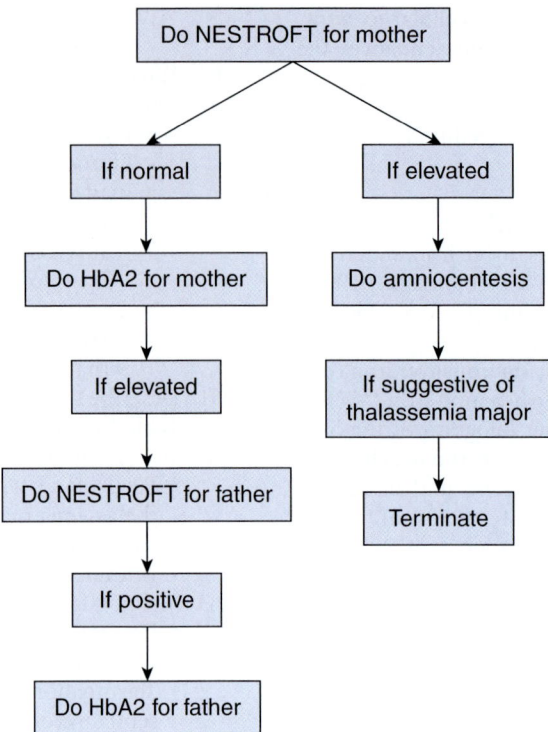

Flowchart 32.1 Antenatal screening for high-risk pregnancy (previous child with thalassemia).

67. What is the gene therapy available for thalassemia?
    Lentivirus vector from human immunodeficiency virus
    (HIV)
68. Discuss the causes of death in thalassemia.
    - Congestive cardiac failure
    - Arrhythmias
    - Sepsis
    - Hemochromatosis
    - Multiorgan dysfunction syndrome (MODS)
69. Mention few points on overall treatment in thalassemia.
    - Treatment of anemia – blood transfusion
    - Removal of iron with iron chelators
    - Treatment of complications
    - Pharmacological measures to increase the fetal hemoglobin
    - Curative by bone marrow transplant
    - Future: Gene therapy
70. What are the types of α-thalassemia syndromes?
    - α-Thalassemia carrier: αα/α-
    - α-Thalassemia trait: αα/— or α-/α-

- HbH: α-/—
- Bart Hb: —/— (γ tetramer) (hydrops fetalis)

71. What are the vaccines to be given in a child with hemolytic anemia?
    - Hepatitis A and B vaccination is important.
    - *Pre-splenectomy vaccination against capsulated organisms*
      - Pneumococcus
      - Meningococcus
      - *H. influenzae*
    - *After splenectomy*
      - Annual flu shot
      - Typhoid polysaccharide vaccine once in 3 years
      - Single dose of pneumococcus polysaccharide vaccine after 5 years
72. What is the schedule for pneumococcus vaccine?
    Flowchart 32.2A and B gives the schedule for pneumococcus vaccine.
73. Name few drugs given after splenectomy.
    - Lifelong penicillin prophylaxis
    - Tablet aspirin to be started if the platelet count goes beyond 8 lakh

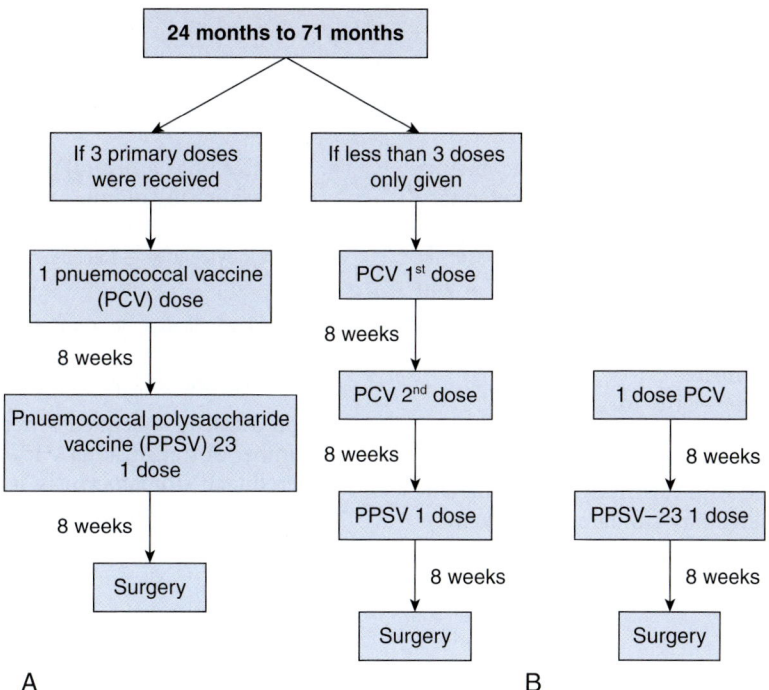

Flowchart 32.2   (A) Schedule for pneumococcal vaccine 24–71 months. (B) Schedule for pneumococcal vaccine >71 months.

Quick Bites

- Examples of neonatal presentation of hemolytic anemia are ABO incompatibility, Rh incompatibility, hereditary spherocytosis, and G6PD deficiency.
- Classification of β-thalassemia is as follows: thalassemia major ($\beta^0\beta^0$), thalassemia intermedia ($\beta^0\beta^+/\beta^+\beta^+$), and thalassemia minor ($\beta\beta^+/\beta\beta^0$).
- α-Thalassemia syndromes are the following:
  - α-Thalassemia carrier: $\alpha\alpha/\alpha$-
  - α-Thalassemia trait: $\alpha\alpha/$— or α-/α-
  - HbH: α-/—
  - Bart Hb: —/— (γ tetramer) (hydrops fetalis)
- Two conditions associated with raised MCHC are hereditary spherocytosis and hereditary stomatocytosis (xerocytosis variety).

- Target cell has a disproportionate increase in membrane area relative to volume – relative membrane excess.
- $$\text{Reticulocyte index} = \text{Reticulocyte count} \times \frac{\text{Patient Hct} \times 1}{\text{Observed Hct} \times \mu}$$
  $$\text{Absolute reticulocyte count} = \frac{\text{Reticulocyte count}(\%) \times 100}{\text{Total RBC count}}$$
  Normal value: 25,000–75,000
- Iron overload is defined by ferritin level $>$1000 µg/L, and number of transfusions $>$15–20 per year.
- Hereditary stomatocytosis is one hemolytic anemia in which splenectomy is contraindicated.

33 Severe Acute Malnutrition

Following introduction, seek permission from the caregiver and introduce yourself to the patient before history elicitation, and identify the case.

Name____Age____Sex____Consanguinity____Order of birth____Place____Informant____

Presenting Complaints and Duration

- Failure to gain weight/lethargy/poor feeding
- Loose stools/vomiting
- Cough/fast breathing
- Edema of both feet
- Skin lesion

History of Presenting Illness

- Describe the presenting complaints in a chronological order.

COMPLICATION HISTORY

- Lethargy/refusal to feed
- Seizures/altered sensorium
- Defective vision/corneal ulcer
- Bony deformity
- Bleeding manifestations
- Recurrent infections
- Behavioral changes

ETIOLOGICAL HISTORY

- Fever/cough/fast breathing
- Vomiting/loose stools
- Exanthematous fever
- Recurrent respiratory tract infection
- Polyuria
- Chronic diarrhea
- Recurrent skin infections/recurrent diarrhea/recurrent respiratory tract infections
- Feeding difficulties: Cleft palate/neuromuscular disorders
- Bad child-rearing practice
- Easy fatigability/recurrent blood transfusion
- Recurrent seizures/vomiting

PAST HISTORY

Comorbidities – any specific system involved

ANTENATAL HISTORY

- Age of the mother at conception
- Maternal immunization
- Iron and folic acid tablets
- Threatened abortion
- Weight gain during pregnancy
- Parity; if multiparous, time interval from the previous pregnancy
- Singleton/multiple gestation
- TORCH infection in the mother
- Chronic illness in the mother
- Maternal complications – PIH (Pregnancy Induced Hypertension)/gestational diabetes mellitus and antepartum hemorrhage
- Antenatal scan

NATAL/POSTNATAL HISTORY

- Preterm
- Birth weight (IUGR (Intra Uterine Growth Restriction), SGA (Small For Gestational Age))
- Home delivery
- Birth asphyxia
- Breastfed or not
- Prelacteal feed
- Time of initiation of feeding
- Hospitalization in the neonatal period

DEVELOPMENT HISTORY

Any developmental delay (transient motor delay)

DIETETIC HISTORY

Younger Than 6 Months

- Prelacteal feed
- Exclusive breastfeeding/breastfeeding on demand
- Formula feeding
- Bottle feeding
- Amount of dilution asked if the child is on formula feeding or cow's milk feeding

Six to 12 Months

- When complementary feeding was started
- Whether breastfeeding was continued during this period

Older Than 1 Year

- By 24-hour recall method – calculate calorie and protein gap.
- Mention whether the mother is aware of hygienic practices before feeding.
- Mention about food fads, if any.

IMMUNIZATION HISTORY

According to the National Immunization or Indian Academy of Pediatrics (IAP) schedule

ALLERGIC HISTORY

- Any adverse reactions to food mentioned

- Cow milk–induced diarrhea (CMPA (Cow's milk protein allergy))

FAMILY HISTORY

- Separated family, neglected child, and social deprivation
- Consanguinity
- Malnutrition in siblings
- Medical illness among family members
- Drug abuse/parental dispute

SOCIOECONOMIC HISTORY

- Socioeconomic class
- Place of residence
- Overcrowding
- Sanitation facilities
- Family fads – any custom or culture fasting and vegetarian diet
- Drinking water

Summary

A _____-year-old child presented with failure to gain weight (mention about other presenting complaints), with/without complications and with/without comorbidities, being a case of malnutrition probably because of _____.

General Examination

- Child's sensorium
- Pallor
- Icterus
- Clubbing
- Cyanosis
- Pedal edema
- Generalized lymphadenopathy

Head-to-Foot Examination

Table 33.1 gives the head-to-foot examination findings in malnutrition.

Vital Signs

- Pulse rate
- Blood pressure
- Respiration: Rate, rhythm, and type of respiration
- Temperature
- JVP (Jugular venous pressure)

Anthropometry (With Interpretation)

- Weight
- Height

TABLE 33.1	Head-to-Foot Examination in a Child With SAM
Head-to-Foot Assessment	**Findings**
1. Head	<ul><li>Microcephaly</li><li>Sunken fontanelles</li><li>Wide open fontanelles</li><li>Delayed closure</li></ul>
2. Hair	<ul><li>Dry</li><li>Lusterless</li><li>Hypopigmented</li><li>Flag sign</li><li>Brittle, easily pluckable hair (to be demonstrated by combing the hair)</li></ul>
3. Face	Moon facies in kwashiorkor, cheeks and temporal regions become hollow in Marasmus
4. Eyes	<ul><li>Pallor</li><li>Bitot spots, corneal ulcers/neovascularization of cornea</li><li>Subconjunctival hemorrhage</li><li>Icterus</li></ul>
5. Oral cavity	Cheilitis, glossitis, atrophic tongue, bleeding gums, oral ulcers, poor dentition, dental caries, tonsillitis
6. Skin	<ul><li>Flaky paint dermatosis</li><li>Crazy pavement skin</li><li>Exanthematous rash</li><li>Skin infections/</li><li>Ulcers/poor wound healing</li></ul>
7. Chest	<ul><li>Rickety rosary</li><li>Scorbutic rosary</li><li>Harrison sulcus</li></ul>
8. Extremities	<ul><li>Edema</li><li>Muscle wasting</li><li>Loose skinfolds</li><li>Koilonychia</li><li>Leukonychia</li><li>Bony deformities</li><li>Pseudoparalysis</li><li>BCG (bacille Calmette-Guerin) scar</li></ul>
9. Signs of child abuse	Multiple bruises in cheeks and buttocks, bruises in various stage of healing, teeth bite mark
10. Look for focus of infection	Upper respiratory tract/lower respiratory tract/loose stools

- Weight/height
- Head circumference
- Mid–upper arm circumference

System Examination

CARDIOVASCULAR SYSTEM

Features of cardiac failure

RESPIRATORY SYSTEM

Look for respiratory tract infection.

ABDOMEN

Ascites, hepatomegaly, and anal excoriation

CENTRAL NERVOUS SYSTEM

Altered sensorium/hypotonia/reduced cognitive function

Diagnosis

- A case of severe acute malnutrition
- With/without complications
- Probable etiology

Frequently Asked Questions

1. Explain the significance of age in malnutrition.
   - Children after 6 months (during complementary feeding) are more prone to malnutrition.
   - Children fall into the "pit of malnutrition" if the transition from liquid diet to solid is not appropriate.
   - Children younger than 5 years are prone to diarrhea and pneumonia.
2. Explain the significance of gender in malnutrition. Neglect is common among female children.
3. List the complication histories elicited in malnutrition.
   - Lethargy/refusal to feed: Hypoglycemia
   - Seizures/altered sensorium: Hypoglycemia and electrolyte disturbances
   - Defective vision/corneal ulcer: Vitamin A deficiency
   - Bony deformity: Rickets
   - Bleeding manifestations: Vitamin K deficiency
   - Recurrent infections: Immunosuppression
   - Behavioral changes
4. List the etiological histories in malnutrition.
   - Fever/cough/fast breathing (LRTI (Lower Respiratory Tract Infection))
   - Vomiting/loose stools (diarrhea)
   - Exanthematous fever
   - Recurrent respiratory tract infections (congestive cardiac failure)
   - Polyuria (Bartter syndrome)
   - Chronic diarrhea/steatorrhea – malabsorption
   - Recurrent skin infections/recurrent diarrhea/recurrent respiratory tract infections – immunodeficiency disorder
   - Feeding difficulties – cleft palate/neuromuscular disorders
   - Bad child-rearing practice
   - Easy fatigability/recurrent blood transfusion – chronic anemia
   - Recurrent seizures/vomiting – metabolic disorder
5. What are the significant antenatal histories in malnutrition?
   - Age of the mother at conception (<19 and >35 – risk for low birth weight)
   - Parity; if multiparous, time interval from the previous pregnancy
   - Singleton/multiple gestations
   - Maternal weight gain
   - History suggestive of TORCH infection in the mother
   - History of chronic diseases in the mother
6. Mention the significance of developmental history in malnutrition.
   - Malnutrition results in transient developmental delay or regression of milestones.
   - If social milestones are predominantly affected, think of neglect.
7. Enumerate the dietetic histories in severe acute malnutrition.
   - Younger than 6 months: Determine whether the child was exclusively breastfed/breastfed on demand, and whether there is a history of formula feeding/history of bottle feeding. If the child is on formula feeds/cow's milk feeding, ask about the amount of dilution.
   - Six to 12 months: Ask when complementary feeding was started/whether breastfeeding was continued during this period.
   - Older than 1 year: The dietetic history is determined by the 24-hour recall method.
   - Mention whether the mother is aware of hygienic practices before feeding.
   - Mention whether the mother is aware of nutritive values of common food items.
   - Mention the history of any adverse reactions to food.
8. List the family and socioeconomic histories in malnutrition.
   - Malnutrition in siblings
   - Medical illness among family members
   - Drug abuse/parental dispute (a risk factor for child abuse)
   - Place of residence/history of overcrowding/sanitation facilities
9. Enumerate the general examination findings in malnutrition.
   - Child's sensorium
     - Altered sensorium because of hypoglycemia, hypothermia, dehydration, shock, and electrolyte disturbances
     - Marasmus (alert)
     - Kwashiorkor (irritable)
   - Pallor: Nutritional anemia and shock
   - Edema: Grading
     1+: Both feet
     2+: Both feet, legs, and both hands
     3+: Generalized edema
*10. List the findings in head-to-foot examination.
   - Head: Microcephaly, sunken fontanelles, and signs of rickets
   - Hair: Dry, lusterless, hypopigmented as shown in Fig. 33.1, flag sign, and brittle, easily pluckable hair

---

*Important question asked in the examination.

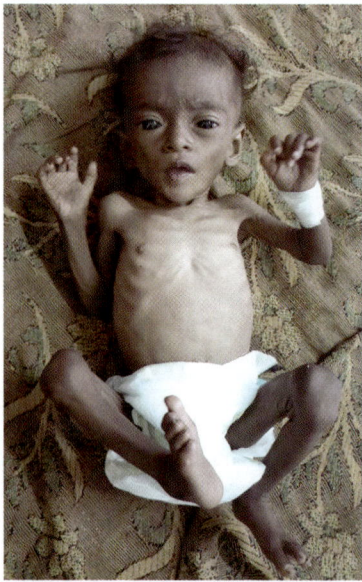

Fig. 33.1 Marasmic facies, dry, lusterless, hypopigmented hair.

(to be demonstrated by combing the hair); occurrence of hair changes because of protein, tyrosine, copper, and zinc deficiency

- Face: Moon facies in kwashiorkor and marasmic facies showing hallow cheeks and temporal regions as shown in Fig. 33.1
- Eyes: Pallor, Bitot spots, corneal ulcers, and subconjunctival hemorrhage
- Oral cavity: Cheilitis, glossitis, atrophic tongue, bleeding gums, oral ulcers, poor dentition, and dental caries
- Skin: Flaky paint dermatosis as shown in Fig. 33.2/crazy pavement skin/exanthematous rash/skin infections/ulcers/poor wound healing
- Chest: Rickety rosary and Harrison sulcus
- Extremities: Edema, muscle wasting, loose skinfolds especially in the gluteal region as shown in Fig. 33.3, koilonychia, leukonychia (white nails because of hypoalbuminemia), and bony deformities

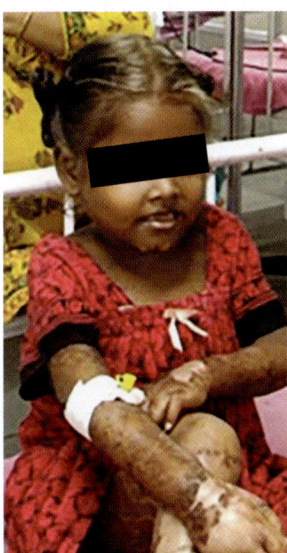

Fig. 33.2 Child with kwashiorkor having flaky paint dermatosis.

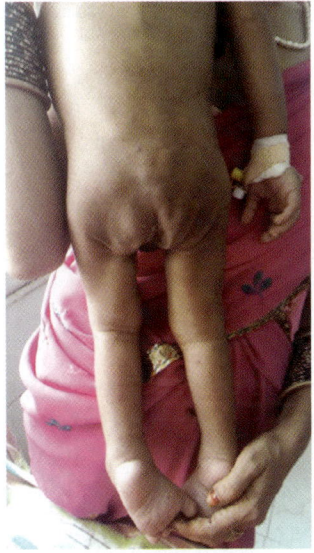

Fig. 33.3 Muscle wasting and loose skinfolds in the gluteal region.

- Signs of child abuse
- Look for the focus of infection

11. Explain the method of weighing a child.
    The child should be weighed on a scale that is built solidly. It should be durable with electronic (digital) reading. The weight is measured to a precision of 10 g.

*12. What is tared weighing?
    - Tared weighing is the weighing in which the scale is reset to zero with the person still on it. Thus, a mother can stand on the scale and be weighed, and the scale is tared now (i.e., reset to zero). The mother can carry her child when she is still on the machine and the scale will show the child's weight alone.
    - Advantages are the following:
    There is no need to subtract the child's weight from that of the mother.
    The child can remain calm while being carried by the mother.
    Fig. 33.4A–C shows tared weighing in children.

13. How should a child's height/length be measured?
    - For a child younger than 2 years old (or less than 87 cm if the age is not available), measure the recumbent length.
    - For a child 2 years or older (or 87 cm or more if the child's age is not available) and able to stand, measure the standing height by a stadiometer.
    - For a child 2 years or older who cannot stand, measure the recumbent length and subtract 0.7 cm to convert it to height.
    - An infantometer has a movable foot piece, whereas a stadiometer has a movable head board. Two persons are needed to measure height/length. Length should be measured to a precision of 0.1 cm.
    - A stadiometer:
    Five points of contact while standing against a stadiometer:
    Occiput
    Shoulder
    Buttocks
    Calf
    Heels
    Fig. 33.5 shows the method of measuring the length.
    Fig. 33.6 shows the method of measuring the height.

*14. Explain the significance of MUAC (Mid-upper arm circumference).
    - Mid–upper arm circumference is suitable in children aged between 6 and 59 months (FIMNCI, 2013). It remains constant in all children in this age group because there is a simultaneous loss of fat and increase in muscle mass. It is one of the age-independent criteria for malnutrition.
    - It is measured to a precision of 0.1 cm.
    Fig. 33.7 shows the method of measuring MUAC.

*15. Describe the WHO classification of acute and chronic malnutrition.
    Table 33.2 shows the WHO (World Health Organization.) classification of acute and chronic malnutrition.

16. What are the signs of shock in SAM (Severe Acute Malnutrition.)?
    Cool peripheries, CRT (Capillary Refill Time) >2 seconds, and weak, thready pulses (FIMNCI (Facility-based Integrated Management of Neonatal and Childhood Illness), 2013)

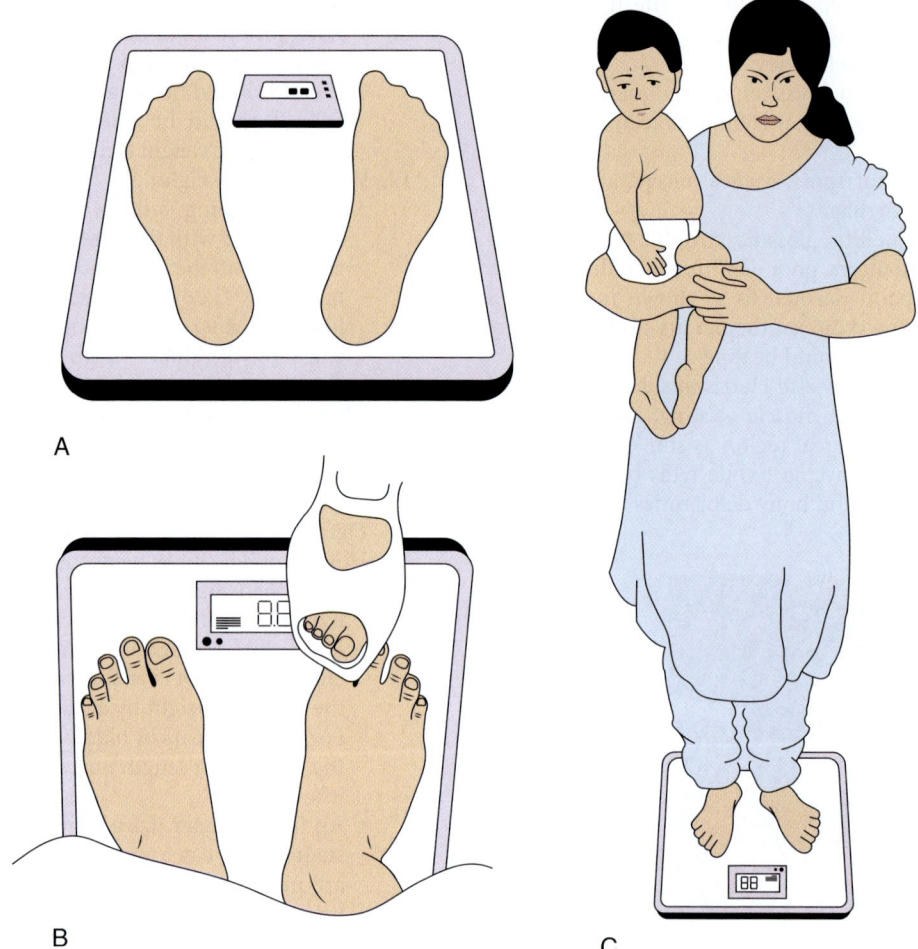

A

B

C

Fig. 33.4 (A) Mother's weight alone. (B) Taring the scale. (C) Machine showing child's weight alone. *(Source: (A–C) https://www.google.com/imgres?imgurl=x-raw-image%3A%2F%2F%2Ff77950ac32d2da200ce7641b60c8ec4661875bc6cfc93ed99a6af2d91ff61dc1&imgrefurl=https%3A%2F%2Fwww.who.int%2Fchildgrowth%2Ftraining%2Fjobaid_weighing_measuring.pdf&tbnid=lNrSMqxQefcmTM&vet=12ahUKEwiijOG4gufuAhUBhEsFHX9GBt8QMygAegUIARC_Q..i&docid=u1Y5UYxJgK-P4M&w=244&h=644&q=tared%20weighing&ved=2ahUKEwiijOG4gufuAhUBhEsFHX9GBt8QMygAegUIARC_AQ.)*

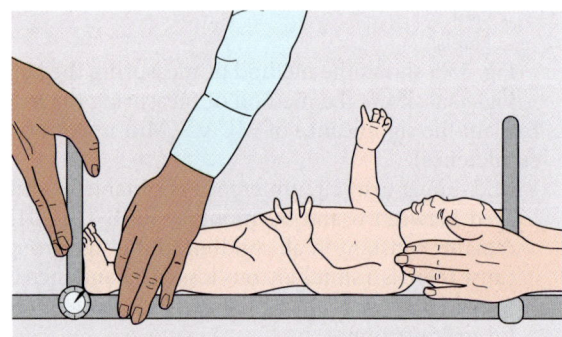

Fig. 33.5 Method of measuring the length using infantometer. *(Source: Reproduced from Tom Lissauer, Will Carroll. Illustrated Textbook of Paediatrics, Sixth Edition, Growth and puberty, Figure 12.3, Oxford, Elsevier Ltd, 2022.)*

17. List the findings to be looked for in system examination.
    Cardiovascular system: Cardiac failure
    Respiratory system: Respiratory tract infection
    Abdomen: Ascites and hepatomegaly
    Central nervous system: Altered sensorium and hypotonia/reduced cognitive function

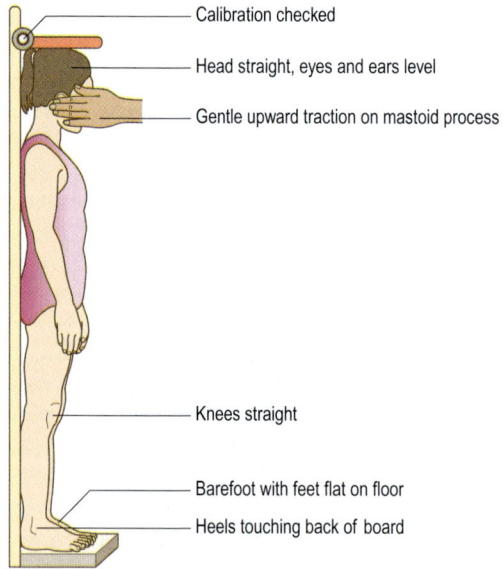

Calibration checked

Head straight, eyes and ears level

Gentle upward traction on mastoid process

Knees straight

Barefoot with feet flat on floor

Heels touching back of board

Fig. 33.6 Method of measuring the height using stadiometer. (Source: Reproduced from Smriti Arora. *Elsevier Clinical Skills Manual: Child Health Nursing*, First South Asia Edition, Paediatric history taking and physical examination, Figure 10-2, New Delhi, Elsevier India, 2020. (Credit line - From J. A. Innes, A. R. Dover, K. Fairhurst. 2018. Macleod's Clinical Examination. 14th ed. Elsevier).

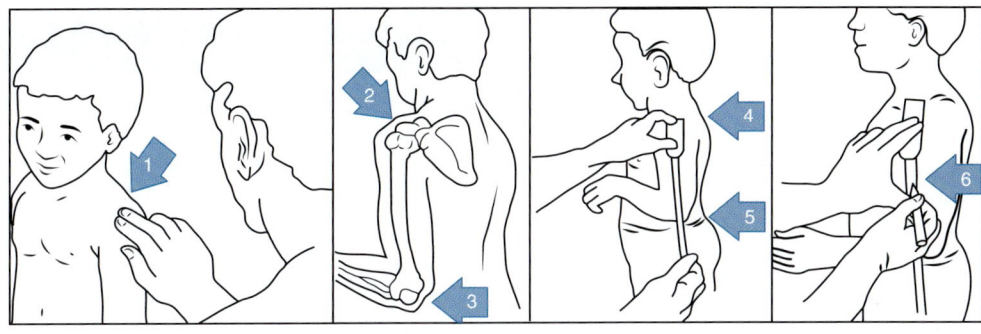

1. Locate tip of shoulder
4. Place tape at the tip of shoulder
2. Tip of shoulder
5. Pull tape past the tip of bent elbow
3. Tip of elbow
6. Mark midpoint

Fig. 33.7 Method of measuring MUAC (**7. After marking the midpoint, measure using arm circumference 'insertion' tape, neither too loose nor too tight with correct tape tension and tape position for arm circumference**). (Source: Reproduced from Rajkumar Patil. *Community Medicine: Practical Manual*, Details of specific clinicosocial cases, Figure 18.4, New Delhi, Elsevier India, 2018. (Credit line -Source: Participant manual for facility based care of severe acute malnutrition. Ministry of Health and Family Welfare, Government of India; 2013.)

TABLE 33.2	WHO Classification of Acute and Chronic Malnutrition			
Weight for age	**Height for age**	**Weight for Height**	**Interpretation**	
Decreased	Normal	Decreased	Acute malnutrition	
Decreased	Decreased	Normal	Chronic malnutrition	
Decreased	Decreased	Deceased	Acute on chronic malnutrition	

TABLE 33.3	Biochemical Changes in Malnutrition
Parameter	**Biochemical Changes**
Proteins	1. Reversal of A:G (Albumin:Globulin) ratio (alpha-2- and beta-globulins are low) 2. Nonessential:essential Amino Acids >3.5 3. Tyrosine, Phenyl Alanine Tryptophan 4. Reduced urine hydroxyproline 5. Reduced beta-lipoproteins
Lipids	1. EFA (Essential fatty acid) reduced 2. Nonessential:essential FA >3 3. Fatty liver (40% of body fat is deposited in liver)
Carbohydrate	Low blood glucose
Electrolytes, minerals	↓ K, Mg, Ca, PO_4, Zn, Cu Dilutional hyponatremia
Enzymes	Low

18. List the causes of abdominal distension in SAM.
    1. Ascites
    2. Hepatomegaly (fatty liver)
    3. Poor tone of abdominal muscles
    4. Ileus because of hypokalemia and sepsis
19. List the investigations to be performed in a child with SAM.
    All children with SAM admitted as inpatients should undergo the following:
    1. Blood glucose
    2. Total leukocyte count and Hb
    3. RFT (Renal function test) and serum electrolytes
    4. Blood cultures, urine routine, and urine cultures
    5. Chest X-Ray
    6. Mantoux
    7. HIV screening
    8. Any other specific test required on the basis of clinical presentation
*20. List the biochemical changes in malnutrition.
    Table 33.3 shows the biochemical changes in malnutrition.
21. What is the prevalence of SAM in India?
    The prevalence of SAM in India is 6.5.
*22. Define severe acute malnutrition.
    - **In infants older than 6 months**
        - Weight-for-height less than −3 SD and/or
        - Visible severe wasting and/or
        - Mid-arm circumference (MUAC) <11.5 cm and/or
        - Bipedal edema
    - **In children younger than 6 months or if length >49 cm**
        - Weight-for-height less than −3 SD and/or
        - Visible severe wasting and/or
        - Edema of both feet

- If length <49 cm, visible severe wasting can be used as a criterion to identify SAM.
*23. Explain the various classification systems in SAM.
    - The classification of nutritional status is based on weight-for-age.
    - The "Indian Academy of Pediatrics (IAP) classification" is as follows:

    - >80% weight-for-age — Normal
    - 71%–80% weight-for-age — Grade I PEM (protein energy malnutrition)
    - 61%–70% weight-for-age — Grade II PEM
    - 51%–60% weight-for-age — Grade III PEM
    - ≤50 weight-for-age — Grade IV PEM

    - When there is edema because of nutritional etiology, letter "K" is added with PEM grade to indicate kwashiorkor.
    Another classification, which is the oldest one (1956), is Gomez's classification:

    - >90% of expected weight — Normal
    - 76%–90% of expected weight — First-degree PEM
    - 61%–75% of expected weigh — Second-degree PEM
    - <60% of expected weight — Third-degree PEM

    - Patients with edema should be included in third-degree PEM, irrespective of weight-for-age.
    - There are various classifications based on age-dependent and -independent criteria available.

24. What is moderate acute malnutrition?
    - Seventy per cent to 80% of expected weight-for-height (Z score of <-3 to <-2 SD (Standard Deviation)) or
    - Mid–upper arm circumference of 115–125 mm and
    - No edema, should have an appetite, and should be alert and clinically well
    - Can be managed in an OP (Out-Patient) basis, setting with the provision of supplementary feeding
25. List the contributing factors for PEM.
    - Increased protein requirement during early infancy and most commonly in the 2nd and 3rd years of life when rapid growth and increase in muscle mass occur
    - Unavailability of protein weaning feeds, which may be because of nonavailability of animal milk or high cost or urbanization, leading to early weaning and poor supplementation
    - Social customs and lack of knowledge, such as prejudice against giving eggs to infants, dietary restriction, purges, and reserving animal proteins for male children, as well as large family size, instability, and illegitimacy
    - Psychological: Maternal deprivation syndrome in which the child is suddenly weaned from the breast and sent to stay with a relative, often living a long way away from the mother
    - Infections and infestations, such as measles, pertussis, diarrhea, respiratory and skin infections, ancylostomiasis, and ascariasis
*26. What is the pathophysiology in SAM?
    - Gopalan's theory of reductive adaptation

    ↓

    Child restricts activity and growth

    ↓

    Mobilisation of fat and proteins which are used for energy. proteins are also used for tissue repair.

    - Marasmus occurs when the child adapts to reduced energy.
    - Kwashiorkor occurs when the child fails to adapt.
    Physiological changes in the body system are the following:
    - GI manifestations: Reduced motility, acid secretion, and absorption
    - Hematological abnormalities: Reduced red cell mass
    Flowchart 33.1 shows the pathogenesis in malnutrition.

TABLE 33.4	Hormonal Changes in SAM		
Hormone	**Marasmus**	**Kwashiorkor**
Cortisol	Very high	High
Insulin	Normal	Low
Growth hormone	Normal/high	Very high

27. List the hormonal changes in PEM.
    - Cortisol: Catabolic hormone (breakdown increases the glucose level; protein lysis increases the amino acid pool; lipolysis increases the fatty acid pool)
    - Insulin: Anabolic hormone (glycogen synthesis and protein synthesis decrease the amino acid pool; lipogenesis decreases the fatty acid pool)
    - Growth hormone: Cortisol-like action in carbohydrate and fat; insulin-like action in protein synthesis
    Table 33.4 gives the hormonal changes in a child with SAM.
28. Why is iron contraindicated in acute phase of malnutrition?
    Iron absorption requires energy. Iron is converted to ferritin, which requires glucose and amino acids, thus aggravating hypoglycemia and amino acid imbalance. Iron also promotes pathogen growth and free radical production.
29. List the criteria for admission in NRC (Nutrition Rehabilitation Center) or health care facility.
    Presence of any of the following emergency signs indicates admission in National rehabilitation center (NRC) or health care facility:
    - Edema
    - Persistent vomiting
    - Very weak and apathetic
    - Fever (axillary temperature >38.5°C)/ Hypothermia (axillary temperature <35°C)
    - Children with fast breathing/chest indrawing/cyanosis
    - Extensive skin lesions, eye lesions, and post-measles states
    - Diarrhea with dehydration on the basis of history and clinical signs
    - Severe anemia, very weak and apathetic
    - Any other general sign that the clinician thinks warrants transfer to an inpatient facility for assessment or care
    - If the caregiver is unable to take care of the child at home

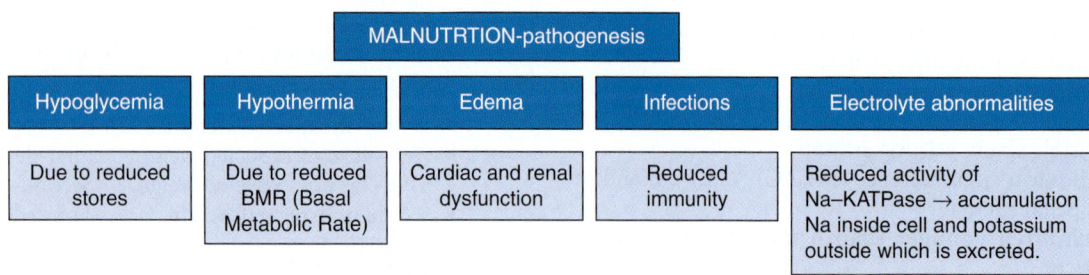

Flowchart 33.1 Pathogenesis in malnutrition.

30. What is NRC? Mention its objectives.

    The acronym "NRC" refers to nutritional rehabilitation center.

    - After treating a life-threatening illness in a hospital, the child with malnutrition can be transferred to NRC for intensive feeding to recover the lost weight, development of emotional and physical stimulation, and capacity building of the caregivers through sustained counseling and behavior-changing activities. NRC is a bridge between hospital and home care.
    - Services provided in NRC include the following:
      a. Treatment and patient management
      b. Nutritional support to inmates
      c. Nutrition education to family members
      d. Capacity building of the caregivers

31. Describe the management of hypoglycemia in a child with SAM.

    - Estimate blood glucose levels by using glucometer or from blood sample collected for lab tests.
    - If blood glucose is low (<54 mg/dL) or suspected hypoglycaemia, immediately the child is given 50 mL bolus of 10% glucose or 10% sucrose (one rounded teaspoon of sugar in three tablespoons of water). Glucose is preferable because it is more easily used by the body. If the child can drink, 50 mL bolus is given orally.
    - If the child is alert but not drinking, give 50 mL bolus by an Nasogastric tube. If the child is lethargic, unconscious, or convulsing, 5 mL/kg body weight of sterile 10% glucose is given by intravenously, followed by 50 mL of 10% glucose or sucrose by Nasogastric tube.
    - If no fluid is available,10% glucose solution with 1 rounded teaspoon of sugar mixed in 3.5 tablespoons of water (10 g in 100 mL) is prepared and given.

32. Describe the treatment of severe hypothermia in a child with SAM.

    - Warm humidified oxygen
    - The child rapidly rewarmed to 34°C within 30 minutes to 1 hour with a radiant warmer
    - The child given 5 mL/kg of 10% glucose i.v.
    - The child given i.v. antibiotics
    - The child given warm feeds immediately

*33. Describe the treatment of dehydration in a child with SAM.

    - The diagnosis of dehydration is on the basis of history because the examination is unreliable.
    - The following history must be present:
      - There should be a definite history of significant recent fluid loss.
      - There should be a history of a recent change in the child's appearance.
      - If the child has sunken eyes, then the mother must say that the eyes have become sunken only after the onset of diarrhea.
    - Assessment of signs of dehydration in SAM
      a. Any history of diarrhea considered as dehydration
      b. Any recent onset of sunken eyes
      c. Absence of tears

      d. Increased thirst
      e. Prolonged CRT, weak/thready pulse, and decreased urine output
    - Treatment of dehydration in SAM
      - Give oral rehydration solution as follows, in amounts based on the child's weight:
        - For every 30 minutes in the first 2 hours, the child is treated with 5 mL/kg weight of oral rehydration solution.
        - For alternate hours up to 10 hours, the child is given 5–10 mL/kg of oral rehydration solution.
        - Reduced osmolarity ORS is used – add 15 mL of potassium chloride to 1 L ORS.
        - The amount offered should be on the basis of the child's willingness to drink and the amount of ongoing losses in stool.

*34. Describe the preparation and constituents of ReSoMal (Rehydration Solution for Malnourished).

    - Add 15 mL of syrup KCl + 1 L of WHO ORS (Oral Rehydration Solution) solution.
    - Or add 1700 mL of water + 1 sachet of WHO ORS solution + 40 g sugar + 1 sachet mineral mix solution.
    - Table 33.5 shows the composition of rehydration solution for children with malnutrition.

35. List the signs of improvement in hydration status.

    - Fewer or less pronounced signs of dehydration
    - Less thirsty
    - Skin pinch not as slow
    - Less lethargic

36. What are the signs of overhydration?

    - Stop ORS if any of the following signs appears:
      - Increase of pulse by 15 and respiratory rate by 5
      - Jugular veins engorged
      - Puffiness of eyes
    - Signs of improved hydration: Three or more of the following:
      - Child no longer thirsty
      - Less lethargic
      - Slowing of respiratory and pulse rates from the previous high rate
      - Skin pinch less slow
      - Tears present
    - **Stop ORS.**

TABLE 33.5	Composition of Rehydration Solution for Children With Malnutrition	
Constituent	**Concentration (mmol/L)**
Glucose	125
Na	45
K	40
Cl	70
Citrate	7
Magnesium	3
Zinc	0.3
Copper	0.045
Total osmolarity	300

*37. Explain the management of shock in a child with SAM.
  - Signs of shock in SAM include cool peripheries, capillary refill time >2 seconds, and weak, thready pulses (FIMNCI, 2013).
  - The fluid of choice is 5% Dextrose with Ringer Lactate or 5% Dextrose with 1/2 NS.
  - The duration of fluid bolus is 1 hour.
  - If there is improvement, give another bolus.
  - If there is no improvement or deterioration, start maintenance and dopamine, review antibiotics, initiate feeding if possible, and give fresh whole blood (10 mL/kg) with furosemide.

*38. What are the indications for blood transfusion in SAM?
  1. Septic shock not responding to fluid therapy
  2. Severe anemia Hb <4 g/dL

39. Mention the types of shock in which initial fluid bolus is given over 1 hour.
  1. SAM with shock
  2. Compensated dengue shock
  3. Diabetic Ketoacidosis with shock

40. What are the causes for cardiac failure in SAM?
  - Microcardia
  - Thiamine, selenium, and PO_4 deficiency
  - Fluid overload
  - Refeeding syndrome

41. Enumerate eye care in patients with SAM.
  - Give single dose of vitamin on day 1 to all patients irrespective of vitamin A deficiency.
  - If there are signs of vitamin A deficiency, give vitamin A on days 1, 2, and 14. If the child's weight is <8 kg, give 1 lakh IU irrespective of age.
  - If there is pus/inflammation, give chloramphenicol/tetracycline eye drops (q.i.d.) for 7 days.
  - If there is corneal ulceration, give the above-mentioned eye drops + atropine eye ointment (t.d.s.).

42. Explain the principles of feeding in a child with SAM.
  - Feeding should include electrolyte/mineral solution (days 1–7), powdered milk, sugar, and oil.
  - The child should be given food that is high in energy, low in protein and iron.
  - The child should be given small, frequent feeds – 130 mL/kg divided every second hour.

*43. Describe the preparation of F-75 starter formula.
  - The F-75 formula contains 75 kcal and 0.9 g protein.
  - It is given as 10-mL/kg/feed every 2 hours.
  - Children are fed with a cup and spoon.
  - Avoid bottle feed.
  - Never leave the child alone while feeding.
  - Use NG-tube feeding if the child does not finish.
  - Eighty per cent of feeds are given as two to three consecutive feeds.
  - Ensure breastfeeding on demand between the started feeds.

  The ingredients of F-75 starter formula are as follows:
  - Milk (30 mL)
  - Sugar – 1 teaspoon (10 g)
  - Water (70 mL)
  - Vegetable oil - 0.5 teaspoon
  - Total calorie/protein - 75 kcal/0.9 g protein per 100 mL

*44. Describe the preparation of F-100 catch-up formula.
  The ingredients of F-100 catch-up formula are as follows:
  - Milk (90 mL)
  - Sugar-3/4 teaspoon (7.5 g)
  - Water (10 mL)
  - Vegetable oil – 11½ teaspoon (20 g)
  - Total calorie/protein - 100 kcal/2.9 g protein per 100 mL.
  - The catch-up formula is usually started from day 2 to 7.
  - In the first 48 hours, catch-up diet is given every 4 hours in the same amount as the last starter diet.
  - On day 3, each feed is increased by 10 mL, as long as the child is finishing feeds. Continue increasing the amount until some food is left.
  - Transition usually takes 3 days. After a transition, the child can feed freely on catch-up diet to an upper limit of 220 kcal/kg/day.

45. What is appetite test?
  - For children aged 7–12 months, 30–35 mL/kg of catch-up diet is given. If the child takes more than 25 mL/kg, then the child should be considered to have a good appetite.
  - For children older than 12 months, feed is locally prepared with the following food items:
    a. Roasted groundnuts - 1000 g
    b. Milk powder - 1200 g
    c. Sugar - 1120 g
    d. Coconut oil - 600 g
  - The test is performed in a separate quiet area.
  - The mother/caregiver should wash her hands and sits comfortably with the child on her lap and offers therapeutic food.
  - The child should not have taken any food for the last 2 hours.
  - When the child has finished taking the food, the amount taken is judged or measured.
  - If the amount of food taken is equal to 5 times child's body weight, then the appetite test is passed.

*46. List the criteria for discharge in a child with SAM.
  The criteria for discharge in a child with severe acute malnutrition are as follows:
  a. Child
    - The child has achieved weight gain of more than or equal to 15% and has satisfactory weight gain for 3 consecutive days (>5 g/kg/day).
    - The child is eating an adequate amount of nutritious food that the mother can prepare at home.
    - After the edema has resolved and all infections and other medical complications have been treated.
    - The child is provided with micronutrients and the Immunization is updated.
  b. Mother
    - Knows how to prepare appropriate foods and feed the child, how to make appropriate toys and play with the child.
    - Knows how to give home treatment for diarrhea, fever, and acute respiratory infections, and how to recognize the signs that the child must seek medical assistance and knows about the follow-up plan.

47. List the criteria for failure to respond in a child with SAM.
    Criteria for failure to respond in approximate time after admission are as follows:
    - Failure to regain appetite and failure to start to lose edema by day 4
    - Edema still present on day 10.
    - Failure to gain at least 5 g/kg/day for 3 successive days after feeding freely on catch-up diet.

48. How is a child with SAM followed up?
    - At 1 week after discharge
    - Every 2 weeks in the 1st month and then monthly thereafter until WHO Z score reaches -1 SD or higher
    - Treatment for helminthiasis: All children at discharge should be given the following:
    Albendazole: 400 mg stat (older than 2 years) and 200 mg stat (younger than 2 years)
    Mebendazole: 100 mg b.d. for 3 days

49. Explain the management of SAM in infants younger than 6 months.
    - The initial assessment and stabilization phase is the same as for older children.
    - Breastfeeding or expressed milk is preferred in place of starter diet.
    - For non-breastfed babies, give starter diet feed prepared without cereals.
    - If breast milk is not enough, give supplementary milk feeds, or if breastfeeding is not possible or the mother is HIV positive, opt for replacement feeds.
    - In the rehabilitation phase, try to establish exclusive breastfeeding.
    - Artificially fed infants should be offered a diluted catch-up diet (catch-up diet diluted by one-third extra water to make volume 135 mL in place of 100 mL).
    - On discharge, the baby should be given locally available animal milk with a cup and spoon.

*50. Describe relactation through supplementary suckling technique (SST).
    - It is a technique that can be used to initiate relactation in mothers who have developed lactation failure.
    - The infant suckles and stimulates the breast at the same time drawing the supplement (expressed mother's milk or therapeutic formula) through the tube.
    - In this technique, one end of a 6 or 8F feeding tube is stuck to the mother's breast close to the nipple and the other end of the tube lies in a bowl of milk (expressed breast milk or diluted F-100) kept lower than the mother's breast while the infant suckles at the mother's breast that stimulates prolactin reflex to secrete more milk as shown in fig 33.8A and B.

51. List the causes of high case fatality rate in children with SAM.
    - Inability to distinguish between acute and rehabilitation phases
    - Excessive use of i.v. fluids
    - Not keeping the child warm and euglycemic during hypothermia
    - Use of diuretics for edema
    - Early use of diet high in protein and sodium
    - Use of iron in the acute phase
    - Failure to monitor signs of overhydration while correcting dehydration
    - Failure to monitor food intake

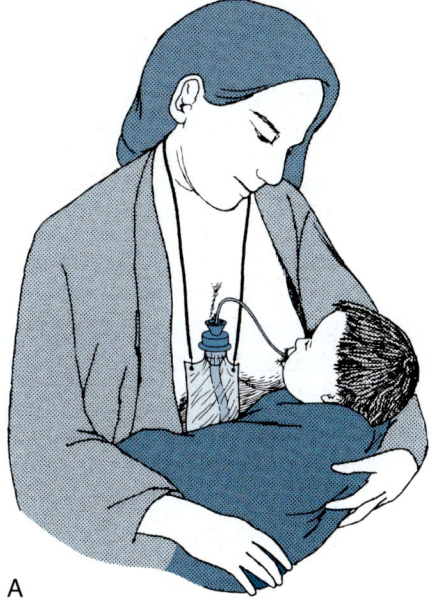

A

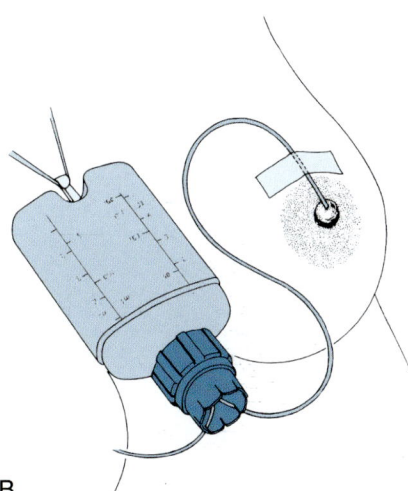

B

Fig. 33.8 A and B Supplementary suckling technique. (Source: *Reproduced* from Ruth Lawrence, Robert Lawrence. *Breastfeeding: A Guide for the Medical Profession*, Ninth Edition, Induced Lactation and Relactation (Including Nursing an Adopted Baby) and Cross-Nursing, Fig. 19.1, Philadelphia, Elsevier Inc., 2022.)

*52. Explain refeeding and nutritional recovery syndrome.
    Table 33.6 shows the refeeding and nutritional recovery syndrome.

53. Enumerate the causes of death in a child with SAM.
    - Hypoglycemia
    - Hypothermia
    - Fluid overload
    - Cardiac failure
    - Infections

54. Explain the acceptable macronutrient distribution range (AMDR) in children.
    Table 33.7 gives AMDR in children.

*55. Mention the normal calorie requirement according to the age (*Nelson*, 20th edition).
    Table 33.8 gives the normal calorie requirement according to the age.

56. Define balanced diet.
    - A balanced diet is a diet with nutrients in the required amount and having the following characteristics:
        - Should have carbohydrate, protein, and fats in ideal proportion as mentioned earlier
        - Should incorporate all foodstuffs (cereals, pulses, legumes, vegetables, fruits, milk, sugar)
        - Should provide micronutrients, fiber, and water.

TABLE 33.7	Acceptable Macronutrient Distribution Range (AMDR) in Children		
Age (years)		1–3	4–18
Energy from fat (%)		30–40	25–35
Energy from carbohydrates (%)		45–65	45–65
Energy from proteins (%)		5–20	10–30

TABLE 33.6	Refeeding and Nutritional Recovery Syndrome
Refeeding Syndrome	**Nutritional Recovery Syndrome**
Because of excess hormones secreted during recovery Characterized by hypertrichosis, parotid swelling, gynecomastia, HSM, encephalitis No special treatment required Monitor the child during therapy	Characterized by hypophosphatemia, hypomagnesemia, hypokalemia leading to myocardial dysfunction, rhabdomyolysis, seizures

TABLE 33.8	Normal Calorie Requirement According to Age	
Age	**Calorie Requirement (kcal/kg/day)**	
0–3 months	115	
3–6 months	110	
6 months to 3 years	100	
Older than 3 years	90–100	

Quick Bites

- Most of the cases of malnutrition in children result from nonorganic causes.
- Children after 6 months (during complementary feeding) are more prone to malnutrition. They fall into the "pit of malnutrition" if the transition from liquid diet to solid is not appropriate.
- The diagnosis of malnutrition is made on the basis of history and examination. Investigations are needed to look for the complications and the underlying etiology.
- A stepwise approach is needed for the management of severe acute malnutrition in children.
- The diagnosis of dehydration in a child with SAM is made on the basis of history because the examination is unreliable.
- I.v. fluids in a child with SAM are used only in a child with shock.
- There is no role of the routine use of diuretics for the treatment of edema in a child with SAM. However, diuretics can be given at the start of blood transfusion to prevent volume overload.
- Iron therapy should be started in the 2nd week of treatment.
- Oral antibiotics can be given in a child with SAM without complications.

34

Diarrhea

Introduce yourself and make the child and the parents comfortable to build a rapport with them.

It is important to identify whether the stool pattern can truly be labeled as diarrhea. Diarrhea is characterized by the following:

1. Increase in the stool frequency
2. Fluidity (liquid consistency is an important characteristic to call it diarrhea)
3. Weight of the stool (more than 10 mL/kg/day amounts to diarrhea)

Always remember to ask the mother about the normal stool pattern of the child especially in the infantile age group.

Name____Age____Sex____Consanguinity____Order of birth____Place____Informant____

Presenting Complaints and Duration

Passing loose stools

History of Presenting Complaints

LOOSE STOOLS

- Duration
- Number of episodes per day
- Consistency and nature of the stools (e.g., rice water, pea soup, oily stools)
- Quantity
- Color of the stool/whether blood stained
- Foul smelling ±
- Associated with borborygmi
- Presence of worms in stools

ASSOCIATED SYMPTOMS

- Crampy abdominal pain ±
- Abdominal distension
- Fever
- Vomiting ±; if present, whether bilious/nonbili-ous and projectile/nonprojectile, and contents of the vomitus

COMPLICATION HISTORY

- Oliguria/edema
- Altered sensorium/seizures
- Cool peripheries/fast breathing
- Limb weakness
- Joint swelling/joint pain
- Failure to gain weight
- Painful skin swellings
- Perianal rash noticed by the mother

ETIOLOGICAL HISTORY

- Fever/exanthematous rash

- Drug intake/toxin
- Failure to gain weight
- Oily stools
- Intake of contaminated foods items such as improperly cooked fried rice (*Bacillus* species), canned foods (*Clostridium botulinum*), street-vended foods, ready-to-eat salads, and raw vegetables (*Salmonella* and *Shigella* species, rotavirus) (mention only the commonly consumed contaminated food items)
- History of any recent travel to diarrhea endemic areas
- Burning micturition/hematuria/cough/fast breathing
- Allergy to any known foods
- Bad child-rearing practice/child neglect
- Going to child care centers
- Recent use of antimicrobial agents (e.g., ampicillin induced) and antineoplastic agents (enteritis)

TREATMENT HISTORY

Medications/i.v. fluids//investigations performed/biopsy performed (for malabsorption syndromes)

PAST HISTORY

- Recurrent episodes in the past
- Long-term drug intake
- Gut surgeries performed (ileal resection)
- Comorbidities

ANTENATAL HISTORY

Infants born to mothers infected with *Listeria monocytogenes* can present with diarrhea in the newborn period.

NATAL/POSTNATAL HISTORY

- Full term/preterm (preterms are more prone to sepsis)
- Birth weight
- Delayed initiation of breastfeeding
- Bottle feeding/formula feeding
- Jaundice in the newborn period
- Gut surgeries performed in the newborn period

DEVELOPMENT HISTORY

Attained age-appropriate milestones or any global developmental delay

DIETETIC HISTORY

Younger Than 6 Months

- Prelacteal feed
- Exclusive breastfeeding/breastfeeding on demand
- Formula feeding

- Bottle feeding
- Amount of dilution asked if the child is on formula feeding or cow's milk feeding

Six to 12 Months

- When complementary feeding was started
- Whether breastfeeding was continued during this period

Older Than 1 Year

By 24-hour recall method, calculate the calorie and protein gap. Mention whether the mother is aware of hygienic practices before feeding.

ALLERGIC HISTORY

Mention about the history of adverse reactions to food.

IMMUNIZATION HISTORY

Immunized up to age according to IAP (Indian Academy of Pediatrics) or Universal Immunization Schedule

FAMILY HISTORY

- Similar illness in sibling
- Sibling death
- Malnutrition in siblings
- Medical illness among family members
- Drug abuse/parental dispute

SOCIOECONOMIC HISTORY

- Socioeconomic class according to the modified Kuppuswamy scale
- Place of residence
- Overcrowding
- Sanitation facilities
- Family fads – any custom or culture fasting and vegetarian diet
- Drinking water

Summary

A _____-year-old _____ child presented with loose stools for _____ days, with/without complications, being a case of acute/persistent/chronic diarrhea, probably because of ___.

General Examination

- Sensorium
- Pallor
- Icterus
- Cyanosis
- Clubbing
- Generalized lymphadenopathy
- Pedal edema

Head-to-Foot Examination

- Head
  - Microcephaly

- Hair: Trichorrhexis nodosa
- Sunken AF (Anterior Fontanelle)
- Bulging AF (raised ICT (Intracranial Tension) secondary to cerebral sinovenous thrombosis)
- Eyes: Pallor, icterus, phlycten, signs of vitamin A deficiency, conjunctivitis, scleritis, and uveitis
- Facial dysmorphism
- Oral cavity: Oral ulcers
- BCG scar
- Arthritis
- Skin: Infections, erythematous serpiginous tracks, erythema nodosum, and pyoderma gangrenosum
- Abdominal distension/anal excoriation/diaper rash
- Signs of malnutrition
- Signs of dehydration

Vital Signs

- Pulse rate
- Blood pressure
- Respiration: Rate, rhythm, and type of respiration
- Temperature

Anthropometry

Weight, height, weight for height, head circumference, and mid–upper arm circumference

System Examination

ABDOMEN

Inspection

- Distended in the upper part/uniform distension
- Skin: Stretched and shiny
- Scars
- Dilated veins
- Umbilicus: Transverse slit and umbilical hernia
- Flanks: Full or free
- Hernia orifices
- Equal movement of all quadrants with respiration
- Perianal excoriation
- Diaper rash
- External genitalia: Micropenis and scrotal edema/vulval edema

Palpation

- Warmth
- Tenderness
- Organomegaly
- Fluid thrill

Percussion

- Shifting dullness
- Liver span

Auscultation

Bowel sounds and bruit

CARDIOVASCULAR SYSTEM

Tachycardia and hypovolemic shock

RESPIRATORY SYSTEM

Signs of pneumonia

CENTRAL NERVOUS SYSTEM

Altered sensorium/signs of raised ICT/focal neurological deficit

Diagnosis

- A case of acute/persistent/chronic diarrhea
- With/without complications
- Probable etiology

Frequently Asked Questions

*1. Explain the significance of age in diarrheal disease.
  - Congenital diarrhea can present at an early age (within the first 6 months).
  - Cow's milk protein allergy usually presents in infancy.
  - Inflammatory bowel diseases can present at an older age.
  - Diarrhea because of infections can present at any age.
  - Diarrhea occurring during introduction of complementary feeding can be the result of malnutrition/food allergy.

2. Explain the significance of gender in diarrheal disease.
  In case of a female child, suspect neglect and autoimmune enteropathy.

3. Enumerate the histories elicited when the mother reports loose stools.
  - Duration: To differentiate between acute/persistent/chronic diarrhea
  - Frequency: Frequent large bowel diarrhea
  - Quantity: Large volume of stools in small bowel diarrhea
  - Color
  - Consistency: Rice water, cholera; pea soup, enteric fever; and oily stools, fat malabsorption

4. Enumerate the complication histories elicited in diarrheal disease.
  - Acute renal failure/hemolytic uremic syndrome: Oliguria/edema
  - Hyponatremia: Altered sensorium/seizures
  - Cerebral sinovenous thrombosis: Headache/vomiting/altered sensorium
  - Hypovolemic shock: Cool peripheries/fast breathing
  - Guillain–Barré syndrome/hypokalemic periodic paralysis: Limb weakness
  - Reactive arthritis: Joint swelling/joint pain
  - Malnutrition: Failure to gain weight
  - Erythema nodosum: Painful skin swellings
  - Complication of osmotic diarrhea: Perianal rash noticed by the mother

5. Enumerate the etiological histories in diarrheal disease.
  - Infective diarrhea: Fever
  - Measles: Exanthematous rash
  - Antibiotic-associated diarrhea: Drug intake (ampicillin, antineoplastic agents, laxatives)/toxin
  - Malnutrition: Failure to gain weight
  - Fat malabsorption: Oily stools
  - Intake of contaminated foods or water-food items such as improperly cooked fried rice (*Bacillus* species), canned foods (*Clostridium botulinum*), street-vended foods, ready-to-eat salads, and raw vegetables (*Salmonella* and *Shigella* species, rotavirus)
  - Recent travel to diarrhea endemic areas
  - Parenteral diarrhea secondary to UTI (Urinary Tract infection)/pneumonia: Burning micturition/hematuria/cough/fast breathing
  - Food allergy: Allergy to any known foods
  - Bad child-rearing practice/child neglect

6. What is the significance of past history in diarrheal disease?
  - Malabsorption: History of recurrent episodes in the past
  - Drug-induced diarrhea: Long-term drug intake
  - Short bowel syndrome: History of gut surgeries performed (ileal resection)
  - Comorbidities: Autoimmune disorders, immunodeficiency disorders, and radiation enteritis

7. List the significance of general examination findings in diarrhea.
  Table 34.1 lists the general examination findings and their significance.

8. List the head-to-foot examination findings in diarrhea and their significance.
  - Head
    Microcephaly: Malnutrition
    Hair: Trichorrhexis nodosa (syndromic diarrhea)
    Sunken Anterior Fontanelle (AF) (severe dehydration)
    Bulging AF (raised ICT secondary to cerebral sinovenous thrombosis)
  - Eyes: Pallor, icterus, phlycten (tuberculosis), signs of vitamin A deficiency, conjunctivitis, scleritis, and uveitis (inflammatory bowel disease)
  - Facial dysmorphism (syndromic diarrhea)
  - Oral cavity: Oral ulcers (inflammatory bowel disease)
  - BCG scar
  - Arthritis (reactive arthritis, arthritis secondary to inflammatory bowel disease)
  - Abdominal distension/anal excoriation/diaper rash
  - Skin: Infections, erythematous serpiginous tracks (cutaneous larva migrans), erythema nodosum, and pyoderma gangrenosum (inflammatory bowel disease)
  - Signs of malnutrition
  - Signs of dehydration

9. *Enumerate the signs of dehydration in diarrhea.
  Table 34.2 lists the signs of dehydration in diarrhea.

10. What is the significance of vital signs in diarrhea?
  - Pulse: Low-volume pulse and tachycardia

TABLE 34.1	General Examination Findings and Their Significance
Clinical Finding	**Significance**
Patient's sensorium	- Altered sensorium in severe dehydration - Shock - Electrolyte imbalance - HUS (Hemolytic Uremic Syndrome) - Cortical vein thrombosis - Sepsis
Pallor	- Malnutrition - HUS - Dysentery - Hemolytic anemia secondary to *Campylobacter* and *Yersinia* - Inflammatory bowel disease - Shock
Icterus	Fat malabsorption secondary to liver disease
Clubbing	Malnutrition, IBD (Inflammatory Bowel Disease)
Generalized lymphadenopathy	TB, HIV, malignancies
Pedal edema	Malnutrition, acute renal failure because of HUS

TABLE 34.2	Signs of Dehydration in Diarrhea		
Sign/Symptom	No Dehydration	Some/Moderate Dehydration	Severe Dehydration
Water loss	<5% in infants <3% in older children	10% in infants 6% in older children	15% in infants 9% in older children
Mental status	Normal	Irritable	Lethargic, unconscious
Thirst	Drinks normally	Thirsty, drinks eagerly	Unable to drink
Eyes	Normal	Slightly sunken	Sunken
Tears	Present	Reduced	Absent
Mouth and tongue	Moist	Dry	Parched
Skin pinch	Goes back immediately	Goes back slowly, <2 s	Goes back very slowly, >2 s
Heart rate	Normal	Normal to increased	Tachycardia Bradycardia in severe cases
Pulse volume	Normal	Decreased	Thready pulse
Capillary refill	<2 s	Prolonged	Prolonged
Extremities	Warm	Cool	Mottled, cyanotic
Urine output	Normal	Decreased	Minimal

- BP
  Hypotension
  Hypertension (Acute Kidney injury because of HUS)
- Respiration: Tachypnea
- Temperature: Suggestive of infection
11. List the systemic findings in diarrhea.
    Abdomen
    - Abdominal distension: Osmotic diarrhea and diarrhea secondary to motility disorders
    - Tenderness: Infection
    - HSM (Hepatosplenomegaly): Infection and malabsorption
    Respiratory system
    - Signs of pneumonia
    Central nervous system
    - Altered sensorium/signs of raised ICT (Intracranial Tension)/focal neurological deficit
12. Enumerate the etiologies of diarrhea.
    Table 34.3 lists the various etiologies of different types of diarrhea.
*13. Describe the etiologies of chronic diarrhea.
    Flowchart 34.1 gives the etiologies of chronic diarrhea.
14. Differentiate between small bowel and large bowel diarrhea.
    Table 34.4 gives the differences between small bowel and large bowel diarrhea.
*15. Describe the features of osmotic diarrhea.
    - Moderate- to large-volume stools
    - Stool quantity proportionate to the intake of offending foods

- Borborygmi
- Bloating present
- Anal excoriation
- Stool pH acidic
- Stool hyperosmolar
- Stool positive for reducing substances
- Resolves on withdrawal of the offending agent
16. List the investigations in acute diarrhea.
    - CBC (Complete Blood Count)
      - Raised TLC (Total Leucocyte Count): Infection
      - Anemia: HUS, dysentery, and worm infestations
    - Renal function test: Features of pre-renal failure and HUS looked for
    - Serum electrolytes: Hyponatremia, hypokalemia, and hypochloremia
    - Stool routine examination
    - Stool culture
17. Enumerate the investigations in chronic diarrhea.
    Table 34.5 gives the investigations in chronic diarrhea.
18. Describe the management of dehydration in diarrheal disease.
    Table 34.6 shows the management of dehydration in diarrheal disease.
*19. Mention some home-available fluids (HAF) for diarrhea.
    - Lemon water
    - Rice water
    - Soups
    - Dal water
    - Lassi
    - Coconut water
    - Plain water
20. Mention the foods to be avoided in diarrheal disease.
    - Foods with high fiber content
    - Carbonated drinks
    - Simple sugar solution
    - Fruit juices
    - Tea/coffee
    - Desserts
    - Milk not a contraindication unless lactose intolerance is suspected
21. Explain the role of zinc in diarrheal disease.
    - Increases gut enzymes
    - Epithelial regeneration

TABLE 34.3	Various Etiologies of Different Types of Diarrhea		
Acute Diarrhea	Persistent Diarrhea	Chronic Diarrhea
- Enteral infections: Viral, bacterial, parasite - Parenteral infections: UTI, pneumonia, sepsis - Drug induced: Ampicillin, *C. difficile* toxins	- Enteral infections - HIV - Primary immunodeficiency disorders	Refer Q. 13

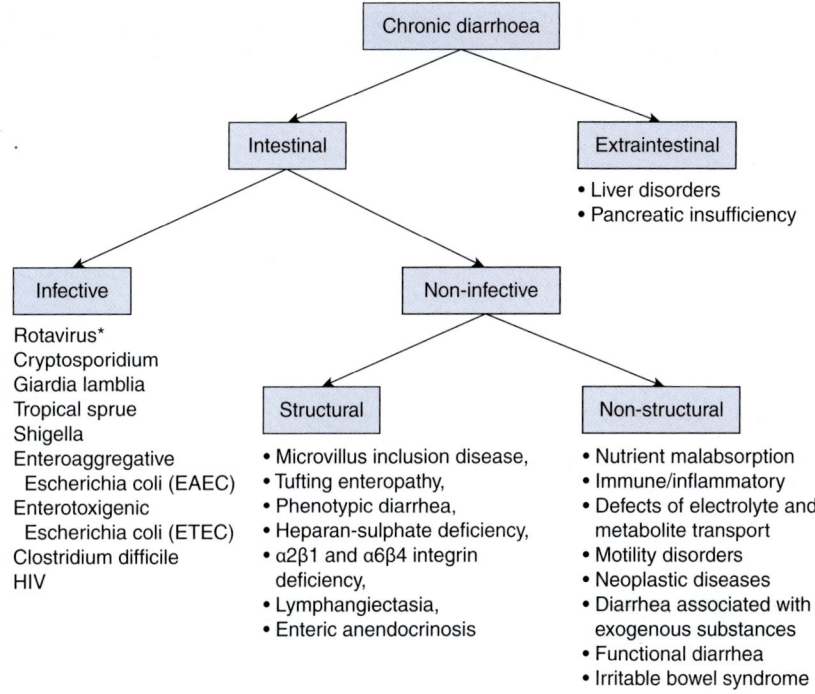

Flowchart 34.1 Etiologies of chronic diarrhea.

TABLE 34.4	Differences Between Small Bowel and Large Bowel Diarrhea	
Feature	**Small Bowel Diarrhea**	**Large Bowel Diarrhea**
Volume of stools	Large	Small
Frequency	Less frequent	Frequent
Nature of stools	Bulky, watery	Associated with blood and mucus
Bloating of abdomen	Present	Absent
Borborygmi and flatulence	Present	Absent
Tenesmus	Absent	Present
Vomiting	Present	Absent
Dehydration	Present	Usually absent

- Reduces purge rate
- Reduces the volume and frequency of stools
- Reduces inflammation

*22. List the indications for antibiotic therapy in acute diarrhea.
The indications for antibiotic therapy in acute diarrhea are as follows:
- Acute dysentery
- Diarrhea in a child with SAM (Severe Acute Malnutrition)
- Diarrhea in an immunocompromised child
- Parenteral diarrhea

The above-mentioned are the indications irrespective of the stool culture reports.

In all other situations, antibiotics should be administered only if a bacterial/protozoal agent is identified.

23. Enumerate the drugs contraindicated in diarrheal disease.
- Antimotility agents
- Antispasmodics
- Antihistamines
- Phenothiazine

24. Enumerate the causes of early onset protracted diarrhea.
- Diarrhea because of structural defects: Microvillus inclusion disease, tufting enteropathy, phenotypic diarrhea, heparin sulfate deficiency, $\alpha2\beta1$ and $\alpha6\beta4$ integrin deficiency, lymphangiectasia, and enteric anendocrinosis
- Diarrhea because of brush border enzyme deficiencies: Congenital lactase deficiency, congenital sucrase-isomaltase deficiency, and congenital maltase-glucoamylase deficiency
- Diarrhea because of defects in membrane carriers: Congenital chloride diarrhea, congenital sodium diarrhea, primary bile acid malabsorption, acrodermatitis enteropathica, Fanconi–Bickel syndrome, and fructose malabsorption
- Diarrhea because of abnormal immune response: Autoimmune polyglandular syndrome type 1 and IPEX (Immune Dysregulation, Polyendocrinopathy, Enteropathy, X-linked)

*25. Explain the role of probiotics in diarrheal disease.
- Probiotics can restore the intestinal flora.
- They also reduce inflammation by downregulation of cytokines and upregulation of anti-inflammatory cytokines.
- They have a definitive role in antibiotic-associated *Clostridium difficile* diarrhea.
- But their routine use in other types of diarrhea has not yet been established, although they have been found to be beneficial in some settings.
- The commonly used probiotics are *Lactobacillus*, *Bifidobacterium*, *Saccharomyces boulardii*, and *Saccharomyces cerevisiae*.

TABLE 34.5	Investigations in Chronic Diarrhea

Investigations to Rule Out Extraintestinal Causes	Investigations for Intestinal Causes

• LFT (Liver Function Test)
• Serum amylase, lipase
• USG (Ultrasonogram) abdomen
	A. **Noninvasive tests**
	  1. Stool routine, culture
	  2. Reducing substances, 72-h fecal fat estimation, occult blood, fecal calprotectin, stool elastase, chymotrypsin
	  3. X-ray abdomen – to rule out diverticula, malrotation, stenosis, blind loop, inflammatory bowel disease
	  4. Serology – antienterocyte antibodies, autoantibodies, serum chromogranin, and catecholamines
	  5. H_2 breath test
	  6. Screening test for celiac disease
	B. **Invasive tests**
	  1. Endoscopy and standard jejunal/colonic histology
	  2. Electron microscopy
	  3. Capsule endoscopy
	  4. Brush border enzymatic activities

TABLE 34.6	Management of Dehydration in Diarrheal Disease

Degree of Dehydration	Type of Treatment	Rehydration Therapy	Replacement of Ongoing Loses	Supportive Care
No/minimal dehydration	Plan A	Home-available fluids	Child weighing <10 kg: 60–120 mL ORS for each loose stool Child weighing >10 kg: 120–240 mL ORS (Oral Rehydration Solution) for each loose stool	Nutrition Zinc supplementation Treatment of electrolyte imbalance
Some dehydration	Plan B	75 mL/kg over 4 h (oral fluids) 50–100 mL/kg ORS over 4 h (Nelson)	Same as above	Same as above
Severe dehydration	Plan C	• 100 mL/kg i.v. fluids Infants: 30 mL/kg in 1 h + 70 mL/kg over next 5 h Older children: 30 mL/kg over 0.5 h + 70 mL/kg over 2.5 h • RL Ringer lactate or Normal Saline 20 mL/kg bolus until perfusion and mental status improves followed by 100 mL/kg ORS over 4 h or DNS (Dextrose Normal Saline) twice maintenance (Nelson)	Same as above If unable to drink, administer through nasogastric tube or DNS + KCl (Nelson)	Same as above

Quick Bites

- The etiologies of diarrhea in children vary according to the age.
- Rotavirus is the most common infective cause of diarrhea in children.
- Malnutrition is one of the most important risk factors as well as complications of diarrhea.
- Correction of dehydration, oral zinc supplementation, and dietary therapy are the mainstay in the management of acute diarrhea.
- Antibiotics should be given irrespective of stool culture reports in the following situations: acute dysentery, diarrhea in a child with SAM, diarrhea in an immunocompromised child, and parenteral diarrhea.
- Probiotics have a definitive role in antibiotic-associated *Clostridium difficile* diarrhea. Their role in other conditions has not yet been established.

Obesity

Model Case Sheet

Following introduction, seek permission from the caregiver and introduce yourself to the patient before history elicitation, and identify the case.

Name____Age____Sex____Consanguinity____Order of birth____Place____Informant____

Presenting Complaints and Duration

Increased weight gain for _____ (duration)

History of Presenting Illness

- Increased weight gain for ____ days/months
- Whether associated with increased gain in height
- Whether associated with hyperphagia

COMPLICATION HISTORY

- Headache/blurring of vision/vomiting
- Behavioral changes
- Snoring/sleep disturbances
- Recurrent episodes of breathlessness/wheeze
- Recurrent abdominal pain/retrosternal burn/retching
- Jaundice with abdominal pain
- Hip/lower limb/musculoskeletal pain
- Skin changes
- Irregular menstrual cycle

ETIOLOGICAL HISTORY

- Lack of physical activity/prolonged television viewing
- Snoring/sleep disturbance
- Constipation/cold intolerance/failure to gain adequate height
- Drug intake
- Facial dysmorphism

PAST HISTORY

- Drug intake
- Surgery
- Comorbidities

PERINATAL HISTORY

- Preterm/IUGR (Intra Uterine Growth Restriction)

DEVELOPMENT HISTORY

- Development delay
- Behavioral changes
- Poor scholastic performance

DIETETIC HISTORY

- Calorie and protein intake
- Salt intake
- Feeding patterns (skipping breakfast/eating extra meals)
- Food items mentioned/any craving for specific food item
- Exclusively breastfed or not
- Formula feeding

FAMILY HISTORY

- Similar illness in family members

Summary

A _____-year-old child presented with increased weight gain since ____ with/without complications, being a case of obesity probably because of ___.

General Examination

- Patient's sensorium
- Pallor
- Cyanosis
- Clubbing
- Icterus
- Edema

Head-to-Foot Examination

- Head: Microcephaly (Cohen syndrome) and craniosynostosis (Carpenter syndrome)
- Dysmorphic facies
- Eyes: Brushfield spots in the iris (Down syndrome), coloboma iris (Biemond syndrome), cataract (Down syndrome, steroid-induced), retinitis pigmentosa (Bardet–Biedl syndrome), and papilledema (pseudotumor cerebri)
- Oral cavity: Macroglossia
- Adenoid hypertrophy
- Skin: Acanthosis nigricans (hyperinsulinism) and generalized hyperpigmentation (POMC (Proopiomelanocortin) deficiency)
- Extremities: Polydactyly (Bardet–Biedl syndrome), syndactyly (Carpenter syndrome), and short metacarpals (pseudohypoparathyroidism)
- Features of hypothyroidism
- Features of Cushing syndrome
- Bowing of tibia
- Restricted hip movements

Vital Signs

- Pulse rate
- Blood pressure
- Respiration: Rate, rhythm, and type of respiration
- Temperature
- JVP (Jugular Venous Pressure)

Anthropometry

- Weight
- Height
- BMI (Body Mass Index)
- Head circumference

Systemic Examination

CARDIOVASCULAR SYSTEM

Features of cardiomyopathy

RESPIRATORY SYSTEM

Features of asthma and chronic obstructive lung disease

ABDOMEN

Epigastric/right hypochondrial tenderness, hepatomegaly, and features of acute pancreatitis

CENTRAL NERVOUS SYSTEM

Signs of raised ICT (Intracranial Tension)

Diagnosis

- A case of obesity
- With/without complications
- Probable etiology

Frequently Asked Questions

1. Explain the significance of age in obesity.
   It gives a clue to etiology. Obesity due to syndromic causes is present since birth. Obesity because of endocrine and dietary causes can present at any age.
2. Why is gender important in obesity?
   Turner syndrome and Prader–Willi syndrome occur in females.
3. List the etiological histories in obesity.
   - Floppiness/developmental delay/cold intolerance/constipation/delayed development of secondary sexual characters: Hypothyroidism
   - Early development of secondary sexual characters/hyperphagia/symptoms of raised ICT: Hypothalamic/pituitary tumors.
   - Binge eating/abnormal eating behaviors, decreased physical activity/increased Television viewing, and disturbed sleep: Sedentary lifestyle
*4. List the complications associated with obesity.
   - Abdominal pain: GERD (Gastroesophageal Reflux Disease)/pancreatitis/gallstones
   - Abdominal distension/jaundice: Nonalcoholic steatohepatitis (NASH)/cirrhosis
   - Hip pain/decreased mobility of the hip and knee pain: Slipped capital femoral epiphysis
   - Headache/vomiting/blurred vision: Pseudotumor cerebri
   - Snoring/apnea: Obstructive sleep apnea
   - Breathlessness/wheeze: Asthma
   - Weakness of limbs: Stroke
   - Polyuria/polydipsia: Diabetes mellitus
   - Abnormal behavior/poor scholastic performance: Syndromic cause (Prader–Willi syndrome)
5. Explain the significance of past history.
   - Parents/caregivers asked whether the child had normal weight gain before this
   - Any comorbidities
   - Drug intake: Hypothyroidism, familial hypercholesterolemia, diabetes mellitus, and GERD/Cushing syndrome
   - Surgery: For gallstones
6. Mention few significant perinatal histories.
   - Maternal weight gain and hypothyroidism in the mother
   - Preterm/IUGR (can develop metabolic syndrome later in life)
   - Mode of delivery: Elective LSCS (Lower Segment Cesarian Section) (large baby)
7. What is the significance of dietetic history?
   - Calorie intake
   - Craving for specific food items – sweetened beverages/potato chips/ice cream/fried items
   - Eating habits – watching TV while eating/picky eating
8. Explain the significance of family history in obesity.
   Syndromic causes/familial hypercholesterolemia/endocrine causes of obesity
9. Enumerate the findings in head-to-foot examination.
   - Features of Bardet–Bidel syndrome, Turner syndrome, and Down syndrome
   - Features of hypothyroidism
   - Eyes: Coloboma/cataract/retinitis pigmentosa/papilledema
   - Moon facies/buffalo hump/abdominal striae
   - Hirsutism
   - Acanthosis nigricans
   - Buried penis (because of increased pad of fat)
   - Tendon/palmar xanthomas
   - Hands: Polydactyly (Bardet–Bidel syndrome) and short metacarpals – pseudohypoparathyroidism
   - Legs: Tibial bowing
   - Skin hyperpigmentation
   - Sexual maturity rating
   Fig. 35.1A–D shows moon facies, buffalo hump, acanthosis nigricans, and buried penis, respectively.
10. List the findings in systemic examination.
   - Cardiovascular system: Features of ASD (Atrial Septal Defect)/VSD (Ventricular Septal Defect)/coarctation of aorta
   - Respiratory system: Tachypnea/intercostal retractions/wheeze
   - Abdomen: Tenderness/features of cirrhosis
   - Central nervous system: Hypotonia/diminished tendon reflexes/signs of raised ICT

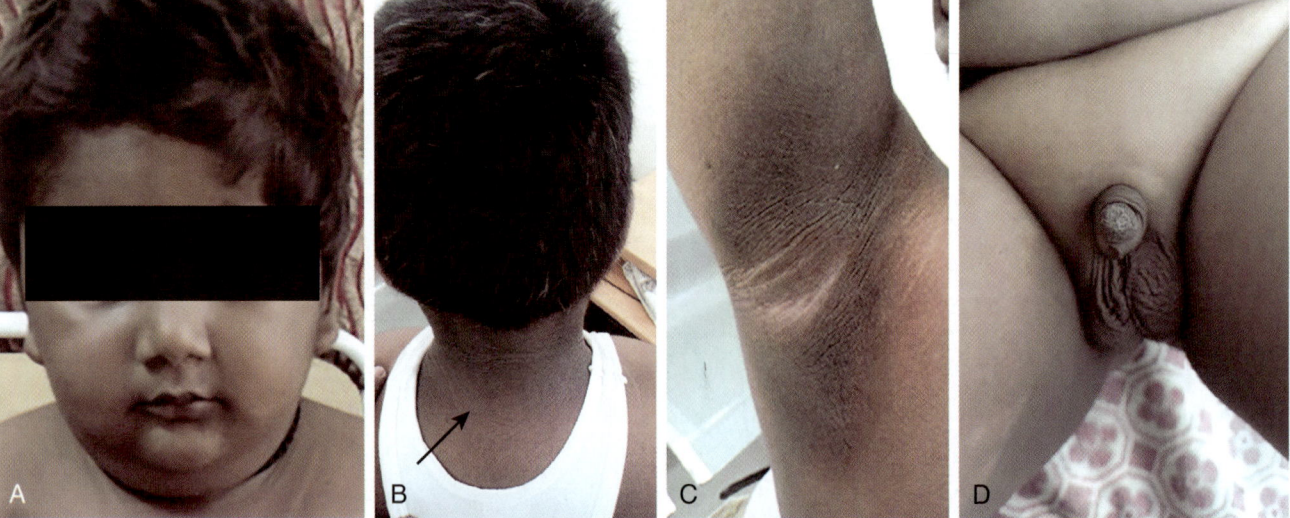

Fig. 35.1   (A) Moon facies. (B) Buffalo hump. (C) Acanthosis nigricans. (D) Buried penis.

11. Define overweight and obesity.
    - BMI (Body Mass Index) ≥95th percentile: Obesity
    - BMI between the 85th and 95th percentiles: Overweight
12. What is adiposity rebound?
    During childhood, levels of body fat change, beginning with high adiposity during infancy, and body fat levels decrease until 5.5 years when they are typically at the lowest level. Adiposity then increases until early adulthood.
13. Enumerate the various etiologies of obesity.
    Flowchart 35.1 shows the various etiologies of obesity
14. What are the comorbidities associated with obesity?
    - Cardiovascular system: Hypertension
    - Respiratory system: Obstructive sleep apnea and asthma
    - Gastrointestinal system: Gallstones, NASH, cirrhosis, GERD, and pancreatitis
    - Central nervous system: Pseudotumor cerebri and migraine
    - Psychological: Depression, anxiety, and poor scholastic performance
    - Musculoskeletal system: Blount disease
    - Metabolic: Dyslipidemia, diabetes mellitus, PCOD, and metabolic syndrome
15. What are the investigations performed in obesity?
    1. **Routinely for all patients**
       - Fasting blood sugar
       - Fasting lipid profile
       - Liver function test
       - Renal function test (to rule out hypertensive nephropathy)
       - Ultrasound abdomen/pelvis (to rule out PCOD)
       - Investigations for complications
    2. **For symptomatic patients**
       - MRI brain and CSF (Cerebrospinal Fluid) opening pressure
       - X-ray hip and knee
       - Polysomnography

    3. **Investigations for etiology**
       - Thyroid function test
       - Dexamethasone suppression test
       - Growth hormone challenge test and IGF-1 (Insulin Like Growth Factor-1) levels
       - Karyotyping
16. Enumerate the management of obesity.
    Flowchart 35.2 gives the management of obesity.
17. Enumerate the various dietary management strategies in obesity.
    - *Initial step*
      The initial step in dietary management consists of motivating the child and parents to reduce the weight.
    - *Traffic signal diet*
      - Calculate the calorie requirement according to Holliday–Segar formula and the required amount of calories can be supplemented by the green light foods and a small quantity of yellow light foods.
      - Similarly, if the mother reports that her child is eating extra meals or snacks because of increased appetite, then those extra meals/snacks can be replaced by green light foods.
      Table 35.1 shows the traffic signal diet.
    Protein-sparing modified fat diet
      - Intensive phase: For 3 months; the child provided with 800–900 kcal/day irrespective of the weight, the goal being to achieve 10% weight reduction in 3 months
      - Continuation phase: 1200 kcal/day for 9 months
      - Along with "rule of 2":
        - 2 g/kg of protein (maximum, 100 g)
        - 2 hours of outdoor activity
        - 2 hours of TV watching
        - 2 L of water per day
    Dietary advice
      - Adopt healthy eating habits.
      - Eat meals as a family at a fixed place and time.

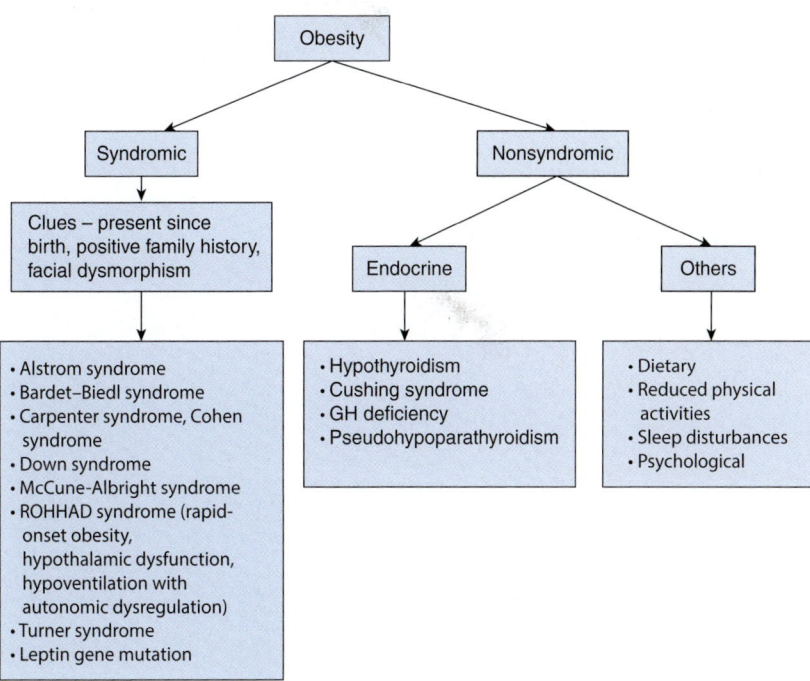

Flowchart 35.1 Etiologies of obesity.

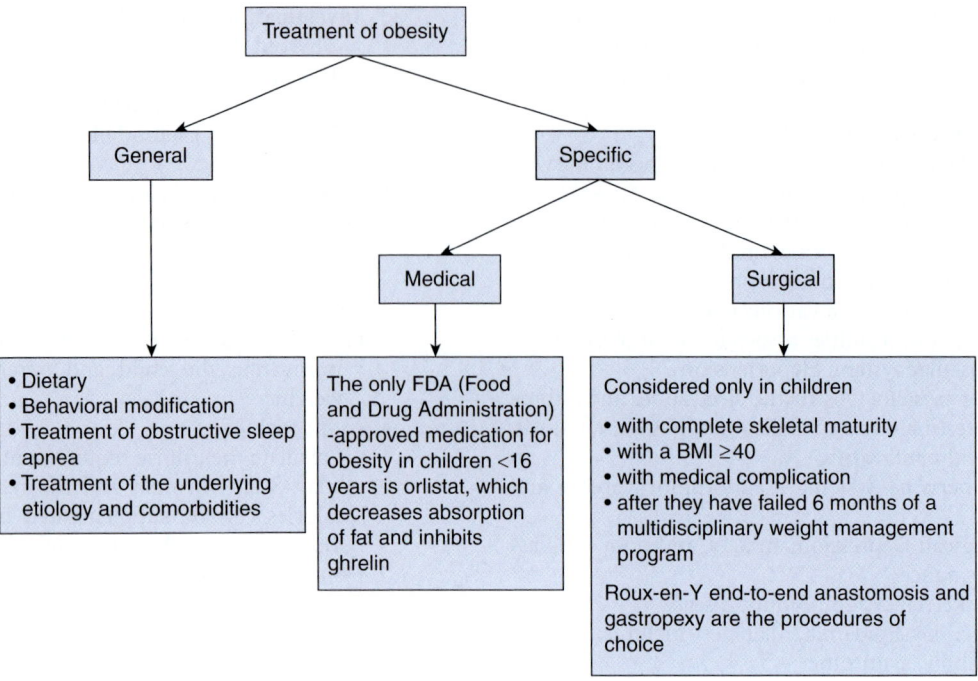

Flowchart 35.2   Management of obesity.

TABLE 35.1	**Traffic Signal Diet**		
Diet	**Quality**	**Type of Foods**	**Quantity**
Green light foods	Low-calorie, high-fiber, low-fat, nutrient-dense	Fruits, vegetables	Unlimited
Yellow light foods	Nutrient-dense, but higher in calories and fat	Lean meats, dairy, starches, grains	Limited
High in calories, sugar, and fat	High in calories, sugar, and fat	Fatty meats, sugar, sugar-sweetened beverages, fried foods	Infrequent or avoided

- Do not skip meals, especially breakfast.
- Do not watch television during meals.
- Use small plates, and keep serving dishes away from the table.
- Avoid unnecessary sweet or fatty foods and sugar-sweetened drinks.

- Remove televisions from children's bedrooms; restrict times for television viewing and video games.
- Do not use food as a reward.

18. Mention the various interventions to prevent obesity.
    - Breastfeeding (BF): Follow exclusive BF for 4–6 months and continue BF with other foods for 12 months.
    - Adopt healthy eating habits.
    - Promote physical activity, including 60 minutes of strenuous exercise five times weekly.
    - Avoid late-night video games/television watching
    - Inculcate the habit of early to bed and early to rise among children.
    - Treat sleep-disordered breathing.

Quick Bites

- The age of presentation of obesity gives a clue to the underlying etiology.
- Family history of obesity can be suggestive of syndromic causes, familial hypercholesterolemia, and endocrine causes of obesity.
- Dietary and behavioral modifications are the mainstay in the management of obesity.
- Orlistat is the only FDA-approved drug for the treatment of obesity in children.

36 Rickets

Following introduction, seek permission from the caregiver and introduce yourself to the patient before history elicitation, and identify the case.

Name_____Age_____Sex_____Consanguinity_____Order of birth_____Place_____Informant_____

Presenting Complaints and Duration

- Progressive bony deformity
- Bone pains and fractures
- Short stature – appears short for age/peers (not gaining adequate height as peers)
- Seizures in young infants and carpopedal spasm in older children
- Delayed dentition and dental deformities
- Proximal muscle weakness
- Delayed motor development

History of Presenting Illness

- Age of onset of symptoms
- Hypotonia and delayed motor development
- Recurrent respiratory tract infections
- Failure to thrive
- Seizures/tetany/stridor
- Delayed dentition/dental caries
- Large head
- Alopecia
- Bone pain/bony deformities
- Sticky, frothy, bulky, greasy, foul-smelling stool
- Jaundice, abdominal distension, and bleeding tendencies
- Polyuria, polydipsia, recurrent vomiting, and lethargy
- Any drug ingestion
- Duration of sunlight exposure and use of any sun screen
- Any visual problems
- Any hard of hearing

PAST HISTORY

Recurrent respiratory tract infections

ANTENATAL HISTORY

- Calcium supplement in an expectant mother
- Consanguinity (autosomal recessive disorder)
- Triradiate pelvis for mothers with osteomalacia
- Any malpresentations

BIRTH HISTORY

- Preterm/full term
- Birth weight
- Prolonged jaundice in the neonatal period

DEVELOPMENTAL HISTORY

Delayed motor milestones

FAMILY HISTORY

- Family history of similar illness – bony deformities especially in lower limbs, alopecia, unexplained short stature, and history of any unexplained sibling death during infancy

DIETETIC HISTORY

- Duration of exclusive breastfeeding
- Detailed history about weaning
- Formula feed – when started and number of times per day
- Any supplementation (vitamin/calcium)

SOCIOECONOMIC HISTORY

Exposure to sunlight – nature, duration, time of the day, and vertical slum

Ventilation and illumination – type of windows, doors, and clothing

General Examination

- Look for irritability.
- Look for pallor/icterus/edema.

Head-to-Foot Examination

HEAD

- Craniotabes
- Macrocephaly
- Hot cross bun
- Frontal bossing
- Delayed closure of anterior fontanelles and posterior fontanelles
- Alopecia
- Delayed dentition/caries
- Enamel dysplasias
- Tooth abscess

CHEST

- Rachitic rosary
- Harrison groove
- Fiddle-shaped chest
- Pectus carinatum
- Chest indrawing because of pneumonia

BACK

- Kyphosis/scoliosis/lordosis

EXTREMITIES

- Widening of wrists and ankles
- Varus/valgus deformities
- Windswept deformity
- Anterior bowing of the tibia and femur
- Coxa vara
- Double malleoli (Marfan sign – palpation of the tibial malleolus gives an impression of double malleoli)
- Intermalleolar distance

SKIN

- Hyperpigmented macules

Vital Signs

- Pulse rate and volume to be noted (in case of anemia in chronic kidney disease, hyperdynamic state is noted)
- Hypertension such as in kidney disease

Anthropometry

Macrocephaly and short stature

Systemic Examination

CARDIOVASCULAR SYSTEM

Congestive heart failure

RESPIRATORY SYSTEM

Chest infections/atelectasis

ABDOMEN

Protuberant abdomen and hepatosplenomegaly

CENTRAL NERVOUS SYSTEM

- Hypotonia, decreased deep tendon reflex, and proximal muscle weakness causing waddling gait
- Other features to look for: Cataract, glaucoma and senso-rineural hearing loss

Diagnosis

A child with rickets probably because of nutritional cause

Frequently Asked Questions

1. What is the adequate sunlight exposure for vitamin D synthesis?

   The adequate sunlight exposure for vitamin D synthesis is 10–30 minutes of exposure to the sunlight between 10 a.m. and 3 p.m. and the amount of Ultraviolet B radiation capable of producing previtamin D3 in the skin is 70 times more effective at 25°C than at 70°C because of the influence of the zenith angle of the sun.

2. Define rickets.

   Rickets is defined as the disease of the growing bone because of unmineralized matrix at the growth plate that occurs in children before the fusion of epiphysis.

3. Why is examination of skin important in rickets?
   - The presence of hyperpigmented macules suggests McCune–Albright syndrome/epidermal nevus syndrome.
   - Epidermal cysts are present in vitamin D–dependent rickets type 2.
   - In dark-skinned children, the production of vitamin D is less (because melanin absorbs the ultraviolet rays essential for vitamin D synthesis).

4. What are the earliest sign and symptom in rickets?

   The earliest symptom is excessive sweating. The earliest sign is craniotabes.

5. Define craniotabes and mention few differentials.

   Craniotabes refers to softening of the skull bones in the occipital and parietal regions along the sutural line because of osteoclasis (pingpong ball appearance).

   Differential diagnoses
   - Rickets
   - Osteogenesis imperfecta
   - Syphilis
   - Hydrocephalus
   - Normally seen in the first few weeks of a preterm

6. What is the reason for the occurrence of hot cross bun appearance?

   The hot cross bun appearance occurs because of uncalcified osteoid (excessive osteoid without remodeling with normally fused sutures).

7. Discuss the reason for the occurrence of hypotonia in rickets.

   Phosphocreatinine: Adenosine Triphosphate (ATP) ratio is altered in rickets and this is the reason for the occurrence of hypotonia.

8. What is Harrison sulcus?

   Harrison sulcus occurs because of the pulling of the softened ribs by the diaphragm during inspiration as shown in Fig. 36.1.

9. What are the differences between rachitic rosary and scorbutic rosary?

Rachitic Rosary (Visible Only When the Upper Limb Is Lifted)	Scorbutic Rosary
Nodular and rounded at the costochondral junction	Angulated with a sharper step-off at the costochondral junction
Nontender	Tender
Because of the widening of the costochondral junction	Because of the formation of subperiosteal hemorrhage and backward displacement of the costochondral junction

10. Discuss the radiological features of rickets and scurvy.

    Rickets:

    X-ray features of rickets are best visualized in the posteroanterior view.
    a. Widening of physis (growth plate)
    b. Loss of sharp border of the edge of metaphysis (fraying)
    c. Loss of the convex or flat surface of the edge of the metaphysis, which becomes concave (cupping) (Fig. 36.2)
    d. Coarse trabeculation of diaphysis
    e. Generalized rarefaction
    f. Absence of provisional zone of calcification

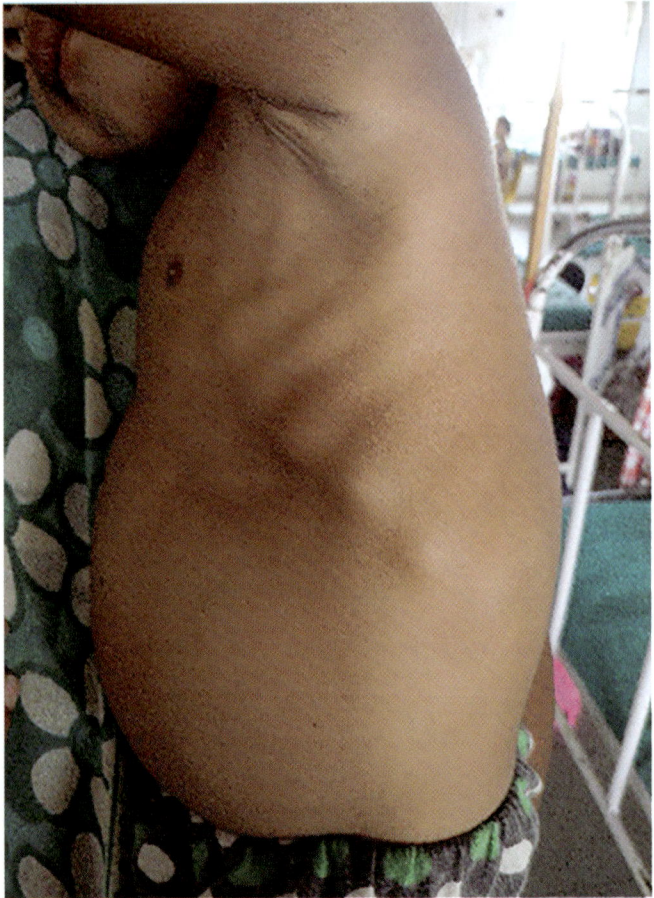

Fig. 36.1 Harrison sulcus.

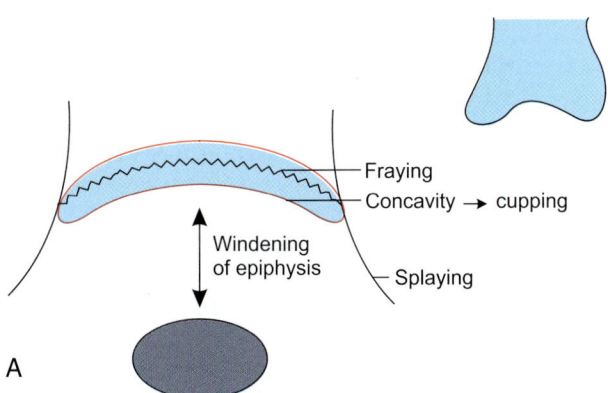

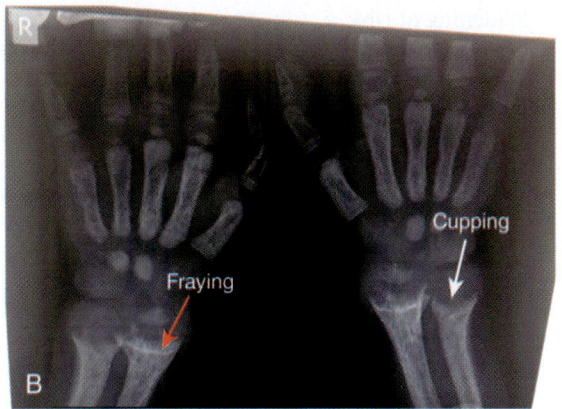

Fig. 36.2   (A) X-ray findings in rickets in long bone – illustration. (B) Cupping, fraying, and coarse trabeculation of diaphysis.

Scurvy

In scurvy, radiological features occur at the distal ends of long bones.

a. Ground glass appearance because of trabecular atrophy

b. Thin cortex called the pencil outlining of the diaphysis and epiphysis

c. An irregular but thickened white line at the metaphysis representing the zone of well-calcified cartilage called "white line of Frankel"

d. A zone of rarefaction, which is a linear break in the bone parallel and proximal to the white line representing an area of debris of broken-down trabeculae and connective tissues, called "Trummerfeld zone" (a late radiological feature)

e. A lateral projection of the white line at the cortical ends, called "Pelkan spur"

f. Ringed epiphysis

g. Possibility of occurrence of calcification on the sides beyond the metaphysis and seeing the broken chips of bone at the corner because of weight bearing, which is called "corner sign"

Fig. 36.3 shows the findings in X-ray in scurvy in an infant.

11. What are the radiological features of osteopenia?

• Prominence of the medial end of the clavicle (head light sign)

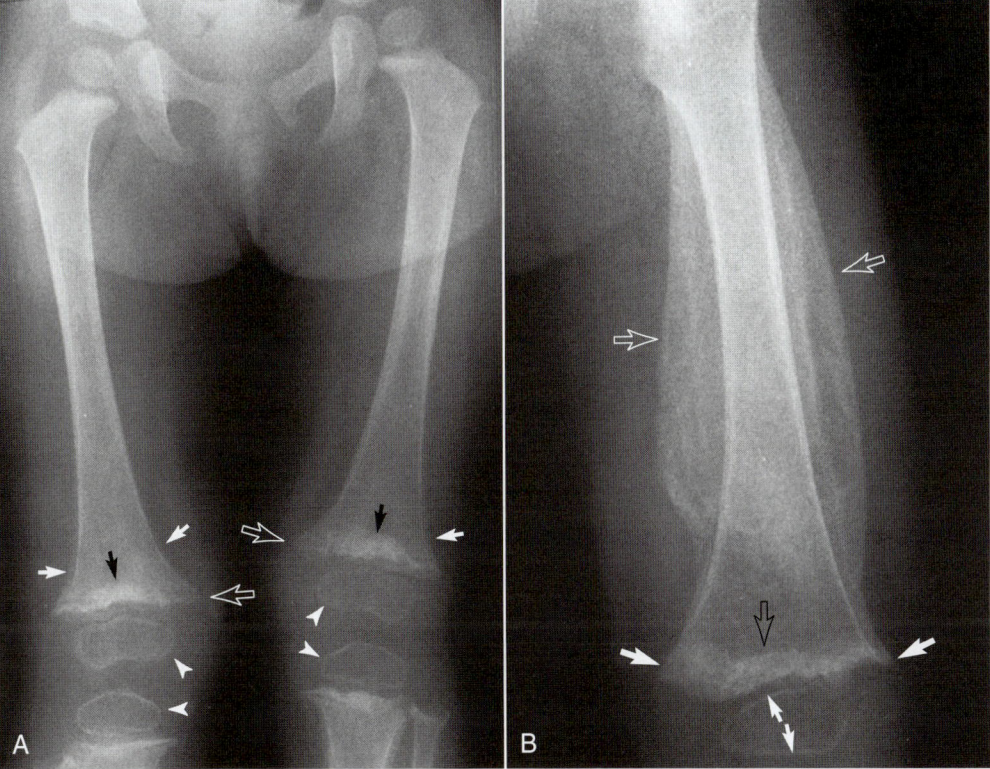

Fig. 36.3   X-ray findings in scurvy. Bilateral femoral radiographs demonstrate subtle periostitis caused by subperiosteal hemorrhage (white arrows), thick, sclerotic metaphyseal lines (black arrows), beaklike excrescences (Pelken spurs) (open arrows), and radiodense shells around the radiolucent epiphyses (Wimberger ring) (arrowheads). *(Source:* Reproduced from John Taylor, Tudor Hughes, Donald Resnick. *Skeletal Imaging: Atlas of the Spine and Extremeties*, Second Edition Femur, FIGURE 8-50, St. Louis, Saunders, 2011.)

- Widening of ribs
- Nonvisualization of spinous processes of the vertebrae
- Lower mineral bone density

12. Mention X-ray feature of rickets in newborn.
   "Mandible mantle sign" – subperiosteal bone formation in the 6th week in rickets of prematurity

13. How do calcipenic and phosphopenic rickets present clinically?
   Table 36.1 shows the differences between calcipenic and phosphopenic rickets.

14. Discuss the differences in the laboratory parameters between calcipenic and phosphopenic rickets.
   Table 36.2 shows the differences in the laboratory parameters between calcipenic and phosphopenic rickets.

15. What are the causes of rickets in a preterm?
   a. Transfer of vitamin D from the mother to the baby more during the third trimester
   b. Rapid growth and higher demand
   c. Breast milk deficient in vitamin D
   d. Prolonged parenteral nutrition
   e. Use of excessive antibiotics, diuretics, and steroids
   f. Cholestatic jaundice

16. What are the clinical features of rickets of prematurity?
   - Commonly manifests in 1–4 months of age
   - Irritability
   - Forehead sweating
   - Nontraumatic fracture of legs, arms, and ribs
   - Softening of ribs → decreased lung compliance → atelectasis and poor ventilation → respiratory distress (rachitic respiratory distress) – develops beyond 5 weeks

- Negative effects on growth >1 year of age (poor linear growth)
- Enamel hypoplasia
- Dolichocephaly, frontal bossing, rachitic rosary, craniotabes, and widening of wrists and ankles
- A screening X-ray taken at 6–8 weeks of age if an infant is at risk

17. Who are at risk of rickets?
   Preterm babies and children with renal and hepatic disorders and malabsorptive states are said to be at risk.

18. Why is ocular examination important in rickets?
   - Pallor
   - Icterus
   - Cataract (Lowe syndrome)
   - Poor visual acuity and visual problems because of cystinosis (Lowe syndrome present as Fanconi syndrome – hypophosphatemic rickets)
   - Fundus examination in Lowe syndrome (Fanconi syndrome) – "circinate irregularities"

19. What are the common causes of alopecia in pediatrics?
   - Vitamin D - dependent rickets (VDDR) type 2
   - Ectodermal dysplasia
   - Children on chemotherapy

20. What is the common age of presentation of nutritional rickets?
   Six to 36 months of age because of the rapid growth

21. Classify 25(OH)-vitamin D as per the recent Indian Academy of Pediatrics (IAP) guidelines.
   - >20 ng/mL (50 nmol/L): Sufficient
   - 12–20 ng/mL (30–50 nmol/L): Insufficient
   - <12 ng/mL (<30 nmol/L): Deficient

22. Discuss the US Institute Of Medicine (IOM) and US Endocrine Society classification of 25-hydroxyvitamin D level.
   US IOM classification
   - Severe deficiency: <5 ng/mL
   - Deficiency: <15 ng/mL
   - Insufficiency: 15–20 ng/mL
   - Sufficient: >20 ng/mL
   - Excess: >100 ng/mL
   US Endocrine Society classification
   - Deficiency: <20 ng/mL
   - Insufficiency: 21–29 ng/mL
   - Sufficiency: >30 ng/mL
   - Toxicity: >150 ng/mL

23. **Classify rickets.**
   Calcipenic rickets
   - Congenital vitamin D deficiency
   - Nutritional vitamin D deficiency
   - Secondary vitamin D deficiency causes such as malabsorption, liver dysfunction, and increased degradation such as drug induced
   - Chronic kidney disease
   - Vitamin D-dependent rickets (VDDR) 1A and B
   - Vitamin D-dependent rickets (VDDR) 2A and B
   - Dietary deficiency of calcium
   Phosphopenic rickets
   Phosphorus deficiency
   - Rickets of prematurity
   - Inadequate intake
   Renal loss
   - X-linked hypophosphatemic rickets
   - Autosomal dominant hypophosphatemic rickets

TABLE 36.1	Differences Between Calcipenic and Phosphopenic Rickets	
Features	Calcipenic Rickets	Phosphopenic Rickets
Muscle weakness	Present	Absent
Bone pain	Common	Uncommon
Extremities involved	Both upper and lower limbs	Lower limb predominantly
Tetany	Present	Absent
Enamel hypoplasia	May be present	Absent
Dental abscess	Absent	May be present

TABLE 36.2	Differences in Laboratory Parameters Between Calcipenic and Phosphopenic Rickets	
Features	Calcipenic Rickets	Phosphopenic Rickets
Serum calcium	Low/normal	Normal
Serum phosphorus	Low	Low
Serum parathormone	Elevated	Normal/slightly elevated
Serum alkaline phosphatase	Markedly elevated	Mild to moderate elevation
Osteopenia and osteitis fibrosa	Present	Absent

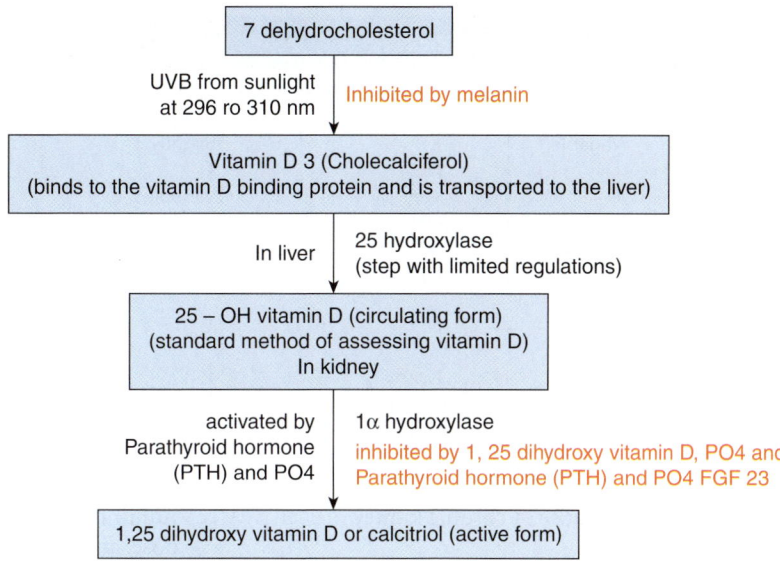

Flowchart 36.1 Physiology of vitamin D formation.

- Autosomal recessive hypophosphatemic rickets types 1 and 2
- Hereditary hypophosphatemic rickets and hyper-calciuria

Overproduction of phosphatonins*
- Epidermal nevus syndrome
- Tumor-induced rickets
- McCune–Albright syndrome
- Generalized disease with phosphaturia
  - Dent disease
  - Fanconi syndrome
  - Distal renal tubular acidosis

24. What is the physiology of the formation of vitamin D?
    Flowchart 36.1 gives the physiology of vitamin D formation.

25. What are the investigations performed for rickets?
    Basic investigations to confirm rickets
    - Serum Ca, P, and Serum alkaline phosphate
    - X-ray of ends of long bones at knees or wrists

    Classical radiological changes
    - Disappearance of the provisional zone of calcification
    - Widening, fraying, and cupping of the distal ends of the shaft

    Second-level investigations
    - Blood urea, creatinine, electrolytes, and Arterial Blood Gas
    - Tubular reabsorption of phosphate (TRP)
    - TRP = 100 − FEP#

      #Fractional Excretion of Phosphate (FEP)

      $$= \frac{\text{Urine phosphate} \times \text{serum creatinine} \times 100}{\text{Serum phosphate} \times \text{urine creatinine}}$$

    - Serum Fibroblast Growth factor-23 (FGF-23)
    - Coagulation profile
    - Urine analysis for specific gravity, glucose, protein, amino acids, potassium, and calcium

- Ultrasound abdomen
- Liver function test
- Stool microscopy for malabsorption
- Inborn error of metabolism studies

Tertiary-level investigations
- Estimation of vitamin D metabolites to differentiate VDDR type 1 from type 2
- Receptor–vitamin D interaction – in vitro study to assess VDDR type 2
- Bone mineral content
- Bone densitometry

26. What are the biochemical markers in different types of rickets?
    Table 36.3 shows the biochemical markers in different types of rickets.

    Points to remember
    - Phosphate (PO_4) level is decreased in all the conditions except chronic kidney disease.
    - PO_4 supplement is given in all the conditions except chronic kidney disease in which PO_4 binders are given instead.
    - 25-Hydroxyvitamin D is normal or slightly increased in all the conditions except nutritional and VDDR-1B.

27. Discuss the similarities and differences between hereditary hypophosphatemic rickets (HHR) and Dent disease.
    Similarities between the two
    The phosphate loss is more; because of hypophosphatemia, the enzyme 1α-hydroxylase is upregulated and hence 1,25-dihydroxyvitamin D is normal.
    Hypercalcemia is present in both the conditions.
    Differences

HHR	Dent Disease
Sodium phosphate cotransporter	Chloride channel transporter defect
Channel defect SLC34A3	Channel defect CLCN5
No low-molecular-weight proteinuria	Low-molecular-weight proteinuria present

---

*Frizzled related protein-4 (FRP-4) and Matrix Extracellular Phosphoglycoprotein (MEPE) have Fibroblast Growth factor 23 (FGF-23) activity.

TABLE 36.3	Biochemical Markers in Different Types of Rickets						
Type	Ca	PO4	25-Hydroxyvitamin D	1,25-Dihy-droxyvitamin D	PTH	Alkaline Phosphatase (ALP)	FGF23
Nutritional	Variable	↓	↓	Slightly ↑	↑	↑	NA
VDDR-1A	↓	↓	N/↑	↓	↑	↑	NA
VDDR-1B	↓	↓	Very ↓	Variable	↑	↑	NA
VDDR-2	↓	↓	N/↑	↑	↑	↑	NA
X-hypophosphatemic rickets	Normal	↓↓	N/↑	↓	Normal	↑	↑
Autosomal recessive hypophosphatemic rickets	Normal	↓↓	N/↑	↓	Normal	↑	↑
Autosomal dominant hypophosphatemic rickets	Normal	↓↓	N/↑	↓	Normal	↑	↑
Hereditary hypophosphatemic rickets	Normal	↓↓	Normal	↑	Normal	↑	Normal
Dent disease	Normal	↓↓	Normal	↑	Normal	↑	Normal
Rickets of prematurity	Variable	↓	Normal	↑	Normal	↑↑	Normal

28. What is peculiar about rickets because of chronic kidney disease?
   - Rickets because of chronic kidney disease occurs because of the decreased activity of 1α-hydroxylase.
   - The serum phosphate levels are high because of poor excretion of the phosphate.
   - Hence, phosphate (PO4) binders are given and dietary restriction of phosphate is advised unlike the other conditions.
   - Frontal bossing and craniotabes are not usually seen here; rather, occipital bossing is prominent.
   - Lower limb involvement is more.

29. Which type of rickets is associated with arterial calcification and associated gene defect?
   Autosomal recessive hypophosphatemic rickets type 2 is associated with arterial calcifications and the gene defect is Ecto-Nucleotide Pyrophosphatase/Phosphodiesterase (ENPP-1).

30. What are the conditions associated with overproduction of FGF23?
   - Tumor-induced osteomalacia
   - McCune–Albright syndrome (triad of polycystic fibrous dysplasia, hyperpigmented macules, and polyendocrinopathy)
   - Epidermal nevus syndrome
   - Neurofibromatosis

31. What is the standard dose of vitamin D supplementation in a child with rickets?
   Administer 1000–2000 IU of vitamin D orally per day until radiographic improvement is seen; then switch to 400 IU/day for <1 year and 600 IU/day for >1 year along with calcium and PO4 supplements.

32. What is Stoss regimen?
   Stoss regimen is as follows:
   a. Administer 600,000 IU of vitamin D orally in six doses (100,000 IU/dose) every 2 hours over a period of 12 hours followed by daily supplementation of vitamin D at a dose of 400 IU/day for <1 year and 600 IU/day for >1 year along with calcium and PO4 supplements started 3 months after Stoss regimen. But this is not applicable for less than 1 year.
   Or
   b. Administer 300,000 IU of vitamin D2 orally in a single dose.
   Or

   c. Administer 600,000 IU intramuscularly as a single dose, and then 400 IU/day.

33. What is resistant rickets?
   - If there is no provisional zone of calcification after 2 weeks of administration of Stoss regimen, repeat one more dose of vitamin D2. If still there is no evidence of provisional zone of calcification by the 4th week, then it is resistant to therapy.
   - Remember that if the child is resistant to the above-mentioned regimen, check for three "Ps," namely, phosphate, pH, and PTH.

34. What is the IAP recommendation for prevention and treatment of vitamin D deficiency?
   The IAP recommendation for prevention and treatment of vitamin D deficiency are as follows:
   - In Preterm neonate, the prevention and treatment dose of vitamin D are 400 IU/day and 1000 IU/day respectively.
   - In Term neonate, the prevention and treatment dose of vitamin D are 400 IU/day and 2000 IU/day respectively.
   - In 2–12 months old infant, the prevention and treatment dose of vitamin D are 400 IU/day and 2000 IU/day respectively. For infants older than 3 months of age, additional dose of 60,000 IU of vitamin D is given weekly for 6 weeks orally.
   - In 1–18 years old children, the prevention and treatment dose of vitamin D are 600IU/day and 3000–6000IU/day respectively. Additionally, a dose of 60,000IU of vitamin D is given weekly for 6 weeks orally.

   The calcium supplementation in vitamin D deficiency are as follows:
   - In Preterm neonate, the prevention and treatment dose of calcium supplementation are 150–220 mg/kg/day and 175–200 mg/kg/day respectively.
   - In Term neonate, the prevention and treatment dose of calcium supplementation are 200 mg/day and 500 mg/day respectively.
   - In 2–12 months of age, the prevention and treatment dose of calcium supplementation are 250–500 mg/day and 500 mg/day respectively.
   - In 1–18 years of age, the prevention and treatment dose of calcium supplementation are 600–800 mg/day and 600–800 mg/day respectively.

35. How is a child on treatment for rickets monitored?
While on calcitriol
- The serum calcium level should be maintained at low normal range and the parathormone level at high normal range so that excess calcitriol and hence nephrocalcinosis and hypercalciuria can be avoided.
- In addition, urine calcium should be monitored (target level is <4 mg/kg/day).
- In X-linked hypophosphatemic rickets, normalization of alkaline phosphate is a better indicator of response to treatment than PO_4 levels because of its variation in levels.
- In rickets of prematurity, periodic measurement of serum bicarbonate is important because metabolic acidosis can cause dissolution of bones.

36. What is the poor prognostic sign in rickets?
Presence of proteinuria

37. What are the mimics of rickets and how are they different from rickets?
- Metaphyseal dysplasia: Here the serum levels of calcium, phosphorus, and vitamin D are normal but the radiological features are always confused with rickets. In this, there is flaring of metaphysis at the end of long bones, often radiolucent, with relative constriction and sclerosis of the diaphysis. In rickets, cupping and fraying in the metaphyseal end, widening of joint space, and decreased bone mineral density – rarefaction – are present.

- Hypophosphatasia: Here, the conspicuous laboratory finding is low alkaline phosphatase level, which is almost never seen in rickets.

38. What is renal osteodystrophy (ROD)? Discuss the radiological findings in ROD.
- In ROD, bone changes occur as a consequence of chronic kidney disease (CKD). The biochemistry and pathogenesis of bone changes are different from those of the vitamin D and phosphorous deficiency rickets.
- Radiological manifestations of ROD are as follows:
  - Widening of epiphysis with cupping and fraying seen in infants
  - Slipped epiphysis and genu valgum, and growth retardation in preadolescents
  - Subperiosteal erosions of the phalanges, proximal end of the tibia, neck of the femur, humerus, and distal end of the clavicle

39. Enumerate stagewise approach to rickets.
Flowchart 36.2 gives the stagewise approach to rickets.

40. How is calcipenic rickets approached?
Flowchart 36.3 shows the approach to calcipenic rickets.

41. How is a case of phosphopenic rickets approached?
Flowchart 36.4 shows the approach to phosphopenic rickets.

42. How is a child with renal rickets approached?
Flowchart 36.5 shows the approach to renal rickets.

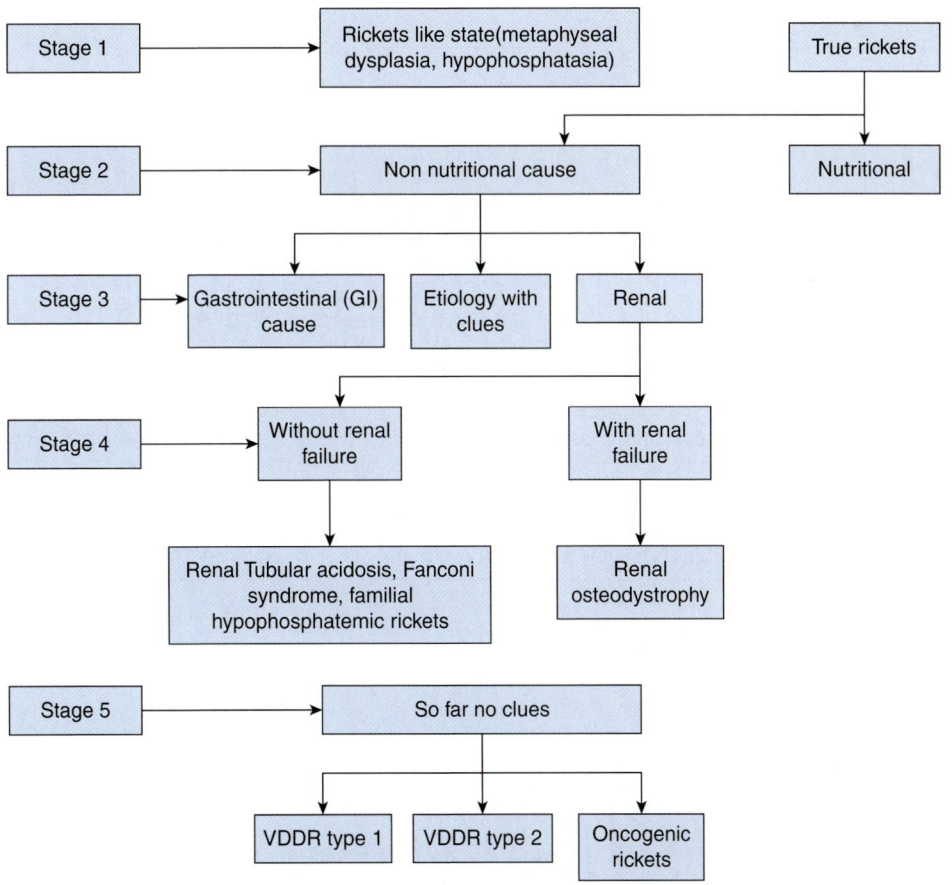

Flowchart 36.2 Stagewise approach to rickets.

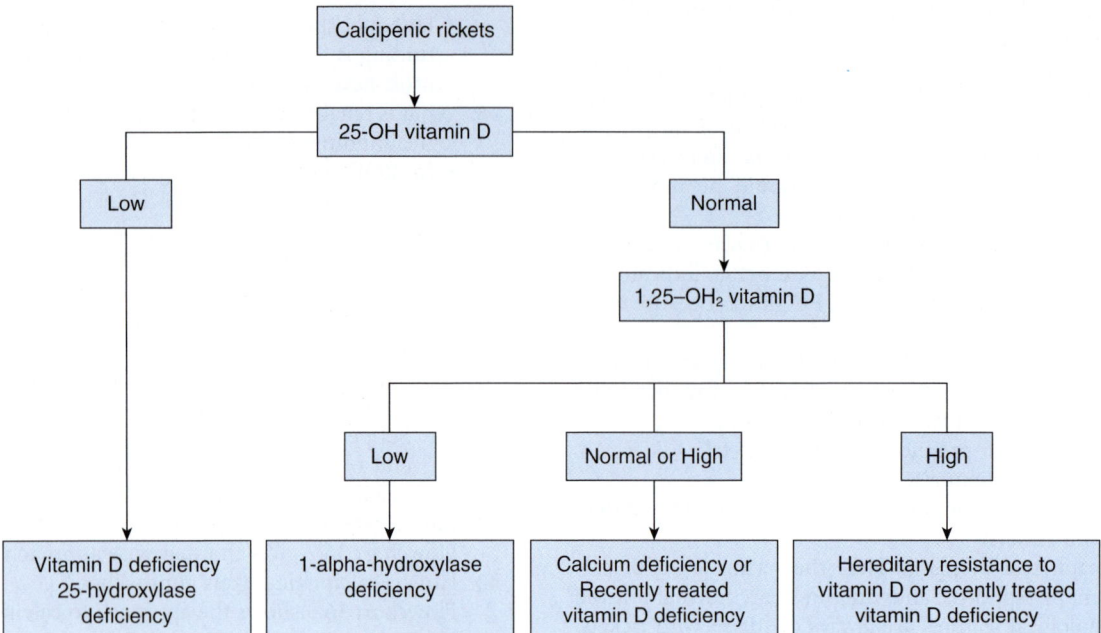

Flowchart 36.3 Approach to calcipenic rickets.

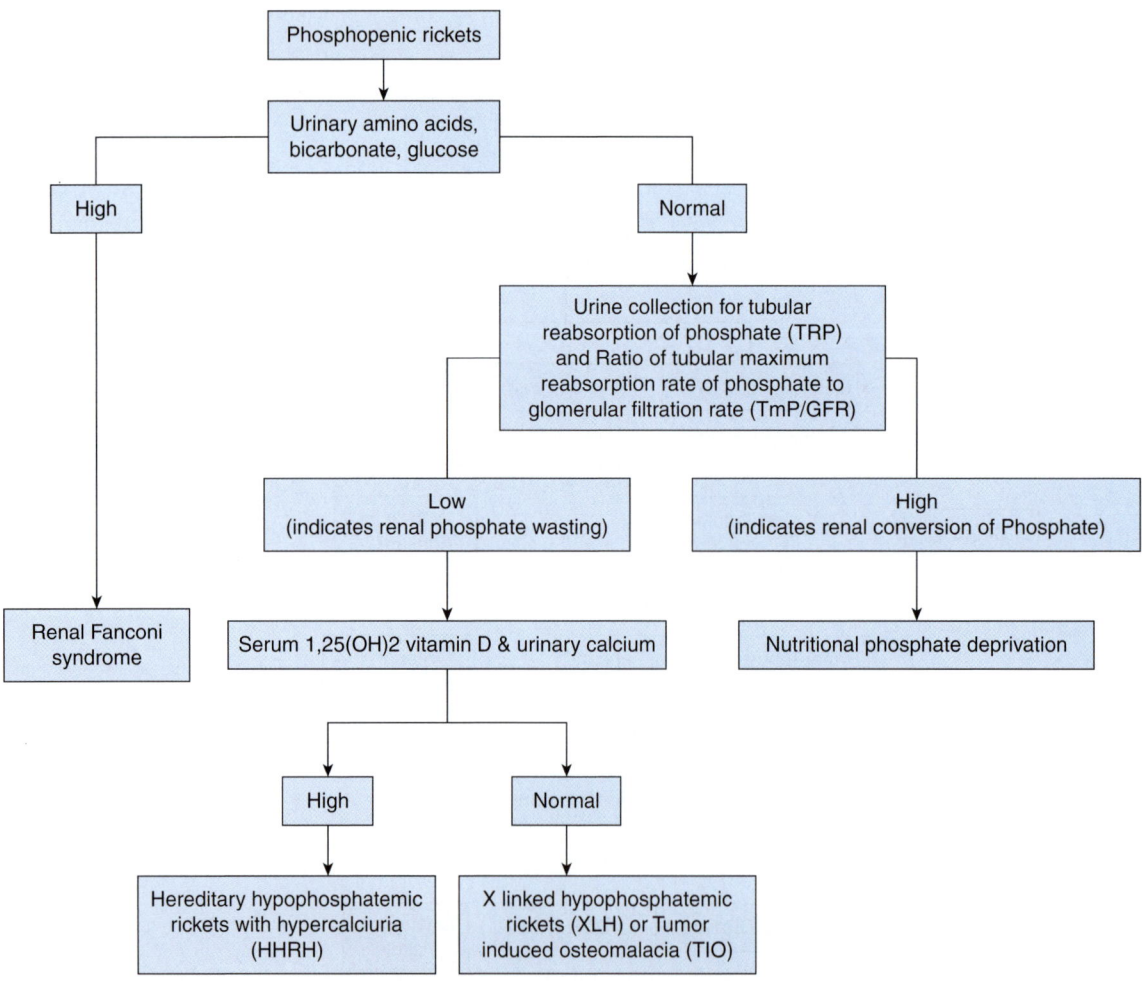

Flowchart 36.4 Approach to phosphopenic rickets.

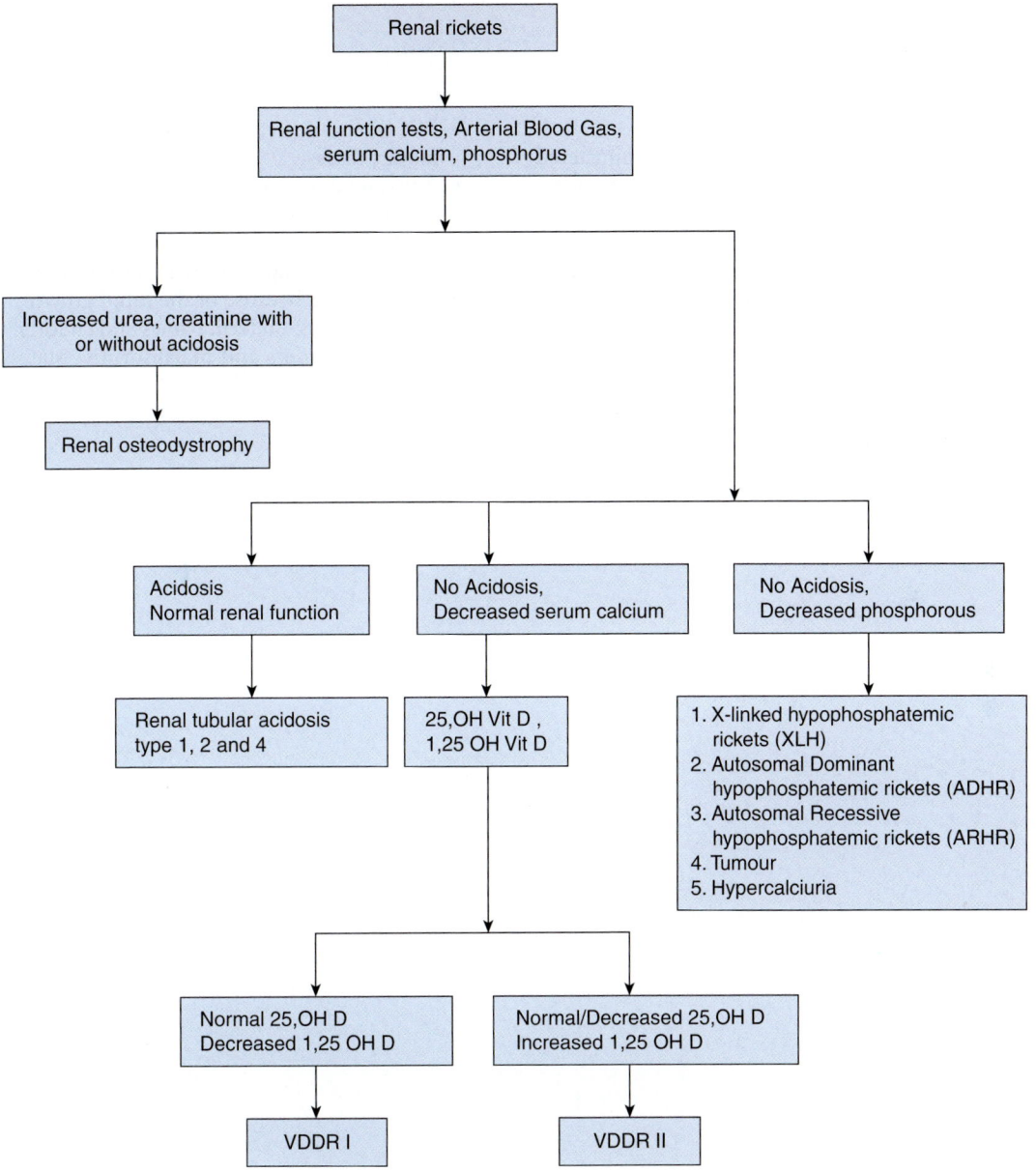

Flowchart 36.5   Approach to renal rickets.

Quick Bites

- Stoss regimen: 600,000 IU of vitamin D2 is administered orally in six doses (100,000 IU/dose) every 2 hours over a period of 12 hours.
- Remember that if the child is resistant to the standard dose in vitamin D treatment after two mega dose in 2-week interval, check for three "Ps," namely, phosphate, pH, and PTH.
- The poor prognostic sign in rickets is the presence of proteinuria.
- 25-Hydroxyvitamin D is normal or slightly increased in all the conditions except nutritional and VDDR-1B.
- PO_4 level is decreased in all the conditions except chronic kidney disease.
- Autosomal recessive hypophosphatemic rickets type 2 is associated with arterial calcifications and the gene defect is ENPP-1
- The common age of presentation of nutritional rickets is 6–36 months because of the rapid growth.
- Risk of rickets: Preterm babies and children with renal and hepatic disorders and malabsorptive states are said to be at risk.

Hypothyroidism

Following introduction, seek permission from the caregiver and introduce yourself to the patient before history elicitation, and identify the case.

Name____Age____Sex____Consanguinity____Order of birth____Place____Informant____

Presenting Complaints and Duration

- Newborn: Poor feeding/lethargy/delayed passage of meconium/jaundice
- Beyond the newborn period: Lethargy/constipation/developmental delay/floppiness of limbs

History of Presenting Illness

- The presenting complaints described in a chronological order
- History for clinical features of hypothyroidism
  - Dry skin
  - Hearing impairment
  - Hoarse cry
  - Delayed dentition
  - Swelling of the neck (older children)
  - Intolerance to cold (older children)
  - Abdominal distension
  - Constipation
  - Limb weakness
  - Edema of limbs

COMPLICATION HISTORY

- Poor scholastic performance/behavioral changes
- Increased weight gain/failure to gain adequate height
- Breathlessness
- Noisy breathing
- Delayed development of secondary sexual characters

ETIOLOGICAL HISTORY

- Drug intake
- Irradiation to the head and neck
- Any neck surgery
- Head trauma

ANTENATAL HISTORY

- Hyperthyroidism/hypothyroidism in the mother
- Antithyroid drugs
- Reduced fetal movements

NATAL/POSTNATAL HISTORY

- Term/preterm
- Birth asphyxia
- NICU (Neonatal Intensive Care Unit) admission
- Passage of meconium
- Hoarse cry/poor feeding
- Jaundice

DEVELOPMENTAL HISTORY

- Delayed milestones
- Poor scholastic performance

DIETETIC HISTORY

- Mention about consumption of iodized salt
- Intake of goitrogens (cabbages, cauliflower, broccoli, millets)

FAMILY HISTORY

- Similar complaints in family members
- Endemic goiter (other family members are also affected)

Summary

A …-year-old child presented with (say history suggestive of hypothyroidism probably) congenital/acquired with/without complications.

General Examination

- Sensorium
- Pallor
- Icterus
- Cyanosis
- Generalized lymphadenopathy
- Edema

Head-to-Foot Examination

- Head: Head size, wide open fontanelles, thick scalp hair, scanty hair, low hairline in forehead, and alopecia
- Facies: Short forehead, widely spaced eyes, depressed nasal bridge, open mouth, protruding tongue, and short neck
- Eyes: Myxedematous swelling of lids/synophrys/pallor/icterus
- Midline cleft palate/midfacial hypoplasia (central hypothyroidism)
- Oral cavity: Delayed dentition/open mouth/protruding tongue/macroglossia
- Neck swelling
- Umbilical hernia
- Skin: Dry and scaly, cool, vitiligo, yellow because of jaundice and carotenemia, and mucocutaneous candidiasis (autoimmune polyglandular syndrome-1 [APS-1])
- Features of Down syndrome, Turner syndrome, and William syndrome looked for
- Calf muscle pseudohypertrophy
- Sexual maturity rating

Vital Signs

- Pulse rate
- Blood pressure
- Respiration: Rate, rhythm, and type of respiration
- Temperature
- JVP (Jugular venous pressure)

Anthropometry

Look for obesity and short stature.

System Examination

CARDIOVASCULAR SYSTEM

Signs of pericardial effusion

RESPIRATORY SYSTEM

Apnea/signs of pleural effusion

ABDOMEN

- Abdominal distension
- Bruit over the liver

CENTRAL NERVOUS SYSTEM

Higher mental functions/hypotonia/weakness/diminished tendon reflexes/choreoathetosis

Diagnosis

- A case of congenital/acquired hypothyroidism
- With/without complications
- Probable etiology mentioned (if it is an acquired hypothyroidism)

Frequently Asked Questions

*1. Explain the significance of age in hypothyroidism.
- The clinical presentation varies according to the age and helps in differentiating between congenital and acquired hypothyroidism.
  - 0–7 days: Poor feeding, lethargy, respiratory problems because of a large tongue, delayed passage of meconium, and wide open fontanelles
  - 7–28 days: Failure to gain weight after 10 days, prolonged cholestasis, and coarse facies
  - Older than 1 month: Above-mentioned features + hypotonia + umbilical hernia
- Age can also help in interpreting the growth and development and to tailor the need of l-thyroxine dose.
- Prognosis is better if the onset of hypothyroidism is after 2 years.

2. Explain the significance of gender in hypothyroidism.
- Autoimmune thyroiditis common in females
- Kocher–Debré–Semelaigne syndrome common in boys

3. Explain the significance of the place of residence.
- People living in hilly areas are prone to iodine deficiency.
- Iodine deficiency is rare in those living in coastal areas.

4. List the findings in general examination.
- Sensorium: Altered sensorium because of mental retardation
- Pallor: Macrocytic anemia/can be because of edema
- Icterus: Cholestatic jaundice/autoimmune hepatitis
- Cyanosis: Because of apnea/airway obstruction
- Generalized lymphadenopathy: Because of LCH (Langerhans cell histiocytosis) (which can cause acquired hypothyroidism)
- Edema

5. List the findings in head-to-foot examination.
Fig. 37.1 shows macroglossia in a child with hypothyroidism.

---

*Important question asked in the examination.

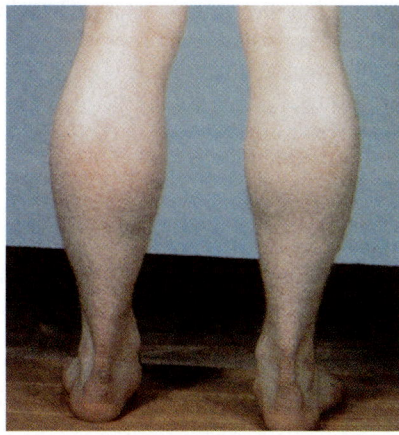

Fig. 37.2 Calf muscle pseudohypertrophy (Kocher–Debré–Semelaigne syndrome). *Source:* Reproduced from Kathryn McCance, Sue Huether. Pathophysiology: *The Biologic Basis for Disease in Adults and Children,* Sixth Edition, Alteration in Conginitive Systems, Cerebral Hemodynamics, and Motor Function, Figure 16.23, St. Louis, Mosby, 2010. (Credit line - From Perkin GD: Mosbys color atlas and text of neurology, London, 1998, Mosby-Wolfe.)

Fig. 37.2 shows calf muscle pseudohypertrophy in a child with Kocher–Debré–Semelaigne syndrome.
- Head
  - Head size may be slightly increased because of myxedema of the brain.
  - Wide open fontanelles, thick scalp hair, scanty hair, and low hairline in the forehead are present.
  - Alopecia is seen in autoimmune polyglandular syndrome-1 (APS-1).
- Facies: Short forehead, widely spaced eyes, depressed nasal bridge, open mouth, protruding tongue, and short neck
- Eyes: Myxedematous swelling of lids/synophrys/pallor/icterus
- Midline cleft palate/midfacial hypoplasia (central hypothyroidism)
- Oral cavity: Delayed dentition/open mouth/protruding tongue/macroglossia
- Neck swelling
- Skin: Dry and scaly, cool, vitiligo, and yellow because of jaundice and carotenemia
Mucocutaneous candidiasis (APS-1)
- Features of Down syndrome (30% of patients develop antithyroid antibodies), features of Turner syndrome (40% of patients develop antithyroid antibodies), and features of William syndrome (50% of patients develop subclinical hypothyroidism) looked for
- Calf muscle pseudohypertrophy: Kocher–Debré–Semelaigne syndrome
- Sexual maturity rating

6. What is the significance of vital signs in hypothyroidism?
- Pulse rate: Bradycardia and low sleeping pulse rate
- Blood pressure: Hypotension
- Tachypnea: Because of pericardial effusion/pleural effusion
- Temperature: Hypothermia
- JVP: Elevated because of pericardial effusion

7. List the findings in systemic examination.
- Cardiovascular system: Signs of pericardial effusion
- Respiratory system: Apnea/signs of pleural effusion

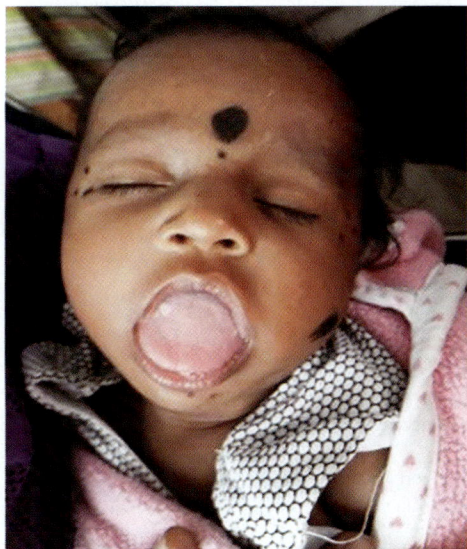

Fig. 37.1 Macroglossia in hypothyroidism.

- Abdomen: Abdominal distension (because of constipation, hypotonia, umbilical hernia) and bruit over the liver (hemangiomas of the liver causing acquired hypothyroidism)
- Central nervous system
  - Higher mental functions
  - Hypotonia
  - Weakness
  - Diminished tendon reflexes
  - Choreoathetosis
  - Ataxia (congenital hypothyroidism because of TTF-1 mutations)

8. Describe the embryology of the thyroid gland.
   - Develops from the floor of the foramen cecum
   - 4 weeks: Start of thyroglobulin synthesis
   - 7 weeks: Bilobed structure formed
   - 10 weeks: Migration to the thyroid cartilage, differentiation of thyroid follicles, and iodide trapping
   - 12 weeks: Beginning of T4 and TSH (Thyroid Stimulating hormone) secretion
   - Second half of gestation to 26 weeks: Maturation of the hypothalamic–pituitary–thyroid axis, which continues postnatally up to 3 months.

9. Enumerate the steps in thyroid hormone synthesis.
   a. Iodide trapping: By Na–I symport (also present in salivary glands, breast, placenta)
   b. Secretion of iodide into colloid by Cl–I antiport (pendrin protein)
   c. Oxidation of iodine by thyroid peroxidase enzyme
   d. Organification of iodine: Iodine attached to tyrosine residue in thyroglobulin molecule
   e. Coupling reaction

   $$\text{Monoiodotyrosine (MIT)} + \text{diiodotyrosine (DIT)} = T3$$
   $$DIT + DIT = T4$$
   $$DIT + MIT = \text{reverse } T3$$

   f. Release of thyroid hormone

10. Describe the physiology of T3 and T4 in the circulation.
    - Only 20% of circulating T3 is secreted by the thyroid gland; the rest is produced locally by deiodination.
    - There are three types of deiodinase enzymes:
      - Type 1, 5′-deiodinase: Converts T4 to T3 in the liver, kidney, and other extrathyroid tissues
      - Type 2, 5′-deiodinase: Converts T4 to T3 in the brain and pituitary
      - Type 3, 5′-deiodinase: Converts T4 to reverse T3
    - T3 is three to four times more potent than T4.
    - Seventy percent of T4 is bound to thyroid-binding globulin, and the remaining is bound to transthyretin (albumin).
    - Free T4 constitutes 0.03% of total T4 in circulation.
    - Fifty percent of T3 is bound to globulin, 50% to albumin, and 0.3% constitutes free T3.

11. What is the normal TSH surge following birth?
    - Within 24–48 hours: 60–70 mIU/L
    - After 48 hours: 5–10 mIU/L

12. Enumerate the drugs causing hypothyroidism.
    - Excess iodide: Amiodarone, nutritional supplements, and expectorants
    - Anticonvulsants: Phenytoin, phenobarbital, and valproate
    - Antithyroid drugs: Methimazole and propylthiouracil
    - Miscellaneous: Lithium, tyrosine kinase inhibitors, interferon alfa, stavudine, thalidomide, and aminoglutethimide

*13. Explain consumptive hypothyroidism.
    In large hemangiomas of the liver, there is increased type 3, 5′-deiodinase that causes increased conversion of T4 to reverse T3. Thyroid secretion is increased, but it is not sufficient to compensate for the large increase in degradation of T4 to reverse T3.

14. List the significant antenatal histories in hypothyroidism.
    - Maternal hypothyroidism
    - Maternal hyperthyroidism (TSH receptor blocking antibody)
    - Drug intake in the mother (lithium, methimazole, antiepileptics, expectorants)
    - Radioiodine administration

15. List the causes of hypothyroidism in a preterm infant.
    - Preterm: Transient hypothyroxinemia of prematurity
    - Sick euthyroidism
    - Exposure to iodine in sick infants (povidone iodine for skin disinfection)

16. What is the normal iodine requirement?
    Incidence of congenital hypothyroidism in India is 1:1000 to 1:1500 live births. Table 37.1 shows the normal iodine requirements in children and adults.

17. What are goitrogens?
    - Substances that act by inhibiting any of the steps in thyroid synthesis
      - Examples of foods: Cabbage, cauliflower, cassava, soy, millets, and broccoli
      - Environmental pollutants: Smoking and perchlorate
      - Micronutrient deficiency: Selenium, iron, and vitamin A

18. What is Quebec scoring?
    Table 37.2 lists the various components of Quebec scoring.

*19. Enumerate the causes of transient hypothyroxinemia.
    - Maternal TSH receptor blocking antibodies
    - Maternal antithyroid drugs
    - Transient hypothyroxinemia of prematurity
    - Sick euthyroid syndrome

TABLE 37.1	Normal Iodine Requirements in Children and Adults
Age	**Requirement**
Infants	30 µg/kg/day
Older children	90–120 µg/day
Adults	150 µg/day
Pregnancy	250 µg/day

TABLE 37.2	Quebec Scoring
Feature	**Score**
Feeding problems	1
Constipation	1
Lethargy	1
Hypotonia	1
Coarse facies	3
Macroglossia	1
Open posterior fontanel	1.5
Dry skin	1.5
Mottling of skin	1
Umbilical hernia	1

Note: If the score is >4/13, hypothyroidism is suspected and the child is investigated accordingly.

20. Describe the method of screening congenital hypothyroidism in newborns.

Flowchart 37.1 gives the screening for congenital hypothyroidism.

21. List the investigations performed in hypothyroidism.

Diagnosis in children is confirmed by measuring serum TSH, T4, and T3 levels.

To evaluate the etiological diagnosis of congenital hypothyroidism the following steps are carried out:

Step 1: Thyroid scan (Tc-99 thyroid nuclear imaging) should be done either before or after 7 days of starting levothyroxine.

Step 2: Ultrasound neck (for thyroid gland).

Step 3: Thyroid antibodies.

Flowchart 37.2 shows the etiological work up in congenital hypothyroidism.

- Other investigations
    a. CBC (Complete Blood count): Anemia
    b. Peripheral smear: Macrocytic anemia
    c. Hypercholesterolemia and elevated CPK (Creatine phosphokinase)
    d. Hyponatremia
    e. ECG Electrocardiogram: Low voltage p-waves and QRS complexes

f. Radiological findings
    - Delayed formation of upper tibial, lower femoral, and cuboidal epiphysis in neonates
    - "Beaking" of the 12th thoracic or 1st or 2nd lumbar vertebra
    - Large fontanels and wide sutures visible on X-rays of the skull, intersutural (Wormian) bones common, and sella turcica often enlarged and round
    - CXR Chest X-Ray: Pericardial effusion and pleural effusion
g. USG Ultrasonogram thyroid: Can determine the nodule dimensions and texture (solid vs. cystic nature)
h. Radioactive iodine uptake
i. Serum antithyroglobulin and antiperoxidase antibodies

22. Describe the treatment and follow-up of hypothyroidism.

- L-Thyroxine is the treatment of choice.
- Treatment with thyroxine should begin as soon as possible and no later than first 2 weeks of life.
- Initial thyroxine dose: 10 -15 microgram/kg/day
- The tablet should be crushed and powdered.
- It should be taken in the morning, on an empty stomach. It should not be mixed with iron, calcium, and soy because this inhibits its absorption.

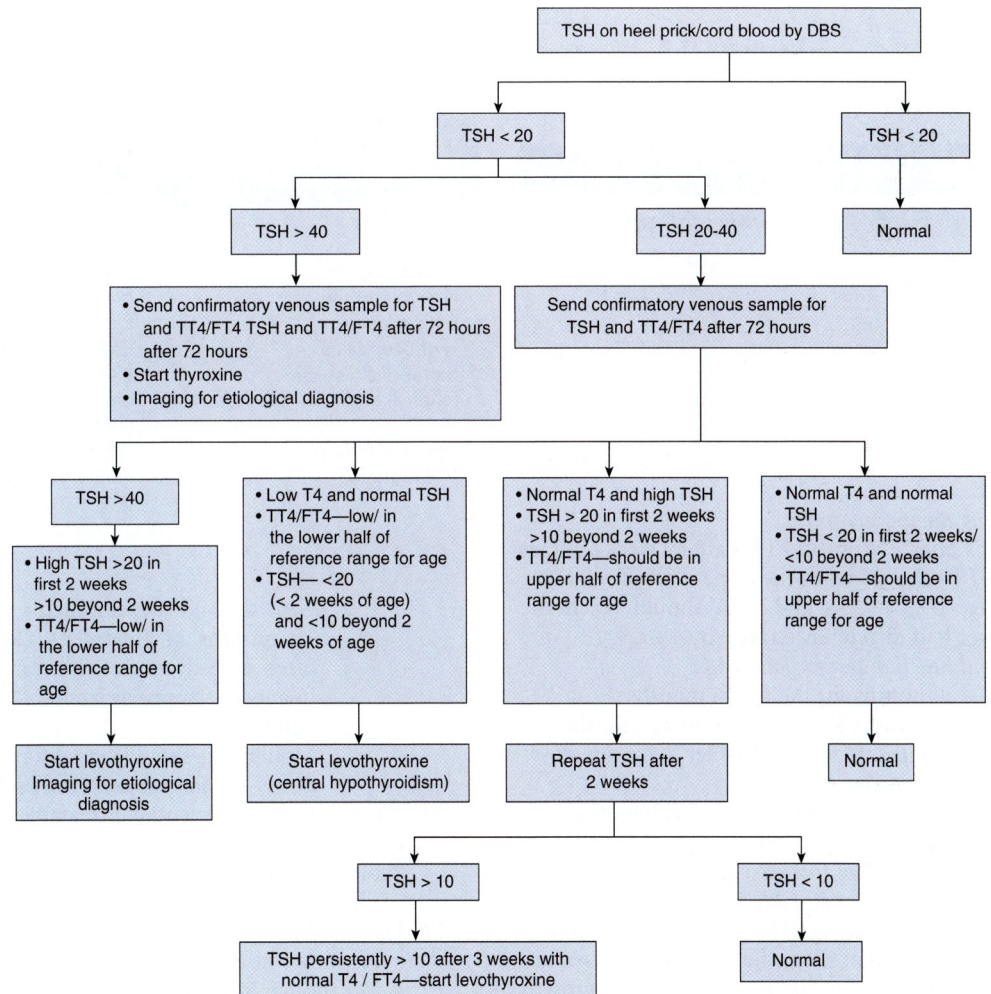

Flowchart 37.1 Screening for congenital hypothyroidism in newborns.

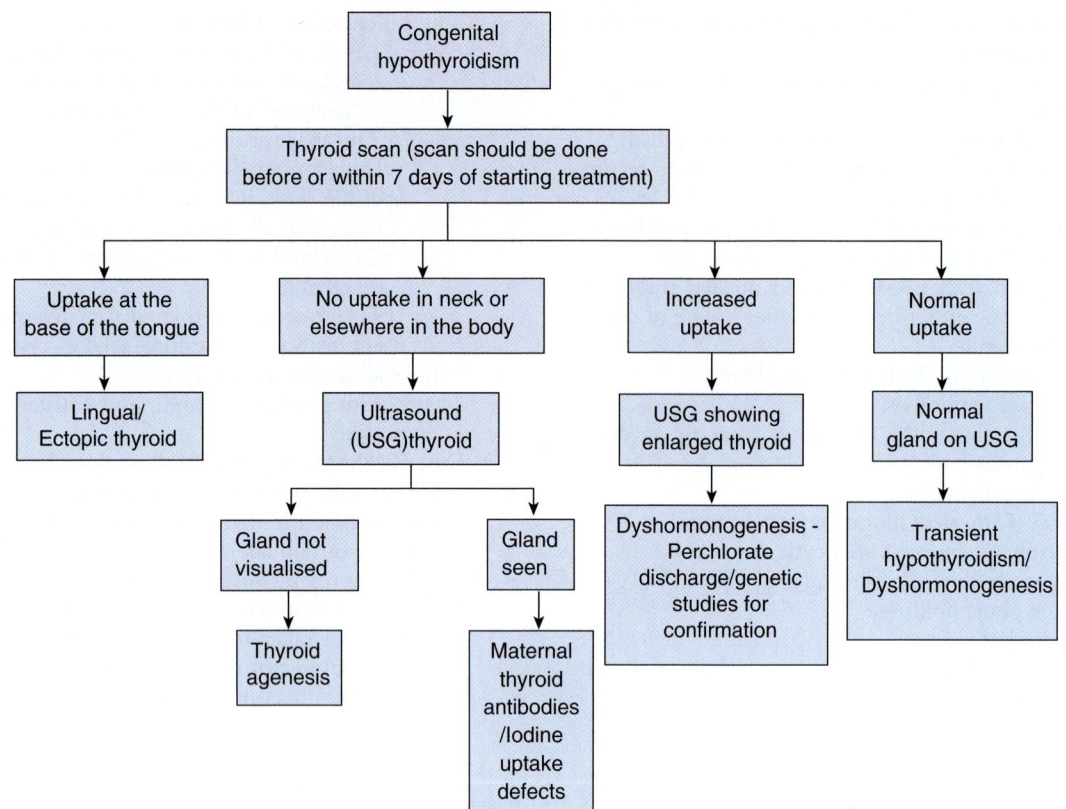

Flowchart 37.2   Etiological work up in congenital hypothyroidism.

TABLE 37.3	Dose of L-Thyroxine
Age	**Dose (μg/kg/day)**
Newborns	10–15
1–3 years	4–6
3–10 years	3–5
Older than 10 years	2–4

TABLE 37.4	Preventable/Treatable Causes of Mental Retardation
Condition	**Interventions**
Birth asphyxia	Improved perinatal care
Hypoglycemia	Early diagnosis and treatment
CNS infections	Early diagnosis and treatment
Hydrocephalus	Early diagnosis and treatment
Metabolic disorders (phenylketonuria, galactosemia)	Early diagnosis + appropriate dietary management + genetic counseling
Hypothyroidism	Early diagnosis and treatment
Malnutrition	Immunization + dietary management

Table 37.3 shows the dose of L-thyroxine according to the age.

Monitoring during treatment

   T4/FT4 after 2 weeks and TSH after 4 weeks. Target T4/FT4 should reach the upper half of reference range by 2 weeks and TSH should reach the lower half of reference range by 4 weeks.

Thyroid function test for follow up:

Every 1-2 months for the first 6 months

Every 2-4 months for the next 6 to 36 months

Every 6 months thereafter (further thyroxine doses are adjusted thereafter)

*   In dyshormonogenetic congenital hypothyroidism (CH), treatment can be stopped for 4 weeks at 3 years of age to reassess whether it is transient or permanent CH. Structural thyroid abnormalities causing CH, require lifelong thyroxine replacement. Periodic bone age X-rays are useful to monitor treatment and future growth potential.

*   Growth and development: During the first 18 months of treatment, skeletal maturation often exceeds expected linear growth, resulting in a loss of approximately 7 cm of the predicted adult height.

*   Monitoring should be performed for complications – craniosynostosis and pseudotumor cerebri.

23. Enumerate the preventable/treatable causes of mental retardation.

    Table 37.4 lists the preventable/treatable causes of mental retardation.

24. List the differential diagnoses of a large tongue.
    *   Hypothyroidism
    *   Metabolic: Mucopolysaccharidoses (MPS) and Von Gierke and Pompe diseases

- Amyloidosis
- Acromegaly
- Lymphangioma/hemangiomas of the tongue
- Down syndrome: Relative macroglossia

25. Describe the mechanism of myxedema in hypothyroidism.

It occurs because of the accumulation of glycosaminoglycan and hyaluronic acid in the skin and subcutaneous tissue.

*26. Explain the prognosis of hypothyroidism.

Delay in diagnosis and treatment can result in considerable brain damage. When the onset occurs after 2 years of age, the outcome is much better even if diagnosis and treatment have been delayed. Twenty percent of patients have a neurosensory hearing defect. Repeat hearing test should be carried out before school age and as required.

Quick Bites

- Age is an important factor in a child with hypothyroidism.
  - It can distinguish between congenital and acquired hypothyroidism.
  - Clinical featuzres vary according to the age.
  - The dose of L-thyroxine is adjusted according to the age.
  - Age is an important prognostic factor.
- Congenital hypothyroidism presents with a failure to gain weight, whereas acquired hypothyroidism presents with an increased weight gain.
- Thyroid dysgenesis is the most common cause of permanent congenital hypothyroidism.
- Hashimoto thyroiditis is the most common cause of acquired hypothyroidism.
- Consumptive hypothyroidism is seen in large hemangiomas of the liver.
- The newborn screening for congenital hypothyroidism can be performed in cord blood (within 24 hours) as well as by the heel prick method (after 48 hours).
- All newborns with hypothyroidism should undergo further evaluation with thyroid scan.
- L-Thyroxine is the treatment of choice for hypothyroidism. It should not be mixed with iron, calcium, and soy because this inhibits its absorption.
- The prognosis for hypothyroidism having onset after the age of 2 years is better.

38

Short Stature

Following introduction, seek permission from the caregiver and introduce yourself to the patient before history elicitation, and identify the case.

Name____Age____Sex____Consanguinity____Order of birth____Place____Informant____

Presenting Complaints and Duration

Not gaining adequate height as peers/sibling

History of Presenting Illness

Failure to gain height since birth or after some illness

ETIOLOGICAL HISTORY

- Lethargy/poor feeding/failure to gain weight
- Recurrent respiratory tract infection, dyspnea, and cyanosis
- Cough/foul-smelling sputum
- Oliguria/edema/polyuria
- Any bony deformity/fractures
- Diarrhea/steatorrhea
- Worms in stools/pica eating
- Constipation/decreased activity/intolerance to cold
- Dysmorphic facies
- Failure of development of secondary sexual characters

PAST HISTORY

- Trauma
- Chronic illness
- Recurrent respiratory tract infection
- Previous hospitalization
- Drug intake – androgens and steroid

ANTENATAL HISTORY

- Fever with rash
- Irradiation in the mother
- Multiple pregnancy
- Chronic illness in the mother
- Pregnancy Induced Hypertension (PIH)/Gestational Diabetes Mellitus (GDM)/any drug intake
- Bleeding per vaginum

NATAL HISTORY

- Birth weight – Appropriate for Gestational Age (AGA)/Small for Gestational Age (SGA)/Intrauterine Growth Restriction (IUGR)
- Birth asphyxia
- Neonatal admission (hypoglycemia)
- External congenital anomalies (midline defect)

DEVELOPMENT HISTORY

Any developmental delay

DIETETIC HISTORY

Decreased diet intake – chronic malnutrition

FAMILY HISTORY

Short stature; ask about the maternal and paternal height, and age of attaining puberty in parents

SOCIAL AND ENVIRONMENTAL HISTORY

- Low socioeconomic class and emotional deprivation

Summary

A …-year-old child with onset of symptoms at … age, with associated problems such as seizures/delayed puberty/poor nutrition/chronic illness, with/without family history of short stature and with/without delayed puberty, probable etiology …, would like to confirm with examination

General Examination

- Conscious
- Oriented
- Dysmorphic facies
- Malnourished
- Pallor
- Cyanosis
- Clubbing
- Generalized lymphadenopathy

Head-to-Foot Examination

- Head: Size and shape
- Hair
- Any dysmorphic facies
- Neck
- Eyes: Icterus, cataract, and epicanthal folds
- Nose
- Oral cavity: No protruding tongue and glossitis
- Ears
- Skeletal deformity
- Chest deformity
- Upper limb
- Nail
- Palm and soles
- Abdomen
- Genu varum/genu valgum
- Skin
- Genitalia

Vital Signs

- Temperature
- Pulse rate
- Respiratory rate
- Blood pressure – can be normal/raised in Chronic Kidney Disease (CKD)

Anthropometry

- Height: <-2 standard deviation (SD)
- Weight: <-2 standard deviation (SD)
- Weight/height <-2 standard deviation (SD)
- Mid-arm circumference
- Upper segment:lower segment
- Arm span
- Mark the following in the growth chart: weight for age, height for age, and mid-parental height (take the mother's and father's height also)

Systemic Examination

RESPIRATORY SYSTEM

- Chest retraction and tachypnea/retraction

CARDIOVASCULAR SYSTEM

- Any murmur

ABDOMEN

- Any organomegaly

CENTRAL NERVOUS SYSTEM

- Any cranial nerve palsy, developmental delay, seizures, and mental retardation

Diagnosis

Proportionate/disproportionate short stature with/without dysmorphism, most probable etiology …

Frequently Asked Questions

1. What is the significance of age and short stature?
   - At birth: Skeletal dysplasia
   - Poor growth in children younger than 2 years: Congenital growth hormone deficiency
   - Pubertal age: Constitutional delay in growth and hypogonadism
2. What is the importance of onset and progression of short stature?
   - Gradual: Chronic diseases, growth hormone deficiency, and hypothyroidism
   - Acute: Intracranial tumors (associated with other symptoms such as visual disturbances)
3. What is the relationship between changes in weight and short stature?
   - Weight gain with short stature: Endocrine disorders
   - Weight loss with short stature: Nutritional and chronic diseases
4. List the etiological history to be elicited in short stature.
   Table 38.1 gives the etiological history in short stature.
5. *What are the syndromes associated with short stature? Mention their salient features.
   Table 38.2 gives the syndromes associated with short stature and their clinical features.
6. What are the causes of rapid growth in height followed by final short height?
   Rapid growth in height followed by reduced growth velocity with short final adult height is seen in hyperthyroidism and precocious puberty leading to early fusion of growth plates.
7. What are the clues in history in diagnosing short stature?
   Table 38.3 gives the clues in history taking.
8. What are the histories to be elicited in psychosocial short stature?
   - Apathetic, temper tantrums, anxiety, and nocturnal enuresis
   - Poor eating habits, purging, and laxative abuse: Anorexia
9. List the clues in head-to-foot examination in a child with a short stature.
   Table 38.4 gives the clues in the head-to-foot examination.
10. What is Archibald sign and where is it seen?
    Archibald metacarpal sign is characterized by a shortening of the 4th or/and 5th metacarpals when the fist is clenched.
    Fig. 38.7A–C shows the short 4th and 5th metacarpals.
11. What is the significance of vital signs and short stature?
    - Bradycardia: Hypothyroidism
    - Hypertension: Cushing disease/intracranial tumor/coarctation of aorta
    - Upper limb and lower limb Blood pressure (BP): Turner syndrome

TABLE 38.1	Etiological History in Short Stature
History	**Etiology**
Shortness of breath, cyanosis, cough, fever	Heart disease, asthma, Tuberculosis (TB)
Diarrhea, steatorrhea, abdominal pain	Malabsorption
Headache, vomiting, visual problems	• Pituitary – hypothalamic mass • Intracranial tumor • Trauma • Surgery
Constipation, lethargy, feeding difficulty	Hypothyroidism
Bony deformity, fractures	Rickets
Polyuria	Renal tubular acidosis, chronic renal failure
History of hepatitis, distension abdomen, melena	Chronic liver disease
Recurrent blood transfusions	Thalassemia and other (chronic anemia)
Chronic infection (TB, HIV)	• Recurrent episodes of fever, cough • Hospital admissions

Endocrine cause	a. Congenital Growth Hormone (GH) deficiency: History starts from newborn
	   Acquired Growth Hormone (GH) deficiency: Any age
	b. Diabetes insipidus: Polyuria/polydipsia/loss of weight
	c. Hypothyroidism
	   Weight gain but poor height
	   Altered school performance, lethargy, constipation, cold intolerance
	d. Prolactinoma: Amenorrhea, galactorrhea
	e. Precocious puberty
	   Early onset of breast maturation before 8 years/testicular enlargement before 9 years, early age of acne, mood variations.
	f. Hyperthyroid: Tremors, diarrhea, restlessness, palpitations, excessive sweating, poor concentration, aggression, mood changes

Dietary history – to elicit weaning practice, calorie and protein intake	Malnutrition
Prolonged use of corticosteroids, amphetamine derivatives	Drug history
Others	Cranial irradiation, chemotherapy

TABLE 38.2	Syndromes Associated With Short Stature
Syndrome	**Features**
Laron syndrome	• Short since birth • Seizures, neonatal hypoglycemia • Facial abnormalities: Epicanthal folds, small palpebral fissure, upturned nose, intellectual difficulties
Prader–Willi syndrome	• Neonatal history: Poor feeding, neonatal intensive care unit (NICU) stay, Nasogastric Tube feeding • Syndromic facies: Railroad track ears, smooth philtrum, thin upper lips • Middle school: Short, obese, learning difficulty, voracious appetite – even steals food • Adolescence: Obese, delayed puberty, discoloration of neck, polyuria (features of type 2 diabetes mellitus)
Turner syndrome	• Poor height since infancy • Learning difficulty • Visual problems • Hearing problems: Sensorineural Hearing Loss (SNHL)/recurrent otitis media, feeding difficulty • Delayed puberty: Primary amenorrhea • Cardiac abnormalities: Breathing difficulty, exercise intolerance, painful muscle cramps after exercise in older children – coarctation of aorta/bicuspid aortic valve
Cushing syndrome	• Excessive hair growth, sudden weight gain • Mood variations, excessive tiredness • Skin discoloration (striae), acne • Prolonged use of steroid cream or oral medication use/alternative medication use

TABLE 38.3	Clues in History Taking
History	**Clues**
Antenatal history	• Substance abuse • Medication • Infections Intrauterine growth restriction (IUGR)
Birth history	• Gestation age Intrauterine growth restriction (IUGR) • History of birth asphyxia (hypopituitarism) • Breech delivery • Low birth weight: Down Syndrome/Turner Syndrome/TORCH- Toxoplasmosis, Other (syphilis, varicella-zoster, parvovirus B19), Rubella, Cytomegalovirus, and Herpes infections/maternal drugs, maternal alcohol, smoking
Neonatal period	• Neonatal hypoglycemia Growth hormone deficiency (GHD) • Prolonged neonatal hyperbilirubinemia (hypothyroidism) • Seizures in newborn period/hypoglycemia: Hypopituitarism • Undescended testes/micropenis: Central cause of short stature • Swelling of the hands and feet at birth: Turner syndrome
Developmental history	a. Delayed milestones: Hypothyroidism, chromosomal/genetic cause b. Delayed puberty in one or both parents (constitutional delay of growth and puberty)
Family history (skeletal dysplasia)	a. Short stature in first/second-degree relatives – familial short stature b. Delayed menarche in mother/delayed voice change/shaving in father: c. Constitutional delay in growth and puberty Previous siblings/relatives with short stature: Systemic disease/skeletal dysplasia d. History of previous sibling death: Skeletal dysplasia e. Poor attachment to parents, not attending school, poor nutrition: Psychosocial dwarfism
Social history	• Child abuse • Family discord • Emotional deprivation (psychosocial dwarfism)

TABLE 38.4	Clues in Head-to-Foot Examination
Etiology	**Clinical Features**
Genetic syndromes	**Syndromic facies** a. Down syndrome b. Noonan syndrome as shown in Fig. 38.1A and B, Russell–Silver syndrome as shown in Fig. 38.2A and B c. Moon facies, cherubic facies: Hypopituitarism d. Laron syndrome as shown in Fig. 38.3 e. Seckel syndrome as shown in Fig. 38.4
Eye findings	• Squint, cataract, color blindness, ptosis • Fundus: Papilledema/optic atrophy

TABLE 38.4	Clues in Head-to-Foot Examination—cont'd
Etiology	**Clinical Features**
Growth hormone deficiency, hypopituitarism	a. Frontal bossing, depressed nasal bridge as shown in Fig. 38.5 b. Midline defects: Crowded teeth, single central incisor, cleft palate c. Micropenis d. Otitis media (conductive hearing loss), sensorineural hearing loss
Malabsorption, rickets	Signs of vitamin deficiencies: Oral ulcers, night blindness, Bitot spots
Chronic liver disease	Jaundice, clubbing
Chronic anemia, renal failure, liver disease	Pallor
Cushing syndrome	Central obesity, striae, proximal weakness
Chronic renal failure	Hypertension
Hypothyroidism	Goiter, coarse and dry skin, delayed relaxation of tendon jerks
Pseudohypoparathyroidism	Round face, short 4th metacarpal
Puberty	Delayed puberty
Turner syndrome	Webbed neck as shown in Fig. 38.6, widely spaced nipples, increased carrying angle in a short girl, edema of hand
Others	Cranial surgical scars/ventriculoperitoneal shunt

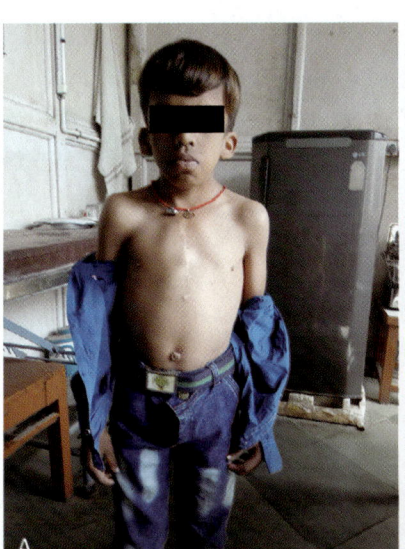
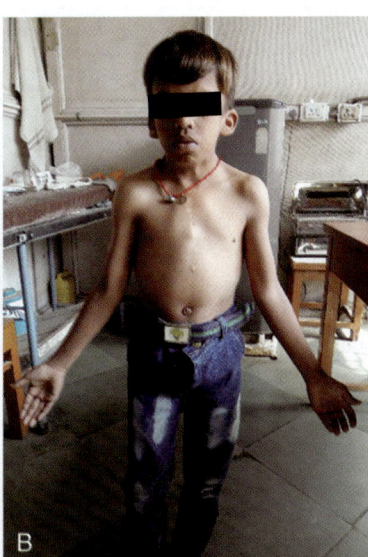

Fig. 38.1 (A) Noonan syndrome: facial dysmorphology – woolly hair, inverted triangle-shaped head, thickly hooded prominent eyes, downward slant of palpebral fissures, low-set ears, deeply grooved philtrum, cupid brow appearance of the upper lip, small chin. (B) Noonan syndrome: pectus sternal deformity (prominent upper sternum and depressed inferior sternum), cubitus valgus deformity of upper extremity (increased carrying angle at the elbow joint), widely spaced nipple, webbed neck.

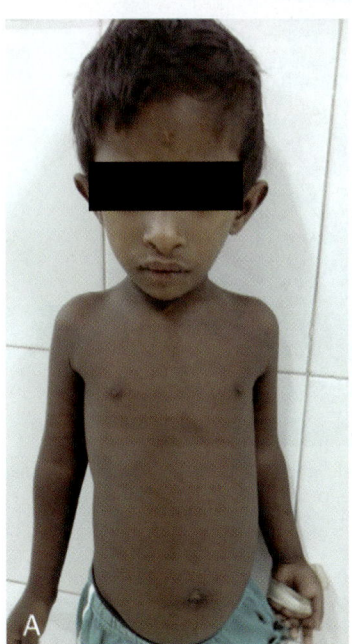
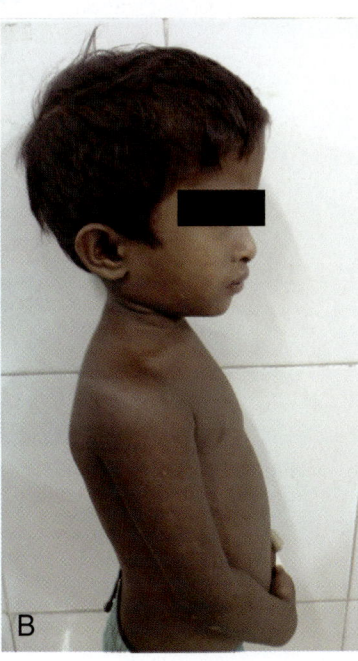

Fig. 38.2 (A) Frontal bossing, broad forehead tapering into narrow chin, micrognathia. (B) Russell–Silver syndrome – pseudohydrocephalus.

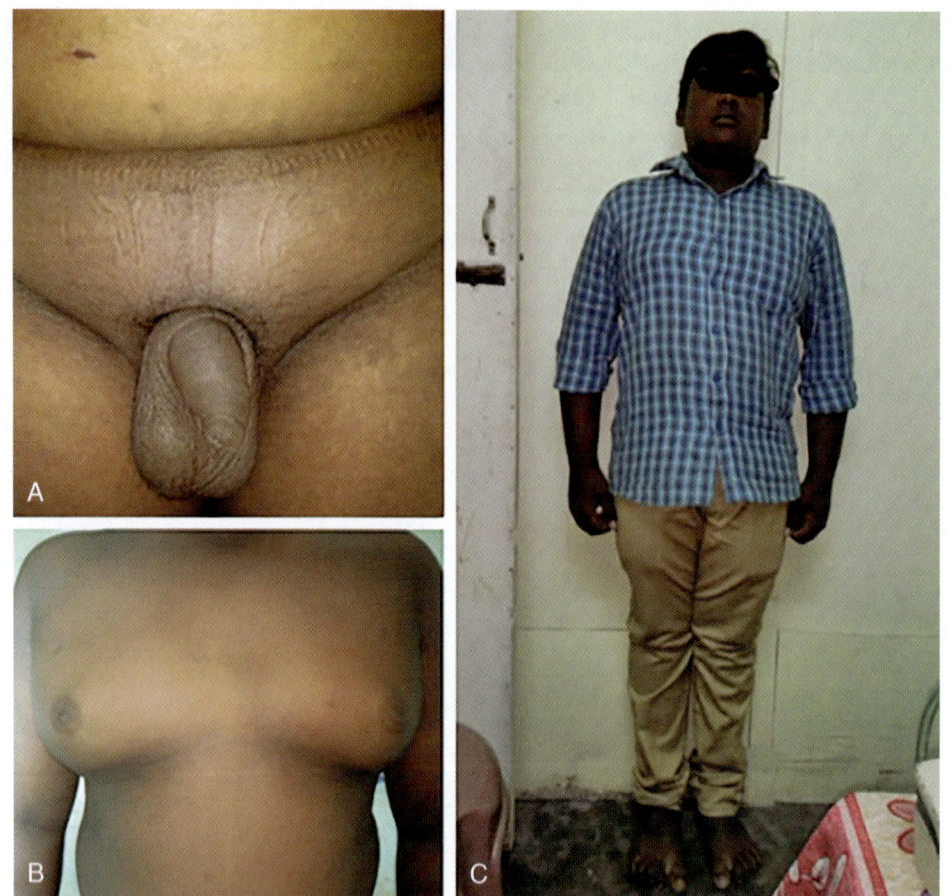

Fig. 38.3   Laron dwarfism with absent secondary sexual characters (A), gynecomastia (B), and short stature (C).

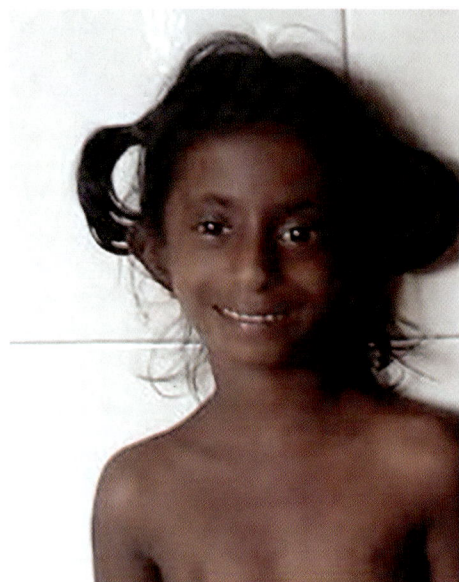

Fig. 38.4   Seckel syndrome – large eyes, beak-like nose, narrow face, receding lower jaw.

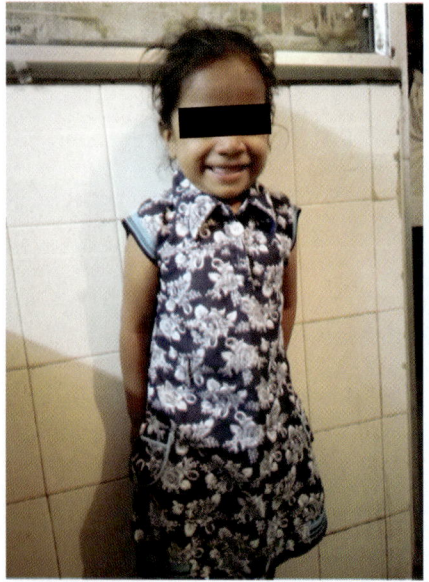

Fig. 38.5   Growth hormone deficiency – prominent forehead, depressed nasal bridge, saddle nose, prominent philtrum.

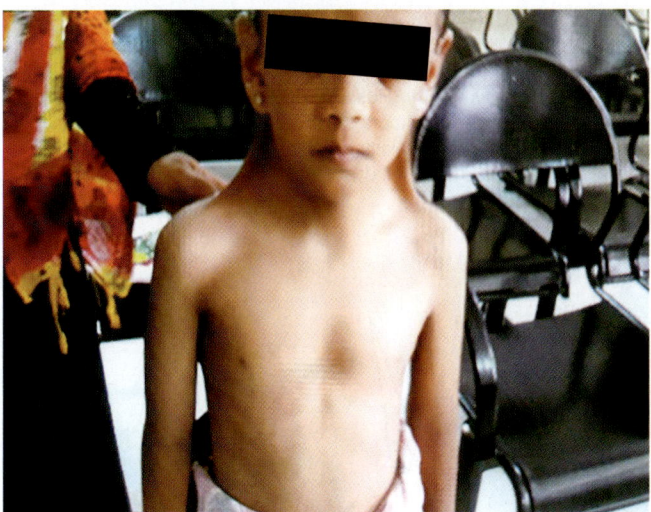

Fig. 38.6 Turner syndrome – webbed neck, widely spaced nipple

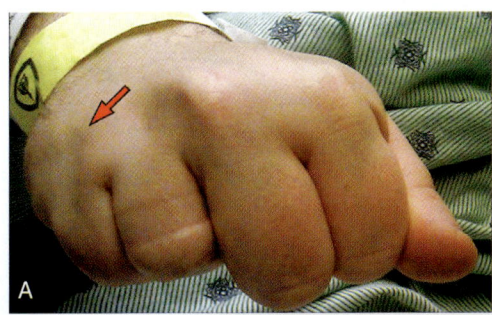

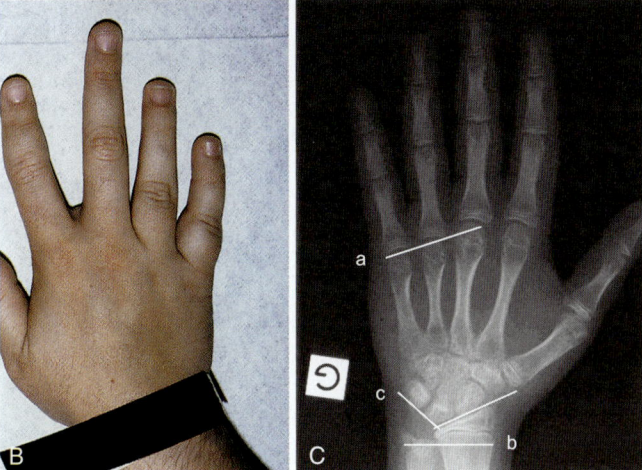

Fig. 38.7 (A) Short 4th metacarpal and absent knuckle when the patient clenches. (B) Short 4th metacarpal – ring finger is shorter. (C) X-ray hand showing short 4th metacarpal – no growth plate in the 4th metacarpal (can be assessed by drawing a line along the heads of the 4th and 5th metacarpals; if this line intersects the head of the 3rd metacarpal, then shortening is present). (Source: (A) Reproduced from Catherine Simpson, Evan Grove, Dr Brian A Houston. Pseudopseudohypoparathyroidism, The Lancet 385(9973):1123. (B) Reproduced from Basil Zitelli, Sara McIntire, Andrew Nowalk. Zitelli and Davis' Atlas of Pediatric Physical Diagnosis, Sixth Edition, Endocrinology, Figure 9-24, Philadelphia, Saunders, 2012. (Credit line - A and B, Courtesy J. Parks, MD, Atlanta, Ga; C, courtesy J. Medina, Pittsburgh, Pa.). (C) Reproduced from S.Cabrol. Le syndrome de Turner☆ Turner syndrome, Annales d'Endocrinologie 68(1):2-9.)

TABLE 38.5	Relationship Between Puberty and Short Stature	
Pubertal Status	**Causes of Short Stature**
Delayed puberty	• Constitutional delayed puberty
	• Pituitary disorder
	• Chronic diseases
Normal puberty	Familial short stature
Advanced puberty	Precocious puberty

12. What is the correlation between puberty and short stature?
    The relationship between puberty and short stature is given in Table 38.5.
13. What are the measurements and maneuvers performed in short stature?
    Fig. 38.8 shows the measurements and maneuvers performed in short stature.
14. Demonstrate height/length measurement and calculate height for age in a child with suspected short stature.
    • For children younger than 2 years, supine length should be measured on an infantometer and two personnel are required to make an accurate measure.
    • For children older than 2 years, standing height is measured on a stadiometer.
    • Plot the value on a reference curve.
    • Calculate the height for age (the chronological age at which this measurement of height is on the 50th percentile of the reference curve). Fig. 38.9 shows the height for age of a child.
15. How is mid-parental height calculated?
    • Mid-parental height (MPH) or target height (TH) range is calculated as follows:

$$\text{Boys: MPH range} = \frac{[(\text{Father's height}) + (\text{Mother's height}) + 13]}{2} \pm 6 \text{ cm}$$

$$\text{Girls: MPH range} = \frac{[(\text{Father's height}) + (\text{Mother's height}) - 13]}{2} \pm 6 \text{ cm}$$

16. What is decimal age?

$$\text{Decimal age} = \frac{[(\text{Age completed in years}) + (\text{Completed age in months})]}{12}$$

    For example, a child aged 5 years and 3 months has a decimal age of 5.25 years.
17. *How is Standard deviation (SD) score calculated?
    Standard deviation (SD) score

$$= \frac{(\text{Child's height}) - (\text{Mean for age})}{\text{SD for age}}$$

18. How is growth velocity calculated and how can one plot in a growth velocity chart?
    • Calculate growth velocity and plot in midpoint between two ages.
    • For example, if height at 5 years is 110 cm and at 6 years is 116 cm, and growth velocity is 6 cm, plot at 6.5 years if growth velocity <25th centile – abnormal.

A. MEASUREMENTS
Height
Lower segment (LS)
Calculate upper segment
  (US) by subtracting LS from
  height
Calculate upper segment (US):
  Lower segment (LS) ratio

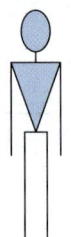

B. MEASUREMENTS
Arm span
Head circumference
Request weight
Assess percentile charts
Calculate height velocity
Request birth parameters
Request parents' percentiles
  and ages of puberty

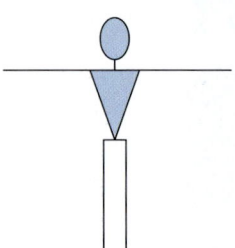

C. HANDS AND FEET
    TOGETHER
To detect:
Asymmetry (Russell-Silver syndrome)
Approximatioonf shoulders
  (absent clavicles in
  cleidocranial dysostosis)

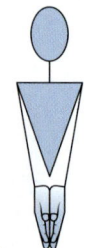

D. ARMS OUT STRAIGHT
To detect:
Cubitus valgus
  (Turner syndrome,
  Noonan syndrome)
  over 15° in girls;
  over 10 in boys

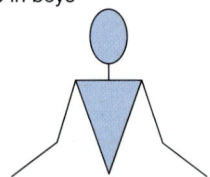

E. THUMBS ON SHOULDERS
To detect:
Proximal segment shortening
  (e.g. achondroplasia,
  hypochondroplasia)
Middle segment shortening
  (e.g. Len-Weill
  dyschondrostenosis,
  Langer mesomelic
  dysplasia)
Distal segment shortening
  (e.g. acromesomelic
  dysplasia)

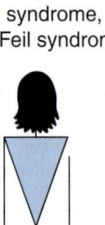

F. PALMS UP
To detect:
Simian crease (Down syndrome,
  Seckel syndrome)
Clinodactyly (Russell-Silver syndrome,
  Down syndrome, Seckel syndrome

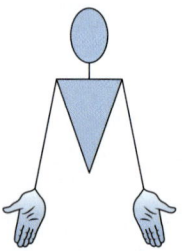

G. MAKE A FIST
To detect:
Short fourth metacarpal
  (pseudohypoparathyroidism,
  Turner syndrome, Fetal alcohol syndrome)

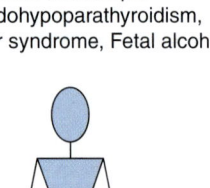

H. BACK
To detect:
Short neck (Klippel-Feil syndrome,
  Noonan syndrome)
Neck webbing (Turner syndrome,
  Noonan syndrome)
Low hairline (Turner syndrome,
  Noonan syndrome,
  Klippel-Feil syndrome)

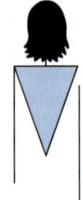

I. BEND OVER AND
    TOUCH TOES
To detect:
Scoliosis (e.g. Noonan syndrome,
  Klippel-Feil syndrome,
  Prader-Willi syndrome)

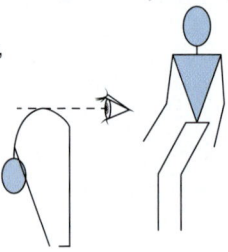

J. SIT UP
To commence systematic
  physical examination

Fig. 38.8 Measurements and maneuvers performed in short stature. (*Source: Reproduced from Wayne Harris, Endocrinology, Fig. 7.3.*)

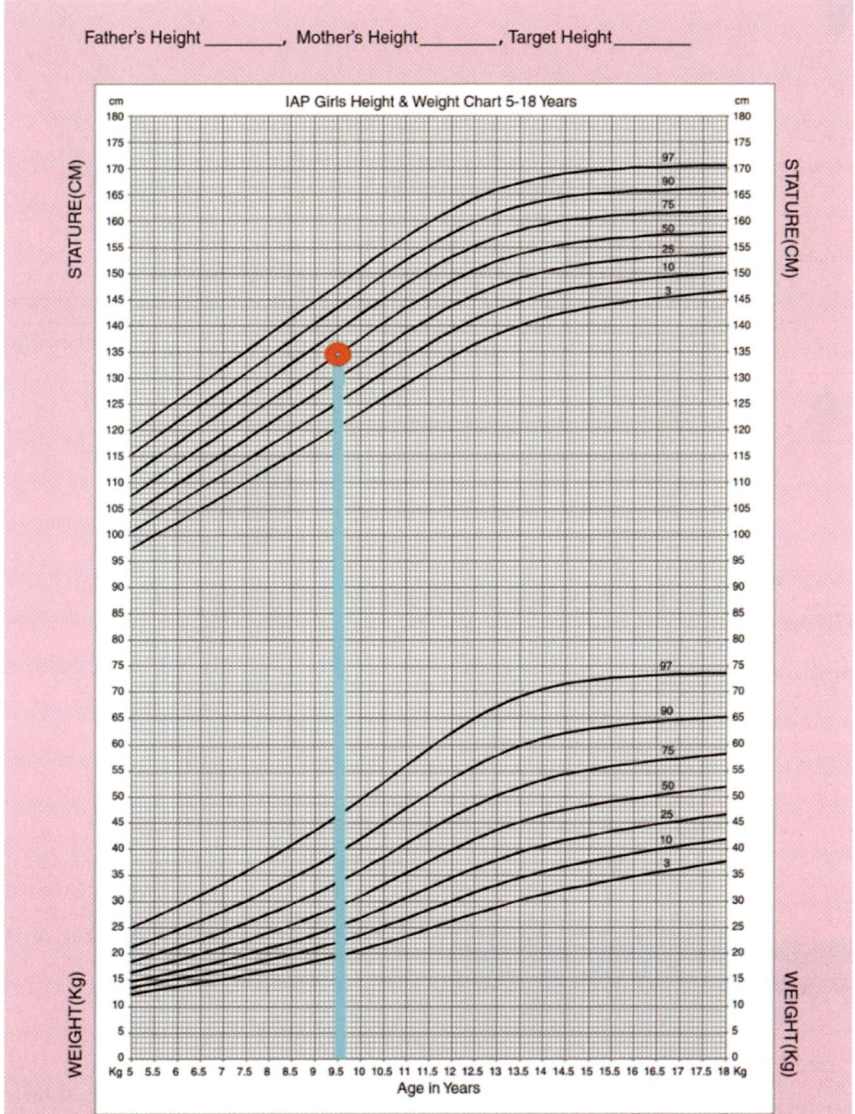

Father's Height _____, Mother's Height _____, Target Height _____

IAP Girls Height & Weight Chart 5-18 Years

Fig. 38.9 Chronological age of a child at which height is at 50th centile. (Source: Modified from Harish Pemde, Vikram Datta, Kamlesh Harish. *Clinical and Practical Paediatrics*, Second Edition, Annexurel 2 l - Growth charts, New Delhi, Elsevier India, 2020.)

19. How is growth velocity calculated in standard deviation (SD) score?

    Specific growth velocity SD score table is available.

    $$\text{SD score} = \frac{(\text{Child's velocity}) - (\text{Mean velocity for age})}{\text{SD for age}}$$

20. How are upper segment and lower segment body proportions measured?
    - Measure the lower segment and subtract it from height to get the upper segment.
      - Upper segment: Vertex to upper border of pubic symphysis
      - Lower segment: Upper border of pubis symphysis to foot
      - Upper segment:Lower segment ratio: Vertex to pubis:pubis to sole of foot and its ratio
    - If the lower segment is longer than the upper segment by more than 5 cm (after completion of puberty), it is considered as disproportionate short stature.

TABLE 38.6	Upper Segment:Lower Segment Ratio	
Age	**Ratio**
At birth	1.7:1
At 3 years	1.3:1
At 8 years	1:1
At 10 years	0.98:1

Table 38.6 gives the normal upper segment:lower segment ratio in children.

21. What is sitting height and how is it measured?
    - It is the distance from the vertex to the base of the sitting surface. Ask the patient to sit on a chair of known height.
    - Measure the sitting height with the stadiometer. Fig. 38.10 gives the sitting height.
    - Repeat the measurement two times. Sitting height = trunk length.

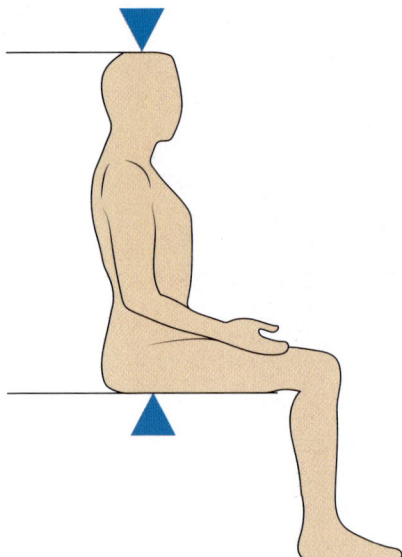

Fig. 38.10 Sitting height. *(Source: https://www.google.com/imgres?img url=https%3A%2F%2Fimage.slidesharecdn.com%2Fgrowthmeasure-140228115514-phpapp01%2F95%2Fgrowth-measures-in-clinical-practice-20-638.jpg%3Fcb%3D1470819038&imgrefurl=https%3A%2F%2Fwww.slideshare.net%2Fmontyshenoy%2Fgrowth-measure&tbnid=CwL36WZRiVUS7M&vet=12ahUKEwji6ryp1fLuAhURSSsKHRL6CuMQMyg DegUIARCpAQ..i&docid=lLrboK849FQVdM&w=638&h=479&q= sitting%20height%20in%20pediatrics&ved=2ahUKEwji6ryp1fLuAhURSSs KHRL6CuMQMygDegUIARCpAQ.)*

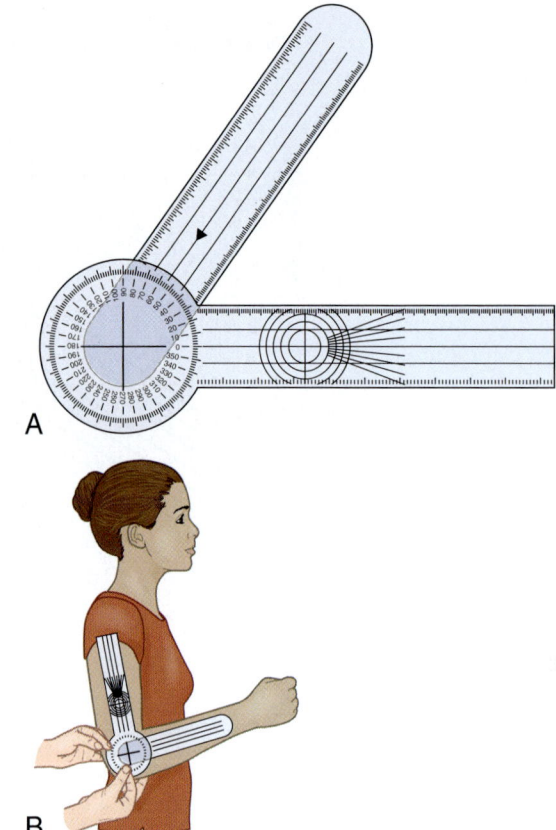

Fig. 38.11 (A and B) Measurement of carrying angle by goniometer at the intersection of long axis of arm and long axis of forearm. *(Source: (B) Reproduced from Brigitte Niedzwiecki, Julie Pepper, P. Ann Weaver. Kinn's The Clinical Medical Assistant: An Applied Learning Approach, Fourteenth Edition, Orthopedics and Rheumatology, Figure 20.13, St. Louis, Saunders, 2020.)*

TABLE 38.7	Clinical Clues in Short Stature
Clinical Features	**Clue to Etiology**
Arms – carrying angle	• Keep the arms straight for carrying angle – wide in Turner syndrome and Noonan syndrome • Normal carrying angle is about 10–15° 1. Fig. 38.11(A and B) shows measurement of carrying angle by goniometer.

Segmental shortening	Ask the child to touch thumb to shoulders to check for short limbs – either distal segment or proximal segment shortening
	  a. Rhizomelic shortening: If the thumb overshoots, there is proximal segment limb shortening, e.g., achondroplasia, chondrodysplasia group, metaphyseal dysplasia
	  b. Mesomelic shortening: If the thumb does not touch the shoulder, there is middle segment shortening, e.g., Leri–Weill disease
	  c. Acromelic shortening: If the thumb does not reach the shoulder, there is distal segment shortening, e.g., Ellis-Van Creveld syndrome
	Fig. 38.12 shows schematic representation of segmental shortening

Limbs – disproportionate short stature	• Measure various limb segments – shoulder-to-elbow (SE) length and the elbow-to-metacarpal length (EMC) • Normally, the SE/EMC ratio is about 1 • Rhizomelia is present if this ratio is lower than 0.98
Back – scoliosis	Adam's forward bend test

• For lower limb length, subtract the sitting height from the standing height. It is more reliable than the upper segment:lower segment ratio.

• Normal values
  - At birth: 70% of the total height
  - At 2 years: 60% of the total height
  - At 10 years: 52% of the total height

22. Mention some special maneuvers that give clues to etiology in short stature.

    Table 38.7 gives the clinical clues in short stature.

23. What is Adam's forward bend test?

    The purpose of this test is to detect structural or functional scoliosis. Ask the patient to bend forward at the waist until the back comes in the horizontal plane, with feet together, arms hanging, and knees extended. The palms are held together. The examiner looks from behind, along the horizontal plane of the column vertebrae. Interpretation: Look for the following:

    • Unlevel shoulders
    • Unlevel hips
    • Head tilting off-center
    • Head not in line with the pelvis
    • Rib prominences/trunk asymmetries
    • Shoulder asymmetry

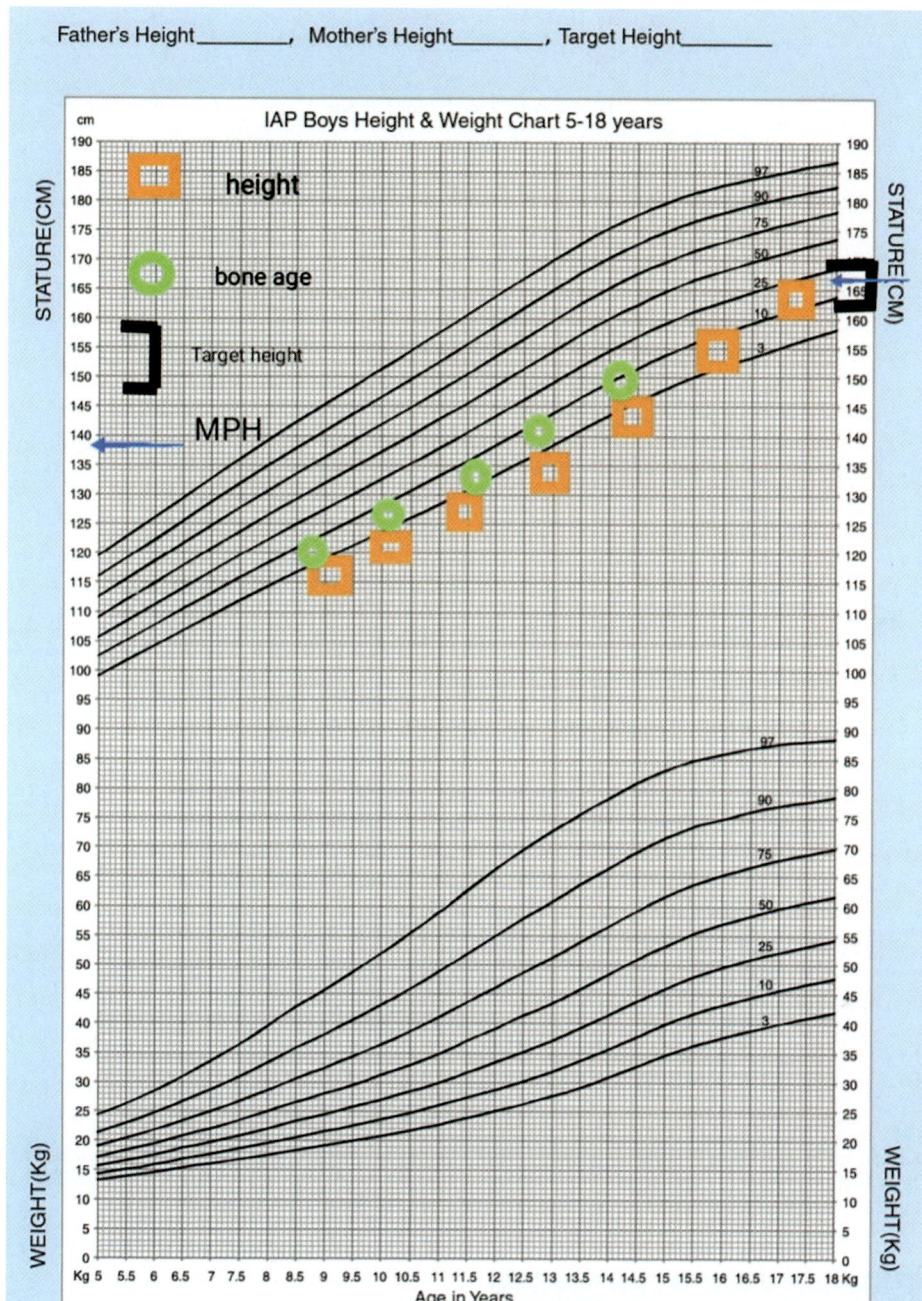

Fig. 38.16 Growth chart showing constitutional growth delay. Note the delayed bone age that does not correspond to the chronological age. Eventual height within mid-parental height and normal percentiles with a catch-up growth. (Source: Modified from Harish Pemde, Vikram Datta, Kamlesh Harish. *Clinical and Practical Paediatrics*, Second Edition, Annexurel 2 I - Growth charts, New Delhi, Elsevier India, 2020.)

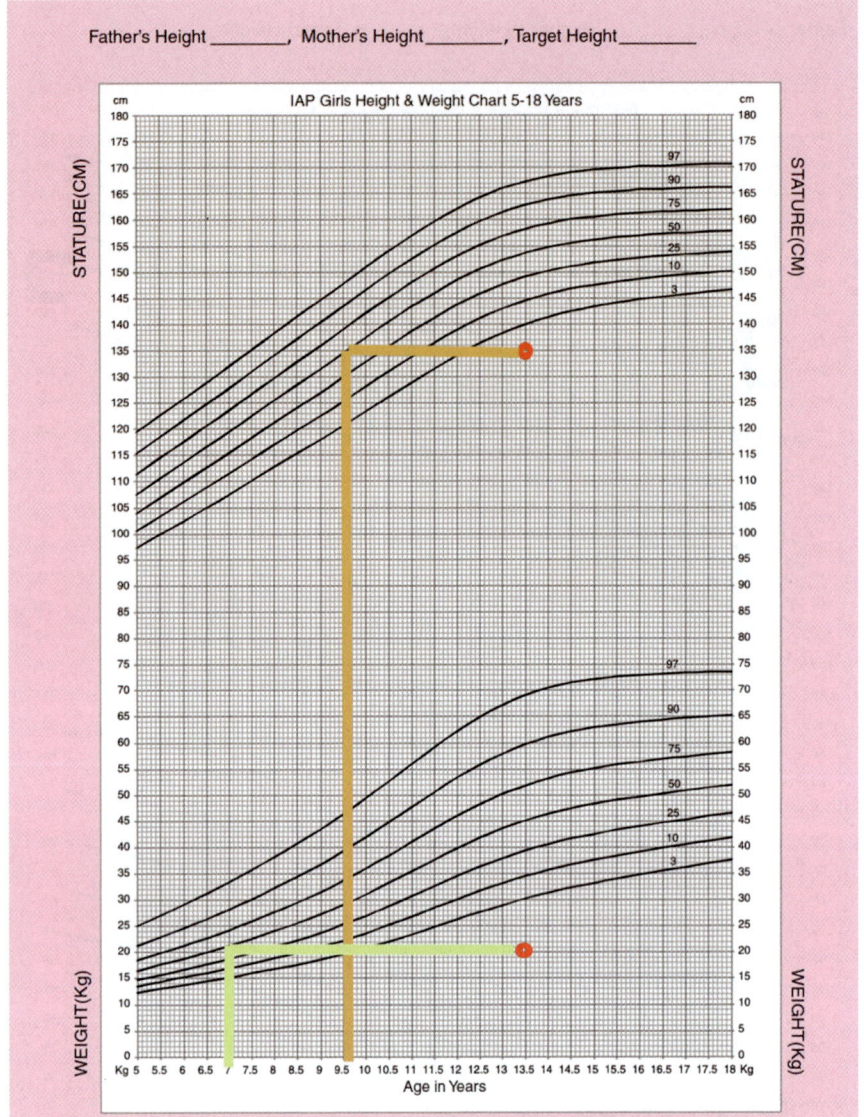

Fig. 38.17 Growth chart of a child with chronic systemic disease – both height and weight are less than third percentile. (Source: Modified from Harish Pemde, Vikram Datta, Kamlesh Harish. *Clinical and Practical Paediatrics*, Second Edition, Annexurel 2 I - Growth charts, New Delhi, Elsevier India, 2020.)

TABLE 38.13	Pathological Causes of Short Stature	
Diagnosis	**Weight**	**Height**
Endocrine	Obese	Short
Systemic/nutrition	Underweight	Short

41. What are the pathological causes of short stature?
    Table 38.13 gives the pathological causes of short stature. Figs. 38.17 and 38.18 give the examples of growth chart of chronic disease and endocrine cause, respectively.
42. Enumerate the treatment of short stature.
    Depending on the underlying etiology, Table 38.14 gives the treatment of specific disorders.
    In case of a confirmed growth hormone (GH) deficiency, Magnetic resonance imaging (MRI) brain is a must before initiating growth hormone. In case of a tumor, growth hormone (GH) will cause growth of the tumor also!

43. What is Madelung deformity?
    - Madelung deformity of the forearm (focal dysplasia of the distal radial physis, leading to a prominent ulna and wrist pain) is commonly seen in Turner syndrome or Short stature Homeobox containing gene (SHOX) mutations.
44. What are the X-ray features in achondroplasia?
    - The calvarial bones are large, whereas the cranial base and facial bones are small.
    - The interpedicular distance, which normally increases from the 1st to the 5th lumbar vertebra, decreases in achondroplasia.
    - The iliac bones are short and round, and the acetabular roofs are flat.
    - The tubular bones are short with mildly irregular and flared metaphyses.
    - The fibula is disproportionately long compared with the tibia. There is protrusion of the epiphysis into the metaphysis of the distal femur, creating the chevron deformity.

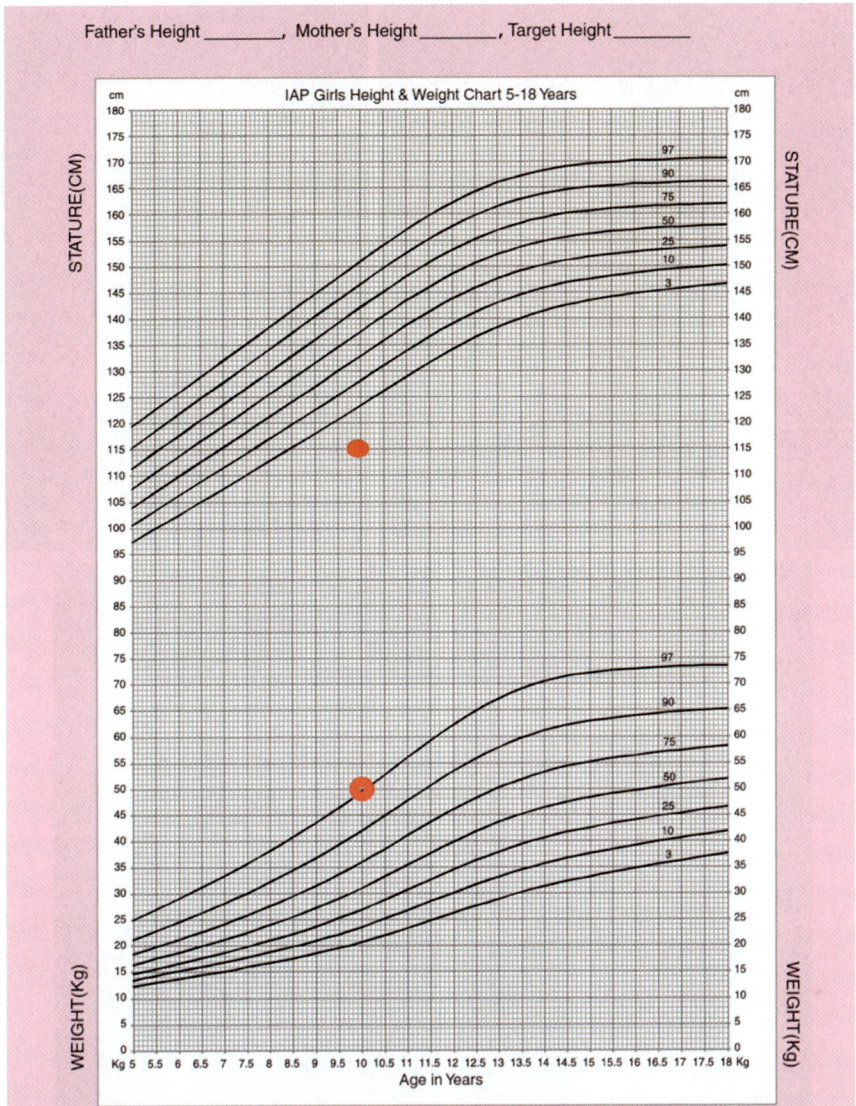

Father's Height _____ , Mother's Height _____ , Target Height _____

Fig. 38.18 Growth chart of a child with endocrine cause: weight – obese (97th percentile); and height <3rd percentile (short stature). Short and obese, endocrine cause. (Source: Modified from Harish Pemde, Vikram Datta, Kamlesh Harish. *Clinical and Practical Paediatrics*, Second Edition, Annexurel 2 I - Growth charts, New Delhi, Elsevier India, 2020.)

TABLE 38.14	Treatment of Short Stature
Chronic disorders	Specific treatment/multidisciplinary approach with other specialties, nutritional supplementation
Malnutrition	Dietary intervention
Familial short stature	Growth velocity monitoring, reassurance
Constitutional short stature	Growth velocity monitoring, reassurance, trial of testosterone to initiate puberty
Growth hormone (GH) deficiency	Growth hormone
Hypothyroidism	Thyroxine

- Fig. 38.19A–C shows the X-ray features of achondroplasia.
45. Where is champagne glass deformity seen?
   - In achondroplasia, the iliac bones are flat, giving rise to a pelvic inlet that resembles a champagne glass pelvis. The acetabular angles are flattened (horizontally,

yellow arrow) and the sacrosciatic notch is small (black arrow) as shown in Fig. 38.20.
46. What is telephone receiver defect?
   In Thanatophoric dysplasia, the femurs are curved and shaped like a telephone receiver.
   Fig. 38.21 shows the telephone receiver defect seen in thanotrophic dysplasia.
47. *How can one interpret abnormal growth with bone age, chronological age, and height for age?
   - Growth formula (CA, chronological age; HA, height for age; WA, weight for age)
   - Normal and abnormal growth interpretation shown in Table 38.15

DISCUSSION ON GROWTH AND GROWTH CHARTS

48. What are growth chart and standard deviation (SD)?
   - Growth chart is a diagnostic tool to measure the deviation of growth from normal.

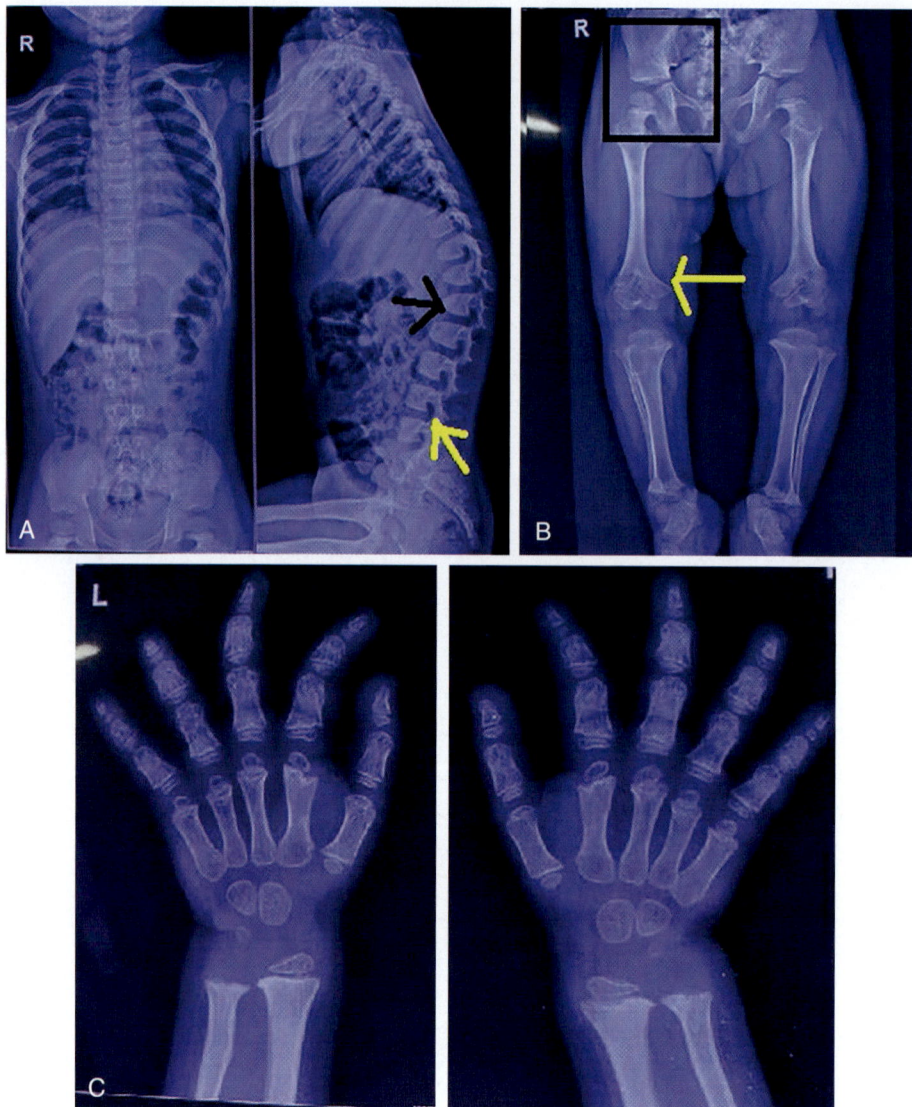

Fig. 38.19   (A) X-ray dorsolumbar spine anteroposterior (AP) and lateral view (black arrow, bullet nose vertebra; yellow arrow, posterior vertebral body scalloping). (B) X-ray pelvis with lower leg anteroposterior (AP) (black, tombstone/square-shaped iliac bone, flattening of acetabular roof; yellow arrow, rhizomelic shortening of femur, flaring of metaphysis). (C) Trident hand short with stubby fingers with separation between the middle and the ring finger.

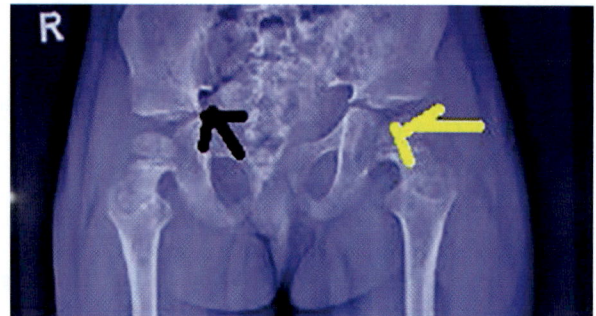

Fig. 38.20   Champagne glass pelvis – achondroplasia.

- The allowed normal range of variations in observations is conventionally taken as between 3rd and 97th percentiles. The percentile curve represents the frequency distribution curve.
- For example, the 25th percentile for height in a population would mean that height of 75% of individuals is greater than this value and that of 24% of individuals is less than this value. Values between 3rd and 97th percentile curves correspond to mean ± 2 SD.

49. What is Z-score?

$$Z\text{-score} = \frac{(\text{Observed value}) - (\text{Mean value})}{\text{Standard deviation}}$$

- In a population with observations in a typical Gaussian (normal) distribution, any individual value can be expressed as how many SDs it lies above or below the mean. This is the Z-score for that observation. Thus, if a child's height is at 2 SD below the mean, it is equivalent to −2 SD.

50. What are growth reference chart and growth standard?
    Table 38.16 gives the differences between growth reference chart and growth standard.

51. What is the normal velocity of growth of height in a child?
    Table 38.17 gives the normal velocity of height.

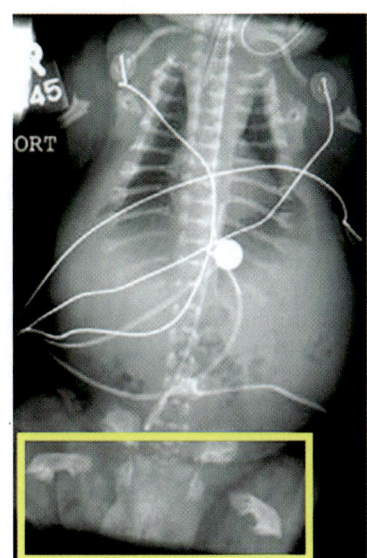

Fig. 38.21 Telephone receiver defect – Thanatophoric dysplasia. (*Source: Nelson, 21st edition, Chapter 716, p. 3726, Fig. 716.2.*)

TABLE 38.15	Normal and Abnormal Growth Interpretation	
Growth	**Interpretation**	**Disorder**
CA = HA = WA	No growth abnormality	Normal child
CA > HA > WA	Poor growth Wasted > stunted	Nutritional/systemic short stature
CA > WA > HA	Poor growth Stunted > wasted	Endocrine/skeletal disorder
WA > CA > HA	Overgrowth, short and obese	Pathological obesity

CA, chronological age; HA, height for age (HA); WA, weight for age (WA).

TABLE 38.16	Differences Between Growth Reference Chart and Growth Standard	
WHO Growth Standard		**Growth Reference (IAP Chart)**
0–5 years		5–18 years
Prescriptive chart		Descriptive chart
Prepared from population in whom all possible environmental and nutritional variables are controlled (children with no environmental, nutrition cosnstraints and without any chronic illness are recruited)		Prepared from population to be growing in optimal health and nutrition (under the influence of social, nutritional, cultural practices of that particular country)
Longitudinal study – same children are measured till 5 years of age		Cross-sectional study

TABLE 38.17	Normal Velocity of Height
Age[a]	**Growth Velocity**
Younger than 3 months	3 cm/month
3–6 months	2 cm/month
6–12 months	1.5 cm/month
1–5 years	6–8 cm/month
6–12 years	5 cm/year

[a]Term newborn, 50 cm; 1 year, 75 cm; 2 years, 86–87 cm; and 2–12 years, 6 cm/year.

52. What is Weech's formula?
    Expected height (cm) = Age (in years) × 6 + 77

53. What is Dine's formula?
    A malnourished baby may have a small head proportionate to the body. Dine's formula is used to avoid false microcephaly in the first 300 days.

    $$\text{Dine's formula} = \frac{\text{Length} + 9.5 \pm 2.5}{2}$$

54. What are the laws of growth?
    The three laws of growth are as follows:
    1. Growth is a continuous and orderly process.
    2. The order of growth is cephalocaudal – during fetal life, growth of the head occurs before that of the neck, and arms grow before legs.
    3. The order of growth is also distal to proximal – that is, the distal parts of the body such as hands increase in size before the upper arms.

55. What are the hormones responsible for growth?
    Growth hormone, insulin-like growth factor-1, thyroid hormones, and sex steroids

56. What are the factors influencing growth?
    • Intrauterine: Maternal nutrition, placental factors, insulin, and insulin-like growth factor-1 (IGF-1)
    • Infancy: Nutrition
    • Childhood: Growth hormone
    • Adolescence: Sex hormones and growth hormone

57. What is the normal growth pattern?
    A sigmoid-shaped curve with maximum growth occurring during infancy (25 cm/year) followed by puberty (10–12 cm/year) as shown in Fig. 38.22

58. What are the causes of growth retardation in the order of frequency?
    • Familial short stature
    • Protein–energy malnutrition
    • Chronic systemic disease
    • Skeletal disorder
    • Constitutional short stature
    • Endocrine disorder
    • intrauterine growth restriction (IUGR)
    • Chromosomal
    • Miscellaneous

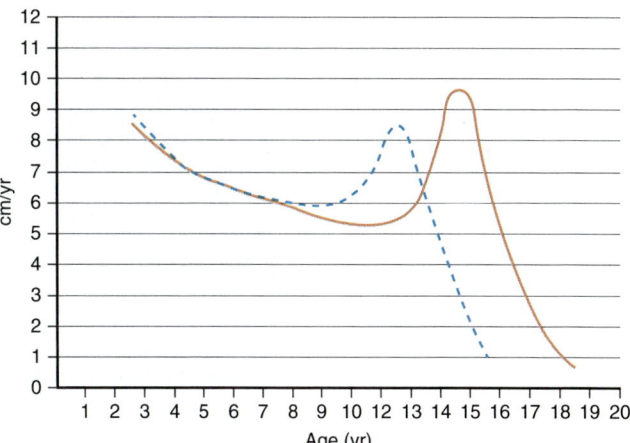

Fig. 38.22 Height velocity shown by solid line (males) and dotted line (females). (*Source: Nelson, 21st edition, volume 1, Chapter 312, p. 1017, Fig. 132.5.*)

59. Classify short stature.

Short stature can be classified as physiological and pathological short stature. Pathological short stature is further divided into proportionate and disproportionate short stature as shown in Flowchart 38.1.

Fig. 38.23 gives the picture of a child with growth hormone deficiency and a child with chronic disease (thalassemia) in comparison with a normal child.

60. What are the endocrine causes of short stature?
    a. Growth hormone deficiency
    b. Hypothyroidism
    c. Cushing syndrome
    d. Rickets
    e. Juvenile diabetes
    f. Pseudohypoparathyroidism
    g. Precocious or delayed puberty
    h. Laron dwarfism

61. What is psychosocial short stature?
    • It is also known as emotional deprivation dwarfism, maternal deprivation dwarfism, and hyperphagic short stature.
    • It occurs because of poor home environment and inadequate parenting.
    • It presents with behavioral manifestations, failure to thrive, social withdrawal, and primitive speech.

    • The child has functional hypopituitarism with decreased Insulin like growth factor-1 (IGF-1) and there is an inadequate response to growth hormone stimulation test.
    • These kids do not benefit from growth hormone replacement therapy.

62. What are the syndromes associated with short stature?
    1. Down syndrome
    2. Seckel syndrome
    3. Russell–Silver syndrome
    4. Seckel syndrome
    5. Gorlin syndrome
    6. Prader–Willi syndrome
    7. Turner syndrome
    8. Noonan syndrome
    9. Aarskog syndrome

63. What are the examples of obesity with short stature?
    • Mostly endocrine cause: Cushing syndrome and hypothyroid
    • Others
        ∘ Prader–Willi syndrome
        ∘ Bardet–Biedl syndrome

64. Who are primordial dwarfs?
    • Primordial dwarfs have a smaller body size in all stages of life – at birth, SGA/IUGR/LBW. After birth, growth

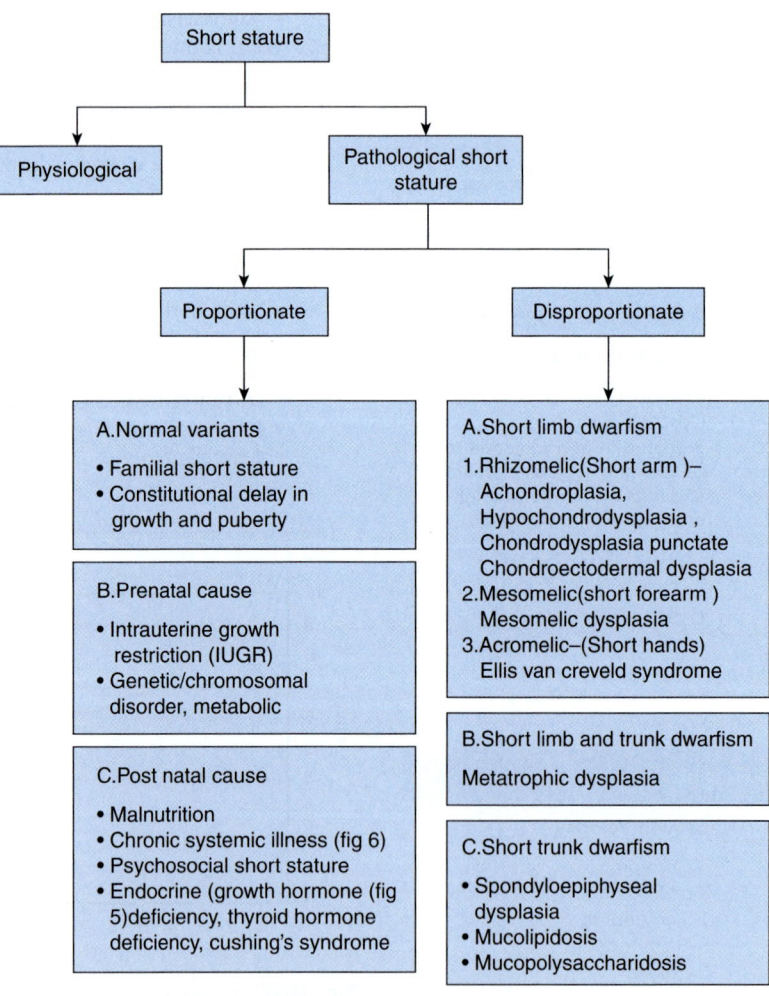

Flowchart 38.1 Classification of Short Stature

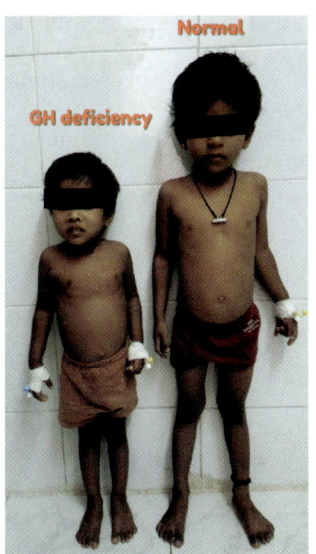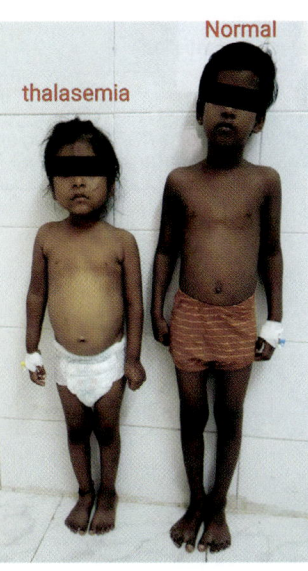

Fig. 38.23 From right to left, growth hormone (GH) deficiency, normal child, thalassemia (short stature because of chronic disease) comparing with normal child.

continues at a much slower rate, leaving individuals with primordial dwarfism perpetually years behind their peers in stature and in weight.

- This condition is difficult to diagnose till 3–5 years of age.
- This condition occurs because of five syndromic causes:
  1. Down syndrome
  2. Russell syndrome
  3. Seckel syndrome
  4. Osteodysplastic primordial dwarfism type 1
  5. Osteodysplastic primordial dwarfism type 2

65. What is the infancy–childhood–puberty (ICP) model of growth?

The infancy–childhood–puberty (ICP) model of growth refers to the infancy–childhood–puberty model of growth. These are times of rapid growth under the influence of nutrition, growth hormone (GH), thyroxine, and sex steroids.

66. What are the criteria to diagnose idiopathic short stature?

Criteria for diagnosing idiopathic short stature are as follows:
  1. Height <-2 SD of age and sex of reference population
  2. Absence of any underlying identifiable systemic or endocrine abnormality
  3. Normal weight for gestational age at birth
  4. Normal body proportion
  5. Presence of adequate food and calorie intake
  6. No psychiatry or severe emotional disturbance
  7. Peak growth hormone response on standard stimulation >10 ng/mL

67. When should growth hormone be started in a child with idiopathic short stature?
  - When the growth is -2 to -3 SD, the growth hormone is started.
  - The time to start is before 5 years or at the least early to puberty.

68. What are the indications for poor response to growth hormone therapy?

Increase in growth of <-1 SD or change in height velocity of -0.3 to -0.5 SD

69. What are the eight Food and drug administration (FDA)-approved indications for growth hormone replacement therapy?
  a. Growth hormone (GH) deficiency
  b. Chronic kidney disease (CKD) post-transplantation
  c. Turners syndrome
  d. Small for gestational age (SGA)/Intra uterine growth restriction (IUGR)
  e. Prader–Willi syndrome
  f. Idiopathic short stature
  g. Short stature Homeobox containing gene (SHOX) gene mutation
  h. Down syndrome

70. What is growth hormone stimulation test and how can one interpret the results?
  - After an overnight fasting for 10–12 hours, the baseline level of growth hormone is taken. It is ensured that free Thyroxine (T4) and cortisol are normal. The sample is taken in the early morning. Then clonidine 150 microgram/m² is given orally (once the previous night and the next dose in the morning) or inj. glucagon subcutaneous 10–15 microgram (mic)/kg is given as stat dose and four samples are taken at 30, 60, 90, and 120 minutes (every 0.5-hour interval for 2 hours).
  - Monitor capillary blood glucose (CBG) and blood pressure every half an hour.
  - If any two values are <10 ng/mL, it is suggestive of growth hormone deficiency.

71. When should one ask for Insulin like growth factor (IGF) values?
  - Insulin like growth factor-1 (IGF-1) levels are used to monitor the response to therapy.
  - They must be measured early morning, fasting sample. If the level is less than the third centile, perform the stimulation test; a level more than the 50th centile makes Growth hormone deficiency (GHD) unlikely.

72. What is the treatment of short stature?

Recombinant human growth hormone replacement therapy is the treatment of choice for pathological short statures. Dose is 0.35 mg/kg/week.

73. How is a child on growth hormone injection followed up?

Table 38.18 gives the follow-up of a child on growth hormone injection.

TABLE 38.18	Follow-Up of a Child on Growth Hormone Injection	
Clinical	**Laboratory (3 Monthly During 1st Year, Annually Later)**	**Radiological**
a. Height	a. Free Thyroxine (T4)	Bone age (if rapid sexual maturation/pubertal age)
b. Height SD score	b. Thyroid stimulating hormone (TSH)	
c. Growth velocity	c. Blood sugar	
d. Any complications – injection site	d. Insulin like growth factor-1 (IGF-1)	
e. Compliance		

SD, standard deviation.

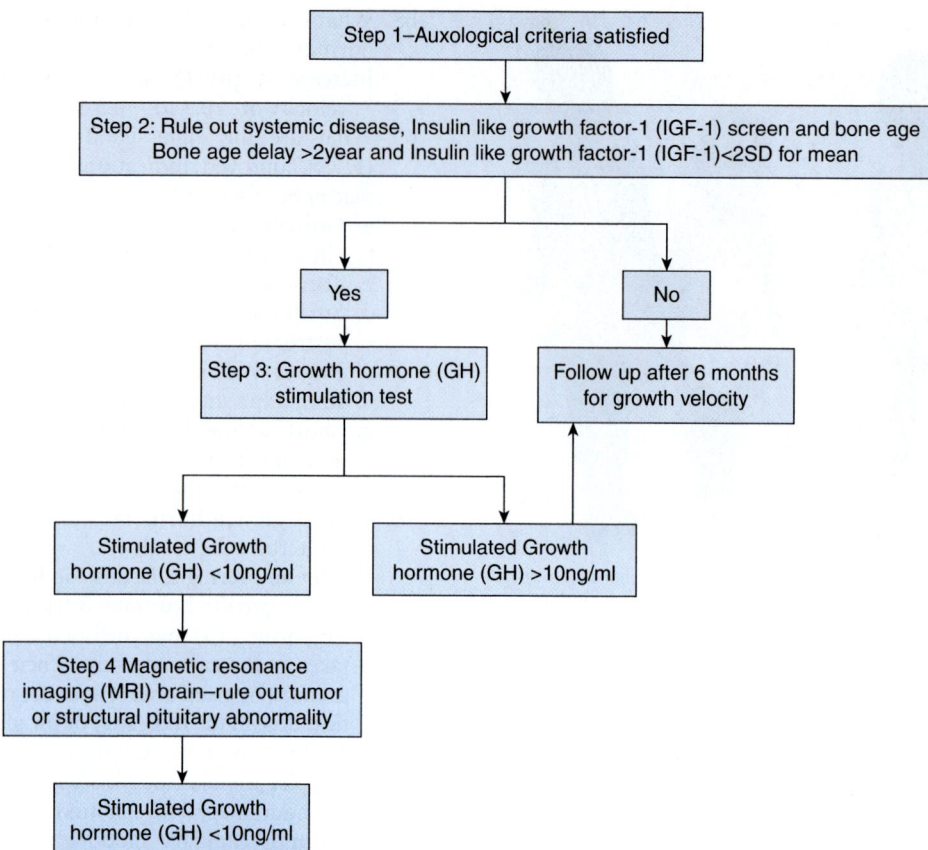

Flowchart 38.2 Approach to proportionate short stature.

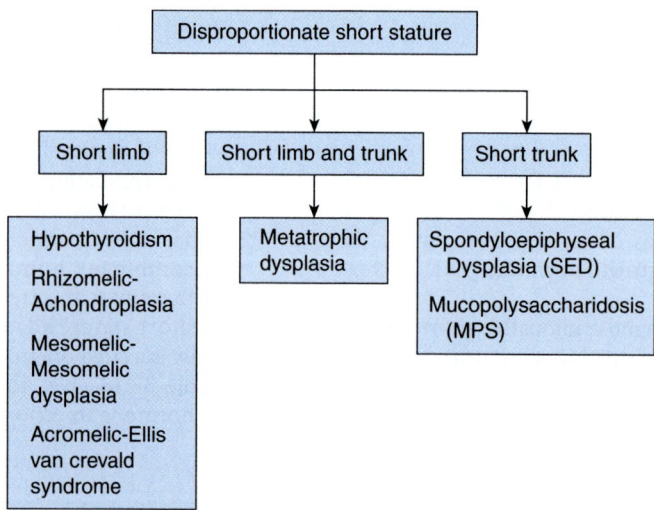

Flowchart 38.3 Approach to disproportionate short stature.

74. When should growth hormone therapy be stopped?
   a. When a child thinks that he or she is tall enough
   b. When height velocity is <1 inch/year
   c. When bone age is >14 for girls and >16 for boys
75. What are the other treatment modalities available for short stature?
   a. Gonadotropin releasing hormone (GnRH) agonists
   b. Aromatase inhibitors (for boys – to retard further growth of puberty and physeal closure)

c. Human chorionic gonadotropin – Gonadotropin releasing hormone (GnRH) analogues in girls
76. Describe the approach to proportionate and disproportionate short stature.
   Flowcharts 38.2 and 38.3 give the approach to proportionate and disproportionate short stature.

Quick Bites

1. CA = HA = WA: Normal child
2. CA > HA > WA: Systemic/nutritional
3. CA > WA > HA: Short stature
4. Short for population but normal for family: Familial short stature
5. Very short for population and family: Endocrine short stature
6. Short for population and short for family: Constitutional or early disease
7. WA > HA > CA: Nutritional obesity
8. WA > CA ≥ HA: Pathological obesity
9. HA > WA > CA: Precocious puberty
10. Any child who crosses two percentile lines in 1-year period: Evaluate
11. Wasted > stunted: Nutritional/systemic short stature
12. Stunted > wasted: Endocrine/skeletal disorder
13. Short and obese: Pathological obesity
14. Tall and obese: Nutritional obesity
15. Younger than 5 years: IAP-modified WHO charts
16. Older than 5 years: IAP 2015 – 5- to 18-year charts

Following introduction, seek permission from the caregiver and introduce yourself to the patient before history elicitation, and identify the case.

Name____Age____Sex____Consanguinity____Order of birth____Place____Informant____

Presenting Complaints and Duration

- Newborn period: Feeding difficulties (because of hypotonia of oral musculatures, cleft palate), vomiting, and delayed passage of meconium/neonatal jaundice
- Beyond newborn period: Feeding difficulties/lethargy/developmental delay/recurrent respiratory tract infections

History of Presenting Complaints

- Elaborate the presenting complaints (most common respiratory illness).
- Ask complication history and etiological history according to the presenting complaints.
- Ask history pertaining to individual systems:
  - Cardiovascular system: Fast breathing/chest indrawing/palpitations (in older children)
  - Respiratory system: Snoring and obstructive sleep apnea
  - Gastrointestinal system
    - Abdominal distention (hypotonia, umbilical hernia, duodenal atresia, pyloric stenosis)
    - Vomiting (duodenal atresia, pyloric stenosis)
    - Constipation
    - Yellowish discoloration of eyes and urine with/without clay-colored stools
    - Aspiration/choking during feeds (tracheoesophageal fistula)
  - Central nervous system: Seizures/flailness of limbs/behavioral abnormalities
  - Hematological system: Easy fatiguability/bleeding gums/bone pain with swelling of joints (leukemia)
  - Others: Impaired vision/impaired hearing

ANTENATAL HISTORY

- Apart from the usual antenatal history, focus on the following:
  - Age of the mother
  - Blood investigations done in the first trimester/second trimester
  - Any anomalies detected in USG Ultrasonogram
  - Karyotyping done or not

NATAL/POSTNATAL HISTORY

- Birth asphyxia (because of hypotonia)
- Delayed passage of meconium
- Neonatal jaundice
- Feeding difficulties
- Vomiting/abdominal distension

DEVELOPMENTAL HISTORY

- Delay in milestones
- Decreased scholastic performance

DIETETIC HISTORY

- Feeding patterns: Direct feeding/spoon/NG feeding
- Choking while feeding
- Regurgitation of feeds

IMMUNIZATION HISTORY

Special vaccine: Pnuemococcal and flu vaccines

FAMILY HISTORY

Similar illness in family members

SOCIOECONOMIC HISTORY

According to the modified Kuppuswamy scale

Summary

A _____-year-old child presented with mention the complaints and history pertaining to Down syndrome

General Examination

- Patient's sensorium
- Pallor
- Cyanosis
- Clubbing
- Icterus
- Generalized lymphadenopathy
- Pedal edema

Head-to-Foot Examination

Table 39.1 gives the head-to-foot examination in Down syndrome.

Vital Signs

- Pulse rate
- Blood pressure
- Respiration: Rate, rhythm, and type of respiration
- Temperature
- JVP (Jugular venous pressure)

Anthropometry

- Wasting
- Stunting
- Microcephaly

TABLE 39.1	Head-to-Foot Examination in Down Syndrome
Region	**Findings**
Skull	• Microcephaly • Flat occiput • Patent metopic suture • Large fontanels with late closure • Sloping forehead • Absent frontal and sphenoid sinuses, and hypoplasia of the maxillary sinuses occur
Eyes	• Upslanting palpebral fissures • Brushfield spots (speckled iris) • Refractive errors (50%) • Strabismus (44%) • Blepharitis (33%) • Acquired lens opacity (30%) • Nystagmus (20%) • Congenital cataracts (3%) • Conjunctivitis • Bilateral epicanthal folds • Tearing from stenotic nasolacrimal ducts • Pseudopapilledema • Keratoconus • Spasmus nutans
Nose	Hypoplastic nasal bone and flat nasal bridge
Mouth and teeth	• An open-mouth tongue protrusion • Microdontia (35%–50%) • Tooth agenesis • Malformed teeth • Delayed tooth eruption • Hypoplastic and hypocalcified teeth • A chapped lower lip • Partial anodontia (50%) • A fissured and furrowed tongue • Angular cheilitis
Ears	• Chronic otitis media • Hearing loss • Overfolded helix
Neck	• Atlantoaxial instability (14%) – laxity of transverse ligaments (which hold the odontoid process close to the anterior arch of the atlas) • The backward displacement of the odontoid process causes laxity, leading to spinal cord compression in 2% of children with Down syndrome
Chest	• The internipple distance is decreased • Short sternum
Hands	• Clinodactyly because of dysplastic middle phalanx of the little finger • Brachydactyly – short and stumpy fingers • Dermatoglyphics – wide ATD angle • Simian crease
Feet	• Wide gap between the first and the second toes (sandal gap)

System Examination

CARDIOVASCULAR SYSTEM

Features of endocardial cushion defect/ventricular septal defect (ventricular septal defect)/atrial septal defect (atrial septal defect)/tetralogy of Fallot (TOF)

RESPIRATORY SYSTEM

Look for features of pneumonia.

ABDOMEN

Umbilical hernia/features of cholestatic jaundice/features of intestinal obstruction

CENTRAL NERVOUS SYSTEM

Hypotonia/poor Moro reflex

Diagnosis

• A case of _____ (mention the primary diagnosis pertaining to the presenting complaints)
• With features of Down syndrome
• With/without complications

Frequently Asked Questions

1. When and who discovered Down syndrome?

   John Langdon Down, an English physician, first described the syndrome in 1866. He is called the "father" of Down syndrome. Down syndrome is the most common trisomy.

2. What is the other name of Down facies?

   Down facies can also be called Mongoloid facies or universal facies (because they have unique facial features throughout).

*3. Explain the correlation between the maternal age and the risk of Down syndrome.

   The risk is inversely related to maternal age.

   Table 39.2 shows the relationship between maternal age and Down syndrome.

4.* Explain the genetics of Down syndrome.

   - It is the most common trisomy.
   - Meiotic nondisjunction is the cause of 95% of cases of Down syndrome.
   - Meiosis I is responsible for 90% of cases of Down syndrome.
   - Robertsonian translocation, which can be inherited or arise de novo, causes 4% of cases of Down syndrome:
     - 14–21 (most common), 21–21, 13–21, and 22–21
   - Mosaicism is the cause of 1% of cases of Down syndrome.
   - Isochromosomes and ring chromosomes are the other rarer causes of trisomy 21.

5. Why is advanced maternal age a risk factor for Down syndrome?

   Because of the older age of the ovum and lack of spindle formation in elderly mothers

*6. Explain Hall's criteria for Down syndrome.

   Hall's criteria aid in the diagnosis of Down syndrome in the neonatal period. They are as follows:

   Flat facial profile - 90%, Poor Moro reflex 85%, Hypotonia-80%, joint hyperflexibility - 80%

   Excessive skin on back of neck - 80%, Slanted palpebral fissures - 80%, pelvis dysplasia - 70%, Unusual ear shape - 60%, Dysplasia of midphalanx of fifth finger - 60%, single transverse palmar crease - 45%, 4 out of 10 suggestive of Down syndrome

   Fig. 39.1 shows Down facies.

7. Mention few causes of Mongoloid and anti-Mongoloid slant.

   - Mongoloid slant: Down syndrome, Prader–Willi syndrome, and ectodermal dysplasia

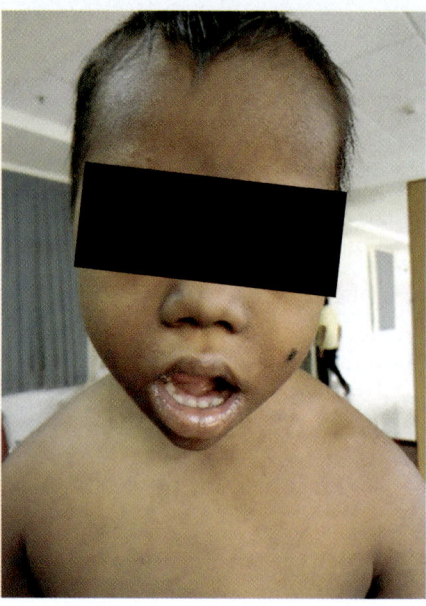

Fig. 39.1 Down facies – Mongoloid slant, epicanthal fold, depressed nasal bridge (flat facial profile), wide open mouth.

   - Anti-Mongoloid slant: Treacher Collins, Sotos syndrome, and Noonan syndrome

*8. Enumerate the surgical conditions associated with Down syndrome.

   A. Gastrointestinal
      - Tracheoesophageal fistula
      - Deudodenal atresia
      - Biliary atresia
      - Annular pancreas
      - Pyloric stenosis
      - Anal atresia
      - Umbilical hernia
      - Hirschsprung disease

   B. Respiratory
      Congenital diaphragmatic hernia

   C. Orthopedic
      - Dislocation of the hip
      - Congenital talipes equinovarus

9. Explain the normal dermatoglyphics.

   - ATD angle: It is a feature of the palm that connects the position of three triradii – a, d, and t. ATD angles are measured for each palm. Two straight lines are drawn through the a and t triradii and the d and t triradii, and the resulting angle is measured. The normal ATD angle is approximately 48° and measured in the adducted palm.
   - Ulnar loop: If the loop opens in the ulnar side, it is an ulnar loop.
   - Radial loop: If the loop opens on the radial side, it is a radial loop.
   - Whorl: It refers to characteristic ridge courses that follow as circuits around the core.
   - Arch: The plain arch is composed of ridges that pass across the finger with a slight bow distally. There are no triradii.

TABLE 39.2	Relationship Between Maternal Age and Down Syndrome	
Age of Mother (Years)		**Risk**
20		1:1925
25		1:1205
30		1:885
35		1:365
40		1:110
45		1:32

Fig. 39.2 shows the normal dermatoglyphics.

*10. Enumerate the dermatoglyphics in Down syndrome.
  - Dermatoglyphics in Down syndrome forms a unique pattern
  - Hand
    - Ulnar loops in digits 1, 2, 3, and 5
    - Radial loops in digit 4
    - Absence of thenar pattern
    - Increased ATD angle
  - Foot
    - 15: Increased fibular loops in the foot
    - 16: Arch tibial loops increased in the hallucal area
    - 17: Small distal loops in the hallucal area
    - 18: Distal loop in area 4 increased in frequency
    - 19: Ridge dissociation

  Fig. 39.3A and B shows the dermatoglyphic pattern of hand and foot, respectively, in babies with Down syndrome

11. Enumerate the hematological complications of Down syndrome.
  - Polycythemia vera
  - Acute myeloid leukemia (AML) (150-fold increased risk; megakaryocytic or erythroblastic type is more common)
  - Acute lymphoblastic leukemia (ALL) (40-fold risk)
  - Transient myeloproliferative disease
  - Neonatal leukemia
  - Good response to AML therapy shown by children with Down syndrome, whereas the response to ALL therapy is same as in normal population.

12. Enumerate the CNS manifestations of Down syndrome.
  - Intellectual disability
  - Seizures
  - Autism spectrum disorders
  - Behavioral disorders (disruptive)
  - Depression
  - Alzheimer disease

*13. Discuss the atlantoaxial instability (AAI) in Down syndrome.
  - Fifteen per cent of individuals with Down syndrome younger than 21 years have AAI.
  - Majority are asymptomatic.
  - Symptomatic AAI can result in spinal cord injury resulting in the following symptoms: neck pain, restricted neck movements, paraplegia, bladder–bowel disturbances, and tingling sensations.
  - Prior to participation in sports that require hyperextension or extreme flexion of the neck (e.g., gymnastics, swimming, high jump, equestrian sports, football, soccer, alpine skinning), X-ray examination (full extension and flexion views) of the neck is required. AAI is diagnosed by an increased atlanto-odontoid interval on flexion/extension lateral radiographs of more than 4.5 mm. Once the diagnosis is confirmed, participation in sports can be

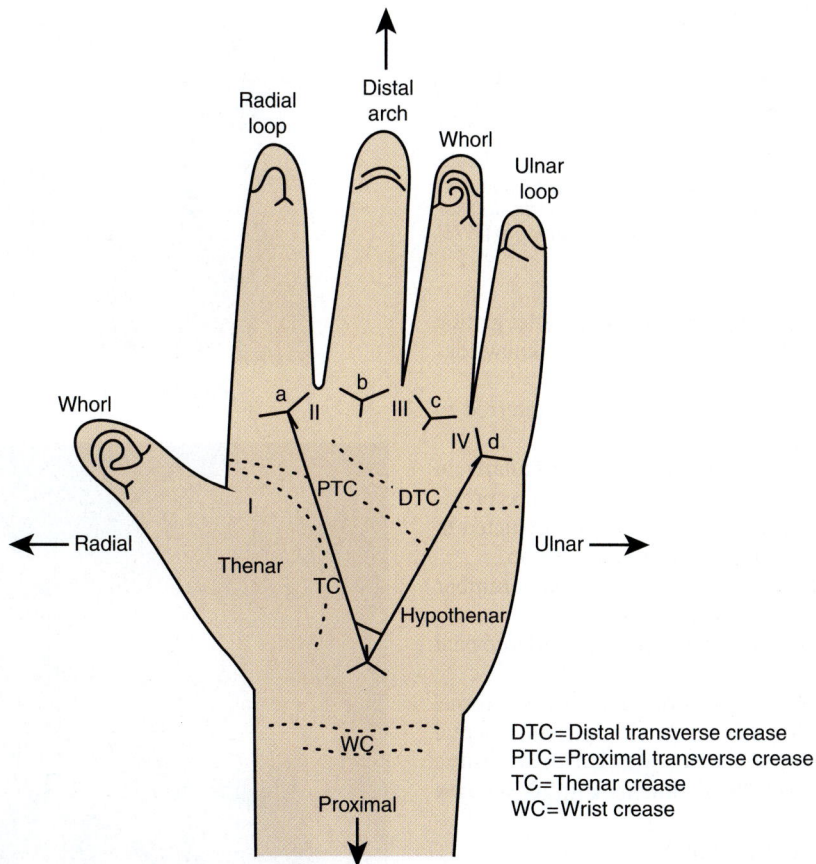

Fig. 39.2 Normal dermatoglyphics in hand. (*Source:* Reproduced from Garima Jindal, Ramesh Kumar Pandey, Sameer Gupta et al. and A comparative evaluation of dermatoglyphics in different classes of malocclusion, *The Saudi Dental Journal* 47(2):88-92.)

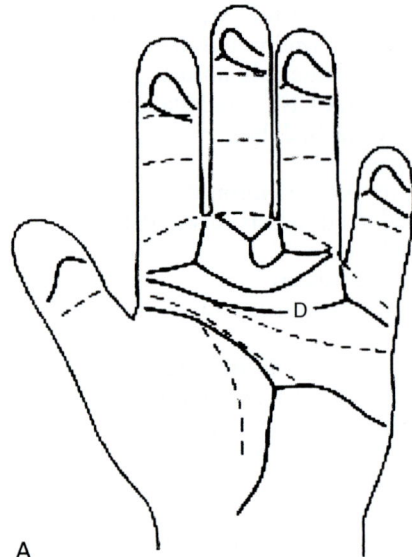

A

Fig. 39.3A Dermatoglyphics in Down syndrome – hand. *(Source: Reproduced from Christine Gleason, Sandra Juul. Avery's Diseases of the Newborn, Tenth Edition, The Dysmorphic Infant, Fig. 19.11, Philadelphia, Elsevier Inc., 2018. Credit Line - (From Holt SB. The Genetics of Dermal Ridges. Springfield, IL: Charles C Thomas; 1968.)*

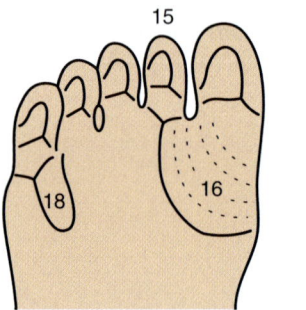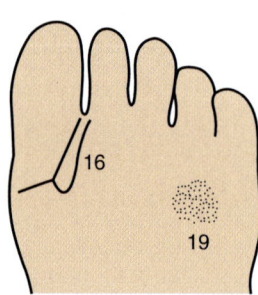

B

Fig. 39.3B Dermatoglyphics in Down syndrome – foot (15 – fibular loops increased in frequency). *(Reprinted/adapted by permission from Springer Nature: Springer-Verlag, Dermatoglyphics in Medical Disorders by Blanka Schaumann and Milton Alter, Copyright Springer (1976). Figure 6.6, p. 148.)*

permitted if the parents or guardians request after getting written certification from a physician and acknowledgment of the risks by the parent or guardian.
- All patients diagnosed with AAI should be referred to an orthopedic surgeon.
- Normal X-ray does not rule out AAI, particularly in young children in whom the radiographic interpretation is difficult. Hence, parents should be instructed to report if any signs of spinal cord injury develop.

14. Discuss the precautions taken while performing lumbar puncture in a child with Down syndrome.
- Avoid hyperflexion of the neck because of atlantoaxial joint instability.

*15. List the cardiovascular complications in Down syndrome.
- Endocardial cushion defects (atrioventricular septal defect [AVSD]; 45% of patients with Down syndrome have AVSD, whereas 50% of patients with AVSD have Down syndrome)
- Ventricular septal defect (VSD)
- Atrial septal defect (ASD)
- Tetralogy of Fallot (TOF)

- Patent ductus arteriosus (PDA)
- Mitral valve prolapse
- Isolated secundum atrial septal defect

16. List the dermatological manifestations of Down syndrome.
- Palmar hyperkeratosis
- Seborrheic dermatitis
- Fissured tongue
- Geographic tongue
- Cutis marmorata
- Xerosis

17. List the endocrinological manifestations of Down syndrome.
- Hypothyroidism
- Type 1 diabetes mellitus

18. Explain the significance of simian crease.
- Simian crease is a single transverse palmar crease.
- Normally, 4% of individuals have a unilateral simian crease and it can be familial.
- It is also found in trisomies 13 and 18, fetal alcohol syndrome, Klinefelter syndrome, and Noonan syndrome.
- Simian crease in an otherwise normal child, whether unilateral or bilateral, does not warrant any investigation.

Fig. 39.4 shows a unilateral simian crease.
Fig. 39.5 shows a bilateral simian crease.

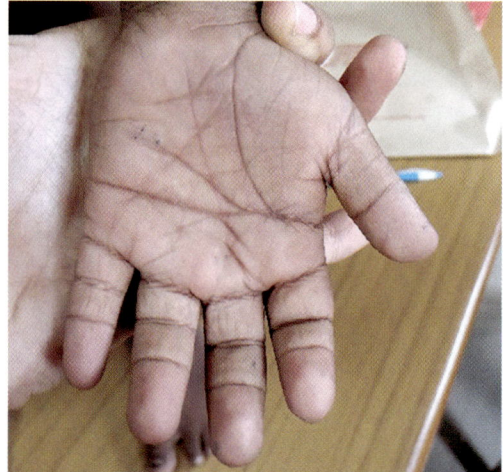

Fig. 39.4 Unilateral simian crease.

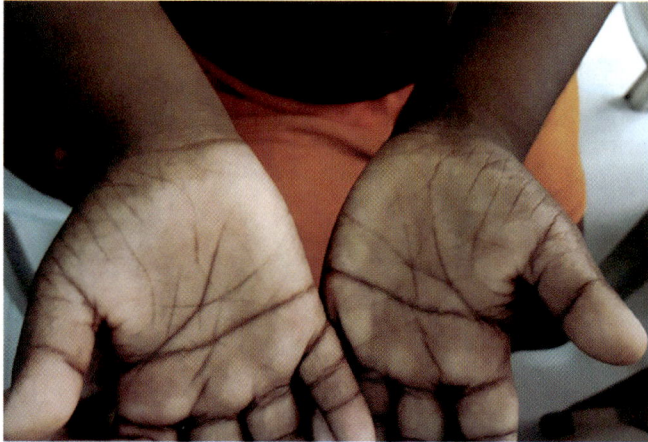

Fig. 39.5 Bilateral simian crease.

*19. Enumerate the antenatal tests to identify Down syndrome.

All women should be offered screening for Down syndrome. Table 39.3 lists the antenatal screening for Down syndrome.

20. Name some screening tests for aneuploidy in maternal serum.
    - Maternal serum alpha-fetoprotein (MSAFP): Decreased in aneuploidy
    - Others: Unconjugated estriol, inhibin, and beta-hCG (Human Chorionic Gonadotropin)
    - Trisomy 21 – Down syndrome: Beta-hCG and inhibin high, and MSAFP and unconjugated estriol decreased
    - Trisomy 18 – Edward syndrome: All four markers low

21. Enumerate various approaches in combined first and second trimester screening.
    - There are two approaches, integrated screening and sequential screening, depending on whether they disclose reports of the first trimester or not while retaining a low screen positive rate.
      a. *Integrated screening*
        - Nondisclosure approach
        - Sensitivity: 97%, low (2%) screen positive rate
        - First trimester ultrasound + results of both first and second trimester maternal serum screening disclosed together
      b. *Sequential screening*: Two types, both of which are disclosure tests
        1. *Stepwise sequential*
          - Results indicating high risk of trisomy 21 in the first trimester are released, and then further screening of the entire remaining population is performed in the second trimester.
          - Screen positive rate is low, 2%–3%, and sensitivity is 95%.
        2. *Contingent sequential*
          - Patients are classified into high-risk, medium-risk, and low-risk groups.
          - Results indicating high risk of trisomy 21 in the first trimester are released but only medium-risk patients are further screened. Low-risk patients do not return for further screening because their risk of fetus with Down syndrome is low.
          - Screen positive rate is low, 2%–3%, and sensitivity is 93%.

22*. What is NIPT?
    - Noninvasive prenatal testing (NIPT) is also called cell-free fetal DNA screening for aneuploidy. Cell-free fetal DNA seen in the maternal serum is of placental origin. It can be detected as early as 9 weeks of gestational age and can be tested throughout the entire pregnancy.
    - This screening test needs a diagnostic test for confirmation.
    - It is not recommended for general population; it is performed only for women considered high risk for aneuploidy:
      - Women older than 35 years
      - Women with a history of fetus or newborn with aneuploidy
      - Carriers of balanced translocation
      - Women with a positive traditional screening test
    - Advantage: The sensitivity of trisomy is 21%–99.3% and specificity is 99.8%.
    - Disadvantage: Cell-free fetal DNA targets specific aneuploidies but misses abnormalities in other chromosomes and those with mosaic karyotype.

23. *What is PGD (Preimplantation genetic diagnosis)?
    - Preimplantation genetic diagnosis is performed for in vitro fertilization process; during the eight-cell stage in humans, prior to transfer, one or two cells are removed and sent for molecular diagnoses. Only those embryos that screen negative for chromosomal abnormality are transferred.
    - PGD is mainly useful for balanced translocation in trisomy 21.

24. Explain the role of antenatal USG in Down syndrome.
    Antenatal (AN) USG findings in Down syndrome
      - First trimester: Nuchal translucency >3 mm thick and abnormal ductal venous flow
      - Second trimester: Echogenic intraventricular foci and ventriculomegaly
      - Nuchal fold thickness >6 mm and hypoplastic or absent nasal bone
      - Aberrant right subclavian artery and echogenic bowel
      - Shortened femur and pelviectasis
      - Cystic hygroma, hydrops, and hepatomegaly
      - Cardiac defects: ASD, VSD, and Truncus Arteriosus
    Role of a USG
      - It estimates the appropriate gestational age on the basis of which the screening test can be decided.
      - Nuchal fold thickness can help in the diagnosis of Down syndrome.
      - It helps to detect fetal anomalies.

*25. What is the definitive diagnosis of Down syndrome?
    The definitive diagnosis is made by karyotyping. If translocation is identified, then both the parents should undergo karyotyping to determine the risk of recurrence in subsequent pregnancy.

26. What are the indications of definitive diagnostic test for genetic disease?
    - *Indications for diagnostic test*
      a. Women with a positive family history of genetic disease
      b. Positive screening test
      c. At risk of ultrasonographic features

TABLE 39.3	Antenatal Screening for Down Syndrome	
First Trimester	**Second Trimester**
1. USG: Nuchal translucency, which is because of fluid collected at the nape of neck >3 mm is positive (also increased in congenital heart disease) Sensitivity <70% 2. NT (Nuchal translucency,) + beta-hCG + PAPP-A (Pregnancy-associated plasma protein A) + maternal age: Sensitivity 80%	1. Quadruple screen: Alpha-fetoprotein (AFP) + beta-hCG + unconjugated estriol + inhibin Sensitivity 80% 2. Combined first trimester + second trimester screening: Sensitivity 95%

TABLE 39.4	**Differences Between Chorionic Villus Sampling and Amniocentesis**	
Features	**Chorionic Villus Sampling**	**Amniocentesis**
Method of analysis	Ultrasonic guidance (transvaginal ultrasound)	Ultrasound-guided needle aspiration
Tissue analyzed	Placental tissue: Trophoblast	Amniotic fluid: 20 mL (replaced within 24 h)
Time of performance	At or after 10 weeks	As early as 10–14 weeks
Pregnancy loss rate	0.5%–1%	• <13 weeks: 1%–2% • 16–20 weeks: 0.5%–1%
Complications	When performed <10 weeks, fetal limb reduction defects and oromandibular malformations	<13 weeks: Increased incidence of clubfoot

d. No need to perform amniocentesis or Chorionic villus sampling for second pregnancy if the first child is trisomy 21

e. Samples of diagnostic test are analyzed for the following:
- Microarray analysis (structural abnormalities)
- Microarray analysis + karyotyping (for aneuploidy)
- DNA analysis: PCR-DNA fragments – alpha-thalassemia, Duchenne and Becker muscular dystrophy, cystic fibrosis, and growth hormone deficiency
- Other compounds: Alpha-fetoprotein (AFP), acetylcholinesterase, bilirubin, and surfactant

Table 39.4 gives the differences between various diagnostic tests performed.

Table 39.5 shows the risk of recurrence according to the karyotype.

27. Explain the frequencies of various clinical findings in Down syndrome.

Table 39.6 lists the frequencies of various clinical findings in Down syndrome.

Fig. 39.6A–C shows clinodactyly, sandal gap, and short neck, respectively.

28. Enumerate the various screening tests for babies with Down syndrome.

Table 39.7 shows the various screening tests for babies with Down syndrome.

29. Compare developmental milestones of children with Down syndrome with those of normal children.

Table 39.8 gives a comparison of developmental milestones of children with Down syndrome with those of normal children.

TABLE 39.5	**Risk of Recurrence According to the Karyotype**	
	RISK OF RECURRENCE (%)	
Type	**Carrier Mother**	**Carrier Father**
14q;21q	15	5
21q;22q	15	5
21q;21q	100	100

TABLE 39.6	**Frequencies of Various Clinical Findings in Down Syndrome**		
Clinical Findings	**Percentage**	**Clinical Findings**	**Percentage**
Mental retardation	99	Short neck	60
Stunted growth	90	Clinodactyly	57
Hypotonia	80	Brushfield spots	56
Large tongue	75	Simian crease	53
Sandal gap	68	Congenital heart disease	40
Short hands	60	Strabismus	35

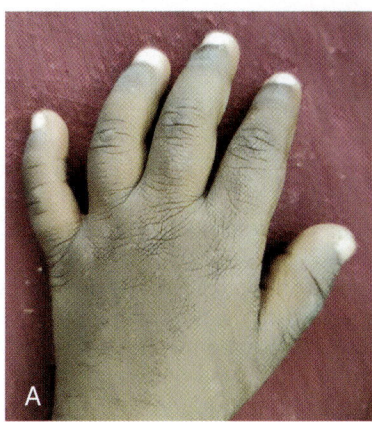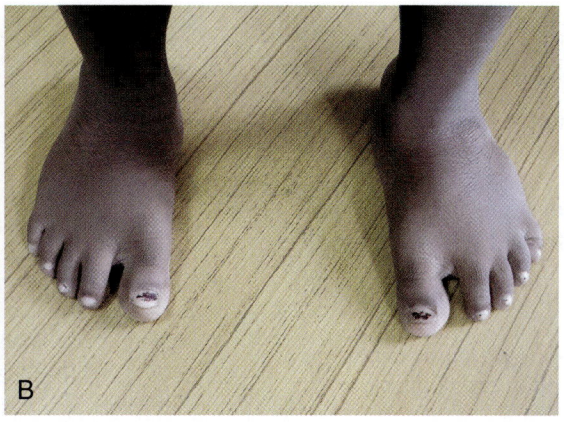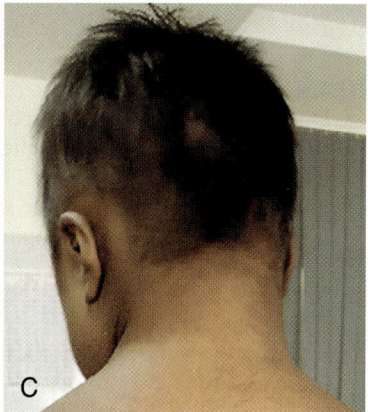

Fig. 39.6A (A) Clinodactyly. (B) Sandal gap. (C) Short neck.

TABLE 39.7	Various Screening Tests for Babies With Down Syndrome		
Testing	**Infants**	**Children**	
Hearing	6 months, 12 months, and then yearly	3–5 years	
T4 and Thyroid Stimulating Hormone)	6 months, and then yearly		
Eyes	6 months, and then yearly	3–5 years	
Teeth	2 years, and then every 6 months		
Hematology	Between 2 and 3 years of age, or earlier if symptoms occur		
Sleep study	3–4 years, or earlier if symptoms of obstructive sleep apnea occur		
Neck X-rays	Between 3 and 5 years of age		
Congenital heart disease	Birth	Young adult for acquired valve disease	
Celiac disease		At 2 years or with symptoms	
Growth and development	At each visit Use Down syndrome growth curves		

Source: Nelson, 21st edition, volume 1, Chapter 98, p. 662, Table 98.8.

TABLE 39.8	Comparison of Developmental Milestones of Down syndrome children with Normal children	
Milestone	**For Normal child**	**For Down syndrome children**
GROSS MOTOR		
Sits alone	5-9 months	6-30 months
Crawls	6-12 months	8-22 months
Stands	8-17 months	1-3.25 years
Walk Alone	9-18 months	1-4 years
SPEECH AND LANGUAGE		
First word	1-3 years	1-4 years
Two- word phrases	15-32 months	2-7.5 years
SOCIAL/SELF-HELP		
Responsive smile	1-3 months	1.5-5 months
Finger feeds	7-14 months	10-24 months
Drinks from cup unassisted	9-17 months	12-32 months
Uses spoon	12-20 months	13-39 months
Bowel control	16-42 months	2-7 years
Dresses self unassisted	3.25 years-5years	3.5-8.5 years

Quick Bites

- Down syndrome is the most common trisomy.
- It is the most common genetic cause of moderate intellectual disability.
- Advanced maternal age is the single most important risk factor and it is inversely proportional to the incidence of Down syndrome.
- Meiotic nondisjunction is the most common cause of Down syndrome.
- Most of the surgical complications of Down syndrome present in the newborn period and in early infancy.

- Hall's criteria are used to aid in the diagnosis of Down syndrome in newborns.
- Children with Down syndrome have a good response rate to AML therapy.
- Atlantoaxial dislocation can result in sudden death in Down syndrome.
- Children with Down syndrome develop Alzheimer disease at an earlier age compared with the normal population.
- Simian crease is also found in trisomies 13 and 18, fetal alcohol syndrome, Klinefelter syndrome, and Noonan syndrome.

Neonatal History Taking and Examination

Short description: A ___-week-old, weighing ___ g, Appropriate for Gestational Age (AGA)/Small for Gestational Age (SGA)/Large for Gestational Age (LGA), male/female, was admitted in view of ___

Antenatal history

Maternal age: ___; height: ___; weight: ___; BMI: ___

Married life: ___ years; ___ parity: Gravida (G), Para (P), Abortion (A), Live Birth (L), Death (D) ___; Last Menstrual Period (LMP) ___; Expected date of delivery (EDD) ___

Conception: Spontaneous or with Rx

Booked at what Gestational age (GA) ___

Antenatal check up (ANC)

Number of check-ups ___

Scans: Details and number of scans

Tetanus toxoid (TT) immunization and iron folic acid

Any history of fever with rashes and joint pains

- History of pregnancy induced hypertension (PIH) (after 20 weeks)/chronic hypertension (HTN) (before 20 weeks of GA)
  - How many drugs? Doses? Since how long?
  - History of value of recent BP recording, proteinuria, edema, oliguria, and any investigations (liver function test (LFT), platelet count)
  - Intrauterine growth restriction (IUGR) – when detected; Doppler – increased resistance; Absent umbilical artery end diastolic flow (AEDF); Reversal of umbilical artery end diastolic flow (REDF); redistribution in middle cerebral artery (MCA); amniotic fluid index (AFI); biophysical profile (BPP)
- History of gestational diabetes mellitus (GDM)/pregestational diabetes mellitus (pre-GDM)/diabetes mellitus (DM) on diet or insulin
  - Controlled or not, recent values? Glycated hemoglobin (HbA1c) values?
  - Compliance with Rx
  - Scans: Targeted Imaging For Fetal Anomalies (TIFFA) and fetal echo?
- History of hypothyroidism: When diagnosed? Medication?
- Any other medical problems: … when detected and drugs?
- Anemia, systemic lupus erythematosus (SLE), jaundice, congenital heart disease (CHD), and heart disease
- History of preterm premature rupture of membrane (PPROM): Duration, uterine tenderness, foul-smelling liquor, Total leukocyte count (TLC), and High vaginal swab (HVS) (if taken)
- History of urinary tract infection (UTI): Recent culture (within 1 month of delivery is significant)
- Any history of drug intake – Non steroidal anti-inflammatory drugs (NSAIDs), antidepressants, etc.

Natal history

- Duration of labor: First stage (>18 hours significant) and second stage (>2 hours after full dilatation)
- Augmentation of labor/induced/assisted vaginal
- Fluids during labor and fever – what antibiotics?
- Cardiotocography (CTG): Normal/suspicious/pathological
- Mecoinium stained liquor (MSL)
- Lower segment cesarean section (LSCS): Indication and elective or emergency (specify the reason)
- Resuscitation: Yes or no ___ Intermittent positive pressure ventilation (IPPV) – how long, Endotracheal tube (ET), medications, and chest compressions?
- APGAR: Cord pH, pCO_2, and Base excess (BE) (acute insult, only pCO_2 will be high; or chronic insult, pCO_2 and Base excess (BE) are high)
- Placenta: Weight, surface, number of cotyledons, calcifications, malformations, clots, etc.

Postnatal/history of present illness

Main reason for admission – elaborate each symptom and **problem oriented**

- **Prematurity**
  - **Reason** (maternal indication or preterm labor or PPROM with chorioamnionitis) – describe each in detail.
  - **Steroids:** What drug? Dosage? How many doses, duration of last dose from the time of delivery, and how many courses?
- **Respiratory distress**

  History of PPROM, UTI, and fever during labor – what antibiotics the mother is on
  - Onset, progression, and course of events
  - Silverman/Downes score
  - Respiratory support: Continuous Positive Airway Pressure (CPAP), ventilation, and oxygen (settings)
  - Surfactant: Doses

  History of pneumonia, Hyaline membrane disease (HMD), Meconium aspiration syndrome (MAS), and Transient tachypnea of newborn (TTNB) (labor before LSCS, excess fluids during labor)
- **IUGR**
  - Reason: Maternal (PIH, SLE, HTN)
  - Placenta
  - Doppler
  - AFI
  - TIFFA scan
- **Jaundice**
  - History of onset and progression
  - Color of stools and urine if prolonged jaundice
  - Maternal blood group and jaundice in the mother

- Family history of jaundice, phototherapy, exchange, early gallstones, splenectomy, and blood transfusion

In all cases, after elaborating the symptom:

Feeding: Nil per oral (NPO) or when started and how much

Past history: In case of readmission

Family history: Number of children

Previous obstetric history

Socioeconomic history: Education and occupation of the mother and father

Kuppuswamy classification

Examination

General disposition

The baby is in level I/II/III/with the mother/placed in an incubator or under a radiant warmer.

The baby is clothed/semiclothed/naked.

Mention all accessories – temperature probe and pulse oximeter probe (on which limb).

Mention i.v. cannula, Peripherally inserted central catheter (PICC) line, Umbilical Venous Catheter (UVC), Umbilical Artery catheter (UAC), any medication drips/infusions, and cling wrap/phototherapy/CPAP/ventilation

Vitals

- **Temperature:** Temperature of the baby, set temperature, heater output, and peripheral to core temperature difference
- **heart rate (HR):** Rate, all pulses (especially femorals), volume, rhythm, and radiofemoral delay
- **respiratory rate (RR):** Rate and **SpO**2 – room air/oxygen – FiO$_2$
- **non-invasive blood pressure (NIBP):** mean arterial pressure (MAP), systole, diastole, pulse pressure, and which limb
- **capillary filling time (CFT)**
- **Color of the extremities:** Pink, cyanosed, and dusky

General examination: Pallor, jaundice, cyanosis, and edema

Head-to-toe examination

Head: Size, shape, and suture – overriding/separation anterior fontanelle (AF)/ posterior fontanelle (PF)/ caput/cephalhematoma)

Face: Dysmorphism, eyes (cataract/coloboma), ears, mouth, and palate (cleft)

Chest, abdomen, genitalia, and limbs

Spine

Whether everything is normal: Can say because no obvious dysmorphism

Gestational age assessment

Anthropometry

Birth weight, length, head circumference (HC), and perfusion index PI: Centiles (Lubchenco chart)

Present weight, Length and OFC (weight – whether following the postnatal growth curve or not?)

Ponderal index

Chest circumference – difference with occipitpofrontal circumference (OFC)

Mid-arm circumference

Systemic examination

Nervous system

- **Higher intellectual functions**
  - Sensorium: Normal, stuporous, lethargic, obtunded, and comatose

- If normal: State of wakefulness and state-to-state variability
- Habituation: To touch (glabellar tap), sound (crumpling paper), and light (on eyes, look for grimace)
- Peak arousablility
- Defense reaction
- Consolability and cudability

- **Cranial nerves**
  - Olfactory (I)
  - Optic (II): Pupillary reflex
  - Oculomotor (III), trochlear (IV), and abducens (VI): Movements of eyes – horizontal (doll's eye) and vertical
  - Trigeminal (V) and facial (VII): Rooting and sucking
  - Auditory (VIII): Response to a bell (turning or change in the heart rate, breathing pattern)
  - Glossopharyngeal (IX): Gag reflex (observe while passing NG tube)
  - Vagus (X) and hypoglossal (XII): Sucking reflex
  - Accessory (XI): Traction reflex

- **Motor system**
  - Passive tone: Posture
    - Axial: Traction (look for head lag), vertical suspension (slipping of the shoulder – for shoulder tone), and ventral suspension (position of the head with relation to the trunk)
    - Appendicular
      Upper limb: Scarf sign
      Lower limb: Popliteal angle (asymmetry, difference in angle), adductor angle, and heel to ear
    - Flappability
    - Feel of the muscles
  - Active tone: Arm recoil and leg recoil
  - Reflexes
    - Grasp: Palmar and plantar
    - Moro's
    - Asymmetrical tonic neck reflex (ATNR)
    - Crossed adductor
    - Deep tendon reflex (DTR)
  - Skull and spine

Respiratory system

Mention whether the baby is on room air/hood box/CPAP/ventilator.

- Settings: Start from either the patient's end or the ventilator/CPAP end.
  - Size of ET tube, fixed at what distance, and visible secretions
  - Inspiratory or expiratory limb of circuit (condensation), humidifier temperature, and temperature at the patient's end
  - Settings: Mode of ventilation
    CPAP/ synchronised intermittent mandatory ventilation (SIMV)/pressure support ventilation (PSV)
    peak inspiratory pressure (PIP)/ poitive end expiratory pressure (PEEP)/ ventilatory ratio (VR)/ inspiratory time (Ti)/ fraction of inspired oxygen (FiO$_2$)/trigger sensitivity/termination sensitivity/graphics (if displayed)
  - Spontaneous respirations

- Synchrony of respirations
- Chest rise: Inadequate, adequate, and more
- respiratory rate (RR)
- Scoring of respiratory distress if present (Silverman or Downes)
- saturation of Peripheral oxygen (SpO_2)
- Auscultation: Bilateral equal air entry and adventitious sounds (wheeze, stridor, crepitations)

Cardiovascular system

- HR
- Peripheral pulses: Rate, volume, femorals, and radio-femoral delay

- Precordial activity
- Murmurs
- Signs of cardiac failure: Hepatomegaly, tachycardia, respiratory distress (RD), and crepts

Abdomen

- Shape: Scaphoid, distended, and visible bowel loops
- Palpation: Soft/tense
- Palpable masses
- Hernial orifice
- Abdominal girth: Whether grossly distended

Genitalia

41 Frequently Asked Questions in Newborn

1. Classify neonates as per the gestational age.
   - Extreme preterm: <28 weeks
   - Very preterm: 28 to 31 6/7 weeks
   - Early preterm: 32 0/7 to 33 6/7 weeks
   - Late preterm: 34 0/7 to 36 6/7 weeks
   - Early term: 37 0/7 to 38 6/7 weeks
   - Full term: 39 0/7 to 40 6/7 weeks
   - Late term: 41 0/7 to 41 6/7 weeks
   - Post-term: >42 weeks (>295 days)

   Source: Cloherty, 8th ed., Chapter 7, p. 80.

2. *What are corrected age, chronological age, and gestational age?

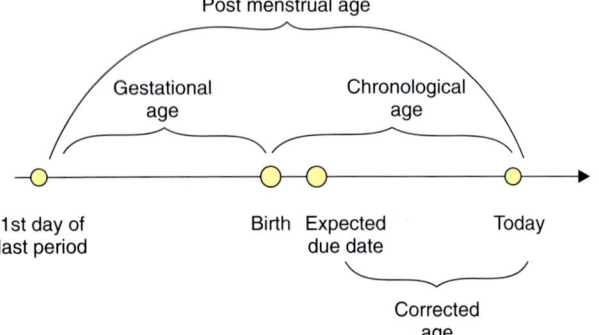

Flowchart 41.1 Postmenstrual age, chronological age, and corrected age.

3. Till how many months can corrections for Gestational age (GA) be made?

   Corrections for GA can be made for the following:
   - For head circumference: Till 18 months of age
   - For weight: Till 24 months of age
   - For length/height: Till 40 months of age

4. Classify newborns as per the weight.
   - The normal weight of a term neonate is ≥2.5 kg irrespective of the gestational age.
   - Low birth weight is 1.5–2.5 kg irrespective of the gestational age.
   - Very low birth weight is <1.5 kg irrespective of the gestational age.
   - Extreme low birth weight is <1.00 kg irrespective of the gestational age.

5. What is postmaturity syndrome?
   - **Stage 1**
     - Dry, peeling, loose, and wrinkled skin
     - Malnourished appearance
     - Decreased subcutaneous fat
     - Open eyed and alert
   - **Stage 2**
     - All features of stage 1
     - Meconium staining of the amniotic fluid
     - Perinatal depression
   - **Stage 3**
     - All the features of stages 1 and 2
     - Meconium staining of the umbilical cord and nails

   - A higher risk of fetal/neonatal death

   Source: Cloherty, 8th ed., Chapter 7, p. 88.

6. *Define Ponderal index.

$$\text{Ponderal index} = \frac{\text{Weight (g)} \times 100}{(\text{Length})^3 \text{ (cm)}}$$

   - A ratio greater than 2.5 is normal.
   - A ratio of 2–2.5 indicates symmetric IUGR.
   - A ratio of less than 2 indicates asymmetric IUGR.

7. What scoring system is used for IUGR?
   It is called clinical assessment of nutritional score (CANS). It includes the following parameters:
   - Hair
   - Cheeks
   - Neck and chin
   - Arms
   - Legs
   - Back
   - Buttocks
   - Chest
   - Abdomen

   The score ranges from 9 to 36.
   A total score of less than 25 indicates IUGR.

8. Define small for gestational age (SGA).
   SGA is defined as birth weight or birth crown–heel length less than 10th percentile for the gestational age or <2 SD below the mean for that gestational age (approximately the third percentile for the gestational age).

9. Define intrauterine growth retardation (IUGR).
   IUGR is defined as the biometry or estimated fetal growth less than the fifth percentile.
   The ultrasound findings can serially show any or a combination of the following:
   - Static interval growth velocity (ideally, scans should be taken at a gap of 2–3 weeks)
   - Increase in the abdominal circumference being less than 1 cm over 2 weeks
   - Biparietal diameter, head circumference, abdominal circumference, femur length, and estimated fetal weight being <10th percentile
   - Reduction in liquor volume
   - Abnormalities in the venous/arterial Doppler of the fetus

10. What are the benign skin changes of a newborn?
    - *Milia:* Distended sebaceous glands are seen over the face as white dots and disappear spontaneously.
    - *Sebaceous hyperplasia:* It is otherwise called "cradle cap" and mainly involves the scalp. Sometimes it is seen as clusters over the nose also. These papules self-resolve in the first few weeks of life.
    - *Erythema toxicum:* It refers to yellowish papules on an erythematous base. It appears on the 2nd or 3rd day of life and disappears within the 1st week of life.

- *Salmon patch:* Small capillary malformations are seen over the forehead (angel kisses), root of the nose, and nape of the neck (stork bites). They mostly disappear by the 1st year of life.
- *Transient pustular melanosis neonatorum (TPMN):* The pustules usually break spontaneously, leaving behind a hyperpigmented macule that takes weeks to months to fade off.
- *Mongolian spots:* Bluish well-demarcated spots appear over the buttocks, trunk, and back of the thighs. They disappear by 1 year of age.
- *Peeling of the skin:* It is commonly seen in post-term infants and some full-term infants also. It needs no intervention.
- *Epstein pearl:* It refers to the epithelial inclusion cysts seen on the hard palate/either side of the median raphe (palatal) and tip of the prepuce at 6-o'clock position (preputial). They are usually round and white in color. They need no intervention.
- *Cutis marmorata:* It refers to an evanescent, lacy, reticulated, red-blue marbled cutaneous vascular pattern because of the exaggerated physiological vasomotor response to cold and disappears with increasing maturity and postnatal age.

11. *Name some physiological changes seen at birth.
    - *Subconjunctival hemorrhage:* The semilunar arcs of subconjunctival hemorrhage located at the outer canthus is a common finding in normal babies. They usually disappear within few days to weeks after birth without any pigmentation.
      - While seeing a case of Sub Conjunctival Hemorrhage (SCH), the following points should be noted:
        - A clear space of sclera should be present between the hemorrhage and the cornea.
        - The temporal aspect of SCH should be visible.
        - If these two are not present, suspect brain pathology.
    - *Epiphora:* Excessive watering of both the eyes without congestion is again a common finding in the newborn. It is because of the obstruction in the nasolacrimal duct. It is treated by giving massage for 15–20 times at a time for three times a day for 1–2 months. If the watering persists beyond 5 months, then syringing through the punctum is indicated.
    - *Breast engorgement (mastitis neonatorum):* This is usually seen on the 3rd or 4th day of life in both male and female babies. Sometimes creamy white discharge can also be seen oozing out from the breasts under the influence of the maternal hormones. They should not be squeezed or massaged because it can lead to breast abscess. It needs no treatment.
    - *Umbilical granuloma:* It is seen as a small flesh-like pale nodule at the base of the umbilicus. It can be managed by application of the rock salt for 48–72 hours. It can also be repeated once every 3–4 days until the base becomes dry.
    - *Bleeding per vaginum:* It is physiological if it starts on the 2nd or 3rd day and persists till the 7th day. It is never seen on day 1 and does not last for more than 5 days. In addition, there should be no bleed from anywhere else in the body.
    - *Vaginal mucoid discharge:* Thick, white, viscid vaginal discharge is present because of the effect of transplacentally acquired estrogen on the vaginal mucosa.
    - *Predeciduous teeth:* These refer to supernumerary teeth that are present at birth or may erupt shortly after birth in the position of lower incisor and they are shed before the primary dentition. They have to be removed if they are loose because of the risk of aspiration/causing difficulty in feeding/causing injury to the mother's breast.

12. What is thermoneutral environment?
    The thermoneutral environment is defined as the narrow range of environmental temperature at which a baby can maintain the normal body temperature with minimum basal metabolic rate and least oxygen consumption.

13. Why are newborns more prone to hypothermia?
    - Large surface area of the babies
    - Limited heat-generating mechanisms
    - Low subcutaneous fat
    - More permeable skin
    - Decreased brown fat
    - Early exhaustion of the metabolic stores such as glucose

14. What happens in response to cold in a newborn?
    - The mechanism of heat generation in newborn is called nonshivering thermogenesis.
    - Exposure to cold in a neonate causes sympathetic surge → rise in catecholamines → uncoupling of β-oxidation of brown fat → release of free fatty acids.
    - Catecholamines increases the metabolic rate that causes hypoglycemia and increase in oxygen requirement.
    - Rise in catecholamines also causes pulmonary and peripheral vasoconstriction, which leads to hypoxemia and metabolic acidosis.

15. What are the 10 steps of warm chain?
    The concept of warm chain is followed from the delivery room to the postnatal ward:
    - Warm delivery room
    - Warm resuscitation
    - Immediate drying
    - Skin-to-skin contact
    - Breastfeeding
    - Bathing/weighing postponed
    - Clothing
    - Rooming in
    - Warm transportation
    - Training and awareness

16. Classify the severity of meconium aspiration syndrome (MAS).
    - Mild MAS: <40% oxygen requirement for less than 48 hours
    - Moderate MAS: >40% oxygen requirement for >48 hours without air leak
    - Severe MAS: Requiring assisted ventilation for >48 hours mostly associated with persistent pulmonary hypertension of newborn (PPHN).

17. Discuss the criteria for therapeutic hypothermia.
    Criteria for therapeutic hypothermia are as follows:
    - Gestational age should be ≥36 weeks and birth weight ≥2000 g.

- Evidence of fetal distress is indicated as one of the following:
  - History of acute perinatal event such as cord prolapse, abruptio placentae, variable/late deceleration, and severe fetal distress
  - Biophysical profile <6/10 or <4/8 within 6 hours of birth
  - Cord pH of ≤7.0 or base deficit ≥16 mEq/L
- Neonatal distress is evidenced by any one of the following:
  - Apgar score of ≤5 at 10 minutes
  - Postnatal blood gas pH at <1 hour ≤7.0
  - Ventilation initiated at birth and continued for at least 10 minutes
  - Evidence of neonatal encephalopathy
  - Abnormal Electroencephalogram with minimum of 20-minute recording
  Source: **Cloherty, 8th ed.,** Chapter 55, p. 804.

18. Name some recently proposed neuroprotective strategies.
    N-methyl-D-aspartate (NMDA) receptor blockers such as ketamine and MK-801; free radical scavengers such as allopurinol, superoxide dismutase, and vitamin E; calcium channel blockers such as nimodipine, nicardipine, and magnesium sulfate; and cyclooxygenase inhibitors such as indomethacin

19. Define asphyxia.
    As per the American Academy of Pediatrics, birth asphyxia is defined as the presence of all of the following criteria:
    - Profound metabolic or mixed academia shown by cord blood pH of <7.00 or base deficit of ≥16 mmol/L
    - Presence of low Apgar scores of less than 3 for more than 5 minutes
    - Signs of neonatal neurological dysfunctioning evidenced by seizures, encephalopathy, and tone abnormalities
    - Evidence of multiple organ involvement such as kidneys, lungs, liver, heart, and intestine

20. Give examples of ambiguous genitalia.
    Examples of disorders of sex development presenting in the newborn period include the infants with the following findings:
    - Bilaterally nonpalpable testis
    - Unilateral cryptorchidism with hypospadias
    - Penoscrotal or perineoscrotal hypospadias with or without microphallus even if testes are descended
    - Female with enlarged clitoris or inguinal hernia
    - Cloacal extrophy
    - Asymmetry of labioscrotal folds with or without cryptorchidism

21. Explain physiological weight loss in newborn.
    - Both the term and the preterm low-birth-weight infants tend to lose weight, about 10%–15%, respectively, in the first 7 days of life and then start gaining weight so that the birth weight is reached by 10–14 days of life.
    - Thereafter, the weight gain should be at least 15–20 g/kg/day for preterm infants and 20–30 g/day for term infants.

22. *Differentiate between facial nerve palsy and congenital absence of depressor angular oris.

Facial Nerve Palsy	Congenital Absence of Muscle
Deviation of angle of mouth to the normal side with absence of nasolabial fold on the affected side	Prominent nasolabial folds will be present on both the sides
The deviation is more laterally	The deviation is more downwards

23. *Classify hemorrhagic disease of the newborn.
    - A moderate decrease in the vitamin K–dependent clotting factors 2, 7, 9, and 10 is seen from 48 to 72 hours after birth and there is gradual return to normal by 7–10 days of life. The following factors cause a drop in vitamin K–dependent clotting factors:
      - When there is lack of free vitamin K from the mother
      - If the bacterial intestinal flora that are normally responsible for the synthesis of vitamin K are absent
    - Table 41.1 gives the **classification of hemorrhagic disease of newborn**.

24. Name some neonatal pain scoring tools.
    CRIES (32–60 weeks)
    - Crying
    - Requiring increased oxygen
    - Increased vital signs
    - Expression
    - Sleeplessness
    Premature Infant Pain Profile (PIPP) (27 weeks to term)
    - Gestational age
    - Behavioral state
    - Heart rate
    - Oxygen saturation
    - Brow bulge
    - Eye squeeze
    - Nasolabial furrow
    Neonatal Infant Pain Scale (NIPS) (28–30 weeks)
    - Facial expression
    - Crying
    - Breathing pattern
    - Arm movement

TABLE 41.1	Classification of Hemorrhagic Disease of Newborn
Onset	**Cause**
Early onset (0–24 h)	drugs such as phenobarbitone, phenytoin, warfarin, rifampicin, isoniazid
Classic disease (2–7 days)	vitamin K deficiency as a result of immaturity of the gut
Late-onset disease (1–6 months)	Cholestasis – malabsorption of vitamin K (biliary atresia, cystic fibrosis, hepatitis) Abetalipoprotein deficiency Idiopathic Warfarin ingestion

- Leg movement
- State of arousal

25. What are nonstress test and contraction stress test?

Nonstress test: It is a noninvasive test that is based on the fact that fetal activity results in a reflex acceleration in the heart rate.

The criteria for a reactive stress test are the following:

- Fetal heart rate between 110 and 160 bpm
- Normal beat-to-beat variability (5 bpm)
- Two accelerations of at least 15 bpm lasting for not less than 15 seconds each within a 20-minute period
- The test is said to be nonreactive if it does not meet the above-mentioned three criteria.

Contraction stress test

This test is based on the fact that uterine contractions can compromise an unhealthy fetus.

- The fetal heart rate begins to decelerate 15–30 seconds after the contraction, reaches the nadir after the peak of contraction, and does not return to baseline until after the contraction ends. This is called late deceleration.
- A contraction stress test is considered complete if uterine contractions have spontaneously occurred within 30 minutes and lasted for at least 40–60 seconds at a frequency of at least three in 10 minutes.
- A contraction stress test is considered positive if late decelerations are consistently seen in association with contractions.
- It is negative if the contractions are not associated with late decelerations.

Source: Based on Sarah Al-Haddab. Antepartum Intrapartum Fetal Monitoring

26. Define Apgar score.

Many features of the Apgar score relate to the cardiovascular integrity and not to the neurological dysfunctioning. The Apgar score tells whether the newborn requires resuscitative measures or not. It does not predict the future neurological outcome.

27. When should resuscitation in a newborn be discontinued?

If there are no signs of life in an infant after 10 minutes of aggressive resuscitative efforts, resuscitation can be discontinued.

28. What is Moro reflex?

- This reflex is elicited when the baby's head is dropped suddenly in relation to the trunk. In addition, the following responses are noted: opening of the hands, abduction and extension of the upper limbs followed by anterior flexion of upper extremities and then an audible cry.
- Development of Moro reflex
  28 weeks: Opening of the hands
  32 weeks: Abduction and flexion of the upper limbs
  37 weeks: Anterior flexion of the upper limbs
- This reflex disappears by 3–6 months of age.

Significance of Moro reflex:

- Absence of Moro reflex: Asphyxia (CNS insult)
- Persisting beyond 3–4 months: Cerebral palsy
- Exaggerated Moro reflex: Kernicterus
- Asymmetrical Moro reflex: Erb palsy, stroke, and humerus fracture

29. Differentiate between Moro reflex and startle reflexes.

Startle reflex is obtained by a loud noise.

The response is similar to Moro reflex except for the following:

- Elbows remain flexed.
- Hands remain closed.
- In addition, in Moro reflex, there is more outward and inward movement.

30. What is red reflex in newborn and its importance?

Red reflex refers to reddish-orange reflection of light from the fundus through a transparent optical media. It is visualised using direct ophthalmoscope, approximately 18 inch away in dim lit room. It is a noninvasive test. Method: Ophthalmoscope is set to +2 (green or black) and focussed on the child's eye. red reflex seen within the pupil. Absent or asymmetrical red reflex is suggestive of a retinal tumor (retinoblastoma)/cataract (Fig. 41.1).

TABLE 41.2 **Apgar scoring system**				
	0 Points	**1 Point**	**2 Points**	**Points totaled**
Activity (muscle tone)	Absent	Arms and legs flexed	Active movement	
Pulse	Absent	Below 100 bpm	Over 100 bpm	
Grimace (reflex irritability)	Flaccid	Some flexion of extremities	Active motion (sneeze, cough pull away)	
Appearance (skin color)	Blue, pale	Body pink, extremities blue	Completely pink	
Respiration	Absent	Slow, irregular	Vigorous cry	

Severely depressed	0–3
Moderately depressed	4–6
Excellent condition	7–10

Source: Reproduced from Nachiket Shankar, Mario Vaz. *Textbook of Applied Anatomy and Applied Physiology*, Second edition, Respiratory changes across the life cycle, FIG. 51.2, New Delhi, Elsevier India, 2022.

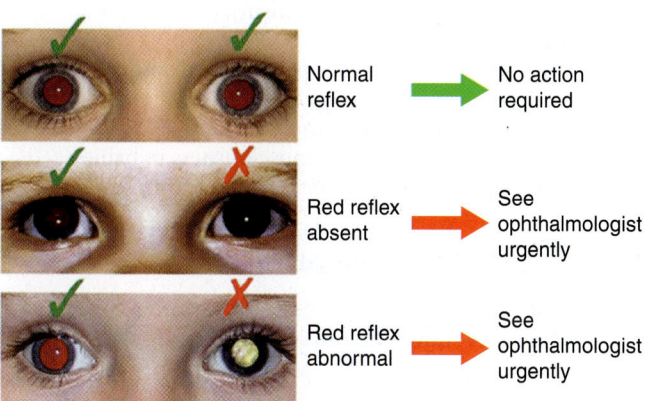

Fig. 41.1 Red reflex and its interpretation. (*Source: Valérie Biousse, Nancy J. Newman, Jonathan A. Micieli: Neuro-Ophthalmology Illustrated. 2020*)

31. What are the "five cleans of safe delivery"?
    Cleans of safe delivery are the following:
    - Clean delivery surface
    - Clean hands of the birth attendant
    - Clean cord cut (blade or instrument)
    - Clean cord tie
    - Clean cord stump without any applicant

32. *What is delivery point screening?
    Child health screening and early intervention services under National Rural Health Mission (NRHM) identify 30 health conditions for early detection, free treatment, and management.

    The following are the Identified health conditions for child health screening and early intervention services:
    Birth defects like
    1. Neural tube defect,
    2. Down syndrome,
    3. Cleft lip and palate/cleft palate alone,
    4. Talipes (clubfoot),
    5. Developmental dysplasia of the hip,
    6. Congenital cataract,
    7. Congenital deafness,
    8. Congenital heart diseases,
    9. Retinopathy of prematurity
    Deficiencies like
    10. Anemia, especially severe anemia,
    11. Vitamin A deficiency (Bitot spots),
    12. Vitamin D deficiency (rickets),
    13. malnutrition,
    14. Goiter,
    Childhood Diseases like
    15. Otitis media,
    16. Rheumatic heart disease,
    17. Reactive airway disease,
    18. Dental caries,
    19. Convulsive disorders and,
    20. Skin conditions like scabies, fungal infection, and eczema,
    Developmental Delay and Disabilities includes
    21. Vision impairment,
    22. Hearing impairment,
    23. Neuromotor impairment,
    24. Motor delay,
    25. Cognitive delay,
    26. Language delay,
    27. Behavior disorder (autism),
    28. Learning disorder,
    29. Attention deficit hyperactivity disorder,
    30. Congenital hypothyroidism, sickle cell anemia, beta-thalassemia (optional).

33. *Discuss the six states of consciousness in babies.
    Table 41.3 gives the six states of consciousness in babies.

DISCUSSION ON NEONATAL SEIZURES

34. Enumerate the causes of neonatal seizures.
    Table 41.4 shows the causes of neonatal seizures.

TABLE 41.3	States of Consciousness in Babies	
State	**Description**	**Level of Consciousness**
State 1	Deep sleep	Lies quietly without moving
State 2	Light sleep	Moves while sleeping, startles at noises
State 3	Drowsiness	Eyes start to close, may close
State 4	Quiet alert	Eyes open wide, face is bright, body is quiet
State 5	Active alert	Face and body move actively
State 6	Crying	Cries, perhaps screams, body moves in disorganized way

Source: Data from Cloherty and Stark's Manual of Neonatal Care 8th edition.

TABLE 41.4	Causes of Neonatal Seizures
Time of Occurrence	**Cause**
<24 h	• Hypoxic ischemic encephalopathy • Subarachnoid hemorrhage • Laceration of tentorium or falx • Local anesthetic injection into the scalp • Inborn error of metabolism – pyridoxine deficiency • Sepsis, meningitis (rare on day 1)
24–72 h	• Intraventricular hemorrhage in preterm babies • Cerebral contusion with subdural hemorrhage (SDH) and subarachnoid hemorrhage (SAH) • Bacterial sepsis and meningitis • Benign familial neonatal seizures • Inborn errors of metabolism – glycine encephalopathy, urea cycle disturbances • Rare causes – drug withdrawal seizures, incontinentia pigmenti, tuberous sclerosis
72 h to 1 week	• Bacterial/fungal sepsis, meningitis • Benign idiopathic neonatal seizures (BINS) – 5th-day fits • Drug withdrawal • Kernicterus • Inborn error of metabolism – organic acidemias, urea cycle disturbances • Others – intracerebral hemorrhage, tuberous sclerosis
1–4 weeks	• Bacterial/fungal sepsis, meningitis • Herpes simplex encephalitis • Storage disorders – GM1 gangliosidosis, Gaucher type 2 • Tuberous sclerosis • Inborn errors of metabolism – organic acidemias, urea cycle disturbances

35. *Differentiate between neonatal seizures and jitteriness.

Neonatal Seizures	Jitteriness
• Predominantly clonic jerky movements	Tremulousness
• Ocular movements will be present	Ocular movements will be absent
• Passive restraint will not halt the movement	Passive restraint can halt the movement
• Autonomic changes will be present	Autonomic changes will be absent
• Stimulation will not induce the activity	Stimulation can induce the activity

36. How are antiepileptics withdrawn in a case of neonatal seizures?

Antiepileptic drugs (AED) can be planned to taper 48 hours after correcting the underlying cause.

Once the child is seizure free for 48 hours, perform a complete neurological examination and EEG. If they are normal, plan to stop AEDs. Flowchart 41.2 shows withdrawal of AED in a child with abnormal CNS examination at discharge.

37. *Demonstrate neonatal reflexes.

Table 41.5 gives the neonatal reflexes and their importance.

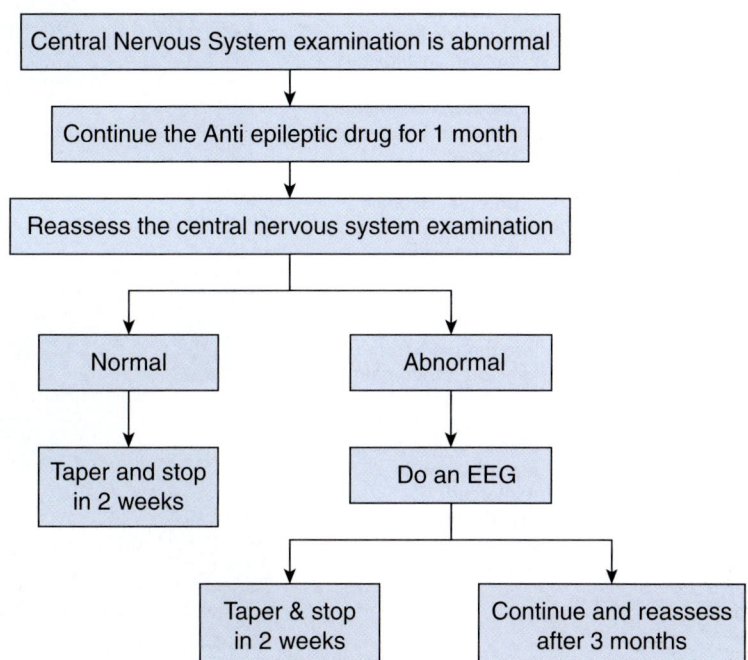

Flowchart 41.2 Withdrawal of AED. AED, antiepileptic drug.

TABLE 41.5	Neonatal Reflexes			
Reflexes	**Appears by**	**Disappearance**	**How to Elicit**	**Clinical Picture**
Moro reflex (Fig. 41.2)	28–37 weeks 1. Opening of hand: 28 weeks 2. Abduction and extension: 32 weeks 3. Adduction and flexion: 37 weeks	3 months	Hold the baby at an angle of 45° from couch and suddenly let the head fall back. Sudden movement of cervical region initiates the reflex. **Reflex:** Abduction and extension of arms, opening of hands (but fingers remain curved) followed by abduction and flexion of upper extremities accompanied by crying, extension of trunk and head with movement of legs. **Significance** Asymmetric Moro reflex: Brachial plexus palsy, cervical rib fracture, hemiplegia Incomplete Moro reflex: Preterm Absent Moro reflex: Hypotonia, Hypoxic Ischemic Encephalopathy (HIE) Exaggerated Moro reflex: Kernicterus	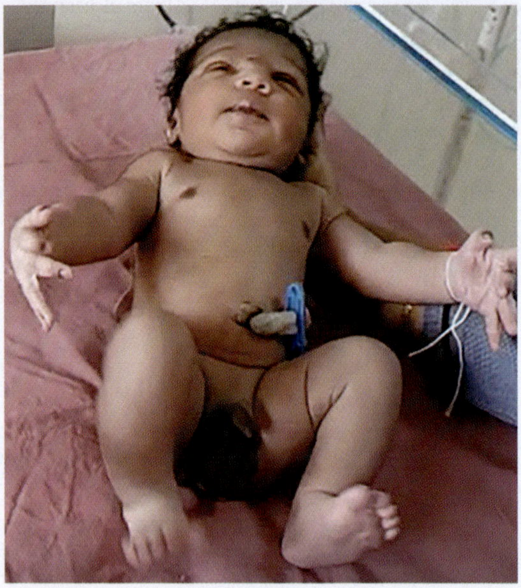
Palmar grasp (Fig. 41.3)	28–37 weeks	3 months	Introduce the finger into the palm from ulnar side. When palm is stimulated, the fingers flex and grasp the object. With attempted removal, grip is reinforced. **Significance:** When it disappears, voluntary grasp appears.	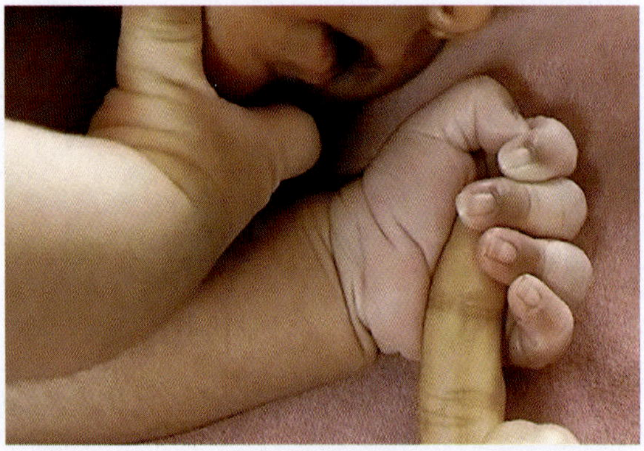
Plantar grasp (Fig. 41.4)	28–37 weeks	6–10 months	Gently stroke the sole of foot behind toes – this causes the infant's toes to curl up tightly.	

Fig. 41.2 First phase of Moro reflex, sudden dropping of infant's head.

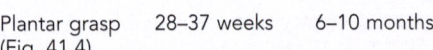

Fig. 41.3 Palmar grasp – flexion of fingers and grasping the object/hand on stimulation.

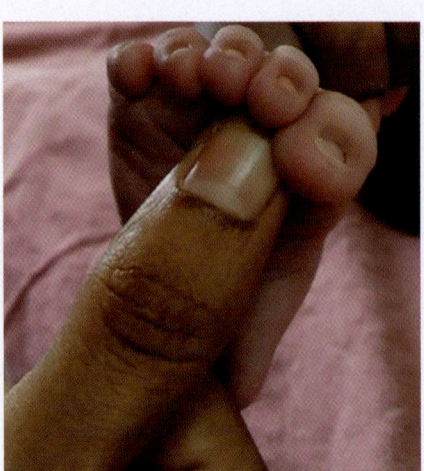

Fig. 41.4 Plantar grasp – curling up of toes on applying firm pressure over the sole of foot.

TABLE 41.5	Neonatal Reflexes—cont'd			
Reflexes	**Appears by**	**Disappearance**	**How to Elicit**	**Clinical Picture**
Crossed extensor reflex (Fig. 41.5)	28–37 weeks	3 months	Hold one leg extended from knee and apply firm pressure to the sole or stroke it from the same side. The free leg flexes, adducts, and then extends, trying to push away from stimulating agents.	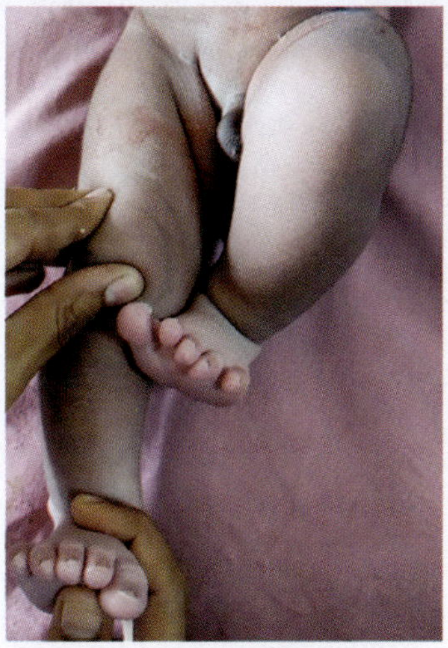
Sucking reflex (Fig. 41.6)	28 weeks	Awake: 3 months Sleep: 6 months	Introduce finger into mouth; vigorous sucking will occur.	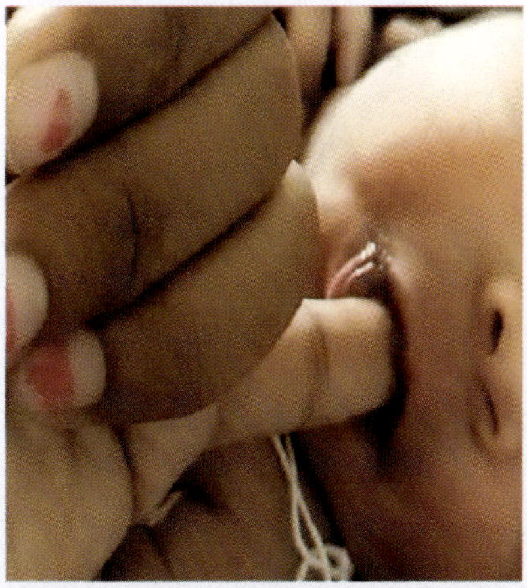
Swallowing reflex	14 weeks		Suck–swallow coordination: 34 weeks.	
Rooting reflex (Fig. 41.7)	34 weeks	1–3 months	When the corner of the mouth is touched, bottom lip is lowered on the same side and tongue moves toward the point of stimulation, and when finger slides away, head turns to follow it.	

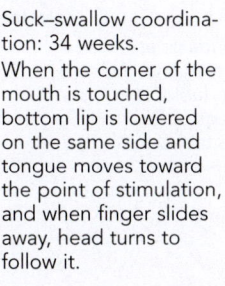

Fig. 41.5 Crossed extensor reflex – on applying firm pressure to the sole, free leg flexes, adducts, and tries to push the stimulating agents away.

Fig. 41.6 Sucking reflex – vigorous sucking on introducing finger.

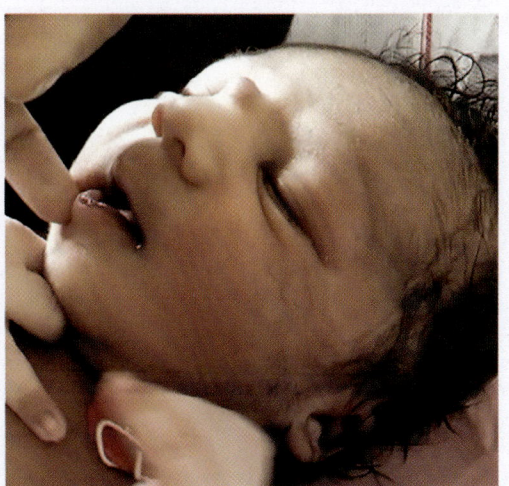

Fig. 41.7 Rooting reflex – lowering of bottom lip and turning of the head toward the point of stimulation.

Continued

TABLE 41.5	**Neonatal Reflexes—cont'd**			
Reflexes	**Appears by**	**Disappearance**	**How to Elicit**	**Clinical Picture**
Asymmetric tonic neck reflex (Fig. 41.8)	35 weeks	3–5 months	With the baby in supine position, when the head is turned to one side, extension of arms on same side to which head turns and flexion of opposite arms occurs. Similar movements occur in legs.	

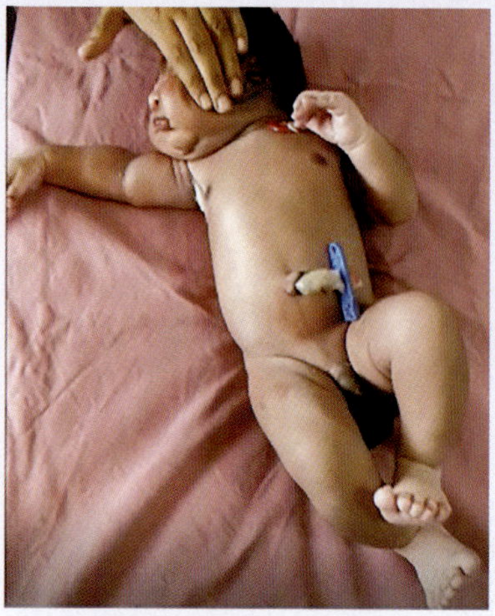

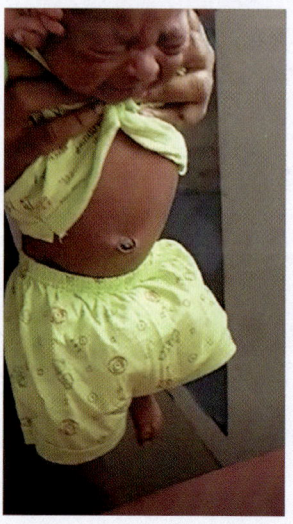

Fig. 41.8   On turning head to one side, extension of arms on same side, and flexion of opposite arms; similar movements occur in legs.

Stepping reflex (Fig. 41.9)	37 weeks	6 weeks	Hold the baby upright over the table, so that sole of foot presses against the table. This causes flexion and extension of legs stimulating walking.	

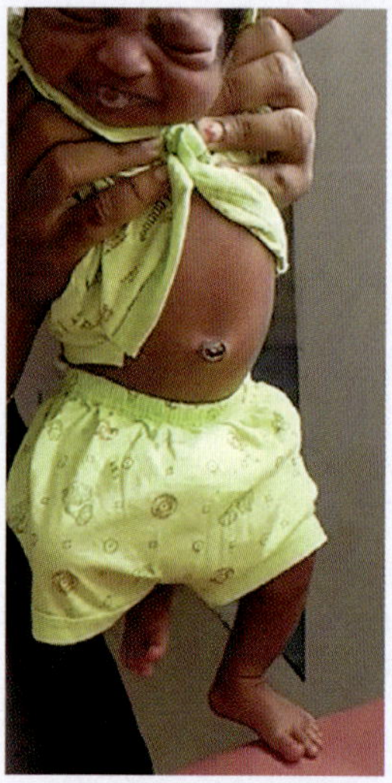

Fig. 41.9   On pressing the sole of the foot upright on the table, there is flexion and extension of legs stimulating walking.

Placing reflex (Fig. 41.10)	Birth	6 weeks	Bring the anterior aspect of tibia against the edge of the table; the baby lifts legs up to step on the table.	

Fig. 41.10   When anterior aspect of tibia is pressed against the table, the baby lifts the legs to step on the table.

TABLE 41.5	Neonatal Reflexes—cont'd			
Reflexes	**Appears by**	**Disappearance**	**How to Elicit**	**Clinical Picture**
Gallant's reflex (Fig. 41.11)	Birth	1 year	With the child in ventral suspension, stimulate the back lateral to spine. This causes flexion of trunk toward the stimulus.	

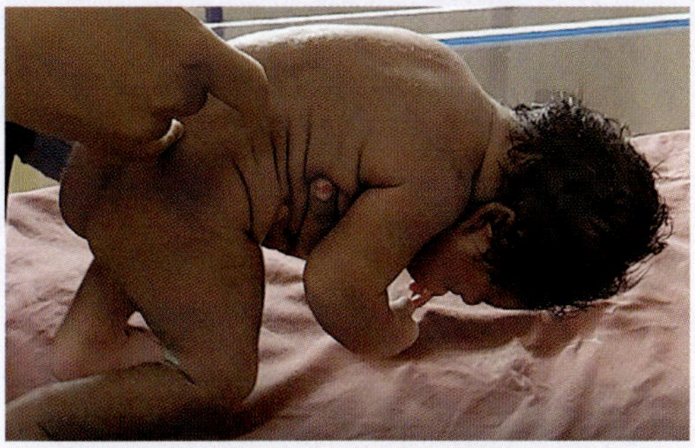

Fig. 41.11 On ventral suspension, stimulation across the back laterally produces flexion of trunk toward the stimulus.

Neck righting reflex (Fig. 41.12A and B)	Birth	6 months	Turn the head to one side; it causes movement of body to same side. **Significance:** This prevents twisting of the baby and asphyxia.	

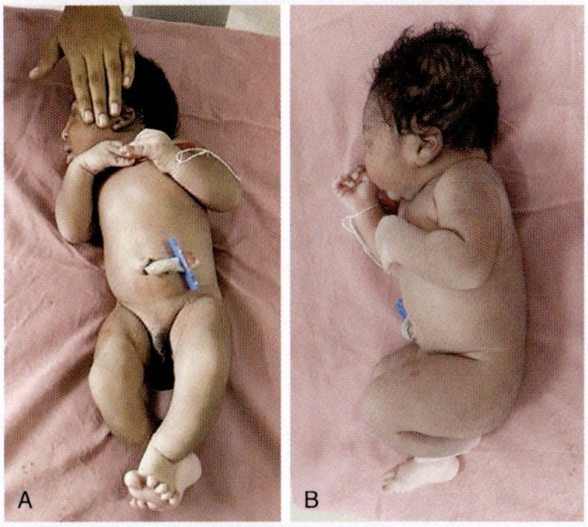

Fig. 41.12 (A and B) Turning the baby's head to one side causes movement of body to same side.

Symmetric tonic neck reflex (Fig. 41.13A and B)(STNR)	3 months	6 months	On flexing the neck, upper limbs flex and lower limbs extend. On extending the neck, upper limbs extend and lower limbs flex.	

Symmetrical Tonic Neck Reflex (STNR)

Onset ~ 4–6 months   Integrates by ~ 8–12 months

Test #1: place in crawling position and flex the head   Test #2: place in crawling position and extend the head

A   Arms flex & legs extend   B   Arms extend & legs bend

Tip: whatever the TOP half of the body does, the BOTTOM does the opposite

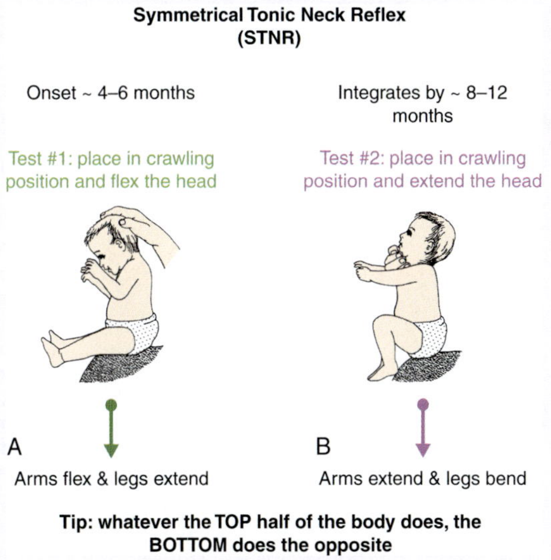

Fig. 41.13 (A) On flexing the baby's neck, upper limbs flex and lower limbs extend. (B) On extending the neck, upper limbs extend and lower limbs flex. (Source: Reproduced from Wanda Webb, Richard Adler. *Neurology for the Speech-Language Pathologist*, Sixth Edition, Pediatrics, FIGURE 11-13, St. Louis, Mosby, 2013. (Credit line - Modified from Capute, A. J., Accardo, P. I., Vining, E. P. G., & Rubenstein, J. E. [1978]. Primitive reflex profile. Baltimore: University Park Press.))

Continued

TABLE 41.5	Neonatal Reflexes—cont'd			
Reflexes	**Appears by**	**Disappearance**	**How to Elicit**	**Clinical Picture**
Landau reflex (Fig. 41.14A and B)	3–6 months	9 months	When the child is in ventral suspension, head, spine, and legs extend. When the head is depressed, hip, knees, and elbows flex. **Significance:** Absent reflex indicates motor weakness.	

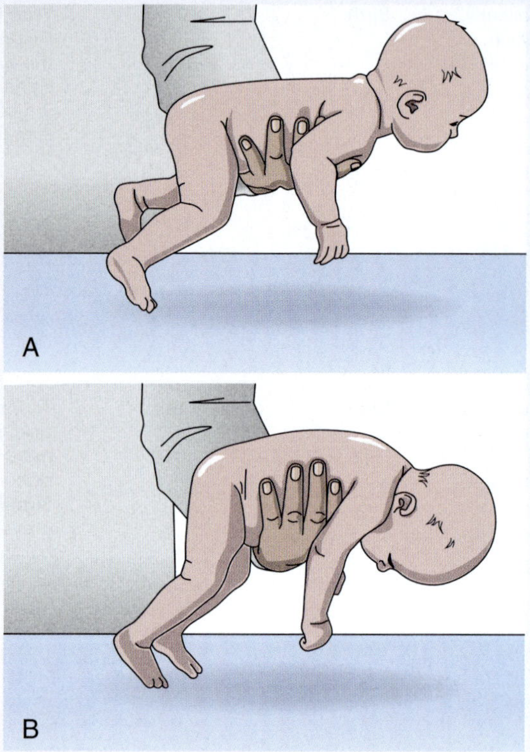

Fig. 41.14 (A) On ventral suspension, head, spine, and legs extend. (B) Head is depressed – hip, knees, and elbows flex. (Source A: Reproduced from Rudolf Schweitzer. Gynäkologie: mit Schwangerschaft, Geburt und Entwicklung des Kindes, 3. Auflage, Schwangerschaft, Geburt und Kindesentwicklung, Abb. 5.43, Munich, Urban & Fischer, 2018. (Credit line - Credit line [L157].) Source B: Reproduced from Rudolf Schweitzer. Gynäkologie: mit Schwangerschaft, Geburt und Entwicklung des Kindes, 3. Auflage, Schwangerschaft, Geburt und Kindesentwicklung, Abb. 5.42, Munich, Urban & Fischer, 2018. (Credit line - Credit line [L157].)).

Reflexes	Appears by	Disappearance	How to Elicit	
Body righting reflex	6 months	1 year	Helps in early attainment of sitting and standing.	
Parachute reflex (Fig. 41.15A–D)	6–9 months	Lifelong	With the child held in ventral suspension, suddenly lower him or her toward the couch; the arm extends as if to protect from falling (forward parachute). **Other ways: Backward, sideward, and downward. Significance:** Absent in cerebral palsy.	

TABLE 41.5	Neonatal Reflexes—cont'd			
Reflexes	Appears by	Disappearance	How to Elicit	Clinical Picture

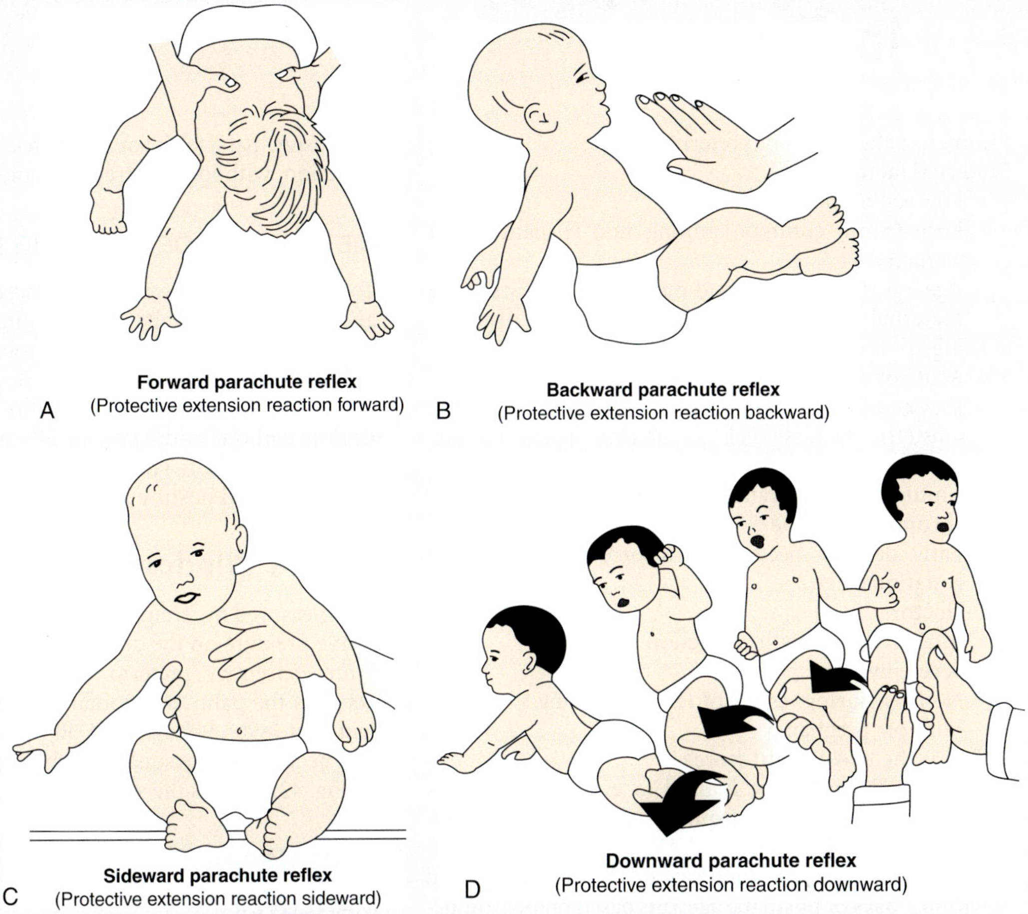

Forward parachute reflex
(Protective extension reaction forward)
A

Backward parachute reflex
(Protective extension reaction backward)
B

Sideward parachute reflex
(Protective extension reaction sideward)
C

Downward parachute reflex
(Protective extension reaction downward)
D

Fig. 41.15   (A) In ventral suspension, on suddenly lowering the infant toward the couch, the arm extends as if to protect from falling. (B) On pushing the infant from the chest side gently toward the ground, the infant responds by extending the arms backward to prevent falling. (C) On making the infant to lower on sidewards toward ground, arms extend to prevent from falling. (D) Baby held around the waist in horizontal prone position; on lowering of the head first to ground, the infant responds by extending the arms and hands to break the fall. (*Source: (A) https:// www.flickr.com/photos/aarbuckle9/8416689077. (B) https://quizlet.com/418513776/developmental-and-vaccines-flash-cards/. (C) https://www. flickr.com/photos/aarbuckle9/8416690039. (D) https://in.pinterest.com/pin/316448311309998546/.*)

Other important reflexes in newborn:

Startle reflex	Obtained by loud voice. Response is similar to Moro reflex but elbow is flexed and hands remain closed.
Perez reflex	When the child is in prone or ventral suspension, pressure is applied along the spine from sacrum toward the head; the infant flexes the arms and legs, extends the neck sometimes with a cry (Fig. 41.16). **Significance:** Stroking the paraspinal muscles in Perez reflex results in urination/defecation.

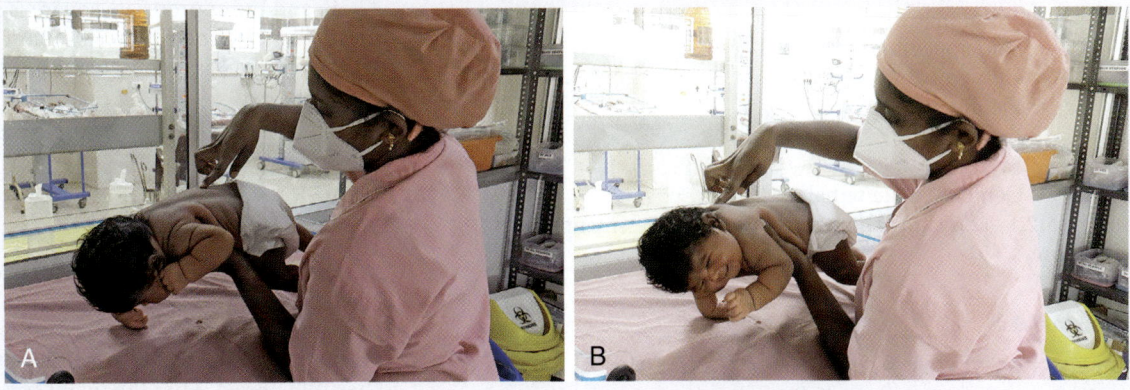

Fig. 41.16   (A) Pressure applied along the spine from sacrum towards head. (B) Infant flexes arms and legs, extends the neck

Magnet reflex	When the child is supine, the examiner's finger is pushed against sole of foot. Knees and hip flex; as the finger is withdrawn, the foot follows finger.
Heel reflex	Pressure on sole of foot causes extension of limb.

1. Enumerate the causes of preterm birth.
   Maternal factors
   - Low socioeconomic factors
   - Race (more common among non-Hispanic black women)
   - Age less than 16 years and more than 35 years
   - Maternal activities requiring long periods of standing
   - Acute or chronic maternal illness
   - Previous history of preterm deliveries
   - Obstetric factors such as uterine malformations, uterine trauma, placenta previa, preterm premature rupture of membranes, cervical incompetence, and abruptio placentae
   - Early delivery because of incorrect estimation of gestational age

   Fetal factors
   - Intrauterine growth restriction
   - Severe hydrops
   - Non-reassuring testing of fetal well-being
   - Multiple pregnancy

2. *What is the new Ballard score?
   - The new Ballard score is used to estimate the gestational age of a neonate from 20 to 44 weeks of gestational age (Table 42.1).
   - The scoring is usually done beyond 24 hours of age and within 7 days of postnatal age. It is based on neuromuscular activity and physical maturity.
   - Score ranges from −10 to 50. The minimum score is −10 and the maximum score is 50. The parameters included in neuromuscular maturity are the following:
     - Posture
     - Square window
     - Arm recoil
     - Popliteal angle
     - Scarf sign
     - Heel to ear
   - Physical maturity
     - Skin appearance
     - Lanugo
     - Plantar surface
     - Breast
     - Eye/ear
     - Genitals (male/female)

Figs 42.1–42.6 show the neuromuscular assessment of Ballard score.

Posture

TO ASSESS TOTAL BODY MUSCLE TONE

The total body muscle tone is assessed in an infant's preferred posture at rest and resistance to stretch of individual muscle groups. As maturation progresses, the fetus gradually assumes increasing passive flexor tone that proceeds in a centripetal direction, with lower extremities ahead of upper extremities.

METHOD FOR DETERMINING MUSCLE TONE

To elicit posture, the infant is placed supine (if found prone) and the examiner waits until the infant settles into a relaxed or preferred posture. If the infant is found supine, gentle manipulation (flex if extended; extend if flexed) of the extremities will allow the infant to seek the baseline position of comfort. Hip flexion without adduction results in the frog-leg position as shown in Fig. 42.1. The figure that most closely depicts the infant's preferred posture is selected.

Square Window

It is measured by straightening the infant's fingers and applying gentle pressure on the dorsum of the hand, close to the fingers. From extremely preterm to post-term, the resulting angle between the palm of the infant's hand and the forearm is estimated at >90°, 90°, 60°, 45°, 30°, and 0°.

The appropriate square on the score sheet is selected.

Fig. 42.2 shows the square window measurement.

Arm Recoil

MANEUVER

- This maneuver focuses on passive flexor tone of the biceps muscle by measuring the angle of recoil following very brief extension of the upper extremity.
- With the infant lying supine, the examiner places hand beneath the infant's elbow for support. Taking the infant's hand, the examiner briefly sets the elbow in flexion, as shown in fig 42.3A and then *momentarily* extends the arm before releasing the hand. The angle of recoil to which the forearm springs back into flexion is noted as shown in fig 42.3B, and the appropriate square is selected on the score sheet. The extremely preterm infant will not exhibit any arm recoil. This is seen in term and post-term infants.

Popliteal Angle

MANEUVER

- This assesses the maturation of passive flexor tone about the knee joint by testing for resistance to extension of the lower extremity.
- With the infant lying supine, and with diaper removed, the thigh is placed gently on the infant's abdomen with the knee fully flexed. After the infant has relaxed into this position, the examiner gently grasps the foot at the sides with one hand, while supporting the side of the thigh with the other hand.

TABLE 42.1	New Ballard Score

(a) Neuromuscular maturity

	−1	0	1	2	3	4	5
Posture							
Square window (wrist)	>90°	90°	60°	45°	35°	0°	
Arm recoil		180°	140°–180°	110°–140°	90°–110°	<90°	
Popliteal angle	180°	160°	140°	120°	100°	90°	<90°
Scarf sign							
Heel to ear							

(b) Physical maturity

Skin	Sticky, friable, transparent	Gelatinous, red, translucent	Smooth pink, visible veins	Superficial peeling and/or rash, few veins	Cracking pale areas rare veins	Parchment, deep cracking, no vessels	Leathery, cracked, wrinkled
Lanugo	None	Sparse	Abundant	Thinning	Bald areas	Mostly bald	
Plantar surface	Heel-toe 40–50 mm: −1 <40 mm: −2	>50 mm no crease	Faint red marks	Anterior transverse crease only	Creases ant. 2/3	Creases over entire sole	
Breast	Imperceptible	Barely perceptible	Flat areola, no bud	Stippled areola 1–2-mm bud	Raised areola 3–4-mm bud	Full areola 5–10-mm bud	
Eye/ear	Lids fused loosely: −1 tightly −2	Lids open Pinna flat, stays folded	Sl. curved pinna; soft; slow recoil	Well-curved pinna; soft but ready recoil	Formed and firm, instant recoil	Thick cartilage, ear stiff	
Genitalia male	Scrotum flat, smooth	Scrotum empty, faint rugae	Testes in upper canal, rare rugae	Testes decending, few rugae	Testes down, good rugae	Testes pendulous, deep rugae	
Genitalia female	Clitoris prominent, labia flat	Prominent clitoris, small labia minora	Prominent clitoris, enlarging minora	Majora and minora equally prominent	Majora large, minora small	Majora cover clitoris and minora	

(c) Maturity rating

Score	Weeks
−10	20
−5	22
0	24
5	26
10	28
15	30
20	32
25	34
30	36
35	38
40	40
45	42
50	44

(*Source:* Reproduced from Tom Lissauer, Will Carroll. *Illustrated Textbook of Paediatrics*, Sixth Edition, Appendix, Figure A.2, Oxford, Elsevier Ltd, 2022. (Credit line - Adapted from: Ballard JL, Khoury JC, Wedig K, et al: New Ballard score, expanded to include extremely premature infants. Journal of Pediatrics 119:417–423, 1991.)).

- Care is taken not to exert pressure on the hamstrings, because this may interfere with their function. The leg is extended until a definite resistance to extension is appreciated. In some infants, hamstring contraction may be visualized. At this point, the angle formed at the knee by the upper and lower leg is measured.
Fig. 42.4 shows the popliteal angle measurement.

Scarf Sign

MANEUVER

- This maneuver tests the passive tone of the flexors about the shoulder girdle.
- With the infant lying supine, the examiner adjusts the infant's head to the midline and supports the infant's hand

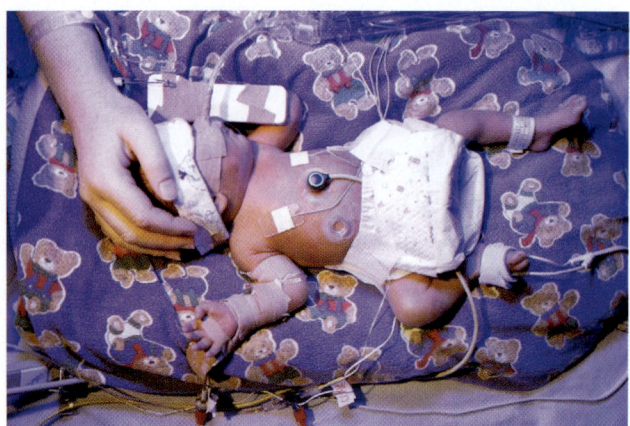

Fig. 42.1 Frog leg posture-Hypotonic posture of premature infant. Without therapeutic positioning, the W configuration of the arms, frogged posture of the legs, and asymmetric head position may lead to positional deformities. (Source: Reproduced from Jane Clifford O'Brien, Heather Kuhaneck. *Case-Smith's Occupational Therapy for Children and Adolescents*, Eighth Edition, Neonatal Intensive Care Unit, Fig. 22.9, St. Louis, Mosby, 2020. (Credit line- Courtesy Infant Special Care Unit, University of Texas Medical Branch, Gasveston, TX. Photograph by Jan Hunter).

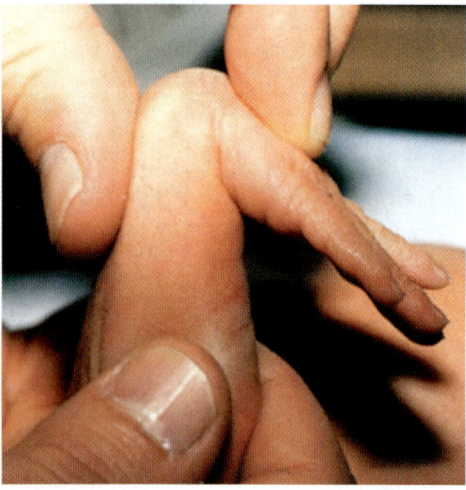

Fig. 42.2 Square window. *(Source:* Reproduced from Basil Zitelli, Sara McIntire, Andrew Nowalk et al. *Zitelli and Davis' Atlas of Pediatric Physical Diagnosis*, Eighth Edition, Neonatology, Fig. 2.10, Philadelphia, Elsevier Inc., 2023.)

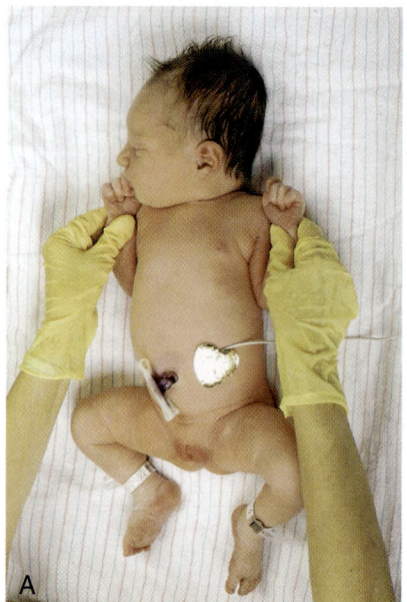

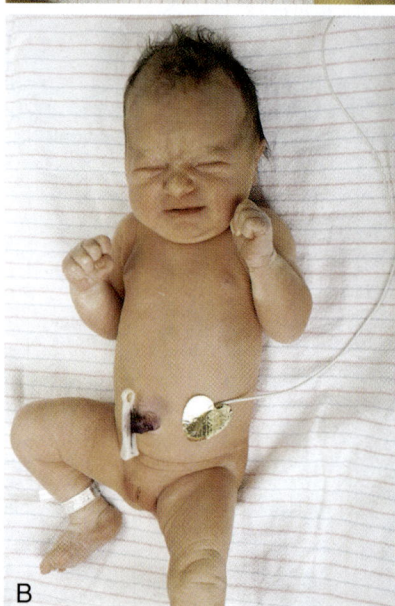

Fig. 42.3 (A and B) Arm recoil. *(Source:* Reproduced from Emily McKinney, Susan James, Sharon Murray. *Maternal-Child Nursing*, Sixth Edition, The Normal Newborn, Fig 21.26, St. Louis, Elsevier Inc., 2022.)

across the upper chest with one hand and the thumb of the examiner's other hand is placed on the infant's elbow.

- The examiner nudges the elbow across the chest of the infant, feeling for passive flexion or resistance to extension of posterior shoulder girdle flexor muscles as shown in Fig. 42.5.

Heel-to-Ear Measurement

- It measures the passive flexor tone about the pelvic girdle by testing for passive flexion or resistance to extension of posterior hip flexor muscles. The infant is placed supine and the flexed lower extremity is brought to rest on the mattress alongside the infant's trunk. The examiner supports the infant's thigh laterally along the side of the body with the palm of one hand. The other hand is used to grasp the infant's foot at the sides and to pull it toward the ipsilateral ear.

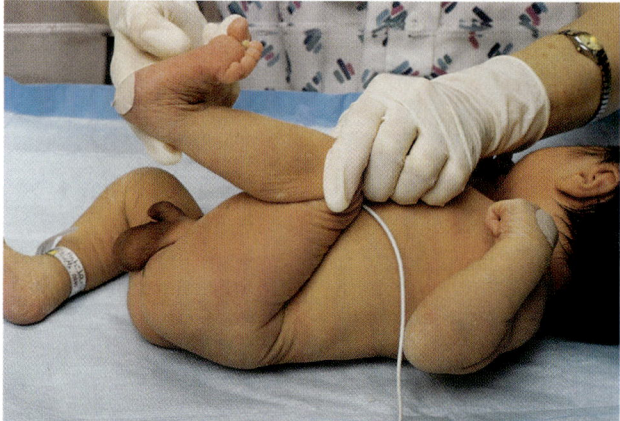

Fig. 42.4 Popliteal angle measurement. *(Source:* Reproduced from Emily McKinney, Susan James, Sharon Murray et al. *Maternal-Child Nursing*, Fourth Edition, The Normal Newborn, Fig 21.27, St. Louis, Saunders, 2013.)

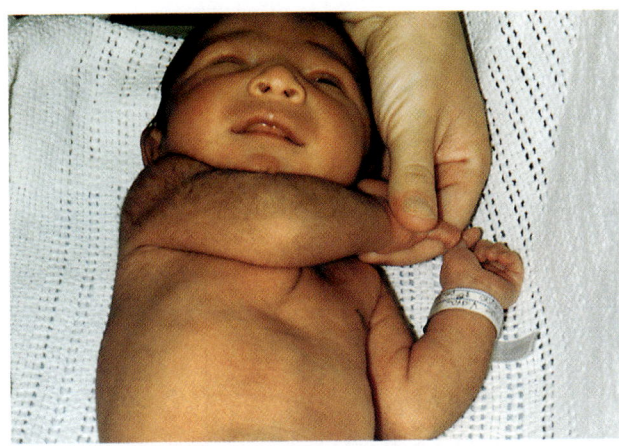

Fig. 42.5 Scarf sign. (*Source:* Reproduced from Debra Price, Julie Gwin. *Pediatric Nursing: An Introductory Text*, Tenth Edition, The New-born Infant, Fig 4.4, St. Louis, Saunders, 2008.)

- The examiner feels for resistance to extension of the posterior pelvic girdle flexors and notes the location of the heel where significant resistance is appreciated as shown in Fig. 42.6. Landmarks noted in order of increasing maturity include the following resistance felt when the heel is at or near the ear (−1), nose (0), chin level (1), nipple line (2), umbilical area (3), and femoral crease (4).

3. What is Dubowitz scoring system?

   It is a scoring system for assessment of gestational age on the basis of 10 neurological and 11 external criteria.

   Dubowitz score is obtained by summing the points for each parameter.

   Interpretation
   - Minimum score: 0
   - Maximum score: 72 (neurological signs, 35; external signs, 37)

   Estimated gestational age: [0.2642 * (total score)] +24.595

   Table 42.2 **gives the Dubowitz scoring system.**

4. *Discuss the complications associated with preterm birth. **Table 42.3 gives the complications associated with preterm birth (head to foot).***

5. Explain the long-term problems associated with preterm birth.
   a. Developmental disability in the form of cerebral palsy and mental retardation

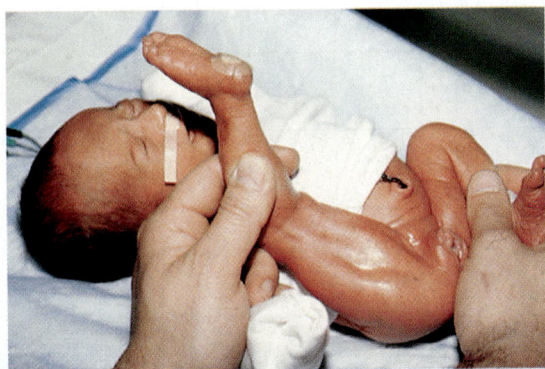

Fig. 42.6 Heel-to-ear measurement. (*Source:* Reproduced from Basil Zitelli, Sara McIntire, Andrew Nowalk et al. *Zitelli and Davis' Atlas of Pediatric Physical Diagnosis*, Eighth Edition, Neonatology, Fig. 2.13, Philadelphia, Elsevier Inc., 2023.)

b. Sensory impairments such as hearing loss and visual impairment

c. Cerebral dysfunctioning such as language disorders, learning disability, hyperactivity, attention deficits, and behavior disorders

d. Retinopathy of prematurity

e. Bronchopulmonary dysplasia

f. Poor growth

g. Increased rate of childhood illness and readmission to the hospital

6. Grade Intraventricular hemorrhage (IVH).

   Papile staging of IVH
   - Grade 1: Isolated germinal matrix hemorrhage (without intraventricular hemorrhage)
   - Grade 2: IVH without ventricular dilatation
   - Grade 3: IVH with ventricular dilatation
   - Grade 4: IVH with parenchymal hemorrhage

   Volpe staging
   - Grade 1: Germinal matrix hemorrhage with no or minimal IVH (<10% ventricular volume)
   - Grade 2: IVH occupying 10%–50% of ventricular volume
   - Grade 3: IVH occupying >50% of ventricular volume
   - Grade 4: Periventricular echodensity

7. Discuss cranial ultrasonography screening in preterm.
   - As per the National Neonatal Forum (NNF) guidelines, routine screening cranial ultrasonography should be performed for all infants weighing less than 1.250 kg or gestational age <30 weeks.
   - It has to be performed at 7–14 days of age and repeated at 36–40 weeks postmenstrual age. However, for unstable babies, the ultrasound can be performed on day 3 also.

8. Define and classify apnea of prematurity.

   Apnea is defined as spontaneous cessation of breathing for 20 seconds or more or accompanied by bradycardia with a heart rate of <100/min or hypoxemia that is detected clinically by cyanosis or oxygen saturation monitoring. It usually presents after 1–2 days of life and within 7 days.

   Apnea is classified as follows:
   - Central apnea (40%) because of immaturity of the central nervous system
   - Obstructive apnea (10%) that occurs when an infant tries to breathe against the obstructed upper airway
   - Mixed apnea (50%), which is most common

9. Enumerate the causes of apnea of prematurity.

   Causes
   - Temperature instability
   - Sepsis
   - Intraventricular hemorrhage
   - Asphyxia
   - Seizures
   - Pneumonia
   - Respiratory distress syndrome
   - Congenital heart diseases (PDA common)
   - Necrotizing enterocolitis
   - Gastroesophageal reflux
   - Anemia of prematurity
   - Hypoglycemia
   - Hypocalcemia
   - Metabolic acidosis

TABLE 42.2　**Dubowitz score**

Neurological sign	Score					
	0	1	2	3	4	5
Posture						
Square window	90°	60°	45°	30°	0°	
Ankle dorsiflexion	90°	75°	45°	20°	0°	
Arm recoil	180°	90–180°	<90°			
Leg recoil	180°	90–180°	<90°			
Popliteal angle	180°	160°	130°	110°	90°	<90°
Heel to ear						
Scarf sign						
Head lag						
Ventral suspension						

Physical (external) criteria

External sign	Score				
	0	1	2	3	4
Oedema	Obvious oedema hands and feet; pitting over tibia	No obvious oedema hands and feet; pitting over tibia	No oedema		
Skin texture	Very thin, gelatinous	Thin and smooth	Smooth, medium thickness Rash or superficial peeling	Slight thickening Superficial cracking and peeling, especially hands and feet	Thick and parchment-like Superficial or deep cracking
Skin colour (infant not crying)	Dark red	Uniformly pink	Pale pink, variable over body	Only pink over ears, lips, palms or soles	
Skin opacity (trunk)	Numerous veins and venules clearly seen, especially over abdomen	Veins and tributaries seen	A few large vessels clearly seen over abdomen	A few large vessels seen indistinctly over abdomen	No blood vessels seen
Lanugo (over back)	No lanugo	Abundant, long and thick over whole back	Hair thinning, especially over lower back	Small amount of lanugo and bald areas	At least half of back devoid of lanugo
Plantar creases	No skin creases	Faint red marks over anterior half of sole	Definite red marks over more than anterior half Indentations over more than anterior third	Indentations over more than anterior third	Definite deep indentations over more than anterior third
Nipple formation	Nipple barely visible, no areola	Nipple well defined, areola smooth and flat, diameter <0.75 cm	Areola stippled, edges not raised: diameter <0.75 cm	Areola stippled, edge raised: diameter >0.75 cm	
Breast size	No breast tissue palpable	Breast tissue on one or both sides <0.5 cm diameter	Breast tissue both sides, one or both 0.5–1.0 cm	Breast tissue both sides, one or both >1 cm	
Ear form	Pinna flat and shapeless, little or no incurving of edge	Incurving of part of edge of pinna	Partial incurving whole of upper pinna	Well-defined incurving whole of upper pinna	
Ear firmness	Pinna soft, easily folded, no recoil	Pinna soft, easily folded, slow recoil	Cartilage to edge of pinna but soft in places, ready recoil	Pinna firm, cartilage to edge, instant recoil	
Genitalia • Male	Neither testis in scrotum	At least one testis high in scrotum	At least one testis right down		
• Female (with hips half abducted)	Labia majora widely separated, labia minora protruding	Labia majora almost cover labia minora	Labia majora completely cover labia minora		

(**Source:** Reproduced from Sue Macdonald, Gail Johnson. Mayes' Midwifery, Fifteenth Edition, The preterm baby and the small baby, Figure 45.1, Oxford, Elsevier Ltd. 2017. (Credit line - Dubowitz LMS, Dubowitz V, Goldberg C: Clinical assessment of gestational age in the newborn infant, J Pediatr 77(1):1–10, 1970.)

TABLE 42.3	**Complications Associated With Preterm Birth (Head to Foot)**
Head to Foot	**Complications in Preterm**
a. Neurological problems	Perinatal depression Intraventricular hemorrhage
b. Ophthalmology	Retinopathy of prematurity
c. Nutritional	Feeding/sucking difficulties
d. Cardiovascular	Patent ductus arteriosus Hypotension because of sepsis-induced vasodilation, cardiac dysfunctioning, hypovolemia
e. Hematological	Anemia of prematurity Hyperbilirubinemia
f. Respiratory	Hyaline membrane disease Apnea of prematurity Bronchopulmonary dysplasia
g. Gastrointestinal	Necrotizing enterocolitis
h. Renal	Immature kidneys are unable to handle the water, solute, and acid loads
i. Temperature regulation	Temperature instability (hypothermia and hyperthermia)
j. Metabolic	Hypoglycemia Hypocalcemia
k. Immunological	Both humoral and cellular responses are poor and hence are prone to sepsis
l. Extremities	Osteopenia of prematurity

10. *How can one prevent apnea of prematurity?
    - Apnea in preterm is prevented by the use of caffeine. Caffeine is given to all the infants weighing less than 1.250 kg and to preterm infants weighing more than 1.250 kg requiring mechanical ventilation; it is initiated 24 hours prior to extubation.
    - Caffeine is started at a loading dose of 20 mg/kg orally or intravenously over 30 minutes followed by a maintenance dose of 5–8 mg/kg once in 24 hours.
    - When should caffeine be stopped? Caffeine is stopped when the infant has reached a postmenstrual age of 34–36 weeks or if he or she is apnea free for 7 days.

11. What is the mechanism of action of caffeine?
    The mechanism of action of the methylxanthines includes the following:
    - Stimulation of the respiratory center (sensitize the central medullary area for hypercapnia)
    - Antagonism of adenosine, which can cause respiratory depression
    - Improvement of the diaphragmatic contractility
    - Increase in minute ventilation
    - Increase in respiratory rate

12. Discuss the adverse events associated with caffeine citrate intake.
    - Tremors, opisthotonus, hyperglycemia, hypokalemia, and jaundice
    - Infrequent adverse events: Tachycardia, gastroesophageal reflex, and constipation

13. When should screening for retinopathy of prematurity (ROP) be performed?
    - ROP screening should be performed for all infants born <34 weeks or with birth weight less than 1750 g; in addition, infants born at 34–36 weeks of gestational age or with birth weight 1750–2000 g should undergo the screening if they have risk factors such as prolonged ventilation.
    - For infants born ≥28 weeks of gestational age, Retinopathy of prematurity (ROP) screening should be performed at 32 weeks of post menstrual age (PMA) or 4 weeks of postnatal age (PNA), whichever is later.

    - For infants born <28 weeks or with birth weight less than 1200 g, ROP screening should be done by 2–3 weeks of age to identify Agressive Posterior ROP (AP-ROP).

14. *Discuss the hearing assessment in preterm.
    - Infants with risk factors such as genetic abnormalities, cytomegalovirus infection, hyperbilirubinemia, asphyxia, meningitis, and preterm should undergo hearing assessment.
    - Remember the schedule as 1, 3, and 6.
      - They should undergo screening at 1 month of age.
      - Infants with a positive screening test should undergo definitive testing by 3 months of age.
      - Intervention for hearing impairment should be performed by the age of 6 months.

15. Discuss the indication of antenatal steroids.
    - This includes preterm labor at 24–34 weeks of gestation even if there is rupture of membranes; steroid is not a contraindication.
    - In case of 34–37 weeks of gestation with risk of preterm delivery within 7 days and not being received steroids earlier, then here chorioamnionitis is a contraindication.

16. Explain the complete course of antenatal steroids.
    Four doses of dexamethasone 6 mg intramuscular should be given once in 12 hours and the last dose should be given 24 hours prior to delivery.

17. What is the rescue course of Antenatal (AN) steroids?
    A pregnant woman with gestational age less than 34 weeks who has completed a full course of antenatal steroids 14 days before and is now at risk for preterm delivery within 7 days can be given one dose of steroids. This is called the rescue course.

18. What are the types of surfactant available?
    Table 42.4 gives the types of surfactant.

19. What is prophylactic and rescue therapy in administering a surfactant?
    - Prophylactic therapy: Administration of a surfactant before the onset of symptoms within minutes after birth is called prophylactic therapy.

TABLE 42.4	**Various Types of Surfactant**	
Trade Name	**Active Ingredient**	**Dose**
Curosurf	Poractant alfa	2.5 mL/kg/dose; two doses 12 hourly
Survanta	Beractant	4 mL/kg/dose; four doses 6 hourly
Infasurf	Calfactant	3 mL/kg/dose; three doses 12 hourly

- Rescue therapy: Administration of a surfactant after the onset of signs and symptoms of respiratory distress syndrome (RDS) is called rescue therapy. It can be early rescue (within 2 hours of birth) or late rescue (after 2 hours of birth).
20. Which antenatal steroid is safe for preterm?
    - The preferred drug in India is dexamethasone.
    - The drug of choice is betamethasone sulfate. But this particular salt of betamethasone is not available in India. The betamethasone available in our country is inferior to dexamethasone. Moreover, dexamethasone is cheaper.
    - It is given intramuscularly rather than intravenously to have a prolonged effect.
21. What are the indications of calcium administration in newborn?
    - Preterm <32 weeks
    - Sick infant of diabetic mother
    - Severe birth asphyxia
22. *What is sepsis scoring?
    - Classification of sepsis
        - Early onset sepsis (< 72 hours)
        - Late-onset sepsis (>72 hours)
    - **Risk factors for early onset sepsis**
        - Low birth weight of less than 2500 g
        - Maternal fever – 2 weeks prior to delivery
        - Foul-smelling liquor
        - Premature rupture of membranes for more than 24 hours
        - One unsterile or >3 sterile per vaginal examinations
        - Prolonged labor for >24 hours
        - Perinatal asphyxia°
    - **Risk factors for late-onset sepsis**
        - Low birth weight
        - Prematurity
        - Intensive care unit admissions
        - Mechanical ventilation
        - Invasive procedures
        - Central lines
    - **Indications for antibiotics**
        - Presence of ≥3 risk factors

- Presence of 2 risk factors + positive sepsis screening
- Strong clinical suspicion of sepsis – two sepsis screenings positive
- Presence of foul smelling liquor
- **Sepsis screening (sepsis screen is said to be positive if >2 parameters are positive)**
- Total leukocyte count <5000 cells/mm³
- Absolute neutrophil count – low counts as per Manroe chart for term and Mouzinho's chart for preterm
- Immature/total neutrophil ratio ≥0.2
- Micro-Erythrocyte sedimentation rate (ESR) >15 mm in the first hour
- C-reactive protein >1 mg/dL

23. Discuss the causes of hypocalcemia in preterm.
    - Occurrence of most of the placental transfer of calcium and parathormone during the last trimester
    - Renal immaturity
    - Low calcium stores
    - Increased stress → increased cortisone → increased tissue → catabolism → increased release of PO_4
24. Define bronchopulmonary dysplasia.
    Table 42.5 gives the definition of bronchopulmonary dysplasia.
25. How is bronchopulmonary dysplasia prevented?
    If the infant is younger than 28 weeks, then injection vitamin A should be administered at a dose of 5000 units/dose intramuscularly three times a week for 4 weeks from birth.
26. *Discuss kangaroo mother care.
    - **Indications**
        - All stable babies weighing <2000 g are eligible for kangaroo mother care (KMC).
        - Babies with birth weight of <1200 g need stabilization if they are suffering from any serious morbidities before initiating KMC.
    - **Duration**
      Sessions that last less than 1 hour should be avoided because frequent handling can cause stress to the baby.
      Skin-to-skin contact can be encouraged for up to 24 hours a day with minimal interruptions only for the change of diapers or for the mother's needs.
    - **Components of KMC**
      Skin-to-skin contact
      Exclusive breastfeeding
      Early discharge
    - **When to discontinue KMC**
      The baby's gestation reaches term or weight is around 2500 g.
      The baby starts to wriggle by pulling the limbs out and crying showing that he or she is uncomfortable.

TABLE 42.5	**Bronchopulmonary Dysplasia**	
	<32 Weeks	**>32 Weeks**
Time of assessment	36 weeks postmenstrual age or discharge	>28 but <56 days postnatal age
Treatment with oxygen	>21% for at least 28 days	>21% for at least 28 days
Mild	Breathing room air at 36 weeks Post menstrual age (PMA)	Breathing room air at 56 days postnatal age
Moderate	<30% FiO_2 at 36 weeks PMA	<30% FiO_2 at 56 days postnatal age

43

Frequently Asked Questions in Neonatal Hyperbilirubinemia

1. Explain the bilirubin metabolism.
   Flowchart 43.1 shows the bilirubin metabolism.
2. *What are the causes of neonatal jaundice?
   Table 43.1 gives the causes of neonatal jaundice.
3. Enumerate relevant points in antenatal history.
   Table 43.2 shows the relevant points in antenatal history.
4. Enumerate examination findings in neonatal jaundice.
   Table 43.3 gives the examination findings in neonatal jaundice.
5. What are the sites to look for icterus?
   - Forehead
   - Tip of the nose
   - Over the sternum
   - Abdomen
   - Knees
   - Palms and soles
6. What is Kramer's rule?
   Kramer's rule is used to note the extent of jaundice. Depth of the jaundice should be carefully noted (light staining as lemon yellow and deep staining as orange yellow) because it indicates the level of jaundice as shown in Fig. 43.1.
   Kramer zones are as follows
   Zone 1 (Face and neck)-Mild jaundice (5-7 mg/dl), Deep jaundice (7-9 mg/dl)
   Zone 2 (Chest and upper abdomen)-Mild jaundice (7-9 mg/dl), Deep jaundice (9-11 mg/dl).
   Zone 3 (Lower abdomen and thighs)-Mild jaundice (9-11 mg/dl), Deep jaundice (11-13 mg/dl).
   Zone 4 (Legs and arms/forearms)-Mild jaundice (11-13 mg/dl), Deep jaundice (14-16 mg/dl).
   Zone 5 (Palms and soles)- Mild jaundice (13-15 mg/dl), Deep jaundice (17 mg/dl or more).
7. Enumerate the causes for physiological hyperbilirubinemia in newborn.
   - Increased bilirubin production
     a. Increased RBC volume per kilogram
     b. Decreased RBC survival (90 days)
     c. Ineffective erythropoiesis
     d. Increased turnover of non-hemoglobin heme proteins
   - Increased enterohepatic circulation
   - Defective uptake of bilirubin because of decreased ligandin
   - Defective conjugation
   - Decreased hepatic excretion of bilirubin
8. What is physiological hyperbilirubinemia?
   - Term babies: The bilirubin level rises up to 6–8 mg/dL from the 3rd to the 5th day of life and then falls. Rise up to 12 mg/dL is physiological.
   - Preterm babies: The bilirubin can rise up to 10–12 mg/dL by the 5th day of life, possibly also >15 mg/dL without any specific abnormality in bilirubin metabolism.

9. *What are the differences between breastfeeding and breast milk jaundice?
   Table 43.4 shows the differences between breastfeeding and breast milk jaundice.
10. What is pathological jaundice?
    - Onset of jaundice before 24 hours of life
    - Any elevation of serum bilirubin that requires phototherapy

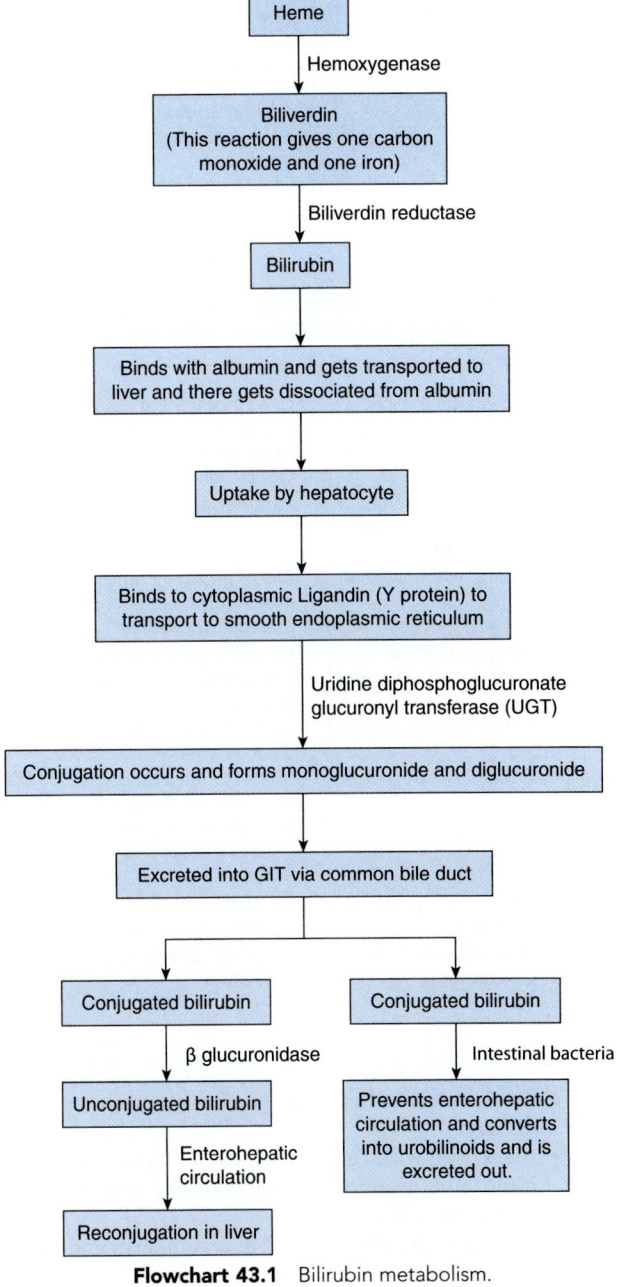

Flowchart 43.1 Bilirubin metabolism.

TABLE 43.1	Causes of Neonatal Jaundice	
Time of Occurrence of Jaundice	**Causes**	
<24 h	*Rh incompatibility*	
	ABO incompatibility	
	Glucose 6 phosphate dehydrogenase (G6PD) deficiency	
	Minor blood group incompatibility	
	RBC membrane defect	
24–72 h	*Rh incompatibility*	
	ABO incompatibility	
	G6PD deficiency	
	Minor blood group incompatibility	
	RBC membrane defect	
	Enclosed hemorrhage	
	Increased enterohepatic circulation	
3–7 days	*Idiopathic*	
	Sepsis	
	G6PD deficiency	
	Enclosed hemorrhage	
	Increased enterohepatic circulation	
>7 days	*Breast milk jaundice*	
	Sepsis	
	Enclosed hemorrhage	
	Increased enterohepatic circulation	
	Hypothyroidism	
	Intestinal obstruction	

TABLE 43.2	Relevant Points in Antenatal History
History	**Relevance**
Maternal drug intake such as nitrofurantoin, sulfonamides, antimalarials	Can displace the bilirubin bound to albumin and also predisposes to hemolysis in a G6PD-deficient infant
History of fever with rashes, lymphadenopathy, and joint pain for the mother	Intrauterine infection (TORCH)
Previous sibling with neonatal jaundice	Blood group incompatibility, breast milk jaundice, Lucey–Driscoll syndrome
Family history of anemia, jaundice, abdominal surgeries	Hereditary spherocytosis, G6PD deficiency, Crigler–Najjar syndrome
History of liver disease in family	α_1-Antitrypsin deficiency, galactosemia
Use of oxytocin in intrapartum	Oxytocin infusion is given in 5% dextrose, so there will be shift of fluid into the Red blood corpuscles (RBCs) and hence hemolysis
History of instrumental delivery	Extravasation of blood
Delayed cord clamping	Polycythemia causing hemolysis
Prolonged parenteral nutrition and use of antibiotics	Increased enterohepatic circulation

- A rise in serum bilirubin by >0.5 mg/dL/h or >5 mg/dL/day
- Associated with any other signs of illness such as vomiting, lethargy, poor feeding, excessive weight loss, and temperature instability
- Jaundice persisting beyond 8 days in term and 14 days in preterm

TABLE 43.3	Examination Findings in Neonatal Jaundice	
Physical Examination	**Relevance**	
Low birth weight, Intrauterine Growth Restriction (IUGR)	Preterm, intrauterine infection	
Small for Gestational Age (SGA)	Polycythemia	
Microcephaly	Intrauterine infection	
Pallor	Hemolytic anemia, extravasation of blood	
Bruises, cephalhematoma	Increased bilirubin formation	
Petechiae	Intrauterine infection, erythroblastosis, sepsis	
Hepatosplenomegaly	Intrauterine infection, hemolytic anemia	
Chorioretinitis	Intrauterine infection	
High-colored urine, clay-colored stools	Cholestatic jaundice	

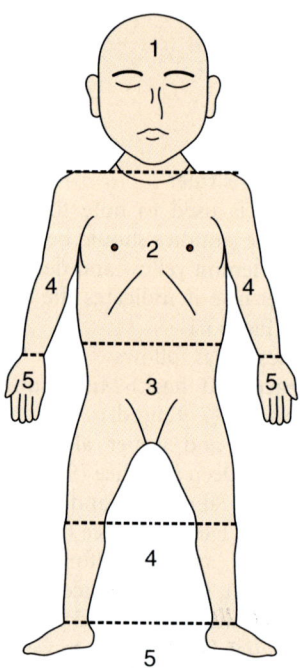

Fig. 43.1   Kramer's rule.

11. What are the indications of phototherapy?
    - Babies with serum bilirubin level above the phototherapy range as per the American Academy of Pediatrics (AAP) chart
    - Prophylactic phototherapy in the following conditions:
        - Extreme low birth weight (<1000 g)
        - Severely bruised infants
        - Babies with direct Coombs test positive and anticipated to have a rapid rise in bilirubin while waiting for exchange transfusion
12. What is Bronze baby syndrome?
    Babies with direct hyperbilirubinemia caused by cholestatic jaundice when administered phototherapy produces bilifuscin like substances due to abnormal

TABLE 43.4	Differences Between Breastfeeding Jaundice and Breast Milk Jaundice	
Breastfeeding Jaundice	**Breast Milk Jaundice**	
Seen in 5%–10% of newborn	Seen in 2%–4% of newborn	
It occurs because of decreased intake of breast milk that leads to increased enterohepatic circulation	It occurs because of some unknown substance present in breast milk that blocks the destruction of bilirubin	
Onset is on days 2–3, peaks by 5th day, and then improves; value does not exceed 15 mg/dL	Onset is by 4–7 days of life	
Disappears by the end of 1st week of life	Jaundice lasts for 3–10 weeks of age and the value can reach up to 20–30 mg/dL	
Treated by adequate breastfeeding	Breastfeeding need not be stopped; can be continued	
Aggravating factor is dehydration	No aggravating factors	

accumulation of photoisomer of bilirubin or due to abnormal hepatic function leading to copper-porphyrin complex which is photo destroyed causing brown pigmentation leading to Bronze baby syndrome. Usually this syndrome is mild resolves after stopping phototherapy.

13. Discuss the mechanism of action of phototherapy.

Phototherapy with a wavelength of 420–470 nm reduces the amount of unconjugated bilirubin (UCB).

The three photochemical reactions are given in Table 43.5.

14. *What is intensive phototherapy?
    - Intensive phototherapy should be provided by delivering irradiance between 400 and 520 nm spectrum of >30 µW/cm²/nm (Compact Florescent Lamp (CFL) 10–30 µW/cm²/nm; Light Emitting Diode (LED) >100 µW/cm²/nm).
    - The distance between the phototherapy unit and the baby should be reduced to 10–15 cm (LED lamps).
    - Double-surface phototherapy can be provided by placing the nude baby on a fiber-optic biliblanket.
    - The light exposure should be uniform over 60 cm × 30 cm area of the skin.
    - White curtains can be used in the room to reflect the light over the baby.

15. Mention some adverse effects of phototherapy.
    - Insensible water loss
    - Redistribution of blood flow
    - Increased fecal water loss
    - Hypocalcemia
    - Retinal damage
    - Tanning of skin for black infants
    - Bronze baby syndrome
    - Reduced mother–baby bond

16. When should phototherapy be stopped?
    - If two total serum bilirubin (TSB) values taken 12 hours apart are below the age-specific cutoff, phototherapy can be stopped.
    - For any hemolytic jaundice, check the total serum bilirubin (TSB) values 12 hours after stopping the phototherapy to see rebound hyperbilirubinemia.
    - Any baby discharged within 3 days should be followed up within 2–3 days.

17. Discuss the peripheral smear finding in ABO incompatibility.

Microspherocytes are seen in peripheral smear. This is because the A antibodies will bind with A antigens. When these antigen–antibody complexes reach the reticuloendothelial system, they are bitten off and these small spherocytes will enter the circulation.

18. Explain the protective mechanism by ABO incompatibility on Rh incompatibility.

The ABO incompatibility protects against the sensitization by an Rh antigen because the maternal antibodies (A/B antibodies) will eliminate the fetal RBCs with A/B antigen before they can encounter the antibody-forming lymphocytes.

19. *Which neonatal hyperbilirubinemia presents more like hemolytic anemia rather than bilirubinemia?

Isoimmune hemolytic anemia caused by Kell antigen presents more like hemolytic anemia.

20. What are the indications of exchange transfusion?

Indications of exchange transfusion are the following:
- When phototherapy fails to prevent a rise in bilirubin
- To correct anemia and features of heart failure in case of hydrops fetalis

TABLE 43.5	Mechanism of Action of Phototherapy	
Photoisomerization	**Structural isomerization**	**Photo-oxidation**
The natural isomer of UCB is converted to less toxic polar isomer and is excreted into bile without conjugation	It is intramolecular cyclization of bilirubin to lumirubin and is rapidly excreted into bile and urine without conjugation	It converts bilirubin to small polar products that are excreted in the urine
Readily converted back to UCB	It is irreversible	It is least important to lower the serum bilirubin levels
Bilirubin levels do not change much	It is the most important pathway to reduce the serum bilirubin	
It occurs at low-dose phototherapy (6 µW/cm²/nm)	It occurs at a dose of 6–12 µW/cm²/nm	

UCB, unconjugated bilirubin.

- To reduce the hemolysis by removing the sensitized RBCs and antibodies
- Cord bilirubin level >4.5 mg/dL and cord hemoglobin <11 g/dL
- Bilirubin rise being >1 mg/dL/h despite phototherapy
- Progressive anemia in hemolytic anemia
- Bilirubin level approximately 20 mg/dL or rapidly rising at such a rate that it will be soon >20 mg/dL

21. How is blood group chosen for exchange transfusion?

    Type of blood used for exchange transfusion in different conditions are as follows:

    For Rh isoimmunisation - Rh negative, blood group "O," or blood group that of the baby suspended in AB plasma cross-matched with baby's and mother's blood is used.

    For ABO incompatibility - Rh compatible and blood group "O"(not that of the baby group), suspended in AB plasma, cross matched with baby's and mother's blood is used.

    For other conditions such as G6PD deficiency - Baby's blood group and Rh type specific cross-matched with baby's and mother's blood is used.

    - The blood should be fresh (<7 days) whole blood, and irradiated and reconstituted with a hematocrit of 45%–50% collected in citrate-phosphate-dextrose.
    - Exchange transfusion usually involves double the volume of the infant's blood, that is, 160–180 mL/kg. This can replace 87% of the infant's blood volume with new blood.
    - After exchange transfusion, phototherapy should be continued and bilirubin levels are measured every 4 hours once.

22. Mention the complications associated with exchange transfusion.
    - Hypoglycemia
    - Hypocalcemia
    - Hypomagnesemia
    - Metabolic alkalosis
    - Hyperkalemia
    - Thrombocytopenia causing bleeding manifestations
    - Embolization into blood vessels, thrombosis, and infarction
    - Hemolysis
    - Infections
    - Temperature instability
    - Necrotizing enterocolitis

23. Explain the other modes of management of hyperbilirubinemia.
    - **Intravenous immunoglobulin**
      - It is used in case of A–O or B–O incompatibility if phototherapy is not effective in lowering serum bilirubin and if the bilirubin is approaching the exchange transfusion levels.
      - It is given at a dose of 0.5 g/kg/day over 2–4 hours for 2 days.
      - It acts by downregulating the Fc receptor–mediated phagocytosis in reticuloendothelial system.
    - **Phenobarbitone**
      - It acts by increasing the concentration of ligandin (protein) and also by inducing the enzyme uridine diphosphoglucuronate glucuronosyltransferase (UGT).

- **Ursodeoxycholic acid (UDCA):** By helping in conjugation of bilirubin
- **I.v. albumin:** Thought to bind with free bilirubin in the serum and hence prevents it from crossing the blood–brain barrier (BBB)
- **Agar and cholestyramine:** Acts by decreasing the enterohepatic circulation
- **Metalloporphyrins/zinc:** Acts by blocking the enzyme heme oxygenase, and is actually useful in Crigler–Najjar

24. What is prolonged jaundice?

    Persistence of significant jaundice for more than 2 weeks in term and more than 3 weeks in preterm is called prolonged jaundice (PJ).

25. Discuss the approach to prolonged jaundice.

    Flowchart 43.2 shows the approach to prolonged jaundice.

26. *What are the stages of Acute bilirubin encephalopathy (ABE)?
    - **Early phase:** Hypotonia, lethargy, high-pitched cry, and poor suck
    - **Intermediate phase:** Opisthotonus, rigidity, oculogyric crisis, retrocollis, irritability, fever, and seizures
    - **Late phase:** Replacement of hypotonia by hypertonia by approximately after 1 week of age, shrill cry, apnea, seizures, coma, and death

27. *What is the tetrad of chronic bilirubin encephalopathy (kernicterus)?
    - Choreoathetoid cerebral palsy
    - Supranuclear gaze palsy
    - Sensorineural hearing loss
    - Dental Enamel Dysplasia

28. *What is BIND score?

    Table 43.6 shows the bilirubin-induced neurological dysfunction (BIND) score.

29. Discuss Bhutani's nomogram.
    - Bhutani's nomogram is an hour-specific bilirubin nomogram (Fig. 43.2). It predicts the ability of subsequent significant hyperbilirubinemia in healthy term and near-term newborn who require follow-up.
      - High-risk zone: >95th percentile
      - Intermediate-risk zone: Two components – upper and lower intermediate-risk zones – divided by 75th percentile
      - Low-risk zone: 40th percentile track

    Source: Publisher Wolters Kluwer, Cloherty, 8th ed., Chapter 26 – neonatal hyperbilirubinemia, p. 338, Fig. 26.1.

30. What are the major risk factors for the development of severe hyperbilirubinemia?

    Risk factors for the development of severe hyperbilirubinemia are the following:

    a. Predischarge total bilirubin (TB) in high-risk zone (>95th percentile for age in hours in Bhutani's nomogram)

    b. Reporting of jaundice within the first 24 hours of birth

    c. 35 -36 weeks of gestational age

    d. Immune or other hemolytic disease

    e. History of jaundice with previous sibling

    f. Cephalhematoma or significant bruising

    g. East Asian race

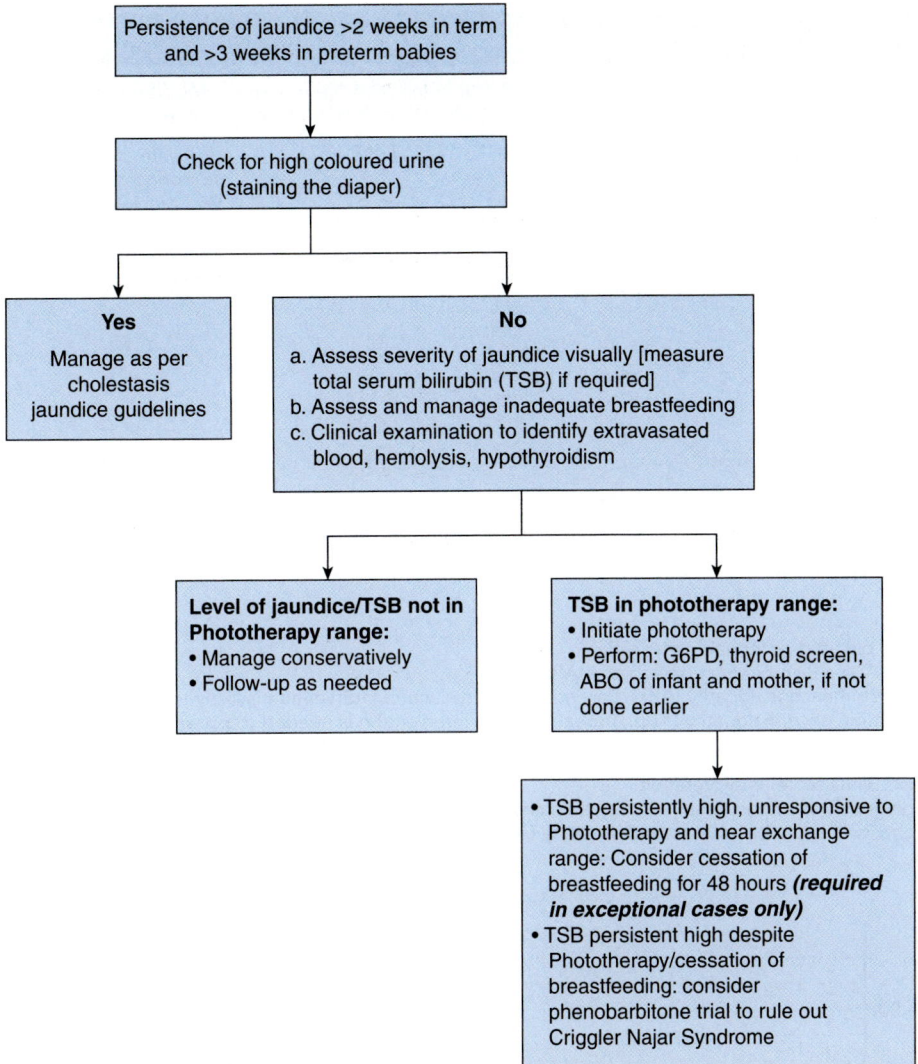

Flowchart 43.2 Approach to prolonged jaundice.

TABLE 43.6	BIND Score and Modified BIND Score (BIND-M Score)		
Item	Bilirubin Induced Neurologic Dysfunction (BIND) score	Modified BIND score	Acute Bilirubin Encephalopathy (ABE)
MENTAL STATUS			
Normal	(0)	(0)	None
Sleepy but arousable; decreased feeding	(+1)	(+1)	Subtle
Lethargy, poor suck and/or irritable/jittery with strong suck	(+2)	(+2)	Moderate
Semi-coma, apnoea, unable to feed, seizures, coma	(+3)	(+3)	Advanced
MUSCLE TONE			
Normal	(0)	(0)	None
Persistent mild to moderate hypotonia	(+1)	(+1)	Subtle
Mild to moderate hypertonia alternating with hypotonia, beginning arching of neck and trunk on stimulation	(+2)	(+2)	Moderate

Continued

TABLE 43.6	BIND score and Modified BIND score (BIND-M score)—cont'd		
Item	Bilirubin Induced Neurologic Dysfunction (BIND) score	Modified BIND score	Acute Bilirubin Encephalopathy (ABE)
Persistent retrocollis and opisthotonos – bicycling or twitching of hands and feet	(+3)	(+3) with crossing or scissoring of arms or legs but without spasms of arms and legs and without trismus	Advanced
CRY PATTERN			
Normal	(0)	(0)	None
High pitched when aroused	(+1)	(+1)	Subtle
Shrill, difficult to console	(+2)	(+2)	Moderate
Inconsolable crying or cry weak or absent	(+3)	(+3)	Advanced
ALTERED GAZE			
Normal gaze	-	(0)	None
Sun-setting; paralysis of upward gaze	-	(+3)	Advanced

BIND score interpretation
0: No indication of acute bilirubin encephalopathy (ABE)
1-3: Subtle signs of mild Acute Bilirubin Encephalopathy (ABE)
4-6: Moderate acute bilirubin encephalopathy (ABE), urgent bilirubin reduction intervention is likely to reverse the acute damage
7-9: Advanced acute bilirubin encephalopathy (ABE), urgent bilirubin intervention is needed to prevent further damage and reduce the severity of sequelae

Bind -M score (Modified BIND score) interpretation
<3: No indication of diagnosis of acute bilirubin encephalopathy (ABE)
> or =3: Positive diagnosis of acute bilirubin encephalopathy (ABE)

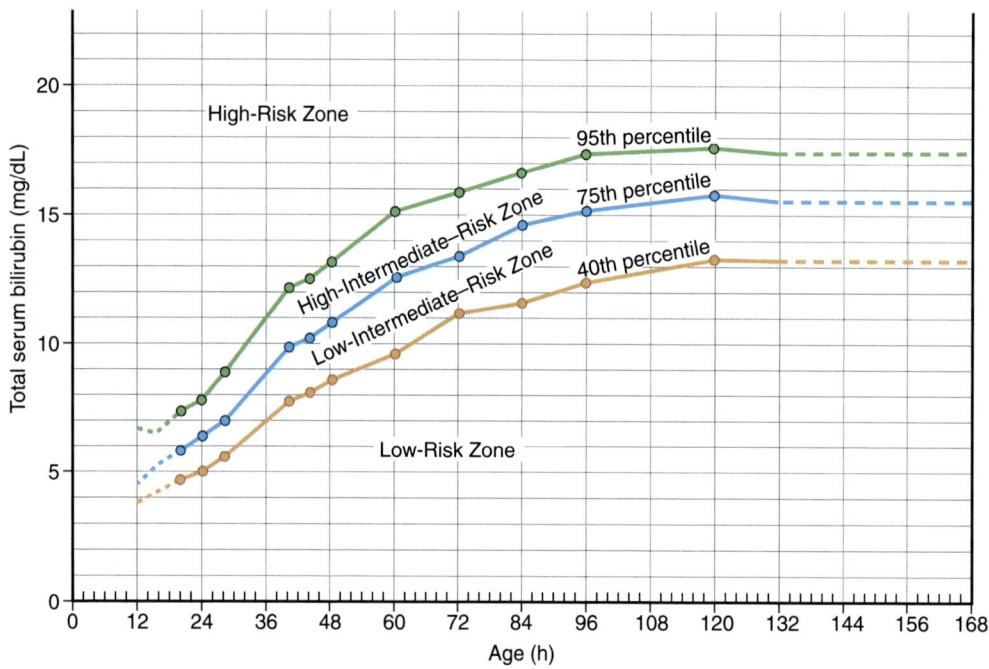

Fig. 43.2 Bhutani's nomogram – risk designation of term and near-term babies on the basis of their hour-specific serum bilirubin values. *(Source:*Reproduced from Christine Gleason, Sandra Juul. *Avery's Diseases of the Newborn*, Tenth Edition, Newborn Nursery Care, Fig. 26.4, Philadelphia, Elsevier Inc., 2018. (Credit line - Modified from Bhutani VK, Johnson L, Sivieri EM. Predictive ability of a predischarge hour-specific serum bilirubin for subsequent significant hyperbilirubinemia in healthy term and near-term newborns. Pediatrics. 1999;103:6–14.).)

Quick Bites

For phototherapy and exchange transfusion chart for term babies, refer AAP guidelines-link – https://pediatrics.aap-publications.org/content/pediatrics/114/1/297.full.pdf.

For hyperbilirubinemia for preterm babies, refer NICE guidelines-link – https://www.nice.org.uk/guidance/cg98/evidence/full-guideline-245411821.

Other Topics of Practical Examination Importance

44 Nutrition

Nutrients (Table 44.1)

TABLE 44.1	Nutrients and Its Nutritive Value				
Ingredient	Calories/ 100 g	Protein/ 100 g	Macronutrients	Micronutrients	Special Features
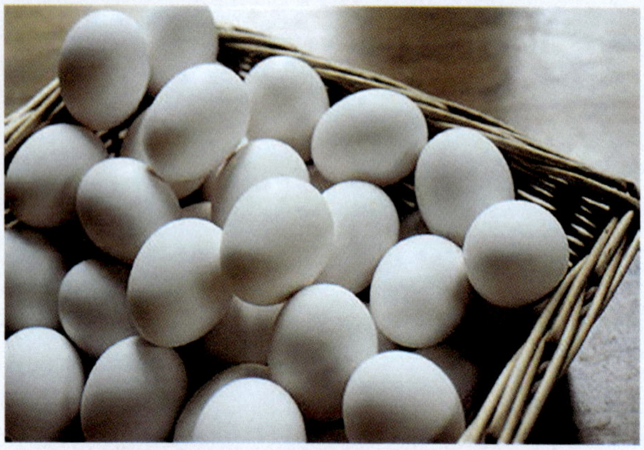 Fig. 44.1 Eggs. (Source: eggs - Bing images)	80 kcal/ 1 egg	6 g/ 1 egg	Fat – 13 g	Iron – 2 mg Calcium – 30 mg	Net protein utilization – 96 Biological value – 96 Protein efficiency ratio – 3.8 Deficient in carbohydrate and vitamin C It is called reference protein It contains all essential amino acids
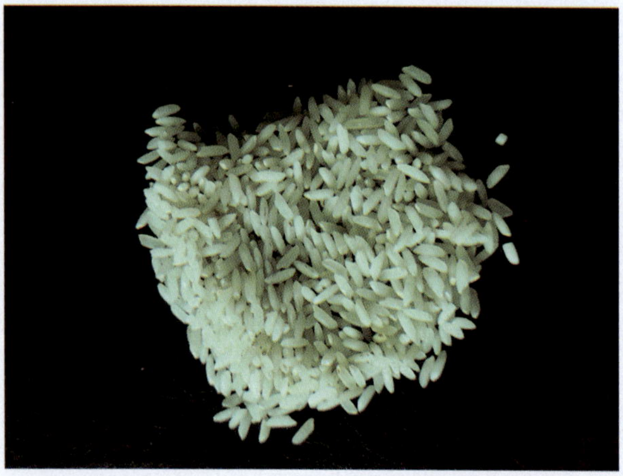 Fig. 44.2 Rice grain.	350	7	Carbohydrate – 78 g Fat – 0.5 g Fiber – 0.2 g	Iron – 0.7 mg	Deficient in lysine and threonine; good source of vitamin B; cooking and washing remove vitamins, especially thiamine

TABLE 44.1	Nutrients and Its Nutritive Value—cont'd				
Ingredient	Calories/ 100 g	Protein/ 100 g	Macronutrients	Micronutrients	Special Features
	350	11	Fat – 1.5 g Fiber – 1.2 g	Iron – 5.3 mg	Deficient in vitamins A and C, and lysine and threonine Cereal:pulse = 3:1 combination provides supplementary effect
	330	7	Fat – 1.3 g Fiber – 3.6 g	Iron – 3.9 mg Calcium – 344 mg	Rich in calcium and good source of essential amino acids
	116/ banana	1.2 g/ banana	Fat – 0.3 g Fiber – 0.3 g	Iron – 0.4 mg	High-fiber content High-iron content High potassium – contraindicated in patients with Chronic kidney disease (CKD)

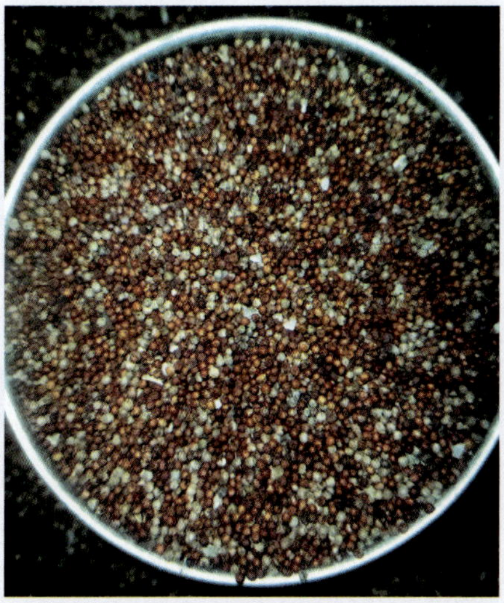

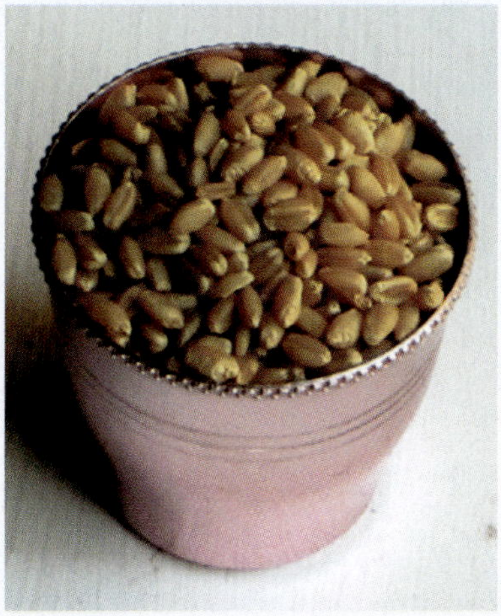

Fig. 44.3   Wheat. (*Source:* Reproduced from C Wrigley, Ian L Batey, Diane Miskelly. *Cereal Grains: Assessing and Managing Quality*, Second Edition, Assessing and Managing Quality at all Stages of the Grain Chain, Figure 1.1, Oxford, Woodhead Publishing Ltd, 2017.)

Fig. 44.4   Ragi.

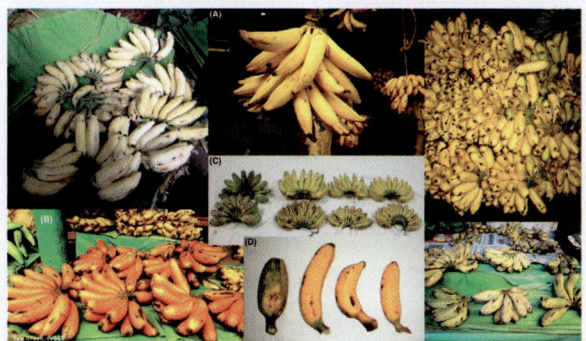

Fig. 44.5   Banana. (Source: Reproduced from Brian Thomas. *Encyclopedia of Applied Plant Sciences*, Second Edition, Banana, Figure 9, Oxford, Academic Press, 2017.)

Continued

TABLE 44.1	Nutrients and Its Nutritive Value—cont'd				

Ingredient	Calories/100 g	Protein/100 g	Macronutrients	Micronutrients	Special Features
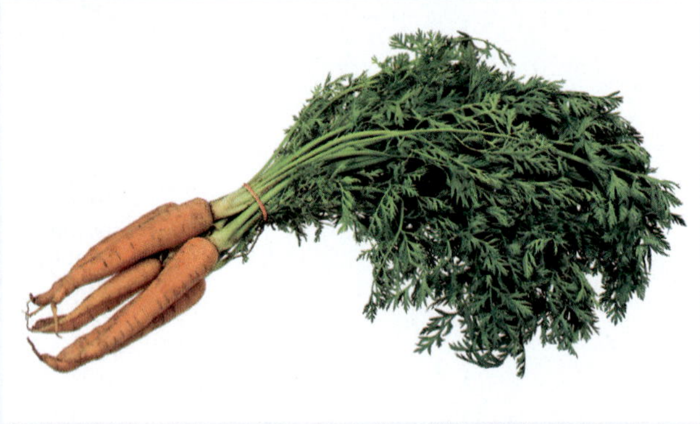 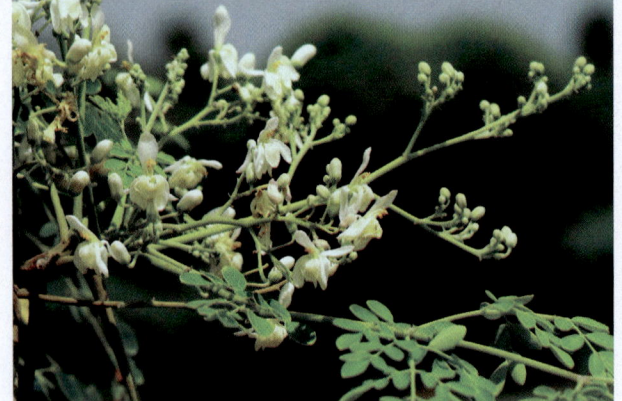	50	3.0	Fat − 0.2 g Fiber − 1.2 g	Iron − 1.0 mg	Rich source of beta-carotene

Fig. 44.6 Carrot. (*Source:* https://en.wikipedia.org/wiki/Carrot#/media/File:Vegetable-Carrot-Bundle-wStalks.jpg)

| | 64 | 9.4 | Carbohydrate − 8.3
Fat − 1.4 g
Fiber − 2 g | Potassium, calcium, folate, vitamin A, vitamin C, iron, magnesium, calcium | Very rich source of vitamin C |

Fig. 44.7 Drumstick leaves. (Source: https://en.wikipedia.org/wiki/Moringa_oleifera#/media/File:DrumstickFlower.jpg)

| | 18 | 0.9 | Carbohydrate − 3.9 g
Fat − 1.5 g | Vitamin A − 42 µg
Vitamin C − 14 mg | Rich source of vitamins A, C, and E. |

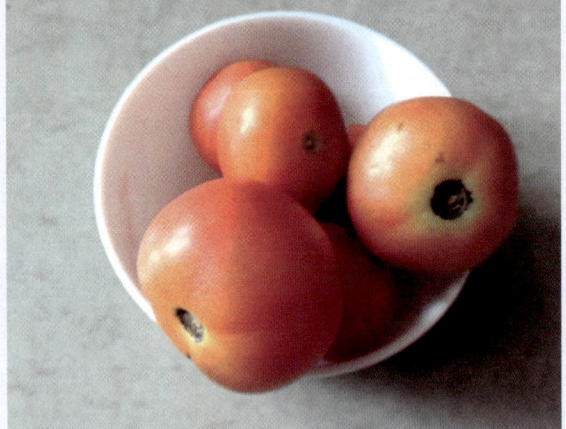

Fig. 44.8 Tomato.

Milk

- Good source of protein, calcium, and vitamins
- Deficient in iron and vitamin C
- Iron and phosphate absorption is affected by high-phosphate content of the milk
- High lactose is present in human milk (7 g%)
- Buffalo milk has high fat content (7 g%)
- Consumption of goat milk causes megaloblastic anemia
- Net protein utilization – 85
- Biological value – 90
- Protein efficiency ratio – 2.8

Table 44.2 shows difference between cow milk and human milk contents.

Table 44.3 gives specific calories and fat content in each milk packet.

Sugar

- Simple sugars – glucose, galactose, and fructose
- Table sugar/granulated sugar – sucrose (glucose + fructose)
- Brown sugar contains 97%, whereas table sugar contains 100% carbohydrate, <2% water, and no fiber, protein, and fat
- Brown sugar has iron (15% of Recommended Dietary Intake (RDI) in 100 g)
    Table 44.4 gives contents of brown sugar and white sugar.
- Health side effects include obesity and metabolic syndrome, cardiovascular disease, addiction, hypoactivity, tooth decay, Alzheimer disease
- Recommendation: <10% of total energy intake

Pulses

Table 44.5 gives contents of various pulses.
    Germinated pulses have vitamin C
    Deficient in vitamin A
    Oligosaccharides can cause flatulence

TABLE 44.2	Differences Between Cow Milk and Human Milk Contents	
Contents	Cow Milk (100 mL)	Human Milk (100 mL)
Energy	67 kcal	67 kcal
Fat	4.1 g	3.4 g
Carbohydrate	4.4 g	7.4 g
Protein	3.2 g	1.1 g
Iron	0.2 mg	0.3 mg

TABLE 44.3	Specific Calories and Fat Content in Each Milk Packet	
Color of the Packet	Calories (100 mL)	Fat (100 mL)
Brown	48 kcal	1.5 g
Blue	60 kcal	3 g
Green	74 kcal	5 g
Orange	96 kcal	6 g

Note: All packets contain approximately 5 g/100 mL of carbohydrate and 3 g/100 mL of protein.

TABLE 44.4	Contents in Brown Sugar and White Sugar	
Contents	Brown Sugar (100 g)	White Sugar (100 g)
Carbohydrate	377 kcal	387 kcal
Protein	—	—
Fat	—	—
Fiber	—	—
Iron	15% of Recommended Dietary Intake (RDI)	—

These belong to legume family and include lentils, peas, beans, and gram, shown in Fig. 44.9A–H. Methionine is limiting amino acid in pulses.

Cereals (Fig. 44.10 A-D)

Cereals are rich in carbohydrates. Lysine is limiting amino acid.

Points to Remember in Cereals and Pulses

- Parboiling: It refers to hot soaking followed by steaming of paddy. Benefits: Vitamins to percolate inside, resistant to insects, increases storage life, and removes toxin BOAA in kesari dal.
- Germination/sprouting: It is a method to enhance vitamin content while decreasing the bulk on cooking (amylase-rich food).
- Fermentation: It enhances vitamin C and digestibility.
- Reference protein:
    The complete protein that provides all amino acids is reference protein. Egg is the reference protein. The quality of dietary protein is based on extent to which it deviates from reference protein.
- Digestibility coefficient = Absorbed nitrogen/Retained nitrogen × 100
- Biological value = Retained nitrogen/Absorbed nitrogen × 100
- Net protein utilization = Retained nitrogen/Retained nitrogen × 100

Total Parenteral Nutrition

Table 44.6 shows total parenteral nutrition.

Diet in Special Situations

1. Chronic kidney disease (CKD)
    1. Calories – liberal calories + 10% extra for illness
    2. Restrict proteins – 0.5–1.25 g/kg
    3. Sodium: Restrict sodium during oliguric phase and during diuretic phase − 1–2 g/dL; increase up to 10 g/dL
    4. Potassium: Restricted
2. Congestive cardiac failure (CCF)
    1. Calories – required daily allowance (RDA) + 10%–30% extra
    2. Fluids – restrict to insensible loss + last day urine output
    3. Protein – RDA or up to 15% of total calories as protein of high biological value
    4. Sodium – restrict to 1/2–1 g/dL

3. Respiratory illness
   1. Asthma – avoid hypoallergic diet – citrus fruits, groundnuts, chocolates, cow milk, egg meat, and fish
   2. Calories – 10%–20% extra calories
   3. Convalescing children – 1–2 extra meal/day at least for 2 weeks

4. Hepatic encephalopathy
   1. Avoid protein by mouth
   2. Sterilize gut by oral ampicillin or neomycin; bowel wash should be given
   3. Lactulose 1–2 mL/kg/day in divided doses
   4. Lactobacilli orally

TABLE 44.5	Contents of Various Pulses		
Contents	Bengal Gram (Kadalai Paruppu)	Black Gram (Ulutham Paruppu)	Green Gram (Payatham Paruppu)
Calorie (kcal)	360	350	340
Protein (g)	17	24	24
Cholesterol (g)	60	60	57
Fat (g)	5.3	1.4	1.3
Fiber (g)	3.9	0.9	4.1
Iron (mg)	4.6	3.8	4.4

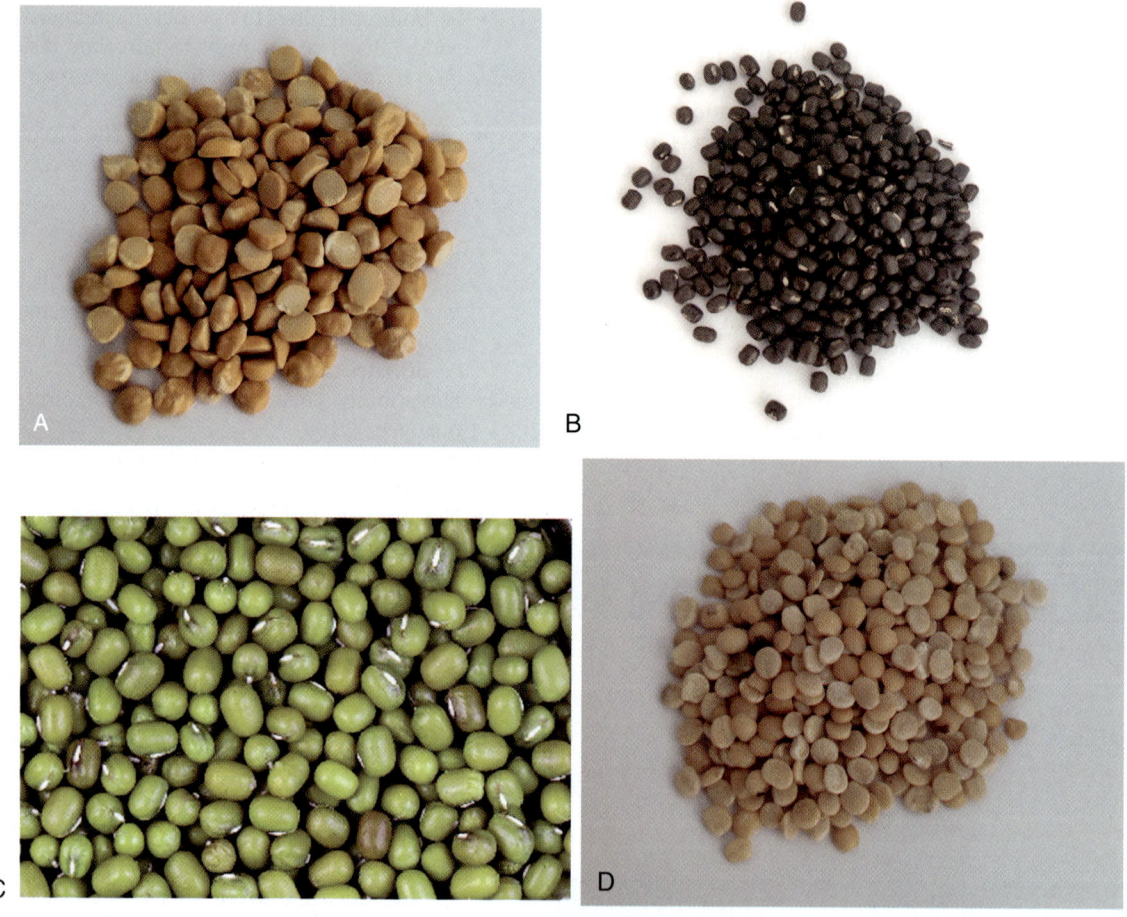

Fig 44.9 (A) Gram dal. (B) Black urad dal. (C) Green gram. Commonly used pulses: (D) Toor dal.

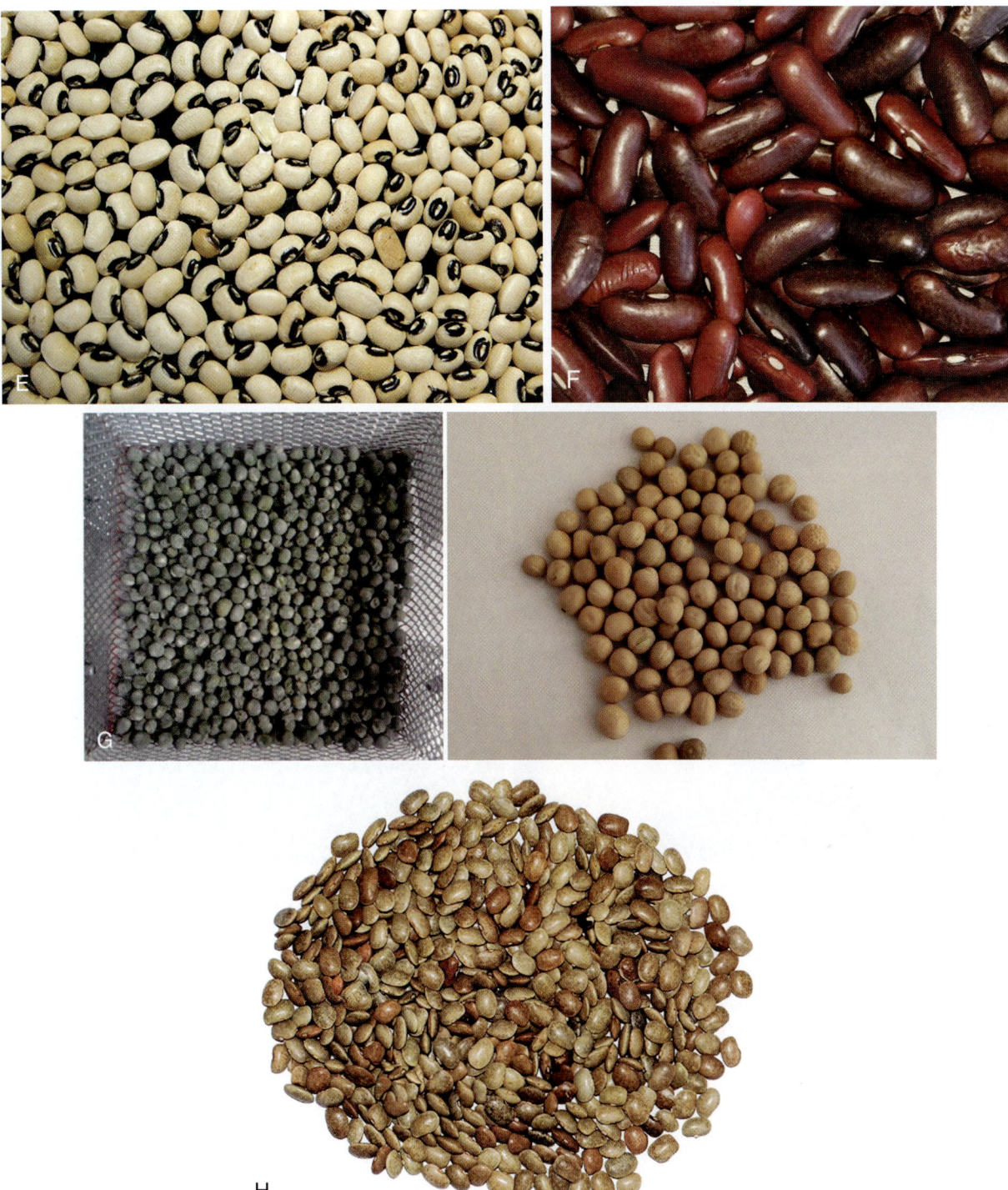

Fig. 44.9—cont'd (E) black-eyed beans, (F) kidney beans, (G) green and white peas, (H) horse gram. (Source C, E, and H: Bing Images); (*Source* F: Reproduced from Rajkumar Patil. *Community Medicine: Practical Manual*, Nutrition, Figure 2.22, New Delhi, Elsevier India, 2018.; Source of dry green peas: Reproduced from Maryam Barzegar, Dariush Zare, Richard L. Stroshine and An integrated energy and quality approach to optimization of green peas drying in a hot air infrared-assisted vibratory bed dryer, *Journal of Food Engineering* 166:302-315.)

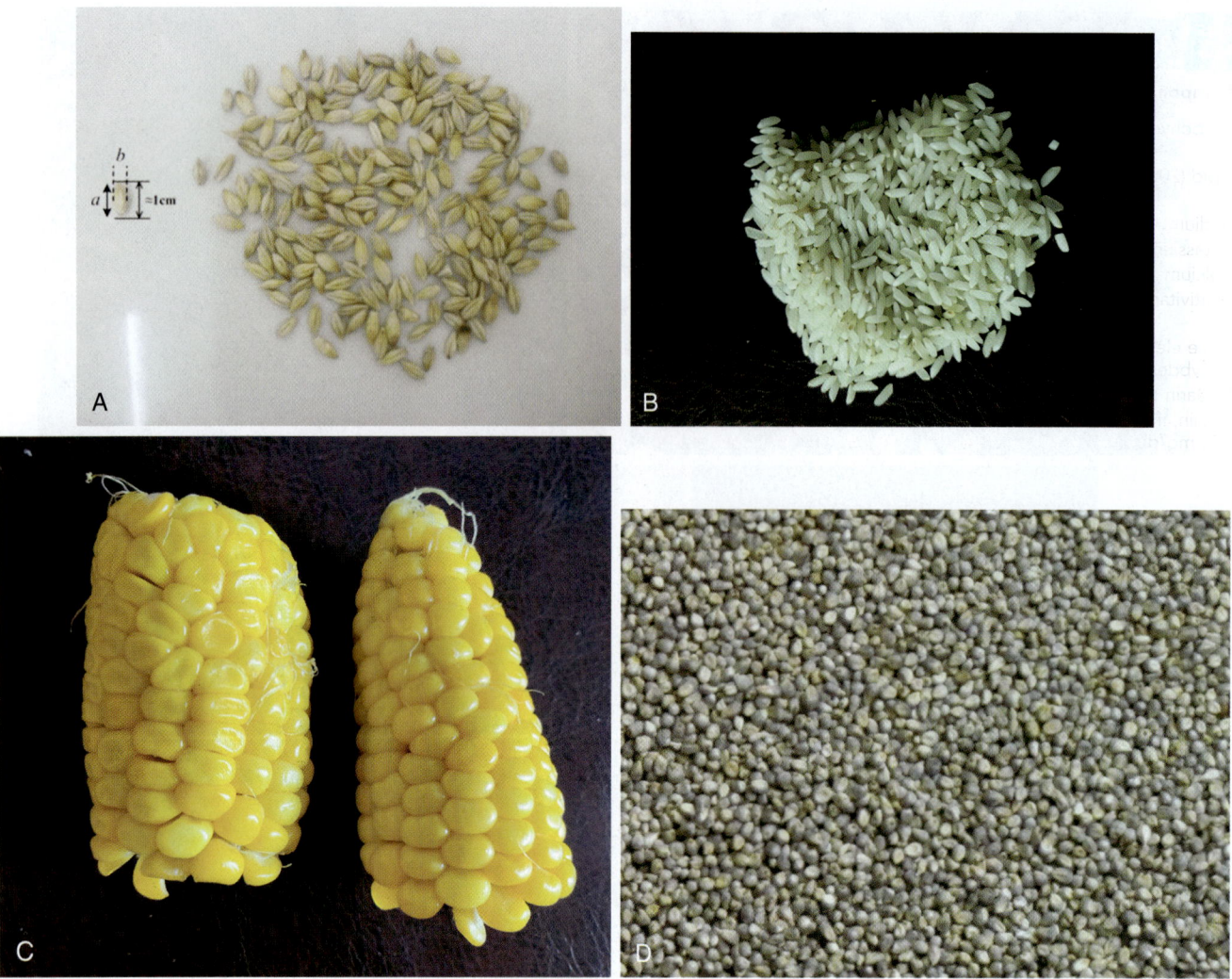

Fig. 44.10 Commonly used cereals: (A) Barley, (B) rice, (C) corn, (D) bajra. (*Source* A: Reproduced from H.C. Werner Muhlbauer, Joachim Muller. Drying Atlas: *Drying Kinetics and Quality of Agricultural Products*, Barley (Hordeum vulgare L.), Fig. 3.1.3, Chennai, Woodhead Publishing, 2020.) (Source D: Bing Images)

TABLE 44.6 Total Parenteral Nutrition		
Component	**How Much to Give**	**What to Monitor**
Carbohydrate (10% Dextrose)	1 mg/kg/min = 0.6 mL/kg/h Start at 4 mg/kg/min	Serum glucose
Lipid (20%) Cover with aluminum foil	1 g/kg – max 3 g/kg	Every 48 h, check cholesterol and triglyceride (TGL) (stop if >200 mg/dL)
Sodium	3–5 mEq	Serum sodium
Potassium	2 mEq/kg	Serum potassium
Calcium	2 mL/kg/dose twice a day	Serum calcium
Multivitamin	<1 kg – 2 mL >1 kg – 5 mL	
Trace elements – zinc, selenium, magnesium, molybdenum	0.2 mL/kg/day	
Heparin	>1 unit/mL	
Insulin, if capillary blood glucose (CBG) > 150 mg/dL	0.05–0.1 IU/kg	CBG

5. Calorie – Recommended Dietary Allowance (RDA) +10%–20% of RDA; glucose-enriched diet
6. Blood transfusion if needed
7. Salt-free albumin
8. Vitamin K and Fresh Frozen Plasma (FFP)
9. Hepatic drip
10. Glucagon – 0.03 mg/kg/day up to 1 mg/dose for 3 days
11. Supplement branched-chain amino acids
12. Hepatic fluid
   The composition of hepatic drip is given in Table 44.7
13. Diet in chronic liver disease
   • Fat malabsorption – Medium chain triglycerides (MCTs) oil
   • Fat-soluble vitamins
     Vitamin A – 10,000–15,000 IU/day
     Vitamin E – 50–400 IU/day tocopherol
     Vitamin D – 5000–8000 IU/day of D3
     Vitamin K – 2.5–3 mg on alternate day orally or 5 mg i.m. twice monthly
   • Water-soluble vitamin – twice the RDA
   • Ursodeoxycholic acid (UDCA) – 15–20 mg/kg/day
5. Diet in diabetes
   1. Meal time should be regular and quantity should be consistent
   2. Fasting should be avoided
   3. Goal: Ensure normal growth with Fasting blood sugar (FBS) < 115 mg/dL, Postprandial blood sugar (PPBS) < 126–140 mg/dL, serum cholesterol < 200 mg/dL, serum Low-density lipoprotein (LDL) < 130 mg/dL, High density lipoprotein (HDL) < 50 mg/dL, Triglycerides(TGL) < 160 mg/dL, and HbA1C – 6%–8%

4. Carbohydrates: Avoid refined sugar, monosaccharide and disaccharide. Complex carbohydrate should be taken. Tubers should be restricted. Whole wheat is preferred as it contains acarbose that slows down absorption.
5. Fiber: Unabsorbed plant polysaccharides delay carbohydrate absorption and hence decrease hyperglycemia. Approximately 25–30 g/day should be taken.
6. Low-fat diet: It increases insulin binding and reduces LDL and Very low density lipoprotein. The polysaturated:unsaturated (P/S) ratio of 1.2:1 is recommended.
7. Fruits: Based on carbohydrate control.
8. Carbohydrate count
   Glycemic index of 70 in 100 g of food – 15 g carbohydrate (except banana, mango, and potato)
   Glycemic index of 40 – pulses/milk – 12 g carbohydrate
   Example: For three idlis in breakfast of weight 75 g
   The carbohydrate count would be 75 + 75 + 75 = 225 g corresponds to 15 + 15 + 3 = 33 g
   1/10th of the carbohydrate count is given as the initial dose of insulin
   This is insulin bolus regime.
9. Glycemic index for 100 g
   More than 70%: Rice, wheat, ragi, maize, potato, banana, and mango
   40%–50%: All pulses, orange, guava, and papaya
   30%–40%: Milk, dairy products, biscuits, and apple
   Less than 20%: Musk melon and green peas (any amount)

Calorie and Protein Values of Common Food Items (Table 44.8)

1 cup = 240 mL, 1 ounce = 30 mL, 1 katori 5 150 mL, 1 glass = 200 mL, 1 tablespoon = 15 mL/15 g, 1 teaspoon = 5 mL/5 g, 1 tumbler average = 200 mL

Intravenous Fluid Calculations

• Water requirements:
   100 cm^3/kg for the first 10 kg
   50 cm^3/kg for the next 10 kg (11–20 kg)
   20 cm^3/kg for the rest (>20 kg)

TABLE 44.7 Hepatic Drip	
Item	**Quantity (mL)**
NS	100
10% dextrose	400
KCl	5
Calcium gluconate	5
Multivitamin	2

TABLE 44.8	Nutritive Values of Common Food Items			
S. No.	Food	Quantity	Calorie (kcal)	Protein (g)
1.	Cooked rice	1 cup	175	4
2.	Egg	1	87	6
3.	Idli, dosa, chapati, poori, vada	1	70	2
4.	Biscuit	1	20	0.5
5.	Upma	1 cup	250	6
6.	Sambhar	1 tablespoon	50	1
7.	Dal	1 teaspoon	10	0.5
8.	Banana	1	100	1
9.	Vegetable	1 cup	100	1
10.	Fish	10 cm piece	80	6
11.	Chicken	3/4 cup	240	6
12.	Oil	1 teaspoon (5 g)	40	2.5
13.	Sugar	1 teaspoon (5 g)	20	0.5
14.	Aavin milk	100 mL	60	3
15.	Formula milk	30 mL water + 1 scoop powder	400–500	12
16.	Butter milk	100 mL	45	2.5
17.	Orange juice	100 mL	100	—
18.	Cereal Pulse Porridge (CPP) kanjee	100 g	320	12
19.	*SAT mix (Precooked ready to mix cereal-pulse)	100 g	360	8
20.	Egg pulp (egg + milk + sugar)	150 mL	200	9
21.	Chicken soup (100 g chicken + 50 g coconut oil + 50 g sugar + 1000 mL water)	100 mL	68	25
22.	Lactose-free diet (1 teaspoon sugar/salt pinch + 3 teaspoon rice powder + 1 teaspoon moong dal + 1/2 teaspoon oil + 100 mL water	100 mL	106	2.2

*This mix is a research and development product of Nutrition clinic, Depatment of pediatrics, Sree Avittom Thirunal (SAT), Hospital Trivandrum

- Sodium requirements:
  3–5 mEq/kg/day
- Potassium requirements
  1–3 mEq/kg/day
- Chloride requirements
  4–6 mEq/kg/day
- To make calculations easier the requirements can be taken as Sodium 4 mEq/kg/day and potassium 2 mEq/kg/day

EXAMPLE

I.v. fluid calculation:
- Consider a 10 kg child
- Total fluid requirement = 10 × 100 = 1000 mL/day
- Sodium = 10 × 4 = 40 mEq/day
- Potassium = 10 × 2 = 20 mEq/day
- Hence, the child should be given 1000 mL of fluid/day with 40 mEq of sodium
- Now next step is to choose an i.v. fluid that gives 40 mEq in 1000 mL.
- NS contains 154 mEq in 1000 mL
- 1/2 NS contains 77 mEq in 1000 mL
- 1/4 NS contains 38 mEq in 1000 mL which is close to the sodium requirement of the child
- To the above-mentioned fluid, add 10 mL KCl which would provide 20 mEq
- Next step is dextrose. Dextrose does not provide adequate calories but it does provide a source of energy for enzymes so that they do not breakdown muscle. D5

provides approximately 252 mOsm/L. Add this to a fluid that contains 80 mOsm/L (40 mEq/L of sodium and 40 mEq/L of chloride). Each is a monovalent ion; therefore, the osmolality is 80.
- Hence, 252 + 80 = 332, which should be greater than the plasma osmolality, which is between 280 and 290. Thus, avoiding a hypotonic solution that would potentially lyse cells.

Glucose Infusion Rate (GIR) (Formulae)

1. GIR = Percentage of dextrose being infused × rate of infusion (in mL/h)/birth weight (kg) × 6 (mg/kg/min)
2. GIR = Rate of i.v. fluids (in mL/kg/day) × percentage of dextrose infused/144 (mg/kg/min)
3. Glucose (in g) = GIR × birth weight × 1.44
4. Example: Percentage of dextrose being infused is calculated as follows:
   The formula for preparing 100 mL of fluid with a desired concentration of glucose by using 5% dextrose and 25% dextrose solutions is as follows: $5X − 25 = Y$, where X is the required percentage of dextrose and Y is the amount of 25% dextrose (in mL) to be made up with 5% dextrose to make a total of 100 mL.

Nutrient Requirements

A balanced diet should consist of the following:
- Carbohydrate 50%; moderate sucrose intake – 10%

- Fat: 30%–35%
- 10% saturated fat, 10% polyunsaturated fat, 10% mono-unsaturated fat
- Omega-6:omega-3 ratio = 5–10:1
- Protein: 20%
- Fiber: Age in years + 5 g (daily requirement) or half the weight
- Salt: 2–3 g/day

ABCDEFG Approach

A − anthropometry
B − biochemical labs
C − clinical
D − dietary
E − environmental/emotional
F − functional
G − growth monitoring

JUNCS

J − junk foods: High in fat, salt, and sugar; low in micronutrients, protein, and fiber; solid fat and added sugar, Dalda, bakery items, frozen desert (SOFAS)
U − ultraprocessed foods: Packaged processed foods − transfat, refined sugar, additives
N − nutritionally inappropriate foods: Tea, coffee, health drinks
C − carbonated/caffeinated/colored foods or beverages
S − sugar: Sweetened beverages

Approximate RDA ICMR (2010)

Table 44.9 gives RDA.

TABLE 44.9	Recommended Dietary Allowances (RDA)
Age Group	**Requirement**
1 year (1/2 of mother's RDA)	1000 kcal
1–3 years (1/2 of father's RDA)	1200 kcal
3–10 years	Add 100 kcal/year
Adolescent boy (equal to father's RDA)	2400 kcal
Adolescent girl (more than mother's RDA)	2200 kcal

Approximate RDA of Micronutrients

Table 44.10 gives approximate RDA of micronutrients.

Role of Zinc in Diarrhea

- Replenishes brush border enzymes
- Regulates fluid electrolyte transport
- Leads to epithelial repair
- Enhances T-helper cell activity
- Improves taste
- Corrects overt/subclinical zinc deficiency

TABLE 44.10	Approximate RDA of Micronutrients
Micronutrients	**Requirement**
B1, B2, B6	0.5–1.5 mg/day
B3 (niacin)	5–15 mg/day
Folic acid (B9, B11)	50–150 µg/day
B12	0.5–1.5 µg/day
Vitamin C	40–50 mg/day
Vitamin A	1500 IU/day
Vitamin D	400 IU/day
Vitamin E	5–15 IU/day
Iron	10–20 mg/day
Zinc	5–15 mg/day
Iodine	50–150 µg/day

45 Vaccination

General Principles of Immunization

1. Immunization at birth means within 48–72 hours but not longer than 1 week.
2. Two live vaccines can be administered simultaneously except oral polio vaccine (OPV), cholera, and yellow fever. There is no such contraindication for inactivated vaccines.
3. Spacing for two different live vaccines
   - Two different live vaccines should be administered within 24 hours.
   - If not, time interval should be at least 4 weeks.
   - If administered less than 4 weeks apart, the second should be repeated after checking antibody titers (does not apply to live oral vaccines).
4. Spacing for doses of live vaccines
   - At least 4 weeks
5. No recommendation for spacing of inactivated vaccines – the minimum interval between two inactivated vaccines is 4 weeks (except rabies).
6. Any number of antigens can be given on the same day.
7. Time interval of vaccines in immunocompromised people should be at least 2 weeks apart. If given <2 weeks, antibody titer should be checked and reimmunized accordingly.
8. Any dose not given at previous visit should be administered at the subsequent visit.
9. A dose is considered valid if it is given up to 4 days before the scheduled date. It is invalid if given >5 days before the scheduled date.
10. Needles need not be changed in between drawing the vaccine into the syringe and injecting it into the child.
11. Different vaccines should not be mixed in the same syringe unless it is specifically licensed and labelled.
12. Any child whose immunization status is unknown should be considered unimmunized and should be given regular course even if already immunized.
13. Route of administration and site
    - Any vaccine with adjuvants should be given by i.m. route.
    - If given intradermally or subcutaneously, it can cause granuloma or abscess formation.
    - All immunoglobulins except rabies are given by intramuscular route.
14. Route and site of vaccination
    - All vaccines with adjuvants should be given by i.m. route.
    - Gluteal region should never be used because of risk of sciatic nerve injury.
    - If they are given by subcutaneous or intradermal route, injection site abscess/granuloma can occur.
      Table 45.1 gives route and site of administration of various vaccine.
      Fig. 45.1A shows various needle sizes and Fig. 45.1B shows angle of administration of vaccine.
15. Key points in selecting the needle for injection

    Needle gauge:
    - Gauge recommendation for intradermal (26−28 G), intramuscular (26−30 G), and subcutaneous (19−27 G) administration
    - The higher the gauge number, the smaller the diameter of the needle
    - The higher the viscosity of the fluid, the lower the gauge size
    - The higher the gauge size, the less the pain or bruise experienced by the patient
    - The lower the gauge number, the stronger the needle; less chance of bending or breaking

    Needle length:
    Recommendations:
    - For intradermal administration: 3/8 to 3/4 inch
    - For intramuscular administration: 7/8 to 1½ inches
    - For subcutaneous administration: 5/8 to 1/2 inch
16. Administration of vaccine
    - Vaccines that are to be given by s.c. route can be given by i.m. but reverse is not possible.
    - Two different i.m. vaccines can be given on the same day and injected on same thigh but at a distance of 1–2 inch.
    - If an i.m. vaccine and an immunoglobulin are to be given on the same day, they have to be given on separate thighs.
    - Following administration of the vaccine, do not withdraw the needle to prevent backflow.
    - Do not rub the site of injection.

TABLE 45.1	Routes and Sites of Administration of Various Vaccines			
Age	Route	Site	Needle	Technique
Newborns	I.m.	Anterolateral aspect of thigh	23 G	Stretch the skin between thumb and index finger
Up to 1 year	I.m.	Anterolateral aspect of thigh	23 G	Bunch the skin, subcutaneous tissue, and muscle
1–12 years	I.m.	Anterolateral aspect of thigh or deltoid	23 G	Same as above
Up to 1 year	S.c.	Thigh	25 G	
1 year	S.c.	Outer triceps	25 G	
All ages	I.d.	Outer deltoid	26 G	

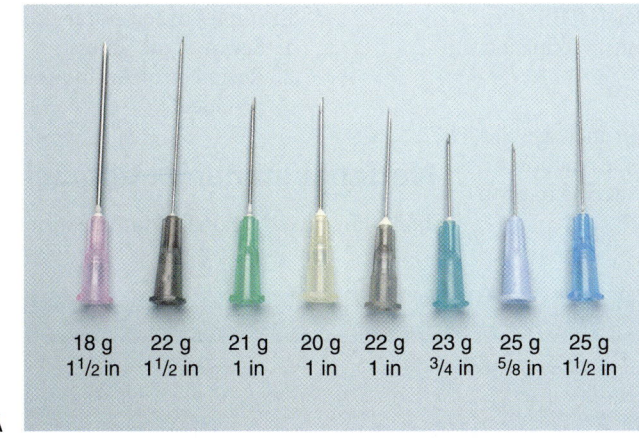

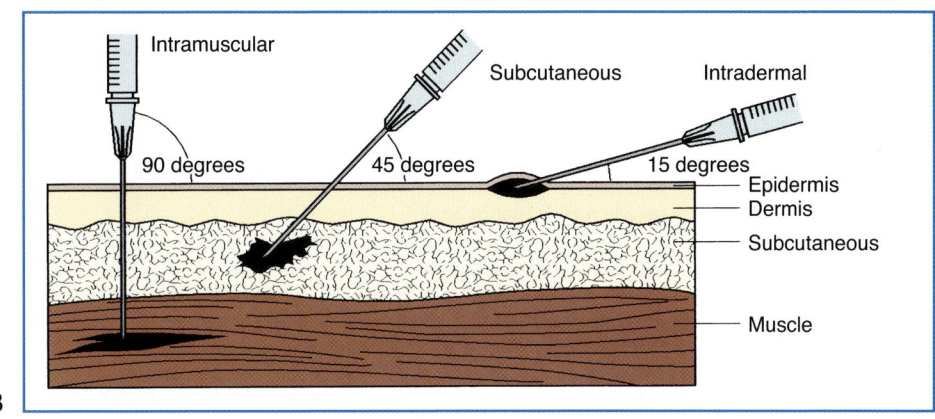

Fig. 45.1 (A) Various size needles. (B) Angle of administration of vaccine. (*Source* (A): Reproduced from Linda Lilley, Shelly Collins, Julie Snyder. *Pharmacology and the Nursing Process*, Tenth Edition, Photo Atlas of Drug Administration, Fig. 9.22, St. Louis, Mosby, 2023. (Credit line - From Rick Brady, Riva, MD.). *Source* (B): Reproduced from Joanna Bassert, Joanna Bassert, Dennis McCurnin. *McCurnin's Clinical Textbook for Veterinary Technicians*, Seventh Edition, Pharmacology and Pharmacy, Fig. 25-5, St. Louis, Saunders, 2010.)

17. *Other important points in vaccination*
    - Basic reproductive number (Ro): It measures the average number of secondary cases generated by one primary case in a susceptible population.
      If Ro < 1: The disease is declining
      If Ro > 1: An outbreak is occurring
    - Vaccine efficacy: It is the ability of the vaccine to protect an individual. It can be assessed through clinical trials, case–control studies, or cohort studies.

$$VE = \frac{ARU - ARV}{ARU}$$

ARU: Attack rate in unvaccinated population
ARV: Attack rate in vaccinated population
VE: Vaccine efficacy
Vaccine effectiveness: It is defined as the ability of the vaccine to protect the community and given as the sum of vaccine efficacy and herd effect.
Cost effectiveness: Expressed as cost per infections/hospitalizations/death prevented.
Herd immunity: Refers to proportion of persons with immunity in a given population.

Herd effect: Reduction of infection or disease in an unimmunized segment resulting in immunizing a proportion of the population. Examples of vaccine having herd effect are conjugated pnuemococcal and Hib vaccines whereas Tetanus and BCG (Bacillus Calmette-Guerin has no herd effect.
Contact Immunity: Refers to the concept of vaccinated individual can 'pass on' the vaccine to another individual through contact.

18. Contraindications and precautions
    - Contraindication: A condition in a recipient which increases the chance of a serious adverse reaction.
    - True contraindications are as follows:
      Permanent complications:
      1. These involve severe allergic reactions to a vaccine component or to a prior dose of vaccine
      2. Encephalopathy that occurs within 7 days of pertussis vaccination
      3. Severe combined immunodeficiency (SCID) as a contraindication to rotavirus vaccine
      Examples of permanent complications:
      1. High fever: 105°F
      2. Persistent crying for >3 hours

3. Hypotonic: Hyporesponsive episodes (HHE) after DPT (Diphtheria, Pertussis and Tetanus) vaccination
4. Seizures within 3 days

Temporary complications:
- These involve conditions that might increase the chance or severity of a serious adverse reaction or that compromise the ability of the vaccine to produce immunity

Examples of temporary complications:
1. Severe acute illness
2. Recipient of Antibody-containing product

National Immunization Schedule

Table 45.2 gives National Immunization Schedule.

TABLE 45.2	National Immunization Schedule		
Vaccine (Site)	**When to Administer**	**Route**	**Dose**
FOR INFANTS			
Bacillus Calmette-Guerin (BCG) (Left Upper arm)	At birth or as early as possible till 1 year of age	Intradermal	0.1 mL (0.05 mL until 1 month of age)
Hepatitis B-birth dose (Anterolateral aspect of mid-thigh)	At birth or as early as possible within the first 24 hours	Intramuscular	0.5 mL
Oral polio vaccine (OPV)-0 dose (Oral)	At birth or as early as possible within the first 15 days	Oral	2 drops
OPV 1, 2 and 3 (Oral)	At 6 weeks, 10 weeks and 14 weeks (OPV can be given till 5 years of age)	Oral	2 drops
Pentavalent 1, 2 and 3 (Anterolateral aspect of mid-thigh)	At 6 weeks, 10 weeks and 14 weeks (can be given till 1 year of age)	Intramuscular	0.5 mL
Rotavirus vaccine (RVV) (Oral)	At 6 weeks, 10 weeks and 14 weeks (can be given till 1 year of age)	Oral	5 drops (liquid vaccine) 2.5 mL (lyophilized vaccine)
Pnuemococcal conjugate vaccine (PCV) (Anterolateral aspect of mid-thigh)	Two primary doses at 6 and 14 weeks followed by booster dose at 9-12 months	Intramuscular	0.5 mL
Inactivated polio vaccine (IPV) (Intra dermal Right Upper arm)	Two fractional doses at 6 and 14 weeks of age	Intradermal two fractional dose	0.1 mL
Measles rubella (MR) vaccine- first dose (Right Upper arm)	9 completed months to 12 months (Measles can be given till 5 years of age)	Subcutaneous	0.5 mL
Japanese encephalitis (JE)-1 Left Upper arm (live attenuated vaccine) Anterolateral aspect of mid-thigh (killed vaccine)	9 completed months to 12 months	Subcutaneous (live attenuated vaccine) Intramuscular (killed vaccine)	0.5 mL
Vitamin A (first dose) (Oral)	At 9 completed months with measles rubella vaccine	1 mL (1 Lakh IU)	Oral
FOR CHILDREN			
Diphtheria, pertussis and tetanus (DPT) booster -1 (Anterolateral aspect of mid-thigh)	16-24 months	0.5 mL	Intramuscular
MR second dose (Right upper arm)	16-24 months	0.5 mL	Subcutaneous
OPV booster (Oral)	16-24 months	2 drops	Oral
JE -2 Left Upper arm (live attenuated vaccine) Anterolateral aspect of mid-thigh (killed vaccine)	16-24 months	0.5 mL	Subcutaneous
Vitamin A (second to ninth dose) (Oral)	16-18 months then one dose every 6 months up to the age of 5 years	2 mL (2 lakh IU)	Oral
DPT booster -2 (Upper arm)	5-6 years	0.5 mL	Intramuscular
Td (Upper arm)	10 and 16 years	0.5 mL	Intramuscular
FOR PREGNANT MOTHER			
Tetanus and adult diphtheria (Td)-1 (Upper arm)	Early in pregnancy	0.5 mL	Intramuscular
Td-2 (Upper arm)	4 weeks after Td-1	0.5 mL	Intramuscular
Td booster (Upper arm)	One dose - If received 2TT/Td doses in a pregnancy within the last 3 years	0.5 mL	Intramuscular

Note:
- JE Vaccine is introduced in select endemic districts after the campaign.
- The 2nd to 9th doses of vitamin A can be administered in 1 to 5 year old children during biannual rounds, in collaboration with ICDS.

IAP Immunization Schedule

Table 45.3 gives IAP immunization Schedule (2020–2021).

The following are the key updates and major changes in IAP Immunization (2020–2021):

- A booster of the inactivated polio vaccine (IPV) is recommended at 4–6 years, importance of IPV in the immunization schedule is reemphasized.
- All children older than 6 months of age are recommended to receive a uniform dose of 15 mg (0.5 mL) of inactivated influenza Vaccine.
- The second dose of varicella vaccine should be preferably administered 3–6 months after the first dose.

Introduction of New Vaccines,they are as follows:

- Tetraxim - DTaP/IPV combination vaccine.
- Menveo - Quadrivalent conjugate meningococcal vaccine.
- Twinrab - Monoclonal antibody cocktail for post exposure prophylaxis of rabies.
- Typhibev - Conjugate (CRM197) typhoid vaccine.
- Pneumosil - 10-valent pneumococcal conjugate vaccine.

The following are the IAP-ACVIP recommendations on newer vaccines:

- Approves the use of Menveo (quadrivalent conjugate meningococcal vaccine) vaccine in the age group of 2–55 years, also reiterates the use of this vaccine only in special situations.
- Approves the use of single dose of Typhibev (conjugate CRM197 typhoid vaccine) vaccine for children older than 6 months to 45 years of age. There is no recommendation for a booster dose.
- Recommends the use of rabies monoclonal antibodies (mAbs) over rabies immunoglobulins (RIGs) in the management of category III bites. For the post exposure management of suspected rabies exposure, both human monoclonal rabies antibody (Rabishield) and murine cocktail monoclonal rabies antibodies (Twinrab) are approved and are available in India.

TABLE 45.3	IAP (Indian Academy of Pediatrics) Immunization Schedule	
Age (completed weeks/months/years.)	**Vaccine**	**Key points**
Birth	BCG OPV Hepatitis B-1	BCG: Before discharge OPV: As soon as possible after birth Hepatitis B should be administered within 24 hours of birth
6 weeks	DTwP/DTaP-1 IPV-1 Hib-1 Hepatitis B-2 Rotavirus-1 PCV-1	DTwP or DTaP may be administered in primary immunization IPV: 6, 10, 14 weeks is the recommended schedule; if IPV, as part of a hexavalent combination vaccine, is unaffordable, the infant should be sent to a government facility for primary immunization as per National Immunization schedule
10 weeks	DTwP/DTaP-2 IPV-2 Hib-2 Hepatitis B-3 Rotavirus-2 PCV-2	RVI: 2-dose schedule; all other rotavirus brands: 3-dose schedule
14 weeks	DTwP/DTaP-3 IPV-3 Hib-3 Hepatitis B-4 Rotavirus-3 PCV-3	An additional fourth dose of hepatitis B vaccine is safe and is permitted as a component of a combination vaccine
6 months	Influenza (IIV)-1	Uniform dose of 0.5 mL for DCGI-approved brands
7 months	Influenza (IIV)-2	To be repeated every year, in pre-monsoon period, till 5 years of age
6-9 months	Typhoid conjugate vaccine	As of available data, there is no recommendation for a booster dose
9 months	MMR-1	
12 months	Hepatitis A	Single dose for live attenuated vaccine
15 months	MMR -2 Varicella -1 PCV booster	
16–18 months	DTwP/DTaP-B1 Hib-B1 IPV-B1	
18–19 months	Hepatitis A-2 Varicella	Only for inactivated hepatitis A vaccine
4–6 years	DTwP/DTaP-B2 IPV-B2 MMR-3	
10–12 years	Tdap HPV (Human Papillomavirus vaccine)	Tdap is to be administered even if it has been administered earlier (as DTP-B2) HPV: 2 doses at 6-month interval between 9 and 14 years; 3 doses: For 15 years and older or immunocompromised of any age (0, 1, 6 months for HPV-2 and 0, 2, 6 months for HPV-4)

- Approves the use of Tetraxim (DTaP/IPV combination vaccine) for the second booster of DPT/IPV at 4–6 years of age.
- Approves the use of Pneumosil (10 valent pneumococcal conjugate vaccine) till 2 years of age in a 3+1 schedule, with the booster administered between 12 and 18 months. Due to the absence of studies in the age group of 2–5 years, the ACVIP does not presently recommend the use of Pneumosil beyond 2 years of age.

The following are the IAP-recommended vaccines for high-risk children:

1. Meningococcal vaccine
2. Japanese encephalitis (JE) vaccines
3. Oral cholera vaccine
4. Rabies vaccine
5. Yellow fever vaccine
6. Pneumococcal polysaccharide vaccine (PPSV-23)

High-Risk Conditions are congenital or acquired immunodeficiency (including HIV infection, immunosuppressive therapy, radiation), Chronic cardiac conditions, Chronic pulmonary conditions (including asthma if treated with prolonged high-dose oral corticosteroids), chronic systemic diseases such as Renal (including nephrotic syndrome), hematological, hepatic diseases, diabetes mellitus, functional/anatomic asplenia/hyposplenia, cerebrospinal fluid leaks, cochlear implants; for pneumococcal infections.

Specific High-Risk Groups are children having pets in home (Rabies vaccine), children in JE endemic areas (Japanese encephalitis vaccine), children in areas with disease outbreaks (Oral cholera vaccine) and for travelers (Rabies vaccine, meningococcal vaccine, yellow fever vaccine).

Individual Vaccine Dose and Its Schedule

Table 45.4 gives individual vaccine, dose, and its schedule.

TABLE 45.4	Vaccine Dose and Its Schedule					
Vaccine	Dose	Route of Administration	Schedule	Minimum Age	Maximum Age (Catch-Up)	Comment
BCG	0.1 mL	Intradermal	Single dose at birth	Birth	5 years	Contraindicated in cell-mediated immune deficiency
OPV	2 drops	Oral	Birth During pulse polio immunization till 5 years age During ring immunization	Birth	4–6 years	Irrespective of age and vaccination, travelers should receive one dose; valid for 1 year
IPV	0.5 mL	Intramuscular (i.m)/sub-cutaneous (s.c) in thigh or deltoid	• 6, 10, 14 weeks • 15−18 months • 4−6 years	6 weeks	4–6 years	Intradermal (Id) schedule 6 and 14 weeks followed in National Immunization Schedule Used for polio switch
Hepatitis B	0.5 mL: Younger than 18 years	I.m.	Birth, 6, 10, 14	Birth	–	Preterm baby weighing <2 kg even if receiving vaccine and immunoglobulin (IG) in HbsAg-positive mothers, three separate doses of vaccine should be given
	1 mL: Older than 18 years		Adult: 0, 1, and 6 months			
DaPT/DwPT	0.5 mL	I.m. thigh/deltoid	• 6, 10, 14 weeks • 18 months • 5 years	6 weeks	7 years	Tdap and Td are used in children older than 7 years and in pregnancy
PCV	0.5 mL	I.m.	6, 10, 14 weeks 15–18 months Younger than 6 months: 3 doses + 1 booster 6–12 months: 2 doses + 1 booster 1–2 years: 2 dose (8 weeks apart, no booster) After 2 years: PCV-13 − single dose PCV-10 − 2 doses (8 weeks apart)	6 weeks	–	Newer recommendation: Pnuemosil (PCV-10) till 2 years (3 + 1 schedule) Preferred: PCV-13 > PCV-10 > PPSV is the order of preference in immunization
PPSV	0.5 mL	S.c.	Single dose; booster 3–5 years later	2 years	–	Not used in healthy individuals; only in high-risk groups
Hib	0.5 mL	I.m.	6, 10, 14 weeks, 15–18 months	6 weeks	5 years	

TABLE 45.4 Vaccine Dose and Its Schedule—cont'd

Vaccine	Dose	Route of Administration	Schedule	Minimum Age	Maximum Age (Catch-Up)	Comment
Rotavirus	1 mL	Oral	6, 10, 14 weeks	6 weeks, first dose not after 15 weeks	8 months	Theoretical risk of intussusception after 8 months
MMR	0.5 mL	S.c.	3 doses: 9 months; 15–18 months; And 5 years	9 months	4–6 years	Standalone measles can be given in epidemics in children older than 6 months but the dose is not considered
Hepatitis A a. Inactivated b. Live attenuated	0.5 mL 0.5 mL	I.m. (inactivated) S.c. (live attenuated)	2 doses at 12 months and 18–24 months Single dose	1 year	18 years	I.m. Ig is given postexposure in children younger than 1 year and adults older than 40 years in immunocompromised and chronic liver disease patients
Varicella	0.5 mL	S.c.	First dose: 15–18 months Second dose: 3–6 months after the first dose	15 months	18 years	• Postexposure 1–12 years – 2 doses, 3 months apart After 12 years – 2 doses, 4 weeks apart • Postexposure vaccine administered: <3 days – 90% efficacy • <5 days – 70% efficacy • Provides 100% protection against severe varicella • Contraindicated in – immunocompromised status, neonates, and pregnancy; in these conditions, VZIG can be given which has an efficacy for 3 weeks
Typhoid (Typbar TCV)	0.5 mL (singles dose)	I.m.	6–9 months	6 months	18 years	No recommendation of booster dose
Typhibev (Biological E vaccine – CRM197): Newer recommendation (typhoid conjugate vaccine)	0.5 mL (single dose)	I.m.	>6 months	6 months	45 years	No booster
Influenza a. TIV (inactivated) b. Live attenuated influenza vaccine (LAIV)	Older than 6 months: 0.5 mL	I.m. Intranasal	Younger than 3 years – 2 doses, 4 weeks apart Older than 3 years – single dose Single dose	6 months 2 years	 49 years	Annual revaccination required
JE (JEEV)	1–3 years: 0.25 mL (3 µg)	Inactivated cell culture	2 doses, 4 weeks apart: 0 and 28 days	1 year	15–18 years	Mandatory for travelers to sub-Saharan Africa
JE (live attenuated): SA 14-14-2	Older than 3 years: 0.5 mL (intramuscular); 0.5 mL (subcutaneous)	Live attenuated	2 doses: 9 months along with measles and second dose 16–18 months with DPT booster	9 months	15–18 years	

Continued

TABLE 45.4	Vaccine Dose and Its Schedule—Cont'd						
Vaccine	Dose	Route of Administration	Schedule	Minimum Age	Maximum Age (Catch-Up)	Comment	
Meningococcal: Menveo – quadrivalent conjugate vaccine (approved in 2020–2021)	0.5 mL	S.c.	Single dose; revaccinate every 10 years	2 years	55 years	High-risk patients: Travelers to Hajj pilgrimage	
Human Papillomavirus (HPV) Vaccine	0.5 mL	S.c.	HPV-2: 9, 14 years: 2 doses, 6 months apart HPV-2: 15, 18 years: 3 doses, 0, 1, 6 months HPV-4: 9–14 years – 2 doses, 6 months apart 15–18 years: 3 doses at 0, 2, and 6 months	9 years for girls	45 years	Male vaccination is currently not recommended	

Rabies Vaccines and Immunoglobulins: Summary of WHO 2018 Updates

VACCINE SCHEDULE

- Post-exposure prophylaxis (PEP) for rabies-exposed individuals of all ages and who were not subject to previous pre-exposure prophylaxis (PrEP) or PEP
- Two-site I.d. vaccine administrations on days 0, 3, and 7 or
- One-site i.m. vaccine administration on days 0, 3, 7 and the fourth dose between days 14 and 28 or
- Two-site i.m. vaccine administration on days 0 and one-site i.m. administration on days 7 and 21.

CATEGORY III DOG BITE

- For individuals with category III exposures, Rabies Immunoglobulin (RIG) is indicated.
- RIG provides passive immunization and is administered only once as soon as possible after the initiation of PEP and not beyond day 7 after the first dose of vaccine.
- The maximum dose is 20 IU Human Rabies Immunoglobulin (hRIG) and 40 IU Equine Rabies Immunoglobulin (eRIG) per kg body weight. There is no minimum dose.
- Infiltrate as much as possible into the wound; the remainder of the calculated dose of RIG does not need to be injected i.m. at a distance from the wound but can be fractionated into smaller, individual syringes to be used for other patients, aseptic retention given
- If Rabies Immunoglobulin is not available, thorough, prompt wound washing, together with immediate administration of the first vaccine dose, followed by a complete course of rabies vaccine, is highly effective in preventing rabies.
- Monoclonal Rabies Immunoglobulin: Human monoclonal antibody (Rabishield) – 3.33 IU/kg.
- Murine cocktail monoclonal antibodies (Twinrab): 40 IU/ kg (approved in 2020–2021) for postexposure prophylaxis.

POST-EXPOSURE PROPHYLAXIS FOR PREVIOUSLY IMMUNIZED INDIVIDUALS

- Post-exposure prophylaxis for rabies-exposed individuals who can document previous PrEP or PEP
- No Rabies Immunoglobulin is indicated
- One-site i.d. vaccine administration on days 0 and 3 or
- Four-site i.d. vaccine administration (equally distributed over the left and right deltoids, thigh, or suprascapular areas) only on day 0 or
- One-site i.m. vaccine administrations on days 0 and 3
- Repeat exposure occurs (i.e., re-exposure within 3 months of completion of PEP), only wound treatment is required, neither vaccine nor Rabies Immunoglobulin are needed.

PRE-EXPOSURE PROPHYLAXIS

- PrEP makes administration of Rabies Immunoglobulin unnecessary after a bite.
- Rabies vaccination likely provides lifetime protection, with vaccine booster in case of an exposure
- Two-site i.d. vaccine administrations on days 0 and 7
- One-site i.m. vaccine administrations on days 0 and 7

SITE OF INJECTION

Vaccine

- For adults, the vaccine should always be administered in the deltoid area of the arm.
- For young children (aged < 2 years), the anterolateral area of the thigh is recommended.
  Source: https://www.who.int/immunization/policy/position_papers/pp_rabies_summary_2018.pdf
  Table 45.5 gives rabies immunization.

Vaccines in Special Situations

IMMUNOCOMPROMISED CHILDREN

The main challenges with these children are as follows:
- They are more prone to infections

TABLE 45.5	**Rabies Immunization**			
Post-exposure prophylaxis Recommendations Based on Category of Exposure	**Category I Exposure**	**Category II Exposure**	**Category III Exposure**	

Immunologically naive individuals of all age groups	Wash exposed skin surfaces; no Post-exposure prophylaxis required	Wound washing followed by immediate vaccination
		Intradermal schedule: 2-sites i.d. on days 0, 3, and 7
		OR
		Intramuscular schedule:
		  a. 1-site i.m. on days 0, 3, 7 and between days 14 and 28
		  b. 2-site i.m. on day 0 and 1-site i.m. on days 7, 21–28
		Rabies Immunoglobulin is not indicated
			Wound washing followed by immediate vaccination
			Intradermal schedule: 2-site i.d. on days 0, 3, and 76
			OR
			Intramuscular schedule:
			  a. 1-site i.m. on days 0, 3, 7 and between days 14 and 28
			OR
			  b. 2-site i.m. on day 0 and 1-site i.m. on days 7, 21–28
			Rabies Immunoglobulin administration is recommended	

Previously immunized individuals of all age groups	Wash exposed skin surfaces; no Post-exposure prophylaxis required	Wound washing and immediate vaccination:
		Intradermal schedule: 1-site i.d. on days 0 and 3
		OR
		Intramuscular schedule:
		  a. 4-site i.d. on day 0
		OR
		  b. 1-site i.m. on days 0 and 3
		Rabies Immunoglobulin is not indicated
			Wound washing and immediate vaccination:
			1-site i.d. on days 0 and 3
			OR
			Intramuscular schedule:
			  a. 4-site i.d. on day 0
			OR
			  b. 1-site i.m. on days 0 and 3
			Rabies Immunoglobulin is not indicated	

Source: https://www.who.int/immunization/policy/position_papers/pp_rabies_summary_2018.pdf

- Immunization will be less effective
- Risk of adverse effects is more.
- We should always weigh the risk-to-benefit ratio before administering vaccines in this group.

Principles of Immunization in Immunocompromised Patients

- All inactivated vaccines can be given.
- All live vaccines are contraindicated in severe immunodeficiency but can be given in mild-to-moderate immunodeficiency if benefits outweigh risks.
- Antibody titers should be checked postimmunization.
- All household contacts should be completely immunized.
- Avoid immunization with transmissible vaccines such as OPV.

HIV

- Asymptomatic patients: All live vaccines can be given, except BCG and OPV
- Symptomatic patients: All live vaccines are contraindicated. MMR and varicella vaccines can be given if CD4 count is >15% of normal.
- Yellow fever vaccine is contraindicated in both of the above-mentioned cases.

Immune-Suppressive Therapy

A. **Systemic steroids**
   - More than 1 mg/kg/day – all live vaccines are contraindicated
   - Less than 1 mg/kg/day – routine immunization
B. **Topical steroids**
   - Routine immunization
   - Other immunosuppressive drugs – all live vaccines are contraindicated

C. **Chemotherapy and radiotherapy**
   - Live vaccines can be given 3 months after stopping chemotherapy or radiotherapy.
   - Inactivated vaccines can be given during therapy.

Hematological Malignancies/Solid Tumors

- Yearly influenza (except induction phase of Acute lymphoblastic leukemia (ALL))
- Pneumococcal conjugate vaccine (PCV) to all newly diagnosed patients

Hematopoietic Stem Cell Transplantation (HSCT) Recipients

- All vaccines to be given after 6 months of completion of therapy
- Inactivated polio vaccine (IPV): Three doses
- PCV: Three doses, fourth dose if there is Graft versus host disease (GvHD)
- Human Papillomavirus (HPV) Vaccine: Three doses in adolescents
- Meningococcal conjugate vaccine (MCV): Two doses in endemic areas
- Pentavalent: Three doses if anti-HbS titer is <10 IU/mL
- MMR and varicella pneumococcal polysaccharide vaccine (PPSV): 1 year later

No live vaccines are given when there is active Graft versus host disease (GVHD).

Solid Organ Transplantation

- All live vaccines should be given 2 weeks prior to the transplant.
- No live vaccine should be given post-transplantation.
- Inactivated vaccines can be given 1–3 months after the transplant.

Splenectomy

- Emergency – 2 weeks after the procedure
- Elective – 2 weeks prior to the procedure
- Vaccines indicated – PCV, Meningococcal conjugate vaccine (MCV), Hib, typhoid, influenza in addition to routine schedule

Primary Immunodeficiency

- B cell and T cell – all live vaccines are contraindicated
- Chronic granulomatous disease (CGD) – live bacterial vaccines are contraindicated
- Complement deficiency – no contraindication

PREGNANCY

- **Tdap** preferably in 26–36 weeks of pregnancy to decrease the incidence of pertussis in the newborn
- **All** live vaccines (yellow fever, MMR, and varicella) are contraindicated – pregnancy should not occur until 4 weeks after receiving the live vaccines

LACTATION

- All live vaccines can be given except yellow fever vaccine. If it is absolutely necessary, yellow fever vaccine can be given, but breastfeeding should be withheld for 10 days following vaccination during postvaccine viremia. In this time, there is chance of virus being excreted in breast milk and causing meningoencephalitis in the newborn infant.

PRETERM LOW BIRTH WEIGHT NEWBORN

- If the mother is HBsAg-positive, the infant should receive vaccine and Hepatitis B immune globulin (HBIg) within 12 hours of birth. After that, three doses at 1, 2, and 6 months are given.
- In infants weighing <2 kg, if status of the mother is not known, they also should be given both vaccine and immunoglobulin.
- All vaccines can be given in preterm low birth weight infants. But hepatitis B vaccine is administered once the infant weighs >2 kg or there is consistent weight gain before discharge.

VACCINES FOR TRAVELERS

Routine Vaccination

DPT (Diphtheria, pertussis, tetanus), hepatitis B, Hib, MMR (Measles, Mumps, rubella), varicella, seasonal influenza, rotavirus, tuberculosis, pnuemococcal vaccine.

Selective Use for Travelers

Few vaccines are must while traveling to endemic areas such as Japanese encephalitis, tick borne encephalitis, meningococcal disease, yellow fever, rabies, cholera, hepatitis A and typhoid fever.

VACCINES FOR ADOLESCENTS

IAP-recommended vaccines for adolescents (10-18 years) are as follows:

- Tdap/Td is given at 10 years of age. Tdap is preferred to Td, followed by repeat dose of Td every 10 years. Tdap to be used once only.
- Human papillomavirus (HPV) vaccine is given only to females aged 10-12 years old.
- It is given in three doses at 0, 1, or 2 (depending on the vaccine used) and 6 months.

Catch-Up Immunization for Adolescents

Catch-Up immunization for adolescents are as follows:

- 2 doses of MMR vaccine at 4–8 weeks interval upto 18 years. one dose is enough, if there is a history of previous immunization with 1 dose of MMR vaccine.
- 3 doses of Hepatitis B vaccine at 0, 1, and 6 months.
- 2 doses of Hepatitis A vaccine at 0 and 6 months. check for anti-HAV prior to vaccination, IgG may be cost-effective. Combination of hepatitis B and hepatitis A may be used in 0, 1, 6 schedule.
- 1 dose of Typhoid vaccine every 3 years. A minimum interval of 3 years should be observed between 2 doses of typhoid vaccine.
- 2 doses of Varicella vaccine in 4–8 weeks interval.

Immunization for Adolescents in Special Situations

Immunization for adolescents in special situations are as follows:

- 1 dose of Influenza vaccine every year.
- Japanese encephalitis vaccine up to 15 years, only in endemic area as catch up immunization.
- 2 doses of PPSV-23 vaccine at an interval of 5 years apart. The maximum number of doses of PPSV-23 vaccine is two.
- Rabies vaccine is given intramuscularly at 0, 3, 7, 14, and 28 days, as soon as possible after exposure.

VACCINATION IN BLEEDING DISORDER

- **Vaccination can be scheduled after administration of clotting factors.**
- When available, subcutaneous route of immunization should be used. If i.m. injections cannot be avoided, they must be given with 23-G needle shortly after administration of clotting factors. The injection site should be compressed for 5–10 minutes with pressure without rubbing.
- Vaccines such as Hib, PCV, and IPV can be given by s.c. route.

VACCINATION IN ACUTE ILLNESS

- Minor illness – continue routine vaccination
- Moderate-to-severe illness – withhold vaccination until illness resolves because worsening can be wrongly attributed to vaccine than to the illness

VACCINATION AFTER IMMUNE PRODUCT ADMINISTRATION

- Blood and other immune products interfere with the production of antibodies to live vaccines, especially measles and varicella. These vaccines not given ≥3 months after the immune product.
- **Exceptions** to this include Live attenuated influenza vaccine (LAIV), Ty21, rotavirus, yellow fever, and zoster vaccines which are all live vaccines but can be given before, during, or after the immune product transfusions or injection.

Principles of Catch-Up Immunization

- Any number of live or inactivated vaccines can be given on the same day maintaining a gap of 5 cm between both vaccination sites if two live injectable vaccines are given in the same site.
- Inactivated vaccines can be given anytime along with any other vaccine.
- Two live injectable vaccines are not given on the same day. A gap of 4 weeks should be present in between two live vaccines, e.g., MMR and varicella, yellow fever and Live attenuated influenza vaccine (LAIV).
- No gap is required in case of OPV, Ty21, and rotavirus vaccines.
- All catch-up vaccines should be given in the minimum recommended interval to entail early immunity.

Adverse Events Following Immunization (AEFI)

DEFINITION

It is defined as any untoward event following vaccination which does not necessarily have a causal relationship with usage of vaccine. The event can be a symptom, sign, or a laboratory finding.

TYPES

- Vaccine product related – due to inherent property of vaccine, e.g., swelling following diphtheria, pertussis, and tetanus (DPT)
- Vaccine quality related – due to defective manufacturing, e.g., improper adjuvant/preservative
- Immunization error related – improper reconstitution/administration
- Immunization anxiety related –vasovagal syncope
- Coincidental event – caused by something other than the vaccine product, immunization error, or immunization anxiety. Example: Fever after vaccination (temporal association) and malarial parasite isolated from blood.

BASED ON SEVERITY

- **Serious AEFI**
  a. Causes hospitalisation, persistent or significant disability /incapacity, death
  b. Usually occurs in clusters
  c. Results birth defect or congenital anomaly
  d. Causes major concern to parents or community
- **Minor AEFI:**
  a. Systemic reactions which results in fever >38°C, irritability, and malaise
  b. Local reactions causing pain, redness and swelling.
- **Severe AEFI:** Increased intensity and severity of minor AEFI results in Severe AEFI.

Table 45.6 shows adverse reaction following specific vaccine administration.

NOTIFICATION OF ADVERSE EVENTS FOLLOWING IMMUNIZATION (AEFI)

- Any event resulting in death or hospitalization

TABLE 45.6	Adverse Reaction Following Specific Vaccine Administration	
Vaccine	**Reaction**	**Time of Onset Since Vaccination**
BCG	Lymphadenitis	2–6 months
	Disseminated BCG	1–12 months
OPV	Vaccine-associated paralytic poliomyelitis (VAPP)	0–30 days
MMR	Febrile seizures, thrombocytopenia	5–12 days 4–30 days
DPT	Incessant cry, seizures, hypotonic hyporesponsive event	0–48 h 0–24 h 0–24 h
Tetanus	Brachial neuritis, sterile abscess	2–28 days 1–6 weeks
JE	Neurological event	0–2 weeks

- Significant unexplained event occurring within 30 days
- AEFI caused by immunization error
- Events of severe parental or community concern

There are two types of reporting formats:
- Case reporting form (CRF)
- Case investigating form (CIF) – preliminary and final

Vaccine Storage

COLD CHAIN

Definition

It is a system of storing and transporting vaccines from point of manufacture to the point of administration in 2–8°C.

Equipment Used for Cold Chain

- Walk-in cold rooms and freezer rooms
- Freezers
- Refrigerators
- Cold boxes
- Refrigerated trucks for transportation
- Vaccine carriers

Recommended Temperature

- Frozen vaccines (varicella, OPV MMRV): In freezer, between −50°C and −15°C
- All other routinely recommended vaccines in refrigerator: Between **2°C** and **8°C**
- Desired average refrigerator vaccine storage temperature is **5°C**.
  Deep freezer - only for Ice packs (-16 degree celsius to -20 degree celsius)
  ILR (Ice Lined Refrigerator) - vaccine storage (+2 to +8 degree celsius)

HEAT-SENSITIVE VACCINES

BCG, OPV, MMR, and Japanese encephalitis (JE)

LIGHT-SENSITIVE VACCINES

BCG and MMR – comes in amber-colored bottles

FREEZE-SENSITIVE VACCINES

DPT, TT, Td, hepatitis B, hepatitis A, pentavalent

STORAGE PROTOCOL IN DOMESTIC FRIDGE

- Freezer compartment — ice cubes, OPV vials
- Main compartment:
  Top — BCG and measles vaccines
  Middle — DTP/DT/TT, typhoid, hepatitis A, hepatitis B, and varicella vaccines
  Lower — diluent
- Door — nothing
- Dial thermometer — top shelf

OPEN VIAL POLICY (OVP) OR MULTI-DOSE VIAL POLICY (MDVP)

To reduce the vaccine wastage as well as Government healthcare costs for immunization, OVP was introduced. Multi-dose vials of OPV, DPT, TT , DT, hepatitis B can be used in subsequent immunization sessions for up to maximum of 4 weeks, if appropriate cold chains are met, vaccine vial monitor (VVM) has not reached the discard point. Open vials of Measles and BCG (freeze dried formulations) as they do not contain preservative after being reconstituted with a diluent must be discarded at the end of each immunization session (maximum of 4-6 hours).

POWER FAILURE

- In case of power failure for <4 hours, the refrigerator doors to be kept closed.
- If back up generator is not available during power failures for >4 hours, vaccine is stored in a cooler, with conditioned ice packs or gel packs.
- If there is no back up facility, identify another available unit nearby site.

46

Drugs

IP and BP

IP stands for Indian Pharmacopoeia, on the basis of which the products are prepared.

BP stands for British Pharmacopoeia.

Common drugs used in Pediatrics

Table 46.1 to Table 46.6 gives common drugs and infusions used in pediatrics and newborn.

TABLE 46.1	Drugs in Pediatrics				
Name of the Drug	Route of Administration	Mechanism of Action	Indication	Adverse Effects	Contraindication
Adrenaline	Intravenous (i.v.)/Intramuscular (i.m.)/nasal/subcutaneous (s.c.)	α_1, α_2, β_1, β_2 and weak β_3 action	1. Bronchial asthma – 1:10,000 (0.1 ml/kg s.c.) 2. Anaphylactic shock – 1:1000 (0.01 mL/kg i.m.) 3. Cardiac arrest – 1:10,000 (0.1 mL/kg i.v.) 4. With local anesthesia 5. Inotrope (0.1–1 mic/kg/min) 6. Bronchiolitis – 1:1000 (0.1 mL/kg nebulization)	Restlessness, palpitation, anxiety, pallor	1. Hypertension 2. Hyperthyroid 3. Angina 4. Children receiving halothane or β-blocker
Noradrenaline	I.v. (action declines after 5 min)	α_1, α_2, β_1, β_3 but no action on β_2 (hence decreases heart rate)	Septic shock	Hypertension, bradycardia, renal failure, skin necrosis due to infiltration	Do not mix with sodium bicarbonate
Dopamine	I.v.	α_1, α_2, D_1, D_2 (no action on β_2)	Low dose: <5 mic/kg/min – dilates renal and mesenteric vessels Moderate dose: 5–15 mic/kg/min – positive inotropic effects Large dose: >15 mic/kg/min – vasoconstriction Used in 1. Distributive shock with normal BP 2. Cardiogenic shock 3. Raised Intracranial Pressure	Palpitations, SVT (Supraventricular Tachycardia), VT (Ventricular Tachycardia), hypertension	
Dobutamine	I.v.	β_1 agonist, α-blocker	Increases cardiac output	Tachyarrhythmias, hypotension, thrombocytopenia	Low BP
Milrinone	I.v.	β_1, $\beta_2 >> \alpha 1$ No α_2 action 5–10 μg/kg/min	1. Compensated shock 2. Myocarditis	Increased myocardial oxygen demand	
Vasopressin	I.v.	V1α receptor 0.0005–0.001 units/kg/min	Should only be used if adequate fluids and noradrenaline at maximum dose have failed in improving MAPS in vasodilatory shock	Digital ischemia Skin necrosis	
Salbutamol	Oral, inhalational	β_1	Asthma Hyperkalemia	Tremors, tachycardia Ventilation–perfusion mismatch Hypokalemia	
Ipravent	Inhalational	M_3 Selectively acts on bronchial muscles; does not depress mucociliary function Peak action – 60–90 min	Acute severe asthma	Dryness of mouth, cough, bad taste, nervousness	

Continued

TABLE 46.1	Drugs in Pediatrics—cont'd				
Name of the Drug	Route of Administration	Mechanism of Action	Indication	Adverse Effects	Contraindication
Hydrocortisone	I.v.	Glucocorticoids and mineralocorticoids action. Major endogenous glucocorticoids	1. Acute adrenal insufficiency 2. Addison disease 3. Anti-inflammatory use in connective tissue disorder 4. Anti-allergic 5. Immunosuppressive uses 6. Anticancer 7. Refractory shock	Peptic ulcer Osteoporosis Cataract Osteoporosis Diabetes mellitus Impaired healing	Renal failure Congestive Heart Failure (CHF) Hyperglycemia Herpesvirus infection Fungal infections
Dexamethasone	I.v./i.m./p.o.	Maximum glucocorticoid activity	1. Croup 2. Meningitis 3. Postextubation 4. Vasogenic cerebral edema 5. Antenatal steroid therapy 6. Antenatally to mother if there is risk of CAH (Congenital Adrenal Hyperplasia) to fetus 7. Allergic reactions 8. Neurocysticercosis/ocular cysticercosis	Peptic ulcer Osteoporosis Cataract Osteoporosis Diabetes mellitus Impaired healing	Renal failure CHF Hyperglycemia Herpesvirus infection Fungal infections
Prednisone	per oral (p.o.)	Maximum both glucocorticoid versus mineralocorticoid	1. Mild croup 2. Acute exacerbation of asthma 3. Tuberculous meningitis, pericardial Tuberculosis (TB), endobronchial TB, miliary TB 4. Bell palsy 5. Duchenne/Becker muscular dystrophy 6. Nephrotic syndrome 7. ITP (Immune Thrombocytopenia), immune hemolytic anemia	Peptic ulcer Osteoporosis Cataract Osteoporosis Diabetes mellitus Impaired healing	Renal failure CHF Hyperglycemia Herpesvirus infection Fungal infections
Calcium gluconate	Slow i.v. under cardiac monitoring	0.5–1 mL/kg 1 mL = 9.8 mg Given with 5% dextrose	1. Hypocalcemia 2. Hyperkalemia 3. Hypermagnesium 4. Calcium channel blocker overdose	Necrosis due to extravasation Bradycardia Hypercalcemia	Bradycardia Should not be mixed with sodium bicarbonate
Potassium chloride	Oral (15 mL = 20 mEq) I.v. (1 mL = 2 mEq)	Potassium channel	1. Hypokalemia 2. DKA (Diabetic Ketoacidosis) 3. Renal Tubular Acidosis 4. Batter syndrome 5. Periodic paralysis	Hyperkalemia Cardiac arrythmia	
Magnesium sulfate	I.v.	Magnesium receptors	1. Hypomagnesemia 2. Acute nephritis 3. Torsades de pointes 4. Bronchospasm (asthma)	1. Respiratory depression 2. Circulatory collapse 3. Pulmonary edema 4. Loss of reflex 5. Drowsiness	Hypercalcemia Cardiac arrest Hypersensitivity
N-acetyl cysteine	Oral I.v.	Increases the levels of glutathione	1. Paracetamol overdose 2. Mucolytic in respiratory infections, especially cystic fibrosis 3. Radiocontrast-induced renal injury	1. Anaphylaxis 2. Vomiting	
Morphine	I.v.	Acts on MU receptors 0.05–0.1 mg/kg	1. Pain 2. Cyanotic spell 3. Persistent Pulmonary Hypertension in the Neonate	Respiratory depression	
Adenosine	I.v.	Prevents presynaptic vesicle release and postsynaptic stabilization of magnesium on N-methyl-D-aspartate receptor 0.1 mg/kg: Increase dose every 2 min by 0.05 mg/kg to max 1.2 mg Rapid saline push	Supraventricular tachycardia	Flushing Respiratory failure Cardiac arrest	Heart block Sick sinus syndrome

TABLE 46.2 Infusions in Pediatrics

Drug	Dosage	Diluent	Infusion Rate
Dopamine (1 mL = 40 mg)	6 × body weight (mL) in 50 mL NS (Normal Saline)	NS/5% D (Dextrose)	5 mL/h = 10 micrograms/kg/min Maximum = 20 micrograms/kg/min
Dobutamine (1 mL = 50 mg)	6 × body weight (mL) in 50 mL NS	NS	5 mL/h = 10 micrograms/kg/min Maximum = 20 micrograms/kg/min
Adrenaline (1 mL = 1 mg)	0.3 mg × body weight (mL) in 50 mL NS	NS	1 mL/h = 0.1 micrograms/kg/min Usually start with 0.3 micrograms/kg/min
Noradrenaline (1 mL = 1 mg)	0.3 × body weight in 50 mL 5% D or 10% D	Only in dextrose fluid (5% D or 10% D)	1 mL/h = 0.1 micrograms/kg/min Usually start with 0.3 micrograms/kg/min
Midazolam (1 mL = 1 mg)	3 × body weight in 50 mL NS	NS	1 mL/h = 1 micrograms/kg/min

TABLE 46.3 Infusions in Newborn

Drug	Dilution	Diluent	Infusion Rate
Dopamine (1 mL = 40 mg)	1 mL in 39 mL NS	NS/5% D	0.6 × body weight = 10 micrograms/kg/min Maximum = 20 micrograms/kg/min
Dobutamine (1 mL = 50 mg)	0.8 mL in 39.2 mL NS	NS	0.6 × body weight = 10 micrograms/kg/min Maximum = 20 micrograms/kg/min
Adrenaline (1 mL = 1 mg)	0.3 mg × body weight (mL) in 50 mL NS	NS	1 mL/h = 0.1 micrograms/kg/min Usually start with 0.3 micrograms/kg/min
Noradrenaline (1 mL = 1 mg)	0.3 × body weight in 50 mL 5% D or 10% D	Only in dextrose fluid (5% D or 10% D)	1 mL/h = 0.1 micrograms/kg/min Usually start with 0.3 micrograms/kg/min
Midazolam (1 mL = 1 mg)	3 × body weight in 50 mL NS	NS	1 mL/h = 1 micrograms/kg/min

TABLE 46.4 Role of Azithromycin in Pediatrics

Condition	Dose (in mg/kg/day)	Durations (in Days)
Enteric fever	10–20	7
Streptococcal pharyngitis	12 – in day 1 6 – from day 2 to day 5	5
Shigellosis	12 – in day 1 6 – from day 2 to day 5	5
Pertussis	0–6 months – 10 mg/kg/day >6 months – 10 mg/kg/day – day 1 5 mg/kg/day – day 2 to day 5	5
Mycoplasmosis	10 mg/kg/day – day 1 5 mg/kg/day – day 2 to day 5	5
Scrub typhus	10	3
Leptospirosis	10	3
Cholera	20	Single dose
Naegleria meningitis	20	14
MAC (Mycobacterium Avium Complex) prophylaxis in AIDS	20 mg/kg weekly Or 5 mg/kg/day daily	

TABLE 46.5 IVIG (Intravenous Immunoglobulin) in Pediatrics

Condition	Dose (g/kg/day)	Duration (in Days)
Neonatal jaundice due to immune hemolytic anemia	0.5–1	Over 6 hrs. doses can be can be repeated.
ITP	0.8–1	2
Primary immunodeficiency disease	0.4–0.8	Once in 30 days
Guillain–Barré syndrome	0.4	5
Acute transverse myelitis	0.4	5
Acute disseminated encephalomyelitis	0.4	5
Autoimmune encephalitis	0.4	5
Myasthenia gravis	0.4	5
West syndrome, Lennox–Gastaut, Landau–Kleffner syndrome	2 g/kg divided over 4 days followed by 1 g/kg monthly	
Postexposure prophylaxis for varicella	0.4	Single dose
Parvovirus-induced aplastic crisis	0.2 (Nelson) 0.4 (IAP)	5
Stevens–Johnson syndrome Toxic epidermal necrolysis	2	2
Kawasaki disease	2	10–12 h
Juvenile dermatomyositis	0.4	5

Other conditions where IVIG can be used are neonatal lupus, immune hemolytic anemia, opsoclonus myoclonus syndrome, and neuromyelitis optica.

TABLE 46.6   Antiepileptic Drugs

Drug	Administra-tion	Mechanism of Action	Adverse Effect
Lorazepam	I.v. 0.05−0.1 mg/kg (maximum 4 mg)	Postsynaptic GABA (Gamma-aminobutyric acid)-A ligand chloride channel	Hypotension Respiratory depression
Midazolam	I.v./i.m./PR (Per rectal) 0.05–0.3 mg/kg	Increase GABA action	Sedation Hypotension Bradycardia
Phenytoin	I.v./p.o. 15–20 mg/kg (maximum 1 g)	Prolongs in-active state of sodium channel	Tachyarrhythmia Dysarthria Ataxia Sedation Purple glove syndrome
Valproic acid	I.v./p.o. 15–20 mg/kg (maximum 25 mg/kg)	Prolongs in-active state of sodium channel Increases GABA action	Hypotension Arrhythmia Pancreatitis Hepatitis
Levetiracetam	I.v. 20–30 mg/kg (maximum 3 g)	Binds to Synaptic vesicle gly-coprotein 2A (SV2A) channel	Behavioral changes
Phenobarbitone	I.v. 15–20 mg/kg (maximum 1 g)	Increases GABA action	Respiratory depression Immunosuppres-sion Hypotension
Thiopentone	I.v. 2–4 mg//kg	Enhances the inhibi-tory action of GABA receptor	Sedation Hypotension Circulatory collapse

Diuretics in Children

1. Loop diuretics
   - Furosemide and bumetanide (most potent)
   - Blocks $Na^+ - K^+ - 2Cl^-$ channel in ascending loop of Henle
   - Potassium reabsorption is reduced – causing hypokalemia
   - Half-life – 12 hours
   - Uses:
     a. For diuresis
     b. Bronchopulmonary dysplasia
     c. Respiratory distress syndrome
     d. Congestive heart failure
     e. Systemic hypertension
     f. With indomethacin for Non-steroidal anti-inflammatory drugs-induced nephrotoxicity
   - Adverse effects – muscle cramps, hypokalemia
2. Thiazide diuretics
   - Blocks Na^+Cl^- in distal convoluted tubule
   - Moderately effective
   - Uses:
     a. Systemic hypertension – has it has mild carbonic anhydrase inhibitory activity so decreases periph-eral vascular resistance
     b. Diuresis
     c. Pulmonary edema
   - Adverse effects – hyperuricemia, cholestasis, hypokale-mia, muscsle cramps
3. Metolazone
   - Acts on both proximal and distal convoluted tubule
   - Blocks Na^+Cl^- channel
   - Ability to produce dieresis in advanced renal failure
   - Minimal potassium loss
4. Spironolactone – potassium-sparing diuretic
   - Inhibits action of aldosterone
   - Enhances potassium secretion and sodium reabsorp-tion of sodium in distal nephron
   - Uses:
     a. Diuresis in ascites, edema
     b. Systemic hypertension
     c. Precocious puberty
     d. Hyperaldosteronism
     e. Barter syndrome
     f. Alport syndrome
   - Adverse effects – hyperkalemia, abdomen pain, azotemia
5. Mannitol
   - Osmotic dieresis
   - Nonelectrolyte
   - Retains water isoosmotically in proximal tubule
   - Inhibits transport processes in thick ascending limb of loop of Henle
   - Expands extracellular volume
   - Uses:
     a. Cerebral edema
     b. Maintains urine output and urine flow in impend-ing renal failure
     c. Dialysis disequilibrium
   - Contraindicated in pulmonary edema, acute tubular ne-crosis, acute left ventricular failure, cerebral hemorrhage

47

Instruments

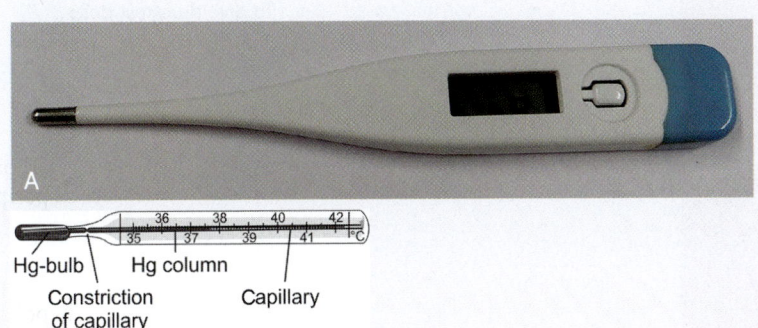

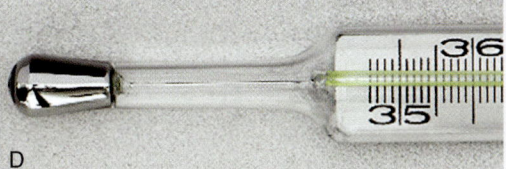

Hg-bulb   Hg column

Constriction   Capillary
of capillary

B

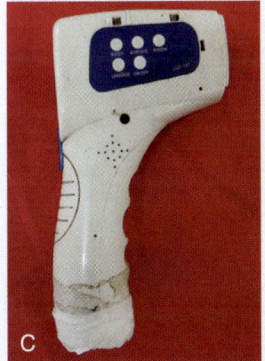

C

D

Fig. 47.1 (A) Digital thermometer. (B) Mercury thermometer. (C) Infrared thermometer. (D) Rectal thermometer. (*Source:* Reproduced from Anders Brahme. *Comprehensive Biomedical Physics*, Measurement of Temperatures of the Human Body, Figure 1, Oxford, Elsevier BV, 2015.)

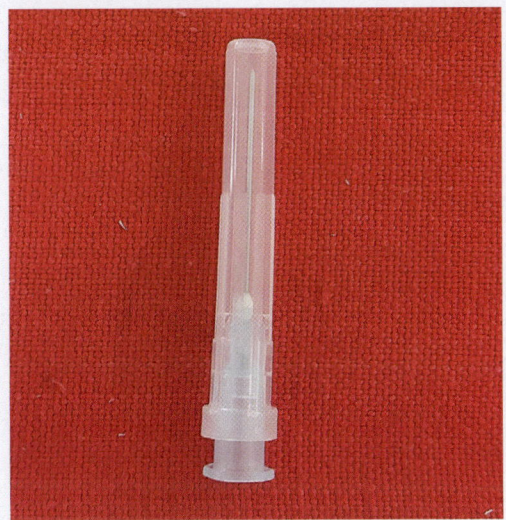

Fig. 47.2 Intramuscular needle.

Thermometer	Used to measure axillary and oral temperatures. Axillary < oral < rectal Rectal temperature >38°C or 100.4°F is defined as fever (Normal: 36.6−38°C or 97.9−100.4°F) Oral temperature + 0.5 = rectal temperature Axillary temperature + 1 = rectal temperature Mild hypothermia: 34−36°C Moderate hypothermia: <34°C (Conversion: Fahrenheit = 1.8 × °C + 32) Fig. 47.1A shows digital thermometer Fig. 47.1B shows mercury thermometers which can measure from 35°C to 42°C (94−108°F) Oral thermometer: Long slender bulb, with blue/green marking Fig. 47.1C shows infrared thermometer with more distance-to-spot ratio; more specific (distance-to-spot ratio is the ratio of distance to the measurement surface and the diameter of temperature measurement area) Fig. 47.1D shows rectal thermometer − lowest measurement 35−42°C (94°108°F) Rectal: Short stubby bulb, red marking
Intramuscular needles (Fig. 47.2)	• Give intra muscular (i.m) injections • Draw blood samples • Lumbar puncture in neonates Length 5/8 inch (deltoid) • 1 inch (anterolateral thigh): 22–25 G

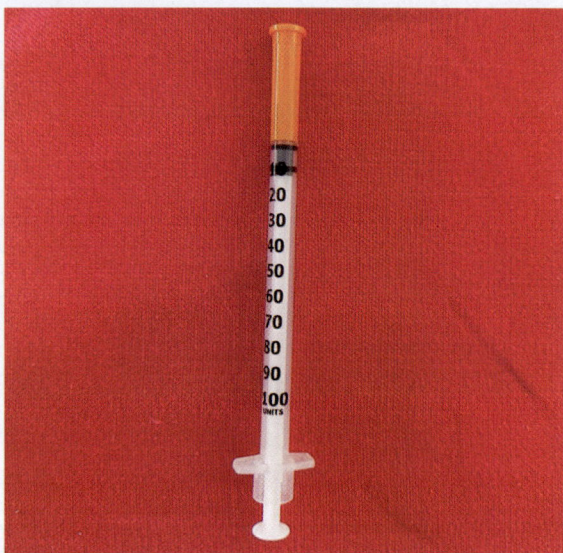

Fig. 47.3   Tuberculin syringe.

Tuberculin sy-ringe (Fig. 47.3)	To perform Mantoux testing; 0.1 mL of purified protein derivative (PPD) is injected intradermally in the forearm and the site is marked; induration of >10 mm is positive
	To administer insulin
	To administer BCG vaccine
	To give drug test dose

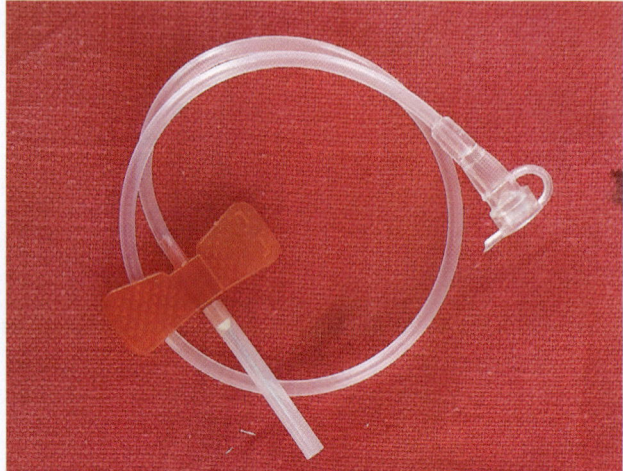

Fig. 47.4   Scalp vein.

Scalp vein set/ butterfly set (Fig. 47.4)	Plastic tubing, metallic needle
	Butterfly-shaped plastic holder
	For administering intravenous infusions such as clotting factors; to administer fluids for a short duration
	Less traumatic, less painful
	Disadvantage: Damages the endothelium
	Not used for thin tortuous veins

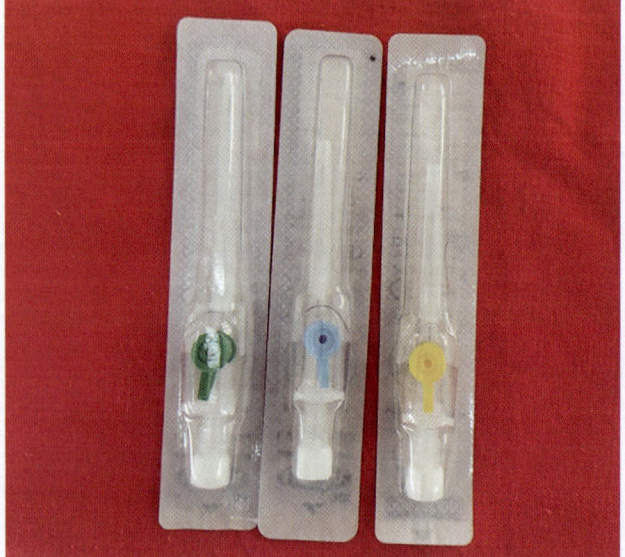

Fig. 47.5   Venflon.

Venflon (Fig. 47.5)	Used to secure a peripheral venous access
	To infuse fluids, boluses, drugs, inotropes, etc.
	Can be left in place for 7 days if maintained properly
	Orange – 14 G
	Grey – 16 G
	White – 17 G
	Green – 18 G
	Pink – 20 G
	Blue – 22 G
	Yellow – 24 G
	Violet – 26 G

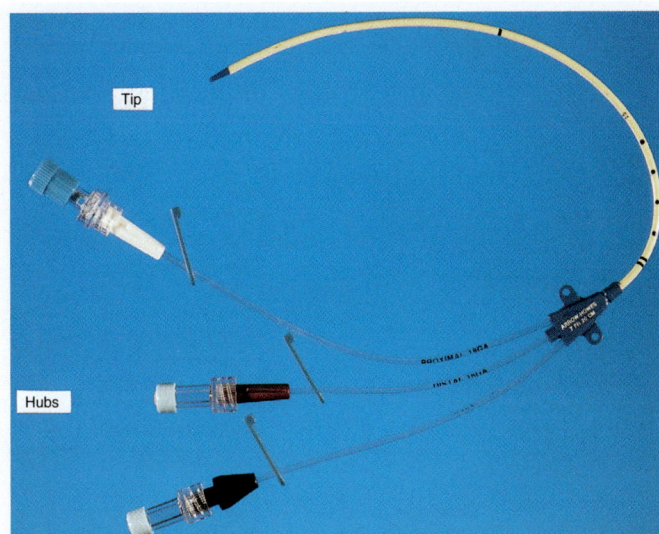

Fig. 47.6 Central vein catheter. (*Source:* Reproduced from Patricia Tille. *Bailey & Scott's Diagnostic Microbiology,* Fourteenth Edition, Bloodstream infections, Figure 67-2, St. Louis, Mosby, 2017.)

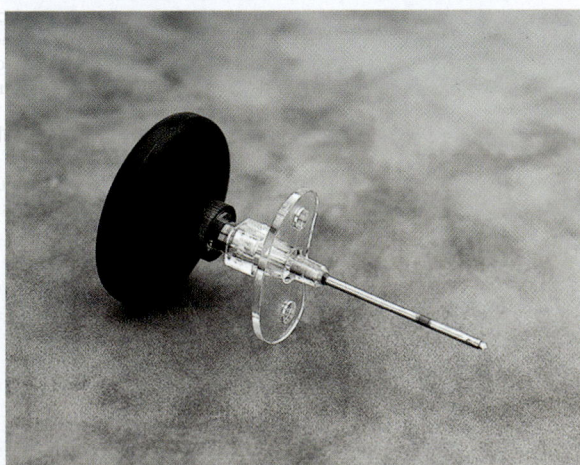

Fig. 47.7 Interosseous needle. (*Source:* Reproduced from Joseph D Tobias, Ross, Allison Kind and Intraosseous Infusions: A Review for the Anesthesiologist with a Focus on Pediatric Use, *Anesthesia & Analgesia* 110(2):391-401. (Credit line - Reproduced with permission from Cook Medical, Bloomington, IN.)

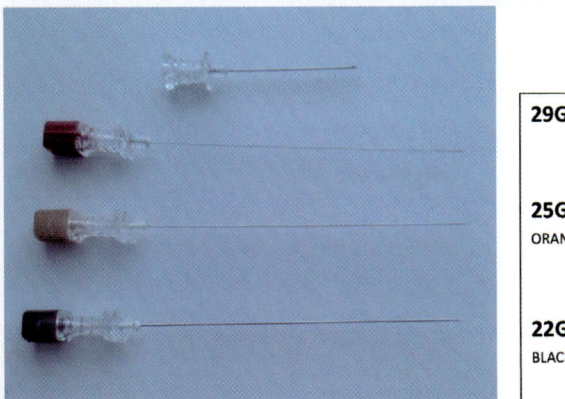

| 29G RED |
| 25G ORANGE |
| 22G BLACK |

Fig. 47.8 Different size Quincke spinal needles. (*Source:* Reproduced from Emad Lotfy Mohammed, Sahar Mohammed El Shal. Efficacy of different size Quincke spinal needles in reduction of incidence of Post-Dural Puncture Headache (PDPH) in Caesarean Section (CS). Randomized controlled study, *Egyptian Journal of Anaesthesia* 33(1):53-58.)

Central line catheter Short-term, triple-lumen central venous catheter. The end from which the catheter is accessed are usually referred to as the hub. After the catheter is inserted, the tip resides within the bloodstream (Fig. 47.6)	Used for central venous access when peripheral line could not be obtained Infusions can be given and blood samples can be drawn through the same catheter through different ports Can be left in place for 10–14 days Sterile precautions to be taken Chances of Central line-associated bloodstream infection (CLABSI) should be considered
Intraosseous needle Cook disposable intraosseous infusion needle with the Dieckmann modification and standard hub design (Cook Medical). Specialized intraosseous needle with circular handle to facilitate placement and stylet to prevent obstruction by bone spicules. (Fig. 47.7)	Used in cases of profound shock when peripheral line could not be secured Inserted at a point 2 cm below and medial to the tibial tuberosity (not to injure the growth plate) Other sites: • Proximal tibia • Distal femur • Iliac crest • Distal tibial Can be left in place and used for 24 h
Lumbar puncture needle	Used to drain cerebrospinal fluid (CSF) for • Therapeutic purposes – analgesics, antibiotics, antineoplastic, anesthesia • Diagnostic purposes • CSF study Post-spinal puncture headache and hypotension are common complications Bleeding diathesis and increased intracranial tension should be ruled out before the procedure 18 G – pink 19 G – ivory 20 G – yellow 22 G – black 23 G – blue 25 G – orange 26 G – brown Types: Dura cutting – Quincke–Babcock needle (Fig. 47.8) Dura separating – Whitacre and Sprotte

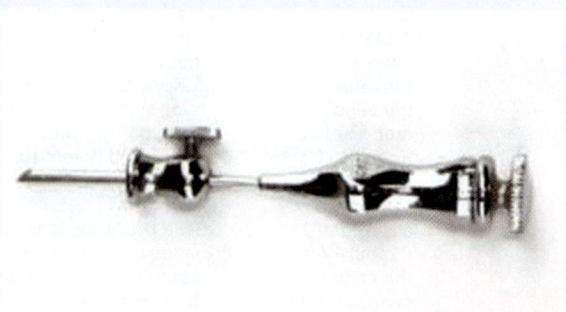

Fig. 47.9 Bone marrow aspiration needle (Salah). *(Source:* Reproduced from RA Trejo-Ayala, M Luna-Pérez, M Gutiérrez-Romero et al. Bone marrow aspiration and biopsy. Technique and considerations, *Revista Médica del Hospital General de México* 78(4):196-201.)

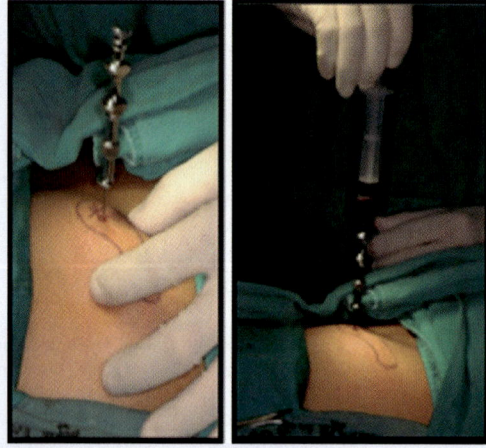

Fig. 47.10 Bone marrow needle (Klima needle). *(Source:* Reproduced from Noel Ye Naung, Srisurang Suttapreyasri, Suttatip Kamolmatyakul. Comparative study of different centrifugation protocols for a density gradient separation media in isolation of osteoprogenitors from bone marrow aspirate, *Journal of Oral Biology and Craniofacial Research* 4(3):160-168.)

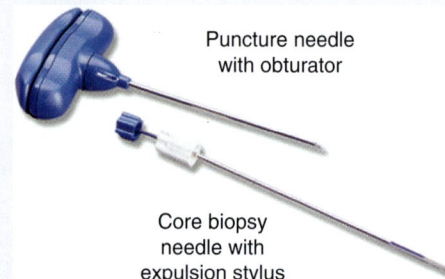

Puncture needle with obturator

Core biopsy needle with expulsion stylus

Fig. 47.11 Bone marrow biopsy (Jamshidi needle). *(Source:* Reproduced from Elaine Keohane, Catherine Otto, Jeanine Walenga. *Rodak's Hematology Clinical Principles and Applications*, Sixth Edition, Bone marrow examination, Figure 14.2, St. Louis, Saunders, 2020. (Credit line - Courtesy Care Fusion, McGaw Park, IL.)

Bone marrow aspiration needle (Salah) (Fig. 47.9)	Used to remove only marrow Used as a diagnostic modality for various hematological conditions such as Immune thrombocytopenic purpura (ITP) and leukemia To diagnose storage disorders, infections such as tuberculosis and kala-azar Therapeutic – bone marrow transplantation Consists of <ul><li>A stylet</li><li>Thick body with nail</li><li>Guard that is 2 cm from tip</li><li>Guard with side screw</li></ul> Posterior iliac crest is the preferred site for aspiration Sternum and tibial tuberosity can also be used
Bone marrow aspiration needle (Klima-Rosegger bone marrow aspiration needle.) (Fig. 47.10)	Klima has a guard which screws along the length of the needle Used mostly Aspiration of bone marrow from anterior iliac crest Can be reused
Sterile Jamshidi Bone Marrow Biopsy and Aspiration Needle. The outer puncture cannula is advanced to the medullary cavity of the bone with the obturator in place to prevent bone coring. The physician removes the obturator and slides the core biopsy needle through the cannula and into the medulla and the expulsion stylus is removed. The core biopsy needle is removed from the puncture needle with the specimen in place. The stylus is used to expel the specimen. (Fig. 47.11)	Used to remove small amount of bone, fluid, and cells Used to diagnose several storage disorders Sites are same as those for bone marrow aspiration Jamshidi needle is longer; can be used both for aspiration and biopsy

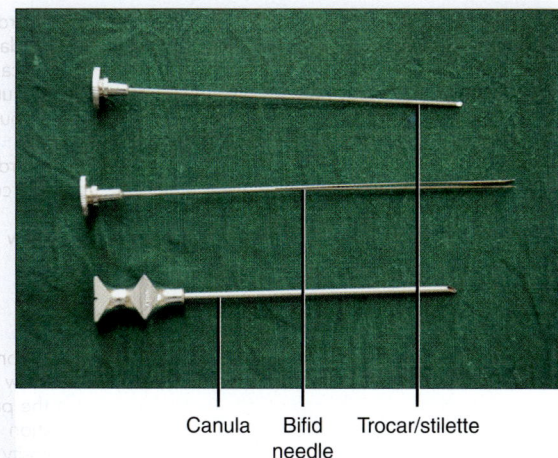

Canula   Bifid   Trocar/stilette
          needle

Fig. 47.12 Liver biopsy needle. (*Source:* Reproduced from G S Sainani. *Manual of Clinical and Practical Medicine*, Procedures, Figure 12.2, New Delhi, Elsevier India, 2010.)

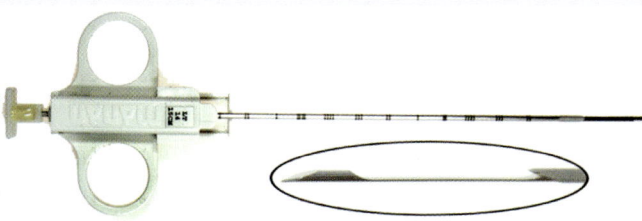

Fig. 47.13 Trucut biopsy needle. (*Source:* Reproduced from S. J. Langley-Hobbs, Jackie Demetriou, Jane Ladlow. *Feline soft tissue and general surgery*, Instruments, Figure 13-4, Chennai, Saunders Ltd, 2014.)

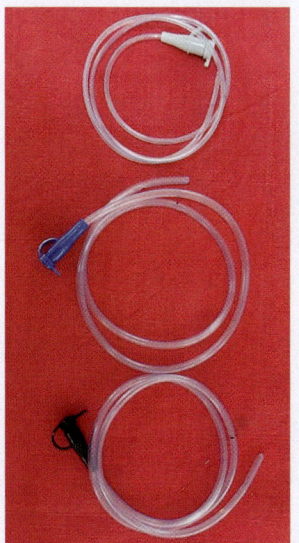

Fig. 47.14 Infant feeding tube.

Vim Silverman liver biopsy needle (needle type: Menghini) (Fig. 47.12)	Bifid type of needle With a trocar and cannula Bleeding diathesis should be ruled out before the procedure Inserted in the 10th Intercostal space (ICS) in midaxillary line on the right side Position: Supine position on firm bed with right flank exposed and right arm drawn upwards Indications: • Storage disorder • Malignancy • Infiltrations: Tuberculosis (TB), Cytomegalovirus infection (CMV), and herpes • Cirrhosis of liver Complications: • Infection • Bleeding in liver • Bile leak • Pneumothorax • Injury to other abdominal organs
Trucut biopsy needle (Fig. 47.13)	Used to take renal biopsy Site of biopsy marked with the help of ultrasound, and ultrasound (USG)-guided biopsy is taken and sent for cytological, Histopathological examinaton (HPE), and immunohistochemical studies
Infant feeding tubes (Fig. 47.14)	Plastic with blunt tip Openings laterally Has radiopaque marker Therapeutic: • Used to decompress the stomach in prolonged Bag Valve Mask (BVM)/ Continuous positive airway pressure (CPAP) ventilation • Used to administer drugs • Used to treat intestinal obstruction • Used to feed and maintain enteral nutrition in newborns and infants who are unable to take oral feeds • Helps in poisoning Diagnostic: • Internal bleeding in Gastrointestinal tract • Gastric lavage in tuberculosis • Diagnose Tracheoesophageal fistula (TEF) • Localize esophageal stricture Complications: • Trauma to nose/pharynx • Tube in trachea • Ulceration/infection • Various sizes are available for different age groups

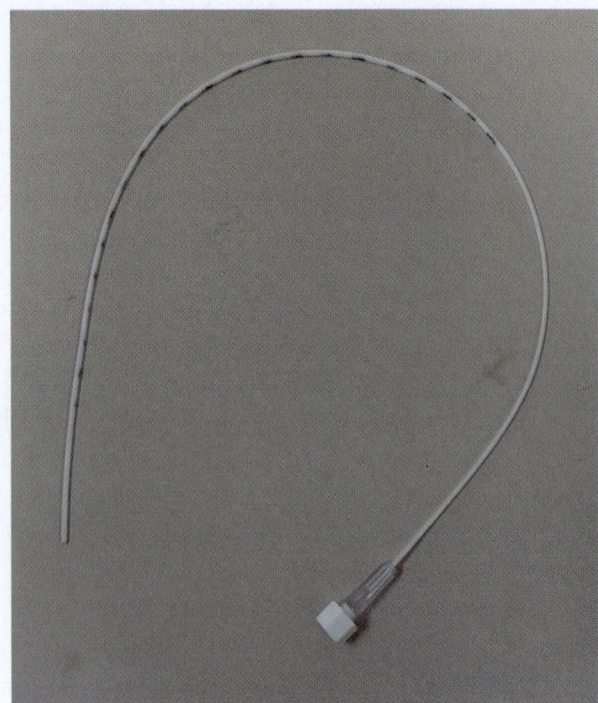

Fig. 47.15 Umbilical vein catheter.

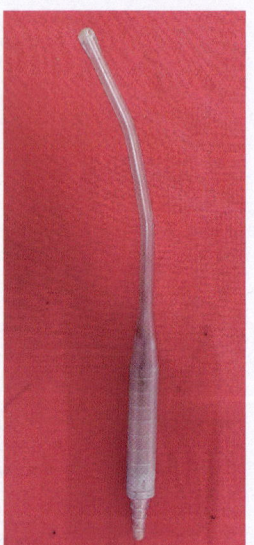

Fig. 47.16 Yankauer suction catheter.

Umbilical vein catheters (Fig. 47.15)	Used to secure central lines in newborns For exchange transfusion For giving adrenaline during newborn resuscitation Used for continuous Arterial blood gas analysis (ABG) monitoring
Yankauer suction catheter (Fig. 47.16)	Used in case of foreign body aspiration which blocks the glottis preventing endotracheal intubation

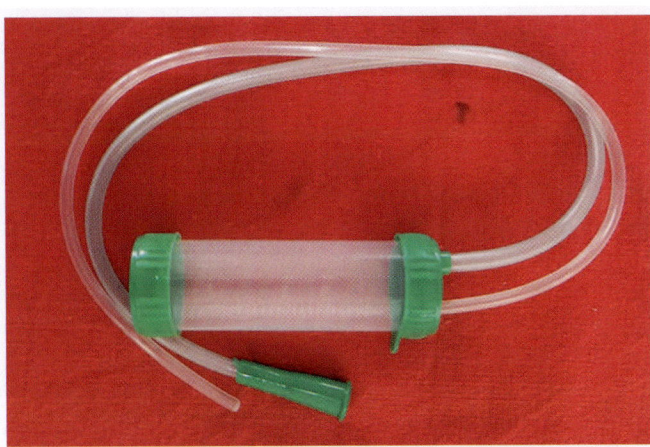

Fig. 47.17 Deleey mucus extractor.

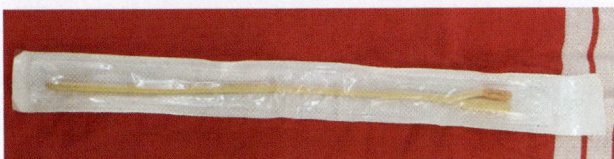

Fig. 47.18 Foley catheter.

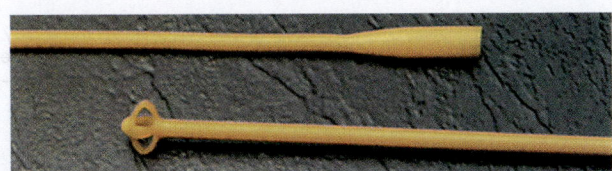

Fig. 47.19 Malecot catheter. (*Source:* Reproduced from Jane Rothrock. *Alexander's Care of the Patient in Surgery*, Sixteenth Edition Genitourinary Surgery, FIG. 15.9, St. Louis, Elsevier Inc., 2019.)

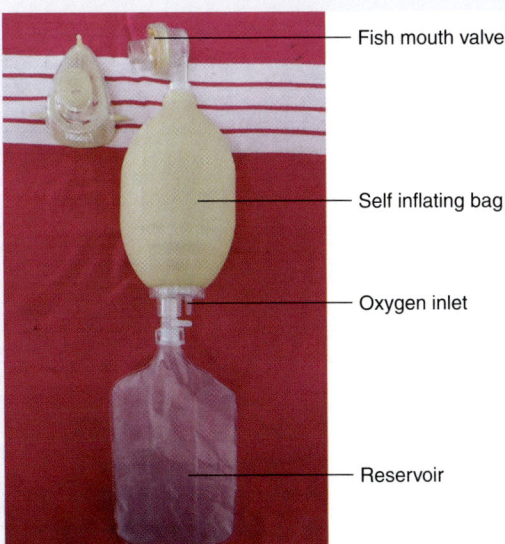

Fish mouth valve

Self inflating bag

Oxygen inlet

Reservoir

Fig. 47.20 AMBU bag.

DeLee mucus extractor (Fig. 47.17)	Used to suck mucus and meconium from the upper airway in newborns during resuscitation Opening at tip
Foley catheter (Fig. 47.18)	Used to drain the bladder and monitor urine output Interactable epistaxis or bleeding esophagus Usually 12 and 14 French catheters are used in pediatrics Parts: • Bladder opening • Balloon port • Urine drainage port • Balloon (only distilled water to be used)
Malecot catheter (Fig. 47.19)	Used to drain pus in case of empyema and loculated effusion Operation drainage in peritoneal cavity Suprapubic cystotomy Side effect: Dermatitis
AMBU (artificial manual breathing unit) bag (Fig. 47.20)	Parts: • Self-inflating bag • O_2 reservoir • Oxygen port inlet • Inlet valve • Outlet valve • Fish-mouth valve • Port for mask • Used in children who cannot maintain spontaneous breathing effectively • Used to improve oxygenation before intubation Disadvantages: • Does not deliver Positive end-expiratory pressure (PEEP) • Cannot deliver free-flow oxygen

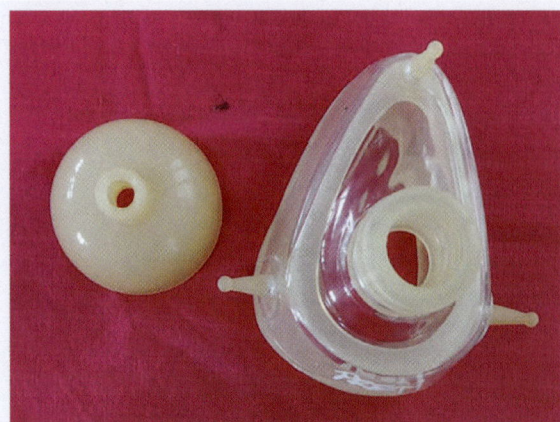

Fig. 47.21 Mask for different age groups: Types — round mask and anatomical mask.

Masks	Used as an interface to give rescue breaths
	Anatomical masks and round masks are available in different sizes for different age groups (Fig. 47.21)
	EC clamping (thumb and index finger holds the mask over the nose and mouth , forming a C while the other three fingers grasp the child's mandible forming an E) technique is used to secure the mask in position
	Appropriate size should cover the bridge of nose and angle of mouth and chin
	Should not cover eyes

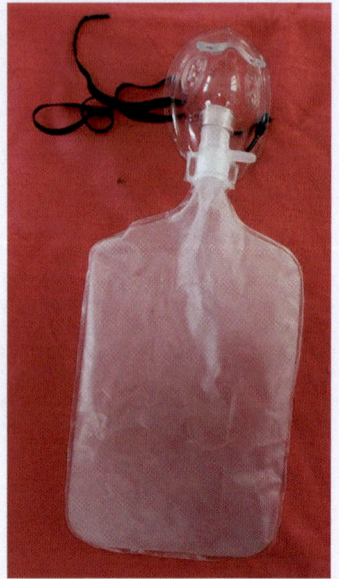

Fig. 47.22 Nonrebreathing mask.

Oxygen mask	Nonrebreathing mask (Fig. 47.22):
	Used to deliver oxygen in children with distress and to correct hypoxia
	Most nonthreatening way of oxygenation
	Delivers FiO_2 at 95%, at 10–12 L/min

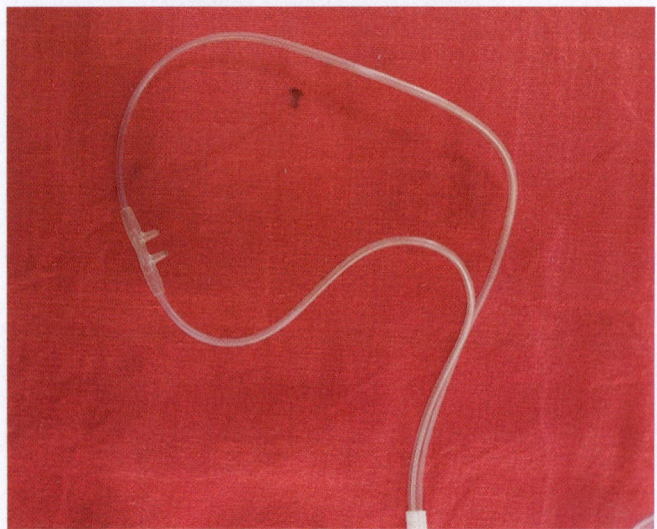

Fig. 47.23 Nasal prongs.

Nasal prongs (Fig. 47.23)	Should not be snugly fitting
	Delivers 40%–60%
	Flow should not be < 4 L/min

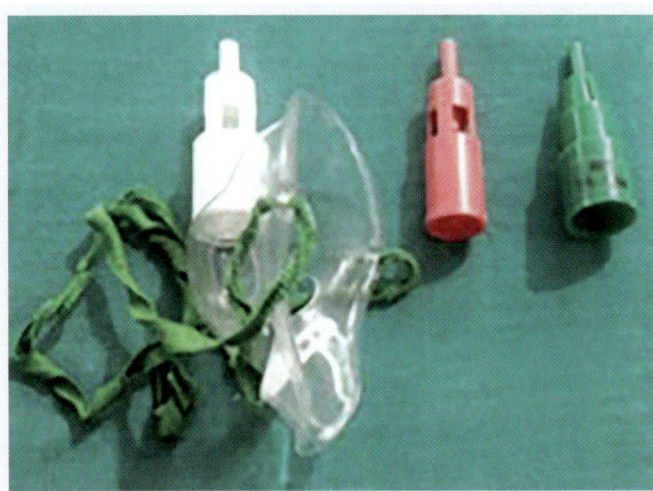

Fig. 47.24 Venturi mask.

Venturi masks with valves (Fig. 47.24)	Delivers controlled FiO_2 Useful for weaning oxygen Blue – 24% Yellow – 28% White – 31% Green – 35% Pink – 40% Orange – 50% (Varies with brand) Flow required: 4–8 L/min

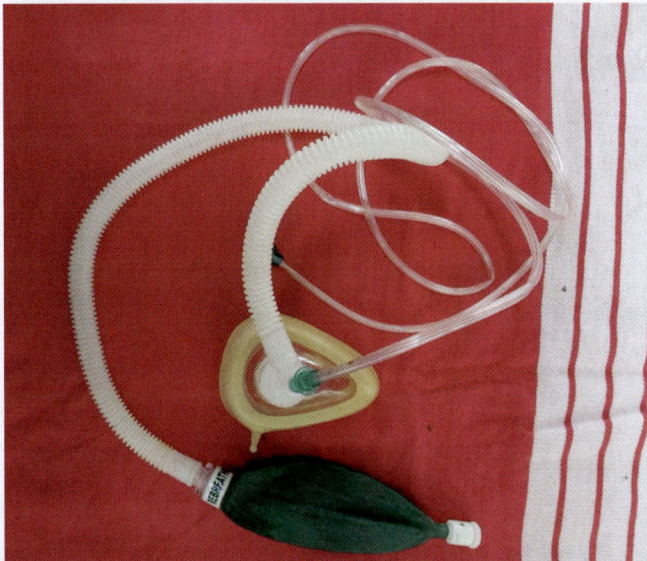

Fig. 47.25 Jackson–Rees circuit.

Jackson–Rees (JR) circuit (Fig. 47.25)	Delivers Positive end-expiratory pressure (PEEP) Useful to support spontaneous breath, weaning mode Disadvantage: Pneumothorax

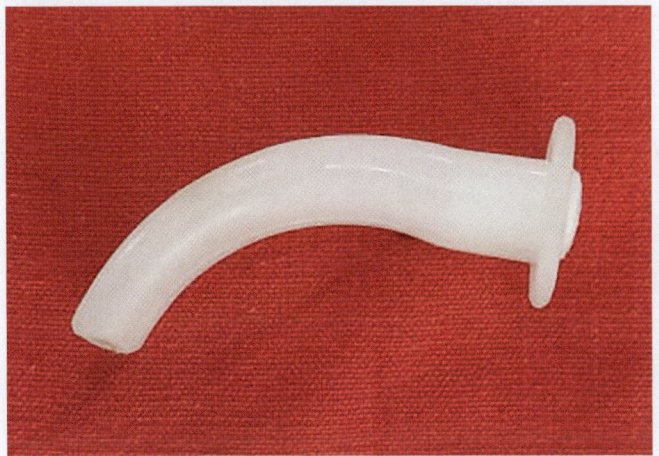

Fig. 47.26 Oropharyngeal airway.

Oropharyngeal airway (Guedel) (Fig. 47.26)	Used to secure airway and prevent tongue bites in case of seizures Used in bilateral choanal atresia in newborns

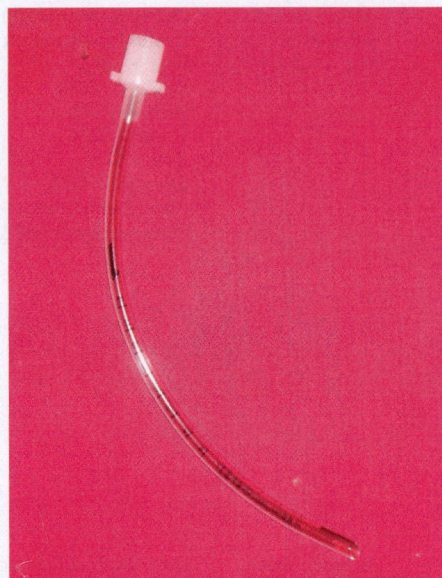

Fig. 47.27 Endotracheal tube (uncuffed).

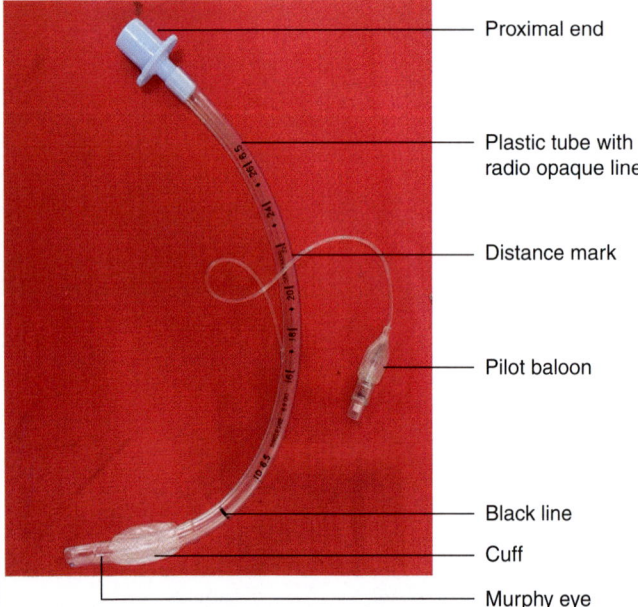

- Proximal end
- Plastic tube with radio opaque line
- Distance mark
- Pilot baloon
- Black line
- Cuff
- Murphy eye

Fig. 47.28 Endotracheal tube (cuffed).

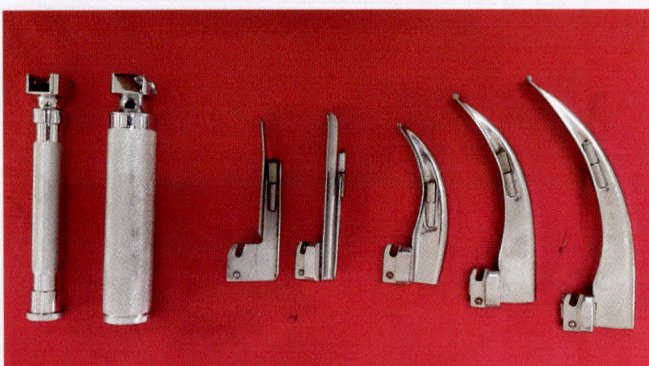

Fig. 47.29 Laryngoscope.

Endotracheal tubes	Used to secure airway in emergency situations
	Different sizes of endotracheal tubes are available for different age groups
	Uncuffed tubes are preferred to prevent pressure necrosis of the airway (Fig. 47.27)
	Cuffed: Used in children older than 8 years; prevents aspiration (Fig. 47.28)
	Parts:
	• Plastic tubes (hypoallergic, disposable, transparent)
	• Proximal end – 15 mm adapter to fit to ventilator
	• Pilot balloon
	• Black line at the vocal cords
	• Radiopaque line to visualize in X-ray
	• Murphy eye to prevent complete blockage of tube
	Distance markings to facilitate placement of tube
	Formula: endotracheal tube (ET) size = (Age/4) + 4 for uncuffed tube
	Cuffed 0.5 size smaller than uncuffed
	Fixation = 3 × tube size
Laryngoscope with blades (Fig. 47.29)	Used to visualize the vocal cord during endotracheal intubation
	Straight blades are used in newborns and infants (McGill)
	Curved blades are used in pediatric patients (Mcintosh)
	Blades are also of different sizes for different age group
	Laryngoscope is held in left hand

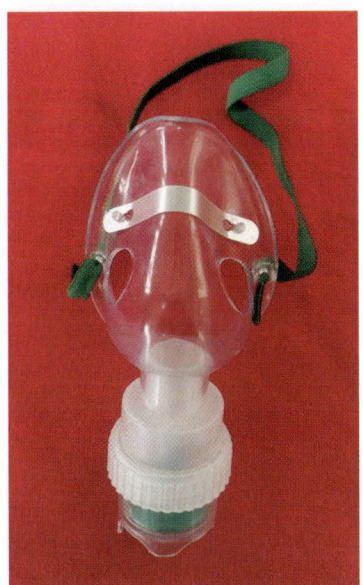

Fig. 47.30   Nebulizer chamber.

Nebulizer chamber (Fig. 47.30)	Used to mix drugs and saline to set up a nebulization current and deliver it through the mask
	Used in acute episodes
	Driven by oxygen
	Works on the Bernoulli's principle
	Normal saline is used with medication
	Can be a potential source of hospital-acquired pneumonia

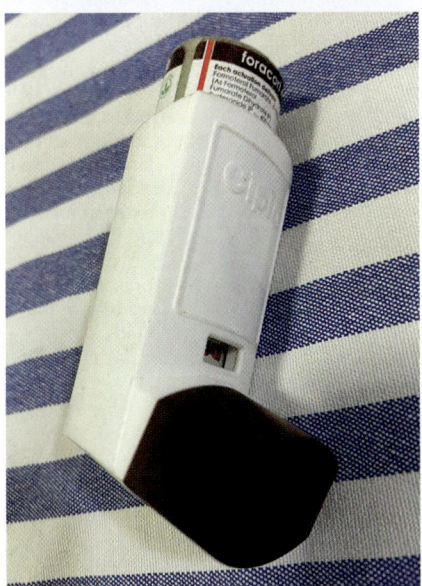

Fig. 47.31   Metered-dose inhaler.

Metered-dose inhaler (Fig. 47.31)	Parts: • Canister – delivers medicine in aerosol • Plastic actuator • Cap
	Disadvantage: Coordination between inspiration and activation of device is necessary
	Used to administer inhaled corticosteroids in children older than 6 years.
	Mask should be used mandatorily in children younger than 6 years

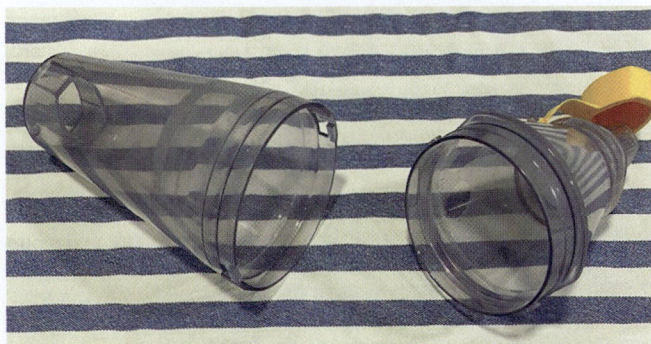

Fig. 47.32   Spacer.

| Spacer (Fig. 47.32) | Used to deliver drugs to low airway |
| | Requires less coordination between inspiration and activation of device |

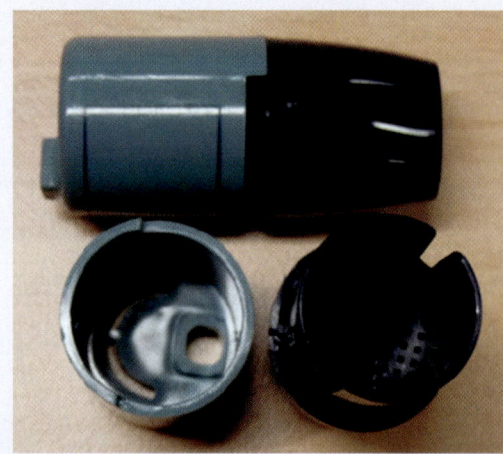

Fig. 47.33 Rotahaler. *(Source:* Reproduced from Srinivas Ravindra Babu Behara, Ian Larson, Paul Kippax et al. An approach to characterising the cohesive behaviour of powders using a flow titration aerosolisation based methodology, *Chemical Engineering Science* 66(8):1640-1648.)

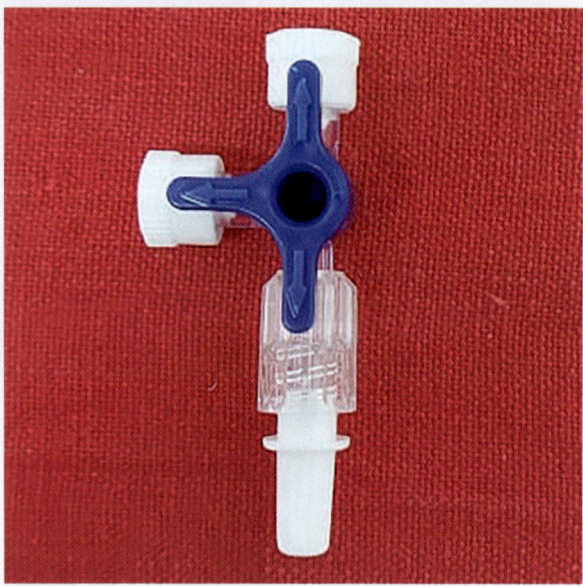

Fig. 47.34 Three-way adapter.

Rotahaler-Dry powder inhaler (DPI) (Fig. 47.33)	Portable No coordination required Disadvantages: • Not used in children younger than 6 years • Dry powder deposits in the pharynx • Dry powder might get affected by humid climate
Three-way adapter (Fig. 47.34)	Provides three-way flow: Inlet to outlet, inlet to side port, and side port to outlet Stopcock can open and close lines Used to infuse fluids in a single venous canula Used to administer drug as in adenosine in Supraventricular tachycardia (SVT) Used in attachment of extension lines Used in exchange transfusion Used in hemodialysis for poisoning Used to tap ascitic or pleural fluid

48

Arterial Blood Gas

Normal Values in Arterial Blood Gas
(Table 48.1)

Table 48.1	Normal Values in ABG	
Normal Parameters	**Arterial**	**Venous**
pH	7.35–7.45	7.32–7.42
$PaCO_2$	35–45	38–52
PaO_2	80–100	30–40
HCO_3	22–28	22–28

Formulas in Arterial Blood Gas
(Table 48.2)

Table 48.2	Formulas in ABG

Winter's formula = $1.5 \times HCO_3^- + 8 + 2$
Anion gap = $Na^+ - (HCO_3^- + Cl^-)$
Δ Anion gap = Measured anion gap – 12
Δ Delta ratio = 24 – Measured HCO_3^-
Delta gap = Δ Anion gap – ΔHCO_3^-
Delta ratio = Δ Anion gap/ΔHCO_3^-

Stepwise Approach to Arterial Blood Gas Analysis (Table 48.3)

Remember: Anticipate the imbalance clinically in a given setting and then proceed for arterial blood gas (ABG) analysis.

STEP 1

Whether it is acidemic or alkalemic
- Normal value: 7.35–7.45
- Any value below 7.35: Acidemic
- Any value above 7.45: Alkalemic

Table 48.3	Stepwise Approach to Arterial Blood Gas
Steps	**Analysis**
Step 1	Whether acidemic, alkalemic or normal
Step 2	Identify primary disturbance is respiratory or metabolic
Step 3	If primary respiratory disturbance, check whether acute or chronic
Step 4	In case of respiratory disorder, whether metabolic compensation is okay
Step 5	If primary metabolic disturbance whether respiratory compensation is okay
Step 6	In case of metabolic acidosis, look for increased anion gap
Step 7	Check if any coexistent metabolic disturbance

STEP 2

Whether the primary disturbance is respiratory or metabolic
- Based on the pH
- Look at the $PaCO_2$ and HCO_3
- For **acidosis:**
  - $PaCO_2$ high − respiratory
  - HCO_3 low − metabolic
- For **alkalosis:**
  - $PaCO_2$ low − respiratory
  - HCO_3 high − metabolic

STEP 3

In case of a primary respiratory disturbance, whether it is acute or chronic
- Acute respiratory acidosis
  - 0.08 ↓ of pH for every 10 ↑ of $PaCO_2$
- Chronic respiratory acidosis
  - 0.03 ↓ of pH for every 10 ↑ of $PaCO_2$
- Acute respiratory alkalosis
  - 0.08 ↑ of pH for every 10 ↓ of $PaCO_2$
- Chronic respiratory alkalosis
  - 0.03 ↑ of pH for every 10 ↓ of $PaCO_2$

STEP 4

In a suspected respiratory disorder, check compensation is okay,
- In an acute respiratory acidosis, HCO_3 increases by 1, for every 10 increase in $PaCO_2$
- In an acute respiratory alkalosis, HCO_3 decreases by 2, for every 10 decrease in $PaCO_2$
- In chronic respiratory acidosis, HCO_3 increases by 3, for every 10 increase in $PaCO_2$
- In chronic respiratory alkalosis HCO_3 decreases by 4, for every 10 decrease in $PaCO_2$.
Remember: 1, 2, 3, 4 begin with respiratory acidosis.

STEP 5

In case of a metabolic disturbance, whether the respiratory compensation is okay
- Metabolic acidosis
  - $PaCO_2 = (1.5 \times HCO_3) + 8 \pm 2 \rightarrow$ "Winter's formula"
- Metabolic alkalosis
  - $PaCO_2$ ↑ by 7 for every 10 ↑ in HCO_3

STEP 6

In case of a metabolic acidosis, whether there is an increased anion gap
- Anion Gap = $Na - (Cl + HCO_3)$
  - Normal value is 12

- In high-anion gap metabolic acidosis (HAGMA), the anion gap is >12
- In normal or nonanion gap metabolic acidosis (NAGMA), anion gap is <12

STEP 7

Whether there are any coexistent metabolic disturbances
- Whether it is pure HAGMA or there is any coexistent NAGMA or metabolic alkalosis
- Delta ratio and delta gap are useful in these scenarios:

$$\text{Delta ratio} = \frac{\Delta \text{ Anion gap}}{\Delta \text{ HCO}_3} = \frac{\Delta \text{ Anion gap} - 12}{24 - \text{HCO}_3}$$

Delta ratio < 1: HAGMA + NAGMA
Delta ratio 1–2: Pure HAGMA
Delta ratio >2: HAGMA + metabolic alkalosis

$$\text{Delta Gap} = \Delta \text{ Anion gap} - \Delta \text{ HCO}_3$$
$$= (\text{Anion gap} - 12) - (24 - \text{HCO}_3)$$

Delta gap:
- Normal: 0
- If delta gap is positive: HAGMA + metabolic alkalosis
- If delta gap is negative: HAGMA + NAGMA or chronic respiratory alkalosis

Special Conditions

HYPOALBUMINEMIA

- Patients with a low serum albumin level, such as in patients suffering from cirrhosis, nephritic syndrome, and malnutrition, will have an anion gap metabolic acidosis, but the measured anion gap will be in the normal range.
- The reason is that albumin has many negative charges on its surface that account for a significant proportion of unmeasured anions.
- Hence, it is believed that in hypoalbuminemia, even normal anion gap is considered as wide.
- Therefore, a formula can be used to calculate the corrected anion gap:

"Figge" formula = Anion gap + [0.25 × (44 − albumin)]

(For every 1 g/dL of fall in albumin level, anion gap falls by 2.5 mEq/L)

HYPOCALCEMIA

- To calculate the correct calcium level in the presence of hypoalbuminemia, the following formula can be used:

Corrected calcium = [0.8 × (normal albumin − patient's albumin)]

(Normal albumin is considered as 4.)

Example Case Scenario

Example: pH = 7.30; pCO₂ = 40; HCO₃ = 16; Na = 145; Cl = 100
- **Step 1:** pH is below 7.35 − **acidemic**
- **Step 2:** Looking at PaCO₂ and HCO₃
  HCO₃ is low and PaCO₂ normal − **metabolic acidosis**
- **Step 3:** Is there compensation?
  Using the Winter's formula:
  Expected PaCO₂ = 1.5 × 16 + 8 + 2 = 32 (30−34)
  No compensation
- **Step 4:** Calculation of anion gap
  Anion gap = 145 − (16 + 100) = 29
  Impression: High anion gap metabolic acidosis
- **Step 5:** Is there any other coexisting disorder?
  Delta ratio = (29–12)/(24–16) = 17/8 = 2.1
  Delta gap = 17–8 = 9
- Delta ratio is >2 and delta gap is positive, hence there is HAGMA + metabolic alkalosis
- *Final impression:*
  High anion gap metabolic acidosis with metabolic alkalosis with respiratory acidosis*

Troubleshooting in Arterial Blood Gas

1. Low pCO₂ and HCO₃ can be seen if excessive heparin is used (dilutional effect)
2. Air bubbles present in sample can falsely show high PO₂ and decreased PCO₂
3. Raised WBC counts can cause decrease in PO₂.

---

*Respiratory acidosis because measured PCO₂ is higher than expected PCO₂.

49

Fluids and Electrolytes

Intravenous Fluid (Table 49.1)

TABLE 49.1	Composition of Normal Intravenous Fluid					
I.v. Fluid	Osmolality (mOsm/L)	Dextrose (g/100 mL)	Sodium (Mmol/L)	Potassium (Mmol/L)	Chloride (Mmol/L)	Others (Mmol/L)
Sodium chloride[a]	308	–	154	–	154	–
Ringer lactate[a]	270	–	131	5	111	Lactate – 29 Calcium – 2
Isolyte-P	368	5	23	20	29	Acetate – 23 Mg – 3 Phosphate – 3
1/2 DNS[b]	154	5	77	–	77	–
10% Dextrose	556	10				
5% Dextrose	278	5				
Plasma-Lyte 148	295	–	140	5	98	Acetate – 27 Gluconate – 23 Magnesium – 1.5

[a]Isotonic fluid – sodium chloride, ringer lactate
[b]If 1/2 DNS is not available readily, it can be prepared by the following method:
- 1/2 DNS is prepared by mixing 250 mL NS + 250 mL 5% D
- 1/3 DNS is prepared by mixing 125 mL NS + 375 mL 5% D

Concentration of Intravenous Fluid (Table 49.2)

TABLE 49.2	Concentration of Intravenous Fluid		
Solution	Concentration	Available	Comments
Sodium bicarbonate	7.5%	10 mL ampoule	1 mL = 1 mEq of HCO_3 + 1 mEq of sodium
Sodium chloride	3%	10 mL ampoule Or 50 mL bottle	1 mL = 0.5 mEq of sodium
Potassium chloride	15%	10 mL ampoule	1 mL = 2 mEq of potassium
Calcium gluconate	10%	10 mL ampoule	1 mL = 9.3 mg of calcium
Magnesium sulphate	50% and 25%	2 mL ampoule	25% magnesium = 4.15 mOsm/dL
25% Dextrose	25 g/100 mL	25 mL ampoule	1389 mOsm/L
50% Dextrose	50 g/100 mL	25 mL ampoule	2525 mOsm/l

Hepatic Drip (Table 49.3)

TABLE 49.3	Hepatic Drip in a Child With Liver disease
Item	Quantity (mL)
NS	100
10% Dextrose	400
KCl	5
Calcium gluconate	5
Multivitamin	2

Maintenance Fluid and Electrolytes in Children and Newborn

MAINTENANCE FLUID AND ELECTROLYTES IN NEWBORN (Table 49.4)

- Use birth weight for all calculations (including antibiotics calculation) as long as the baby's postnatal weight remains below the birth weight. Once the birth weight is regained, use actual body weight for calculations.
- First 48 hours for baby's weight >1000 g, use 10% dextrose as maintenance fluid; <1000 g – 5% dextrose as maintenance fluid (no electrolyte supplementation in first 48 hours)
- More than 48 hours – for all birth weight neonate – Isolyte-P
- If the neonate has the same body weight as yesterday, continue the same amount of fluid as the present-day fluid volume
- If the neonate has an increased body weight than the previous day, restrict the fluid as the previous day
- If the neonate has normal weight loss as in the first 7–10 days, continue with increasing the fluid requirement each day

Daily Fluid Requirement in a Newborn (ml/kg/day) (Table 49.4)

TABLE 49.4	Daily Fluid Requirement in a Newborn (ml/kg/day)						
Birth Weight (g)	Day 1	Day 2	Day 3	Day 4	Day 5	Day 6	Day 7
<1000	80	100	120	130	140	150	160
1000–1500	80	95	110	120	130	140	150
>1500	60	75	90	105	120	135	150

ELECTROLYTE SUPPLEMENTATION IN NEWBORN

- Electrolyte supplementation in a newborn usually starts after 48 hours (after the onset of diuresis) (Table 49.5).

MAINTENANCE FLUID AND ELECTROLYTES IN CHILDREN

- Maintenance fluid requirement in children is calculated by **Holliday–Segar formula** as given in Table 49.6.
- Flow of fluid: For microdrip set: mL/h = Number of microdrops/minute (assume 1 mL = 60 microdrops); and for conventional i.v. set: divide the above by 4 (1 mL = 15 drops)

Electrolyte Requirement in a Newborn (Table 49.5)

TABLE 49.5	Electrolyte Requirement in a Newborn		
Neonate	Sodium (mEq/kg/day)	Potassium (mEq/kg/day)	Calcium[a] (mL/kg/day)
Term	2–3	2–3	4
Preterm	3–5	2–3	4

[a]Calcium in the first 3 days in high-risk neonate (birth asphyxia, Infants of diabetic mothers (IDM) preterm, sick neonate).

Daily Maintenance Fluid Requirement in Children (Table 49.6)

TABLE 49.6	Daily Maintenance Fluid Requirement in Children	
Body Weight (kg)	Fluid Rate	Fluid Volume (per 24 h)
<10	4 mL/kg/h	100 mL/kg
10–20	40 mL + 2 mL/kg/h for each kilogram more than 10 kg	1000 mL + 50 mL/kg for each kilogram more than 10 kg
>20	60 mL + 1 mL/kg/h for each kilogram more than 20 kg	1500 mL + 20 mL/kg for each kilogram more than 20 kg

ELECTROLYTE REQUIREMENT IN CHILDREN

- Sodium: 3–5 mEq/kg/day
- Potassium: 2–3 mEq/100 mL
- Glucose: 5 g/100 mL

Electrolyte Imbalance

APPROACH TO HYPONATREMIA

- Normal serum sodium: 135–145 mEq/L
- Hyponatremia (serum sodium): <135 mEq/L
- Step 1: Determine whether it is true hyponatremia (rule out pseudohyponatremia)
  - Pseudohyponatremia:
    1. Improper sampling (blood taken from the vein proximal to an infusion of hypotonic saline), normal osmolality
    2. Factitious hyponatremia: Hyperglycemia; mannitol therapy – increased osmolality
    3. Pseudohyponatremia: Laboratory artifact – hyperlipidemia, hyperproteinemia, low osmolality
- Step 2: Whether the child is symptomatic (seizures, irritability, Altered level of consciousness (ALOC)) or asymptomatic
- Step 3: Acute and symptomatic – treat with bolus (3% NaCl: 3–5 mL/kg over 30 minutes to 1 hour); chronic and asymptomatic – no bolus
- Step 4: If asymptomatic – categorize according to volume status (Table 49.7)

Approach to Asymptomatic Hyponatremia (Table 49.7)

TABLE 49.7	Approach to Asymptomatic Hyponatremia		
Condition	Hypovolemic Hyponatremia	Euvolemic Hyponatremia	Hypervolemic Hyponatremia
Volume status	Dehydration present	No dehydration No edema	Edema present
Causes	1. Extrarenal (vomiting, diarrhea, third space loss) 2. Renal – renal tubular acidosis, diuretic therapy, endocrine (adrenal insufficiency, Congenital adrenal hyperplasia (CAH)) 3. Cerebral salt wasting	1. Syndrome of inappropriate antidiuretic hormone (ADH) secretion (SIADH) – respiratory cause (pneumonia, bronchiolitis) CNS – traumatic brain injury, CNS infection 2. Water intoxication – use of 5% dextrose 3. Psychogenic water drinking	1. Renal failure 2. Nephrotic syndrome 3. Congestive heart failure 4. Liver failure
Investigation: Urine sodium	Urine Na > 20 mEq/L – renal Urine Na < 20 mEq/L – nonrenal	Urine Na > 20 mEq/L – Syndrome of inappropriate antidiuretic hormone (ADH) secretion (SIADH) Urine Na < 20 mEq/L – water intoxication	Urine sodium > 20 mEq/L – renal failure Urine Na < 20 – all others
Treatment	Correction = Deficit + maintenance Deficit = (135 – measured sodium) × body weight × 0.6, over 24 h or First 50%: 8 h Next 50%: 9–16 h	Treat the underlying cause Syndrome of inappropriate antidiuretic hormone (ADH) secretion (SIADH) – fluid restriction (two-third fluid)	Treat the underlying cause Restriction of water and sodium Diuretics

Approach to Hypernatremia (Table 49.8)

TABLE 49.8	Approach to Hypernatremia
Hypernatremia	**Serum Sodium > 145 mEq/L**
Causes	1. Disproportionate water loss than electrolytes – diarrheal dehydration with predominant vomiting or reduced intake; infants – increased body surface area relative to body weight and renal immaturity 2. Electrolyte-free water loss – in diabetes insipidus, inaccessibility to water (infants, child with mental retardation, depressed level of consciousness) 3. Sodium excess – improper mixing (formula feeds, ORS), salt poisoning, mineralocorticoid excess (hyperaldosteronism)
Clinical features	CNS – lethargy, convulsions, high-pitch cry, doughy feel of abdomen
Investigations	Serum electrolytes, urine electrolytes, serum osmolality, other arterial blood gas analysis
Management	One-fourth to one-half normal saline in 5% dextrose at the rate of 150% (1.25−1.5 times maintenance) = isotonic deficit + free water deficit + maintenance fluid
Monitor	Serum Na, every 4–6 h
Rate of fall: Optimal – 0.5 mEq/h 12 mEq/24 h	If rapid fall >0.5 mEq/h: Increase Na concentration − 1/4 to 1/3 to 1/2 Decrease rate: 1.5 to 1.25 times to 1.0 maintenance fluid Optimal fall – 0.5 mEq/h – continue same fluid at same rate Slow fall <0.5 mEq/h Decrease Na TO 1/2 to 1/3 to 1/4 Increase rate of IVF 1.0 to 1.25 to 1.5 times

Approach to Hypokalemia (Table 49.9)

TABLE 49.9	Approach to hypokalemia		
	SERUM POTASSIUM LEVEL < 3.5 mEq/L		
Hypokalemia	**Reduced Intake**	**Transcellular Shift**	**Loss**
Causes	a. Rare cause – i.v. fluid without potassium supplementation b. Malnutrition	a. Insulin therapy b. Beta-2 agonist − salbutamol c. Bicarbonate correction – correction of acidosis d. Poisoning − rodenticide/insecticide poisoning	1. Renal loss − Renal tubular acidosis (RTA) Bartter syndrome, Gitelman syndrome 2. Gastrointestinal loss − vomiting, diarrhea
Clinical features	Hypotonia, proximal muscle weakness, respiratory paralysis GIT − ileus, phantom hernia Cardiac arrhythmia Polyuria − decreased concentrating ability		

Investigations	Four investigations – arterial blood gas, urine potassium, transtubular potassium gradient (TTKG), blood pressure
	Hypokalemia with one of the following:
	• Scenario 1:
	  • Metabolic acidosis
	  • Check urine potassium if urine K > 20 mEq/L − renal loss − Renal tubular acidosis (RTA)
	  • If urine K <20 mEq/L − GIT loss − diarrhea
	• Scenario 2: Metabolic alkalosis
	  • Check urine chloride, if urine chloride >20 mEq/L − renal loss − Bartter syndrome
	  • If urine chloride <20 mEq/L − GIT loss − vomiting
	• Scenario 3: With hypertension
	  • Check plasma aldosterone concentration (PAC); plasma renin activity (PRA); and plasma aldosterone:plasma renin ratio (PAC:PRA ratio)
	    a. PAC increased, PRA increased, and PAC:PRA < 10 = renovascular hypertension
	    b. PAC increased, PRA decreased, and PAC:PRA > 20 = primary hyperaldosteronism
	    c. Decreased PAC and decreased PRA = congenital adrenal hyperplasia, 11-beta hydroxyl deficiency, Liddle syndrome
	• Scenario 4:
	  • Transtubular potassium gradient (TTKG)
	• Formula:
	  $$\dfrac{\text{Urine K/plasma K}}{\text{Urine Osm/plasma Osm}}$$
	• TTKG < 4 – extrarenal loss; TTKG > 4 – renal loss (e.g., renal artery stenosis and hyperaldosteronism)		

Management	1. Severe hypokalemia – serum K < 2.5 mEq/L, presence of paralysis, cardiac arrythmia, ECG changes
	  • I.v. potassium – 0.5–1 mEq/kg given at a rate of 0.3 mEq/kg/h (1 mEq/kg is given over 3 h) – not to exceed 10 mEq/h
	  • For example, in a 10 kg child, potassium correction of 1 mEq/kg is given as
	    Total potassium required = 10 mEq = 5 mL (1 mL = 2 mEq)
	    Dilute this 5 mL with 10 times the amount in normal saline – 50 mL NS (do not mix with dextrose to prevent further transcellular shift)		

Continued

TABLE 49.9	Approach to hypokalemia—cont'd

SERUM POTASSIUM LEVEL < 3.5 mEq/L

Hypokalemia

That is, 50 mL given over 3 h, i.e., around 16 mL/h for 3 h
Maximum potassium concentration
    Peripheral line = 40 mEq/L
    Central line = 60 mEq/L
2. Moderate hypokalemia
- Serum K = 2.5–3.0, no cardiac involvement, no paralysis
- Add 10 mL of i.v. potassium in 500 mL of maintenance fluid (double potassium in maintenance)
3. Mild hypokalemia = 3–3.5 mEq
- Oral potassium (15 mL = 20 mEq): Mix it with juice to prevent gastric irritation
- Dietary supplements – orange juice, coconut water

Approach to Hyperkalemia (Table 49.10)

TABLE 49.10	Approach to Hyperkalemia

SERUM POTASSIUM > 5.5 mEq/L				
Hyperkalemia	**Spurious**	**True Hyperkalemia**		
Causes	Difficult sampling Squeezing of limb Leukocytosis, thrombocytosis	*Increased release* Acute hemolysis Trauma Rhabdomyolysis	*Transcellular shift* Acidosis Hyperkalemic periodic paralysis	*Decreased excretion* Acute or chronic renal failure Primary or secondary hypoaldosteronism	*Others* ACE inhibitors, NSAIDs

Clinical features
Respiratory failure, cardiotoxicity
Signs: Cardiac arrythmia − Ventricular fibrillation asystole

Investigations
1. Serum potassium level
2. ECG – tall peak T wave, prolonged PR, low voltage QRS, prolonged QRS with sine wave pattern

Management
Step 1: Stop potassium-containing fluid; use potassium-sparing drugs
Step 2: Stabilizing membrane/managing cardiotoxicity
I.v. 10% calcium gluconate
- Dose: 0.5–1 mL/kg
- Time of onset: 1–3 min
- Duration of action: 30–60 min

Step 3: Shift of potassium Extracellular fluid (ECF) to Intracellular fluid (ICF)
  a. I.v. sodium bicarbonate (7.5%)
    Dose: 1–2 mL/kg over 10 min
    Time of onset: 20–30 min
    Duration of action: 2 h
  b. Insulin and glucose = 1 g/kg of dextrose + 0.1 units/kg short-acting insulin as infusion over 1 h or add 6 units of short-acting insulin + 100 mL of 25% dextrose, infuse at the rate of 2 mL/kg as slow i.v. for 1 h
    Time of onset: 20–30 min
    Duration: 2–4 h
  c. Nebulized salbutamol (beta-2 agonist): 0.05 mL/kg
    Time of onset: 20–30 min
    Duration of action: 4–6 h

Step 4: Elimination of potassium from the body
  a. Frusemide: 1–2 mg/kg i.v.
  b. Potassium exchange resin (Kayexalate)
    Dose: 1 g/kg/dose, oral/rectal
    Time of onset: 4 h
    Duration of action: 4–6 h
  c. Dialysis: Renal failure – excretion of potassium

Approach to Hypocalcemia (Table 49.11)

TABLE 49.11	Approach to Hypocalcemia		
	Total Calcium		**Ionized Calcium**
Hypocalcemia Mg/dL to mmol/L = mg/dL/4	Children: <8.5 mg/dL Term neonate: <8 mg/dL or 2 mmol/L Preterm: <7 mg/dL or 1.75 mmol/L		Children: <2.1 mmol/L Term: <4.8 mg/dL <1.2 mmol/L Preterm: 4 mg/dL <1 mmol/L
Causes	Neonatal hypocalcemia Early: <72 h of birth a. Prematurity b. Birth asphyxia c. Infant of diabetic mother d. IUGR	Late: Onset within 3–7 days a. Phosphate-rich cow's milk, formula feeding b. Transient hypoparathyroidism of newborn c. Magnesium deficiency d. Hypoparathyroidism	Hypocalcemia of infants and children a. Vitamin D deficiency b. Hypoalbuminemia c. Metabolic alkalosis d. Hypoparathyroidism e. Pancreatitis f. Renal failure
Clinical features	Lethargy, poor feeding, seizures, apnea, tetany, cramps, laryngospasm, stridor		
Investigations	1. Serum calcium level (ionized calcium), 25-(OH)-D$_3$ level 2. Alkaline phosphatase, magnesium, Parathyroid hormone (PTH) level 3. ECG – corrected QT interval > 0.46 s		

Management	1. Newborn
	  a. Symptomatic newborn – i.v. 10% calcium gluconate: 2 mL/kg (dilute with 1:1 ratio with 5% dextrose) as bolus under cardiac monitoring followed by maintenance – 80 mg/kg/day (4 mL/kg/day) for 48 h and then 40 mg/kg/day (2 mL/kg/day)
	  b. Asymptomatic newborn – i.v./p.o. calcium gluconate 80 mg/kg/day – for 48 h, followed by maintenance same as mentioned for symptomatic newborn
	2. Children
	  a. Sick children: i.v. 10% calcium gluconate: 1-2 mL/kg i.v. over 3–5 min, maximum of 10 mL
	  b. Not sick: oral 100–200 mg/kg/day		

Approach to Hypercalcemia (Table 49.12)

TABLE 49.12	Approach to Hypercalcemia		
	SERUM CALCIUM > 12 mg/dL **SYMPTOMS PRESENT > 15 mg/dL**		
Hypercalcemia	**Neonate**	**Infant**	**Older Children**
Causes:	a. Excess calcium supplementation b. Secondary hyperparathyroidism (maternal hypocalcemia) c. Primary hyperparathyroidism	a. Subcutaneous fat necrosis b. Vitamin D excess c. Williams syndrome d. Blue diaper syndrome	a. Vitamin D excess b. Primary hyperparathyroidism c. Thiazide diuretics d. Immobilization e. Milk alkali syndrome
Clinical features	Constipation, polyuria, and polydipsia (impairs the ability of the renal tubule to respond to ADH) Signs: Bradycardia, hypertension, proximal muscle weakness, cardiac arrest, and death		
Investigations	1. Serum calcium level (ionized calcium) 2. Serum phosphorous, alkaline phosphatase, magnesium, Parathyroid hormone (PTH) level, 25-(OH)-D$_3$ 3. Urinary calcium estimation – nephrocalcinosis		
Management	Step 1: Diuresis – 1.5–2 times maintenance fluid Step 2: I.v. frusemide Step 3: If serum calcium level > 14 mg/dL – calcitonin 2–4 units/kg every 6–12 h Bisphosphonates – 0.5–1 mg/kg/dose over 4–5 h for 2 days Step 4: Oral steroid 1–2 mg/kg/day Step 5: Refractory hypercalcemia – dialysis If hypercalcemia is due to primary hyperparathyroidism – subtotal parathyroidectomy		

Approach to Hypomagnesemia (Table 49.13)

TABLE 49.13	Approach to Hypomagnesemia			
	SERUM MAGNESIUM < 1.8 mEq/L			
Hypomagnesemia	**Extrarenal**		**Renal**	
Causes	a. Diarrhea b. Vomiting c. Nasogastric suctioning d. Inflammatory bowel disease		a. Drugs – diuretics b. Aminoglycosides c. Tubular injury d. Congenital defect in reabsorption of magnesium	
Clinical features	Central Nervous System (mental changes, tremors)/neuromuscular irritability Signs: Exaggerated Deep tendon reflexes (DTR) carpopedal spasm, tetany			
Investigations	1. Serum magnesium level (spectrophotometry) 2. ECG – ST depression, altered T wave, prolonged PR, widened QRS			
Management	Mild asymptomatic Oral replacement: 10–20 mg/kg/day in three to four divided doses	Moderate symptomatic (hypomagnesemic tetany) I.v./i.m.: 0.4–0.8 mEq/kg (5–10 mg/kg) with 50% $MgSO_4$ (50% $MgSO_4$ = 4 mEq/mL = 48 mg)	Severe symptomatic (hypomagnesemia) I.v. (total = 4 mEq/kg): Day 1: 1 mEq/kg over 2–6 h Days 2–5: 0.5 mEq/kg over 2–4 h	

Approach to Hypermagnesemia (Table 49.14)

TABLE 49.14	Approach to Hypermagnesemia	
	SERUM MAGNESIUM > 2.5 mEq/L	
Hypermagnesemia	**Newborn**	**Children**
Causes	Mother with Pregnancy-induced hypertension (PIH) received $MgSO_4$	a. Intake: Medications, magnesium-containing enemas b. Trauma, shock, burns, cardiac arrest
Clinical features	Nausea, vomiting, lethargy Signs: Hypotonia, absent Deep tendon reflex (DTR), respiratory depression, hypotension, Altered level of consciousness (ALOC)	
Investigations	1. Serum magnesium level (spectrophotometry) Associated electrolyte abnormality – hyperkalemia and hypercalcemia 2. ECG – atrial fibrillation, widening of QRS, conduction delays – heart block	
Management	• I.v. calcium gluconate – 1 mL/kg under cardiac monitoring • Saline diuresis • I.v. frusemide • Nonmagnesium enemas • Refractory – dialysis	

Fluids in Special Situations (Table 49.15)

TABLE 49.15	Fluids in Special Situations
Condition	**Fluid Requirement**
Newborn – warmer/phototherapy	Maintenance fluid + additional fluid (20 mL/kg/day)
Newborn Patent ductus arteriosus (PDA)	Restrict maintenance fluid 120 mL/kg/day
Newborn Bronchopulmonary dysplasia (BPD)	Total fluid = 120–140 mL/kg/day
Newborn necrotizing enterocolitis	Total fluid = 200 mL/kg/day
Acute renal failure	Acute renal failure + oliguria = replacement of insensible water loss (400 mL/m²/day) or 25%–40% of maintenance fluid) with D5 1/2 NS Replace urine output milliliter for milliliter with D5 1/2 NS ± KCl (Nelson)
Polyuria	Replacement of insensible water loss (25%–40% of maintenance) with D5 1/2 NS ± KCl + Measure urine electrolytes + Replace urine output milliliter for milliliter with solution based on measured urine electrolytes (Nelson)
Fever	10%–15% for each rise of 1°C
Ventilated child	Two-third maintenance fluid restriction (humidification of gases)

TABLE 49.15	Fluids in Special Situations—cont'd
Diarrhea	WHO guidelines: Some dehydration – 75 mL/kg over 4 hours(h) Severe dehydration – total 100 mL/kg <1 year – 30 mL/kg over 1 h 70 mL/kg over 5 h year >1 year −30 mL/kg over 30 min 70 mL/kg over 2.5 h
Tachypnea/respiratory problem	Two-third maintenance fluid restriction (Syndrome of Inappropriate Anti-diuretic hormone-SIADH)
Diabetic ketoacidosis (DKA)	Deficit + maintenance fluid over 48 h
Diabetes insipidus (hypernatremic dehydration)	Dehydration % with 0.45% saline
Surgery Preferred – isotonic – crystalloid	• Major (thoracic/abdominal): 10 mL/kg/h of surgery • Others: 2–5 mL/kg/h of surgery • Stromal losses (jejunostomy/ileostomy): Ringer lactate – volume by volume
Idiopathic hypertrophic pyloric stenosis (IHPS)	Dehydration % correction Preferred fluid – 0.45% normal saline in dextrose
Trauma	1 mL of blood can be replaced with 3 mL of crystalloid Blood transfusion for major bleeding with shock
Burns	*Parkland formula* • 4 mL/kg + % of burns + maintenance fluid • 50% of calculated fluid: First 0–8 h • Next 50% of calculated fluid: 9–24 h • Half of the total calculated fluid in 24–48 h
Renal disease	Previous day urine output + insensible water loss (400 mL/m^2)
Replacement fluid for emesis/nasogastric losses	Normal saline + 5 mL (10 mEq KCl) Replace output volume by volume (milliliter for milliliter every 1–6 h)

50 Development

Development

Definition: It is the process of maturation of functions and acquisition of new skills.

Principles of Development

Many a times, developmental milestones may be difficult to remember and many of us have the tendency to cram it quickly and forget it just as fast. However, it is very easy to remember if the principles of development are known, which are as follows:

1. Development is a continuous process from the conception to maturity.
2. Developmental milestones are directly proportional to the myelination of the brain.
3. The sequence of development is same in all children but the rate at which it occurs varies.
4. Generalized mass activity is replaced by specific individual response, e.g., initially child grasps with the entire palm and later pincer grasp occurs indicating that actions become finer.
5. Development occurs in cephalocaudal direction, e.g., first neck holding occurs, then only sitting followed by standing occurs.
6. Certain primitive reflexes have to be lost to achieve voluntary movement, e.g., plantar grasp has to be lost before the baby starts to walk.

Developmental Milestones

These can be split into four domains:

a) Gross motor – development of locomotion
b) Fine motor and vision – development of eye−hand control
c) Speech and hearing – development of language
d) Social and personal – use of acquired abilities to reflect understanding of the environment

According to latest edition of *Illingworth's The Development of the Infant and the young child, 11e*, there are five domains in development milestones which are Motor, Language, Cognitive, Social and Adaptive, and Activities of Daily Living. Tables 50.1 and 50.2 enlist the developmental milestones. For easy remembrance, we can use "Rule of 3," such as 3 months, 6 months, 9 months, and so on until 24 months for the major milestones (Table 50.1). Other months such as 2 months and 5 months have been given in **bold font** to keep these distinct from this rule. Table 50.2 enlists the milestones for the ages 2, 3, 4, and 5 years.

Table 50.3 shows the pictorial depiction of a few gross motor and fine motor milestones.

HEARING

- When a sound is heard, newborn responds by crying, blinking, startling, becoming quiet, or change in the ongoing activity is noticed
- Turns head to source of sound: 3–4 months

TABLE 50.1	Developmental Milestones From Birth up to 2 Years of Age			
Age (Months)	Gross Motor	Fine Motor	Language	Social
2		**Hand regard – observes his or her own hand intently**		**Social smile**
3	Neck holding	Bidexterous approach	Cooing	Recognizes mother
4–5	**Rolling over**	**Mouthing of objects**		
6	Sitting with support	Unidexterous approach	Monosyllables (ma, ba, da, pa)	Mirror play
7		**Transfers objects**		**Stranger anxiety**
8	**Sitting without support**	**Radial palmar grasp**		
9	Crawling	Immature pincer grasp (tries using thumb and index finger for holding objects)	Bisyllables (mama, baba, dada)	Says "bye-bye" Plays peek-a-boo Object permanence
12	Standing without support	Mature pincer grasp, casting of objects (throwing it away), pointing using index finger	Two to three words with meaning	Plays ball game
15	Walking	Scribbling Tower of two	Four to six words Jargon, responds to name calling, names familiar objects	Points for objects, indicates wet pants
18	Running	Tower of three	10 words with meaning, names pictures, identifies body parts by name	Domestic mimicry
21	Climb up the staircase with two feet per step	Tower of six	Speaks simple two-word sentences	Dry by day
24	Climb down the staircase Jumps	Tower of seven, turns single page, unscrews lids, turns door knobs, draws a circular stroke	Two- to three-word sentences	Parallel play, names at least two to three objects, points to two to three body parts

- Turns head to one side and downwards for sounds from below: 5–6 months
- Localizes the sound from above the level of ears: 7 months
- Looks at the source of sound diagonally: 10 months

VISION

- Newborn fixates on and can follow a moving person or bright-colored ring held at 8–10 inches up to a range of 45°
- Can move up to 90°: By 1 month
- Can move up to 180°: By 3 months

- Binocular vision: Begins by 6 weeks and well developed by 4 months
- Adjusting of position to follow objects: 6 months
- Following of rapidly moving objects: 1 year

Red Flag Signs for Developmental Delay

AT ANY AGE

1. Maternal concerns
2. Persistent primitive reflexes
3. Persistent squint

TABLE 50.2	Developmental Milestones Between 2 and 5 Years of Age			
Age (Years)	Gross Motor	Fine Motor	Language	Social
2	Jumping, climbs down the staircase with support, two feet per step	Draws a straight line Tower of seven Forms train	Two- to three-word sentences, knows ~50–100 words	Holds spoon well, parallel play, names at least two to three objects, points to two to three body parts Dry by day
3	Rides tricycle, stands on foot for a few seconds, goes up with one foot per step but comes down two feet per step	Draws a circle Tower of nine Forms a bridge	Says name, age, sex; knows ~250 word	Handedness is established; dresses and undresses but needs help for buttons Dry by night
4	Hops, comes down also with one foot per step	Draws a square/plus/rectangle Forms a gate	Able to tell a poem, story, or song Uses past tense Mention four colors	Goes to toilet alone, role playing, differentiate between right and left
5	Skipping with rope	Draws a triangle/multiplication sign Forms steps (5–6 years)	Ask questions Uses future tense	Dresses and undresses on own, ties shoelaces

Note: Drinks from cup and feeds with spoon but rotates it near mouth: 12–18 months; feeds with spoon without rotation: 18–24 months

TABLE 50.3	Pictures of a Few Gross Motor and Fine Motor Milestones	
	Image	Milestone and Age of Appearance

GROSS MOTOR MILESTONES

1.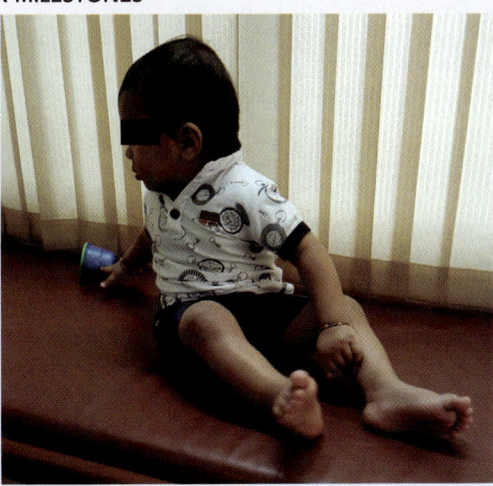

- Pivoting – turns diagonally (Fig. 50.1)
- Seen between 7 and 9 months

Fig. 50.1 Pivoting. (Source: Reproduced from O P Misra, Karen Marcdante, Shakuntala Prabhu et al. *Nelson Essentials of Pediatrics*, First South Asia Edition, Growth and development, FIG. 13-14, New Delhi, Elsevier India, 2016.)

Continued

TABLE 50.3	Pictures of a Few Gross Motor and Fine Motor Milestones—cont'd
Image	**Milestone and Age of Appearance**

2.

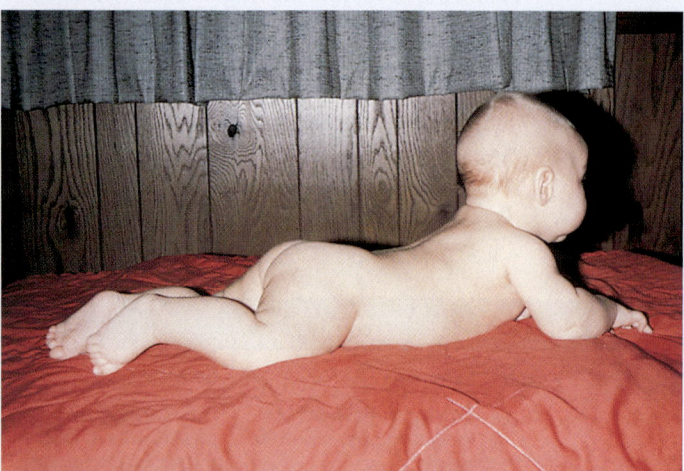

Fig. 50.2   Crawling. (Source: Reproduced from Basil Zitelli, Holly Davis. *Atlas of Pediatric Physical Diagnosis*, Fifth Edition, Developmental-Behavioral Pediatrics, Figure 3-10, Philadelphia, Mosby, 2007.)

- Crawling – abdomen on the ground (Fig. 50.2)
- Seen between 8 and 9 months

3.

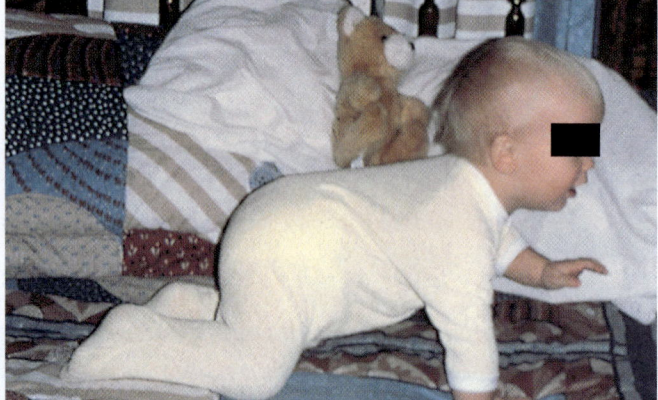

Fig. 50.3   Creeping. (Source: Reproduced from Basil Zitelli, Holly Davis. *Atlas of Pediatric Physical Diagnosis*, Fifth Edition, Developmental-Behavioral Pediatrics, Figure 3-10, Philadelphia, Mosby, 2007.)

- Creeping – abdomen off the ground but knee on the ground (Fig. 50.3)
- Seen between 9 and 10 months

4.

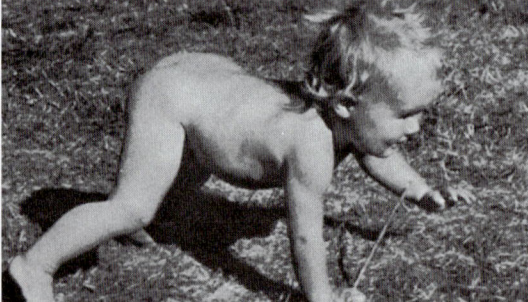

Fig. 50.4   Bear walking. (Source: Reproduced from Robert Palisano, Margo Orlin, Joseph Schreiber. *Campbell's Physical Therapy for Children*, Fifth Edition, Motor Development and Control, FIG. 3.18, St. Louis, Saunders, 2017. (Credit line - ([A] From van Blankenstein M, Welbergen UR, de Haas JH: Le développement du nourrisson: Sa première année en 130 photographies. Paris: Presses Universitaires de France; 1962. p 54.)

- Bear walking – abdomen and knee off the ground (Fig. 50.4)
- Seen at 11 and 12 months

TABLE 50.3	Pictures of a Few Gross Motor and Fine Motor Milestones—cont'd
Image	**Milestone and Age of Appearance**

5.

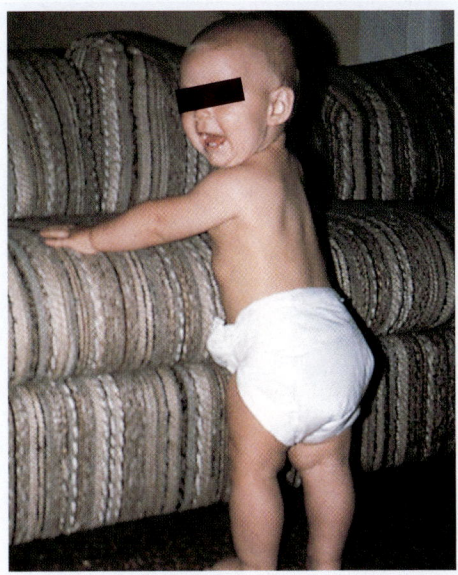

Fig. 50.5 Cruising. (Source: Reproduced from Basil Zitelli, Holly Davis. *Atlas of Pediatric Physical Diagnosis*, Fifth Edition, Developmental-Behavioral Pediatrics, Figure 3-10, Philadelphia, Mosby, 2007.)

- Cruising – holding onto furniture and walking (Fig. 50.5)
- Seen between 11 and 12 months

FINE MOTOR MILESTONES

6.

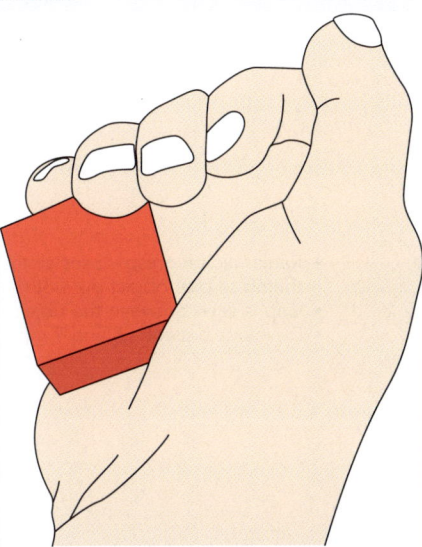

Fig. 50.6 Ulnar grasp.

- Ulnar grasp – the cube is picked up by using the ulnar side of hand (Fig. 50.6)
- Develops between 4 and 6 months

7.

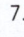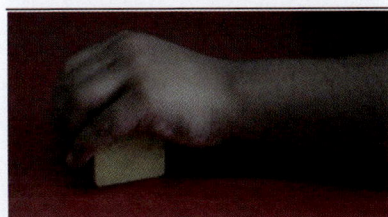

Fig. 50.7 Palmar grasp. (Source: Reproduced from Giovanni Baranello, Davide Rossi Sebastiano, Emanuela Pagliano. Hand function assessment in the first years of life in unilateral cerebral palsy: Correlation with neuroimaging and cortico-spinal reorganization, *European Journal of Paediatric Neurology* 20(1):114-124.)

- Palmar grasp – picks up the cube by using the central portion of the palm without use of thumb finger (Fig. 50.7)
- Develops between 4 and 6 months

Continued

TABLE 50.3	Pictures of a Few Gross Motor and Fine Motor Milestones—cont'd
Image	**Milestone and Age of Appearance**

8.

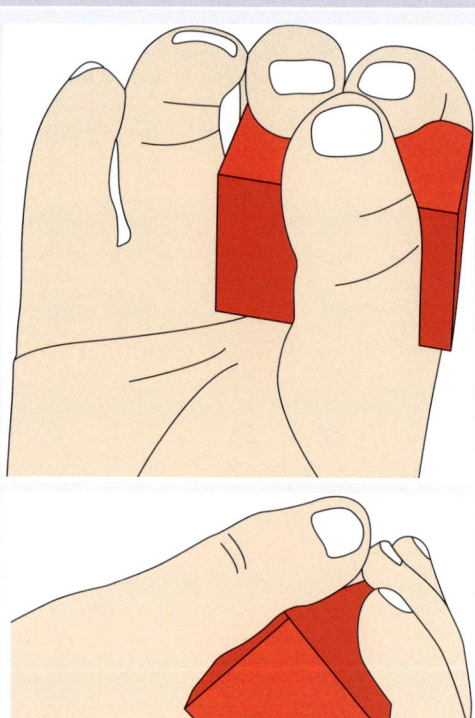

Fig. 50.8   Radial palmar grasp.

- Radial palmar grasp – picks up objects by using the thumb in addition to the central portion of palm (Fig. 50.8)
- No gap seen between the object and palm
- Develops between 6 and 7 months

9.

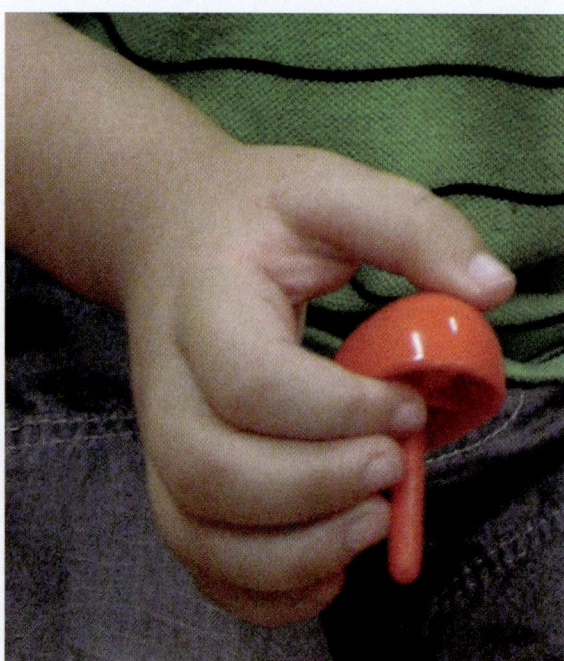

Fig. 50.9   Radial digital grasp. (Source: Reproduced from Emily S. Ho, Measuring Hand Function in the Young Child, *Journal of Hand Therapy* 23(3):323-328.)

- Radial digital grasp – uses all the fingers including thumb to pick object but not the palm (Fig. 50.9)
- Gap is seen between the object the palm
- Develops between 8 and 9 months

TABLE 50.3	Pictures of a Few Gross Motor and Fine Motor Milestones—cont'd
Image	**Milestone and Age of Appearance**

10.

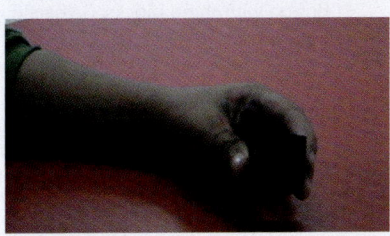

Fig. 50.10 Immature pincer grasp. (Source: Reproduced from Giovanni Baranello, Davide Rossi Sebastiano, Emanuela Pagliano. Hand function assessment in the first years of life in unilateral cerebral palsy: Correlation with neuroimaging and cortico-spinal reorganization, *European Journal of Paediatric Neurology* 20(1):114-124.)

- Immature pincer grasp (Fig. 50.10)
- Develops by 9 months

11.

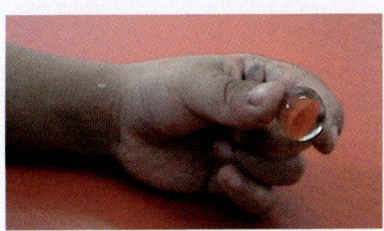

Fig. 50.11 Mature pincer grasp. (Source: Reproduced from Giovanni Baranello, Davide Rossi Sebastiano, Emanuela Pagliano. Hand function assessment in the first years of life in unilateral cerebral palsy: Correlation with neuroimaging and cortico-spinal reorganization, *European Journal of Paediatric Neurology* 20(1):114-124.)

- Mature pincer grasp (Fig. 50.11)
- Develops by 12 months

12.

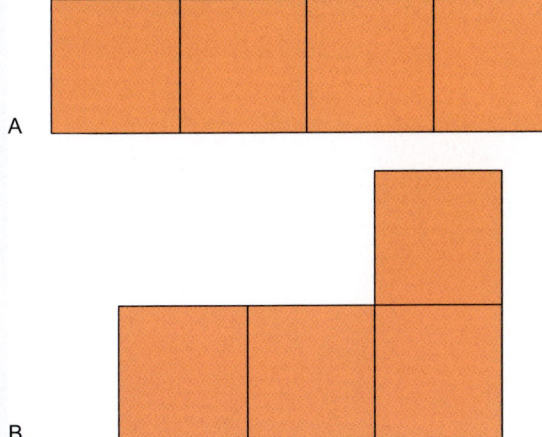

Fig. 50.12 (**A**) Train and (**B**) train with chimney.

Train with four blocks: 2 years of age (Fig. 50.12A)
Train with chimney with four blocks: Seen by 2.5 years of age (Fig. 50.12B)

Continued

TABLE 50.3	Pictures of a Few Gross Motor and Fine Motor Milestones—cont'd
Image	**Milestone and Age of Appearance**

13

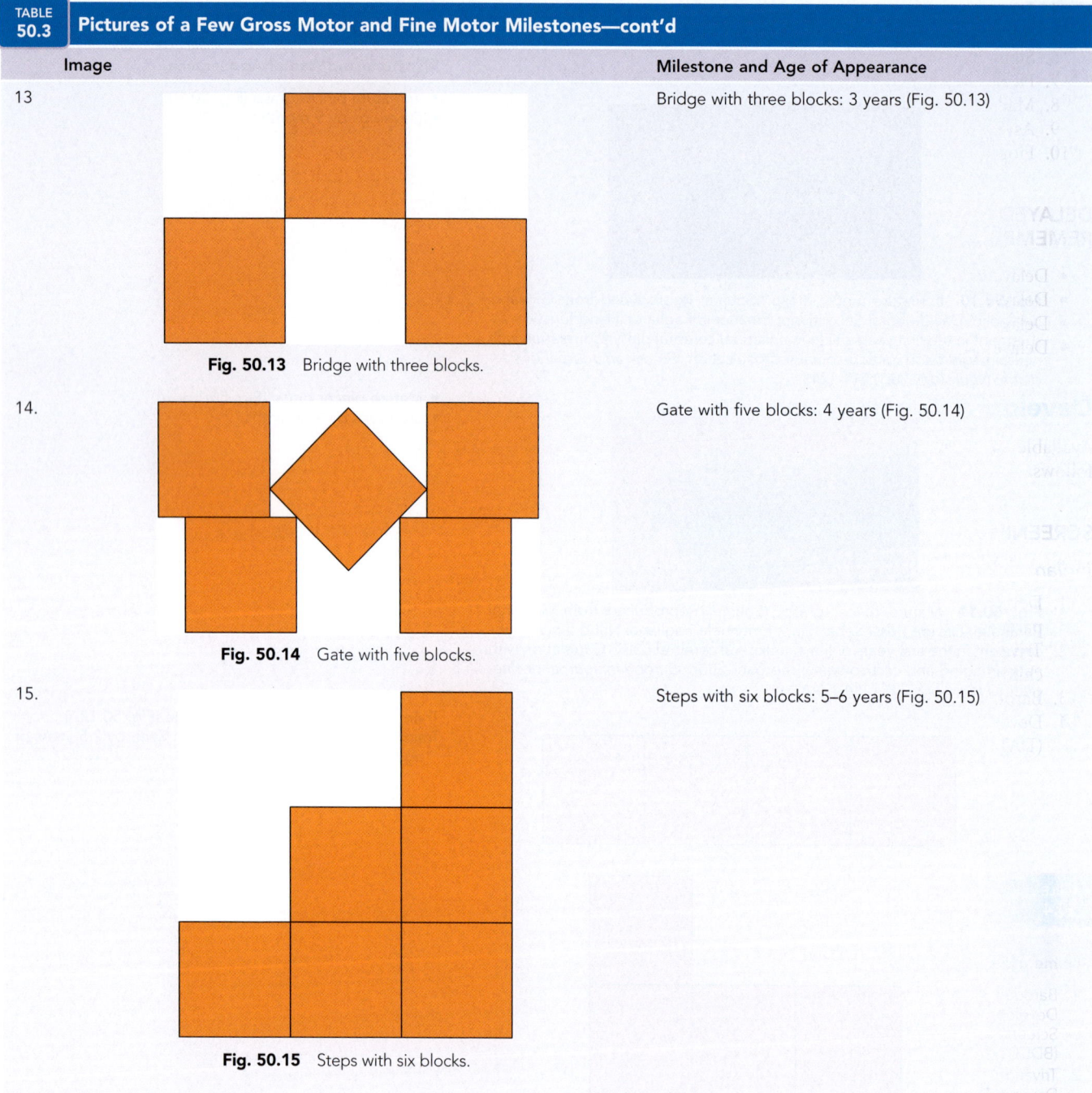

Fig. 50.13   Bridge with three blocks.

Bridge with three blocks: 3 years (Fig. 50.13)

14.

Fig. 50.14   Gate with five blocks.

Gate with five blocks: 4 years (Fig. 50.14)

15.

Fig. 50.15   Steps with six blocks.

Steps with six blocks: 5–6 years (Fig. 50.15)

4. Discordance in development in different domains
5. Regression of previously acquired skills
6. Significant family history
7. Hearing loss at any age
8. Macrocephaly or microcephaly
9. Asymmetry of movements, persistent toe walking
10. Floppiness or increased tone

DELAYED MOTOR MILESTONES (CAN BE REMEMBERED WITH RULE OF 5)

- Delayed neck control by 5 months
- Delayed sitting by 10 months
- Delayed standing by 15 months
- Delayed walking by 20 months

Development Assessment Tools

Available development assessment tools can be divided as follows.

SCREENING TOOLS

Indian

1. Development Observation Card (DOC) – can be used by parents and Anganwadi workers
2. Trivandrum Development Screening Chart (TDSC) – for children between the age of 0 and 2 years
3. Baroda Developmental Screening Test (BDST)
4. Development Assessment Tool for Anganwadi Workers (DATA)

5. ICMR Psychosocial Developmental Screening Test
6. INCLEN Neurodevelopmental Screening Test

International

1. Denver Developmental Screening Test II (DDST) – for children between the age of 2 weeks and 6 years
2. Bayley Infant Neurodevelopmental Screen (BINS)
3. Ages & Stages Questionnaire (ASQ)
4. Parents Evaluation of Developmental Status (PEDS)
5. Developmental Profile I/II
6. Gesell Development Schedule

ASSESSMENT TOOLS

Indian

1. Developmental Assessment Scale for Indian Infants (DASII)
2. Child Development Center (CDC), Kerala, grading for motor milestones

A few of the above-mentioned tests are described in detail in Table 50.4.

Intelligence Assessment Tests and Autism Screening

1. Indian adaptation of Vineland Social Maturity Scale
2. Indian adaptation of Stanford–Binet Test.
3. Revised Wechsler Intelligence Scales
4. M-CHAT-R/F – Modified Checklist for Autism in Toddlers, revised with follow-up
5. Social Communication Questionnaire (SCQ) for autism

TABLE 50.4 Developmental Screening and Assessment Tools

Name of Test	Adaptation	Age Group Assessed	Components	Interpretation	Comments
1. Baroda Developmental Screening Test (BDST)	From Bayley Scale for Infants by P. Phatak	0–30 months	22 motor items 32 mental items Total = 54 items	The total number of items passed is plotted against chronological age; more than 97% is considered pass	Easy to use; adapted for Indian population; sensitivity 66%–93%; specificity 77%–94%
2. Trivandrum Development Screening Chart (TDSC) (Fig. 50.16)	Selected from Baroda norms	Older: 0–2 years Newer: 0–3 years, 3–6 years	17 components (0–2 years) 27 components (0–3 years) 24 components (3–6 years) Contains motor, mental items, hearing and visual function assessment as well	• Each item is shown as a horizontal block which represents 3% and 97% passing the Baroda norms • A vertical line is drawn at chronological age • If a child does not achieve any item to the left side of the line, then assessment for developmental delay should be carried out	• Take only a few minutes • Easy to use • No special training required • Sensitivity – 67%, specificity – 79%
3. DASII	Revision of Baroda norms	0–30 months	67 motor items, 163 mental items Total = 230 items	Based on the number of items passed, development quotient (DQ) is calculated separately for motor and mental items; DQ > 85 is considered normal	• Can be used for detailed assessment • Needs special training, requires special test kit • Takes up to 30–40 min

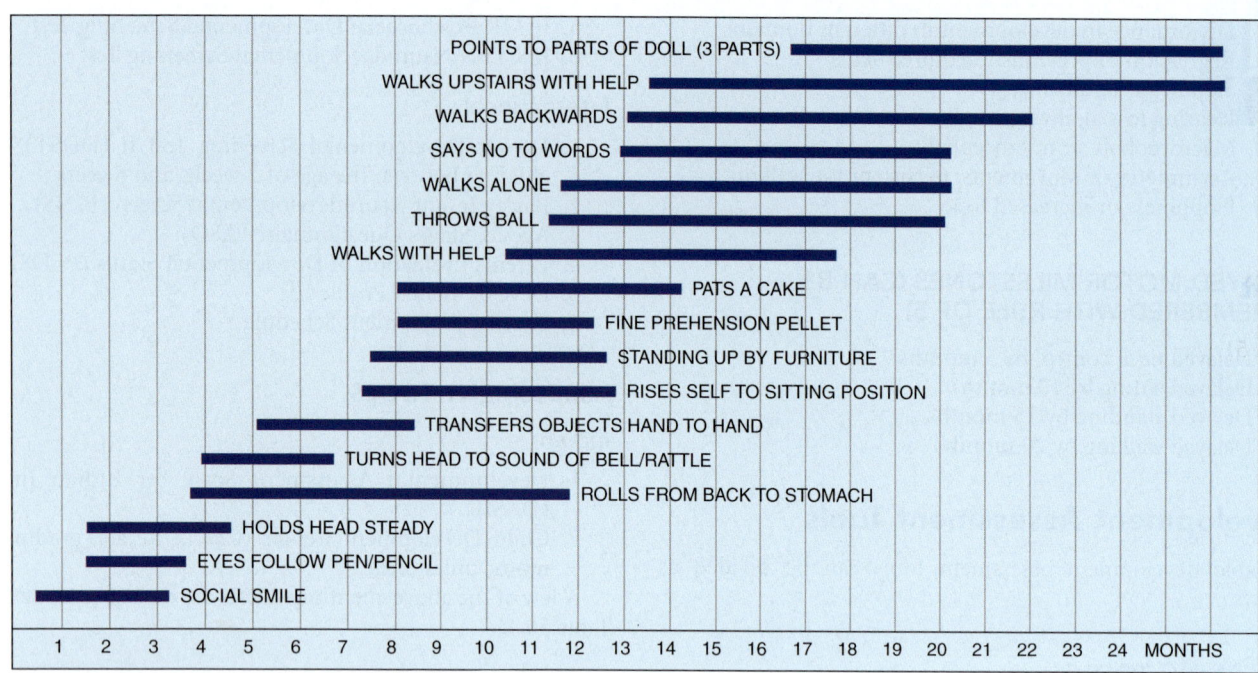

NOTE : To use this chart, keep a pencil vertically on the age of the child. All milestones falling to the left of the pencil should have been achieved by the child. Based on BSID Baroda norms & Trivandrum Developmental Screening Chart (TDSC)

▬▬▬▬ This represents normal range

Fig. 50.16 Trivandrum Developmental Screening Chart. (*Source:* Reproduced from O P Misra, Karen Marcdante, Shakuntala Prabhu. *Nelson Essentials of Pediatrics*, First South Asia Edition, Growth and development, Fig. 13-3, New Delhi, Elsevier India, 2016.)

Development Kit Needed for Examination (Fig. 50.17)

1. A red ring
2. A small bell
3. 10 cubes of 1 inch each
4. Shape form board
5. A picture book of common objects
6. Paper and pen
7. Ball
8. Thread
9. Cards with circle, cross, square, and triangle drawn
10. Color pencils/crayons
11. Tic Tac candies
12. Doll for naming body parts
13. Coloring book

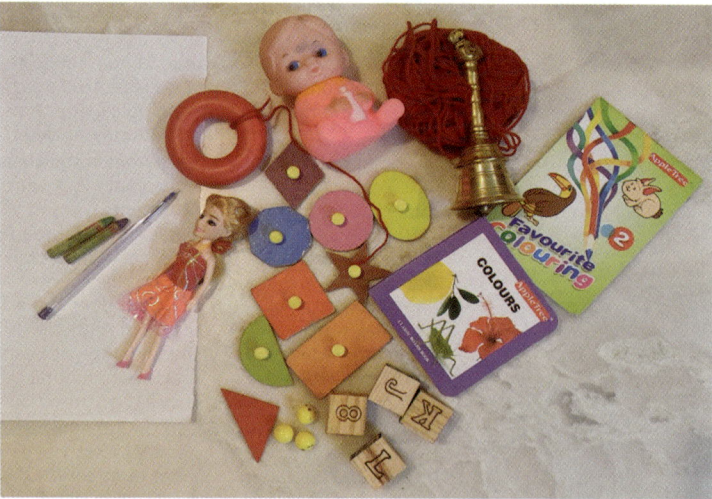

Fig. 50.17 Items to be included in a development kit.

pGALS (paediatric Gait Arms Legs and Spine)

Gait

Fig. 51.1A-B

A.

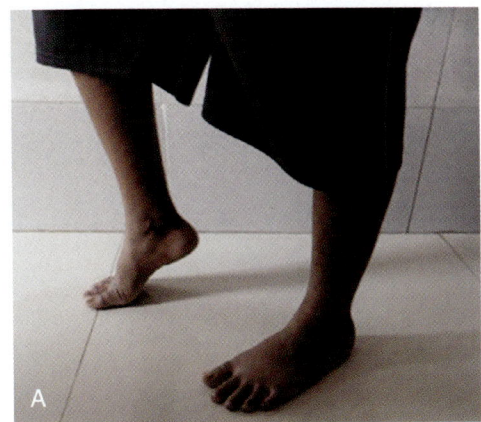

A. "Walk on your tiptoes." Observe the child walking on tiptoes.

B.

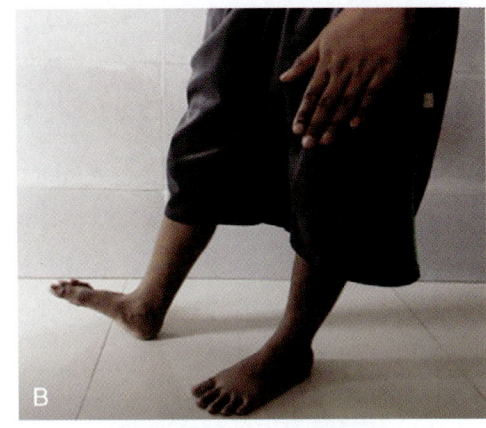

B. "Walk on your heels." Observe the child walking.

Arms

Fig. 51.2A-H

A.

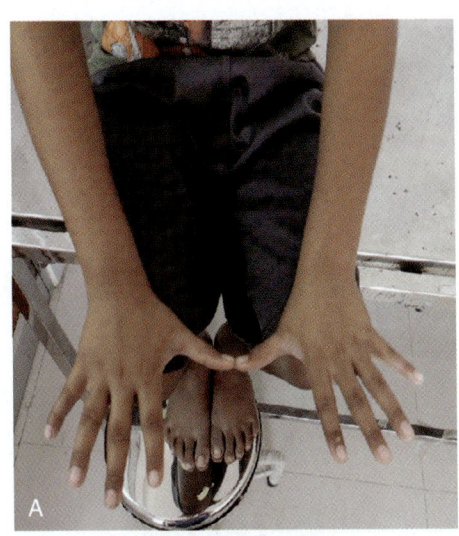

A. "Put your hands out in front of you."

B.

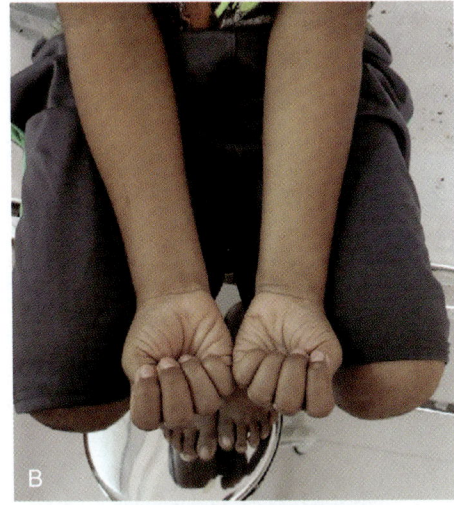

B. "Turn your hands over and make a fist. Pinch your index finger and thumb together."

C.

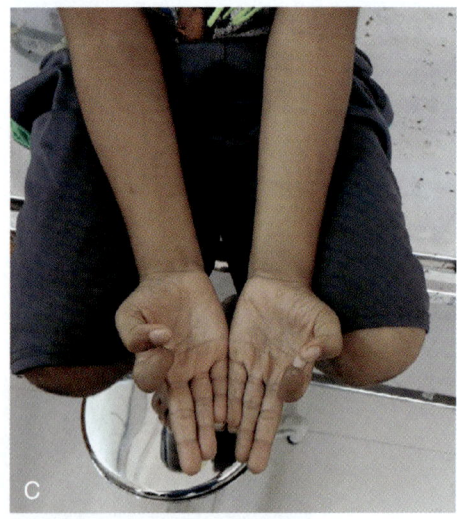

C. "Touch the tips of your fingers with your thumb."

D.

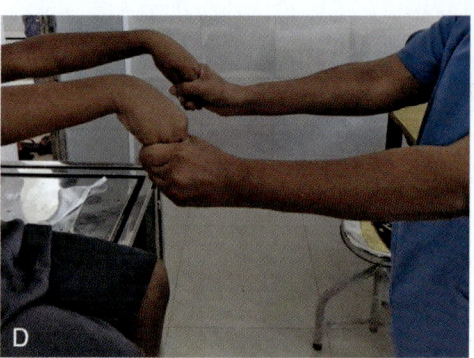

D. Squeeze the metacarpophalangeal joints.

E.

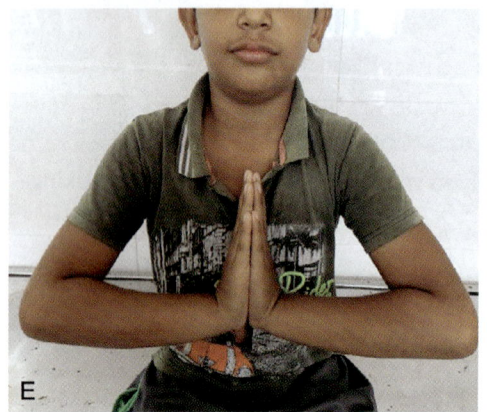

E. "Put your hands together."

F.

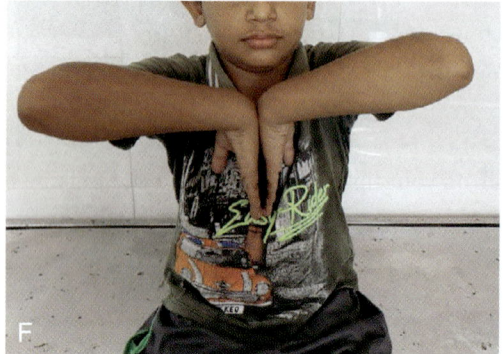

F. "Put your hands back-to-back."

G.

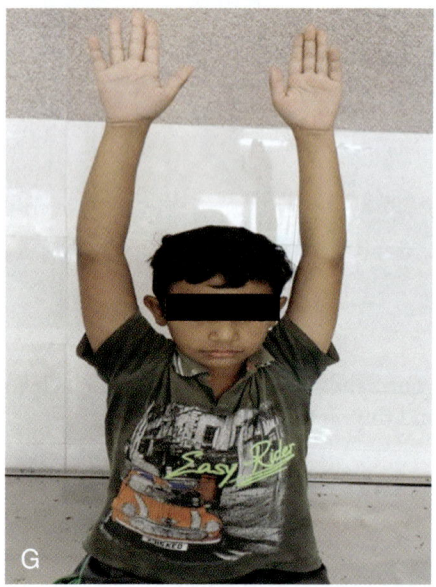

G. "Reach up and touch the sky. Look at the ceiling."

H.

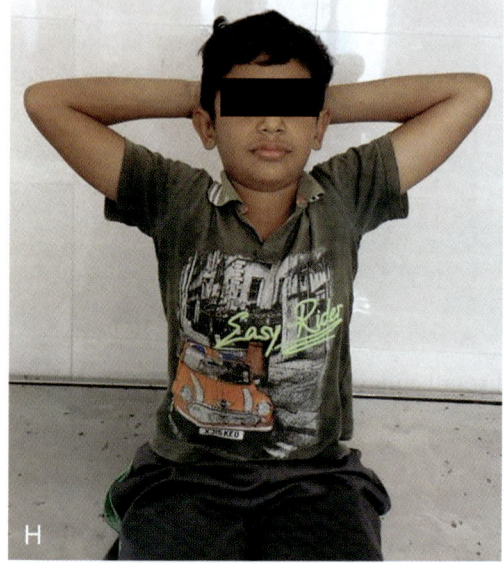

H. "Put your hands behind your neck."

Legs

Fig. 51.3A-C

A.

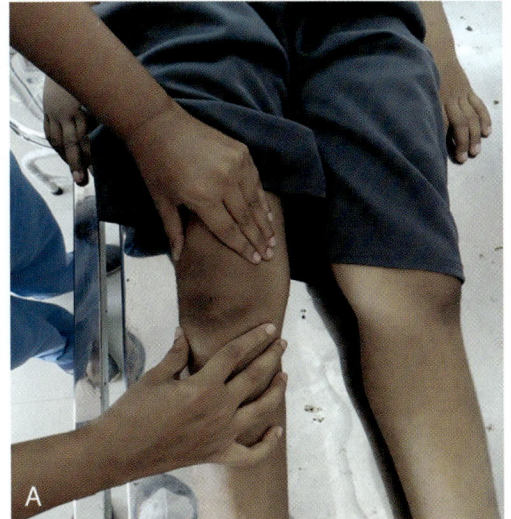

A. Feel for effusion at the knee.

B.

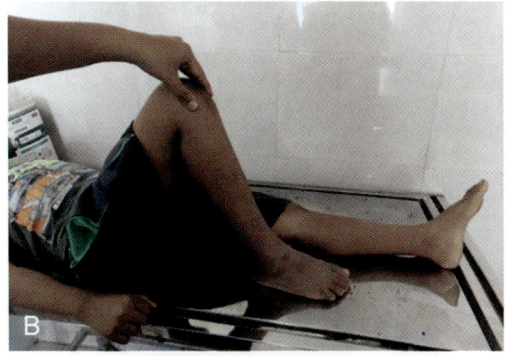

B. "Bend and the straighten your knee."

C.

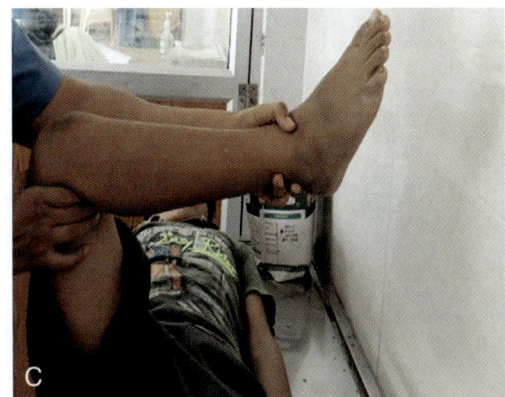

C. Passive flexion (90°) with internal rotation of hip.

Spine

Fig. 51.4A-D

A.

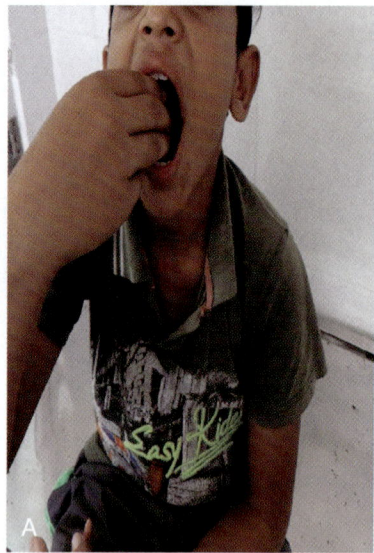

A. "Open your mouth and put three of your (child's own) fingers in your mouth."

B.

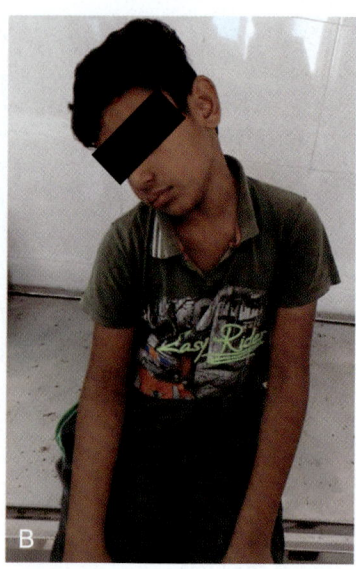

B. Lateral flexion of cervical spine: "Try and touch the shoulder with your ear."

C.

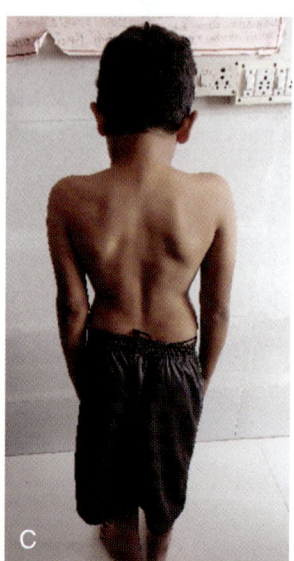

C. Observe the spine from behind.

D.

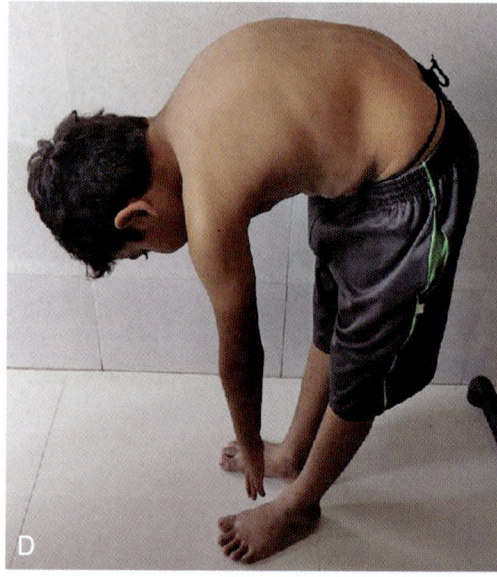

D. "Can you bend and touch your toes?" Observe the spine from side and behind.

Health programs is a vast topic. This chapter is compiled to help students revise their portions in a quick and concise manner before their examinations. This chapter covers the highlights of each program which is important from examination point of view. Textbook reading is mandatory for thorough understanding of the content. Hope this tabular format helps in easy and crisp revision.

Schemes Under National Rural Health Mission (NRHM) (Table 52.1)

Child Nutrition Programs (Table 52.2)

Universal Immunization Programme

1. 1978: Expanded Programme on Immunization (EPI) – limited reach – mostly urban
2. 1985: Universal Immunization Programme (UIP)
   - For reduction of mortality and morbidity due to 6 Vaccine Preventable Disease (VPD)s
   - Indigenous vaccine production capacity enhanced
   - Cold chain established

TABLE 52.1	NRHM Programs			
S. No.	Program	Beneficiaries	Service Provided	Special Feature
1.	Janani Suraksha Yojana (JSY) (April 12, 2005)	Antenatal and postnatal mothers	A) Cash assistance for institutional deliveries and postnatal care in government institutions; mother and Accredited Social Health Activist (ASHA) both get cash B) Vande Mataram Scheme: Any private obstetrician/maternity home/MBBS doctor can volunteer to provide safe motherhood services C) Safe abortion services: Medical method by using mifepristone followed by misoprostol; manual vacuum aspiration is available in Primary Health Centre (PHC)	1. Organizing Health and Nutrition Day once a month at Anganwadi center to provide antenatal/postnatal care and health education to pregnant women 2. Maternal death review at community and facility level 3. Each beneficiary has a JSY card and her pregnancy will be tracked
2.	Janani Shishu Suraksha Karyakram (JSSK) started on June 1, 2011	Pregnant women and children	A) Free transport to hospital and back home for pregnant women and newborn up to 30 days of life and free medical and food services during the hospital stay B) Nutritional Rehabilitation Centers (NRCs) for severe acute malnutrition (SAM)	Services at the NRCs a) Treatment of medical complications b) Therapeutic feeding c) Sensory stimulation and emotional care d) Counselling on preparation of nutritious food hygienically by using locally available food items e) Follow-up of the children after discharge
3.	Integrated Management of Neonatal and Childhood Illness (IMNCI) It is one of the main interventions under Reproductive and Child Health (RCH)-II/National Rural Health Mission (NRHM)	• Sick newborn and children • Young infants up to the age of 2 months • Children aged 2 months to 5 years	Focus on most common cause of mortality Nutrition assessment and counselling for all sick infants and children Individual signs to classify the severity of illness which calls for Specific action (pink — referral; yellow — initiation of treatment in health facility; and green — management at home) Home visit for all newborns: Three visits (within 24 h of birth, days 3–4 and days 7–10); for newborn with low birth weight – three more visits on days 14, 21, and 28	• C-IMNCI (community IMNCI): To empower communities and household to adopt healthy and safe practices to protect health of children younger than 5 years • F-IMNCI: IMNCI + facility-based care package Continuum of quality care for severely ill newborn and children (includes asphyxia management, sepsis, pneumonia, meningitis, and severe malnutrition) • IMNCI + ETAT (IMNCI + Emergency Triage Assessment and Treatment) includes triage, maintain temperature, ABC (Airway, Breathing, Circulation) oxygen, coma, convulsions, and dehydration management

Continued

TABLE 52.1	NRHM Programs—cont'd			
S. No.	Program	Beneficiaries	Service Provided	Special Feature
4.	Rashtriya Bal Swasthya Karyakram (RBSK): February 2013	Newborn and children (1–18 years)	The main idea here is to screen children for the 4 Ds and aid in early detection and management; the 4 Ds are as follows: Defect at birth: Neural tube defect, congenital heart disease, cleft lip and palate, development dysplasia of hip, talipes, Retinopathy of prematurity (ROP), congenital cataract, club foot, Down syndrome Deficiencies: Severe Acute Malnutrition (SAM) anemia, vitamin A deficiency, vitamin D deficiency, goiter Diseases of childhood: Rheumatic heart disease, asthma, convulsive disorders, dental caries, otitis media, skin conditions (scabies, fungal infection, and eczema) Developmental delays including disabilities: Vision and hearing impairment, motor delay, cognitive delay, autism, Attention Deficit Hyperactivity Disorder (ADHD) learning disorder, congenital hypothyroidism, sickle cell anemia, thalassemia	Services offered are as follows: For newborn: At public health facilities, home visits by ASHAs till 6 weeks of age For children aged 6 weeks to 6 years: Screening at Anganwadi by the mobile medical teams For children aged 6–18 years: School health camps once a year by the medical teams
5.	Rashtriya Kishor Swasthya Karyakram (RKSK) (National Adolescent Health Programme) (January 7, 2014)	Adolescents	1. Adolescent nutrition: Weekly iron and folic acid supplementation 2. Information and counselling on adolescent sexual reproductive health and other health issues 3. Menstrual hygiene 4. Adolescent health clinics (reproductive and sexual health services) 5. Preventive health check-ups	Other services provided are as follows: Distribution of sanitary napkins, contraceptives, HIV testing and counselling, abortion facilities, management of sexual abuse, de-addiction facilities
6.	RMNCH + A strategy (2013)	Reproductive, Maternal, Newborn, Child, and Adolescent Health strategy	Reproductive and maternal health: Postpartum Intra-uterine contraceptive device (IUCD) provision of contraceptives, free pregnancy test kits, sterilization services, booking pregnancies in their early antenatal period, management of high-risk pregnancies Newborn health: Essential newborn care at the delivery points, supporting breastfeeding, home-based newborn care, special newborn units with good infrastructure Child health: Complementary feeding, immunization, management of illness (diarrhea and pneumonia) Adolescent health: Prevent adolescent pregnancy, menstrual hygiene, weekly iron and folic acid supplementation, Adolescent Reproductive and Sexual Health Programme (ARSH)	
7.	Weekly Iron and Folic Acid Supplementation (WIFS) Programme (under Adolescent Health Programme)	Adolescent girls and boys	1. Weekly elemental iron (100 mg)/folic acid (500 µg) 2. 52 weeks/year – in school every Monday 3. Biannual deworming – albendazole 400 mg, 6 months apart 4. Improvement in nutrition and prevention of anemia	

TABLE 52.1	NRHM Programs—cont'd			
S. No.	Program	Beneficiaries	Service Provided	Special Feature

8.	Indian Newborn Action Plan (INAP)	Started on September 18, 2014. Root to tertiary care involving girls, women, mother, newborn, children – adolescents. Target – single digit NMR and stillbirths by 2030. Consists of Home based newborn care (HBNC), Newborn Stabilization Unit (NBSU), Facility based newborn care (FBNC), Special newborn care unit (SNCU)	• Six pillars:
			  • Preconception and Antenatal care (ANC)
			  • Care during labor/childbirth
			  • Care of newborn at birth
			  • Care of healthy newborn
			  • Care of small and sick newborn
			  • Care beyond newborn survival	

TABLE 52.2	Child Nutrition Programs				
S. No.	Program	Beneficiaries	Service Provided	Duration	Special Care
1.	Integrated Child Development Services (ICDS)	Children younger than 6 years, pregnant and lactating mothers. Women aged 15–45 years. Adolescent girls	For children 1–6 years: 300 kcal, 15 g protein. Pregnant women: 500 kcal, 25 g protein	300 days/year	Iron and Folic acid, iodine salt
2.	Immunization	Children – six vaccines. Ante-Natal Care (ANC) mothers	Vaccination		ANC health check-ups
3.	Health check-ups and treatment of minor illness	Children younger than 6 years, ANC, malnourished people	Referral service, education plan. Adolescent scheme	1. Aganwadi center (1000 population in rural and 750 in urban) 2. Mukhya Sevika: 20–25 centers supervision 3. Child development project officer	1. Decrease rural communicable disease 2. Tribal development block 3. Urban group slum
4.	Nutrition deficiency prevention: Vitamin A deficiency	RCH programme – 5 megadoses of vitamin A. Children younger than 3 years	First dose – 9 months. Second dose – 15–18 months. 6 months – 3 doses		
5.	National Nutritional Anaemia Prophylaxis Programme	Children aged 1–5 years. Pregnant and lactating mothers. Family planning	1. 1 tablet (100 mg iron + 0.5 mg folic acid): ANC 2. Preschool: 20 mg iron + 0.1 mg folic acid 3. Deworm to prevent hookworm infestation 4. Anemic pregnant mothers: 200 mg iron + 1 mg folic acid		
6.	National Iodine Deficiency Disorders Control Programme (NIDDCP)		Iodated salt (15 ppm) at the household level		
7.	Mid Day Meal Scheme	Children aged 6–11 years	300 kcal/8–12 g proteins	200 days/year	
8.	Special Nutrition Programme	Children aged 1–3 years	6–72 months: 300 kcal with 10 g protein. SAM: 600 kcal/20 g proteins. Mother: 500 kcal with 20 g protein		

Continued

TABLE 52.2	**Child Nutrition Programs—cont'd**				
S. No.	Program	Beneficiaries	Service Provided	Duration	Special Care
9.	Balwadi Nutrition Programme.	3–5 years	300 kcal 10 g protein	270 days/year	
10.	Applied Nutrition	Children aged 3–6 years	Health education training for mass population Staff training		
11.	Prime Minister's Overarching Scheme for Holistic Nutrition or POSHAN Abhiyaan (earlier called National Nutritional Mission): Malnutrition-free India by 2022	Infants and young children	To reduce stunting Improve utilization of Anganwadi services		Early childhood development (ECD) Early childhood care and education (ECCE)

- Phased implementation – all districts covered by 1989–1990
- Monitoring and evaluation system implemented

3. 2014: India which was declared as free of wild poliovirus transmission in the year 2014 (last case was reported on January 13, 2011), and is currently following the Polio Eradication Endgame Strategic Plan as follows:
   a. India has switched from trivalent OPV (tOPV) to bivalent OPV (bOPV) on April 25, 2016, both in polio campaigns and routine immunization.
   b. As a risk mitigation measure, country has introduced inactivated polio vaccine, two fractional doses, given intradermally at 6 and 14 weeks.

4. *Pulse Polio Programme in India*: National Immunization Days (NIDs) commonly known as Pulse Polio Immunization Programme was launched in India in 1995 and is conducted twice in early part of each year. In addition, multiple rounds (at least two) of sub-NIDs have been conducted in high-risk areas.

5. Japanese encephalitis (JE) vaccine is being given as a routine in 179 endemic districts.

6. MR vaccine was introduced through a campaign in 2017 and slowly introduced in the routine immunization program by replacing two doses of measles vaccine

7. *Mission Indradhanush*:
   Government of India had launched it as a flagship on December 25, 2014.
   Aim: To improve the full immunization coverage in the country from the current 65% to more than 90% through special immunization drives.
   Focus: Districts with poor immunization coverage were identified and covered in a phased manner where children would receive all the due vaccines.
   Participants: ANM, health supervisors and ASHAs, Anganwadi workers, and link workers.
   Vaccines under Mission *Indradhanush*: Diphtheria, pertussis, tetanus, childhood TB, polio, hepatitis B, and measles are included here. In addition to this, vaccines for JE and *Haemophilus influenzae* type b (Hib) are also being provided in certain states.

X-ray Head and Neck

Approach to head and neck X-ray is shown in Flowchart 53.1.

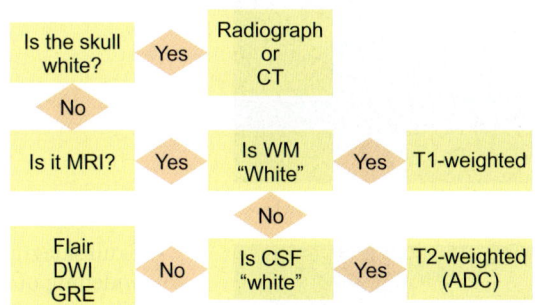

Flowchart 53.1 Approach to head and neck X-ray.

X-RAY HEAD

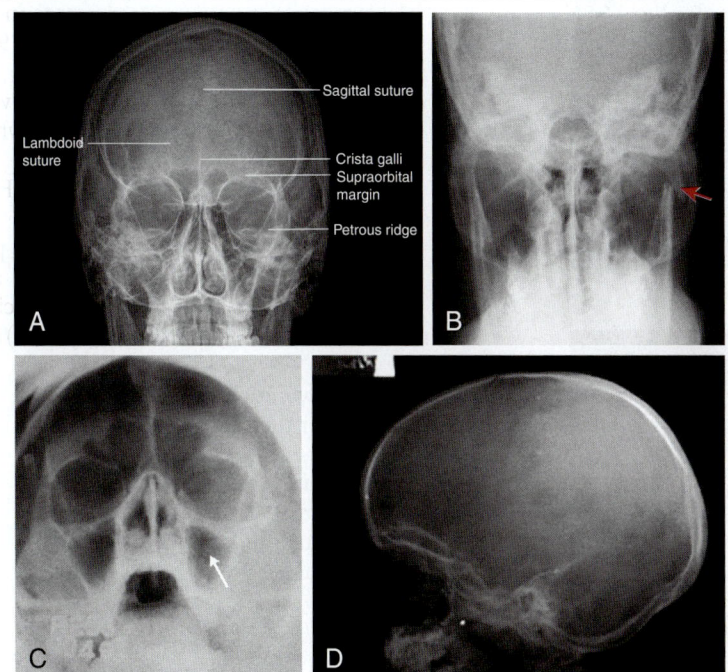

(A) Cadwell view – PA view.
(B) Towne view.
(C) Waters view.
(D) Lateral view.

Commonest view – lateral view

Fig. 53.1 (A to D) Various views of skull X-ray. *(Source (A) http://www.wiki-radiography.net/page/Skull_Radiographic_Anatomy. (B) Reproduced from Raymond Fonseca. Oral and Maxillofacial Surgery: 3-Volume Set,* Third Edition, Imaging of the Temporomandibular Joint, Figure 37-3, St. Louis, Saunders, 2018. *(C) Reproduced from P. L. Dhingra, Shruti Dhingra. Diseases of Ear, Nose and Throat & Head and Neck Surgery,* Eighth Edition, Some imaging techniques in ENT, Fig. 96.3, New Delhi, Elsevier India, 2022.)*

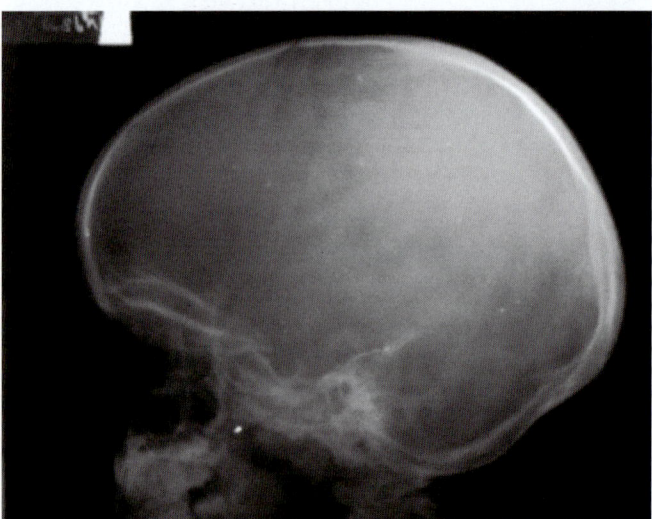

Fig. 53.2 Normal skull X-ray – lateral view (commonest view).

Examine for
  a. Size and shape
  b. Thickness and density of the bone
  c. Sutures and vascular markings
  d. Calcification
  e. Lucent or sclerotic defects
  f. Base of the skull and cranial cavity

Normal skull skiagram

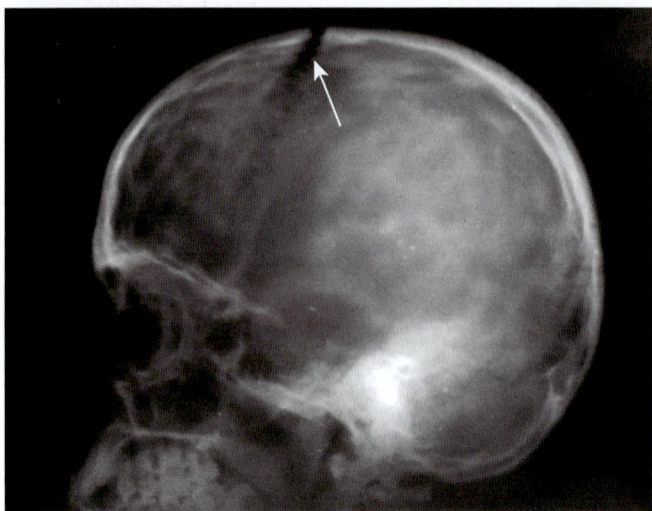

Fig. 53.3 Silver-beaten appearance (raised ICP).

- Skull skiagram showing widening of sutures
- Silver-beaten appearance

- Seen in **raised intracranial tension**

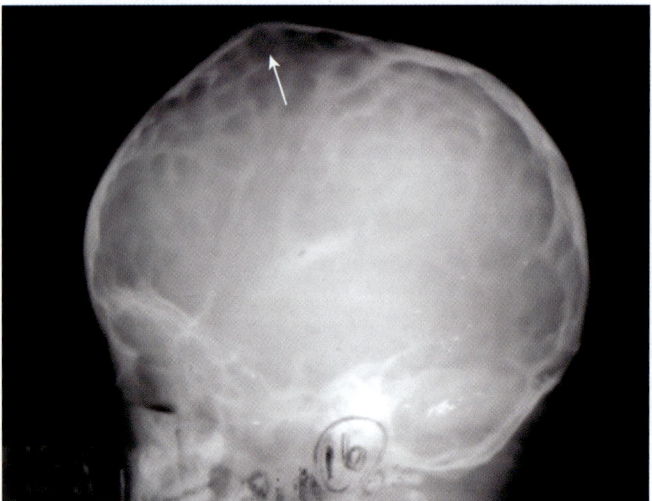

Fig. 53.4 Craniosynostosis.

- Premature closure of sutures
- Exaggerated convolutional markings all over the skull vault
- None of the sutures seen
- Sutures do not fuse regularly, resulting in irregular skull shape

Craniosynostosis

- Copper-beaten appearance
- Mandibular prognathism, maxillary hypoplasia

Crouzon syndrome

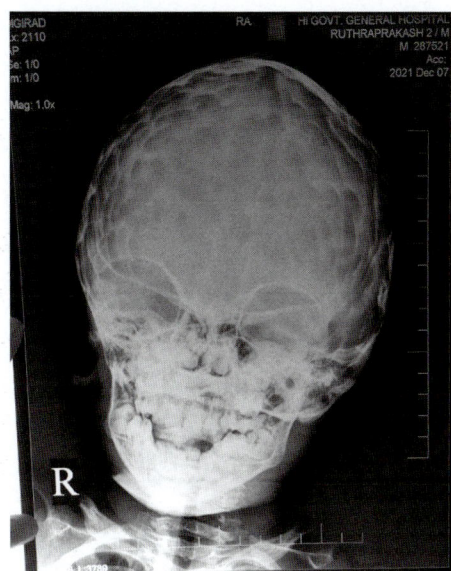

Fig. 53.5   Crouzon syndrome.

Overriding of sutures

Microcephaly with overriding of sutures

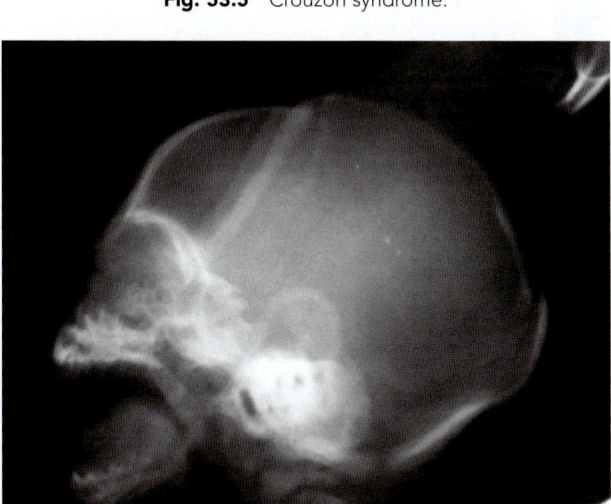

Fig. 53.6   Microcephaly with overriding of sutures.

- X-ray skull shows widening of the diploic spaces of the cranial bones
- Coarsened trabeculae
- Hair on end appearance indicating extramedullary hematopoiesis

- **Anemic changes**
- Classically occurs in beta thalassemia Diagnosed in late or improperly managed children

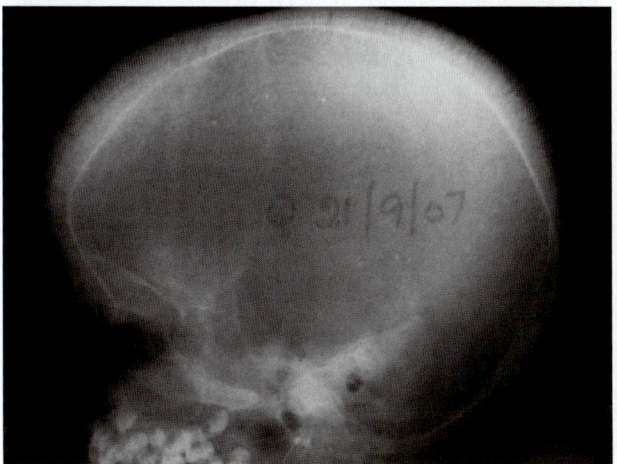

Fig. 53.7   Hair on end appearance – beta thalassemia.

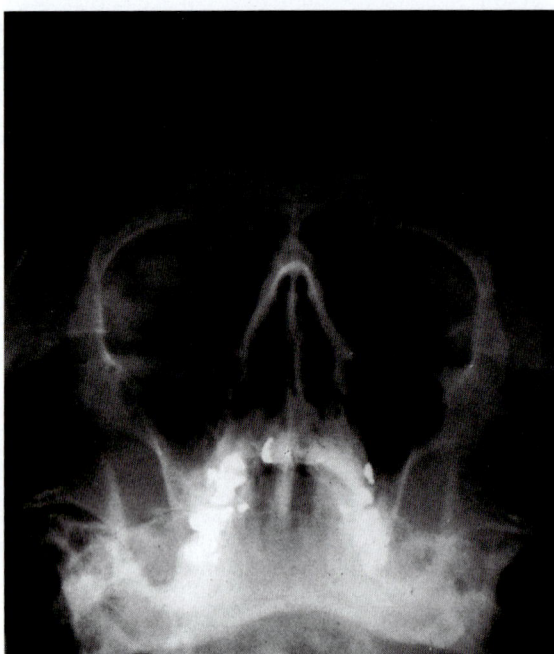

Fig. 53.8 *(Source:* Reproduced from Joen Iannucci, Laura Jansen Howerton. *Dental Radiography: Principles and Techniques*, Fifth Edition, Extraoral Imaging, FIG 23-8, St. Louis, Saunders, 2017. (Credit line -From Whaites and Drage: Essentials of dental radiography and radiology, ed 5, London, 2013, Churchill Livingstone.)

- Waters view shows bilateral maxillary antrum, frontal sinuses, ethmoid sinuses and lower margin of sphenoid sinuses

Other name: **Occipitomental view** – to identify maxillary sinus pathology – sinusitis, polyp

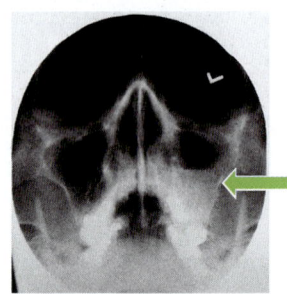

Fig. 53.9   Maxillary sinusitis. *(Source:* Modified from Nina Kowalczyk. *Radiographic Pathology for Technologists*, Eighth Edition, Respiratory System, FIG. 3.50, St. Louis, Saunders, 2022.)

- Opacification of maxillary sinus (air-fluid level in left maxillary sinus suggestive of maxillary sinusitis)

Maxillary sinus pathology

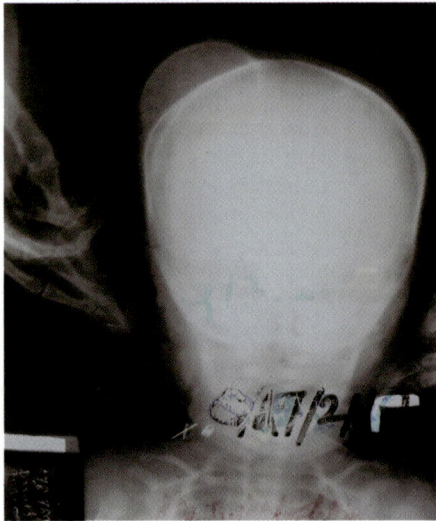

Fig. 53.10   Cephalhematoma.

- X-ray skull PA view – cephalhematoma.
- Right parietal region with linear skull fracture with soft tissue swelling

Cephalohematoma

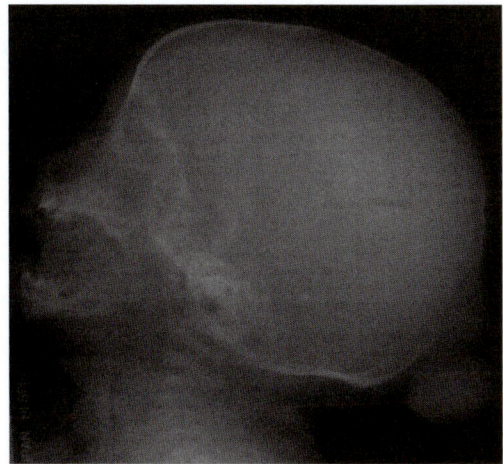

Fig. 53.11 Occipital encephalocele.

- Lucent area seen in the occipital region

Occipital encephalocele

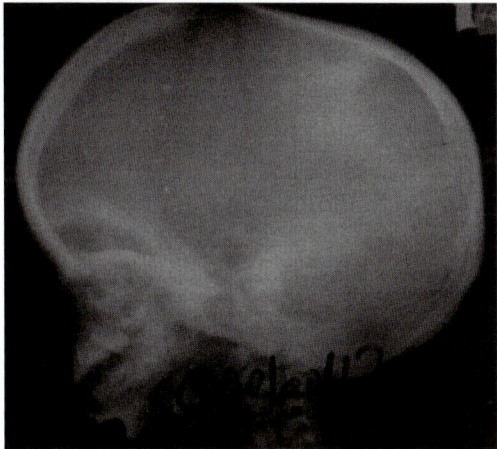

Fig. 53.12 Dermoid scalp.

- Well-circumscribed lucency over the coronal suture

Dermoid scalp

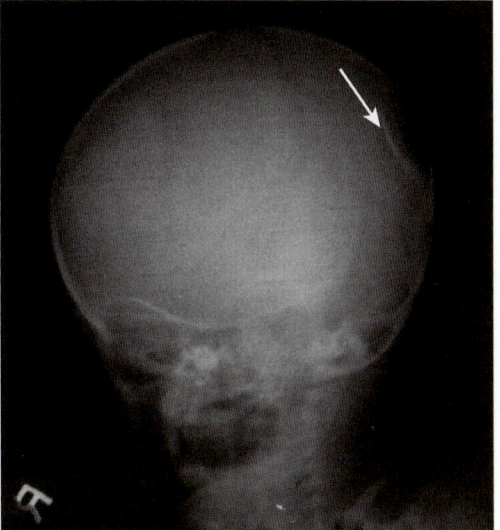

Fig. 53.13 Depressed skull fracture.

- Frontal radiograph shows parallel dense lines due to depressed bone fragments and associated lucency due to absence of bone

Depressed skull fracture

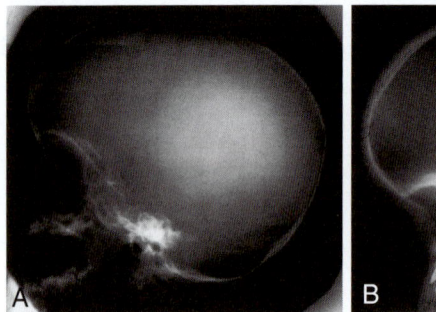 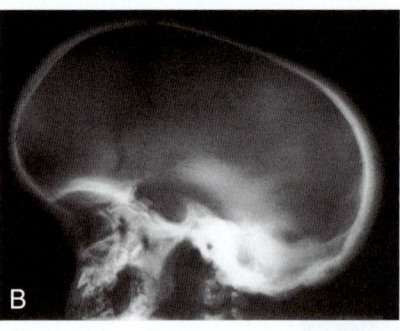

(A) Lateral radiograph of skull shows relatively large cranial vault with narrow skull base

(B) Prominent forehead with depressed nasal bridge

Achondroplasia skull X-ray

Fig. 53.14 A Large cranial vault with narrow skull base. B. Prominent forehead with depressed nasal bridge. *(Source:* (A) Reproduced from Thomas Pope, Hans Bloem, Javier Beltran et al. *Imaging of the Musculoskeletal System,* Dysplasias, FIGURE 103-1, Philadelphia, Saunders, 2008. *(B)* Reproduced from Donald Ortner. *Identification of Pathological Conditions in Human Skeletal Remains,* Second Edition, Skeletal Dysplasias and Related Diseases, FIGURE 19-10, London, Academic Press, 2003.)

X-RAY NECK

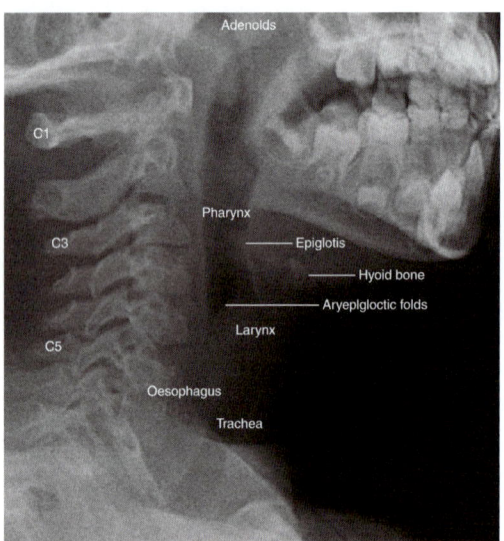

- X-ray lateral view of the neck

Normal lateral view of neck

Fig. 53.15 Normal lateral view of neck. *(Source: Analysing lateral soft tissue neck radiographs | Semantic Scholar)*

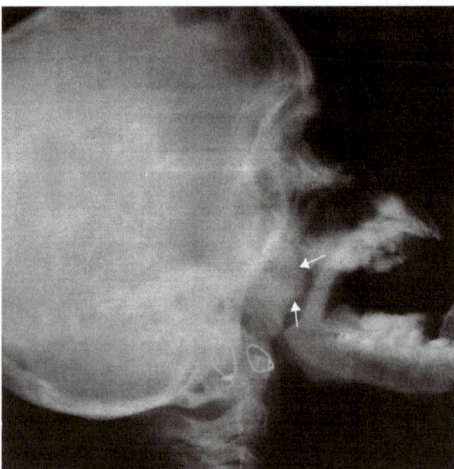

- X-ray nasopharynx showing enlarged adenoids (taken in full extension of head and full inspiration)
- Adenoids are invisible in less than 6 months and regress after 6 years of age
- Improper positioning results in false positive due to pseudosubluxation

Adenoids

Fig. 53.16. Adenoids. *(Source:* Reproduced from P. L. Dhingra, Shruti Dhingra. *Diseases of Ear, Nose and Throat & Head and Neck Surgery,* Eighth Edition, Adenoids and other inflammations of nasopharynx, Fig. 48.4, New Delhi, Elsevier India, 2022.)

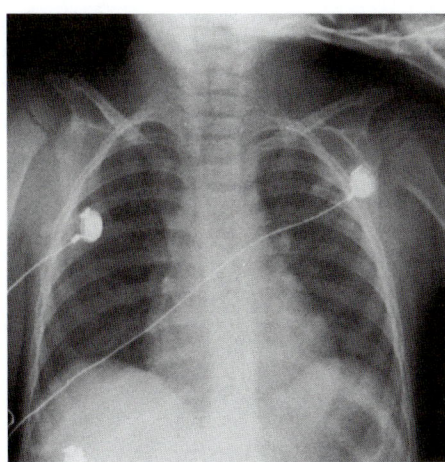

- X-ray of a child with croup showing typical subglottic narrowing (steeple sign)

Steeple sign – acute laryngotracheal bronchitis (croup)

Fig. 53.17. Steeple sign – acute laryngotracheal bronchitis (croup). *(Source:* Modified from Nelson Textbook of Pediatrics. Acute Inflammatory Upper Airway Obstruction (Croup, Epiglottitis, Laryngitis, and Bacterial Tracheitis, Fig. 412.1, 2020.)

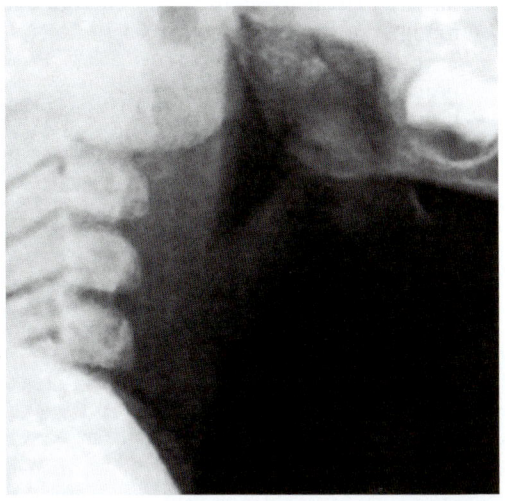

- Lateral X-ray of upper airway shows swollen epiglottis (thumb sign)

Thumb sign – acute epiglottitis

Fig. 53.18. Thumb sign – acute epiglottitis. *(Source:* Reproduced from Nelson Textbook of Pediatrics. Acute Inflammatory Upper Airway Obstruction (Croup, Epiglottitis, Laryngitis, and Bacterial Tracheitis, Fig. 412.2, 2020.)

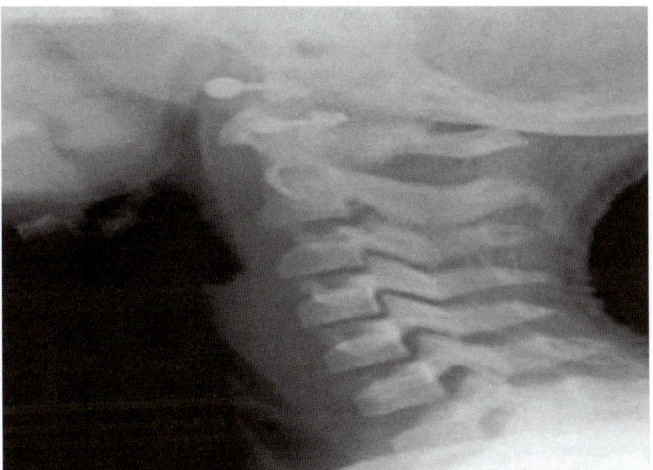

- Lateral radiograph of neck of a child with bacterial tracheitis showing pseudomembrane detachment in trachea

Bacterial tracheitis

Fig. 53.19. Bacterial tracheitis. *(Source:* Reproduced from Nelson Textbook of Pediatrics. Acute Inflammatory Upper Airway Obstruction (Croup, Epiglottitis, Laryngitis, and Bacterial Tracheitis, Fig. 412.3, (c) 2020.)

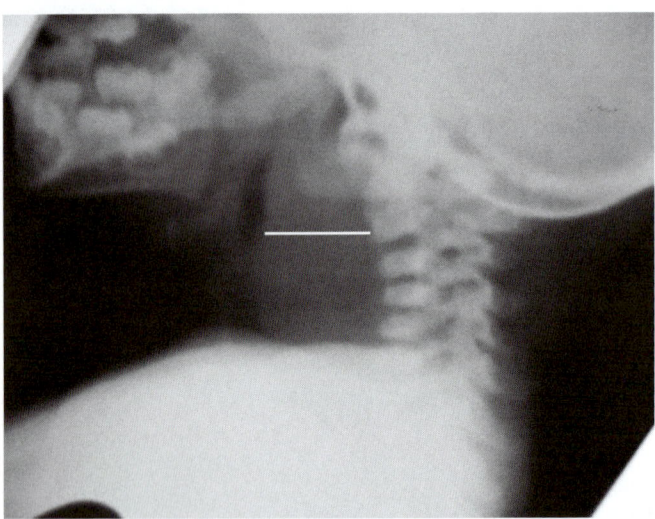

Fig. 53.20. Retropharyngeal abscess.

- Prevertebral soft tissue varies with age and location
- In children
  - Normal: At C3 – <7 mm (or less than 1/3rd of the vertebral body)
  - At C6 – <14 mm (less than that of the vertebral body)
- Prevertebral space is grossly widened
- Cervical vertebra appears normal

Retropharyngeal abscess

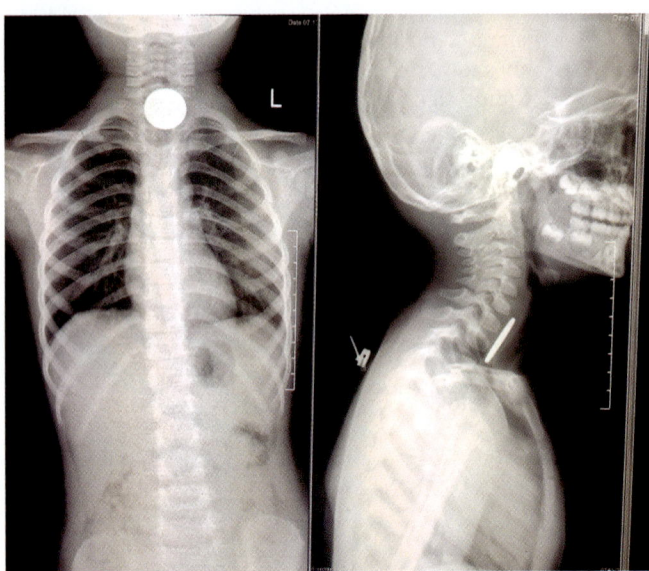

Fig. 53.21. Foreign body – coin.

To differentiate between the foreign body in esophagus or in trachea – look for the appearance of the coin in X-ray
- If the foreign body is seen in full surface in AP film, it is in esophagus and not in trachea

Foreign body – coin

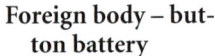

Fig. 53.22. Foreign body – button battery.

- Lateral X-ray helps to distinguish between a button battery and coin
- Immediate removal: Nose, ear, pharynx, esophagus
- Esophageal ulceration can occur within 4 hours
- >15 mm unlikely to pass pylorus
- If they pass pylorus, 90% pass out within 3 weeks

Foreign body – button battery

Chest X-ray

General principles in chest X-ray:
- Name, hospital number, date and time, and side mark
- Plain or contrast
- Projection AP or PA
- Phase of respiration
- Any rotation: Symmetry of medial ends of clavicle
- Exposure

HOW TO READ A CHEST X-RAY

AP view
- Usually taken in infant and preschool children
- Clavicle horizontal – notch seen in the middle of the clavicle
- Scapula away from lung shadow
- No lung tissue above the clavicular shadow
- Vertebral bodies more prominent

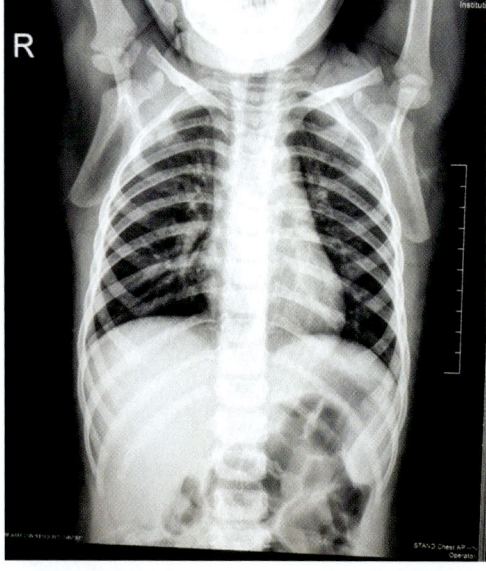

Fig. 53.23.   Chest X-ray AP view.

PA view
- Usually taken in older children
- Clavicle oblique – no notch seen in the middle of the clavicle
- Scapula within lung shadow
- Lung tissue seen above the clavicular shadow

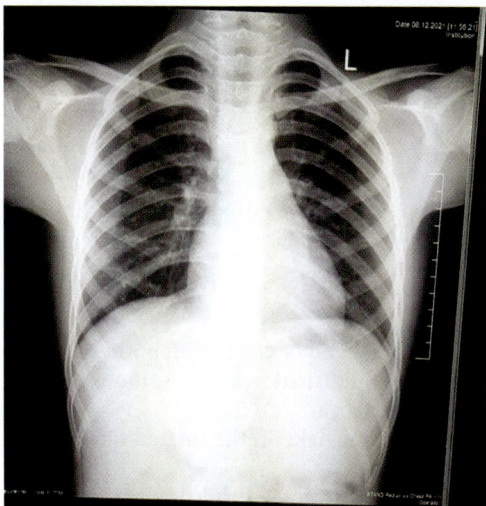

Fig. 53.24.   Chest X-ray PA view.

Phases of respiration
- At full inspiration (A), Dome of diaphragm corresponds to the anterior ends of 5th–7th rib and posteriorly 8th–10th rib
- Expiratory film (B) exaggerates the heart size and bronchovascular markings
- Inspiratory film: Anterior rib – 6th
- Midinspiratory film: Anterior rib – 5th
- Expiratory film: Anterior rib – 4th

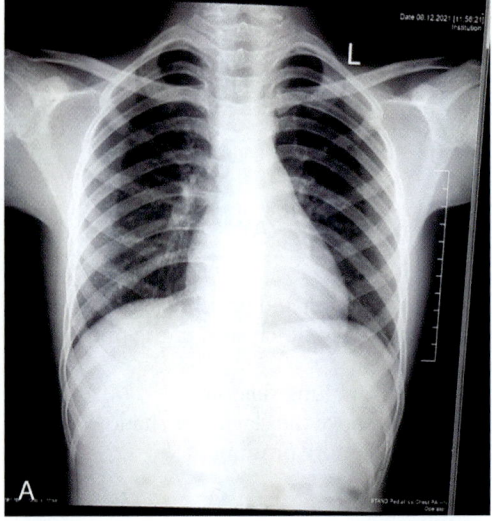

Fig. 53.25A.   (A) Inspiratory film.

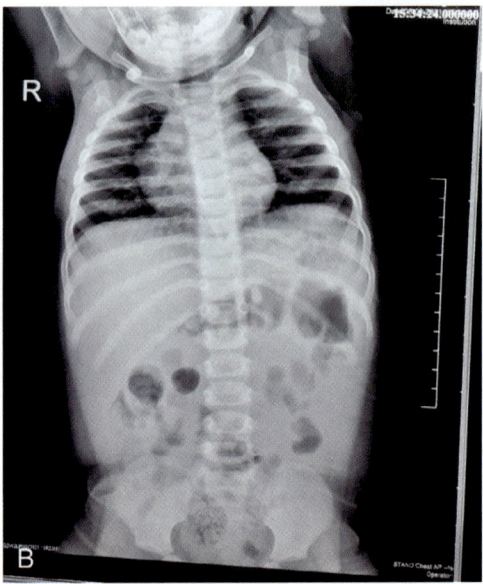

Fig. 53.25B.   (B) Expiratory film.

Normal film – medial end of clavicle on both sides should be equidistant from the spinous process of the vertebra

Rotated film – the lung field on the rotated side looks hyperlucent

Medial end of clavicle on rotated side is closer to vertebra

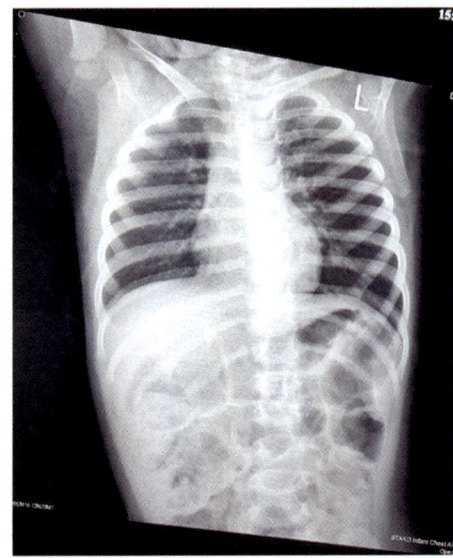

Fig. 53.26.   Rotated film.

- Proper exposure/Properly penetrated CXR: Lower thoracic vertebra should be visible through the heart; detailed spine, intervertebral disk, and pulmonary vessels are seen behind the heart
- Underexposed film (A): Cardiac shadow is opaque with little or no visibility of thoracic vertebra; the spine is not visible; lungs become whiter and denser, they appear as if infiltrates are present
- Overexposed film (B): Heart becomes more lucent; lungs become proportionately darker; only the spine is visible, not the pulmonary vessels; lung peripheries become extremely radiolucent as in emphysema

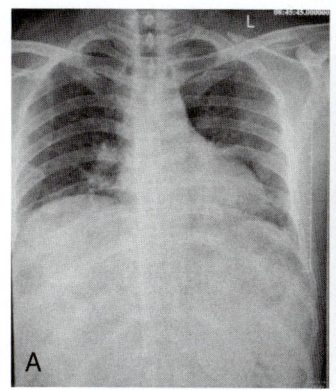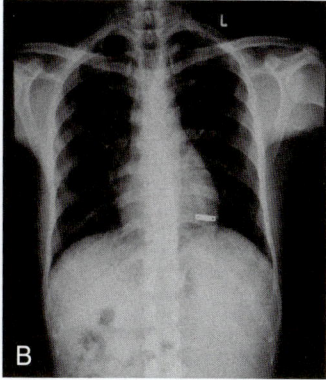

Fig. 53.27.   (A) Underexposed. (B) Overexposed.

A TO E IN CHEST X-RAY

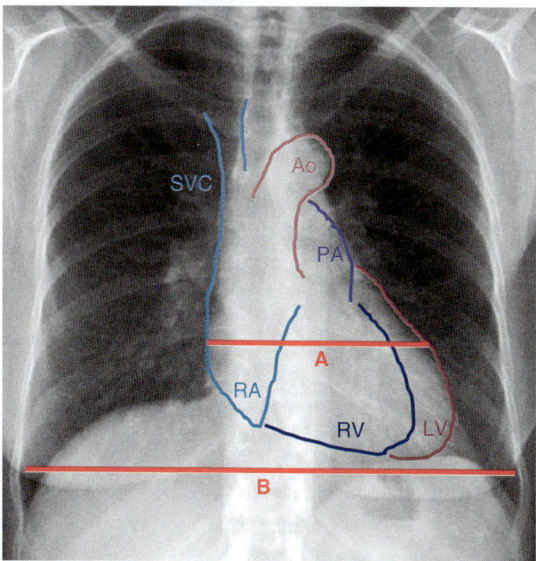

Fig. 53.28.   Chest X-ray – markings. *(Source: Modified from Sarah Sarvis Milla, Shailee Lala. Problem Solving in Pediatric Imaging,* Imaging the Child With Respiratory Distress, Fig. 1.7, Philadelphia, Elsevier Inc., 2023.)

A: Airway	1. Position of clavicle
	2. Trachea position – carina at the level of T4–T5
	3. Lung volume – increased or decreased (Compare on both side)
	4. Air outside the lung (pneumothorax, pneumomediastinum)
	5. Air under the diaphragm
B: Bones	1. Ribs
	2. Horizontal – anterior ribs
	3. Oblique – posterior ribs
	4. Check for crowding of ribs – collapse
	5. Fracture
	6. Increased or decreased density of bones
	7. Flail chest (fracture of two or more consecutive ribs in two or more segments)
	8. Any bifid ribs
	9. Vertebral body density
	• Hemivertebra (errors of segmentation)
C: Cardiac shadow	1. Cardiothoracic angle
	2. Cardiac shape
	• Egg shape (TGA), money bag appearance (pericardial effusion), boot-shaped heart (TOF), figure of 8 (TAPVC)
D: Diaphragm	Position (elevated – eventration)
	Air under the diaphragm – visceral perforation
E: Extra	Thymic shadow, mediastinal node, soft tissue swelling

NORMAL CHEST X-RAY

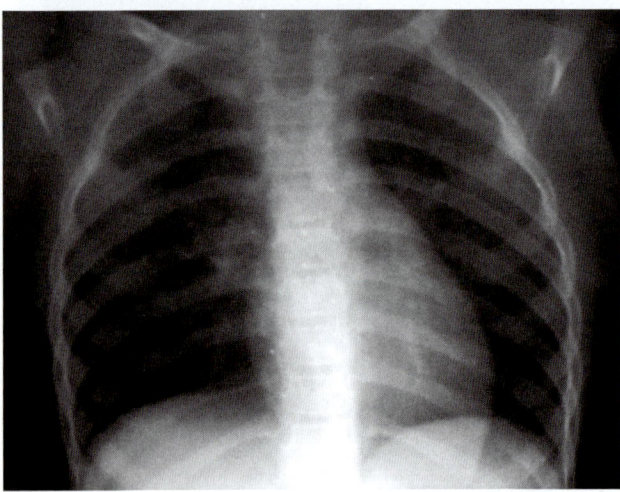

Fig. 53.29.   Normal chest X-ray.

- Whether readable quality
- Look for symmetry – medial end of clavicles
- Both sides – equal in volume
- Equal in aeration (translucency)
- Penetration

Always go by the following eight questions while reading a chest X-ray:

1. Color or lucency (more white or black)
2. Volume of hemithorax (small or large)
3. Mediastinal shift
4. Costophrenic angle (obliterated)
5. Tubes – tracheal tube, NG tube, chest tube, VP shunt
6. Lines
7. Above the diaphragm
8. Below the diaphragm

WHITE SHADOWS

- Varying density, air bronchogram – pneumonia
- Uniform density, decreased volume, mediastinal shift, rapid change – collapse
- Triangular, uniform density – segmental collapse
- Uniform density, CP angle lost – pleural fluid
- Bilateral – pulmonary edema, ARDS
- Foreign body
- Tumor and fibrosis rare in children

Examples of White Shadows in X-ray

X-ray	Interpretation	Diagnosis
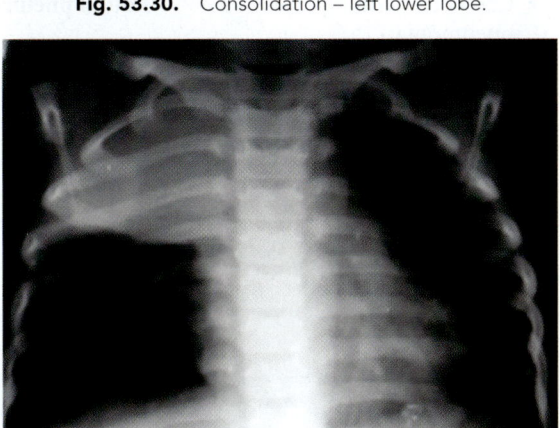 **Fig. 53.30.** Consolidation – left lower lobe.	• Uniform haziness in left lower hemithorax • No mediastinal shift • No loss of lung volume • Costophrenic angle free and left dome of diaphragm not pulled up	**Consolidation – left lower lobe**
Fig. 53.31. Consolidation – right upper lobe.	• Uniform haziness in right upper hemithorax • No mediastinal shift • No loss of lung volume	**Consolidation – right upper lobe**
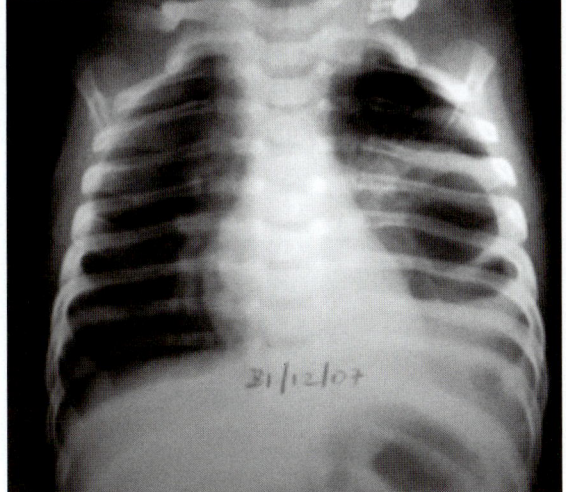 **Fig. 53.32.** Pneumonia with pneumatocele – left lower lobe.	• Small lucent areas within the left lower zone haziness • No air fluid level	**Pneumonia with pneumatocele –** left lower lobe

X-ray	Interpretation	Diagnosis

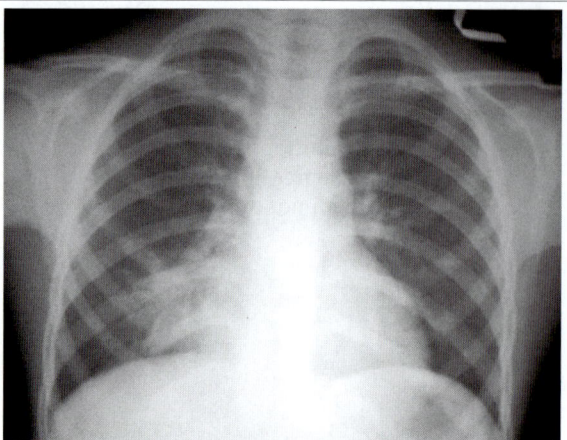

Fig. 53.33.   Pneumonia – right middle lobe.

- Haziness in right lower hemithorax
- Right heart border not clearly seen (patch merging with right heart border)
- No loss of lung volume

Pneumonia – right middle lobe

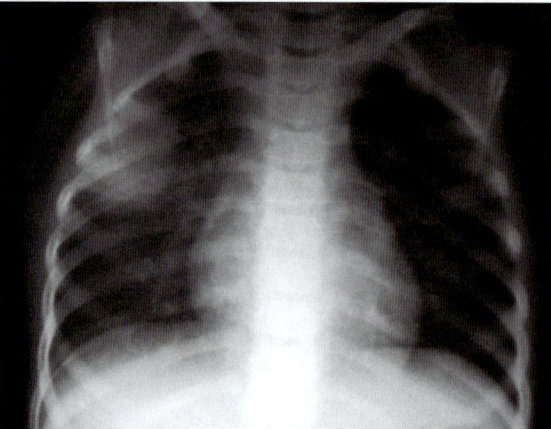

Fig. 53.34.   Round pneumonia.

- Can occur with mycoplasma pneumonia
- Round homogenous opacity in periphery of right upper zone
- No mediastinal shift
- No loss of lung volume

Round pneumonia

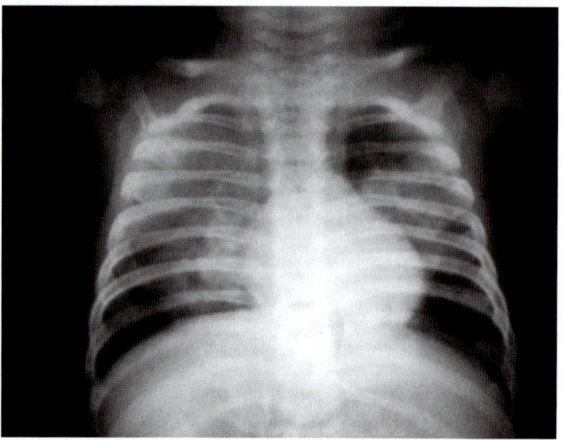

Fig. 53.35.   Extensive bronchopneumonia.

- Patchy heterogenous opacities seen in both lung fields
- No mediastinal shift
- No loss of lung volume

Extensive broncho-pneumonia

X-ray	Interpretation	Diagnosis
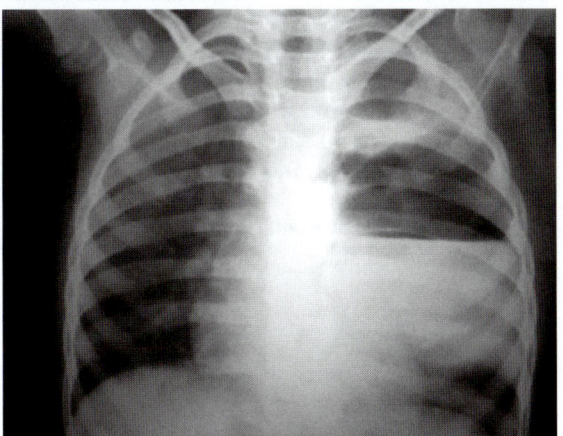**Fig. 53.36.** Lung abscess – left upper lobe.	• Air fluid level in the left hemi-thorax merging with the upper cardiac silhouette • Left costophrenic and cardio-phrenic angles are free • Normal bronchovascular markings on the right side	**Lung abscess – left upper lobe**
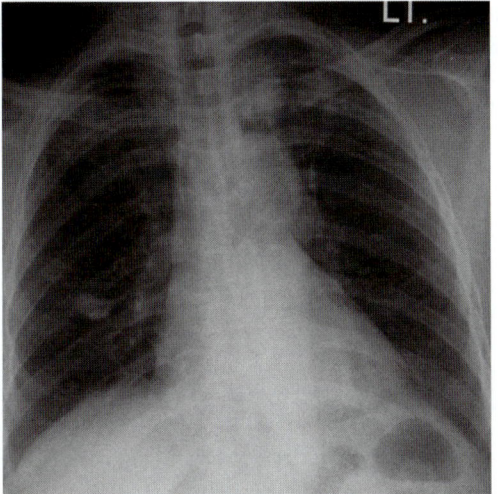**Fig. 53.37.** Gohn focus. *(Source: Reproduced from* Patricia Walker, William Stauffer, Elizabeth Barnett et al. *Immigrant Medicine*, First Edition, Tuberculosis, Fig. 19.5, Edinburgh, Saunders, 2007.	Well-circumscribed small opacity – Gohn focus	**Gohn focus**
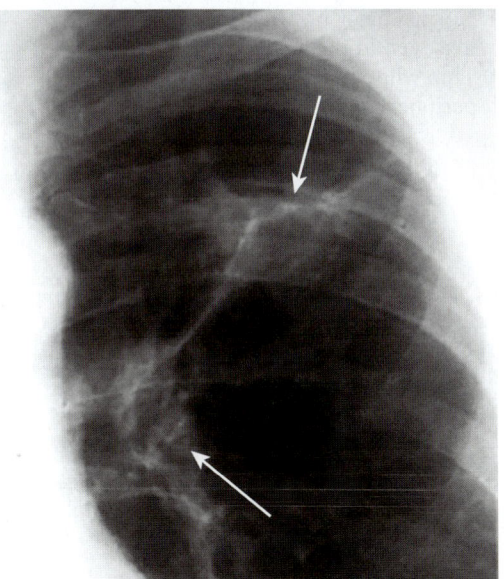**Fig. 53.38.** Gohn complex. *(Source: https://en.wikipedia.org/wiki/ File:Chest_x-ray_of_Gohn%27s_complex_of_active_tuberculosis.jpg)*	• Gohn complex consist of Gohn focus + pulmonary lymphadenopathy	**Ranke complex =** Calcified Gohn complex

X-ray	Interpretation	Diagnosis

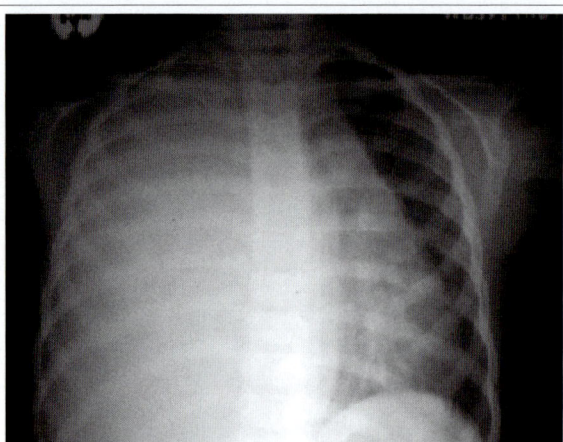

Fig. 53.39. Empyema thoracis – right.

Interpretation:
- Homogenous opacity in the right hemithorax with absent bronchovascular markings
- Widening of the intercostal spaces on the right side
- Shift of mediastinum to the left side
- Normal bronchovascular markings in the left side

Diagnosis: **Empyema thoracis – right**

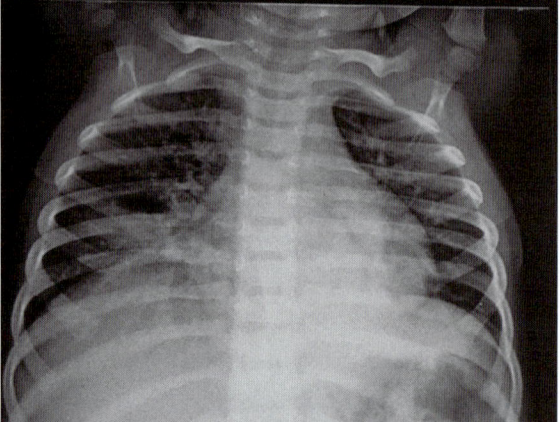

Fig. 53.40. Subpulmonic effusion.

Interpretation:
Right lower lobe haziness
Elevation of right diaphragm

Diagnosis: **Subpulmonic effusion**

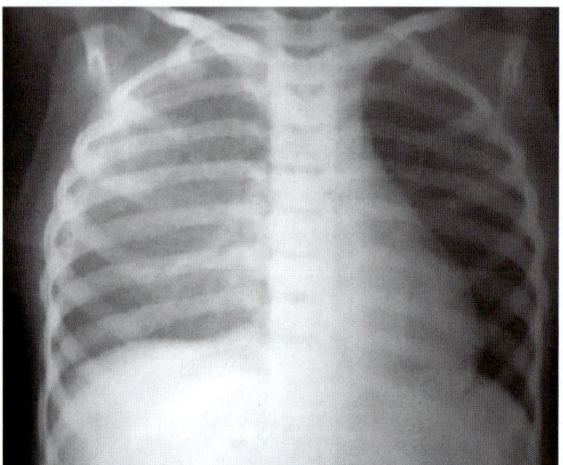

Fig. 53.41. Pleural fluid – right.

Interpretation:
- Right hemithorax appears more white when compared to left hemithorax
- No mediastinal shift
- Normal bronchovascular markings seen in the left side
- Thin white line seen in the periphery of right hemithorax

Diagnosis: **Pleural fluid – right**

X-ray	Interpretation	Diagnosis

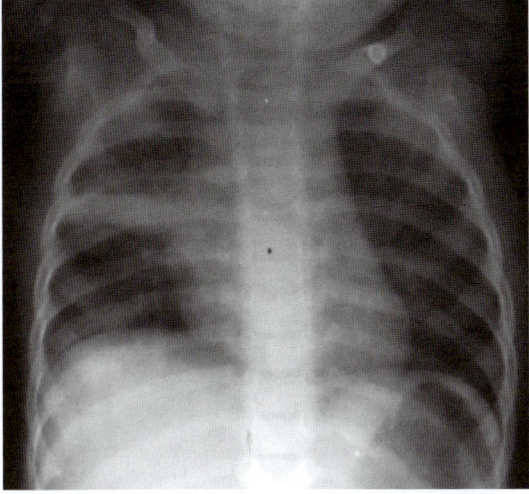

- Band-like opacity in the right mid-zone
- Bronchovascular markings seen normally in both lung fields
- Can occur in some pneumonias, congestive cardiac failure

Minor fissure effusion – right side

Fig. 53.42.   Minor fissure effusion – right side.

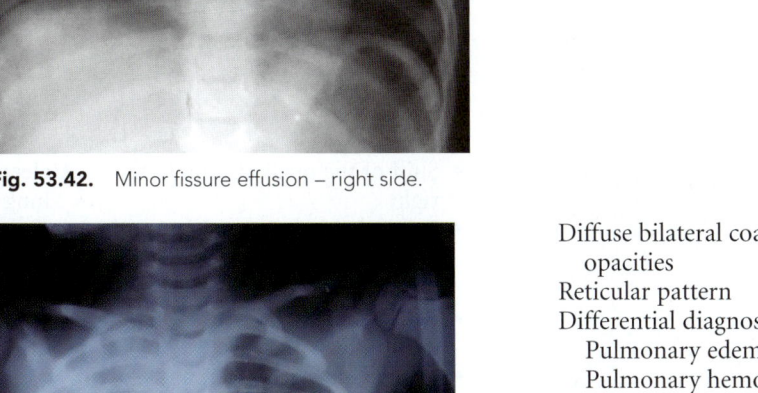

Diffuse bilateral coalescent opacities
Reticular pattern
Differential diagnoses:
   Pulmonary edema
   Pulmonary hemorrhage

ARDS

Fig. 53.43.   ARDS.

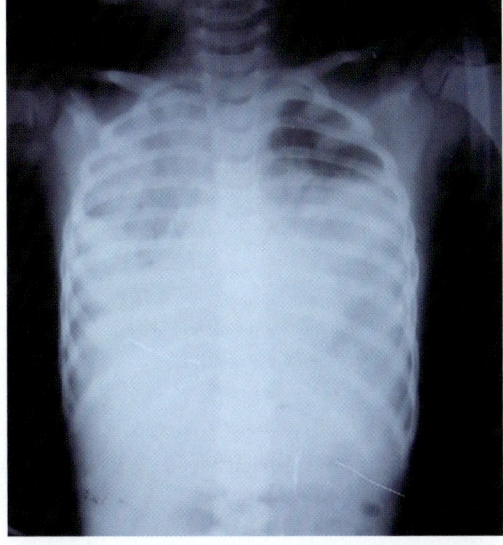

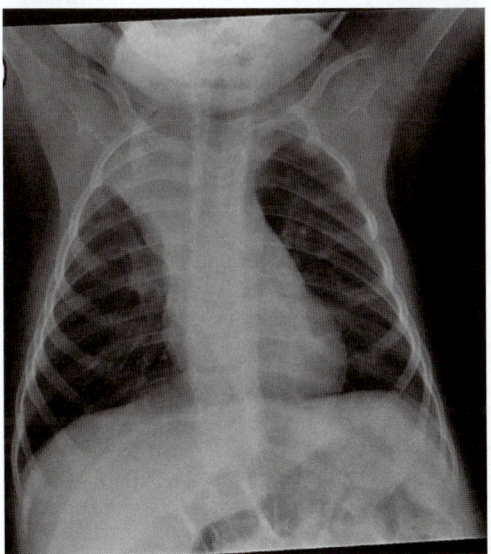

- Homogenous opacity seen in right upper lobe
- Crowding of ribs

Segmental collapse

Fig. 53.44.   Segmental collapse – right upper lobe.

X-ray	Interpretation	Diagnosis

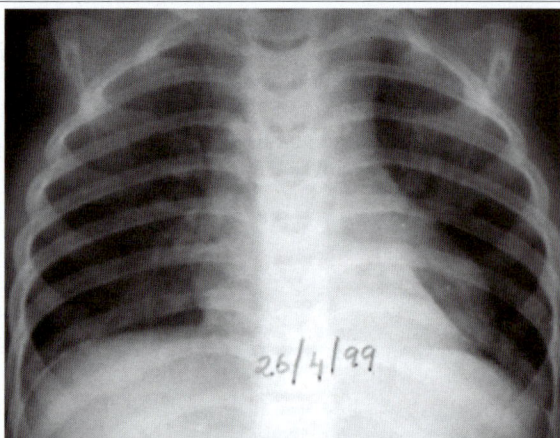

Fig. 53.45. Atelectasis – left lower lobe.

- Increased opacity with absent bronchovascular markings with a concave border seen through the cardiac silhouette near the left border
- Normal bronchovascular markings on the right side and left upper zone

Atelectasis – left lower lobe

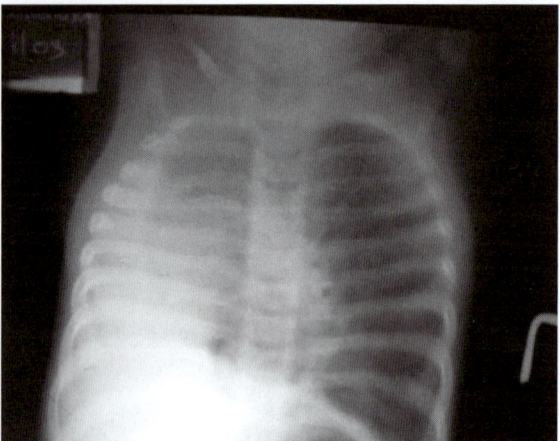

Fig. 53.46. Atelectasis – right lung (if the child is in distress). Agenesis – right lung (if the child is not in respiratory distress).

- Shift of the mediastinum to the right
- Left lung has larger volume and wide intercostal spaces compared to the right
- Normal bronchovascular markings in the left lung
- Cardiac silhouette seen in the extreme right hemithorax

Atelectasis – right lung (if the child is in distress)
Agenesis – right lung (if the child is not in respiratory distress)

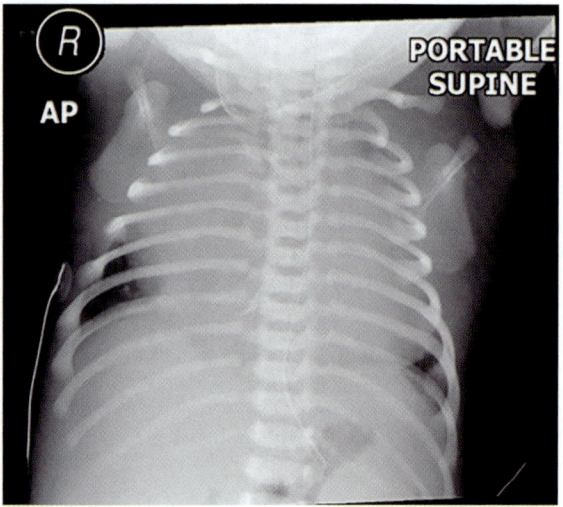

Fig. 53.47. Diffuse homogenous opacity – both lungs.

Diffuse homogenous opacity seen throughout the thorax
Differential diagnoses:
Massive cardiomegaly
Empyema

Examination of the child, insertion of ICD – no fluid drained, probably **tumor – teratoma**

X-ray	Interpretation	Diagnosis

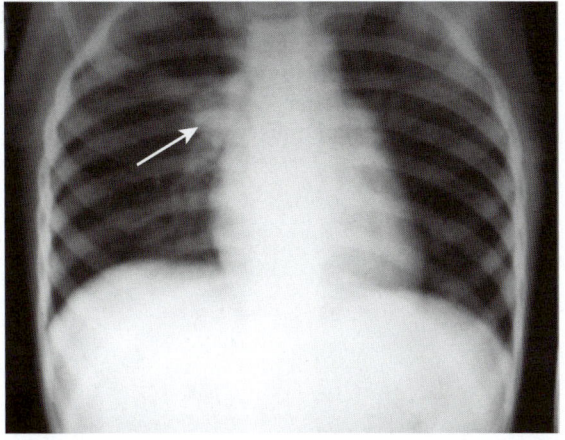

Fig. 53.48.   Mediastinal node.

- Circumscribed opacity
- Smooth convex outer margin
- Trachea not indented

Mediastinal node

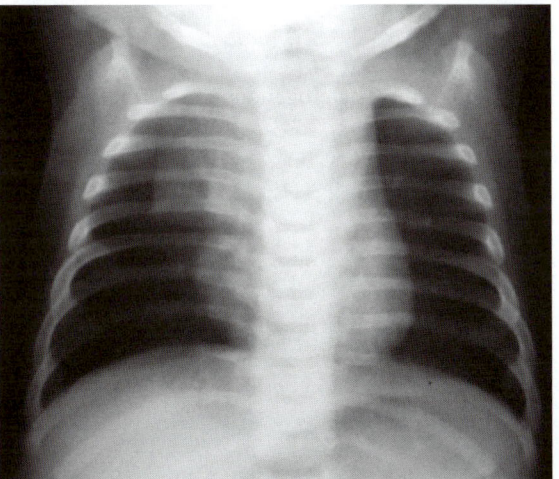

Fig. 53.49.   Normal thymus.

- Homogenous opacity in the right upper zone with sharp border having a sail-like appearance
- Normal lung volume on both sides
- Normal bronchovascular markings on both sides

Normal thymus

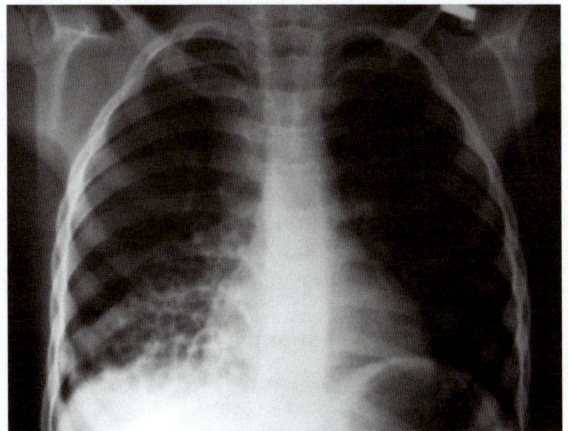

Fig. 53.50.   Bronchiectasis – right lower lobe.

- Multiple small cavities (soap bubble appearance) of varying size seen in the right lower zone
- Normal bronchovascular markings in the right upper zone and in left lung
- No shift of mediastinum

Bronchiectasis – right lower lobe

X-ray	Interpretation	Diagnosis
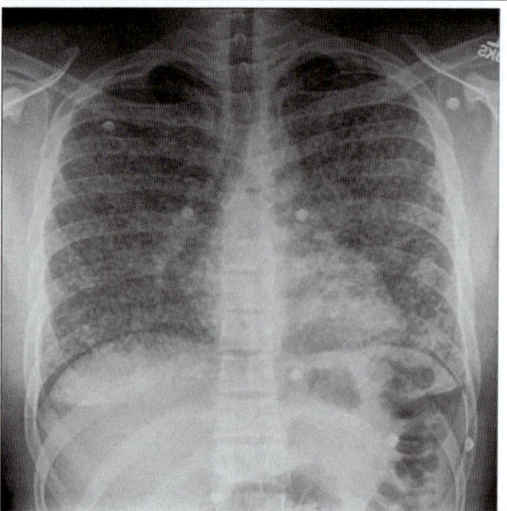 **Fig. 53.51.** Miliary mottling.	• Uniform pinhead-size discrete opacities distributed symmetrically in both lung fields extending up to the periphery • Commonly seen in miliary tuberculosis	**Miliary mottling**
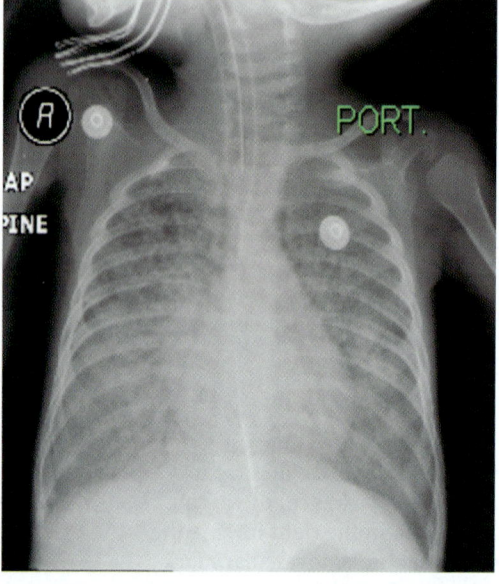 **Fig. 53.52.** Interstitial lung disease.	Bilateral diffuse heterogenous opacity Diffuse infiltrates seen	**Interstitial lung disease**
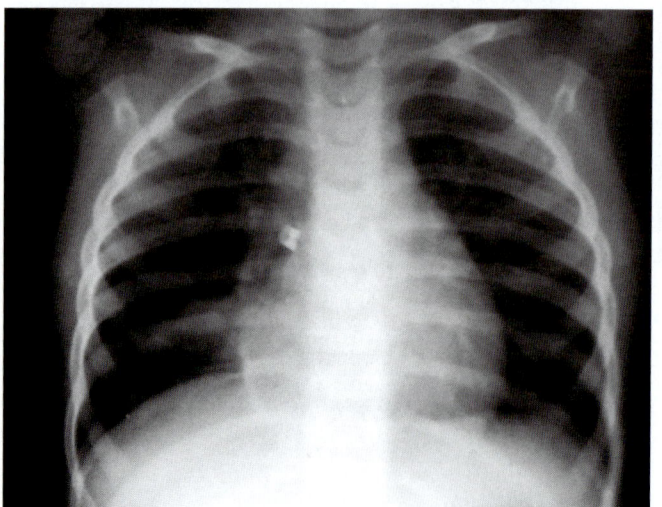 **Fig. 53.53.** Foreign body in the right main bronchus, with pneumonia in the right lower lobe.	• Normal volume lungs on both sides with normal bronchovascular markings • Small heterogenous patch in the right lower zone • Metallic foreign body in the right hilum	**Foreign body** in the right main bronchus, with pneumonia in the right lower lobe

BLACK SHADOWS

- Collapsed lung margin, no BV markings, mediastinal shift – pneumothorax
- No collapse of lung, BV markings – normal
- Emphysema (compensatory)
- Collapsed lobe, BV markings, emphysema of one lobe – congenital lobar emphysema
- Attenuated BV markings, large hyperinflated hemithorax – obstructive emphysema

Air Collection in Specific Places Have Different Diagnosis

- Normal: In alveoli in correct volume
- Pleura: Pneumothorax
- In the whole lung (alveoli): Obstructive emphysema (disease on the same side)
- In the whole lung (alveoli): Compensatory emphysema (disease on the opposite side)
- In one lobe: Congenital lobar emphysema; lower lobe collapse
- Pneumatocele: One area of lung
- Mediastinum: Pneumomediastinum
- Sliding hernia, Morgagni hernia, diaphragmatic hernia: Air in the right structure but that (organ) structure is in abnormal location

Examples of Black Shadow in X-ray

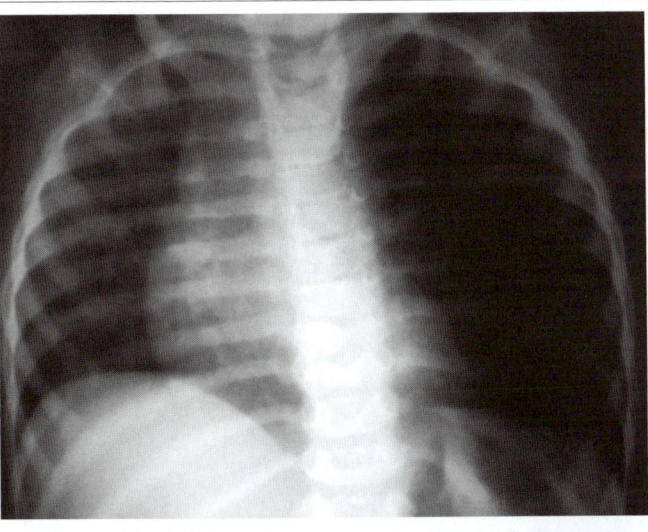

Fig. 53.54. Obstructive emphysema – left.

- Larger in volume – one side (left)
- Darker, but bronchovascular markings seen
- Collapsed lung not seen

Obstructive emphysema – left

- Intercostal spaces widened out
- Straitening of ribs
- Increase translucency in both lung fields
- Flattened diaphragm on both sides
- Squaring of both apex

Bilateral hyperaeration

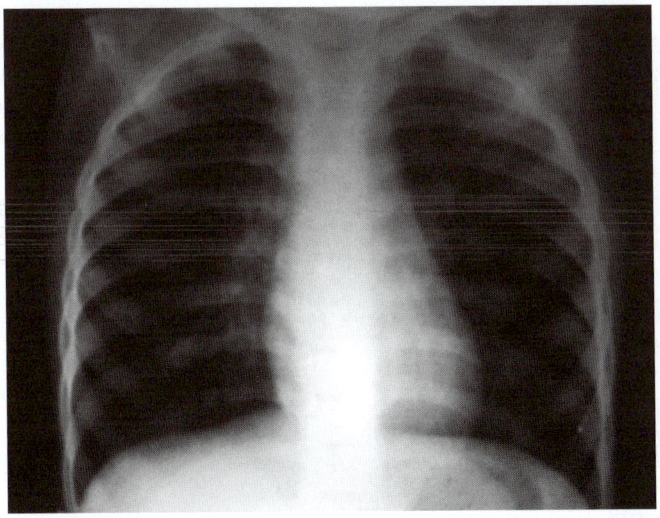

Fig. 53.55. Bilateral hyperaeration.

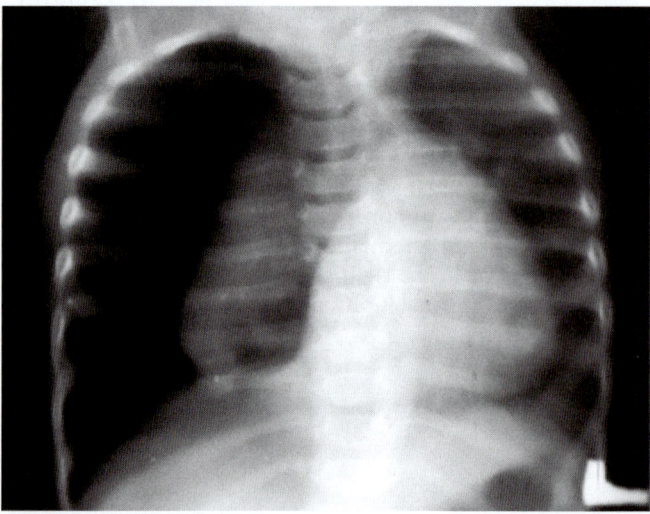

- Larger in volume – one side (right)
- Darker in color
- Vessel markings absent
- Collapsed lung seen on right side

Pneumothorax – right

Fig. 53.56.   Pneumothorax – right.

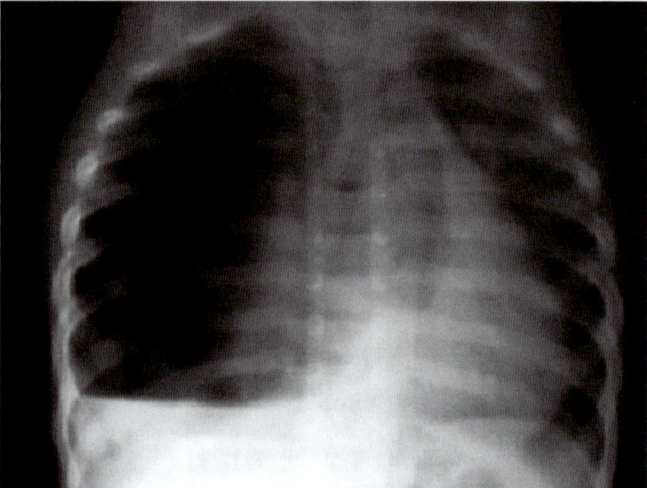

- Air and fluid level on the right side
- Absence of bronchovascular markings on the right side
- Collapsed right lung close to the hilum
- Shift of mediastinum to left

Pyopneumothorax – right

Fig. 53.57.   Pyopneumothorax – right.

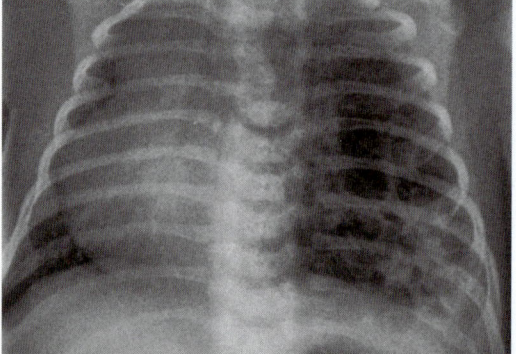

- Shift of the mediastinum to the right
- Left hemithorax has larger volume

Congenital cystic adenomatoid malformation of the left lung

Fig. 53.58.   Congenital cystadenomatoid malformation of the left lung. *(Source: Reproduced from Rajiv PK, Satyan Lakshminrusimha, Dharmapuri Vidyasagar. Essentials of Neonatal Ventilation,* Hypoxic Respiratory Failure, Fig. 8.15, New Delhi, Elsevier India, 2018.)

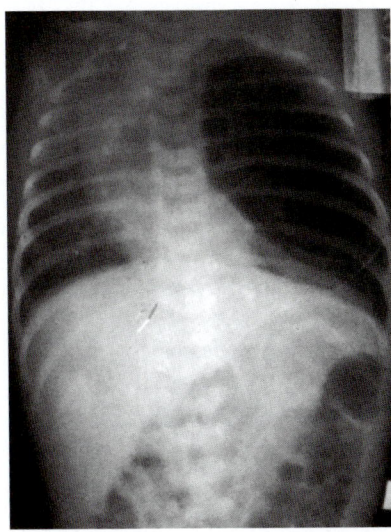

- Shift of mediastinum to the right
- Left hemithorax has larger volume
- Normal bronchovascular markings in the left upper lobe with atelectasis of the left lower lobe
- Normal bronchovascular marking on the right lung

Congenital lobar emphysema of the left upper lobe

Fig. 53.59. Congenital lobar emphysema of the left upper lobe.

TUBES IN CHEST X-RAY

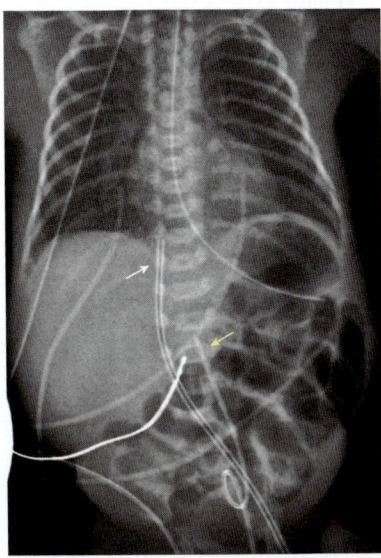

Fig. 53.60. Umbilical venous catheter (UVC) and Umbilical arterial catheter (UAC). (Source: Reproduced from Martin Keszler, Gautham Suresh, Jay P. Goldsmith. *Goldsmith's Assisted Ventilation of the Neonate*, 7e, Fig 9.6, Philadelphia, Elsevier Inc., 2022.)

Fig 53.60. UVC and UAC: The umbilical venous catheter (UVC) takes a normal straight course superiorly from the umbilicus. The UVC tip is just above the diaphragm in the right atrium at the T8 level. The UAC tip (white arrow) lies at T7-T8, below the ductus arteriosus (DA) & above the celiac axis and the tip of a "low" lying umbilical arterial line (yellow arrow) is just above the L3 vertebral body (The UAC tip lies at T7-T8, below the ductus arteriosus (DA) & above the celiac axis). Note that both catheters enter the patient at the same level (through the umbilicus) but the UAC follows the umbilical artery inferiorly before coursing superiorly in the iliac system to the aorta.

Normal position of **Umbilical venous catheter (UVC) and Umbilical arterial catheter (UAC)**

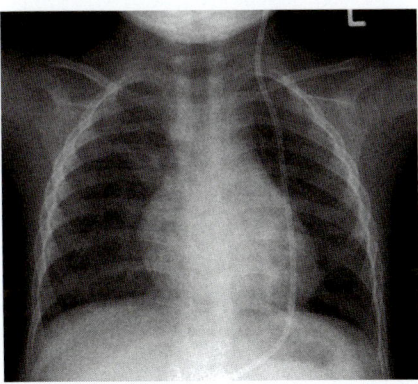

Fig. 53.61. Ventriculoperitoneal shunt catheter. (Source: Reproduced from Ania Carolina Muntau. *Die 50 wichtigsten Fälle Pädiatrie*, Abb 43.1, Munich, Urban & Fischer, 2012.)

Fig 53.61. Ventriculoperitoneal shunt-frontal catheter insertion, subcutaneous passage of shunt and distal catheter tip in the abdomen.

Ventriculoperitoneal shunt

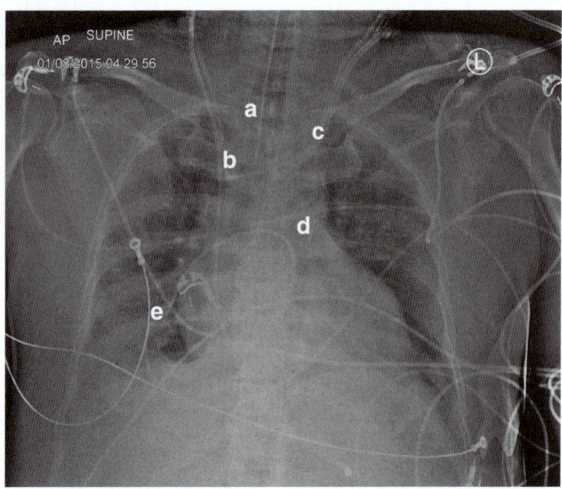

Fig. 53.62. Various tubes in chest X-ray. (Source: Reproduced from Adam Feather, David Randall, Mona Waterhouse. *Kumar and Clark's Clinical Medicine*, 10e, Fig 10.16, Edinburgh, Elsevier Ltd, 2021.)

Fig 53.62. The X-ray shows
(a) Endotracheal tube (Tip of ETT – ideal at T2 or T3, should be midway between clavicle and carina)
(b) End of central venous line
(c) Double-lumen catheter for continuous renal replacement therapy placed via the left internal jugular vein
(d) Tip of the intra-aortic balloon pump travelling superiorly from a femoral artery and
(e) Pulmonary artery catheter

Various tubes in chest X-ray

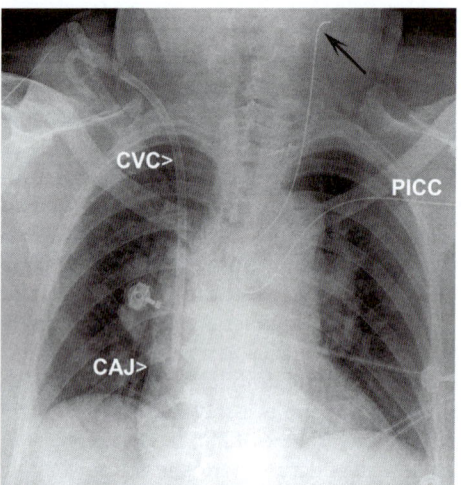

Fig. 53.63. PICC and CVC. (Source: Reproduced from Jean-Louis Vincent, Frederick Moore, Mitchell Fink. *Textbook of Critical Care*, 7e, Fig 66.9, Philadelphia, Elsevier Inc., 2017.)

Fig 53.63. Chest x-ray AP view: Left peripherally inserted central venous catheter (PICC) courses cephalad from the left brachiocephalic vein into the left internal jugular vein, with its tip (arrow) residing in the mid neck. Right internal jugular Central venous catheter (CVC) tip in a good position at the cavoatrial junction (CAJ).

Peripherally inserted central venous catheter (PICC) and Central venous catheter (CVC).

OTHER EXAM-ORIENTED CHEST X-RAY

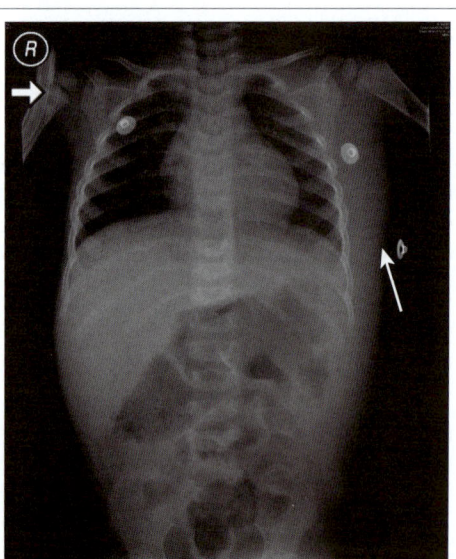

Fig. 53.64. Cellulitis/necrotizing fasciitis.

- Unilateral soft tissue swelling
- Chest wall edema

Cellulitis/necrotizing fasciitis

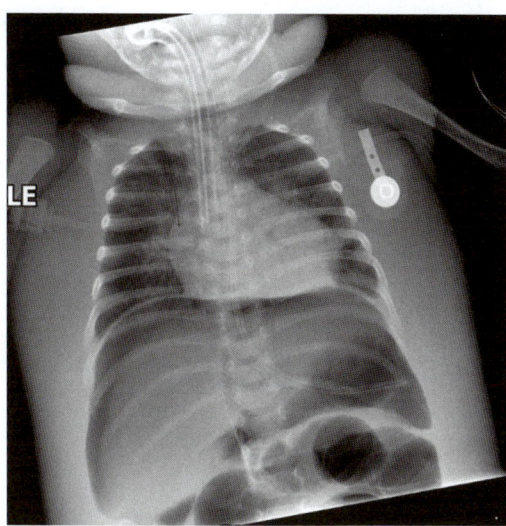

- Bilateral soft tissue swelling
- Chest wall edema

Probably capillary leak

Fig. 53.65. Capillary leak.

Cardiac

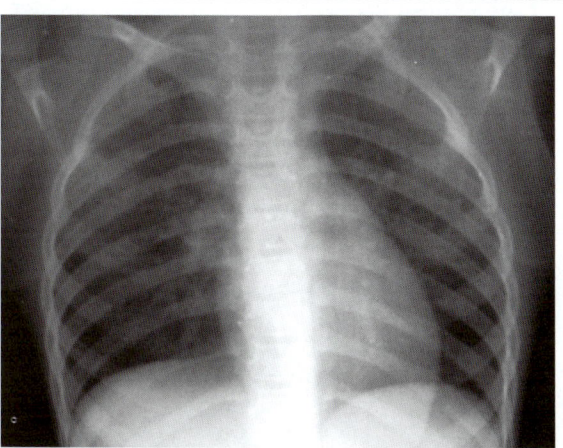

- Cardiac silhouette normal
- CT ratio normal <0.5

Normal cardiac shadow

Fig. 53.66. Normal cardiac shadow.

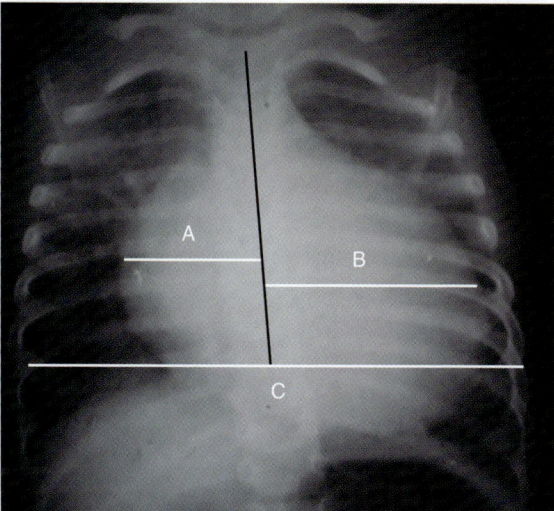

- Use two scales
  Place one scale in the midpoint of the vertebral bodies
  Take two points
  1st: Measure the maximum convexity of left heart border from the midpoint of the vertebral borders
  Add with the maximum convexity of right heart border from the midpoint of the vertebral borders
    2nd: Transthoracic diameter (maximum curvature of chest wall
- Cardiothoracic ratio – normal
  <0.5 – children
  <0.6 – newborn and infancy

Cardiomegaly

Fig. 53.67. Cardiomegaly.

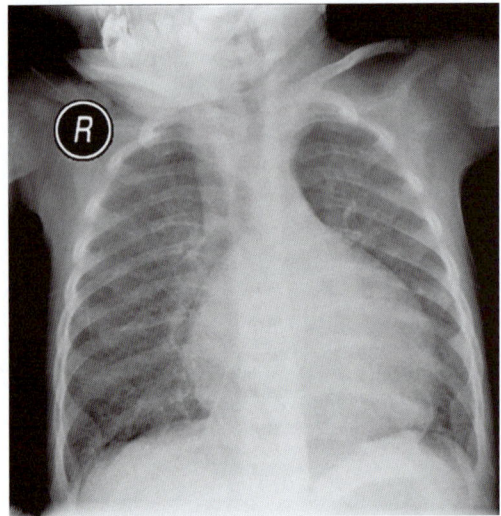

Fig. 53.68. Cardiomegaly with congestion.

- Increased cardiothoracic ratio
- Heterogenous opacity seen on both lung fields

Cardiomegaly with congestion

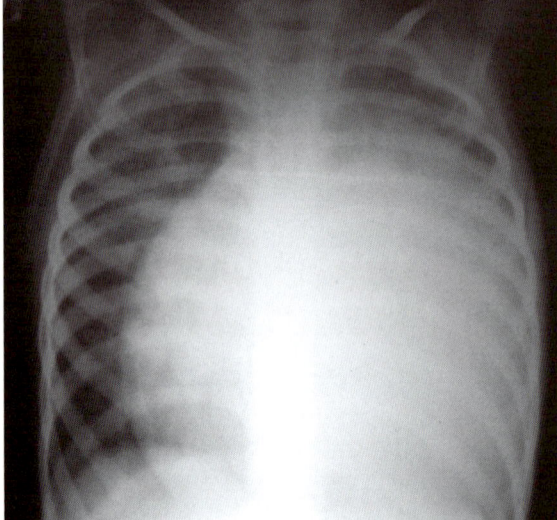

Fig. 53.69. Pericardial effusion.

- Cardiac silhouette is large, almost occupying the entire chest – gross cardiomegaly
- Money bag appearance

Pericardial effusion

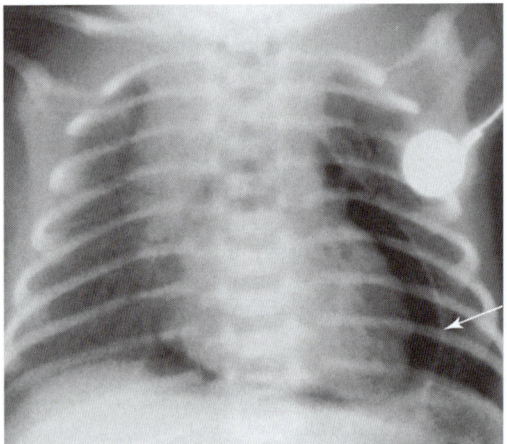

Fig. 53.70. Pneumopericardium. (*Source:* Reproduced from Terry Des Jardins, George Burton. *Clinical Manifestations and Assessment of Respiratory Disease*, Eighth Edition, Pulmonary Air Leak Syndromes, Fig 38.5, St. Louis, Mosby, 2020. (Credit line - From Gleason, C. A., & Juul, S. E. [2018]. Avery's diseases of the newborn [10th ed.]. Philadelphia: Elsevier.)

- Clear hyperlucent area around the cardiac silhouette
- Lower border of cardiac silhouette appears distinctively above the diaphragm separated by hyperlucent area

Pneumopericardium

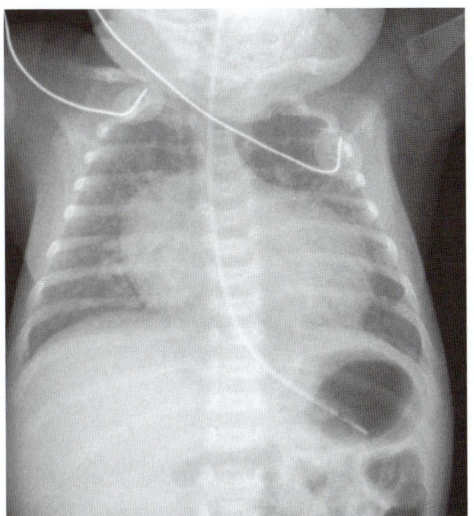

Fig. 53.71. Transposition of great arteries. *(Source:* Reproduced from Lane Donnelly. *Fundamentals of Pediatric Imaging*, Second Edition, Cardiac, Fig 4.20, Philadelphia, Elsevier Inc., 2017.)

- Egg on side or egg on string appearance
- Heart appears globular due to abnormal convexity on right atrial border and left atrial enlargement
- Also, superior mediastinum appears narrow due to thymic atrophy and hyperinflated lungs, which gives the picture of egg suspended on a string

Transposition of great arteries

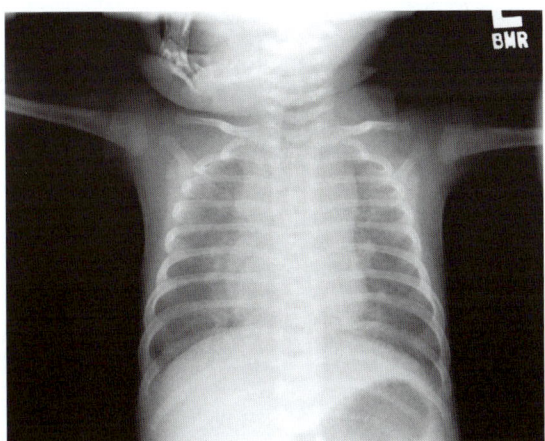

Fig. 53.72. TAPVC (total anomalous pulmonary venous connections). *(Source:* Reproduced from Michael Crawford, John DiMarco, Walter Paulus. *Cardiology*, Third Edition, Abnormalities of the Pulmonary Veins, Fig 107B.2, Philadelphia, Mosby Ltd, 2010.)

- Figure of eight appearance/ snowman sign
- Paratracheal region shows
  Right – prominent SVC
  Midline – innominate vessel
  Left – vertical vein

TAPVC Total Anomalous Pulmonary Venous Connections

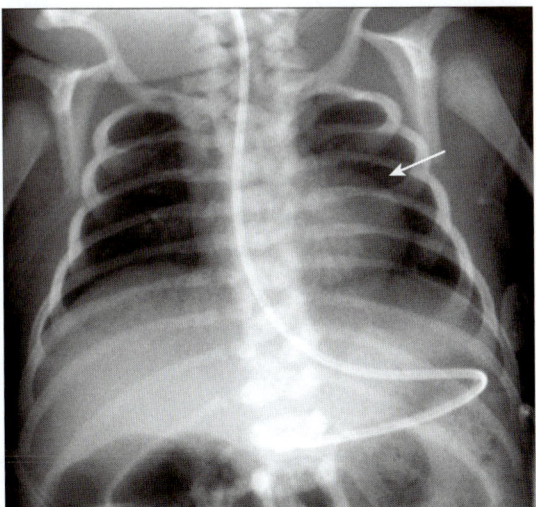

Fig. 53.73. Tetralogy of Fallot. *(Source:* Reproduced from Terry Des Jardins, George Burton. *Clinical Manifestations and Assessment of Respiratory Disease*, Eighth Edition, Congenital Heart Diseases, FIGURE 42.7, St. Louis, Mosby, 2020. (Credit line - Courtesy Dayton Children's Hospital, Dayton, Ohio).)

- The "boots toe" corresponds to a elevated cardiac apex, while the broad "foot" portion corresponds to an increased prominence of the left cardiac border caused by right cardiac hypertrophy.

Tetralogy of Fallot

Newborn

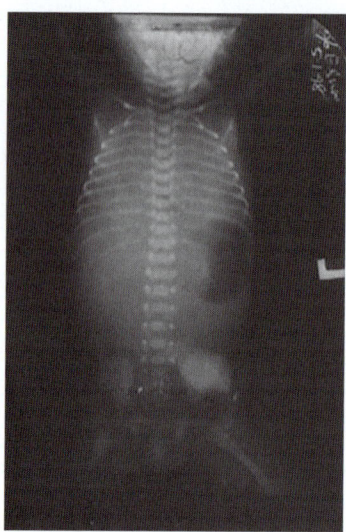

- Bilateral symmetrical diffuse ground glass opacity
- Low lung volume
- Lung whiteout

Respiratory distress syndrome

Fig. 53.74. Respiratory distress syndrome (bilateral symmetrical diffuse ground glass opacity).

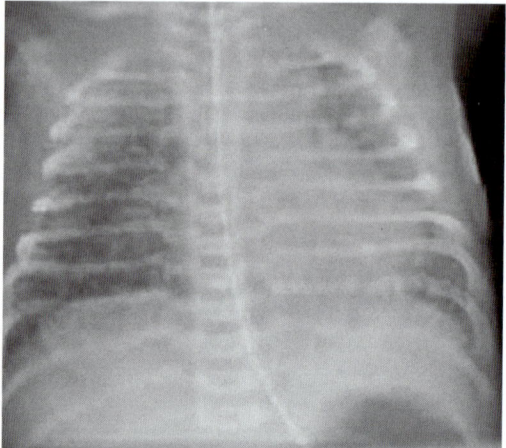

- Asymmetric heterogenous patchy opacities
- Hyperinflated lung
- Flattened hemidiaphragms

Meconium aspiration syndrome

Fig. 53.75. Meconium aspiration syndrome (asymmetric heterogenous patchy opacities).

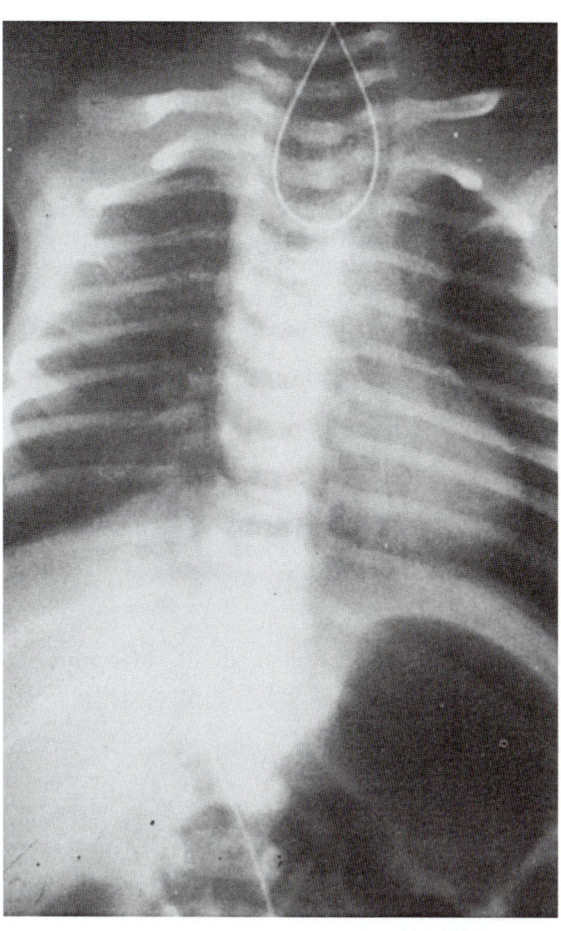

- Nasogastric tube is seen coiling near the 5th thoracic vertebra
- Fundal gas shadow is seen below the left dome of diaphragm
- Both domes of diaphragm are normal
- Heart and lung appear normal

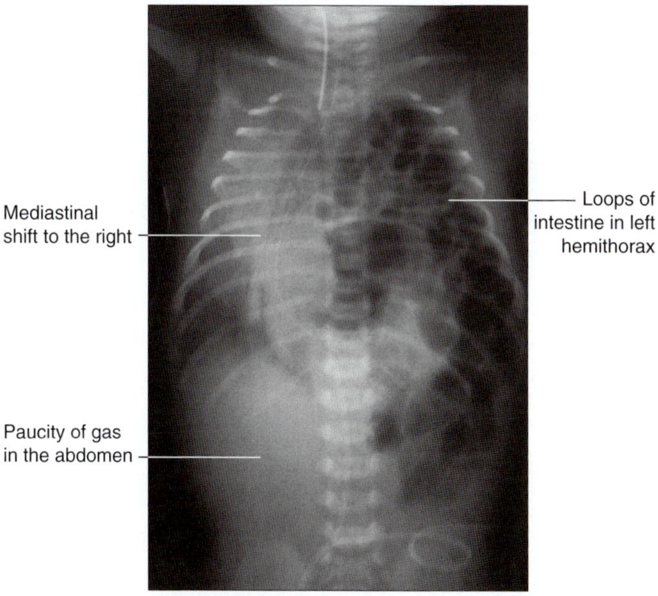

Esophageal atresia with tracheo-esophageal fistula

Fig. 53.76. Esophageal atresia with tracheoesophageal fistula. *(Source: Reproduced from Robert Kliegman, Heather Toth, Brett Bordini et al. Nelson Pediatric Symptom-Based Diagnosis: Common Diseases and their Mimics,* Second Edition, 15 - Vomiting and Regurgitation, Fig. 15.3, Philadelphia, Elsevier Inc., 2023.)

Mediastinal shift to the right

Loops of intestine in left hemithorax

Paucity of gas in the abdomen

- Left hemithorax has multiple air-filled loops of intestine
- Shift of mediastinum to right
- Left dome of diaphragm has a defect through which intestinal loops are entering left thoracic cavity
- Right dome of diaphragm is normal
  (NG tube seen in the abdomen)

Diaphragmatic hernia left

Fig. 53.77. Congenital diaphragmatic hernia (left). *(Source: Reproduced from Susan Standring. Gray's Anatomy: The Anatomical Basis of Clinical Practice,* Forty Second Edition, Development of the lungs, thorax and respiratory diaphragm, Fig. 20.3, London, Elsevier Ltd, 2021. (Credit line - Courtesy of Mr G Jawaheer, Great North Children's Hospital, Newcastle upon Tyne.).

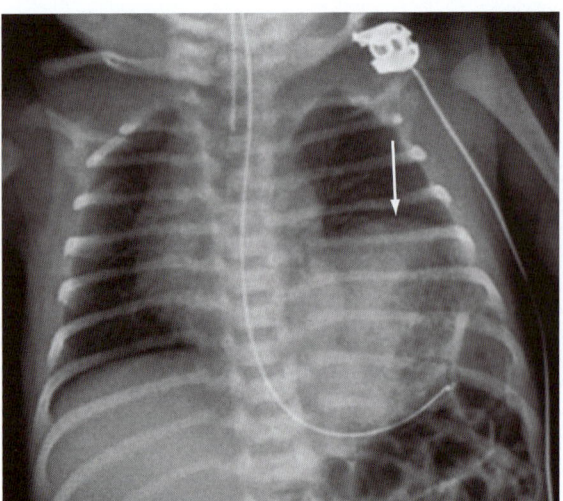

- Fundal gas shadow is seen beneath the left dome of diaphragm in the left thoracic cavity
- Nasogastric tube seen coiling back into left thoracic cavity (in the stomach)
- Mediastinal shift to right
- Left dome of diaphragm is highly placed
- Right dome of diaphragm is normally placed

Eventration left dome of diaphragm (right eventration of diaphragm can wait, but left-side eventration of diaphragm requires immediate surgical intervention as stomach can goes for malrotation/volvulus)

Fig. 53.78. Eventration left dome of diaphragm. *(Source: Reproduced from* Courtney Townsend. *Sabiston Textbook of Surgery: The Biological Basis of Modern Surgical Practice,* Twenty First Edition, Pediatric Surgery, Fig. 67.2, Philadelphia, Elsevier Inc., 2022.)

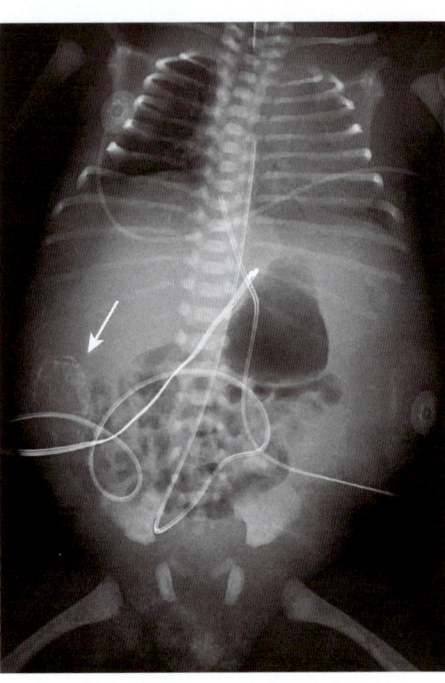

- Radiopaque density (calcification) noted in the right side of the abdomen
- Heart and lungs appear normal
- Bones are normal

Meconium peritonitis

Fig. 53.79. Meconium peritonitis. *(Source: Reproduced from Lane Donnelly. Fundamentals of Pediatric Imaging,* Second Edition, Gastrointestinal, Fig 5.23, Philadelphia, Elsevier Inc., 2017.)

Abdomen

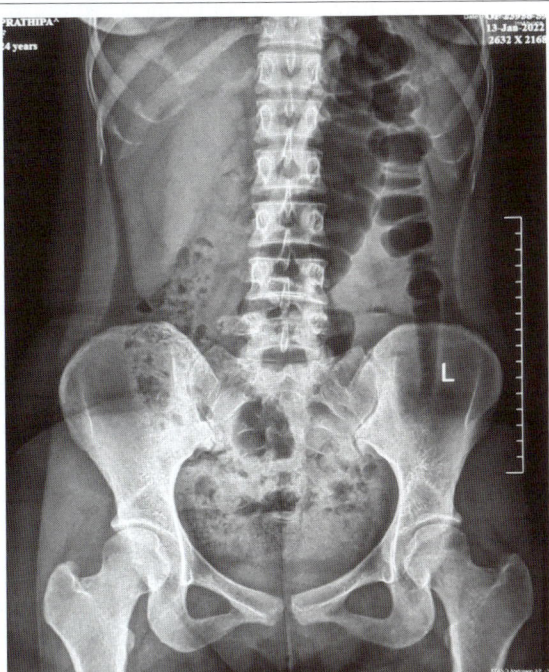

Fig. 53.80.   Normal plain X-ray of abdomen.

- X-ray Abdomen
- Stomach (Air and fluid filled)
- Small bowel (central, valvulae conniventes across lumen and closely spaced)
- Large bowel(peripheral, Haustral markings seen)
- Normal diameter of bowel- 3, 6, 9 Rule (Small bowel-3cm, Large bowel- 6cm, Caecum -9cm)

Normal plain X-ray of abdomen

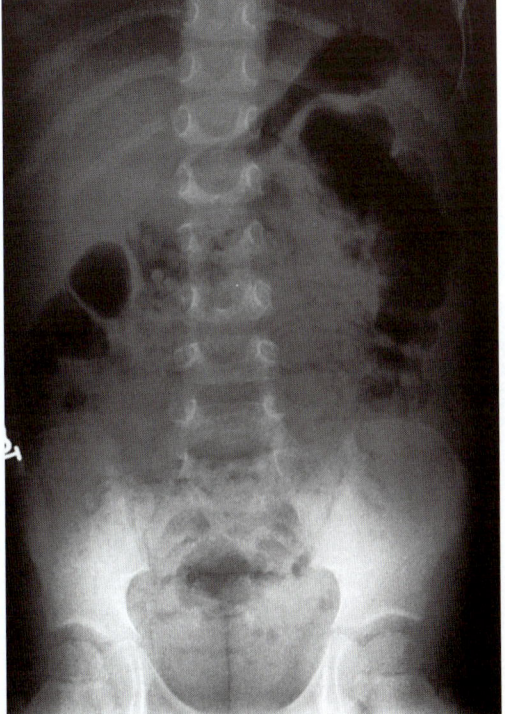

Fig. 53.81.   Ascariasis in plain X-ray abdomen. (*Source: Reproduced from* Richard Gore, Marc Levine. *Textbook of Gastrointestinal Radiology*, Third Edition, Diseases of the Pediatric Stomach and Duodenum, Figure 119-23, Philadelphia, Saunders, 2008.)

- Unusual gas pattern in the middle duodenum and jejunum.

Worm infestation in plain X-ray abdomen

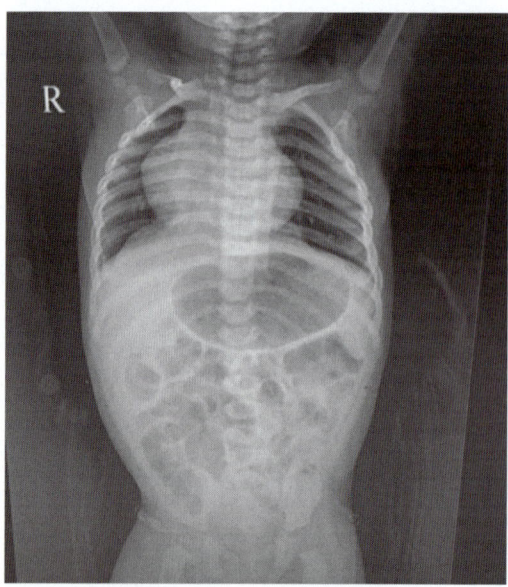

- Normal bronchovascular markings in both lung fields
- Heart position is reversed – apex in the right hemithorax
- Domes of the diaphragm are normal
- Stomach is overdistended

Acute gastric dilatation with dextro-cardia

Fig. 53.82. Acute gastric dilatation with dextrocardia.

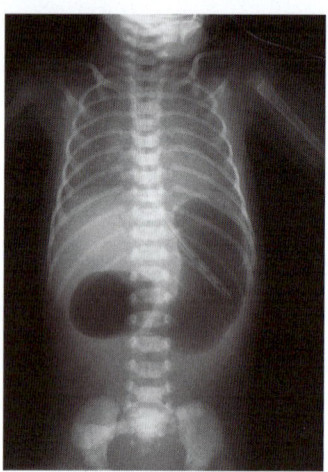

- Normal bronchovascular markings in both lung fields
- Cardiac silhouette is normal
- Domes of the diaphragm are normal
- Double bubble seen in the abdomen

Duodenal atresia

Fig. 53.83. Duodenal atresia. *(Source: Reproduced from* Richard Polin, Mark Ditmar. *Pediatría. Secretos, Séptima edición, Gastroenterología,* Figura 7.15, Madrid, Elsevier ESP, 2022. (Credit line - Tomado de Zitelli BJ, Davis HW. Atlas of Pediatric Physical Diagnosis. 5th ed. Philadelphia, PA: Mosby; 2007:637.))

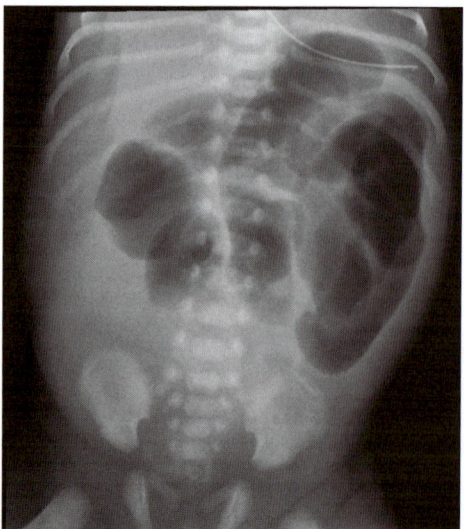

- Multiple distended small intestinal loops seen (pile of coin appearance)
- Large bowel loops are not visualized (no haustrations in any of the distended loops)
- Both domes of diaphragm appear normal

Small bowel obstruction, probably **ileal atresia**

Fig. 53.84. Ileal atresia. *(Source:* Reproduced from Lucinda GC Tullie, Michael P Stanton, and Bilious vomiting in the newborn, *Paediatric Surgery* 34(12):603-608.)

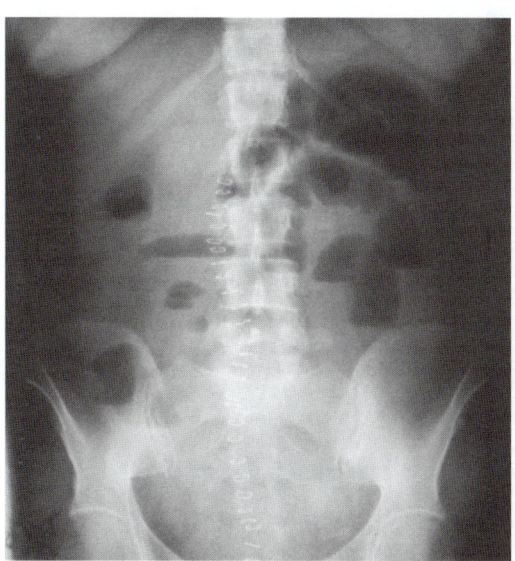

- Dilated bowel loops
- Air fluid level

Abdomen erect –
ileus

Fig. 53.85. Abdomen erect – ileus. (*Source:* Reproduced from James M.Messmer and Gas and Soft Tissue Abnormalities, *BS:RADCON*, Fig. 3, © 2008.)

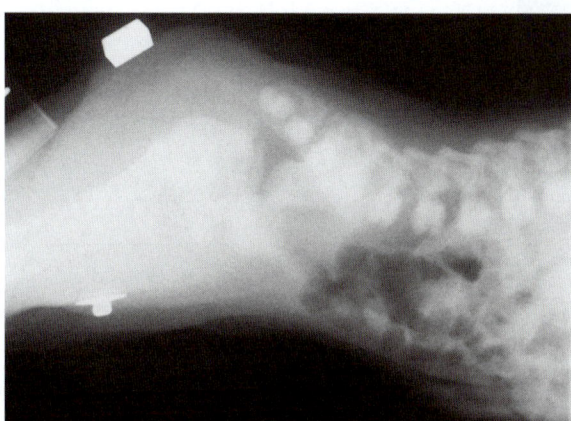

- Prone cross-table lateral view (otherwise called as Invertogram), with pelvic elevation at 24–36 hours of age in babies with high anorectal malformations. A radiopaque marker (i.e. a coin) is placed over the expected anus using radiolucent tape. The distance between the air filled distal rectal pouch and the anal dimple marked by radioopaque coin is noted.

Ano-rectal
malformation

Fig. 53.86. Prone translateral – intestinal obstruction. In cross table view, baby is placed in prone position and X-ray beam is passed horizontally from sideward. (*Source: Reproduced from Janet Rennie. Rennie & Roberton's Textbook of Neonatology,* Fifth Edition, Gastroenterology, Fig. 29.82, Chennai/Oxford, Churchill Livingstone, 2012.)

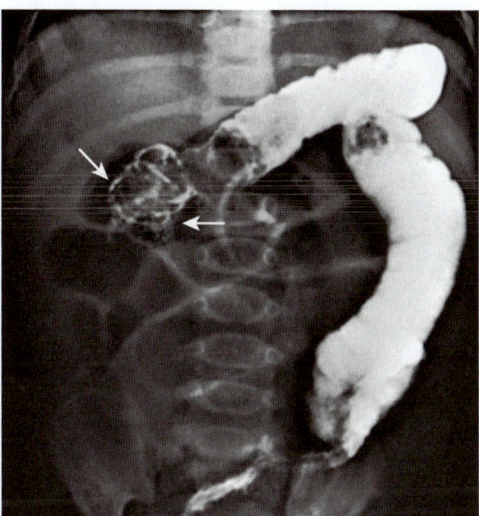

Contrast material seen between the intussusceptum and intussuscipiens

Cutoff sign
(coiled spring
appearance)
intussus-
ception

Fig. 53.87. Cutoff sign – intussusception. (*Source: Reproduced from* Robert Kliegman, Bonita Stanton, Joseph St. Geme. *Nelson Textbook of Pediatrics,* Twentieth Edition, Ileus, Adhesions, Intussusception, and Closed-Loop Obstructions, Figure 333-2, Philadelphia, Elsevier Inc., 2016).

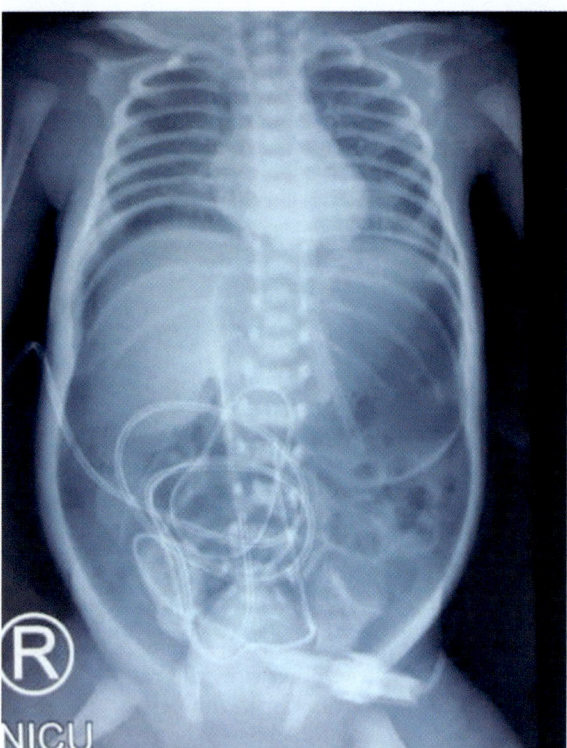

Fig. 53.88. Pneumoperitoneum. *(Source: Reproduced from* Aminuddin Harahap, Agus Harianto, Risa Etika et al., and Spontaneous Ileum Perforation in a premature twin with Coronavirus-19 positive mother, *J Pediatr Surg Case Rep* Apr;67:101807.)

- Air under the diaphragm
- Air on both side of the bowel wall – football sign

Pneumoperito-neum

RADIOPAQUE SHADOW IN THE ABDOMEN

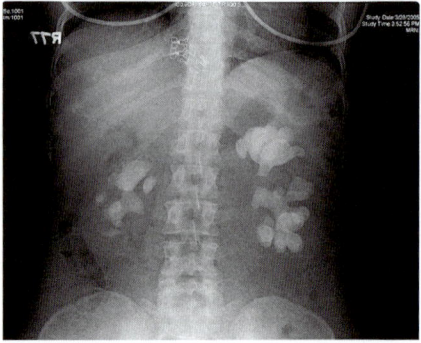

Fig. 53.89. Calculi in urinary tract on right side. *(Source: Reproduced from* Theodore O'Connell. *USMLE Step 2 Secrets,* Sixth Edition, Nephrology, Fig. 22.4, St. Louis, Elsevier Inc., 2022. (Credit line - From Wein AJ, Kavoussi LR, Novick AC, et al. Campbell-Walsh Urology. 9th ed. Philadelphia: Saunders; 2007 [fig. 43.9]).)

Bilateral staghorn calculi composed of struvite. in a child with recurrent urinary tract infections.

staghorn calculi

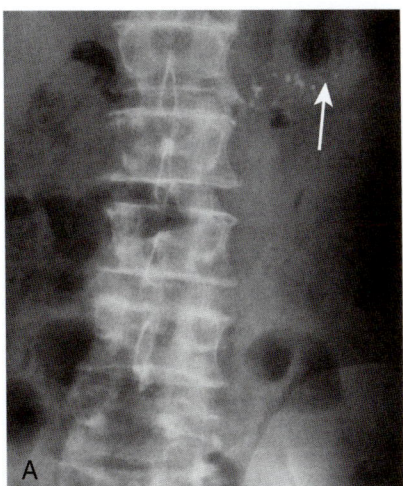

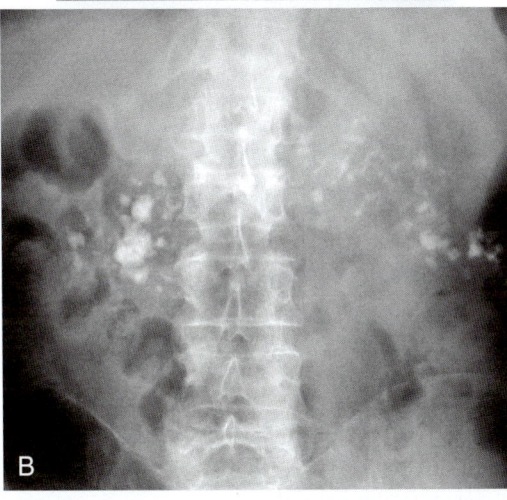

Numerous dense, discrete opacities that cross the midline at the level of L1 to L2 (arrow). The normal pancreas is not visible on abdominal plain films.

Pancreatic calculi (A and B)

Fig. 53.90. (A and B) Pancreatic calculi. *(Source: Reproduced from Dennis Marchiori. Clinical Imaging: With Skeletal, Chest and Abdomen Pattern Differentials, Third Edition, Abdomen Patterns, FIG 32.3, St. Louis, Mosby, 2014.)*

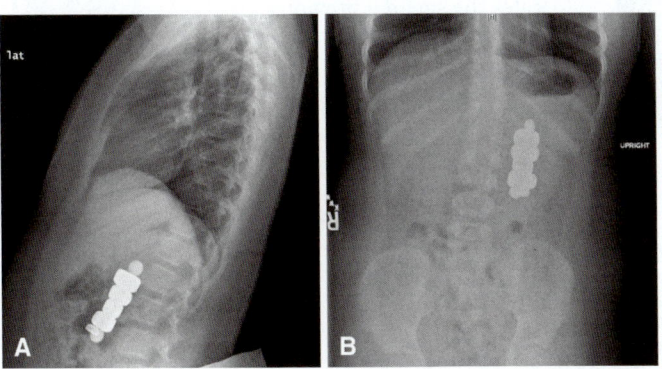

Radiopaque structures seen in the abdomen suggestive of foreign body (Pica)

Pica

Fig. 53.91. Pica. *(Source: Reproduced from Julie C Brown, Karen F Murray, Patrick J Javid, and Hidden Attraction: A Menacing Meal of Magnets and Batteries, The Journal of Emergency Medicine 43(2):266-269.)*

ABDOMEN CONTRAST

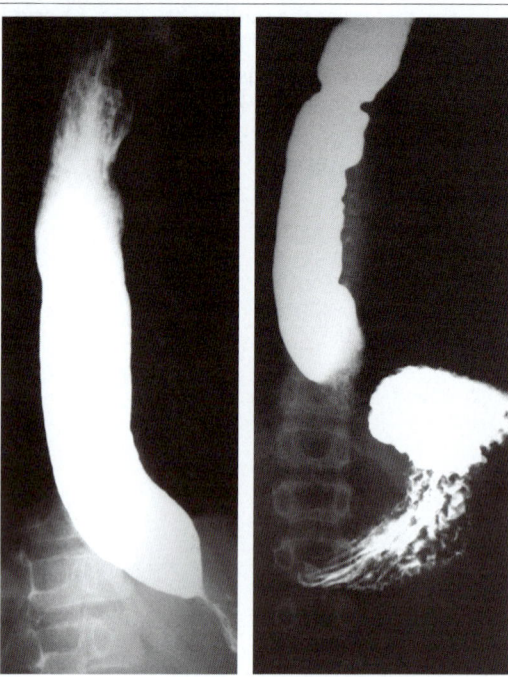

- Barium swallow showing enlarged esophagus, stagnant fluid before the contrast was administered. Emptying is very slow and the cardia has a typical "carrot" or "bird's beak" pattern (left).

  Note the smooth eccentric narrowing at D 10 level

Achalasia cardia

Fig. 53.92. Achalasia cardia. *(Source: Reproduced from* Jay Grosfeld, James O'Neill, Arnold Coran et al. *Pediatric Surgery*, Sixth Edition, Disorders of Esophageal Function, Fig 70.5, Philadelphia, Mosby, 2006.)

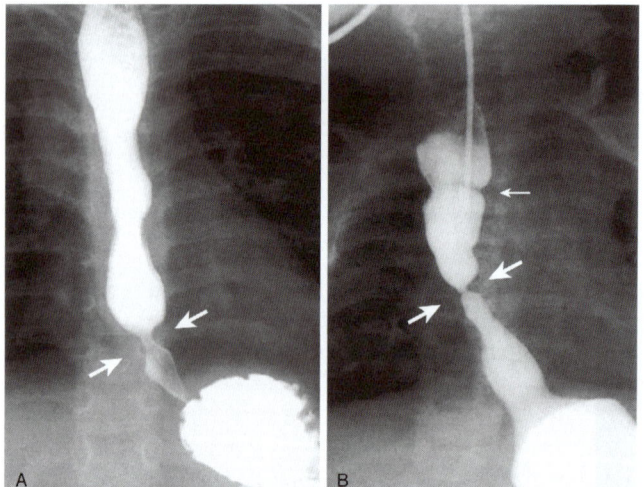

- A, Barium esophagogram with a tapered narrowing in the distal esophagus and dilatation of the proximal esophagus. B, Barium esophagogram with an abrupt narrowing in the mid-esophagus (large arrows). The small arrow indicates the site of a previous repair for esophageal atresia

Congenital esophageal stenosis

Fig. 53.93. Congenital esophageal stenosis. *(Source: Reproduced from* Mark Feldman, Lawrence Friedman, Lawrence Brandt. *Sleisenger and Fordtran's Gastrointestinal and Liver Disease: Pathophysiology, Diagnosis, Management*, Eleventh Edition, Anatomy, Histology, Embryology, and Developmental Anomalies of the Esophagus, Fig. 43.10, Philadelphia, Elsevier Inc., 2021. (Credit line - A and B, From Usui N, Kamata S, Kawahara H, et al. Usefulness of endoscopic ultrasonography in the diagnosis of congenital esophageal stenosis. J Pediatr Surg 2002; 37:1744.)

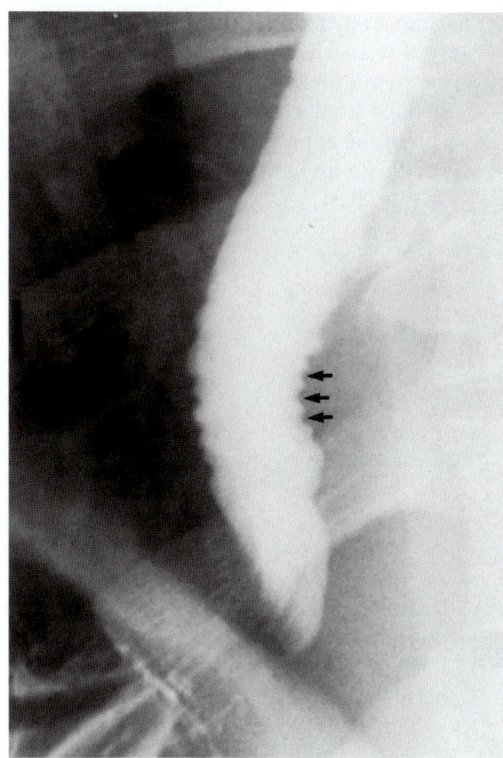

A moderately long stricture seen in the upper thoracic esophagus, with multiple distinctive ringlike indentations (arrows) in the region of the stricture.

Congenital esophageal stricture

Fig. 53.94. Congenital esophageal stricture. *(Source: Reproduced from BS:RADCON, Esophagitides, Other, Fig 13, © 2008.)*

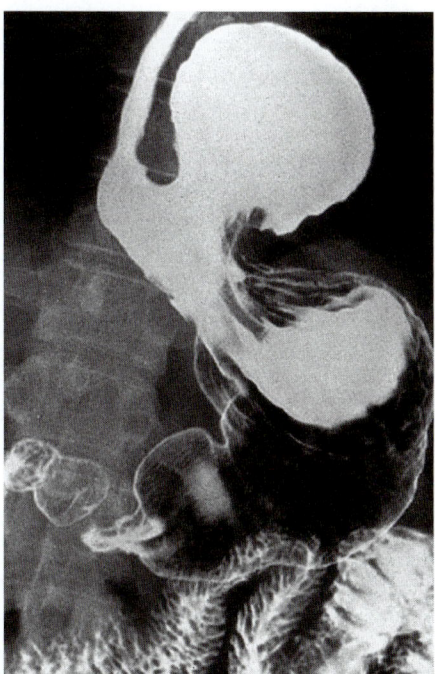

Barium study done in the Trendelenburg position showing hiatus hernia

Hiatus hernia

Fig. 53.95. Hiatus hernia. *(Source: Reproduced from O. James Garden, Andrew Bradbury, John Forsythe et al. Principles and Practice of Surgery: Adapted International Edition, Sixth Edition, The oesophagus, stomach and duodenum, Fig.13.7, Oxford, Churchill Livingstone, 2012.)*

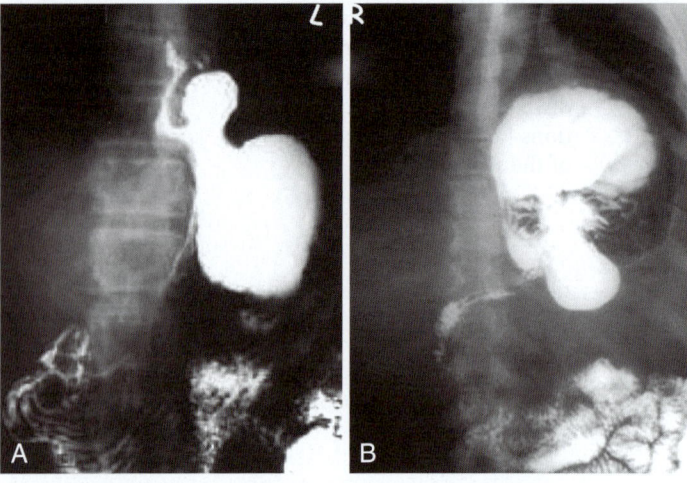

Fig. 53.96. Hiatus hernia (paraesophageal hernia). *(Source: Reproduced from A B M Abdullah. Radiology in Medical Practice*, Fifth Edition, Contrast X-ray, PLATE 3.18, New Delhi, Elsevier India, 2020.)

- Barium study reveals greater part of stomach in the right lower hemithorax

  Air-filled stomach has given the appearance of cystic lesion in the plain X-ray chest

  Hiatus hernia (paraesophageal hernia)

(A) Radiolucent area appears on right side thorax

(B) Barium swallow shows herniation of stomach

Morgagni hernia (A and B)

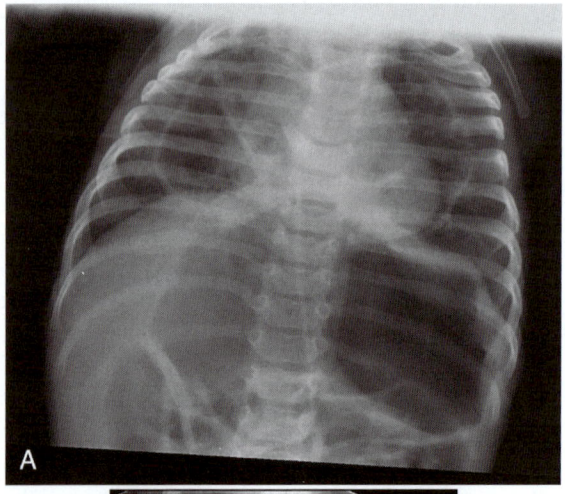

Fig. 53.97. (A) Plain X-ray – Morgagni hernia.(B) Barium swallow – herniation of stomach in Morgagni hernia.

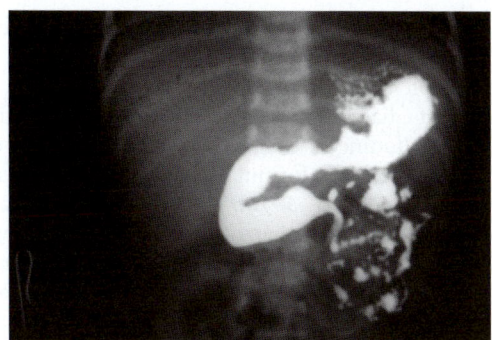

Fig. 53.98. Normal barium study.

- DJ flexure seen on the right
- Small bowel loops on the left
- Large bowel loops on right side of abdomen

Normal barium study

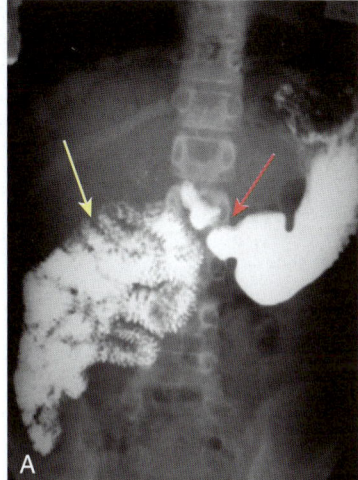

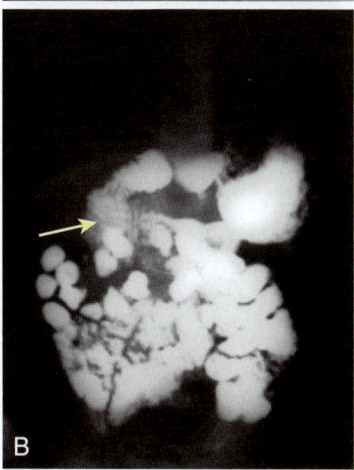

Fig. 53.99. (A) Malrotation.(B) Subhepatic position of cecum (malrotation).

- (A) DJ flexure does not cross the spine (red arrow) and the bowel loops are seen to be on the right side of spine (yellow arrow)
- (B) The subhepatic position of cecum

Malrotation

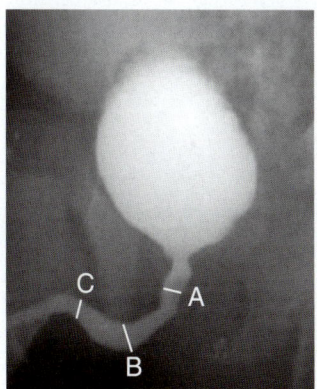

Fig. 53.100. Normal MCU.

Normal MCU
  (a) Posterior urethral diameter
 (b and c) Anterior urethral diameter consists of proximal and distal bulbar urethra

Normal micturating cysto-urethrogram (MCU)

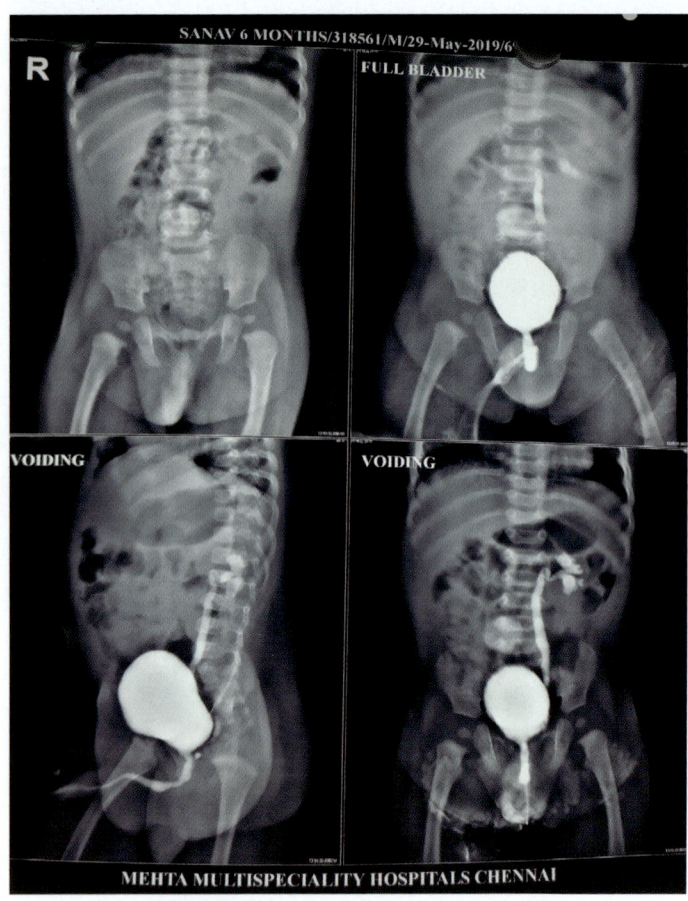

Fig. 53.101. (A–D) Series of images in MCU.

- MCU
- Procedure: Child in fluoroscopic table – diluted contrast (diatrizoate meglumine/iodine)
- Volume: Koff's formula: (Age in years + 2) × 30 mL
  - MCU showing narrow anterior urethral stream, dilated posterior urethra, dilated and trabeculated bladder with diverticulae, and secondary VUR on left

Posterior urethral valves
(A) Before dye administration
(B) Image of full bladder in AP view taken
(C) Voiding phase – oblique view – delineating entire urethra
(D) End of voiding – full frontal view – abdomen including kidney regions/amount of postvoid residue noted

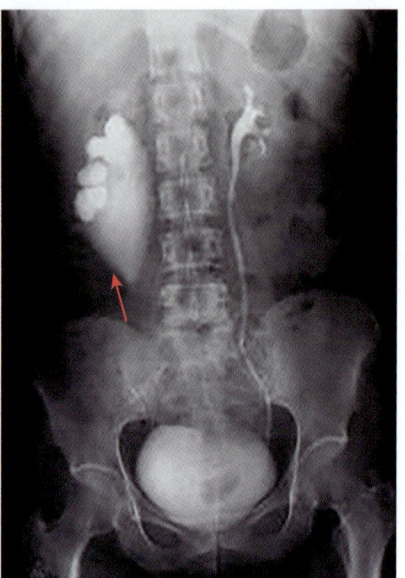

Fig. 53.102. PUJ obstruction.

Dilation of renal pelvis on right (red arrow)

PUJ obstruction

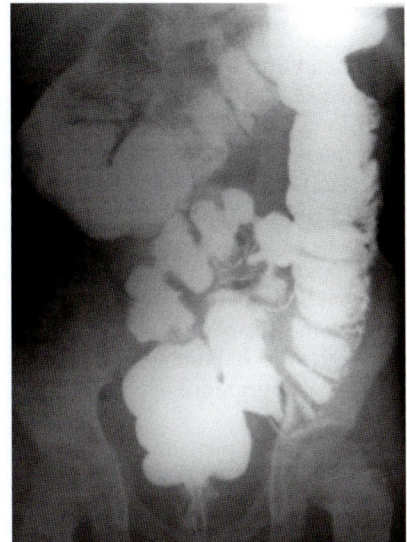

Colon visualized up to hepatic flexure

Normal barium enema

Fig. 53.103. Normal barium enema.

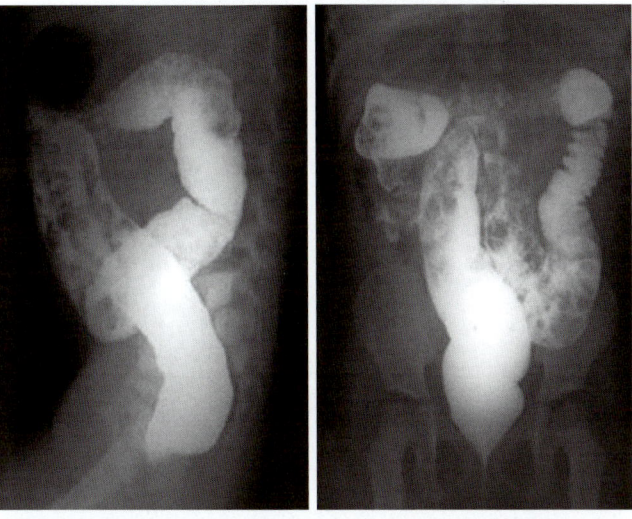

- Barium enema – lateral and AP views
- Note the uniform dilatation of the colon right from the anal verge without any narrow segment

Habitual constipation

Fig. 53.104. Barium enema – lateral and AP views showing habitual constipation.

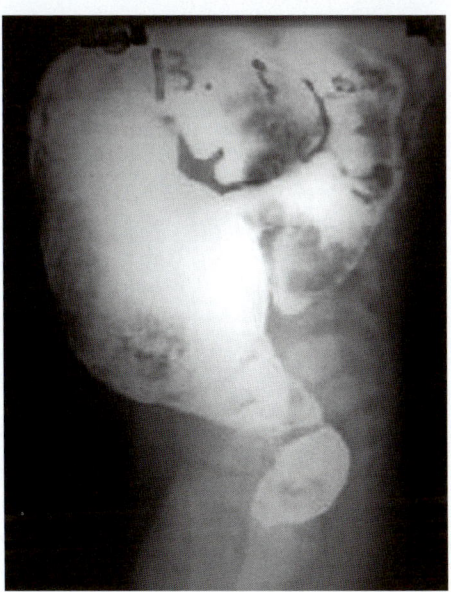

- Barium enema
- Well-defined narrow segment and dilated proximal segment

Hirschsprung disease

Fig. 53.105. Barium enema – Hirschsprung disease.

Skeletal Dysplasia

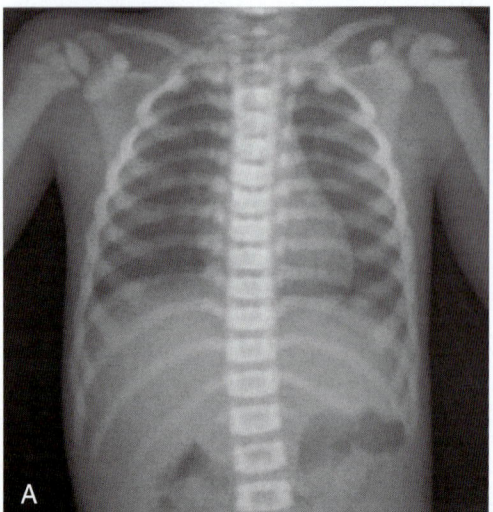

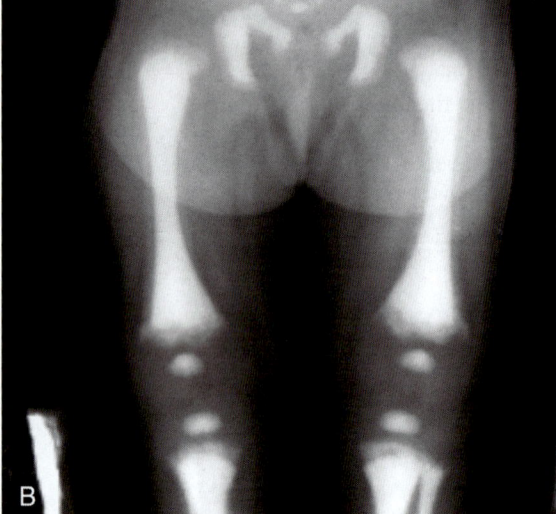

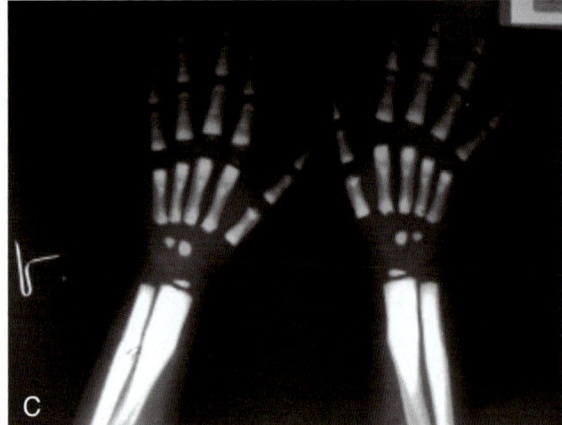

Osteopetrosis

(A) Lateral end of clavicle and ribs show dense lines
(B) X-ray long bones – cortex and inner medulla both are darker (uniformly dense and no differentiation between cortex and medulla)
(C) X-ray hand
  Increased bone density (absence of corticomedullary differentiation), smoothening of bone surfaces
  Cylindrical appearance of the metacarpals
  Normal terminal phalanges

Fig. 53.106. **(A) Dense lines** – osteopetrosis. *(Source: Reproduced from* Robert Kliegman, Joseph St. Geme. *Nelson Textbook of Pediatrics, 2-Volume Set,* 21st Edition, Disorders Involving Defective Bone Resorption, Fig 719.1, Philadelphia, Elsevier Inc., 2019. (From Campeau P, Schlesinger AE: Skeletal dysplasias (Fig. 14). [Updated 2017, Jan 30]. In De Groot LJ, Chrousos G, Dungan K, et al, editors. *Endotext [internet].* South Dartmouth, MA, 2000, *MDText.com, Inc. https://www.ncbi.nlm.nih.gov/books/NBK279130/.))* **(B) X-ray long bones – absent corticomedullary differentiation – osteopetrosis. (C) Increased bone density – osteopetrosis.**

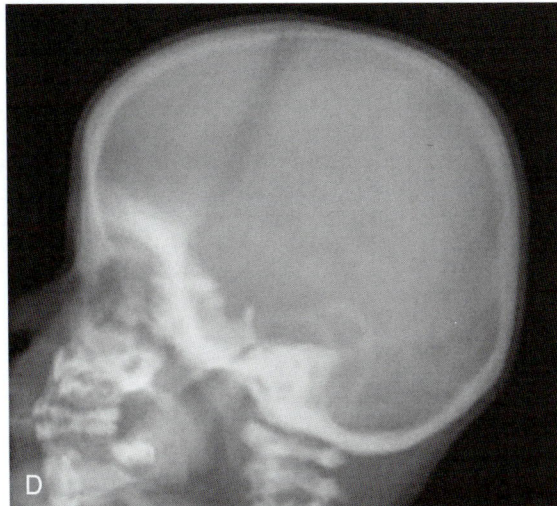

(D) X-ray mandible showing **increased density with maintenance of the normal angle of the mandible**

(E) X-ray lower limb – flaring and elongation of distal femoral and proximal tibial epiphyses funnel-like shape (**Erlenmeyer flask deformity**) **with** uniform increased density of bone

(F) X-ray spine – dense sclerotic band adjacent to the vertebral endplates with normal mid-body (**sandwich vertebra**)/**rugger jersey spine** – alternating dense–lucent–dense appearance

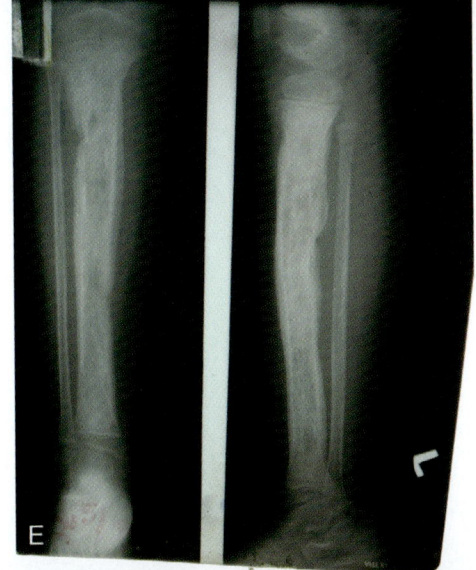

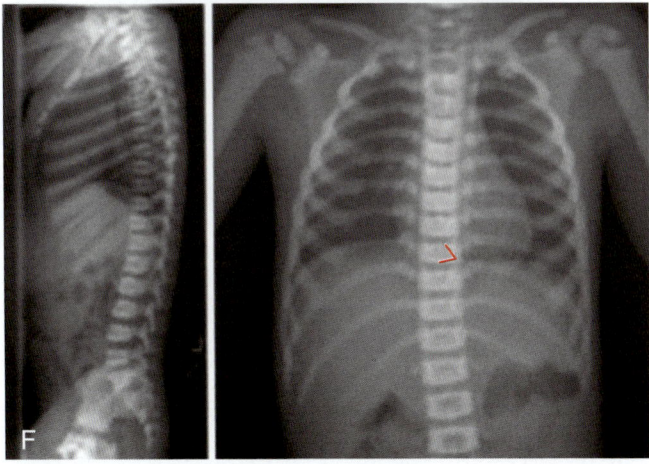

Fig. 53.106., Cont'd (D) Mandible showing increased density with maintenance of the normal angle of the mandible. **(E) Erlenmeyer flask deformity. (F) Sandwich vertebra/rugger jersey spine.** (Source D and F: Reproduced from Robert Kliegman, Joseph St. Geme. *Nelson Textbook of Pediatrics, 2-Volume Set*, 21st Edition, Disorders Involving Defective Bone Resorption, Fig 719.1, Philadelphia, Elsevier Inc., 2020. (From Campeau P, Schlesinger AE: Skeletal dysplasias (Fig. 14). [Updated 2017, Jan 30]. In De Groot LJ, Chrousos G, Dungan K, et al, editors. Endotext [internet]. South Dartmouth, MA, 2000, MDText. com, Inc. *https://www.ncbi.nlm.nih.gov/books/NBK279130/.)*

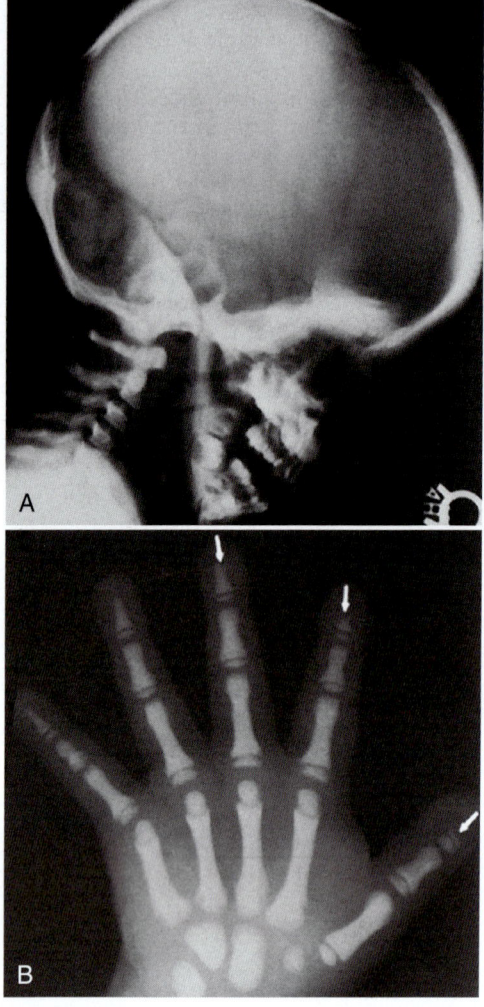

(A) Widely open cranial sutures, dense bones, prognathism (loss of mandibular angle), lack of normal development of mastoids, and paranasal sinuses.

(B) Generalized osteosclerosis, with acro-osteolysis-resorption of terminal phalanges (arrows).

Pyknodysostosis

Fig. 53.107. (A) Loss of mandibular angle and increased density of cranial vault (pyknodysostosis). *(Source Reproduced from* Dennis Marchiori. *Clinical Imaging: With Skeletal*, Chest, and Abdomen Pattern Differentials, Second Edition, Congenital Diseases, Fig. 8.38, St. Louis, Mosby, 2005. (Credit line - From Taybi H, Lachman RS: Radiology of syndromes, metabolic disorders, and skeletal dysplasias, ed 4, St. Louis, 1996, Mosby.))

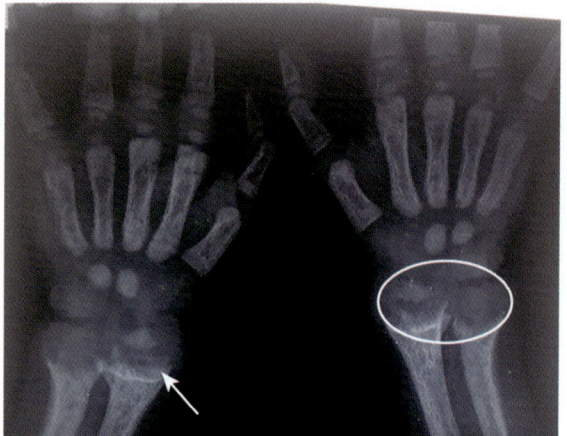

Epiphyseal widening (circle)
Flaring of metaphysis
Cupping and fraying (arrow)

Rickets

Fig. 53.108.   Flaring of metaphysis, cupping, and fraying in rickets.

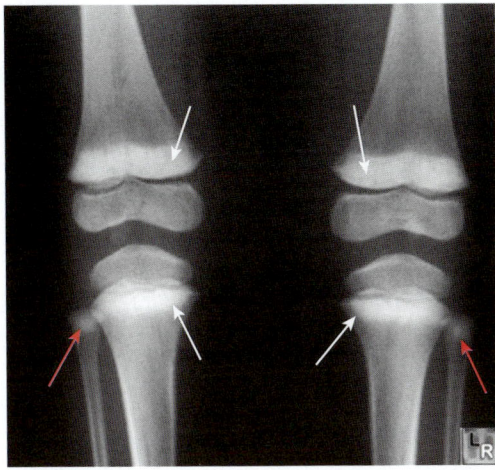

(A) Lead lines in long bones – these are dense metaphyseal bands at the distal femurs and proximal tibias (white arrow); similar dense bands at the heads of both fibulas (shown by red arrows)

Lead poisoning (Other features include)
- Prominence of manubrium sternum
- Medial border of scapula prominent and visualized
- Lead lines seen in ribs and upper end of humerus)

Fig. 53.109. Lead lines in long bones (lead poisoning). *(Source: Reproduced from* Richard Polin, Mark Ditmar. *Pediatric Secrets*, Seventh Edition, Emergency medicine, Fig. 5.6, Philadelphia, Elsevier Inc., 2021. (Credit line- From Dapul H, Laraque D. Lead poisoning in children. Adv Pediatr. 2014:61:313-333.))

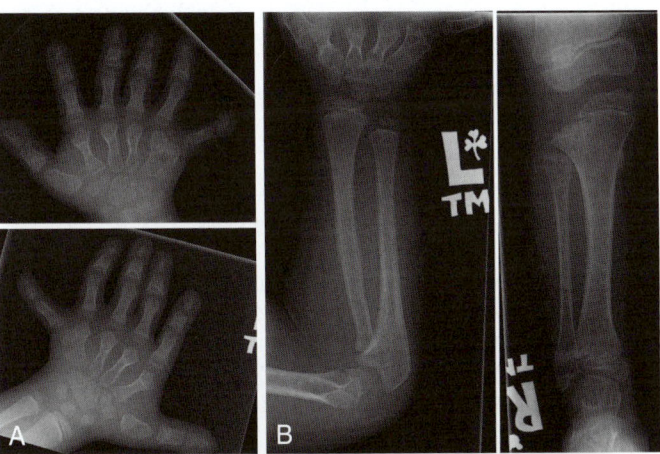

(A) Bilateral postaxial polydactyly in the hands
(B) Characteristic mesomelic limb shortening typically involving forearms and lower legs. Note fibular shortening and dysplastic epiphyses secondary to cartilage dysplasia.
(C) Bell-shaped chest

- **Chondroecto-dermal dysplasia** (Ellis–Van Creveld syndrome)

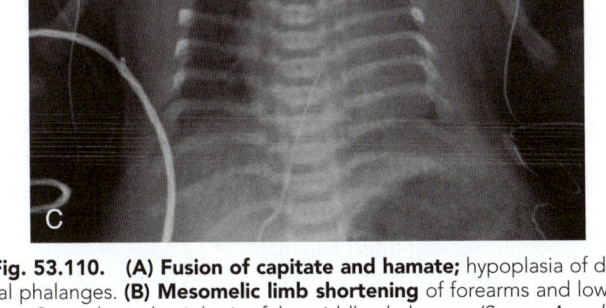

Fig. 53.110. **(A) Fusion of capitate and hamate;** hypoplasia of distal phalanges. **(B) Mesomelic limb shortening** of forearms and lower legs Cone-shaped epiphysis of the middle phalanges. *(Source A and B: Reproduced from* Sarah Sarvis Milla, Shailee Lala. *Problem Solving in Pediatric Imaging*, Skeletal Dysplasias, Fig. 11.11, Philadelphia, Elsevier Inc., 2023. **(C) Bell-shaped chest.** *(Source: https://www.researchgate.net/figure/Anteroposterior-portable-chest-radiograph-in-a-newborn-infant-with-Ellis-van-Creveld_fig4_47754642)*

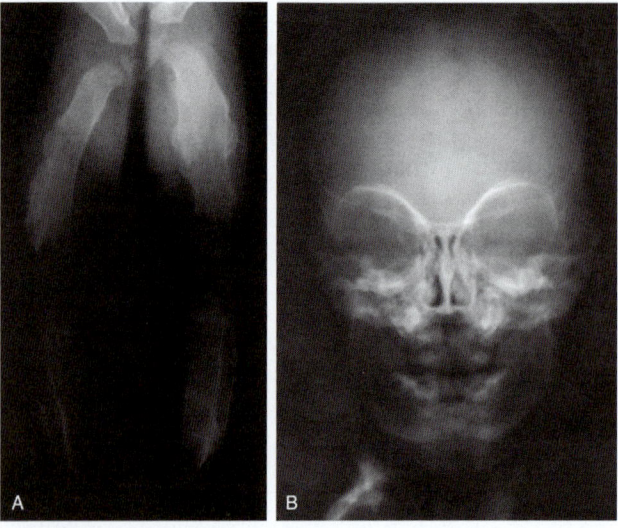

(A) Cortical hyperostosis of both legs   **Caffey disease**
(B) Hyperostosis of mandible

Fig. 53.111. (A) Cortical hyperostosis of right leg. *(Source: Reproduced from* Robert Kliegman, Joseph St. Geme. *Nelson Textbook of Pediatrics, 2-Volume Set*, 21st Edition, Other Inherited Disorders of Skeletal Development, Fig 720.7, Philadelphia, Elsevier Inc., 2020. (From Kamoun-Goldrat A, le Merrer M: Infantile cortical hyperostosis (Caffey disease): a review. J Oral Maxillofac Surg 66:2145–2150, 2008, Figs. 1 and 2.)) (B) *Hyperostosis of mandible.*

ᵃDiscussion on MPS X-ray is given in neurodegenerative disorder Chapter 6.

X-ray Pelvis

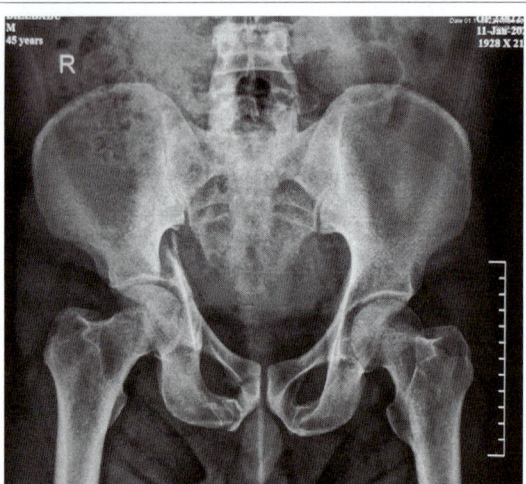

- X-ray pelvis is the looking glass of bony dysplasia   **Normal pelvis**
- Ileum is smooth and round
- Sacrosciatic notch is a big smooth curve
- Interpedicular distances increases from L1 to L5
- Crests
- ASIS
- AIIS
- Greater trochanter
- Lesser trochanter
- Ischial tuberosity

Fig. 53.112. X-ray pelvis AP view (from top to down).

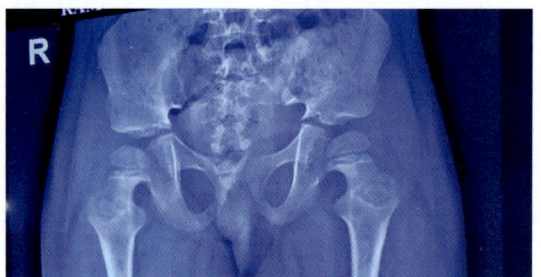

Squared ileum   **Achondroplasia**
Narrow sacrosciatic notch
Decreasing interpedicular
    distance from L1 to L5

Fig. 53.113. Achondroplasia.

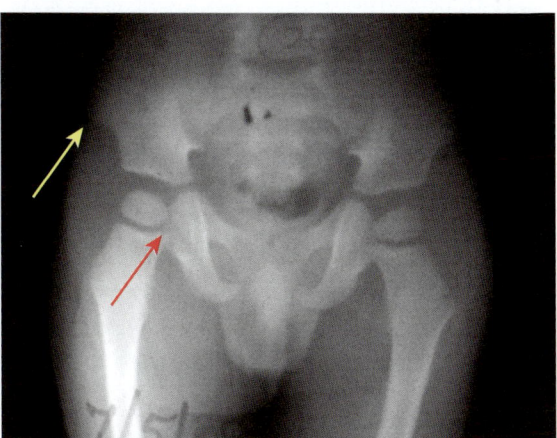

Fig. 53.114.   Down syndrome X-ray pelvis.

- Flared out ileum
- Prominent anterior-superior iliac spine (yellow arrow)
- Flattened acetabular roof (red arrow)

Down syndrome

AP and lateral view for SCFE

(A) **Klein's line** – straight line drawn along the superior cortex of the femoral neck on AP radiograph intersects some portion of the femoral neck; in progressive displacement of epiphysis, Klein's line no longer intersects the epiphysis

(B) **Frog-leg lateral view** – displaced femoral epiphysis

Slipped capital femoral epiphysis (SCFE)

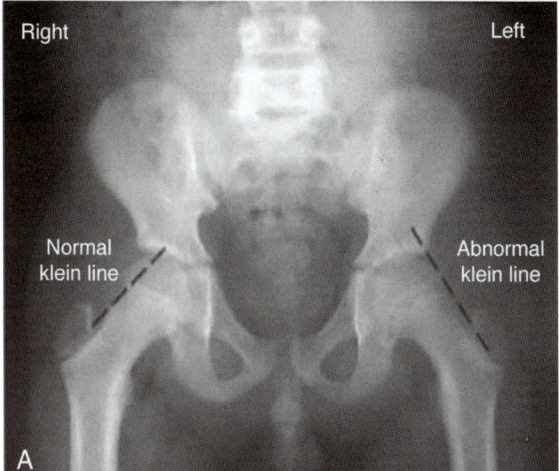

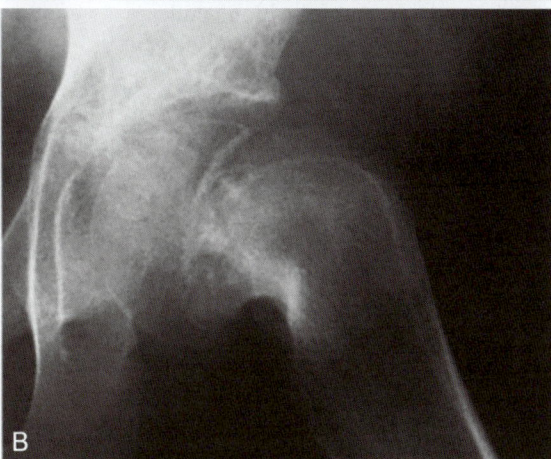

Fig. 53.115.   (A) Normal Klein's line. *(Source: Reproduced from* Robert Kliegman, Joseph St. Geme. *Nelson Textbook of Pediatrics, 2-Volume Set,* 21st Edition, Disorders Involving Defective Bone Resorption, Fig 698.15, Philadelphia, Elsevier Inc., 2020.)* **(B) Frog-leg lateral view** *– displaced femoral epiphysis in SCFE. (Source: Reproduced from* Robert Kliegman, Joseph St. Geme. *Nelson Textbook of Pediatrics, 2-Volume Set,* 21st Edition, Disorders Involving Defective Bone Resorption, Fig 698.16b, Philadelphia, Elsevier Inc., 2020. (From Herring JA: Slipped capital femoral epiphysis. In Herring JA, editor: Tachdjian's pediatric orthopaedics, ed 5, Philadelphia, 2014, WB Saunders, Fig. 18.1, p. 632.))*

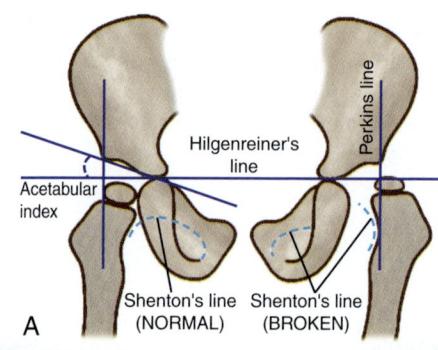

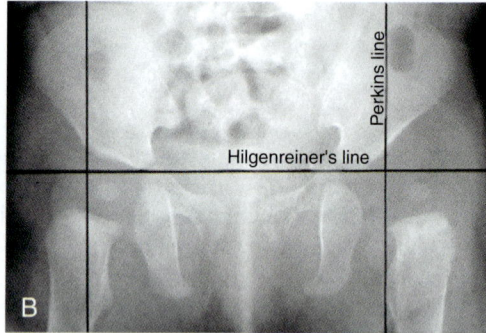

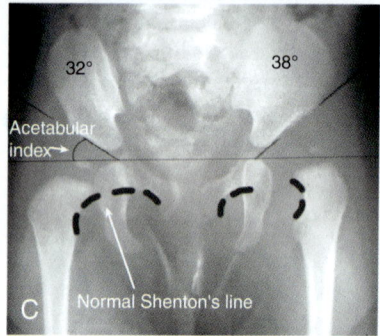

Fig. 53.116. A to C *(Source: Reproduced from Robert Kliegman, Joseph St. Geme. Nelson Textbook of Pediatrics, 2-Volume Set, 21st Edition, Disorders Involving Defective Bone Resorption, Fig 698.8 A-C, Philadelphia, Elsevier Inc., 2020).*

(A–C) Radiographic measurements of development dysplasia of hip

> **Hilgenreiner line** is drawn through the triradiate cartilages
>
> **Perkins line** is drawn perpendicular to Hilgenreiner line at the lateral edge of the acetabulum (**both lines shown in Fig. A and B**)
>
> The ossific nucleus of the femoral head should be located in the medial lower quadrant of the intersection of these two lines
>
> **Shenton's line** curves along the femoral metaphysis and connects smoothly to the inner margin of the pubis
>
> In a child with hip subluxation or dislocation, this line consists of two separate arcs and is described as broken (**as shown in Fig. C**)
>
> The **acetabular index** is the angle between a line drawn along the margin of the acetabulum and Hilgenreiner line
>
> In normal newborns, it averages 27.5° and decreases with age

- **Putti's triad** for developmental dysplasia of the hip include:
  1. Superolateral displacement of proximal femur
  2. Increase in acetabular angle
  3. Small capital femoral epiphysis

Developmental dysplasia of hip (DDH)

Well-formed lower femoral and upper tibial epiphysis

Term baby – normal knee joint

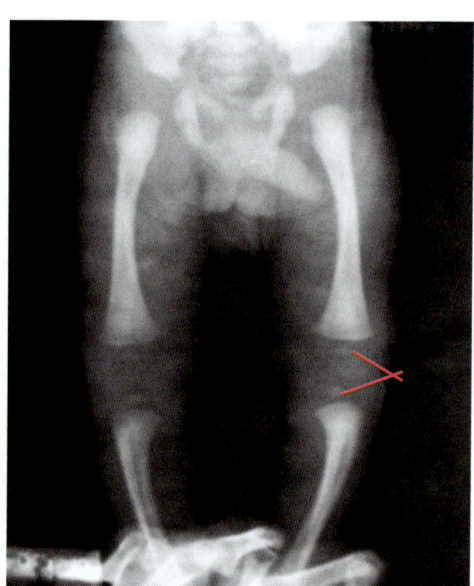

Fig. 53.117. Term baby – normal knee joint.

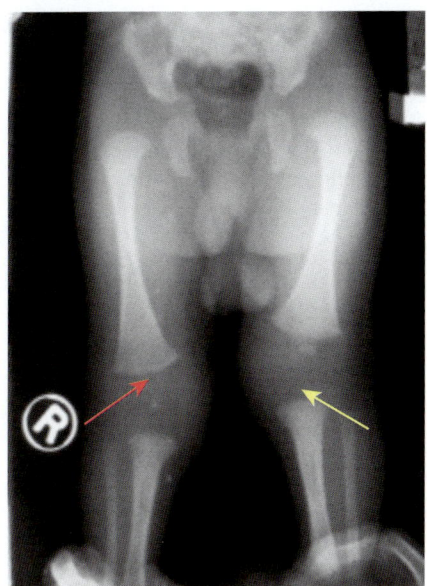

Small lower femoral epiphysis (red arrow) and absent upper tibial epiphysis (yellow arrow)
- X-ray knee (neonate) Femoral and tibial epiphysis are absent or small
- X-ray pelvis (above 1 year) Dysgenesis or absence of upper femoral epiphysis

X-ray knee joint in a term baby with **hypothyroidism**

Fig. 53.118. Femoral and tibial epiphysis are absent or small (hypothyroidism).

X-ray Lower Limb

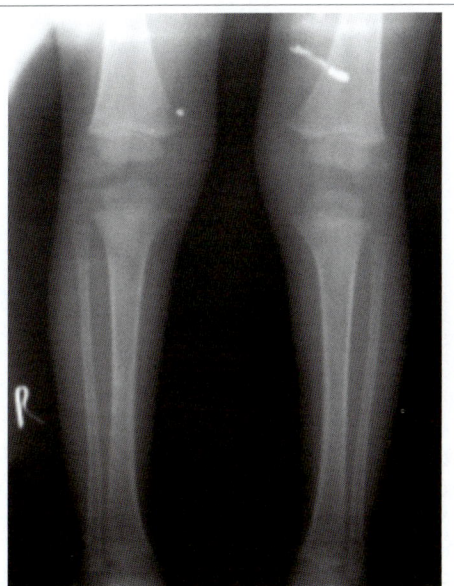

From outer to inner
1. Skin
2. Subcutaneous fat (light density)
3. Muscle (denser area around bone)
4. Bone (in the center)

Normal appearance of lower limbs

Fig. 53.119. Normal appearance of lower limbs.

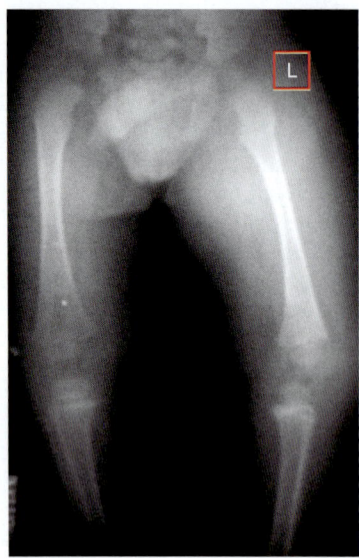

Fig. 53.120.   Acute osteomyelitis – left.

- X-ray of both lower limbs – AP:
  Compare both sides.
  Normal versus abnormal
- Wide muscle mass seen all around the
  bone on the left side (earliest changes –
  soft tissue swelling, loss or blurring of
  normal fat planes)

**Acute
osteomyelitis
– left**

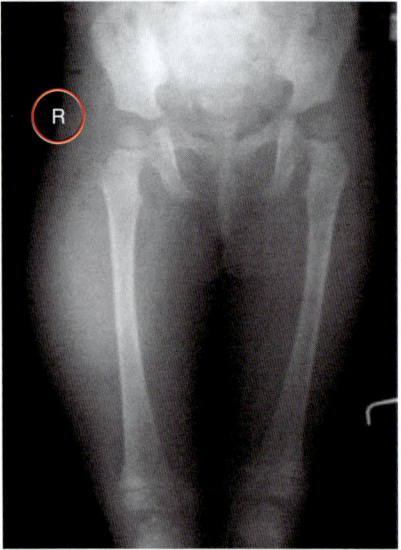

Fig. 53.121.   Deep muscle abscess – right.

- X-ray of both lower limbs – AP:
  Compare both sides
  Normal versus abnormal
- Muscle mass increased on one side of the
  limb only (denser area around
  the bone on right side)

**Deep muscle
abscess – right**

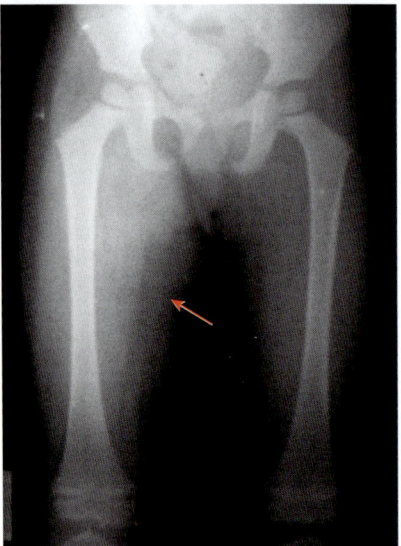

Fig. 53.122.   Cellulitis.

- X-ray of both lower limbs – AP:
  Compare both sides
  Normal versus abnormal
- Wide subcutaneous tissue on right side
  (increased mass in light density)

Cellulitis

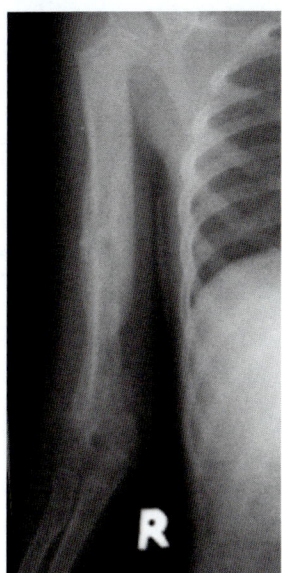

Fig. 53.123.   Pyogenic osteomyelitis humerus.

Sequestration with exuberant new bone formation

Pyogenic osteomyelitis humerus

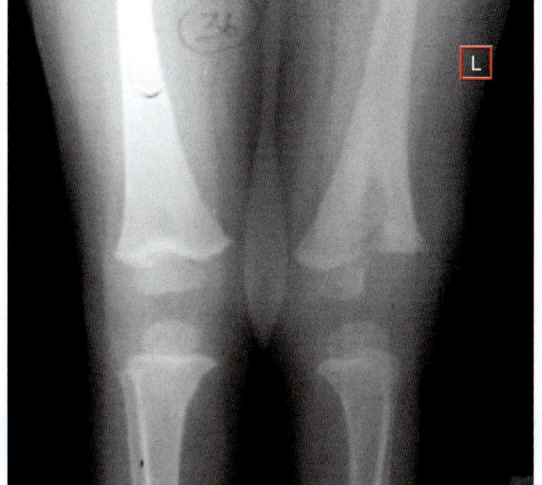

Fig. 53.124.   Tuberculous osteomyelitis of left femur.

Osteolytic lesions involving the epiphysis

Tuberculous osteomyelitis of left femur

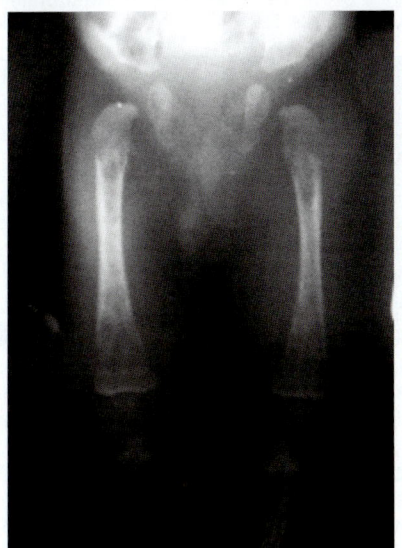

Fig. 53.125.   Syphilitic osteomyelitis.

Bilateral symmetrical periostitis and metaphysitis

Syphilitic osteomyelitis

How to Read CT and MRI

Introduction

- With increasing use of neuroimaging, a pediatric post-graduate must know at least how to identify normal and abnormal findings. This chapter gives an overall view of interpreting CT/MRI.
- Certain diseases are better identified in CT than MRI. One should know what to order for certain neurological disorder. Table 54.1 lists diseases that are identified in CT/MRI.

How to Differentiate Between CT and MRI

Table 54.2 lists the differences between CT and MRI.

TABLE 54.1	Diseases Identified in CT/MRI
CT	**MRI**
• Fracture • Trauma bleeding • Hemorrhage • Calcification • Hydrocephalus • Infections – meningitis, Tuberculous Meningitis (TBM), Neurocystecercosis (NCC), tuberculoma, Acute Disseminated Encephalomyelitis (ADEM)	• Congenital malformations • Neuronal migration disorders • Neurometabolic disorders • Infections • Neoplasms

Various Shades in CT/MRI – White and Black Shadow

Table 54.3 shows various shades in CT/MRI.

CT Images

Table 54.4 shows various CT images.
Table 54.5 shows abnormal CT images.

Black shadows in CT

1. Hydrocephalus (dilated ventricle)
2. Infarct
3. Cerebral edema
4. Abscess

Table 54.6 shows abnormal black shadows in CT.

MRI

Overall approach to MRI

Flowchart 54.1 shows overall approach to MRI.
Table 54.7 shows MRI images of the brain.
Which sequence to look for each abnormality?

Table 54.8 shows abnormality identified in each MRI sequence.

TABLE 54.2	Differences Between CT and MRI			
Features	**CT**	**MRI Brain – T1 (Similar to CT: Anatomy Maintained; Gray Matter – gray; White Matter – White)**	**MRI Brain – T2**	**MRI Brain – T2-FLAIR (Marble-Like Appearance)**
Image		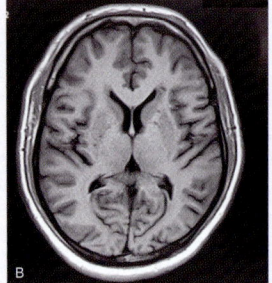	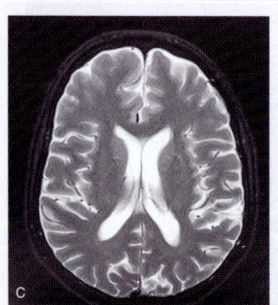	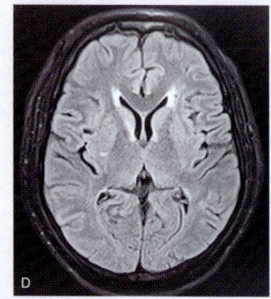

Fig. 54.1 A-D. (A) Normal CT. (B) T1W. (C) T2. (D) T2-FLAIR. *(Source: https://radiopaedia.org/cases/normal-ct-brain-7-years) (Source: Axial T1W MRI of the brain. Though the entire image occupies hard disk... | Download Scientific Diagram (researchgate. net)) (Source: T2 weighted image | Radiology Reference Article | Radiopaedia.org) (Source: T2-FLAIR - Questions and Answers in MRI (mriquestions.com))*

Features	CT	MRI Brain – T1	MRI Brain – T2	MRI Brain – T2-FLAIR
Scalp	Black	White	White	White
Bone	White	Black	Black	Black
CSF	Black	Black	White	Black
Gray matter	Gray	Gray	White	White
White matter	White	White	Gray	Gray

TABLE 54.3	Various Shades in CT and MRI	
Description	**CT**	**MRI**
Lesions of gray matter White shadows	Called density • Hyperdense • Examples: Hemorrhage, calcification, tumors, tuber, and contrast enhancement	Called intensity • Hyperintense – high signal intensity • Examples: • MRI T1: Fat, contrast enhancement • MRI T2: Cyst, tumor, CSF, demyelination, edema, abscess • Fluid-attenuated inversion recovery (FLAIR): Same as T2 (black CSF) • Diffusion-weighted imaging (DWI): Infarct, abscess
Black shadows	Hypodense Examples: Edema, infarct, and abscess	Hypointense – low signal intensity Examples: Brain abscess and infarct

ABNORMAL MRI OF THE BRAIN

a. **Pediatric tumor** – astrocytoma, medulloblastoma, craniopharyngioma, ependymoma, choroid plexus tumor
b. **Infarct/Hypoxic ischemic encephalopathy (HIE)**
c. **Neurocysticercosis/tuberculoma**
c. **Congenital malformation**
d. **Demyelination**
   Table 54.9 shows abnormal MRI images in pediatric patients.

DEMYELINATION

Normally in T2W, CSF appears white, gray matter appears white, and white matter appears gray

In demyelination, white matter appears white in T2W.
In an MRI T2W, one can identify neurodegenerative disorder depending on which site is involved.
Flowchart 54.2 shows approach to demyelination.
Table 54.10 shows demyelinating disease in MRI.

MR SPECTROSCOPY

Table 54.11 shows MR spectroscopy images.

TABLE 54.4	CT Images
Views/cut	• For head CT – bone window and brain window are two important window settings • **Bone window** – for visualizing bony structures – skull and bone lesion (to identify any fracture) • **Brain window** – visualizing brain parenchyma

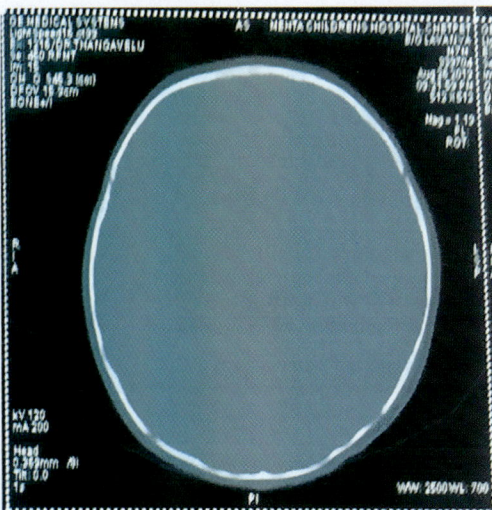

Fig. 54.2 CT bone window.

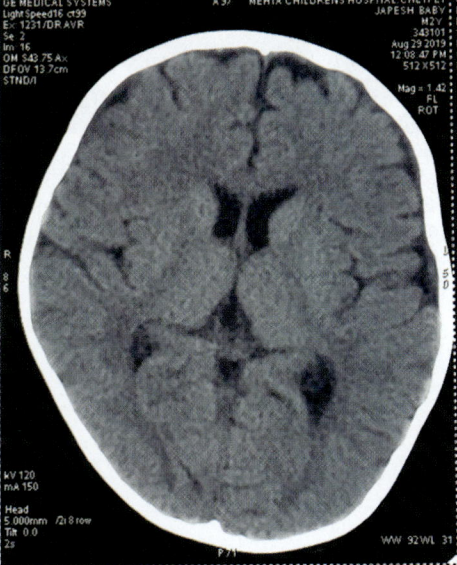

Fig. 54.3 Normal CT brain window.

TABLE 54.5	Abnormal CT Images

Abnormal image

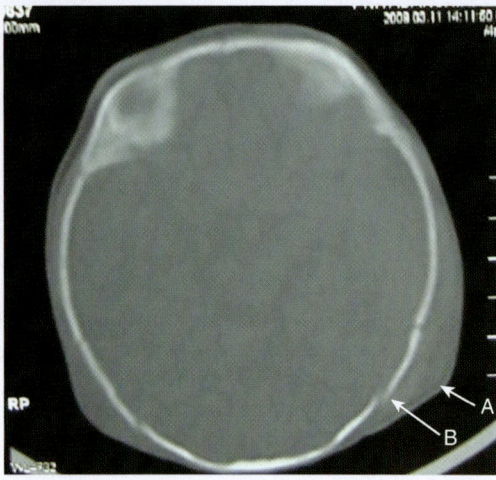

Fig. 54.4 Fracture skull: (A) Soft tissue swelling and (B) fracture.

White shadows in CT brain

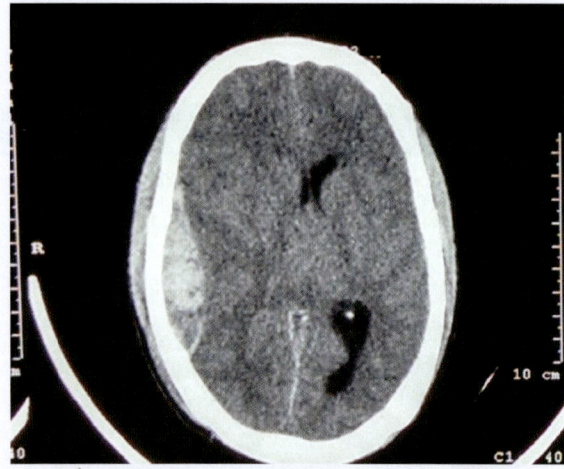

Fig. 54.5 Extradural hemorrhage (Right temporoparietal extradural hemorrhage with midline shift). (*Source:* Reproduced from Hemanshu Prabhakar. *Essentials of Neuroanesthesia*, Neurotrauma, Figure 32.2, Oxford, Academic Press, 2017.)

Fracture

1. Sharp margins
2. Cortical discontinuity ± displacement
3. Soft tissue swelling

Suture Line

1. Zigzag line
2. No cortical discontinuity/displacement
3. No soft tissue swelling

1. Acute hematoma
2. Acute hemorrhage Subarachnoid hemorrhage (SAH), Subdural hemorrhage (SDH), Extradural hemorrhage (EDH)
3. Hemorrhagic contusion
4. Calcification
5. Postcontrast study – blood vessels, meningeal enhancement, inflammatory lesions, neoplasm

Extradural hematoma (biconvex shaped)
- Blood between the skull and dural layer of brain (due to tear or injury in the middle meningeal artery)
- Do not cross the suture line
- Always associated with skull fracture

TABLE
54.5 | **Abnormal CT Images—cont'd**

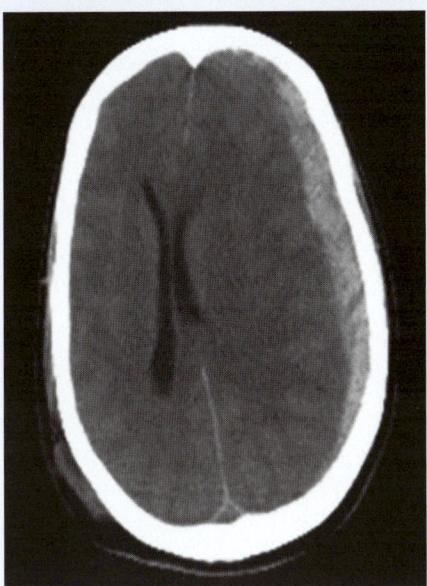

Fig. 54.6 Subdural hemorrhage. *(Source: https://www.sciencedirect. com/topics/neuroscience/subdural-hematoma)*

Subdural hematoma
- Collection of blood in between dura and arachnoid layers of the brain
- Crescent shaped
- Can cross suture line
- Tear in bridging veins in subdural space

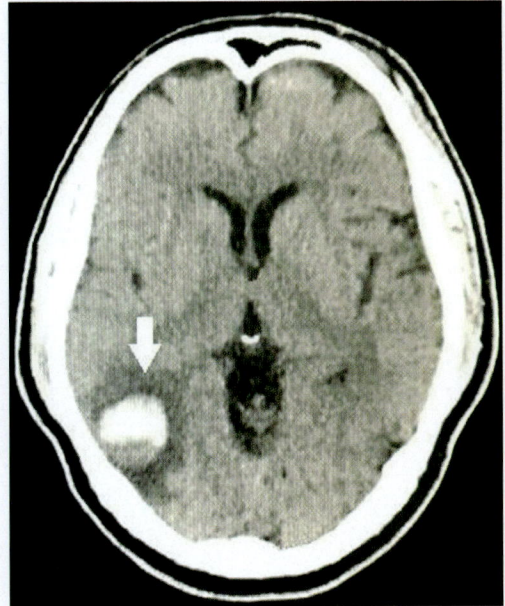

Fig. 54.7 Intraparenchymal bleeding. *(Source:* Reproduced from Leonardo C Welling, Nicollas Nunes Rabelo, Mateus Gonçalves de Sena Barbosa et al. Intracerebral Hemorrhage and Ferroptosis: Something Else that STICH Should Know?, *World Neurosurgery* Jun;150:211-212;2021.)

Intraparenchymal bleeding
- Intraparenchymal hemorrhage in temporopatrietal region. The hyperdense (bright image) area represents acute bleeding, and the hypodense area shows hematoma absorption and penumbra area (arrow).

Continued

TABLE 54.5 | **Abnormal CT Images—cont'd**

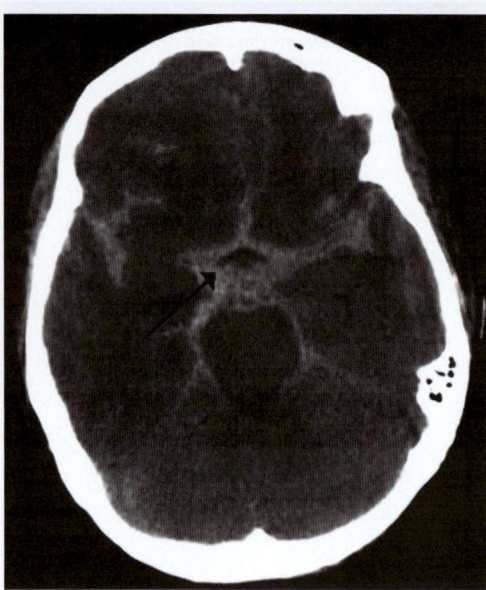

Fig. 54.8 Subarachnoid hemorrhage. *(Source-https://en.wikipedia. org/wiki/File:SubarachnoidP.png)*

Subarachnoid hemorrhage
Bleeding in the subarachnoid spaces
Subarachnoid hemorrhage — white area in the center stretching into the sulci on either side

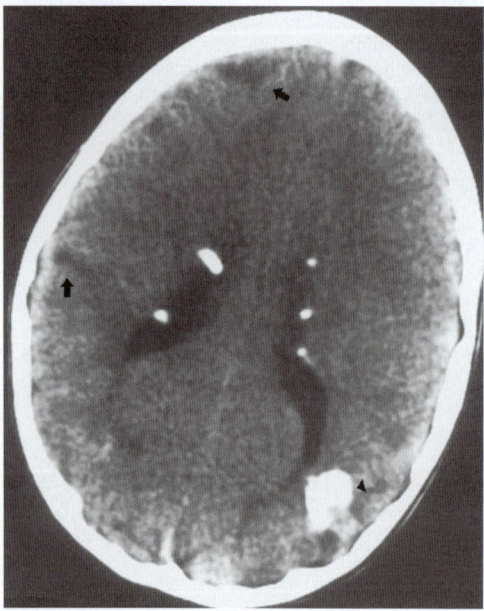

Fig. 54.9 Subependymal nodule. *(Source:* Reproduced from Robert Daroff, Joseph Jankovic, John Mazziotta et al. *Bradley's Neurology in Clinical Practice*, Seventh Edition, Neurocutaneous Syndromes, Fig. 100.3, London, Elsevier Inc., 2016. (Credit line - Reprinted with permission from Roach, E.S., Kerr, J., Mendelsohn, D., et al., 1991. Diagnosis of symptomatic and asymptomatic gene carriers of tuberous sclerosis by CT and MRI. Ann N Y Acad Sci 615, 112–122.)

Subependymal nodules: (Tuberous sclerosis)
typical calcified subependymal nodules; a large calcified parenchymal lesion (arrowhead) and low-density cortical lesions (arrows) are seen

TABLE 54.5   **Abnormal CT Images—cont'd**

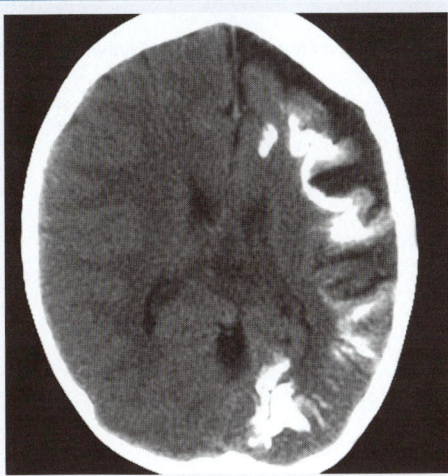

Fig. 54.10   Subcortical calcification along the left frontal, parietal occipital lobe depicting tram-track–like appearance. (*Source:* Reproduced from Anne Osborn. *Essentials of Osborn's Brain: A Fundamental Guide for Residents and Fellows*, Vascular Neurocutaneous Syndromes, 40-4A, Elsevier Inc., 2020.)

Sturge–Weber syndrome
Cortical atrophy and extensive calcifications in the cortex and subcortical white matter throughout most of the left cerebral hemisphere, depicting Tram track lines

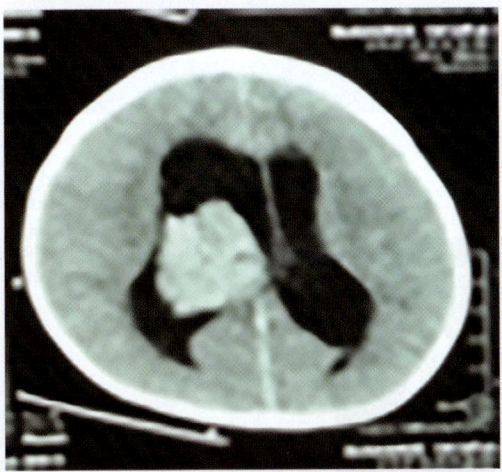

Fig. 54.11   Choroid plexus tumor.

Choroid plexus tumor
Intraventricular enhancing mass suggestive of choroid plexus tumor in the right lateral ventricle

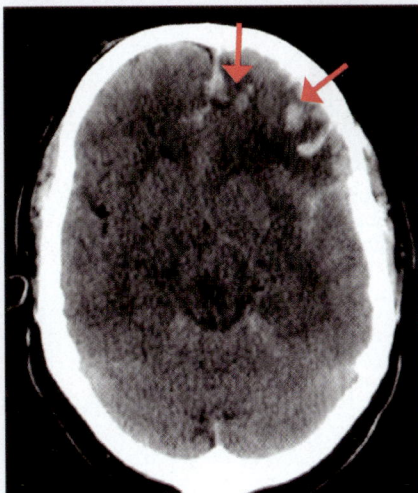

Fig. 54.12   Cortical contusion. (*Source:* Reproduced from G. Omar Enríquez. Imaginología en trauma, *Revista Médica Clínica Las Condes*, 24(1):68-77;2013).

Cortical contusion – hypodense area in the left frontal region
Imaginological (brain CT classification) of cerebral contusion
    1a: Lobar microcontusion or cerebral contusion < 1 cm
    1b: Bilateral lobar microcontusion or cerebral contusion
    2a: Unilateral lobar contusion
    2b: Bilateral lobar contusion
    3a: Hemispheric contusion with severe unilateral mass effect
    3b: Hemispheric contusion with severe bilateral mass effect

Continued

TABLE 54.5	Abnormal CT Images—cont'd

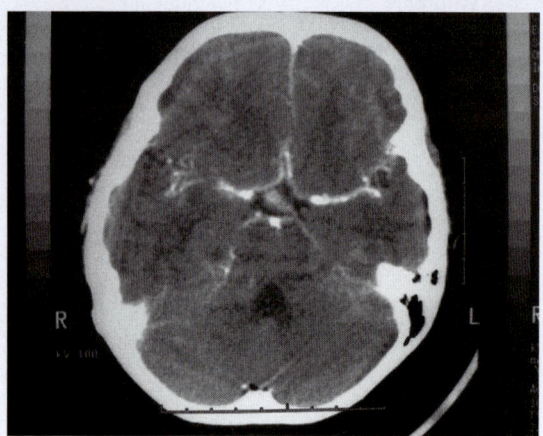

CT brain contrast:
CT brain contrast showing increased meningeal enhancement suggestive of CNS infection

Fig. 54.13 CT brain contrast showing increased meningeal enhancement. (Source: Reproduced from Ming-Han Tsai, Yhu-Chering Huang, Tzou-Yien Lin. Development of tuberculoma during therapy presenting as hemianopsia, *Pediatric Neurology*, 31(5):360-363;2004).

TABLE 54.6	Abnormal Black Shadows in CT

CT Picture	Findings

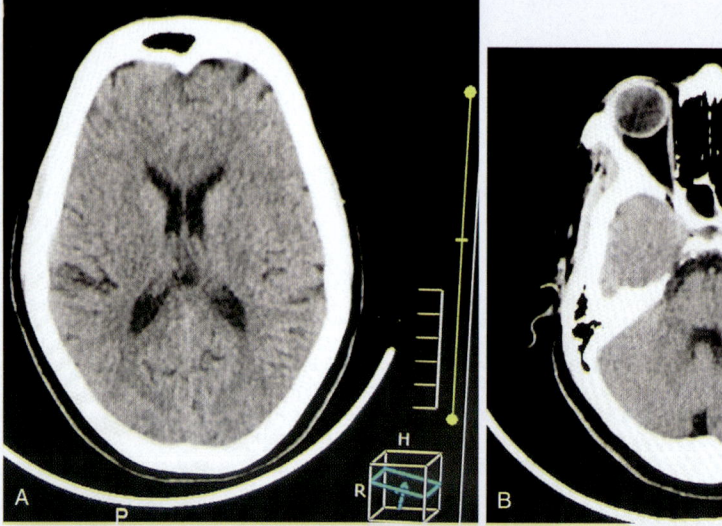
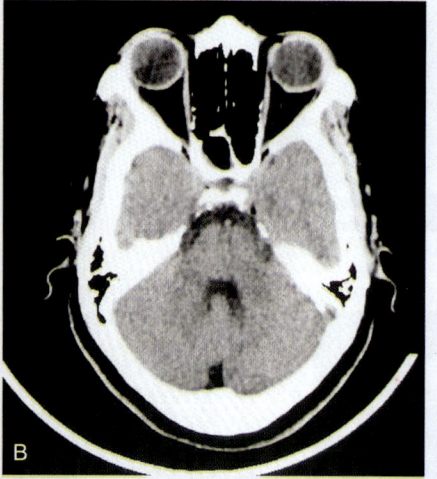

(A and B) **Normal ventricle**
(C) **Hydrocephalus (aqueductal stenosis)** — symmetrical dilatation of lateral and 3rd ventricle

Fig. 54.14 A-D (A and B)- Normal ventricles. (C) Aqueductal stenosis. (*Source C-MedPix Case - Aqueductal stenosis. (nih.gov)*)

TABLE 54.6	**Abnormal Black Shadows in CT—cont'd**

CT Picture	Findings

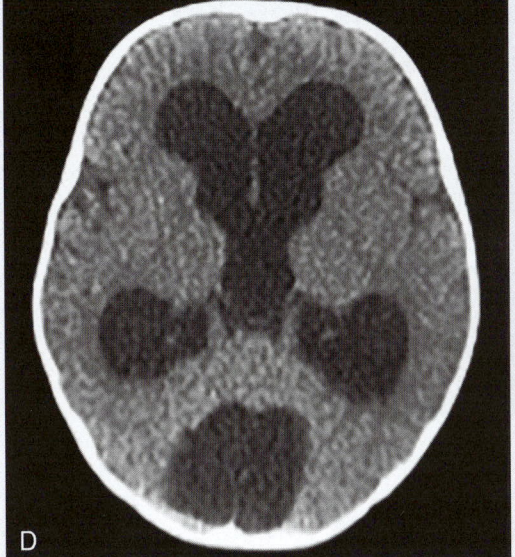

(D) **Tetrahydrocephalus** with posterior fossa cyst

Fig. 54.14, cont'd (D) Tetrahydrocephalus (*https://www.google.com/url?sa=i&url=https%3A%2F%2Fwww.researchgate.net%2Ffigure%2Fa-b-Preoperative-CT-scan-showing-the-tetraventricular-hydrocephalus-posterior-fossa_fig1_263130753&psig=AOvVaw2i8qddbizIsefmTq4kGSf2&ust=1610251144796000&source=images&cd=vfe&ved=0CAIQjRxqFwoTCMD9ypH7je4CFQAAAAAdAAAAABAD*)

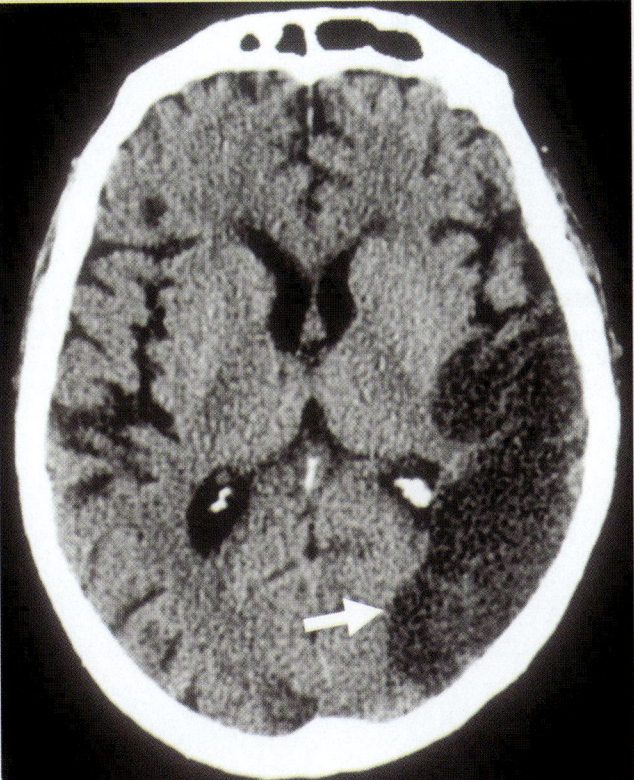

Infarct (hypodense area-arrow) in parietal region Middle cerebral artery (MCA) territory

Fig. 54.15 Infarct in the MCA territory. (*Source:* Reproduced from Grant Liu, Nicholas Volpe, Steven Galetta. *Liu, Volpe, and Galetta's Neuro-Ophthalmology: Diagnosis and Management,* Third Edition, Retrochiasmal Disorders, Figure 8.15, London, Elsevier Inc., 2019).

Continued

TABLE 54.6	Abnormal Black Shadows in CT—cont'd

CT Picture	Findings

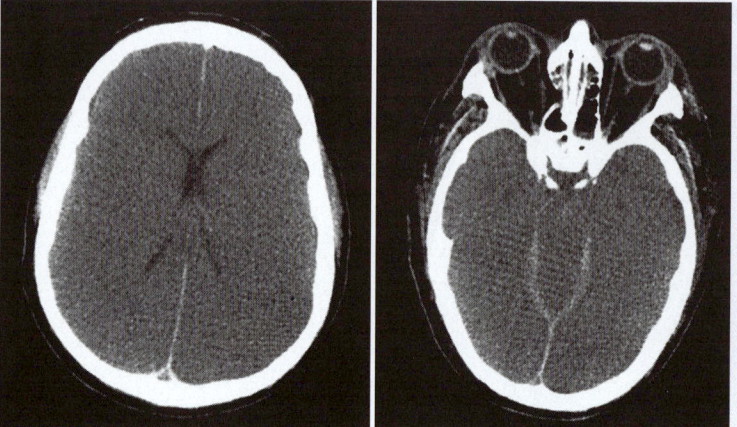

Features of diffuse cerebral edema:
- Loss of differentiation between white and gray matter
- Loss of sulci and gyri
- Slit-like ventricles
- Effacement of cisterns

Fig. 54.16 Cerebral edema. (*Source:* Reproduced from Nancy Newman, Joseph Jankovic, John Mazziotta. *Bradley and Daroff's Neurology in Clinical Practice,* Eighth Edition, Anoxic-Ischemic Encephalopathy, Fig. 83.5, Philadelphia, Elsevier Inc., 2022.)

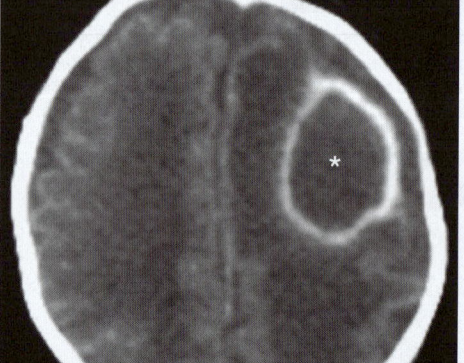

Brain abscess
Hypodense ring enhancing lesion seen in left frontal lobe

Fig. 54.17 Brain abscess. (*Source:* Reproduced from Michele Walters, Richard Robertson. *Pediatric Radiology: The Requisites,* Fourth Edition, Brain Imaging, Figure 8.52, Philadelpha, Elsevier Inc., 2017.)

Discussion on MRI brain

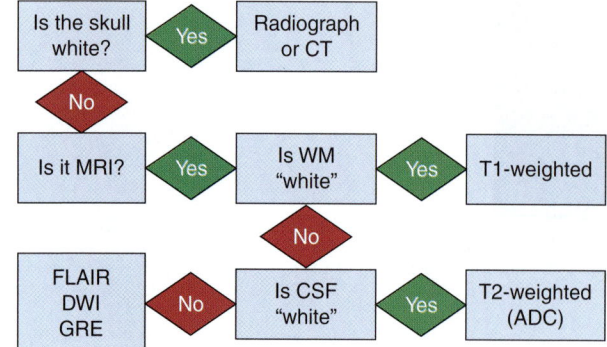

Flowchart 54.1   Overall approach to MRI.

| TABLE 54.7 | MRI Images |

Normal MRI

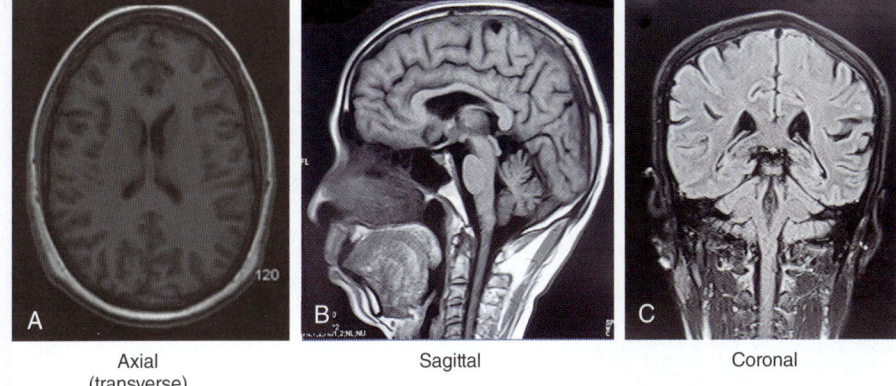

Axial
(transverse)

Sagittal

Coronal

Fig. 54.18 (A–C) Different planes.

Different planes:
- Axial or horizontal
- Sagittal
- Coronal

Normal MRI images – parts identified in different plane

Normal MRI images – parts identified in each plane (A, axial, B, sagittal, and C, coronal view)

Normal

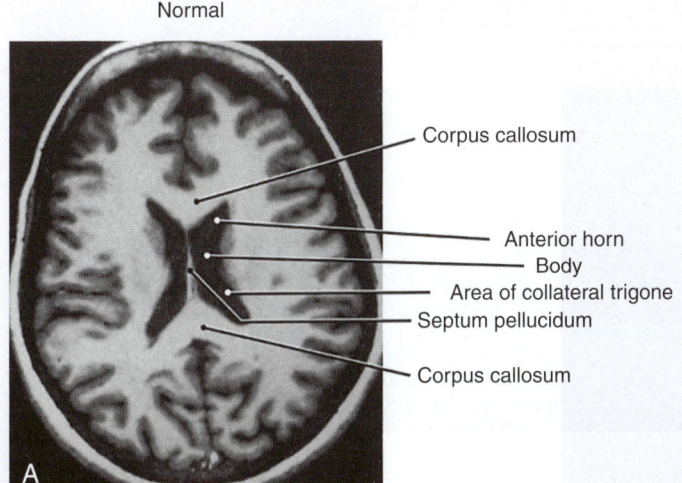

- Corpus callosum
- Anterior horn
- Body
- Area of collateral trigone
- Septum pellucidum
- Corpus callosum

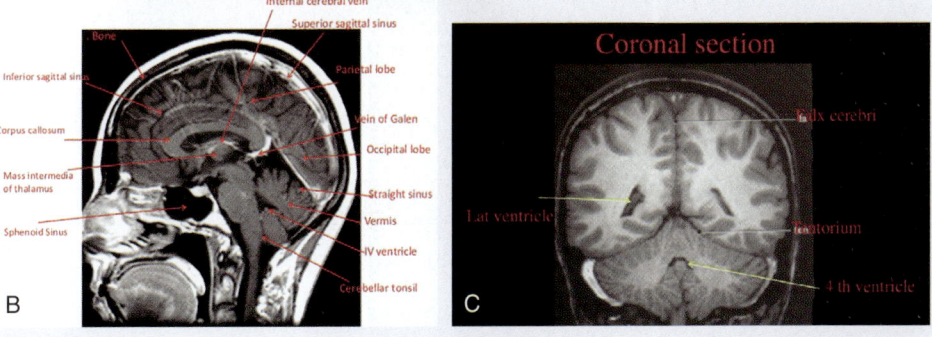

Fig. 54.19 (A) Axial view. (B) Sagittal view. (C) Coronal view. (*Source:* Reproduced from Kathryn McCance, Sue Huether. *Pathophysiology: The Biologic Basis for Disease in Adults and Children*, Eighth Edition, Alterations in Cognitive Systems, Cerebral Hemodynamics, and Motor Function, Fig 17.21, St. Louis, Mosby, 2019. (Credit Line - From Haines DE, editor: Fundamental neuroscience for basic and clinical applications, ed 4, Philadelphia, 2013, Saunders.)

Continued

TABLE 54.7	MRI Images—cont'd

MRI sequences

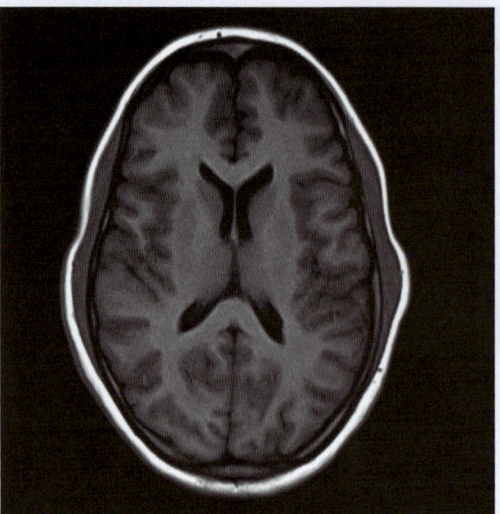

Fig. 54.20   T1W. (*Source: Axial T1W MRI of the brain. Though the entire image occupies hard disk... | Download Scientific Diagram (researchgate.net)*)

Sequences or images:
T1W, T2W, fluid-attenuated inversion recovery (FLAIR), diffusion-weighted imaging (DWI), apparent diffusion co-efficient (ADC)

T1W
Resembles CT brain
- Gray matter is gray
- White matter is white
- CSF is black
- Gray/white differentiation is sharp
- Fat is bright
- Bone is black
- Contrast studies only on T1

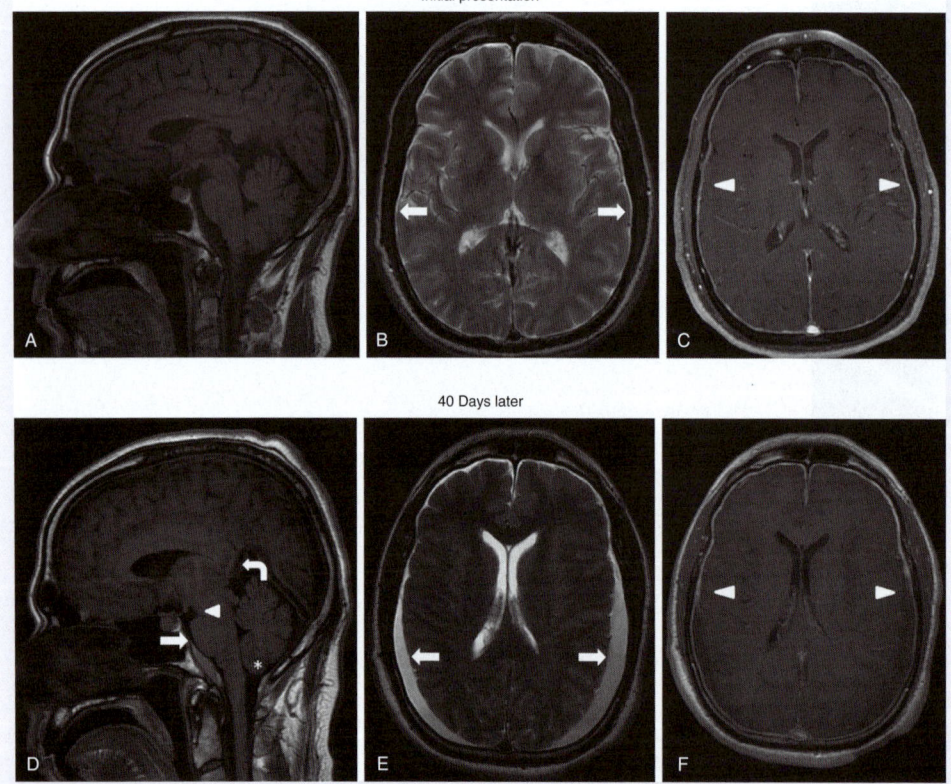

Fig. 54.21   T1 contrast. (*Source: Reproduced from Juan Small, Daniel Noujaim, Daniel Ginat. Neuroradiology: Spectrum and Evolution of Disease*, Intracranial Hypotension, Figure 17.1, Philadelphia, Elsevier Inc., 2019.)

Contrast studies are done in T1 to identify infection, inflammation, brain tumor, vascular pathology Fig 54.20 T1W post contrast image shows diffuse, smooth pachymeningeal enhancement

TABLE 54.7	MRI Images—cont'd

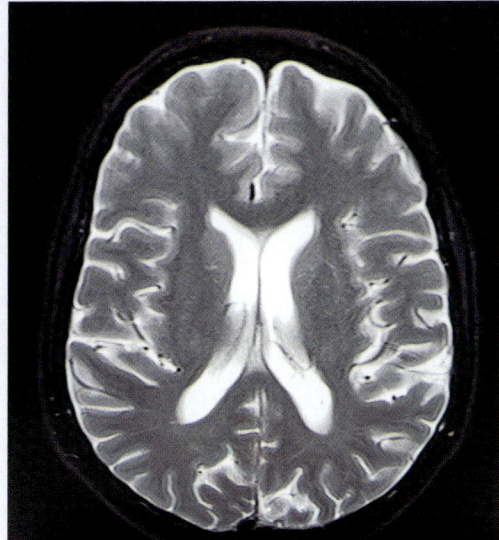

Fig. 54.22   T2W images.

T2W image:
Gray matter dark
White matter gray
CSF bright
Fat intermediate
Bone dark
Most of cystic/solid appear bright
Advanced techniques are done in T2

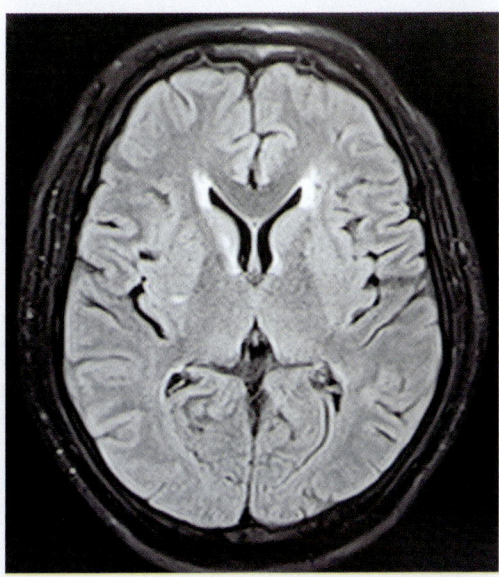

Fig. 54.23   T2-FLAIR. *(Source: T2-FLAIR - Questions and Answers in MRI (mriquestions.com))*

T2-FLAIR
1. Similar to T2 except CSF
2. CSF − dark
3. All tissues other than CSF − bright

Continued

TABLE 54.7	MRI Images—cont'd

What are **ADC and DWI**?
DWI – normal

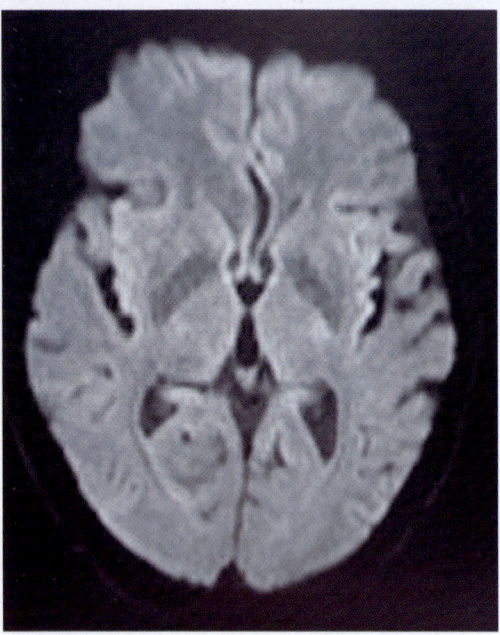

Fig. 54.24 Normal DWI. *(Source: MR Terminology - postgraduate training (google.com))*

ADC

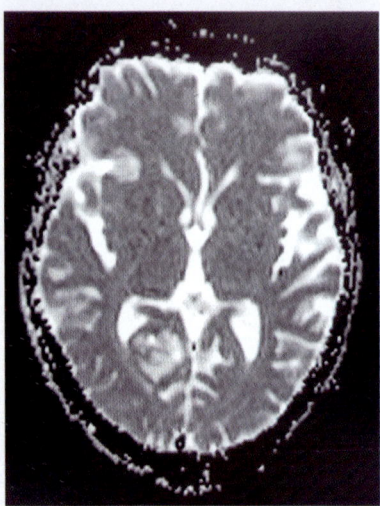

Fig. 54.25 ADC mapping. *(Source: https://www.slideshare.net/RobertCruz23/dwi-adc-mri-principles-applications-in-veterinary-medicine -slide 22)*

- **DWI**
  - In DWI, skull and scalp layers will not be shown
  - CSF – black, gray, and white difference is not distinct
  - DWI – a newer technology in MRI; useful in identifying acute ischemia and infarct very early
  - In cytotoxic edema due to acute ischemia, diffusion is restricted; because of swelling of the cell, there is no space for the diffusion to occur so diffusion is restricted; hence, areas of reduced diffusion appear brighter on DWI and darker on ADC

- **ADC**
  - ADC (a diffusion coefficient map) is a measure of magnitude of diffusion within the tissue and it is calculated by combining at least two DWI images that vary in diffusion but all other parameters are normal
  - An ADC of a tissue is expressed in units of mm^2/s
  - ADC and DWI work as positive and negative pictures of each other

  ADC is used to differentiate false-positive (T2 shine through – artifact) or real lesion (acute infarct)

TABLE 54.8	Abnormality Identified in Each MRI Sequence

Imaging	Defects
T1W Image	For anatomical details; subacute hemorrhages
T2W images	Edema, demyelination, infarct, chronic hemorrhage
FLAIR image	Edema, demyelination, infarct in periventricular region
ADC and DWI ((DWI and ADC are done only in axial view)	It is called "the stroke sequence" 1. Acute infarct – in DWI, it is bright (high signal intensity), and in ADC, it is dark (restricted diffusion) 2. Arachnoid cyst – dark in DWI and bright in ADC

TABLE
54.9
Abnormal MRI Images

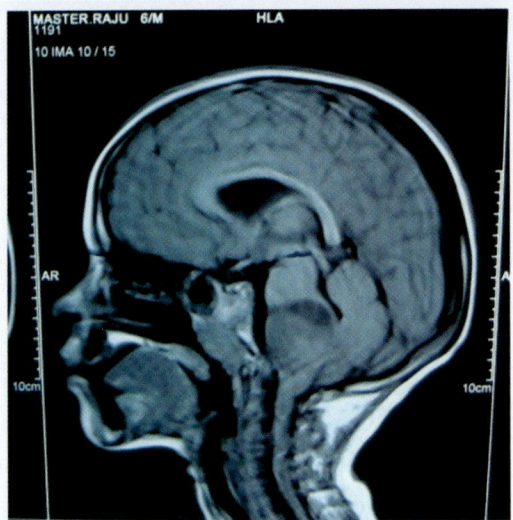

Fig. 54.26 Plain MRI – posterior fossa tumor.

Posterior fossa tumor
Hypodense lesion seen in posterior fossa

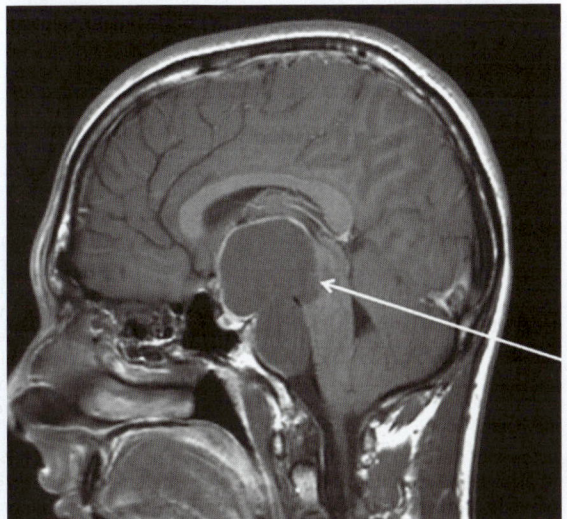

Fig. 54.27 Plain MRI – sagittal view – craniopharyngioma.

Craniopharyngioma
• Bilobed hypointense lesion in suprasellar region with peripheral enhancement

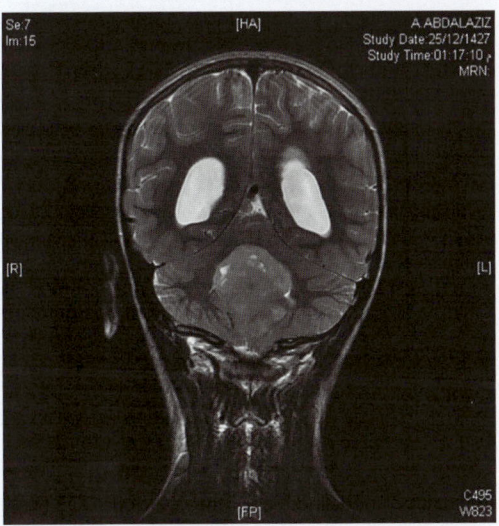

Fig. 54.28 Fourth ventricular tumor.

4th ventricular tumor
MRI showing 4th ventricular mass with markedly dilated 4th ventricle

Continued

TABLE
54.9 **Abnormal MRI Images—cont'd**

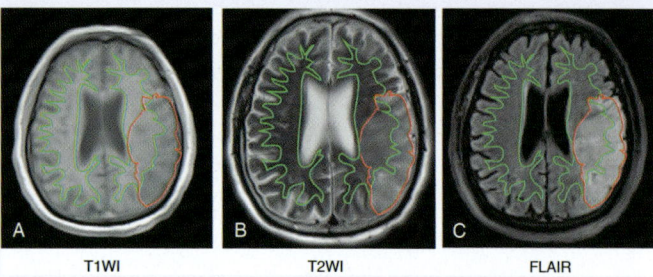

T1WI   T2WI   FLAIR

Fig. 54.29 Infarct. (*Source:* Reproduced from Yuan Wang, Gang Liu, Dandan Hong et al. White matter injury in ischemic stroke, *Progress in Neurobiology* 141:45-60;2016.)

Infarct

T1 WI (a) shows mixed areas of abnormal signal intensity in the Gray and White Matter(WM) of the temporal lobe. T2 WI (b) and FLAIR (c) images demonstrate high intensity signal in the infarct zone with subtle prominence of White matter.

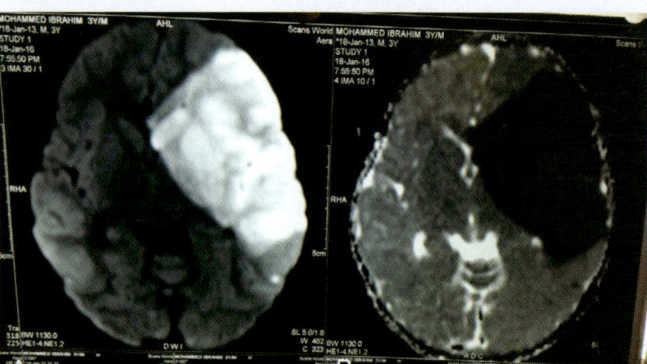

Fig. 54.30 Infarct: (A) DWI and (B) ADC.

Diffusion-weighted image (DWI):
- To visualize an area of acute ischemia
- MRI diffusion-weighted images shown as bright signal
- ADC sequence – appears as dark area
- Suggestive of acute infarct when the infarct in DWI is white (hyperintense or high signal); it will be black (low signal) in ADC
- Rule: High signal DWI + low signal ADC = True abnormality
High signal DWI + high signal ADC = False-positive

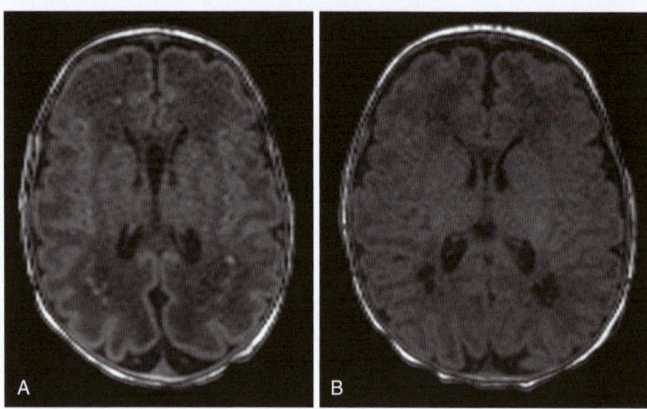

Fig. 54.31 A, and B (*Source:* Reproduced from Jeffrey Perlman. *Neurology: Neonatology Questions and Controversies*, Second Edition, Magnetic Resonance Imaging's Role in the Care of the Infant at Risk for Brain Injury, Figure 16.24, Philadelphia, Saunders, 2012.)

HIE sequelae

A: White matter abnormalities in the frontal and parieto-occipital characterized by chainlike T1 hyperintensities in a -week preterm infant with small adjacent cysts on axial T1-weighted images at 2 weeks of life. B: The cysts have evolved on the second MRI at term-equivalent age into significant bilateral periventricular cysts consistent with cystic periventricular leukomalacia.

TABLE 54.10	Demyelinating Disease in MRI—cont'd

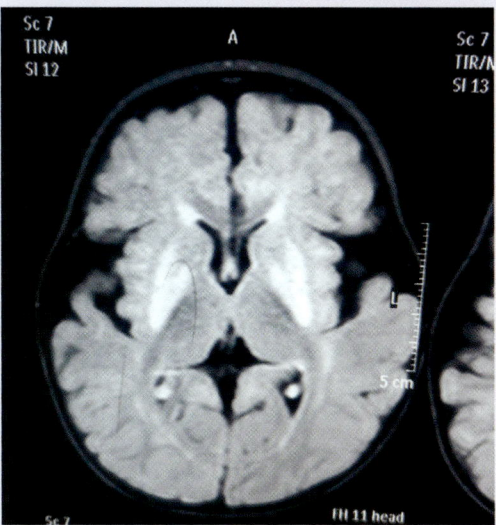

Fig. 54.42 Glutaric aciduria type 1.

Glutaric aciduria type 1:
Bilateral symmetrical signal alteration in the basal ganglion and symmetrical cerebral volume loss in frontal and temporal lobes with prominent CSF space suggestive of glutaric aciduria type 1

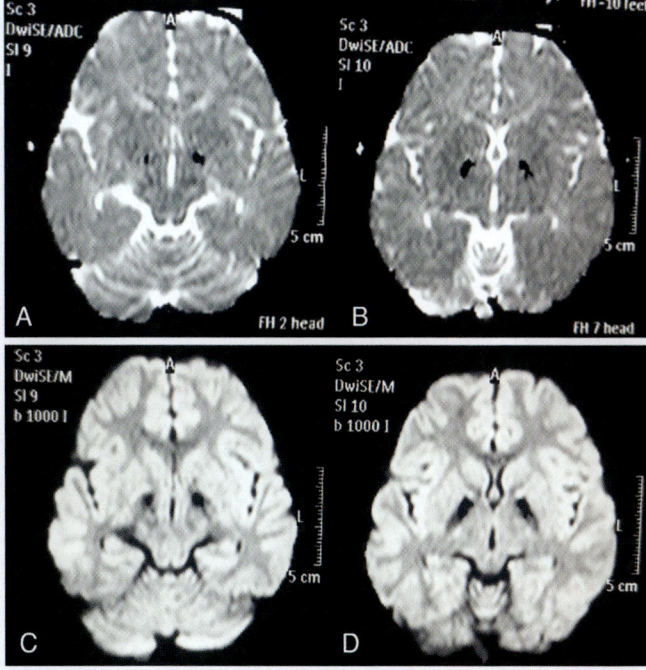

Fig. 54.43 (A and B) ADC mapping. (C and D) DWI.

Pantothenate kinase disorder:
Bilateral symmetrical dark signal foci with hyperintense foci on T2-FLAIR; ADC and DWI in the globus pallidus suggestive of pantothenate kinase disorder

Continued

TABLE 54.10	Demyelinating Disease in MRI—cont'd

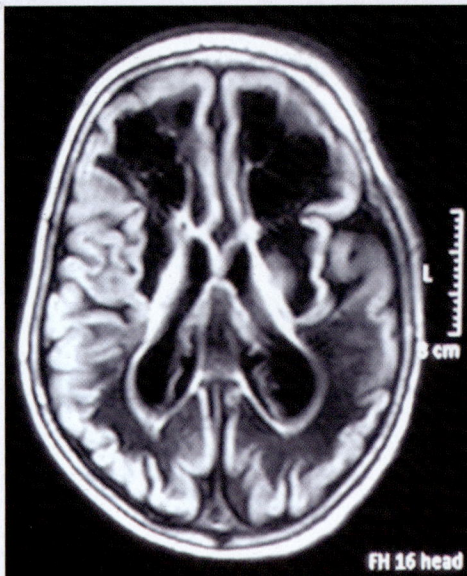

Complete loss of white matter in bilateral cerebral hemisphere with diffuse cortical thinning suggestive of **Vanishing white matter disease**

Fig. 54.44   Vanishing white matter disease (T1 FLAIR-loss of white matter).

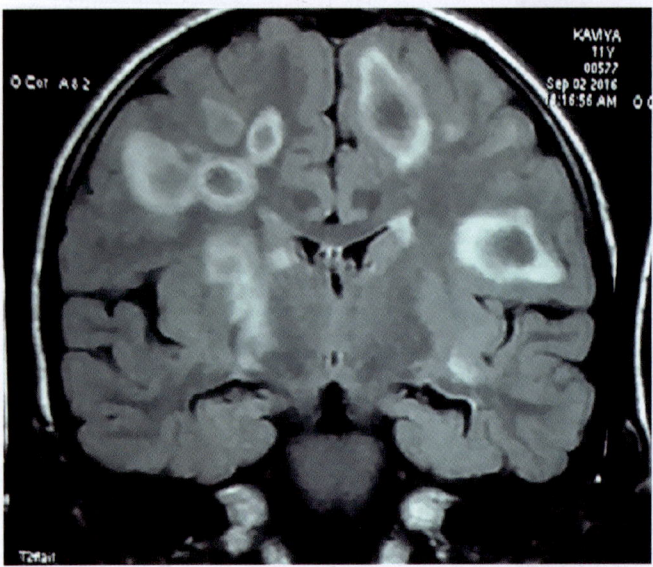

Fig. 54.45   Coronal view T1 — multiple open-ring-enhancing zesion.

Acute Disseminated Encephalomyelitis (ADEM)
Multiple open-ring-enhancing lesion (Fig. 54.45-T1W- Coronal view and Fig. 54.46- T2W-Axial view) Suggestive of Acute Disseminated Encephalomyelitis (ADEM)

TABLE 54.10	Demyelinating Disease in MRI—cont'd

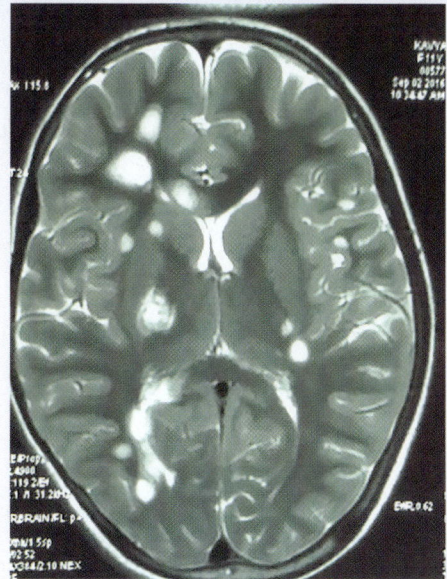

Fig. 54.46 Axial view T2W — multiple open-ring-enhancing lesion.

MR SPECTROSCOPY

TABLE 54.11	MR Spectroscopy

Normal peak

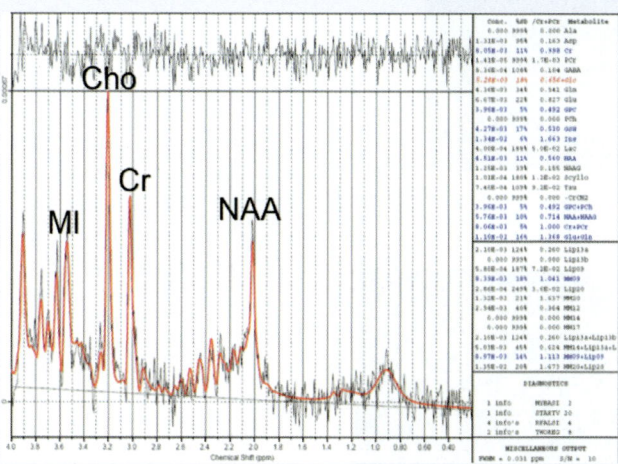

Normal magnetic resonance spectroscopy (MRS) peak: *N*-acetyl aspartate (NAA), choline, creatinine and myo-inositol highest peak being NAA (healthy neuronal marker)
- Choline is a marker of cellular turnover
- Other primary markers are lipid and lactate

Fig. 54.47 MRS spectrum of major metabolites in a normal brain. (*Source:* Reproduced from Richard Martin, Avroy Fanaroff, Michele Walsh. *Fanaroff and Martin's Neonatal-Perinatal Medicine, 2-Volume Set: Diseases of the Fetus and Infant*, Eleventh Edition, The Role of Neonatal Neuroimaging in Predicting Neurodevelopmental Outcomes of Preterm Neonates, Fig. 61.3, Philadelphia, Elsevier Inc., 2020. (Credit line - With permission from Parikh NA. Advanced neuroimaging and its role in predicting neurodevelopmental outcomes in very preterm infants. Semin Perinatol. 2016;40(8):530-541.)

Continued

TABLE 54.11	MR Spectroscopy—cont'd

Glioma

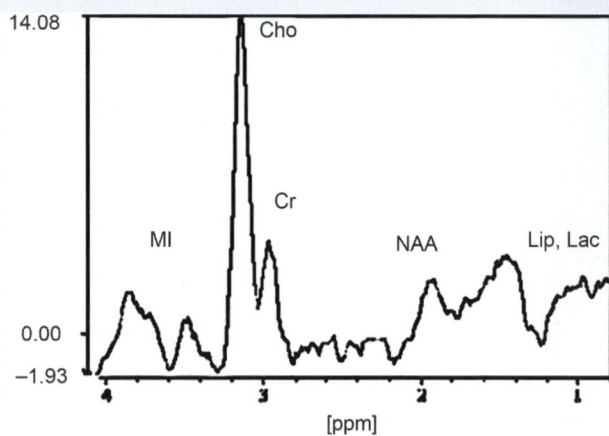

Fig. 54.48 Glioma. (Source: Reproduced from Muhammad Arshad Javid, Ume Habiba, Quratul Ain Rashid et al. Age-related metabolic study of glioma brain using magnetic resonance spectroscopy, *Materials Today: Proceedings* 47(Supp):S116-S120; 2021.)

Glioma:
High choline peak (due to increased turnover) absent NAA (N-acetylaspartate) peak, reversed lipid and lactate peak
Suggestive of – **glioma**

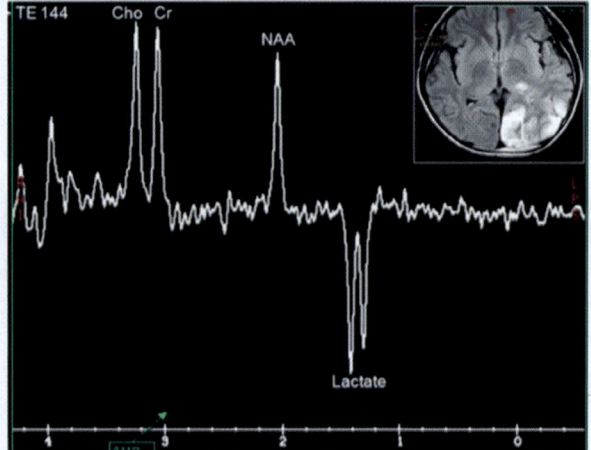

Fig. 54.49 Mitochondrial disorder. (*Source:* Reproduced from Ching-Shiang Chi, Hsiu-Fen Lee, Chi-Ren Tsai et al. Lactate peak on brain MRS in children with syndromic mitochondrial diseases, *Journal of the Chinese Medical Association* 74(7):305-309; 2011.)

Mitochondrial disorder
Lactate peak on brain MRS in mitochondrial encephalopathy, lactic acidosis, and stroke-like episodes
Lactate inverted doublet in mitochondrial cytopathy

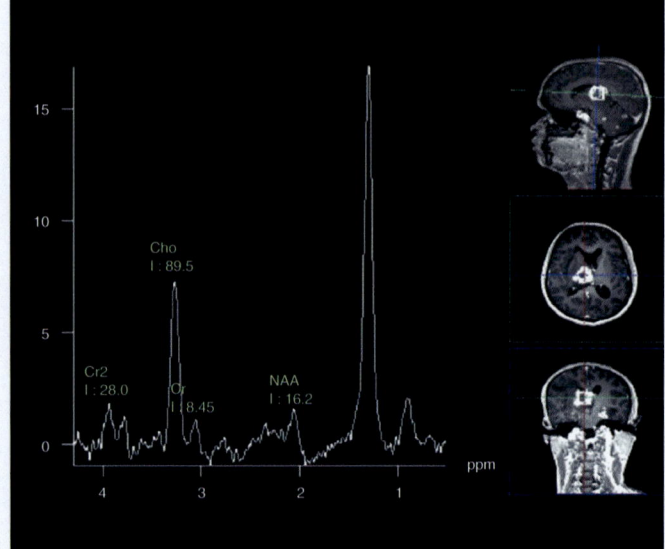

Fig. 54.50 Tuberculoma. (*Source:* Reproduced from Alfredo Quinones-Hinojosa. *Schmidek and Sweet Operative Neurosurgical Techniques: Indications, Methods, and Results,* Seventh Edition, Management of Tuberculous and Fungal Infections of the Nervous System, Fig 132.11, Philadelphia, Elsevier Inc., 2022).

Tuberculoma
a. High lipid peak (specific for tuberculoma)
b. Reduce N-acetylaspartate (NAA), creatinine, choline/creatinine ratio > 1

TABLE 54.11	MR Spectroscopy—cont'd

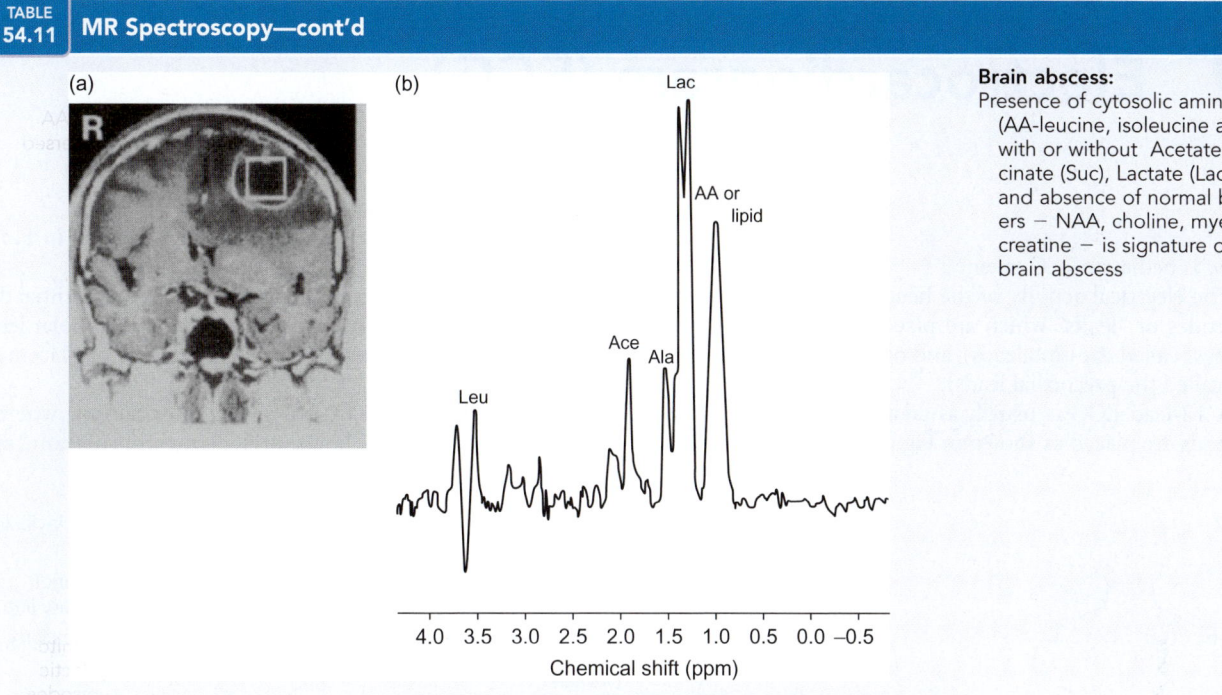

Brain abscess:
Presence of cytosolic amino acid (AA-leucine, isoleucine and valine) with or without Acetate (Ac), Succinate (Suc), Lactate (Lac), Lipid and absence of normal brain markers — NAA, choline, myeline, and creatine — is signature of bacterial brain abscess

Fig. 54.51 Brain abscess. *(Source:* Reproduced from Madan Kaila, Rakhi Kaila. *Quantum Magnetic Resonance Imaging Diagnostics of Human Brain Disorders,* Magnetic Resonance Imaging Diagnostics of Human Brain Disorders, Figure 3.91, London, Elsevier Inc., 2010.)

Electrocardiogram (ECG)

ECG

1. How is pediatric ECG taken?
   - The electrical activity of the heart is captured by electrodes or "leads" which are placed on both arms and legs (called the limb leads), and on the chest in six areas (called the precordial leads).
   - A 12-lead ECG is usually is taken in a child, and the leads are placed as shown in Fig. 55.1A and B.

2. What are the leads in a 12-lead ECG?
   - The types of ECG leads placement are given in Flowchart 55.1.
   - Bipolar leads help in the measurement of potential difference between two electrodes, whereas unipolar leads help measure the true voltage at the site of placement of the electrode.
   - Limb leads give frontal plane information, whereas chest leads give horizontal plane information, and

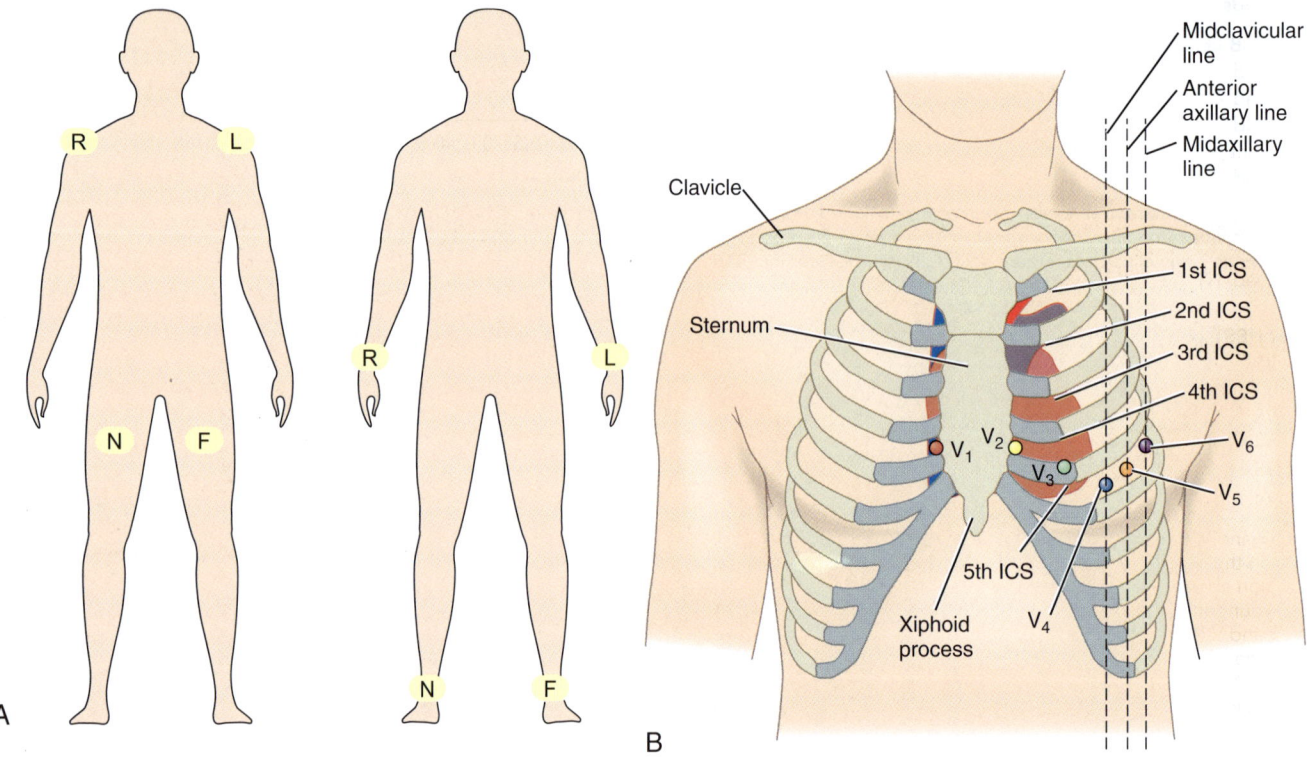

Fig. 55.1 (A) Limb leads (remember as traffic signal lights: Red, yellow, and green). (B) Chest leads. (Source: Reproduced from Brigitte Niedzwiecki, Julie Pepper, P. Ann Weaver. *Kinn's The Medical Assistant: An Applied Learning Approach*, Fourteenth Edition, Principles of Electrocardiography, FIGURE 26.12, St. Louis, Saunders, 2020.)

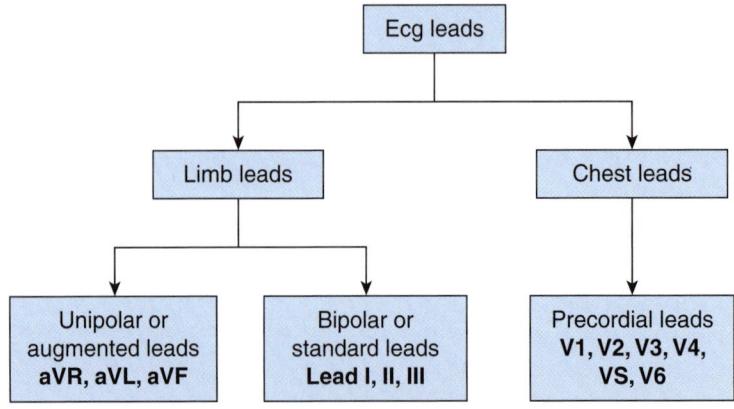

Flowchart 55.1 Types of ECG leads.

together the electrical events of all parts of the heart with the exception of posterior surface of heart are obtained.

- The locations of leads are given in Table 55.1.

3. What are the differences between pediatric ECG and adult ECG?

   The findings seen in a pediatric ECG are given in Table 55.2.

4. How do the ECG findings differ during the various ages of a child?

   Table 55.3 shows the ECG difference among various age groups.

5. What are the components of pediatric ECG?

   The components of pediatric ECG are given in Table 55.4.

6. What are the normal waves and interval in an ECG and which leads are they best seen in?

   Fig. 55.3 represents the waves and intervals present in an ECG.

   Table 55.5 describes the physiology behind the waves and intervals along with normal values and the leads in which they are best seen.

7. What are the conditions that require ECG in pediatrics?

   ECG is taken in pediatrics for the following conditions:
   1. Disproportionate tachycardia (sinus tachycardia, Supraventricular tachycardia (SVT), etc.)
   2. Bradycardia (conduction blocks)
   3. Suspected electrolyte disturbance
   4. Myocarditis/pericarditis
   5. Congenital heart disease
   6. Life-threatening arrhythmias

8. How to read a pediatric ECG?

   The steps given in Table 55.6 give a simple way to read a pediatric ECG.

9. How to interpret axis in ECG and what are the abnormalities in axis?

   There are two methods to the assessment of QRS axis:
   a. **Quadrant method/thumb rule (using lead 1 and aVF) (Fig. 55.6):**

      The steps are as follows:
      - Observe R wave in lead 1 and aVF (can use left thumb for lead 1 to represent left side and right thumb for aVF to represent the right side)
      - Identify how is the deflection of R wave in these two leads – whether positive or negative
      - If positive in lead 1, raise the left thumb up. If positive in aVF, raise the right thumb. If both thumbs up, it is normal axis.
      - If positive in lead 1 (left thumb up) but negative in aVF (right thumb low), this indicates left axis deviation (LAD) (left thumb higher than right thumb) and vice versa is the right axis deviation (RAD).
      - This is best shown in Table 55.7.
   b. **Isoelectric lead analysis:**

      This method requires understanding of the hexaxial reference system (Fig. 55.7).

TABLE 55.1	Location for leads placement
Leads	**Position**
LIMB LEADS	
Lead 1	Right arm to left arm
Lead 2	Right arm to left leg
Lead 3	Left arm to left leg
Right leg	Neutral
Lead aVR	The average of left arm and left leg electrodes to the right arm
Lead aVL	The average of the right arm and left leg electrodes to the left arm
Lead aVF	The average of the right arm and left arm electrodes to the left leg
CHEST LEADS	
V1	4th intercostal space, right sternal border
V2	4th intercostal space, left sternal border
V3	Midway between V3 and V4
V4	5th intercostal space, left midclavicular line
V5	5th intercostal space, anterior axillary line
V6	5th intercostal space, midaxillary line

V3R and V4R: Lead placement similar to V3 and V4, respectively, but on the right side like mirror image. These are used to get information about the right ventricle. V4R must be included in children younger than 5 years.

V1 and V2, right-side leads; V3 and V4, septal leads; V5 and V6, left-side leads.

Lead 1, aVL, and V3−V6: anterolateral region; lead 2, 3, aVF: inferior region.

TABLE 55.2	Normal Findings in Pediatric ECG
ECG	**Findings**
Heart rate	Children usually have higher heart rates in comparison to adults; there is a gradual decrease in heart rate as the age advances
Axis	• **At birth:** Right axis deviation (between 70° and 180°) and dominant R waves in right precordial leads (tall R waves in lead V1 and deep S waves in lead V6 indicate right ventricular dominance) • **By 1 year of age:** As the LV mass grows, dominant axis gradually shifts to left side (+10 to +100)
T waves	• **At birth:** T waves are positive in all precordial leads. • **Beyond day 3 of life:** T waves become negative in lead V1 and upright T wave in lead V6; it remains this way up to 8 years of age (juvenile T wave pattern) • **At 8–10 years:** T wave in V1 lead becomes upright; rarely may remain inverted throughout adolescence (juvenile T wave inversion) • T waves are of low voltage as well
Q wave	Deep Q wave in inferior leads and V5 and V6
PR interval	Shorter PR interval (because of rapid heart rate in children)
QRS duration	QRS duration is shorter because of decreased muscle mass
R/S progression	Adult type R/S progression in the precordial leads (deep S waves in V1 and V2 and tall R waves in V5 and V6) is rarely seen in first month of life

TABLE 55.3 ECG Findings Through Various Age Groups

Preterm Infant	Full-Term Newborn	One Week to One Month	Adolescent
1. RV dominance but more left-ward forces due to presence of PDA; axis is toward left 2. More chance of deep Q in V6 3. Low voltage QRS and T in limb leads 4. Shorter PR, QT intervals, and QRS duration	1. Right axis deviation 2. RV dominance in precordial leads (tall R in V1 and deep S in V6) 3. QRS and T waves voltage slightly low 4. T wave upright up to 3rd day of life	1. Right axis deviation 2. R wave dominance across precordial leads, but S may become normal 3. T wave negative in V1 4. Higher T wave voltage	1. Normal axis 2. LV dominance (deep S in V1, tall R in V5 and V6) 3. Upright T in all precordial leads; rarely juvenile T wave inversion may persist

TABLE 55.4 Components of Pediatric ECG

Pediatric ECG	Standard Components
Initial step	Name, age, hospital ID, date
Standardization (Fig. 55.2)	Normal: Two large squares (1 mv = 10 mm)

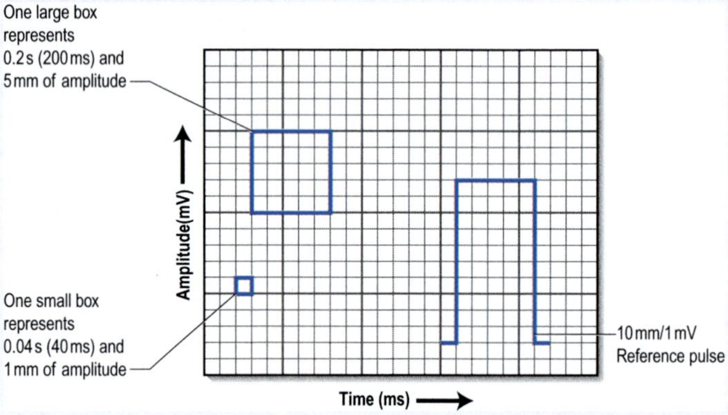

One large box represents 0.2 s (200 ms) and 5 mm of amplitude
One small box represents 0.04 s (40 ms) and 1 mm of amplitude
Amplitude (mV)
Time (ms)
10 mm/1 mV
Reference pulse

Fig. 55.2 Standardization of ECG. (Source: Reproduced from Nisha Patel, Daniel Knight. *CHURCHILL'S POCKETBOOKS OF Clinical Practical Procedures for Junior Doctors*, First Edition, PERFORMING AN ELECTROCARDIOGRAM (ECG), Fig. 14.2, Edinburgh, Churchill Livingstone, 2009.)

Speed	25 mm/s
Horizontal axis	Time: Each small square = 0.04 s; each big square = 0.2 s
Vertical axis	Voltage: Each small square = 0.1 mV = 1 mm

R
RR interval
R
PR interval
ST interval
TP interval
QT interval
P
Q
S
J
T
U
P wave duration
PR segment
QRS duration
ST segment
0.04s 40ms
0.20s 200ms
Speed: 25 mm/sec

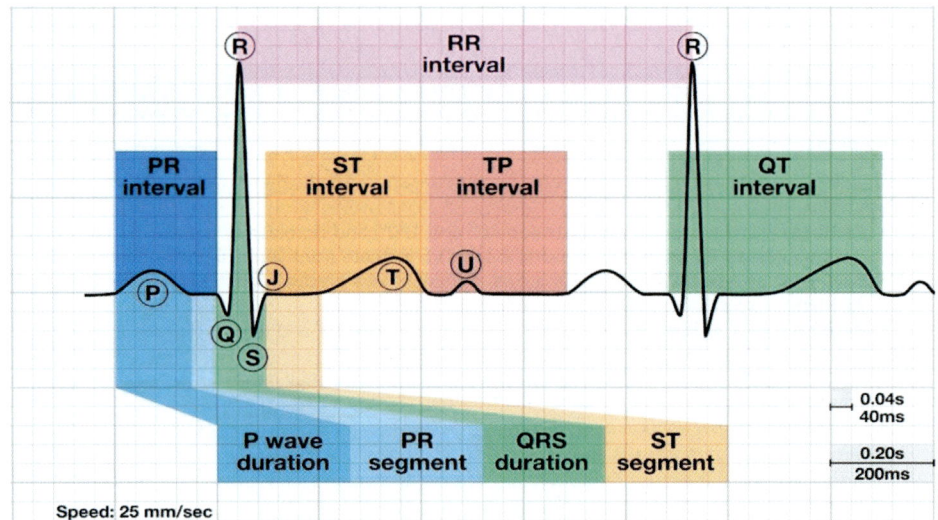

Fig. 55.3 Waveforms and intervals in ECG. (Source: Reproduced from Barbara Mukami Maweu, Sagnik Dakshitm, Rittika Shamsuddin et al. and CEFEs: A CNN Explainable Framework for ECG Signals, *Artificial Intelligence in Medicine* 115: 102059.)

TABLE 55.5	ECG Waveforms, Intervals, Normal Values, Best Lead for Assessment		
Waves and Intervals	**Physiology**	**Normal Values**	**Best Lead for Assessment**
P wave	Atrial repolarization	Width: <25 mm Height: <25 mm	• Lead 2 (mainly) • V1 (to assess negative component of P) • Normally negative in aVR
Q wave	Septal activation	Duration: <0.04 s Depth: <1/4th of succeeding R wave (<4 mm)	• Lead 1, aVL, V4−V6, aVF (normally seen) • Normally not seen in V1−V3
QRS	Ventricular muscle depolarization	0.09 s (2 small squares)	• RS progression seen in chest leads (transition leads) • R/S ratio measured in V1/V2 and V5/V6
T wave	Ventricular repolarization	>1/8th to <2/3rd of preceding R wave (maximum height 6 mm in limb leads and 10 mm in precordial leads)	• Amplitude to be seen in V5/V6 • Normally inverted in V1 between 3 days of life to 8 years
PR interval	Measured from beginning of P to beginning of Q or R if Q is isoelectric	0.12–0.20 s (~0.16 s) (3–5 small squares)	Longest PR interval in any lead is taken as the PR interval
QRS duration	Measured from beginning of Q to end of S	0.09 s (2 small squares)	Duration is best measured in leads with lower QRS amplitude (limb leads) or V1 and V2
QT interval	Measured from onset of Q to end of T wave Represents the total duration of electrical activity of the ventricles	0.40–0.44 s (11 small squares)	Best measured in a lead where Q is seen
ST segment	Measured from J point to beginning of T wave	Normally curves into the proximal limb of T wave and not perfectly horizontal (deviation < 1 mm) Loss of this normal concavity is abnormal	• Best seen in precordial leads • Normally some ST elevation seen in V1−V4 (<1 mm)
R-R interval	Measured from the complex preceding the QRS whose QT interval has been measured Represents the ventricular cardiac cycle (an indicator of ventricular rate)	• Depends on the heart rate of the child • Only mild variation is usually present between R-R intervals (<3 small divisions)	• Lead 2

PR segment is measured from end of P wave to beginning of QRS but it is not a clinically useful measurement.
QT dispersion: This is the difference in QT interval in different leads which occurs because of inherent differences in duration of action potential in different parts of the myocardium.
J point is the point of end of S wave and beginning of ST segment – not much useful in pediatrics.

TABLE 55.6	Steps in Reading Pediatric ECG
Step 1: Standardization (calibration) (Fig. 55.4)	• Normal is 1 mv = 10 mm, seen in the beginning or end of ECG tracing • If deflections are too big, standardization can be reduced to half (1 mv = 5 mm), in which case measured heights of the waves should be multiplied by 2 • If deflections are too small, it can be doubled (1 mv = 20 mm); therefore, measured heights should be reduced by half

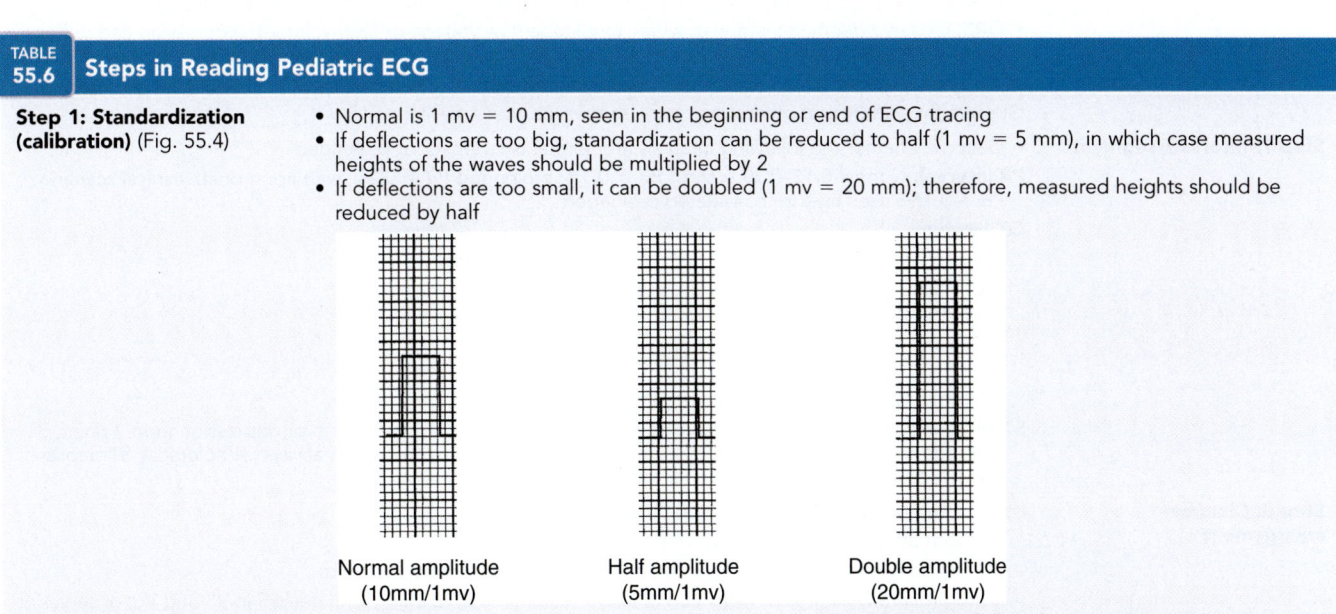

Normal amplitude (10mm/1mv)   Half amplitude (5mm/1mv)   Double amplitude (20mm/1mv)

Fig. 55.4 Various standardization in ECG. (Source: Modified from Bruce Long, Eugene Frank, Ruth Ann Ehrlich. *Radiography Essentials for Limited Practice*, Sixth Edition, Additional Procedures for Assessment and Diagnosis, Fig. 25.20, St. Louis, Elsevier Inc., 2021.)

Continued

| TABLE 55.6 | **Steps in Reading Pediatric ECG—cont'd** |

Step 2: Speed

• Normal – 25 mm/s (Fig. 55.5)

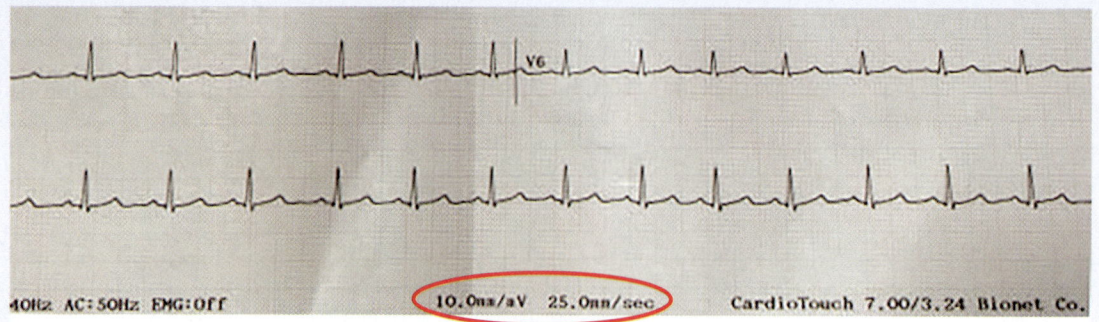

Fig. 55.5   ECG strip showing speed of 25 mm/s.

Step 3: Rate

• R–R interval is used to calculate the heart rate
• Either of the two formulas can be used:

$$\frac{1500}{\text{No. of small squares}} \quad \text{OR} \quad \frac{300}{\text{No. of large squares}}$$
$$\text{(R–R interval)} \qquad\qquad \text{(R–R interval)}$$

Step 4: Rhythm

• Usually seen in lead 2
• Sinus rhythm is described as:
  a. PQRST sequence maintained (P followed by Q)
  b. P wave axis and morphology – normal
  c. PR interval – constant
  d. Atrial rate and ventricular rate are almost the same
  e. R-R interval can vary according to HR; usually on inspiration, there is narrowing and on expiration it is wide (variation is usually < 3 small squares)
• If R-R interval variation is >3 squares, while the rest 4 criteria are normal, it is called sinus arrhythmia

Step 5: Axis

• There are two methods to see the axis of QRS:
  a. Quadrant method
  b. Isoelectric lead analysis
• Identify if the axis is normal or right axis deviation (RAD) or left axis deviation (LAD) or extreme axis deviation (EAD).

Step 6: Waves

• Look if P, QRS, T waves are normal or whether any abnormalities present
• **P waves**: Observe morphology; normally, 25 mm wide × 25 mm tall; "P" pulmonale is seen in right atrial enlargement (>25 mm tall), "P" mitrale is seen in left atrial enlargement (>25 mm width)
• **QRS**: Observe duration (narrow or wide), amplitude (low voltage or high voltage), progression and deflection; look for any deep Q waves; look for relationship between R and S wave, R/S ratio
• **T waves:** Look for T wave inversion, concordance or disconcordance with QRS, flattening or tall T waves
Observe for presence of other waves such as J waves and U waves

Step 7: Intervals/segment

• Observe whether the following intervals are normal, shortened, or prolonged
PR interval: Normal 0.12–0.20 s; short PR < 0.1 s, prolonged PR > 0.2 s; with appropriate clinical scenario, PR > 0.16 s itself may be considered prolonged
QT interval:
  • Varies inversely with the heart rate; hence, usually corrected QT (QTc) is used; it is calculated by using Bazett formula:

$$QTc = \frac{QT\,(\text{in ms})}{\sqrt{RR\,(\text{in s})}}$$

  • Normal QTc is 0.40–0.44 s; prolonged if > 0.44 s; short QTc is < 0.30 s
ST segment: Observe if normal concavity is maintained; look for ST elevation or depression from J point; ST elevation may be mildly present (<1 mm) in children but ST depression is always pathological; ST depression because of J point depression from isoelectric line is not abnormal

Step 8: Chamber enlargement

Look for the presence of the following chamber enlargement:
  1. Right atrial enlargement (RAE): P pulmonale (>25 mm tall)
  2. Left atrial enlargement (LAE): P mitrale (>25 mm width, wide and bifid)
  3. Right ventricular hypertrophy (RVH): RAD + tall R in V1, V2 along with deep S in V5 and V6; observe for RV strain pattern as well
     • Left ventricular hypertrophy (LVH): LAD + tall R in V5 and V6, deep S in V1 and V2; observe for LV strain pattern as well

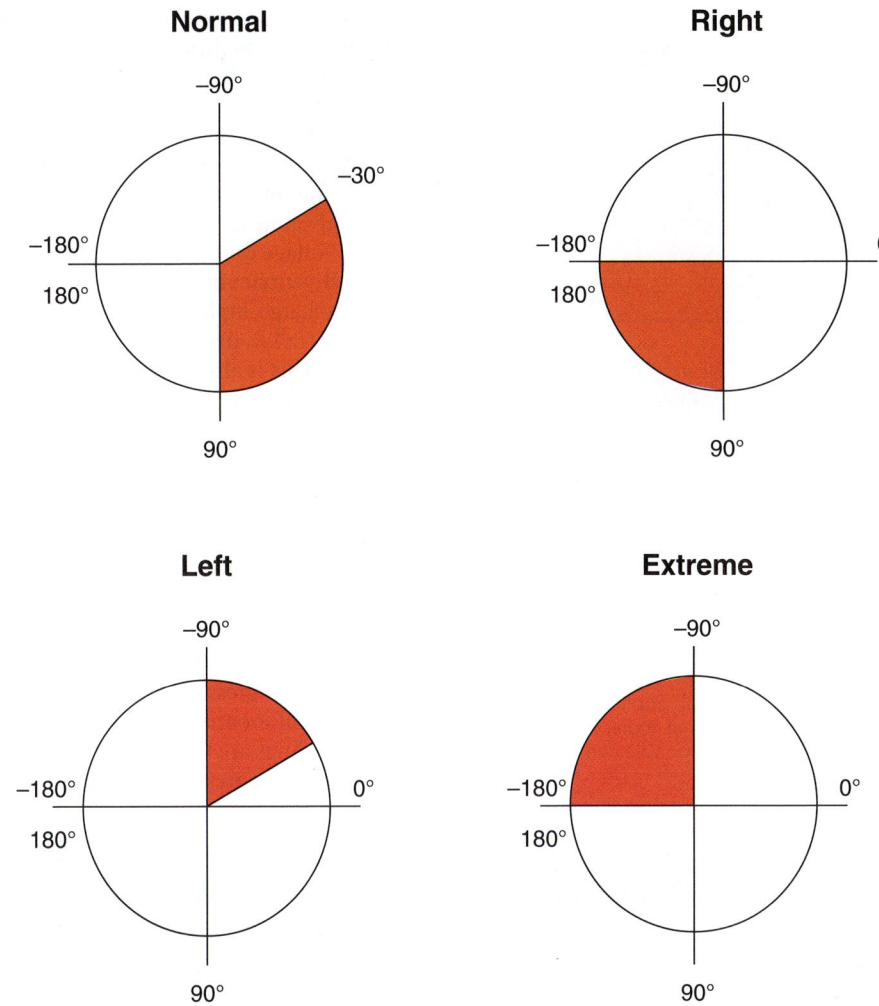

Fig. 55.6 Schematic representation of various quadrants. (Source: Reproduced from Sascha Fulde, Gordian W. O. Fulde. *Emergency Medicine: The principles of practice*, Sixth Edition, Quick reference, Figure 6.2, Sydney, Churchill Livingstone, 2013. (Credit line - Figures 6.1 and 6.2 adapted from Goldberger AL, Clinical electrocardiography: a simplified approach, 7th edn, Philadelphia: Mosby, 2006: Figs 5-2 and 5-13. Available: www.mdconsult.com/books/bbmapAsset?appID=MDC&isbn=0-323-04038-1&eid=4-u1.0-B0-323-04038-1..50006-8..gr13&assetType=full.).

TABLE 55.7	Interpretation of Axis by Using Quadrant Method		
		LEAD AVF	
Leads and Deflection		**Positive**	**Negative**
LEAD 1	Positive	Normal axis (0° to +90°)	Left axis deviation (0° to −90°)
	Negative	Right axis deviation (+90° to +180°)	Extreme axis or northwest deviation (−90° to +180°)

* In this, lead 1 is perpendicular to aVF, lead 2 is perpendicular to aVL, lead 3 is perpendicular to aVR, and vice versa.
* The steps of interpretation by using this method are as follows:
  - First, choose the lead which is most isoelectric in your ECG trace (i.e., Q and R are of the same height). The axis is at 90° to this lead.
  - Next choose the lead which is perpendicular to the isoelectric lead. This lead will give the direction of the axis.
  - If QRS is positive in the second lead, then axis is roughly in the same direction as this lead.
  - On the contrary, if QRS is negative in the second lead, then axis is in the opposite direction to this lead.
  - For example, if isoelectric lead is aVL (Q = R), the perpendicular lead to this is lead 2. Now, if QRS is positive in lead 2, then it points toward the same direction as in the reference system, hence normal axis. However, if QRS is negative in lead 2, then it points toward opposite direction, hence extreme axis deviation (EAD).

Abnormalities in axis are discussed in Table 55.8.

10. What are the abnormalities in waves of a pediatric ECG?
    The abnormalities waves of a pediatric ECG are given in Table 55.9.

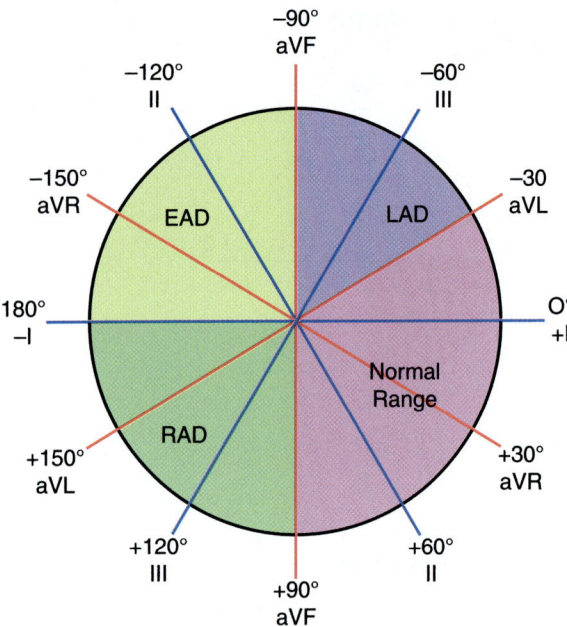

Fig. 55.7 Hexaxial reference system. (Source: Reproduced from Mario Vaz, Anura Kurpad, Tony Raj. *Guyton and Hall Textbook of Medical Physiology*, Third South Asia Edition, Clinical applications of the electrocardiogram, Fig. 34.28, New Delhi, Elsevier India, 2020. (Credit line - Source: modified from https://sites.google.com/site/cardiacchaos/axis-deviation-1.))

11. What are the abnormalities of intervals in ECG?

The abnormalities of intervals in ECG are given in Table 55.10.

Short QTc is not a common finding but may be seen in hypercalcemia, hypermagnesemia, digitalis effect, etc.

12. What are the ECG findings of ventricular hypertrophy?
   - The ECG findings of ventricular hypertrophy are given in Table 55.11.
   - Voltage criteria for LVH are given in Table 55.12.
   - **Biventricular hypertrophy:**
     - Large biphasic QRS complexes are seen in V2–V5 (tall R, deep S).
     - This is also known as Katz−Wachtel phenomenon.

13. What are the ECG findings in common electrolyte disturbances?

The ECG findings in common electrolyte disturbances are given in Table 55.13.

14. What are the ECG changes in myocarditis and pericarditis?

The ECG changes in myocarditis and pericarditis are given in Table 55.14.

15. What are the ECG changes in a patient with dextrocardia?
   - All waves − global negativity in lead 1 and aVL
   - All waves, P, QRS, T are positive in aVR
   - Nonprogression of R waves from V1 to V6
   - To differentiate between wrong leads placement – all findings are the same as in dextrocardia but there is R wave progression from V1 to V6 (Fig. 55.14)

TABLE 55.8	**Abnormalities in Axis**	
ECG Picture With Diagnosis	**ECG Findings**	**Conditions Seen in**

1. **Right axis deviation (RAD)** (Fig. 55.8A)	• Using quadrant method:
	Lead 1 − negative
	aVF − positive
	• Using isoelectric method:
	  • aVR is isoelectric so lead 3 is perpendicular
	  • QRS in lead 3 is positive, hence RAD
		• Tetralogy of Fallot
		• Atrial septal defect
		• D-Transposition of great vessels (D-TGV)
		• Total anomalous pulmonary venous connection (TAPVC)

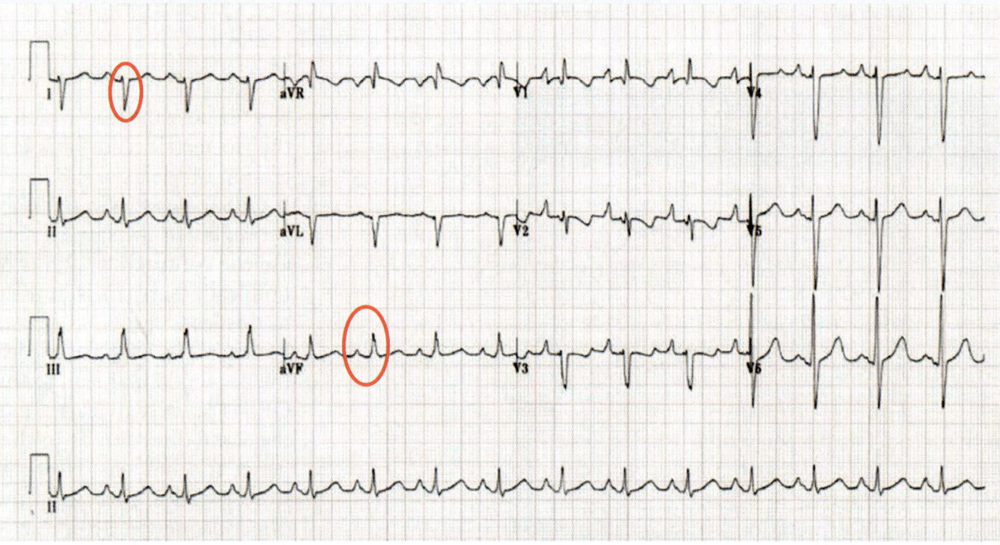

A

Fig. 55.8 (A) ECG with right axis deviation (RAD). (Source: Modified from Dr. Scott Dougherty, Jonathan Carapetis, Liesl Zuhlke. *Acute Rheumatic Fever and Rheumatic Heart Disease*, Clinical Evaluation and Diagnosis of Rheumatic Heart Disease, Fig. 5.6, San Diego (CA), Elsevier Inc., 2021.)

TABLE 55.8	Abnormalities in Axis—cont'd

2. **Left axis deviation (LAD)** (Fig. 55.8B)

- Using quadrant method:
  Lead 1 − positive
  aVF − negative
- Using isoelectric method:
  - Lead 2 is isoelectric so lead aVL is perpendicular
  - QRS in lead aVL is positive, hence LAD

- Atrioventricular septal defect
- Pulmonary atresia with intact ventricular septum
- Tricuspid atresia

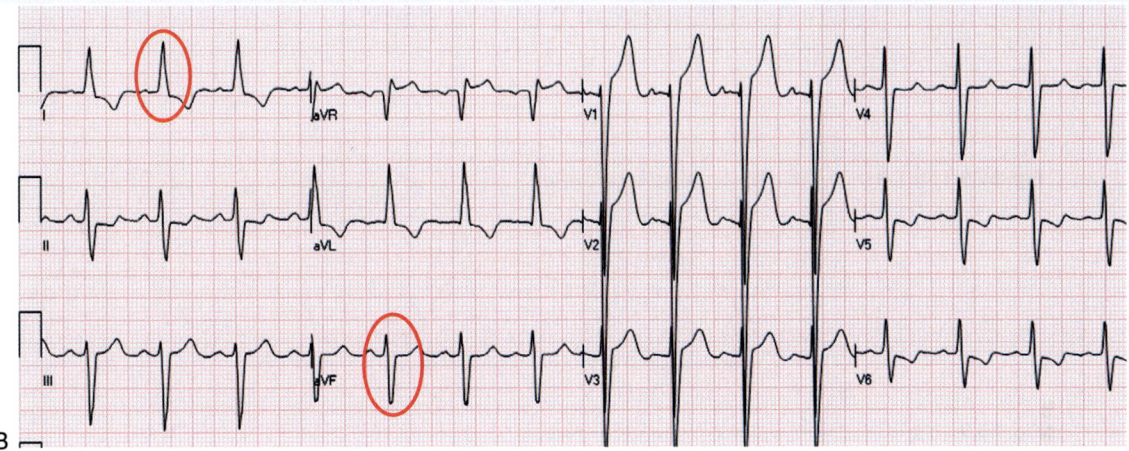

B

Fig. 55.8 (B) ECG with left axis deviation (LAD). (Source: Reproduced from Henry D Huang, Yochai Birnbaum, and ST elevation: differentiation between ST elevation myocardial infarction and nonischemic ST elevation, *J Electrocardiol* 44(5):494.e1-494.e12.)

3. **Extreme axis deviation (EAD)** (Fig. 55.8C)

- Using quadrant method:
  Lead 1 − negative
  aVF − negative
- Using isoelectric method:
  - Lead 1 is isoelectric so lead aVF is perpendicular
- QRS in lead aVL is negative, which when seen in opposite direction, it is EAD or north-west deviation

- Endocardial cushion defect or atrioventricular septal defect (AVCD)
- Before infancy

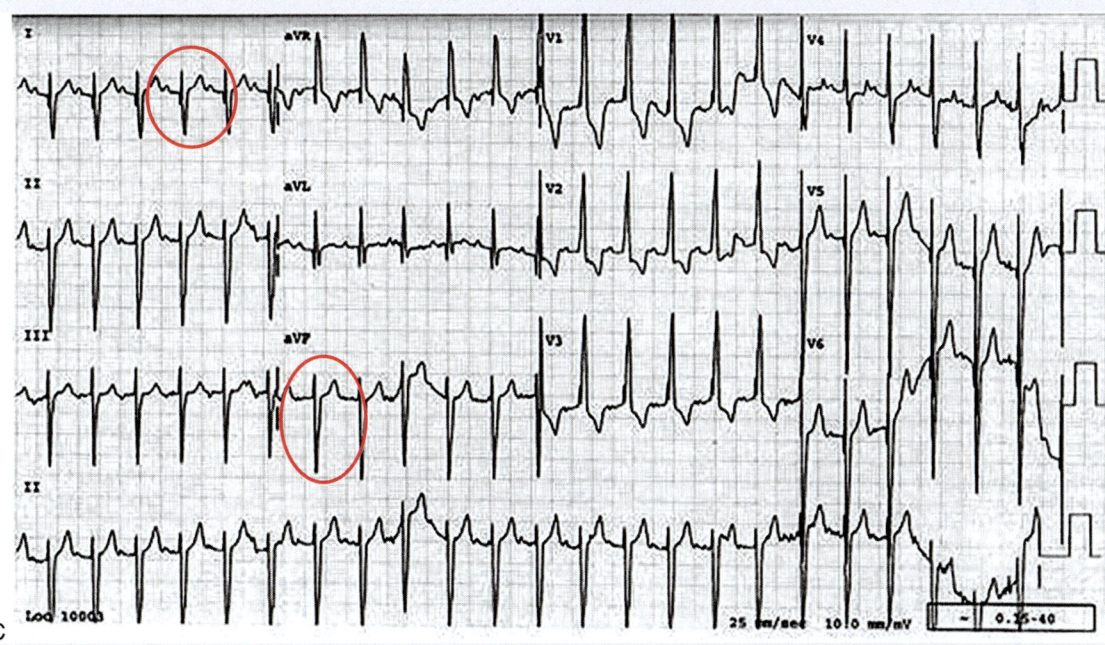

C

Fig. 55.8 (C) ECG with extreme axis deviation (EAD). (Source: https://ekg.md/content/right-axis-deviation/; (C) https://www.semanticscholar.org/paper/Cardiac-emergencies-in-the-first-year-of-life.-Yee/aaf1045b4df831f28f5c4eeab978a7103bf4d890/figure/3)

TABLE 55.9	**Abnormalities in Waves of ECG**	
Abnormalities in Waves	**ECG Picture/Findings**	**Condition in Which It Is Seen**

P WAVE
P pulmonale
(Fig. 55.9A)

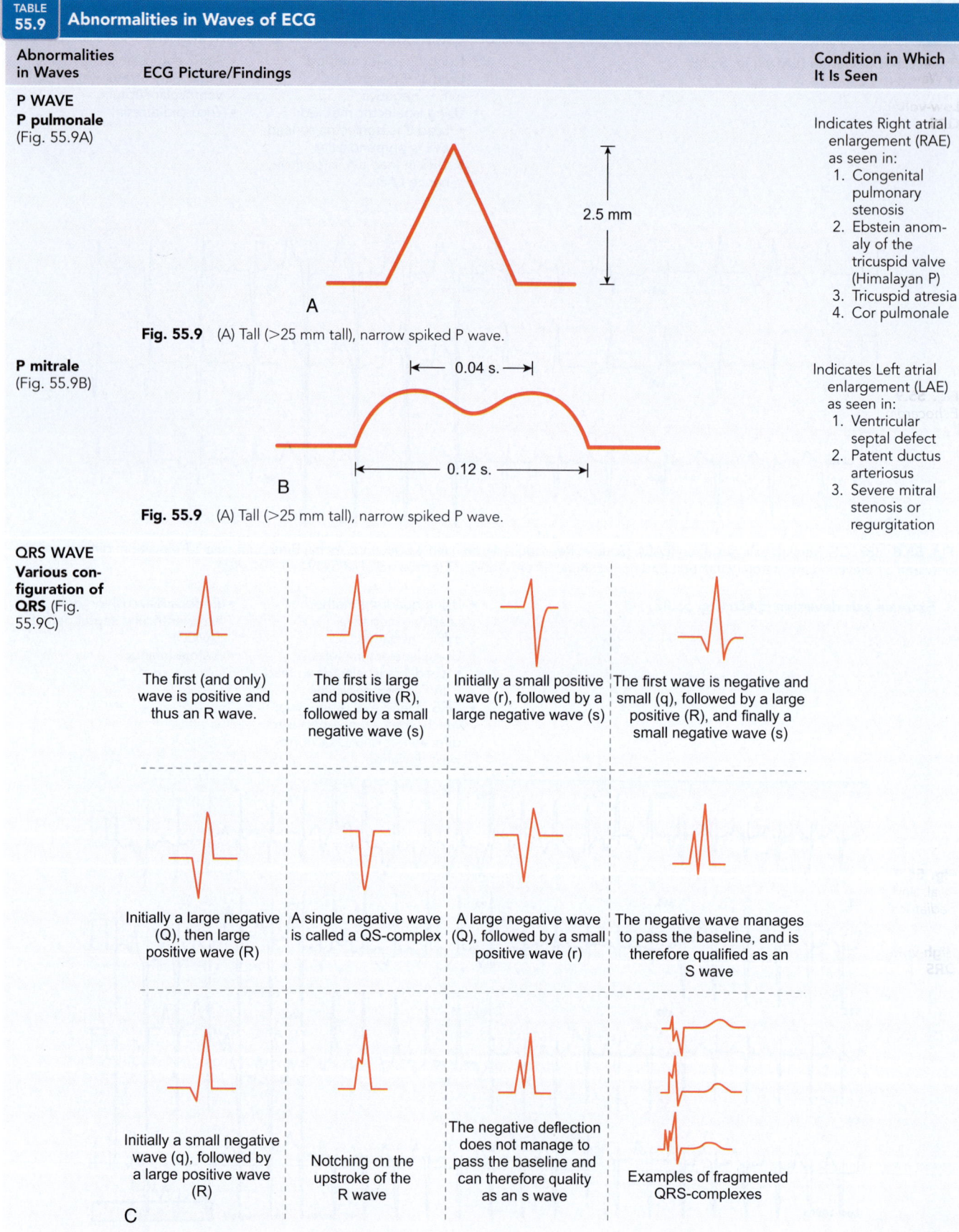

2.5 mm

A

Fig. 55.9   (A) Tall (>25 mm tall), narrow spiked P wave.

Indicates Right atrial enlargement (RAE) as seen in:
1. Congenital pulmonary stenosis
2. Ebstein anomaly of the tricuspid valve (Himalayan P)
3. Tricuspid atresia
4. Cor pulmonale

P mitrale
(Fig. 55.9B)

0.04 s.

B

0.12 s.

Fig. 55.9   (A) Tall (>25 mm tall), narrow spiked P wave.

Indicates Left atrial enlargement (LAE) as seen in:
1. Ventricular septal defect
2. Patent ductus arteriosus
3. Severe mitral stenosis or regurgitation

QRS WAVE
Various configuration of QRS (Fig. 55.9C)

The first (and only) wave is positive and thus an R wave.

The first is large and positive (R), followed by a small negative wave (s)

Initially a small positive wave (r), followed by a large negative wave (s)

The first wave is negative and small (q), followed by a large positive (R), and finally a small negative wave (s)

Initially a large negative (Q), then large positive wave (R)

A single negative wave is called a QS-complex

A large negative wave (Q), followed by a small positive wave (r)

The negative wave manages to pass the baseline, and is therefore qualified as an S wave

Initially a small negative wave (q), followed by a large positive wave (R)

Notching on the upstroke of the R wave

The negative deflection does not manage to pass the baseline and can therefore quality as an s wave

Examples of fragmented QRS-complexes

C

Fig. 55.9   (C) Various configurations of QRS complex.

TABLE 55.9	Abnormalities in Waves of ECG—cont'd	
Abnormalities in Waves	**ECG Picture/Findings**	**Condition in Which It Is Seen**
Low-voltage QRS	Definition: Total amplitude of R + S < 5 mm in limb leads and <10 mm in precordial leads (Fig. 55.9D and E) 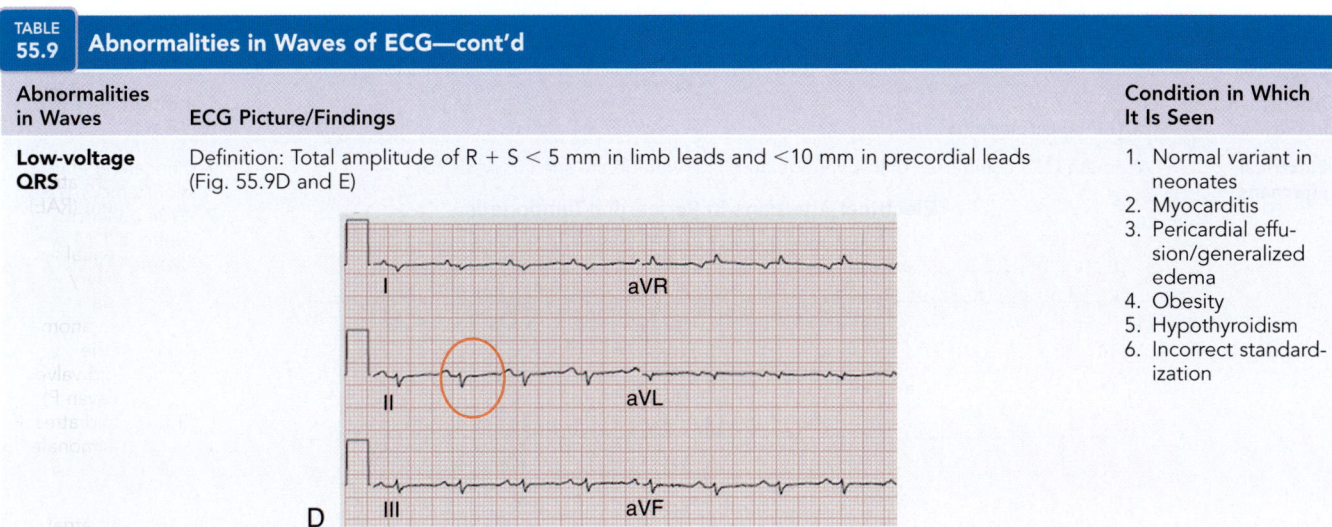	1. Normal variant in neonates 2. Myocarditis 3. Pericardial effusion/generalized edema 4. Obesity 5. Hypothyroidism 6. Incorrect standardization

Fig. 55.9 (D) Limb lead 2. (Source: Modified from American Society of Echocardiography. *ASE's Comprehensive Echocardiography*, Third Edition, Amyloid, Figure 153.1, Philadelphia, Elsevier Inc., 2022.)

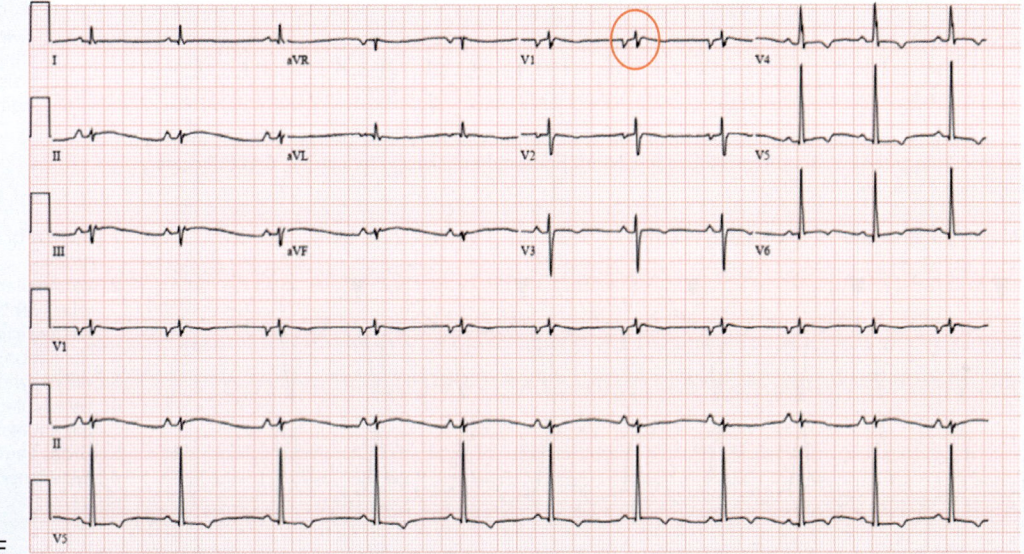

Fig. 55.9 (E) Precordial lead V1 and V5. (Source: Modified from Nak Hyun Choi, Leonardo Liberman, Eric S Silver et al. and Arrhythmogenic left ventricular cardiomyopathy in an adolescent patient with DSP mutation, *Progress in Pediatric Cardiology* 62: 101405.)

High-voltage QRS	Definition: Total amplitude of R + S > 20 mm in limb leads and <30 mm in precordial leads (Fig. 55.9F) 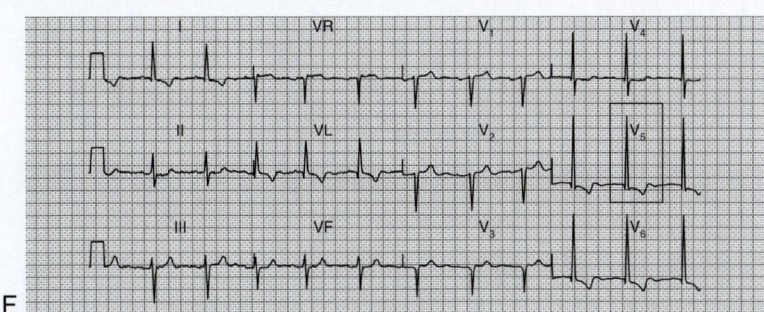	1. Thin chest wall in children 2. Ventricular hypertrophy (right or left) 3. Conduction disturbances Note: High voltage as a single abnormality need not be given pathological significance

Fig. 55.9 (F) Limb lead 2. (Source: Reproduced from Miles Witham, Mudher Al-Khairalla. *100 Plus Diseases for the MRCP PART 2*, Second Edition, Cardiology, Figure 1.3, Edinburgh, Churchill Livingstone, 2008. (Credit line - Reproduced with permission from Hampton (2003) The ECG in Practice, 4th edn. Churchill Livingstone.).

Continued

TABLE 55.9	Abnormalities in Waves of ECG—cont'd		

Abnormalities in Waves	ECG Picture/Findings		Condition in Which It Is Seen
Electrical alternans	Alternate QRS complexes of low voltage and high voltage are seen (Fig. 55.9G) **Electrical Alternans in Pericardial Tamponade** 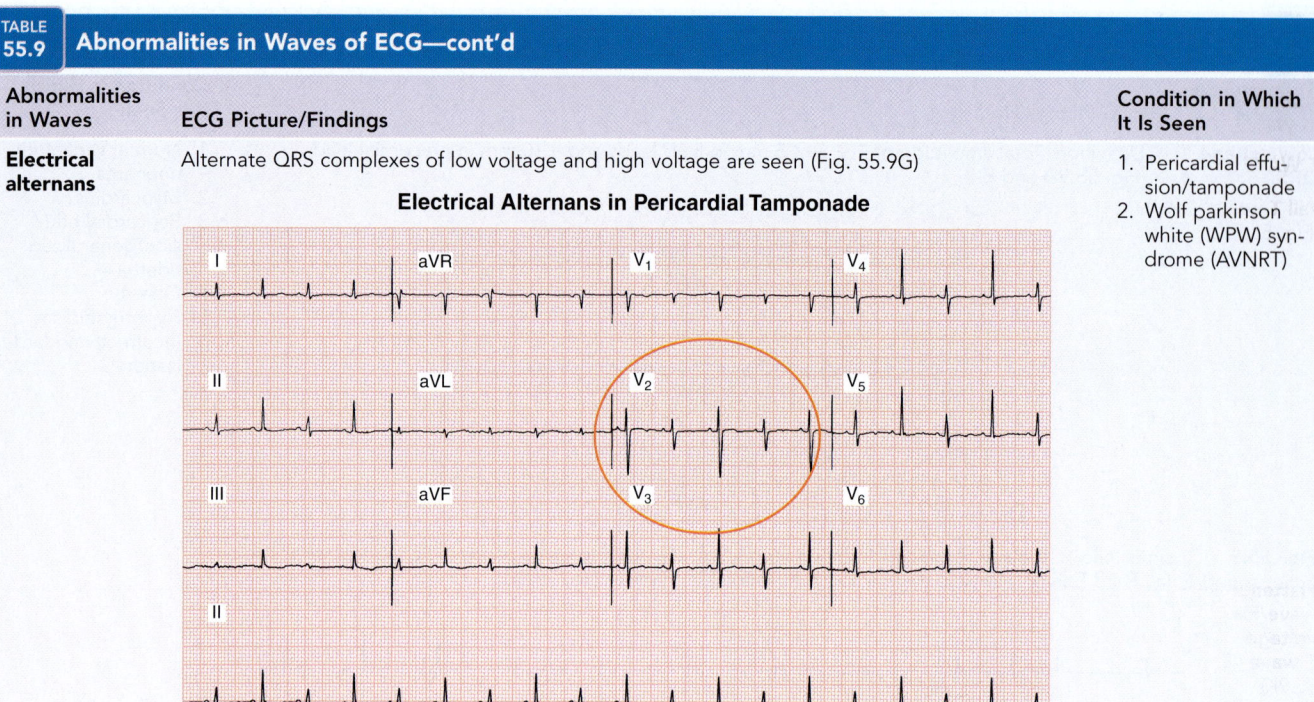		1. Pericardial effusion/tamponade 2. Wolf parkinson white (WPW) syndrome (AVNRT)

Fig. 55.9 (G) Electrical alternans. (Source: Reproduced from Ary Goldberger, Zachary Goldberger, Alexei Shvilkin. *Goldberger's Clinical Electrocardiography: A Simplified Approach*, Ninth Edition, Pericardial, Myocardial, and Pulmonary Syndromes, Fig. 12.3, Edinburgh, Elsevier Inc., 2018.)

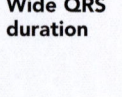 **Wide QRS duration**	Definition: QRS duration > 0.09 s (Fig. 55.9H) 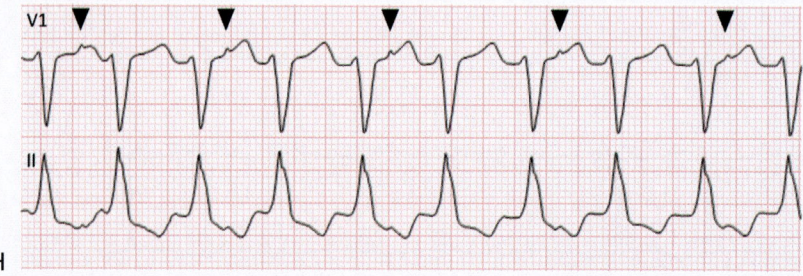		1. Bundle branch blocks 2. Ventricular arrhythmias (ventricular tachycardia/fibrillation) 3. WPW syndrome 4. Ventricular pacemaker 5. Gross ventricular hypertrophy

Fig. 55.9 (H) Lead 2 with QRS of 0.4 s (Wide QRS). (Source: Modifed from Douglas Sawyer, Ramachandran Vasan. *Encyclopedia of Cardiovascular Research and Medicine*, Wide QRS Complex Tachycardia: What is the Diagnosis?, Fig. 12, Oxford, Elsevier Inc., 2018.)

Narrow QRS duration	Definition: QRS duration < 0.09 s (Fig. 55.9I) 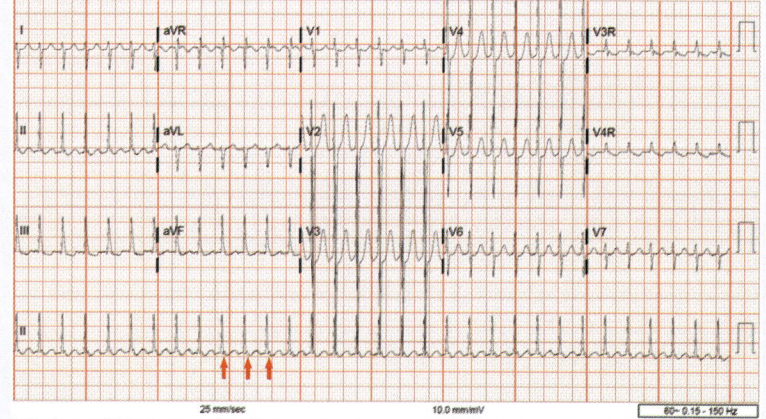		Depending on origin: 1. SA node: Sinus rhythm with normal P wave (sinus tachycardia) 2. Atria: Abnormal P wave, atrial flutter, atrial fibrillation 3. AV node/junction: No P wave or abnormal P wave with short PR – supraventricular tachycardia

Fig. 55.9 (I) Lead 2 with QRS of 0.04 s (Narrow QRS). (Source: Modified from Vincent Thomas, Balaji Seshadri. *Arrhythmias in Children: A Case-Based Approach*, 9-month-old with recurrent episodes of supraventricular tachycardia despite medical therapy, Figure 6.1, Chennai, Elsevier Inc., 2022.)

TABLE 55.9	Abnormalities in Waves of ECG—cont'd	

Abnormalities in Waves	ECG Picture/Findings	Condition in Which It Is Seen

T WAVE

Tall T wave (Fig. 55.9J)

Tall T wave is >2/3rd of the preceding R wave

1. Hyperkalaemia
2. May be normal variation in chest leads
3. Ventricular strain pattern in volume overload

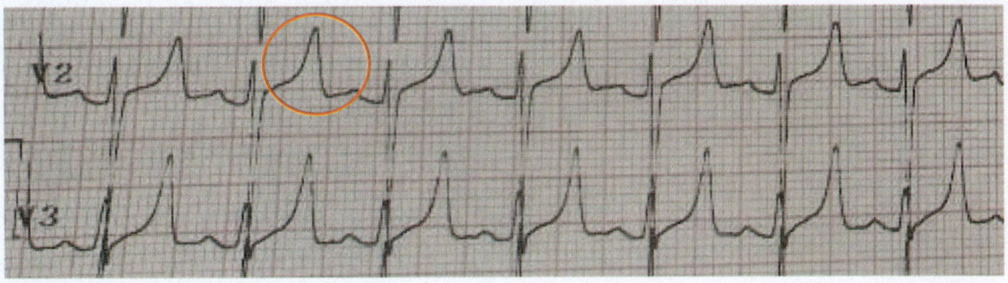

Fig. 55.9 (J) Tall T wave.

Flattened T wave/low-voltage T wave (Fig. 55.9K)

Small T wave is <1/8th of preceding R wave

1. Hypokalemia
2. Digitalis effect
3. Low voltage – hyothyroidism, myocarditis, effusion

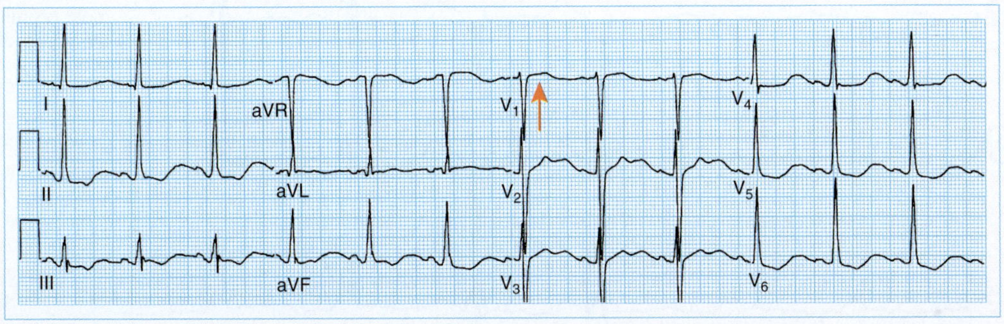

Fig. 55.9 (K) Flat T wave. (Source: Modifed from Brian Olshansky, Mina Chung, Steven Pogwizd, et al. *Arrhythmia Essentials*, Second Edition, Drug Effects and Electrolyte Disorders, Figure 9.5, Philadelphia, Elsevier Inc., 2018.)

T wave inversion (Fig. 55.9L)

1. Ischemia/infarction
2. Myocarditis
3. Conduction disturbances (pre-excitation or bundle branch block (BBB)
4. Ventricular strain pattern
5. Juvenile T wave inversion
6. Physiological in athletes, fever, anxiety but rarely

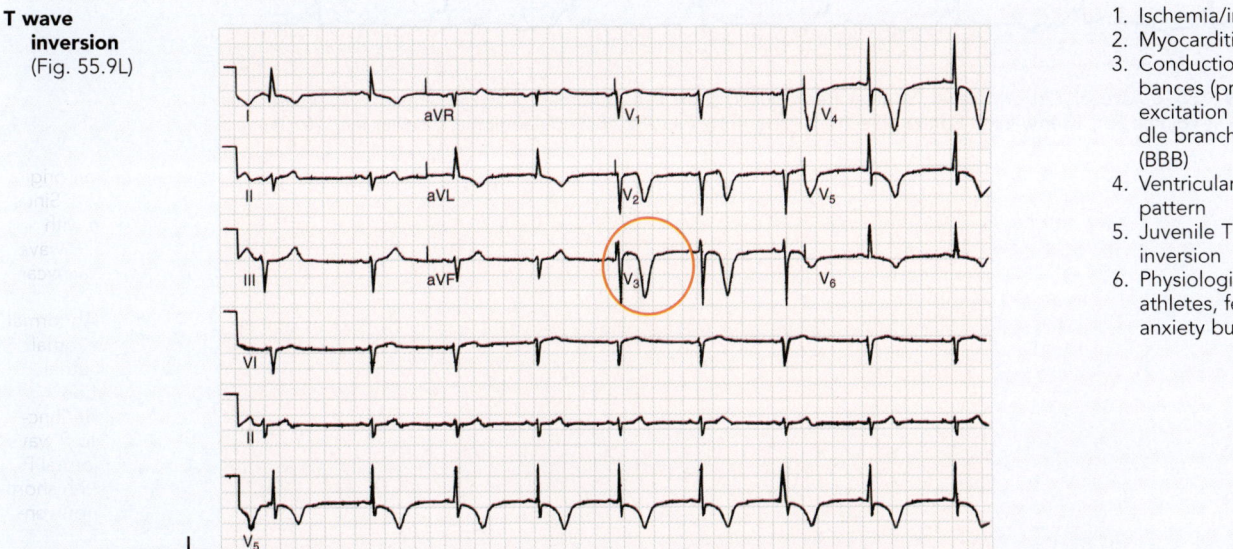

Fig. 55.9 (L) Inverted T wave. (Source: Modified from Peter Libby, Robert Bonow, Douglas Mann et al. *Braunwald's Heart Disease: A Textbook of Cardiovascular Medicine*, Twelfth Edition, Neuromuscular Disorders and Cardiovascular Disease, FIGURE 100.18, Philadelphia, Elsevier Inc., 2022. (Credit line - Courtesy Dr. Charles Fisch, Indiana University School of Medicine, Indianapolis.))

Continued

TABLE 55.9	Abnormalities in Waves of ECG—cont'd	

Abnormalities in Waves	ECG Picture/Findings	Condition in Which It Is Seen
OTHER WAVES **U wave** (Fig. 55.9M)	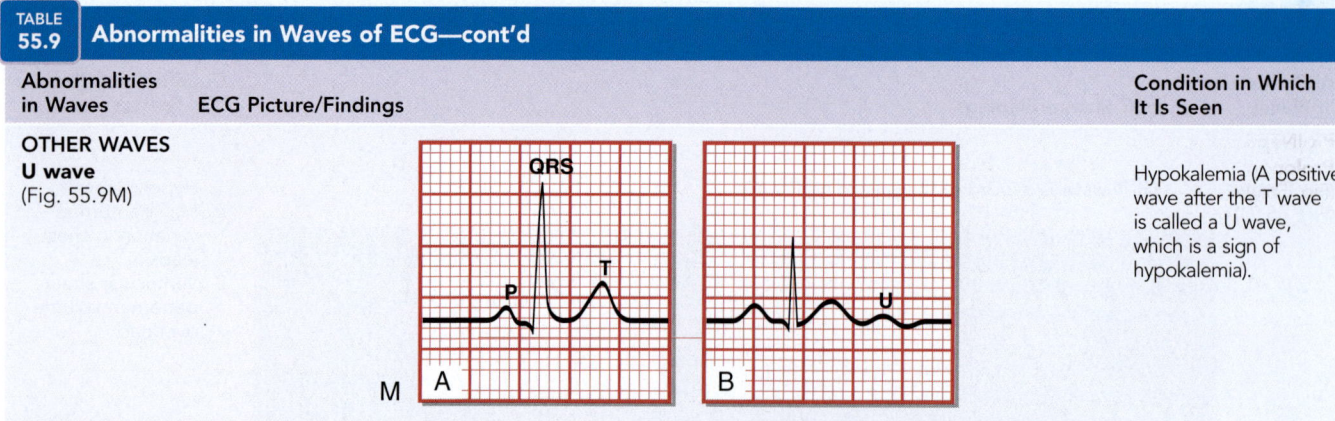	Hypokalemia (A positive wave after the T wave is called a U wave, which is a sign of hypokalemia).

Fig. 55.9 (M) U wave. (Source: Reproduced from Edward Goljan. *Rapid Review Pathology*, Fifth Edition, Water, Electrolyte, Acid-Base, and Hemodynamic Disorders, Fig 5.13, Philadelphia, Elsevier Inc., 2019. (Credit Line - From Gaw A, Murphy MJ, Srivastava R, Cowan RA, O'Reilly DSJ: Clinical Biochemistry: An Illustrated Colour Text, 5th ed, Churchill Livingstone Elsevier, 2013, p 22, Fig. 11.2.).

J wave (Fig. 55.9N)	Also known as Osborn wave 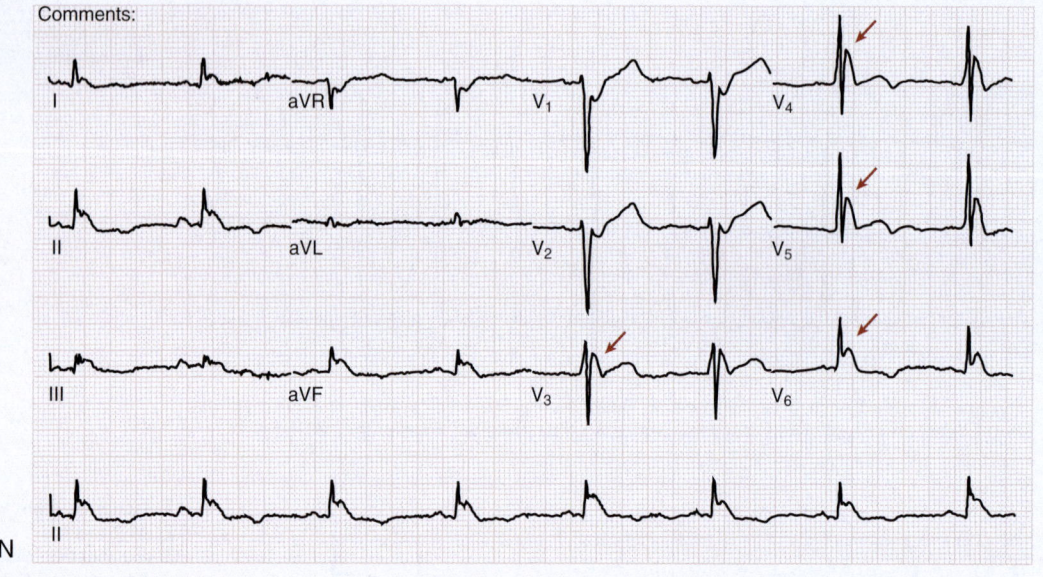	The Osborn wave (J wave) is a positive deflection at the J point (negative in aVR and V1); it is usually most prominent in the precordial leads, seen in hypothermia

Fig. 55.9 (N) J wave or Osborn wave. (Source: Reproduced from Lee Goldman, Andrew Schafer. *Goldman-Cecil Medicine, 2-Volume Set*, Twenty-Sixth Edition, Electrocardiography, FIGURE 48-3, Philadelphia, Elsevier Inc., 2020.)

TABLE 55.10	Abnormalities of Interval in ECG	
Abnormalities in Intervals	**ECG Picture/Findings**	**Condition in Which It Is Seen**
PR INTERVAL **Prolonged PR** (Fig. 55.10A)	Prolonged PR is >0.20 s 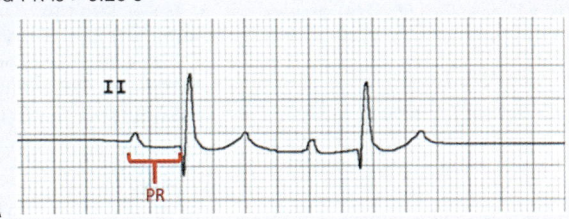 **Fig. 55.10** (A) Lead 2 with PR interval of 0.32 s. The interval should be measured in the *lead* with the largest, widest P wave and the longest QRS duration. (Source: Reproduced from Joanna Bassert. *McCurnin's Clinical Textbook for Veterinary Technicians and Nurses*, Tenth Edition, Emergency and Critical Care Nursing, Fig. 25.31, St Louis, Saunders, 2022.)	1. First-degree heart block 2. Myocarditis 3. Drugs: Calcium channel blockers, beta-blockers, digoxin toxicity, opioid clonidine 4. Hyperkalemia 5. Certain congenital heart diseases (Ebstein anomaly, ASD, ECD)
Short PR (Fig. 55.10B)	Short PR is <0.12 s 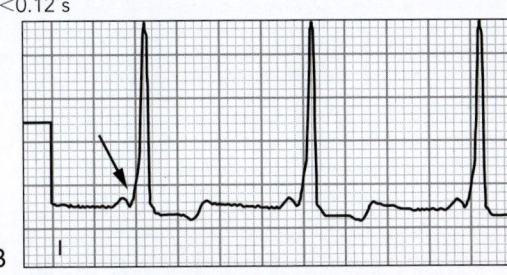 **Fig. 55.10** (B) Short PR interval of 0.08 s. (Source: Reproduced from Rick Kellerman, David Rakel, KUSM-W Medical Practice Association. *Conn's Current Therapy 2022*, Tachycardias, Figure 37.4, Philadelphia, Elsevier Inc., 2022.)	1. WPW syndrome 2. Glycogen storage disease (Pompe disease)
QTC INTERVAL **Long QT** (Fig. 55.10C)	• QTC >0.46 s is abnormal 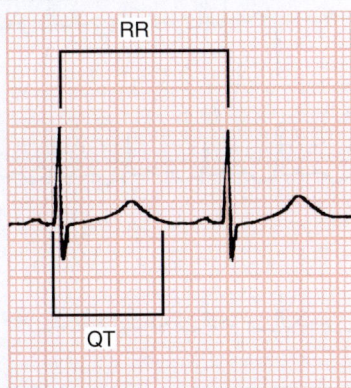 **Fig. 55.10** (C) Prolonged QTc of 0.63 sec. (Source: Reproduced from Ary Goldberger, Zachary Goldberger, Alexei Shvilkin. *Goldberger's Clinical Electrocardiography: A Simplified Approach*, Ninth Edition, How to Make Basic ECG Measurements, Fig 3.9, Edinburgh, Elsevier Inc., 2018.) QTc is calculated here as follows: $$QTc = \frac{600\,(QT\ in\ ms)}{\sqrt{0.92\,(RR\ in\ s)}}$$ $$= 670\,ms\ or\ 0.67\,s$$	1. Congenital causes: • Long QT syndrome, Romano−Ward syndrome (Autosomal dominant), Jervell−Lange syndrome (Autosomal recessive) 2. Acquired causes: • Drugs: Terfenadine, astemizole, ketoconazole, quinidine, erythromycin, etc. • Hypocalcemia, hypomagnesemia • Subarachnoid hemorrhage • Myocardial dysfunction

TABLE 55.11	**ECG Findings of Ventricular Hypertrophy**	
	Right Ventricular Hypertrophy	**Left Ventricular Hypertrophy**
Axis	Marked right axis deviation	Left axis deviation
Voltages	• Dominant R wave in V1–V3 (>5–7 mm tall) and dominant S wave in V5 and V6 (>7 mm deep) • R in V1 + S in V6 is >11 mm Fig. 55.11(A) shows right ventricular hypertrophy	• Increased voltage of the S wave V1 and V2, III, aVR and dominant R wave in V5, V6, 1, and aVL as shown in Fig. 55.11(B) • S in V1/V2 + R in V6 is >35 mm (or 45 mm if only this is taken – Sokolow–Lyon criteria) • Voltage criteria for LVH are described later
R/S progression	Neonatal precordial RS pattern or reversal of adult pattern.	Adult type of RS progression
R/S ratio	>1 in V1 or <1 in V6 (more useful in children older than 6 years)	Decrease R/S ratio in V1 and V2
Strain pattern	RV strain pattern; ST depression and T wave inversion in V1–V3	LV strain pattern: ST depression and T wave inversion in V5 and V6
Abnormal T waves	Positive T in V1 in children between the age of 3 days to 6 years (provided it is upright elsewhere also); this alone indicates significant RVH	Inverted T waves in lead 1 and aVL
Abnormal Q waves	qR pattern in V1; presence of Q in right side leads indicates severe RVH	Deep Q wave in the left precordial leads
Other points	RBBB pattern may be present: rsR' in V1–V3 (M-shaped QRS)	Increase in QRS duration

Fig. 55.11C shows ECG of biventricular hypertrophy

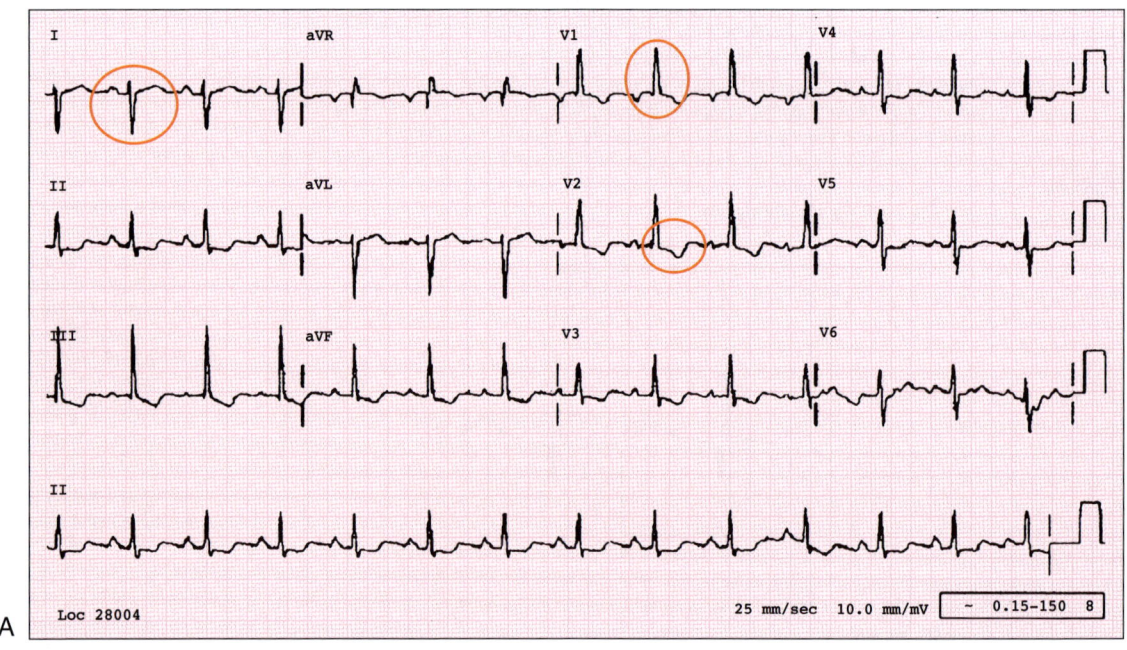

Fig. 55.11   (A) ECG showing right ventricular hypertrophy (RVH) – right axis deviation dominant R in V1 and V2 with deep S in V5 and V6 R + S > 11 mm, ST depression and T wave inversion in V1–V3 s/o RV strain pattern. (Source: Modifed from Nancy Koster. *Cardiovascular Imaging Review*, Electrocardiography, Figure 1-49, Philadelphia, Saunders, 2011.)

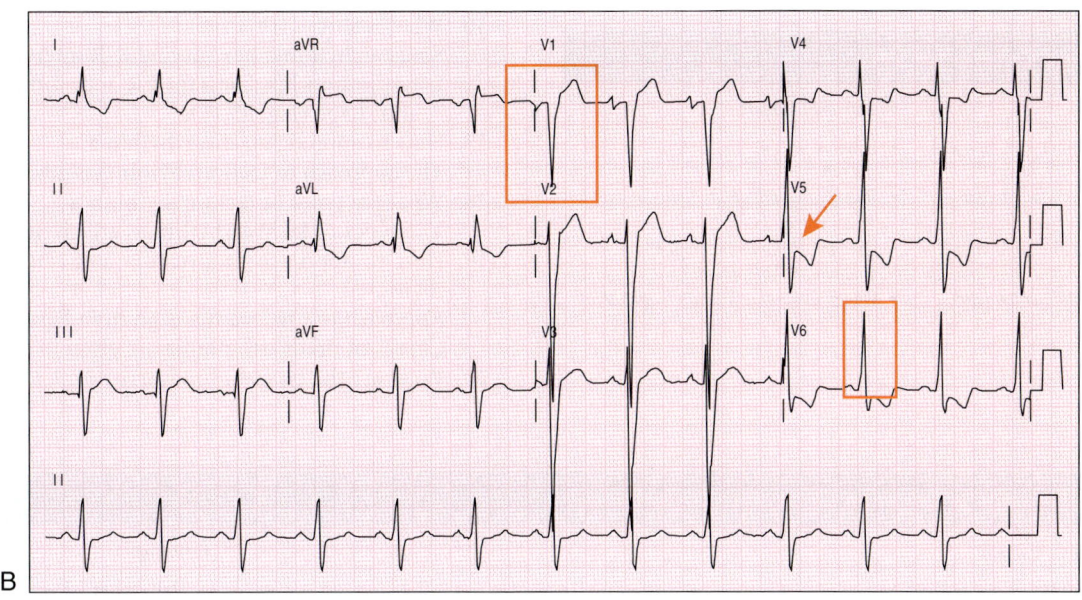

Fig. 55.11   (B) ECG showing left ventricular hypertrophy (LVH) – left axis deviation dominant R in V5 and V6 with deep S in V1 and V2 ST depression in V5 and V6 and T wave inversion in aVL s/o LV strain pattern. (Source: Modifed from Nancy Koster. *Cardiovascular Imaging Review*, Electrocardiography, Figure 1-11, Philadelphia, Saunders, 2011.)

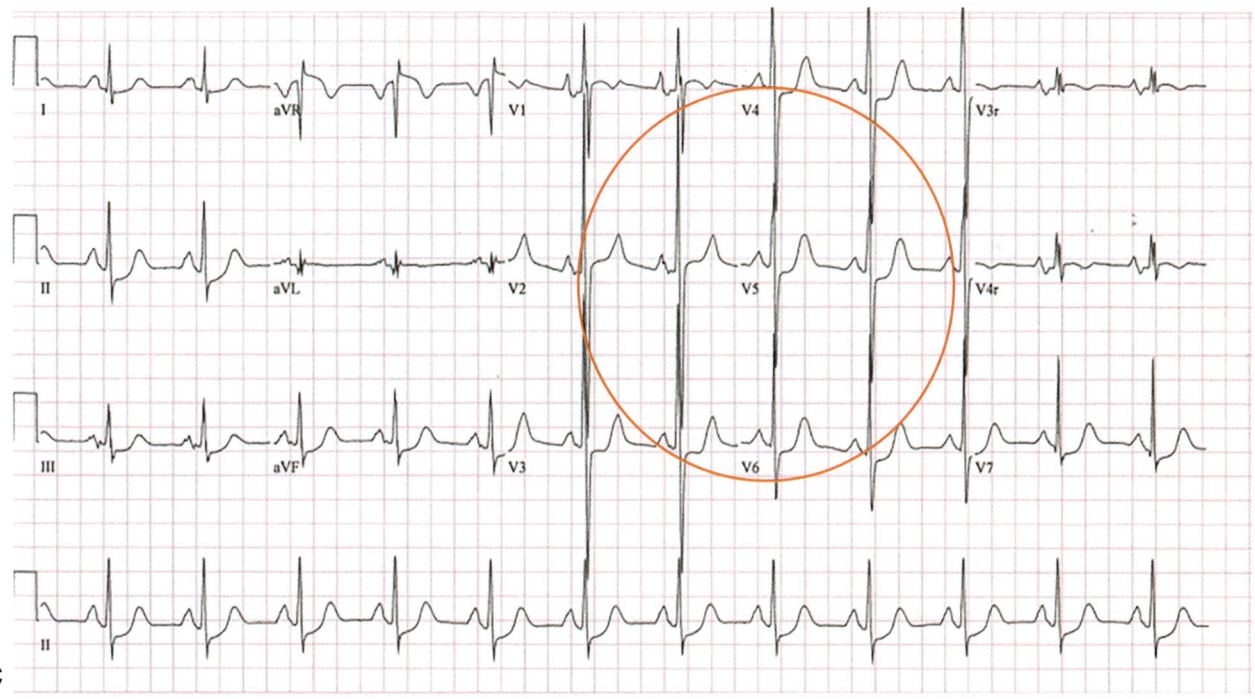

Fig. 55.11   (C) ECG showing biventricular hypertrophy (biphasic QRS in V2–V5 seen). (Source: Modified from Susan W. Denfield and Overview of pediatric restrictive cardiomyopathy - 2021, *Progress in Pediatric Cardiology* 62:101415.)

TABLE 55.12	Voltage Criteria for LVH	
Limb Leads		**Precordial Leads**
• R wave in lead 1 + S wave in lead 3 > 25 mm		• R wave in V4, V5, or V6 > 26 mm
• R wave in aVL > 11 mm		• R wave in V5/V6 + S wave in V1 > 35 mm
• R wave in aVF > 20 mm		• Largest R wave + largest S wave > 45 mm
• S wave in aVF > 14 mm		• Deep Q (>4 mm) in V5 and V6

16. What is sinus arrhythmia?

    Sinus arrhythmia has varying R-R interval according to respiration but constant PR and normal P wave size and shape (Fig. 55.15).

17. How to approach tachyarrhythmia?

    The approach to tachyarrhythmia is given in Fig. 55.16.

18. What are types of tachyarrhythmias?

    The types of tachyarrhythmias are given in Table 55.15.

19. How to approach bradycardia and causes of bradyarrhythmia?

    Approach to bradycardia is given in Fig. 55.18.

    Causes of bradyarrhythmia are given in Table 55.16.

20. What are the types of bradyarrhythmia?

TABLE 55.13	ECG Findings in Common Electrolyte Disturbances
Condition With ECG	**Findings**

1. **Hyperkalemia** (Fig. 55.12A)

1. Tall, tented T waves (red circle)
2. P waves flatten with prolonged PR; P wave disappears later
3. Broad QRS
4. ST elevation
5. Sine wave pattern (when K^+ levels rise higher)
6. Finally ventricular fibrillation if left untreated

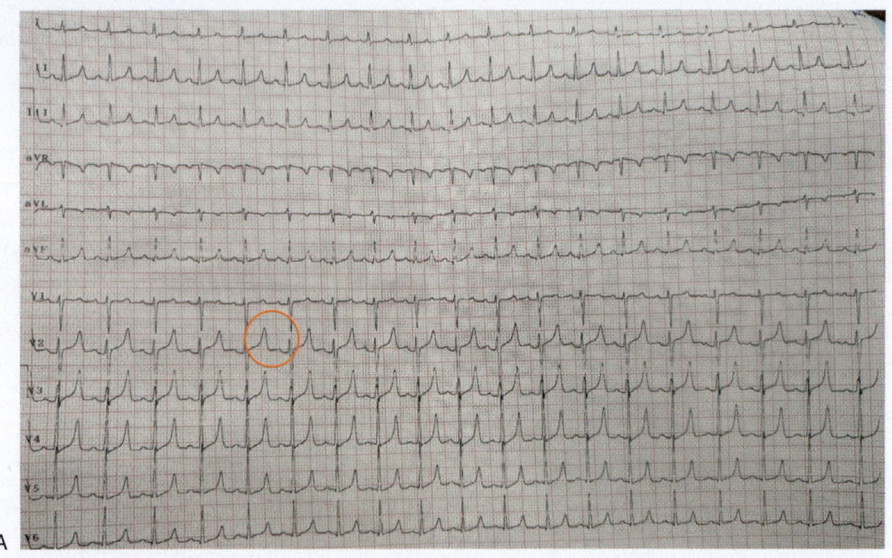

A

Fig. 55.12 (A) ECG showing features of hyperkalemia.

2. **Hypokalemia** (Fig. 55.12B)

1. Short PR
2. T wave flattening (A - red arrow) or low-amplitude T wave or inversion
3. Prominence of U wave (B)
4. QTc prolongation (because T wave duration is prolonged)
5. ST depression (C)

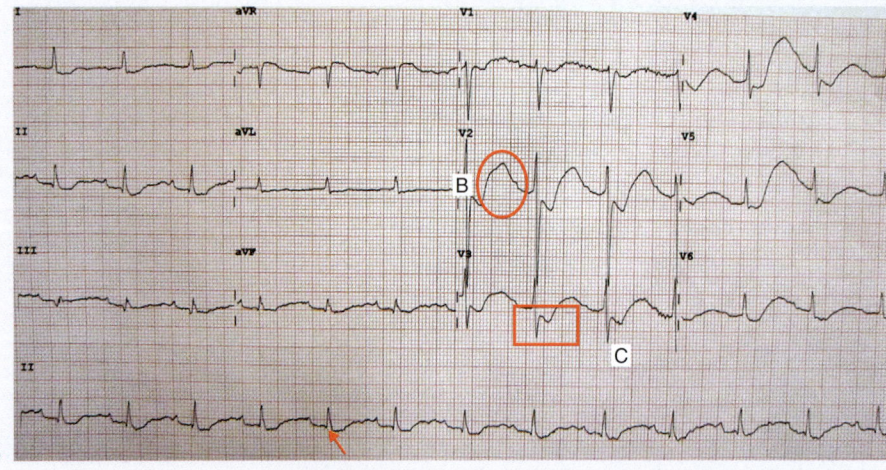

B

Fig. 55.12 (B) ECG showing features of hypokalemia.

TABLE 55.13	ECG Findings in Common Electrolyte Disturbances—cont'd

Condition With ECG	Findings
3. **Hypocalcemia/hypomagnesemia**	Prolonged QTc (due to prolongation of ST segment; T wave duration is normal) (Fig. 55.12C)

Fig. 55.12   (C) ECG showing QTc prolongation. (Source: Modified from Mithilesh Das, Douglas Zipes. *Electrocardiography of Arrhythmias: A Comprehensive Review*, Second Edition, Polymorphic Ventricular Tachycardia and Ventricular Fibrillation in the Absence of Structural Heart Disease, Fig. 13.28, Philadelphia, Elsevier Inc., 2022.)

TABLE 55.14	ECG Changes in Myocarditis and Pericarditis

Condition With ECG	Findings
1. **Myocarditis** (Fig. 55.13A) 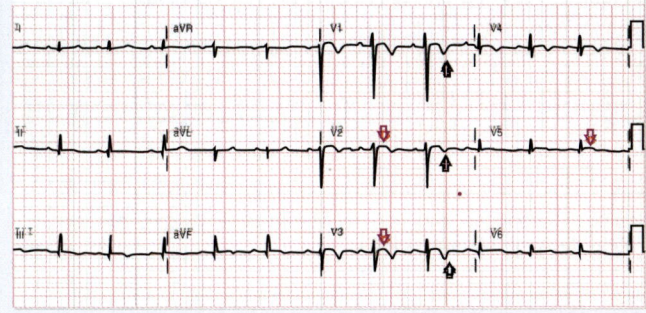	1. Sinus tachycardia 2. Diminished QRS voltage 3. Nonspecific ST and T wave changes 4. Any degree of AV block may be seen

Fig. 55.13   (A) ECG findings in a patient with myocarditis (T wave inversion in all Leads). (Source: Modified from Mark Miller, Stephen Thompson. *DeLee & Drez's Orthopaedic Sports Medicine: Principles and Practice*, Fourth Edition, Comprehensive Cardiovascular Care and Evaluation of the Elite Athlete, FIGURE 15-11, Philadelphia, Saunders, 2015. (Credit line - From Battle RW, Mistry DJ, Malhotra R: Cardiovascular screening and the elite athlete: advances, concepts, controversies, and a view of the future. Clin Sports Med 30:503–524, 2011.))

Continued

TABLE 55.14	ECG Changes in Myocarditis and Pericarditis—cont'd

Condition With ECG	Findings
2. **Pericarditis** (Fig. 55.13B) 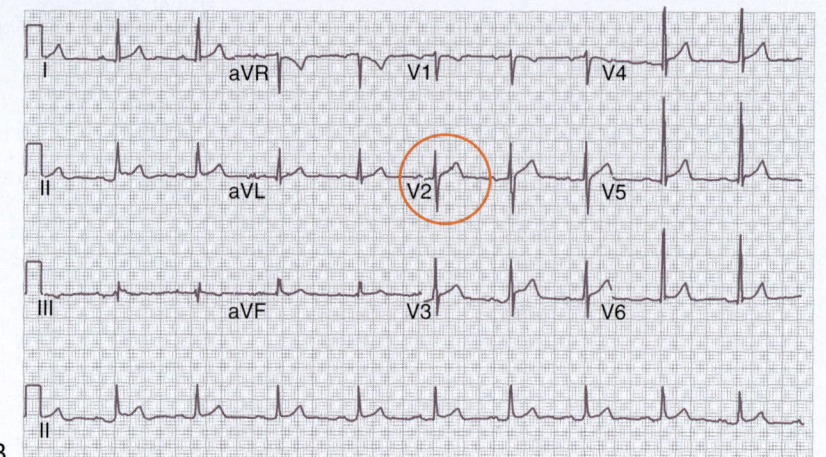	1. ST/T changes seen – may vary depending on time of presentation: • Acute phase (stage 1): ST elevation with concavity upwards along with downsloping of TP line as shown in Fig. 55.13C • Subacute phase (stage 2): ST back to baseline, T wave amplitude decreases (within few days) • Chronic phase (stage 3): T wave inversion occurs after a few weeks (Fig. 55.13D) • Stage 4: ECG becomes normal in a couple of months

Fig. 55.13 (B) ECG findings in a patient with pericarditis. (Source: Modified from Catherine Otto, Rebecca Schwaegler, Rosario Freeman. *Echocardiography Review Guide: Companion to the Textbook of Clinical Echocardiography*, Second Edition, Pericardial Disease, Figure 101, Philadelphia, Saunders, 2011.)

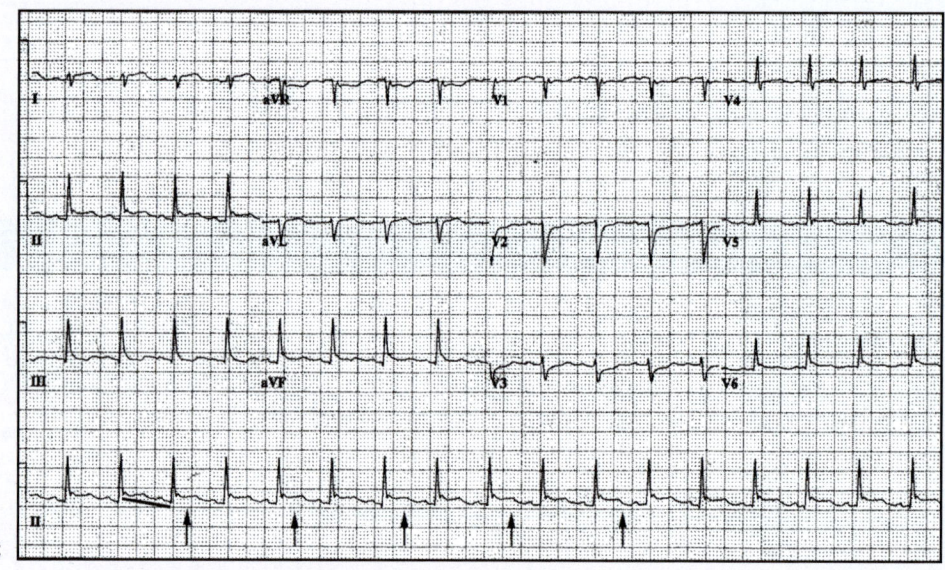

Fig. 55.13 (C) Spodick sign – stage 1 pericarditis. (Source: Reproduced from John N Makaryus, Amgad N Makaryus, Bernard Boal, and Spodick's Sign, *The American Journal of Medicine* 121(8):693-694.)

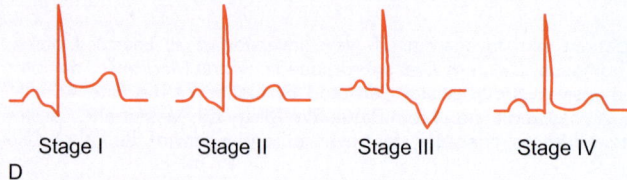

Fig. 55.13 (D) ST/T changes in pericarditis.

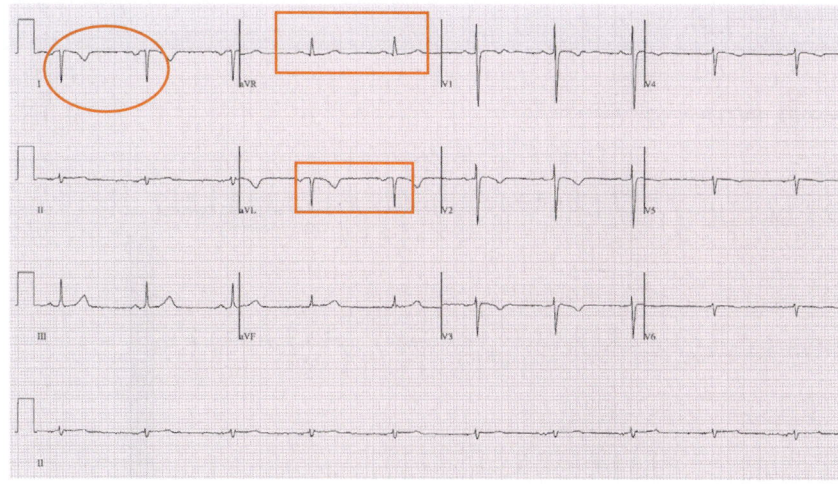

Fig. 55.14 ECG findings in dextrocardia. (Source: Modified from Mithilesh Das, Douglas Zipes. *Electrocardiography of Arrhythmias: A Comprehensive Review: A Companion to Cardiac Electrophysiology: From Cell to Bedside*, Important Concepts, FIGURE 1-3, Philadelphia, Saunders, 2012.)

Sinus arrhythmia

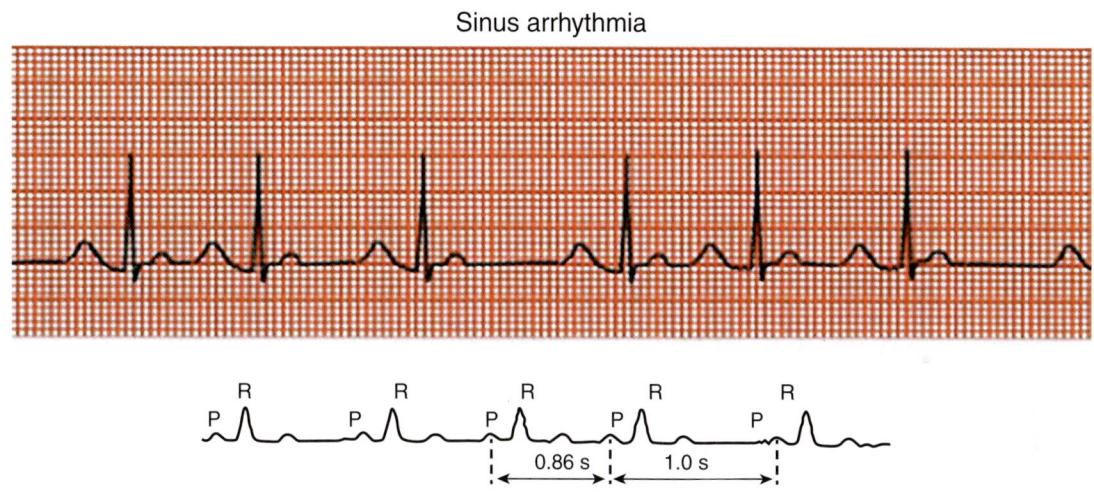

Fig. 55.15 ECG showing varying R-R with respiration (sinus arrhythmia). Note: Interval P−P is different. The longest P−P interval differs from the shortest P−P interval by more than 0.12 s. (Source: https://en-wiki.cardio-cloud.ru/index.php?title=Sinus_arrhythmia)

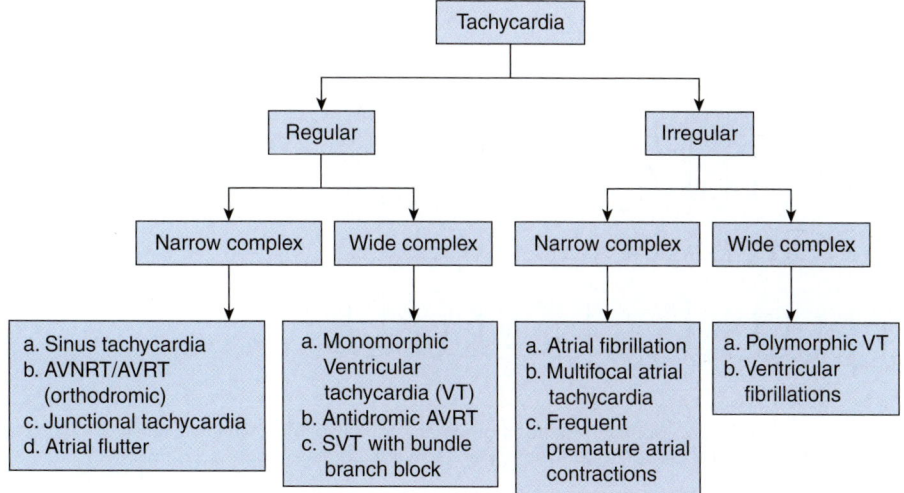

Fig. 55.16 Approach to tachycardia.

TABLE 55.15	Types of Tachyarrhythmia

ECG	Findings
1. **Supraventricular tachycardia (SVT)** (Fig. 55.17A)	1. HR > 220/min in infancy, >180/min in children older than 1 year 2. Narrow QRS < 0.09 s 3. Absent P wave

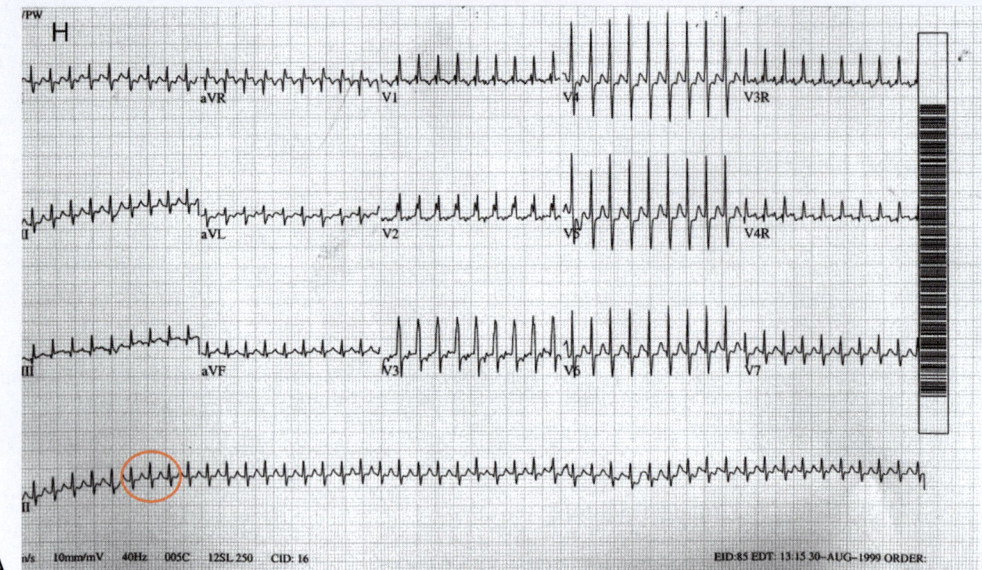

Fig. 55.17 (A) ECG showing supraventricular tachycardia. (Source: Modified from Victoria Vetter. *Pediatric Cardiology: THE REQUISITES IN PEDIATRICS*, First Edition, Pediatric Evaluation of the Cardiac Patient, Figure 1-3, Philadelphia, Mosby, 2006.)

ECG	Findings
2. **Atrial flutter** (Fig. 55.17B)	1. Narrow complex tachycardia 2. Flutter waves with sawtooth configuration – best seen in leads 2, 3, aVF 3. Rate 240–360 with varying blocks (2:1, 3:1, 4:1) with normal QRS

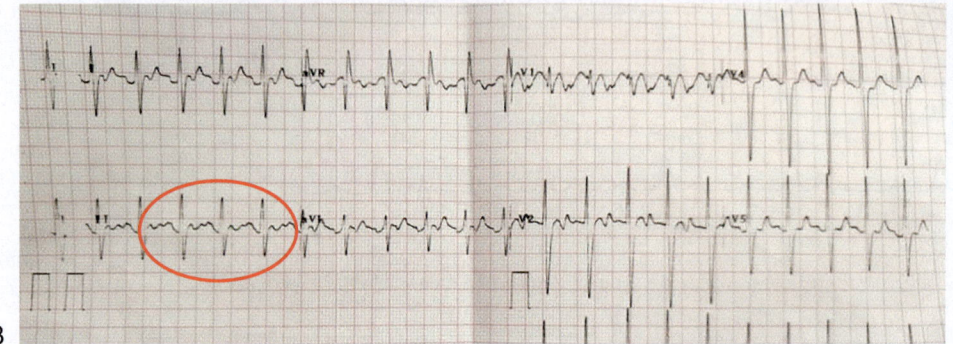

Fig. 55.17 (B) ECG showing atrial flutter.

ECG	Findings
3. **Atrial fibrillation**	1. Fibrillatory waves as shown in Fig. 55.17C 2. Rate fast – 350–600 3. Irregular ventricular response with normal QRS (irregularly irregular rhythm)

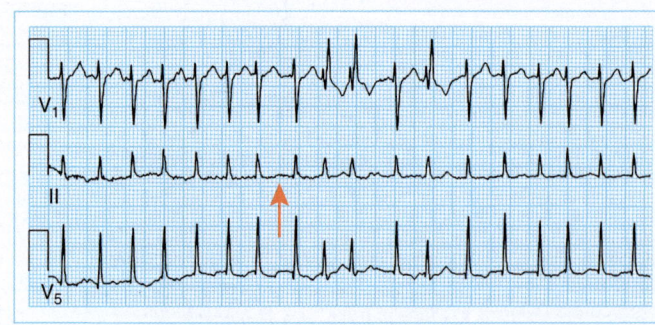

Fig. 55.17 (C) ECG showing atrial fibrillation. (Source: Modifed from Brian Olshansky, Mina Chung, Steven Pogwizd et al. Arrhythmia Essentials, Second Edition, Supraventricular Tachyarrhythmias, Figure 5.12, Philadelphia, Elsevier Inc., 2018.)

TABLE 55.15	Types of Tachyarrhythmia—cont'd

ECG	Findings

4. **Junctional rhythm** (Fig. 55.17D)

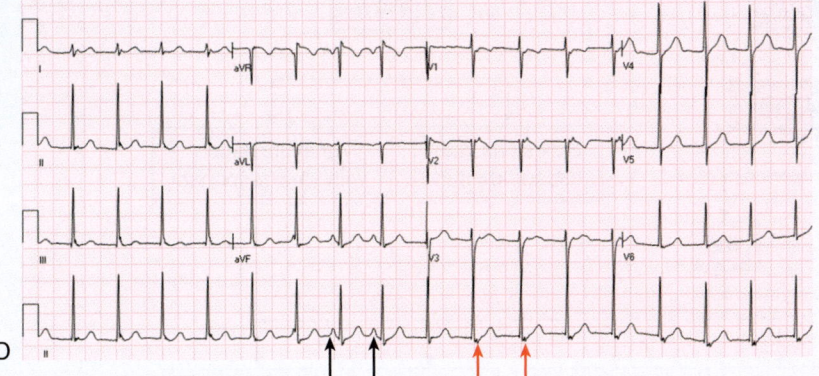

1. Narrow complex
2. P waves may be absent or inverted or hidden by QRS complex (red arrow)
3. Short PR

Fig. 55.17 (D) ECG showing junctional rhythm. (Source: Modifed from Mithilesh Das, Douglas Zipes. *Electrocardiography of Arrhythmias: A Comprehensive Review*, Second Edition, Atrioventricular Conduction Abnormalities, Fig. 3.37, Philadelphia, Elsevier Inc., 2022.)

5. **Ventricular tachycardia (VT)** (Fig. 55.17E)

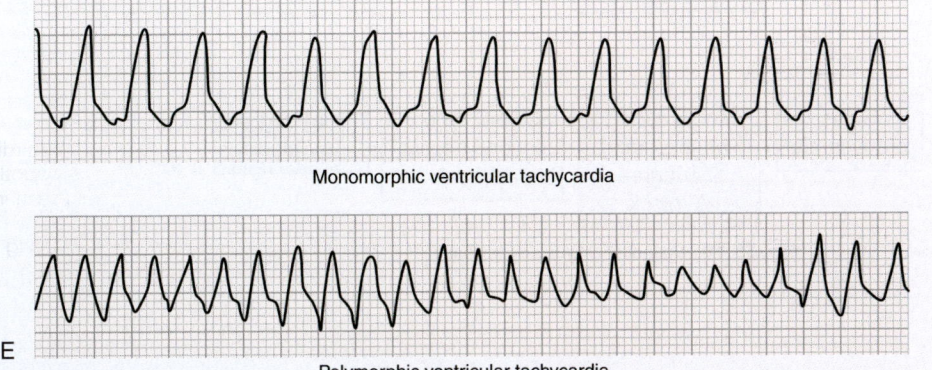

Monomorphic ventricular tachycardia

Polymorphic ventricular tachycardia

1. Wide QRS (>0.9 s)
2. HR – 120–200/min
3. No P wave
4. Fast and regular
5. T wave opposite to the direction of QRS
6. Three or more ventricular premature contractions (VPC) QRS bizarre and wide and T pointing in opposite direction
7. Monomorphic VT: QRS morphology similar in all beats, indicating a single arrhythmogenic focus
8. Polymorphic VT: QRS morphology Varies in each beat, indicating multiple arrhythmogenic foci

Fig. 55.17 (E) ECG showing monomorphic VT (above) and polymorphic VT (below). (Source: Reproduced from Roberta Hines, Katherine Marschall. *Stoelting's Anesthesia and Co-Existing Disease*, Seventh Edition, Abnormalities of Cardiac Conduction and Cardiac Rhythm, FIG. 8.6, Philadelphia, Elsevier Inc., 2018.)

6. **Ventricular fibrillation** (Fig. 55.17F)

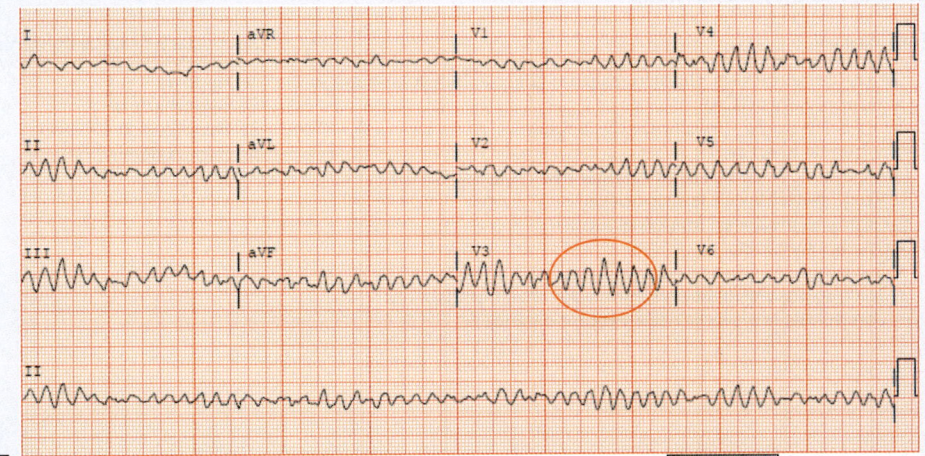

1. Chaotic and irregular waves
2. Fibrillatory waves
3. Wide QRS

Fig. 55.17 (F) ECG showing ventricular fibrillation. (Source: Modifed from Douglas Sawyer, Ramachandran Vasan. *Encyclopedia of Cardiovascular Research and Medicine*, Ventricular Fibrillation and Defibrillation, Fig. 1, Oxford MRW, Elsevier Inc., 2018.)

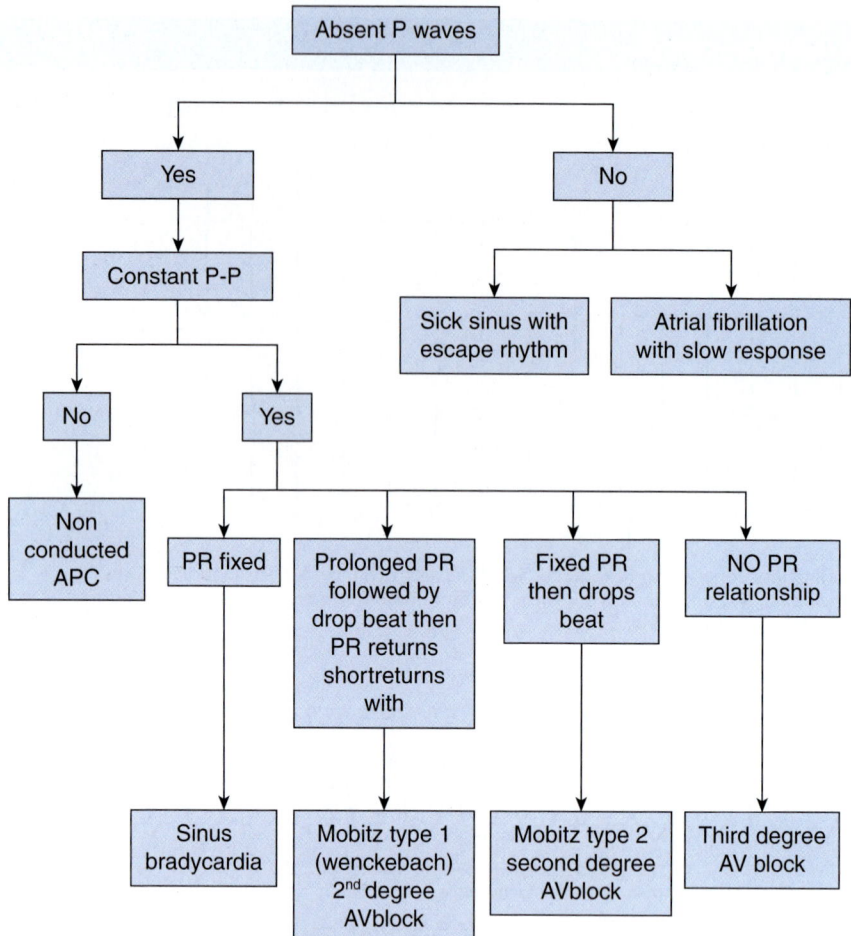

Fig. 55.18 Approach to bradycardia.

TABLE 55.16	Causes of Bradyarrhythmia	
PRIMARY BRADYARRHYTHMIA		
Physiological	**Pathological**	**Secondary Bradyarrhythmia**

Increased vagal tone (athletes, airway interventions, IC injury)	1. Drugs (beta-blockers, digoxin, calcium channel blockers, tricylcic antidepressants (TCA))
	2. Sinus bradycardia, sinus node dysfunction
	3. Congenital heart block
	  (a) Anatomic – complex congenital heart disease (CHD) (e.g., heterotaxy, L-transposition)
	  (b) Immune mediated (maternal lupus)
	4. Acquired AV block
	  • Surgical
	  • Toxin exposures (carbonmonooxide, organophosphate compunds, scorpion, snake venom, oleander)
		1. Hypoxia
		2. Hypothermia
		3. Hypotension (severe)
		4. Hyperkalemia

ECG	Findings

1. **Sinus bradycardia** (Fig. 55.19A)

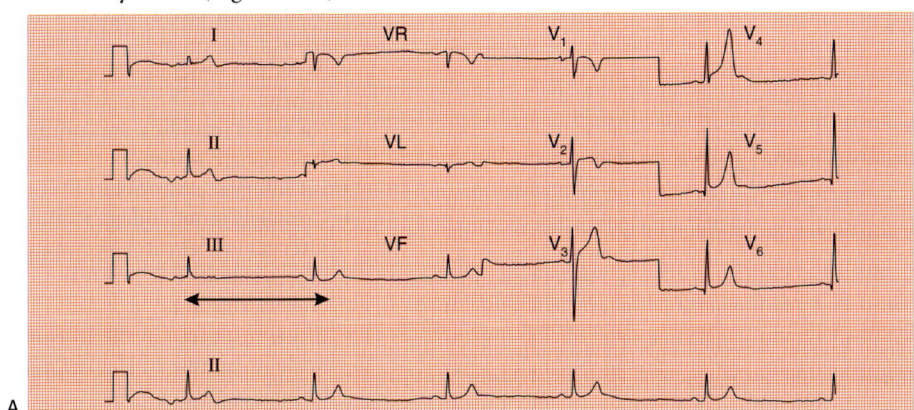

A

Fig. 55.19 (A) ECG showing sinus bradycardia (PR less than 60, normal PR interval – red arrow). (Source: Modified from John Hampton. *The ECG Made Easy*, Eight Edition, The ECG in Healthy Subjects, Edinburgh, Churchill Livingstone, 2013.)

1. Bradycardia, normal PR interval, sinus rhythm
2. Causes:
   a) Well child – athlete and on beta-blocker therapy
   b) Sick child – Intracranial pressure (ICP), poisoning(beta-blocker, calcium channel blocker (CCB), digoxin, oleander)

2. **First-degree heart block** (Fig. 55.19B)

First-degree AV block

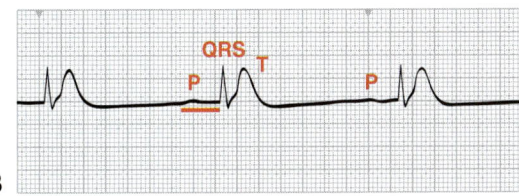

B

Fig. 55.19 (B) ECG showing first-degree heart block (prolonged PR).

1. PR interval prolonged
2. Causes:
   a) Atrioventricular (AV) septal defects
   b) Corrected TGA
   c) Rheumatic carditis
   d) Diphtheria
   e) Digoxin toxicity
3. Patients are usually asymptomatic
4. No specific treatment, primary disease management

3. **Second-degree heart block – Mobitz I** (Fig. 55.19C)

Second-degree AV block
(type I AV block [Wenckebach's])

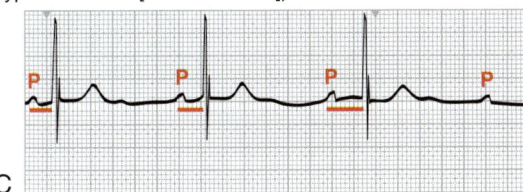

C

Fig. 55.19 (C) ECG showing Mobitz type I heart block.

1. Progressive increase in PR interval until a P wave is not conducted; in the next cycle, PR interval normalizes
2. Block at the level of the AV node so the QRS is narrow
3. It often *spontaneously* resolves, and typically responds to atropine
4. It is also known as Wenckebach phenomenon

4. **Second-degree heart block –Mobitz II** (Fig. 55.19D)

Second-degree AV block
(type II AV block)

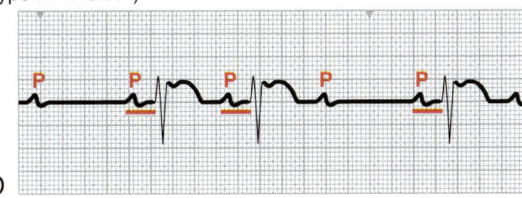

D

Fig. 55.19 (D) ECG showing Mobitz type II block.

1. Constant PR interval for consecutively conducted beats until one or more beats are dropped
2. Block occurs low down in the conduction system – the QRS is wide
3. It does not respond to atropine, and is important to recognize because pacing will be needed

ECG	Findings

5. Third-degree/complete heart block (Fig. 55.19E)

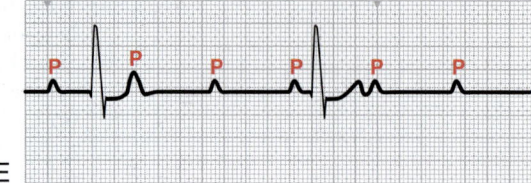

Third-degree AV block
(complete AV block)

E

Fig. 55.19   (E) ECG showing third-degree/complete heart block. (Source: Reproduced from Maureen Barry, Donna Goodridge, Sharon Lewis et al. *Medical-Surgical Nursing in Canada: Assessment and Management of Clinical Problems*, Third Edition, Nursing Management, Figure 38-16, Toronto, Mosby Canada, 2014. (Credit line - Source: Wesley, K. (2011). Huszar's basic dysrhythmias and acute coronary syndromes: Interpretation and management (4th ed.). St. Louis: Mosby.)

- Atrial rate 1500/15 = 100 (P–P)
- Ventricular rate 1500/55 = 18 (R–R)
- Atria and ventricles beat independently
- No atrial impulses are conducted
- P waves are normal
- PR interval is variable
- Constant independent P–P interval (atrial rate) and regular independent R–R interval (ventricular rate)
- Block can occur at the level of AV node or bundle of His (BOH) or bundle branches
- QRS maybe narrow if the block is above BOH or wide (at or below BOH)
- P waves not related to QRS complex

6. Wolff−Parkinson−White (WPW) syndrome (Fig. 55.19F)

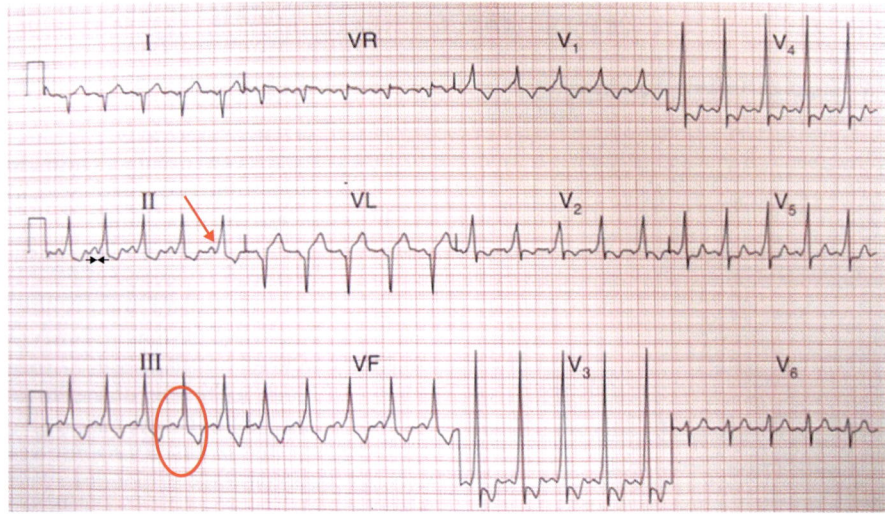

Fig. 55.19   (F) ECG of Wolff−Parkinson−White (WPW) syndrome.

- WPW syndrome
- Short PR (less than lower limit of N for age) − black arrow
- Delta wave (initial slurring of QRS) − red arrow
- Wide QRS (more than upper limit of normal) − red circle
- Usually present clinically during episodes of supraventricular tachycardia
- It is a type of pre-excitation due to abnormal conduction pathway bundle of Kent, connecting between atrium and ventricle; treatment − radiofrequency ablation

Clue: Wide + short PR+ delta − WPW

ECG	Findings
7. Right bundle branch block (RBBB) (Fig. 55.20)	• rSR′ pattern in V1, V2, V3 wide QRS • Widened and slurred S in V6: Suggestive of RBBB • Seen in atrial septal defect (ASD), postcardiac surgery • Clue: Remember as MARROW — M pattern in V1, V2, and V3; W pattern — widened and slurred S in V6 suggestive of RBBB

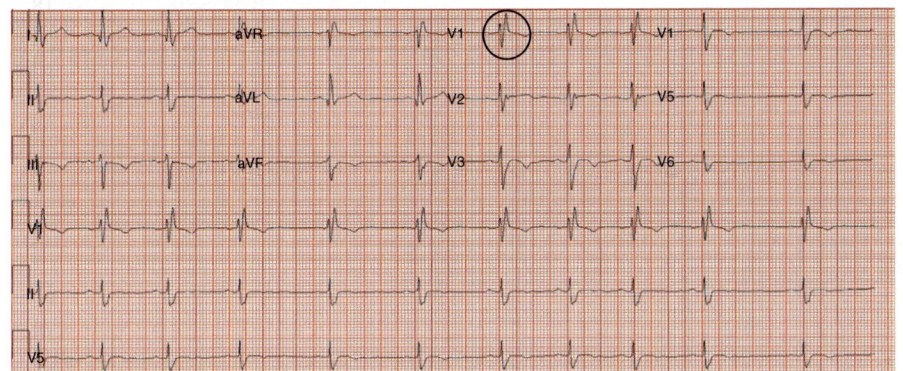

Fig. 55.20 Right bundle branch block. (Source: Modifed from American Society of Echocardiography. *ASE's Comprehensive Echocardiography*, Third Edition, Chagas Cardiomyopathy, Figure 157.1, Philadelphia, Elsevier Inc., 2022.)

9. Left bundle branch block (Fig. 55.21)	• Left bundle branch block: rS pattern in V1 (tiny R and deep S — red circle), monophasic R wave in lateral lead (lead 1, aVL, V5 and V6 — blue circle) • Clue: WILLIAM – W pattern (dominant S wave) in V1 and M pattern (broad and notched R wave) in V5 and V6

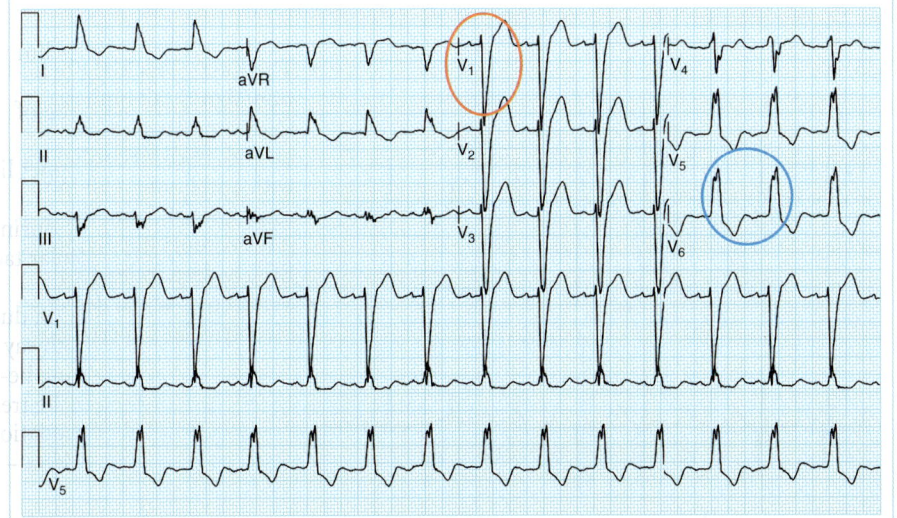

Fig. 55.21 Left bundle branch block. (Source: Modified from Brian Olshansky, Mina Chung, Steven Pogwizd et al. *Arrhythmia Essentials*, Second Edition, Bradyarrhythmias—Conduction System Abnormalities, Figure 2.13, Philadelphia, Elsevier Inc., 2018.)

21. What are the findings in ECG in congenital heart disease?

Atrial septal defect (ASD) (Fig. 55.22)

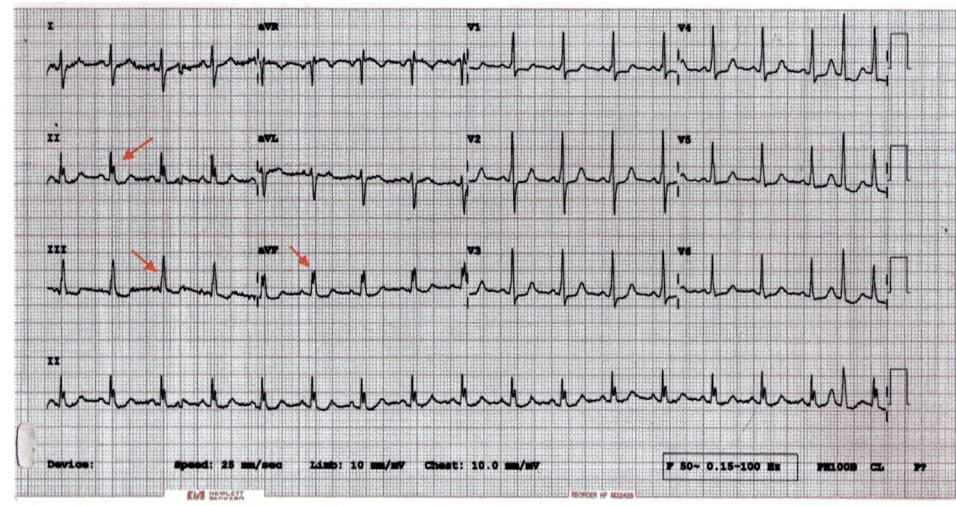

- Right axis deviation
- Crochetage sign (red arrow): A notch near the apex of R wave in inferior limb leads (lead 2 and aVF);inferior leads show notched R wave
- Right ventricular hypertrophy
- Partial RBBB

Fig. 55.22   Atrial septal defect. (Source: Reproduced from Jeet Ram Kashyap, Suraj Kumar, and A forgotten notch: Crochetage sign, *IHJ Cardiovascular Case Reports* 3:77-78.)

Ventricular septal defect (VSD) (Fig. 55.23)

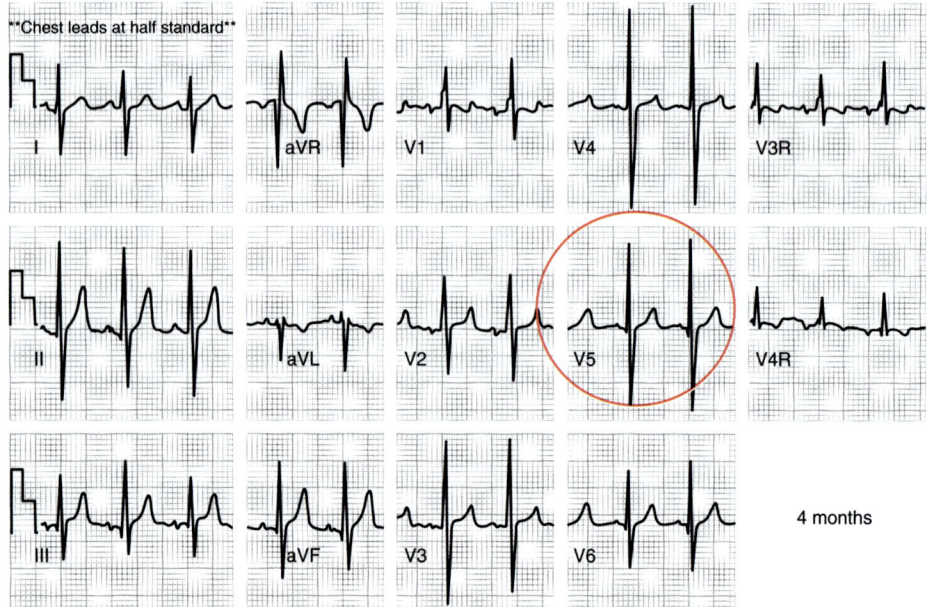

- The **Katz−Wachtel phenomenon/sign** is tall biphasic (R = S); QRS complexes in lead V2, V3, or V4 − mid-precordial leads with amplitude >50 mm; because the QRS amplitude is high, it overshoots the margins of ECG as seen in lead V4
- Ventricular septal defect with biventricular hypertrophy

Fig. 55.23   Ventricular septal defect. (Source: Modified from Borys Surawicz, Timothy Knilans. *Chou's Electrocardiography in Clinical Practice: Adult and Pediatric*, Sixth Edition, The Electrocardiogram in Congenital Heart Disease, Figure 30-6, Philadelphia, Saunders, 2008.)

ALCAPA (Fig. 55.24)

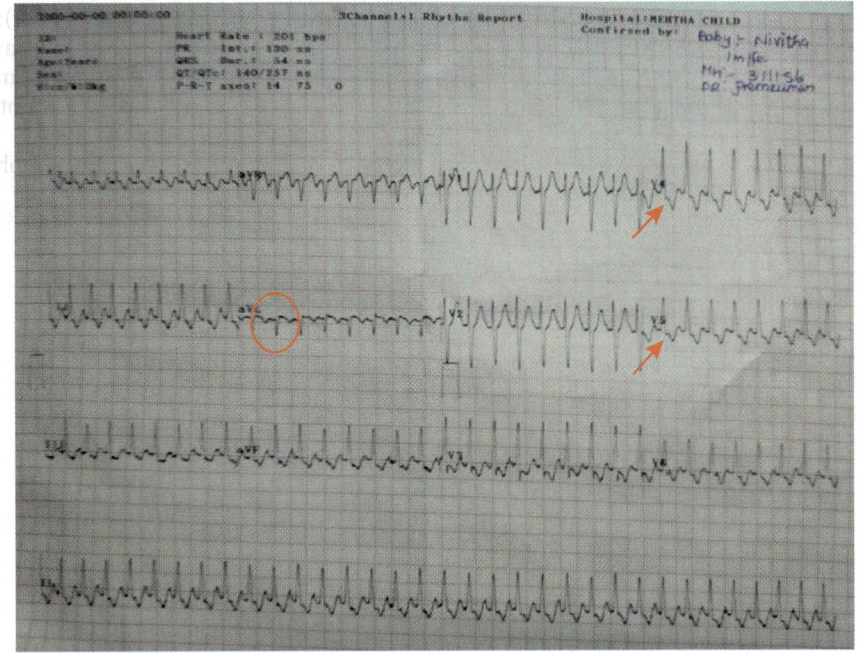

Fig. 55.24 ECG of a child with ALCAPA.

- Myocardial infarct pattern in ECG
- ST segment depression in V3–V6 (red arrow)
- T wave inversion in all chest leads
- Pathological Q in aVL (red circle)
- Rule of 4 for pathological Q wave
  >4 mm height
  >0.04 s
  >1/4th of the preceding R wave

Tricuspid atresia (Fig. 55.25)

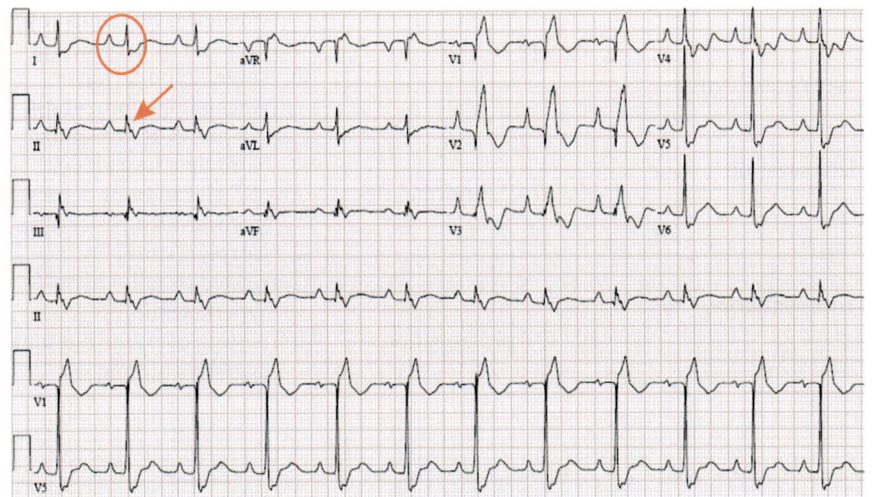

Fig. 55.25 Tricuspid atresia. (Source: Modified from Margaret M Fuchs, Heidi M Connolly, and Ebstein Anomaly in the Adult Patient, *Cardiol Clin* 38(3):353-363. (Credit line - From Das MK, Zipes DP. Fragmented QRS: a predictor of mortality and sudden cardiac death. Heart Rhythm. 2009;6(3 Suppl):S8-14.))

- Himalayan P waves (RT atrial enlargement) − P > half of the preceding R wave; right axis deviation; notched R wave in lead 2, lead 3, aVF, and V1 suggestive of fragmented QRS due to abnormal conduction in atrialized right ventricle seen in Ebstein anomaly
- Present with cyanosis and multiple clicks CXR − massive cardiomegaly, box-shaped heart due to left atrial enlargement
- Associated with ASD and patent foramen ovale in 90% of the cases

Quick bites

A. Key for analysis of rhythm disturbances
1. Slow or fast
2. Regular or irregular
3. Narrow or wide
4. P present or absent

B. Points to differentiate between congenital and acquired heart block

Congenital Heart Block	Acquired Heart Block
• QRS duration normal because pacemaker of the ventricular complex at a level higher than the bifurcation of BOH	• Prolonged QRS because the pacemaker of the ventricular complex is below the bifurcation of BOH
• Ventricular rate is faster compared to acquired heart block (50–80 per min)	• Ventricular rate is 40–50 per min (idioventricular rhythm)
• Rate is somewhat variable under physiological conditions	• Ventricular rate is relatively fixed

C. Clues for tachycardia and bradycardia
1. Wide + tachycardia – VT
2. Wide + bradycardia – Congenital heart block (CHB)
3. Intermittent wide – VPC
4. Wide + short PR+ delta – WPW

D. How to differentiate between atrial and ventricular extrasystole?

Atrial Extrasystole	Ventricular Extrasystole
• Narrow	• Wide bizarre
• Preceded by abnormal P and PR	• No preceding P
• Incomplete compensatory pause	• Complete compensatory pause

E. Always go by the steps.

1. Rate	<60 − bradyarrhythmias >180/220 − tachyarrhythmias
2. Look at the QRS: >0.09	a. Wide + tachycardia – VT b. Wide + bradycardia – CHB c. Intermittent wide – VPC d. Wide + short PR + delta – WPW
3. Look at the P wave: (n − 2.5 × 2.5) prominent in lead 2 and V1	a) Tall P - Right Atrial Enlargement b) Broad Bifid P - Left Atrial Enlargement c) Absent in lead 2 (not a sinus rhythm) d) Bizarre look? Inverted in lead 2 (junctional [nodal] rhythm)
4. Any Q wave? Lead 2, aV1, V5, V6?	4. Rule of 4; ALCAPA
5. Look at the aVR: If positive, monophasic	a. Dextrocardia b. Right axis deviation c. RV hypertrophy
6. Look at P–R: (Normal is 0.12 to 0.20 seconds i.e., 3–5 small squares)	a. Short PR – WPW b. Long PR– first-degree heart block
7. Look at PQRS	If PQRS sequence is not maintained, it is not sinus rhythm
8. Fast or slow	a. Very fast or very slow? b. Large R and S (Katz− Wachtel phenomenon) c. P-P and R-R not similar (complete heart block)
9. ST/T abnormalities	Any ST elevation or depression (myocarditis, pericarditis, scorpion sting) T inverted or tall – hypo-/hyperkalemia
10. QT prolongation	If T sitting over one big square, suggestive of long QT

Electroencephalogram (EEG)

Definition

Electroencephalogram (EEG) measures the electric potential difference between two points on the scalp, which helps to study the neuronal dysfunction and abnormal excitation of the cortex in children with seizures. It helps in recognition of the type of seizure along with localization of the epileptogenic focus.

Basics of EEG Reading

ELECTRODE PLACEMENT

- When reading EEG, it may be noted the alphabets and numbers on the right side of the paper represent the electrodes from which each wave is originating. Fig. 56.1 shows normal EEG waveforms.
- EEG electrode placement is done per the International 10–20 system, i.e., 10%–20% gap between the electrodes.
- EEG electrodes are labeled per the underlying area of the brain, as shown in Fig. 56.2.
- Central electrodes are labeled with z, e.g., Fz, Cz, and Pz.
- Right-sided leads are depicted with even numbers (2, 4, 6, 8), e.g., P4.
- Left-sided leads are depicted with odd numbers (1, 3, 5, 7), e.g., F3.

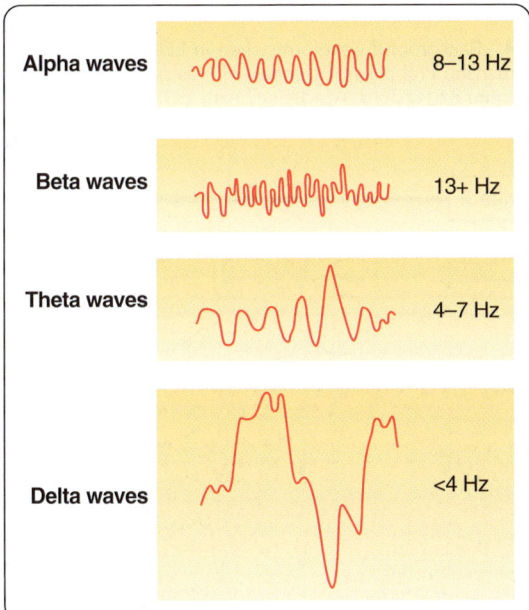

Alpha waves		8–13 Hz
Beta waves		13+ Hz
Theta waves		4–7 Hz
Delta waves		<4 Hz

Fig. 56.1 Normal EEG Waveforms. (*Source:* Reproduced from Kevin Patton, Gary Thibodeau, Andrew Hutton. *Anatomy & Physiology,* Adapted International Edition. Central nervous system, Unf in box 20.6, London, Elsevier Ltd, 2019)

EEG WAVEFORMS

These can be classified as shown in Fig. 56.3.

Background Activity

- This gives information about the neurologic state of the child.
- Normal wave forms: During normal awake state, alpha waves can be seen, and during normal sleep state sleep spindles, K complexes and vertex waves can be seen.
- Other background abnormalities include beta waves, theta waves, and delta waves. When describing abnormal background activity, the frequency and voltage should be mentioned along with whether it is intermittent or continuous, right, or left and which region of the brain it is arising from.
- Fig. 56.4 shows the background abnormalities seen in EEG
- Fig. 56.5 represent a normal EEG at awake and sleep state. The straight lines running across vertically represent the duration, and between two lines the duration is considered to be 1 second.

Epileptiform Discharges

The following should be observed when describing EEG waveforms:

- Shape of waveform – spike/sharp/spike wave/polyspike
- Frequency in Hz
- Amplitude or voltage
- Localization – right/left, region of brain
- Incidence and duration – rare/intermittent/occasional/frequent/continuous
- Pattern – run/rhythmic/periodic

Fig. 56.6 shows various morphology of epileptiform discharges that can be observed in an EEG.

Fig. 56.7 shows EEG during seizure activity.

Common EEG Patterns in Practical Examination

Having understood the basics of EEG, let us see some of the EEG patterns commonly encountered in the examinations. It is to be noted that this chapter only gives a clue to recognizing the common EEG patterns; pathophysiology and treatment aspects are not covered here.

BENIGN CHILDHOOD EPILEPSY WITH CENTROTEMPORAL SPIKES (BECTS)

- This is also known as Rolandic epilepsy.
- This is activated by drowsiness and sleep. Seizure wakes the child from sleep; consciousness is preserved.

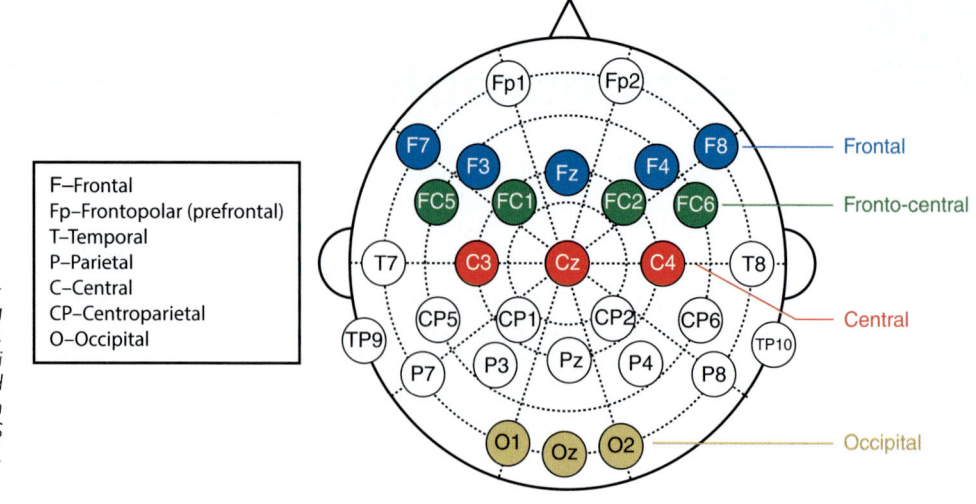

Fig. 56.2 The EEG electrode placement over skull. (*Source: Yang, Weiping & Yang, Jingjing & Gao, Yulin & Tang, Xiaoyu & Yanna, Ren & Takahashi, Satoshi & Wu, Jinglong. (2015). Effects of Sound Frequency on Audiovisual Integration: An Event-Related Potential Study. PLOS ONE. 10. e0138296. 10.1371/journal. pone.0138296.*)

F—Frontal
Fp—Frontopolar (prefrontal)
T—Temporal
P—Parietal
C—Central
CP—Centroparietal
O—Occipital

EEG waveforms

Background abnormalities

Alpha waves(8–13Hz)– Normal awake record

Beta waves (>12Hz) seen with drowsiness, barbiturates, BZD

Theta waves (4–7Hz)– Mild slowing, during wakefulness in children

Delta waves (1–3Hz)– Marked slowing

Abnormal epileptiform discharges

Spikes

Sharps

Spike waves

Polyspikes

Fig. 56.3 Different EEG waveforms.

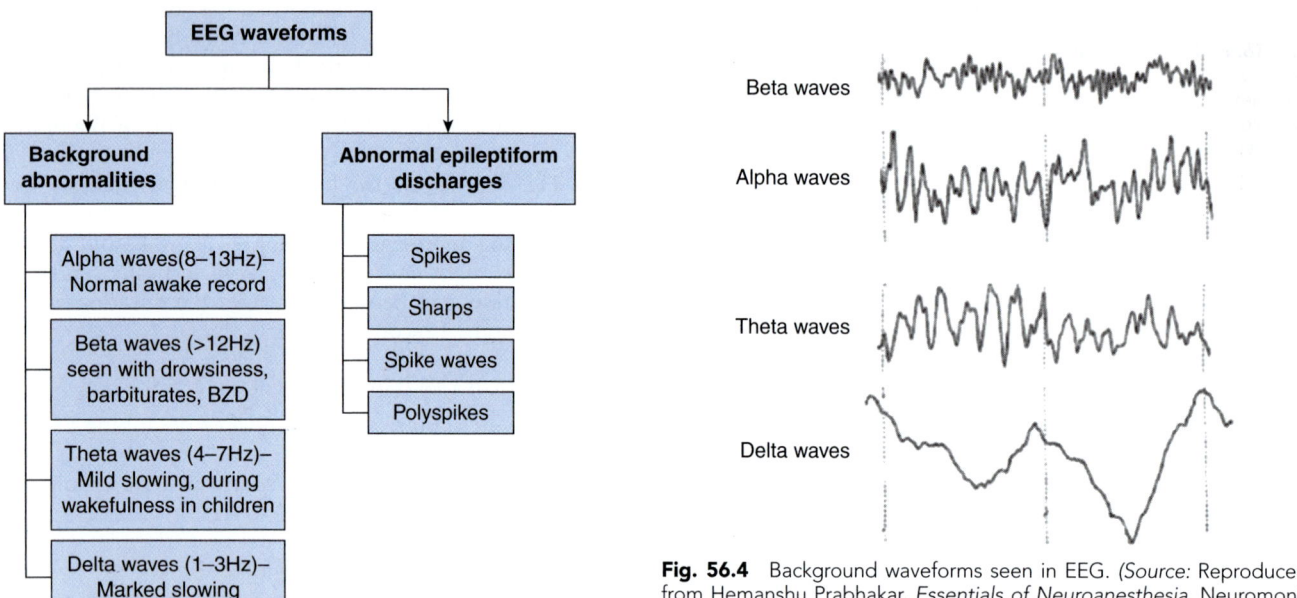

Beta waves

Alpha waves

Theta waves

Delta waves

Fig. 56.4 Background waveforms seen in EEG. (*Source: Reproduced from Hemanshu Prabhakar. Essentials of Neuroanesthesia. Neuromonitoring, Figure 8.8, Oxford, Academic Press, 2017.*)

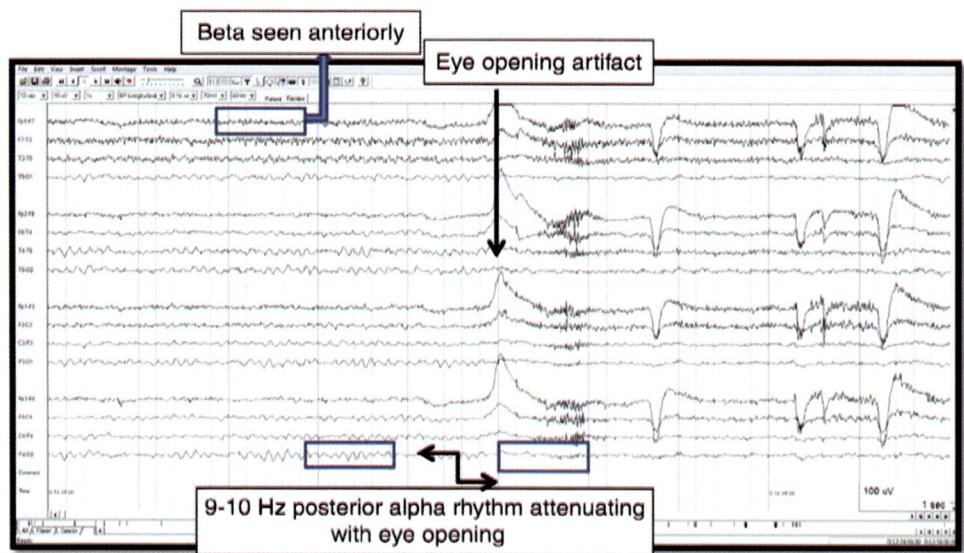

Beta seen anteriorly

Eye opening artifact

9-10 Hz posterior alpha rhythm attenuating with eye opening

Fig. 56.5 Normal EEG at awake and sleep states. (*Source: Sazgar M., Young M.G. (2019) Normal EEG Awake and Sleep. In: Absolute Epilepsy and EEG Rotation Review. Springer, Cham. https://doi.org/10.1007/978-3-030-03511-2_6*)

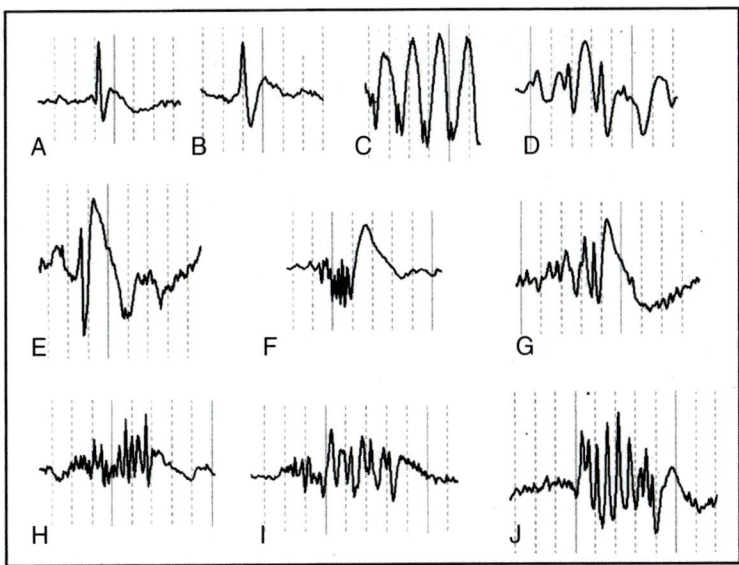

Fig. 56.6 Various morphology of epileptiform discharges. Epileptiform discharges. A, spike; B, sharp wave; C, spike-and-wave complexes; D, sharp-and-slow-wave complexes; E, slow-spike-and-wave complex; F, polyspike-and-wave complex; G, multiple-sharp-and-wave complex; H, polyspike complex; I & J, multiple sharp wave complexes. Even though spikes and sharp waves usually have after-going slow waves, the term spike-and-wave complex is usually reserved for the situation in which the slow wave is very prominent, higher in voltage than the spike. The interval between vertical lines represents 200 msec. *(Source:* Reproduced from Theodore Stern, Maurizio Fava, Timothy Wilens et al. *Massachusetts General Hospital Comprehensive Clinical Psychiatry*, Second Edition. Laboratory Tests and Diagnostic Procedures, Figure 3-15, London, Elsevier Inc., 2016. *Credit line (From Abou-Khalil B, Misulis KE: Atlas of EEG & seizure semiology. Philadelphia, 2006, Butterworth-Heinemann.)*

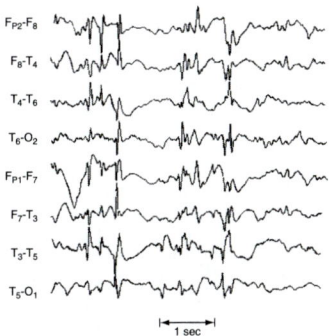

Fig. 56.7 EEG with seizure activity. *(Source:* Reproduced from Fred Ferri. *Ferri's Clinical Advisor 2022*, Seizures, Generalized Tonic Clonic, FIG. 2, Philadelphia, Elsevier Inc., 2022).

- **EEG finding**: Unilateral or bilateral spike discharges of high voltage in the central or centrotemporal region, as shown in Fig 56.8 (A) and (B).

CHILDHOOD ABSENCE SEIZURES

- Absence seizures usually last for a few seconds in the form of usually staring episodes. They do not have an aura, no postictal state; and post seizure the child continues to do the activity as prior to seizure without realizing the interruption.
- Precipitated by hyperventilation for 3–5 minutes.
- **EEG finding**: 3-Hz spike and wave pattern is typical; 3 Hz means within 1 second 3 wave forms can be seen, as encircled in the Fig. 56.9.

GENERALIZED TONIC-CLONIC SEIZURE (GTCS)

- **EEG finding**: Generalized repetitive spikes in the tonic phase and periodic bursts of spikes in the clonic phase are seen, as shown in Fig. 56.10A and B.

INFANTILE SPASM

- This is a type of seizure that occurs as sudden stiffening of body with briefly bending forward or backward of the arms, legs, and head, lasting for a second or two and usually occurs in clusters. It is commonly seen during wakefulness or active sleep.
- Triad of infantile spasms occurring in clusters with developmental delay and hypsarrhythmia is seen in West syndrome.
- **EEG finding**: Hypsarrhythmia is the characteristic finding. These are high-voltage, chaotic, disorganized, and asynchronous slow background discharges superimposed with multifocal or sharp waves, as shown in Fig. 56.11. Spikes may vary in location, are generalized but never repetitive.
- In infantile spasms, in addition to hypsarrhythmia, slow spike and wave pattern, burst suppression may also be seen, especially during quiet sleep.

JUVENILE MYOCLONIC EPILEPSY (JME)

- This is also called Janz syndrome. This is characterized by myoclonic jerks in the morning hours; the child ends up dropping things and may have GTCS while waking up.
- Precipitated by photic stimulation, sleep deprivation, alcohol (older children), and certain cognitive activities.

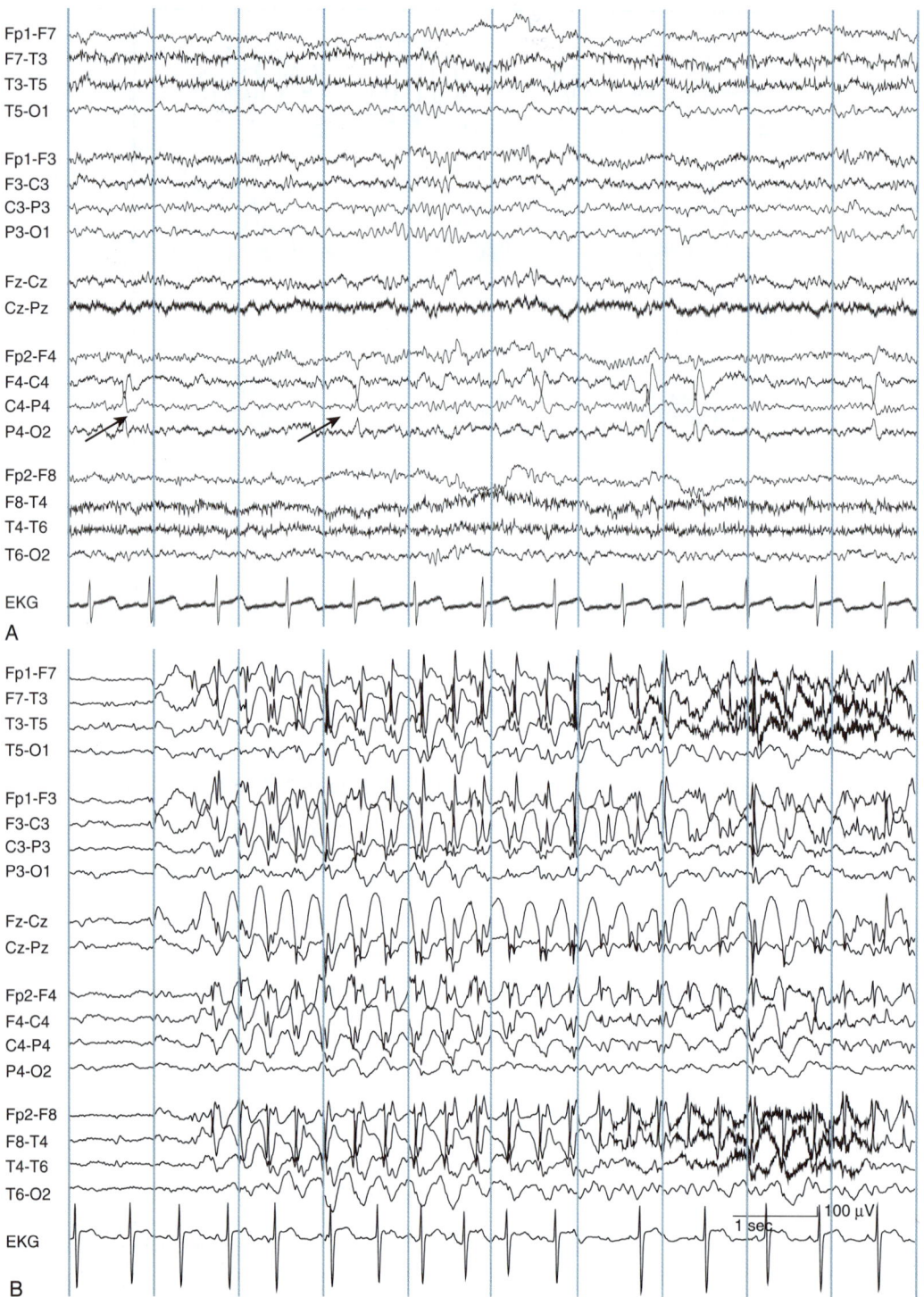

Fig. 56.8 Fig 56.8 (A) Shows right central spike-wave complexes (arrows) in a patient with rolandic epilepsy. The Fig 56.8 (B) is recorded later in the same patient at sleep onset showing a run of generalized spike-wave discharges. *(Source:* Reproduced from Mark Libenson. *Practical Approach to Electroencephalography,* First Edition, The EEG in Epilepsy, Figure 10-32, Philadelphia, Saunders, 2010.)

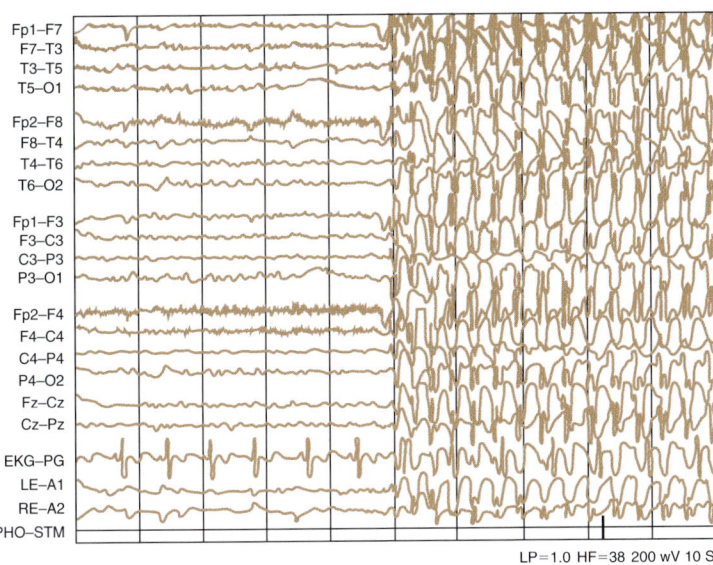

Fig. 56.9 EEG showing 3 Hz Generalized spike-and-wave discharges characteristic of absence seizures. (*Source*: Reproduced from Basil Zitelli, Sara McIntire, Andrew Nowalk et al. *Zitelli and Davis' Atlas of Pediatric Physical Diagnosis*, Eighth Edition, Neurology, Fig. 16.65, Philadelphia, Elsevier Inc., 2023.)

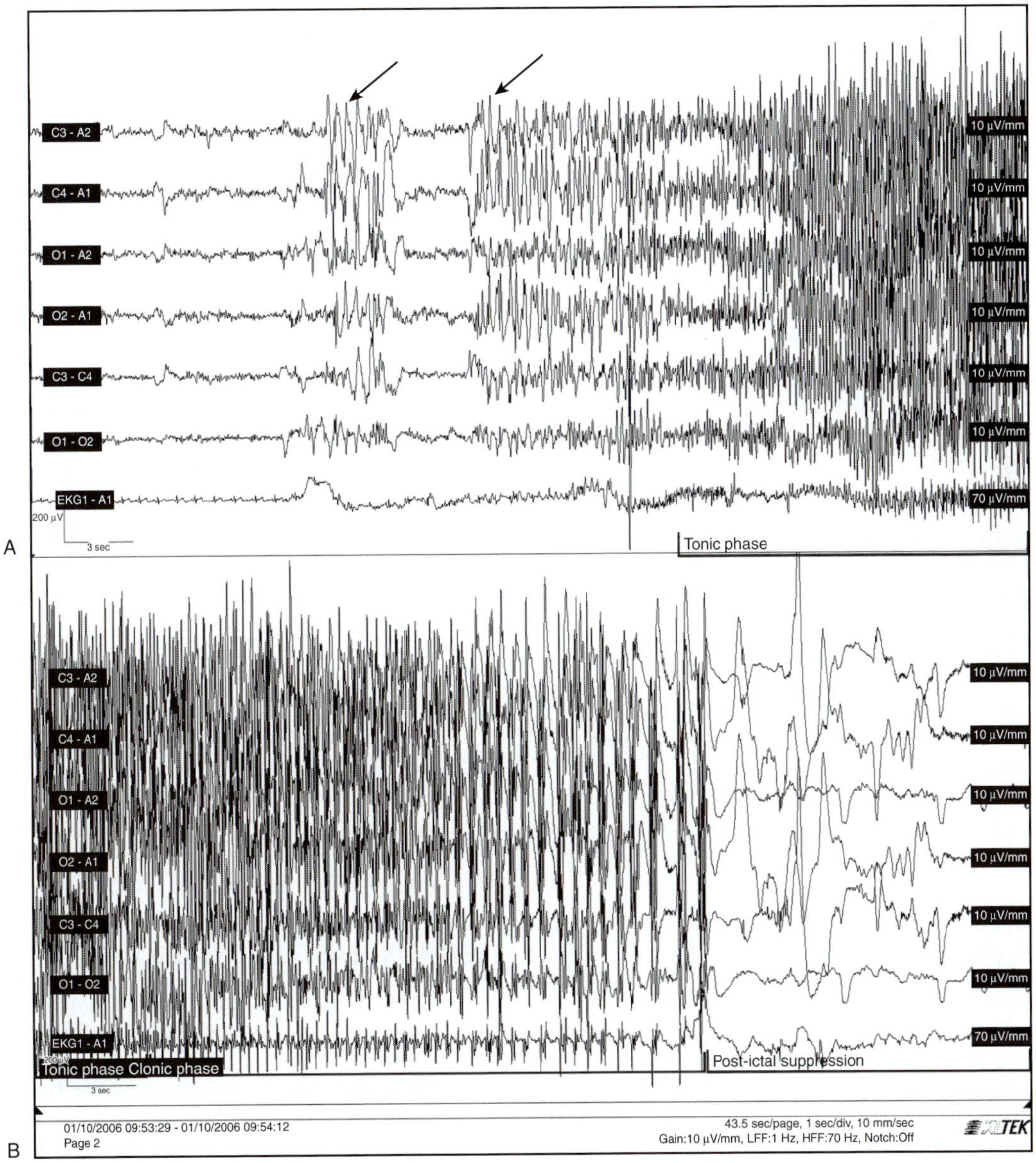

Fig. 56.10 (A) EEG showing epileptiform discharges during the tonic phase of GTCS. (B) EEG showing epileptiform discharges during the clonic phase of GTCS, where ictal discharges are changed to periodic spike-wave discharges followed by postictal suppression of activity. (*Source*: Reproduced from Alon Avidan. *Review of Sleep Medicine*, Fourth Edition, Overview of Electroencephalography and Epilepsy, Figure 18.19, Philadelphia, Elsevier Inc., 2018.)

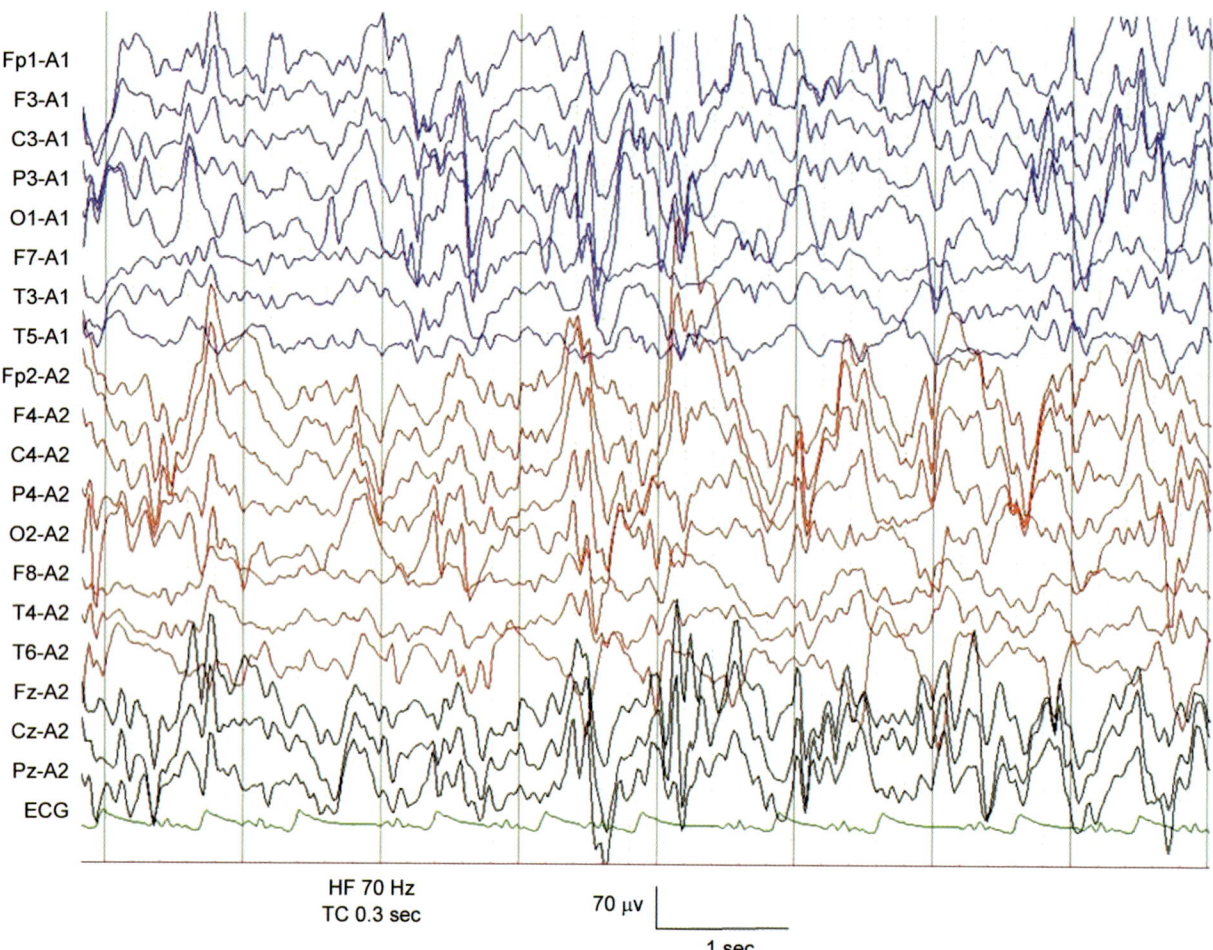

Fig. 56.11   EEG showing hypsarrhythmia. The background is disorganised, chaotic with high voltage spike and slow wave discharges. *(Source: Reproduced from U. V. Misra, J Kalita. Clinical Electroencephalography, Second Edition, Epileptiform and nonepileptiform paroxysmal EEG abnormalities, FIG. 5.18, New Delhi, Elsevier India, 2018.)*

- **EEG finding**: Generalized interictal epileptiform discharges – bilateral, symmetrical spike and polyspike, and wave discharges of 3.5–6 Hz, as shown in Fig. 56.12.

BURST SUPPRESSION PATTERN

- This pattern may be seen in subacute sclerosing panencephalitis (SSPE), phenobarbital coma, general anesthesia, hypothermia.
- **EEG finding:** Comprises alternating long intervals of amplitude suppression interrupted by bursts of mixed frequencies, as shown in Fig. 56.13.

PERIODIC LATERALIZED EPILEPTIFORM DISCHARGES (PLEDS)

- Usually this occurs due to acute neuronal injury.
- This can be seen in brain infections such as herpes encephalitis, strokes, tumors, hematomas, metabolic conditions such as hepatic encephalopathy, and hypoxia.
- **EEG finding**: These are repetitive (relatively uniform waves), periodic (occurring at regular intervals), focal,

or localized to a hemisphere.; epileptiform discharges that may be spikes, spikes and waves, polyspikes, or sharps commonly recurring every 1–2 seconds, as shown in Fig. 56.14.

EXTREME DELTA BRUSH PATTERN

- This pattern is characteristic of anti N-methyl-D-aspartate (NMDA) receptor encephalitis.
- **EEG findings**: Extreme delta brush pattern consists of generalized rhythmic delta waves with superimposed bursts of rhythmic beta waves giving the brush appearance on EEG, as shown in Fig. 56.15.

LENNOX–GASTAUT SYNDROME

- Lennox–Gastaut syndrome is a triad of atypical absence, atonic, and myoclonic seizure with intellectual disability.
- **EEG findings:** Characteristic EEG findings are 1–2 Hz spike and slow waves, polyspike bursts in sleep, and a slow background while awake, as shown in Fig. 56.16.

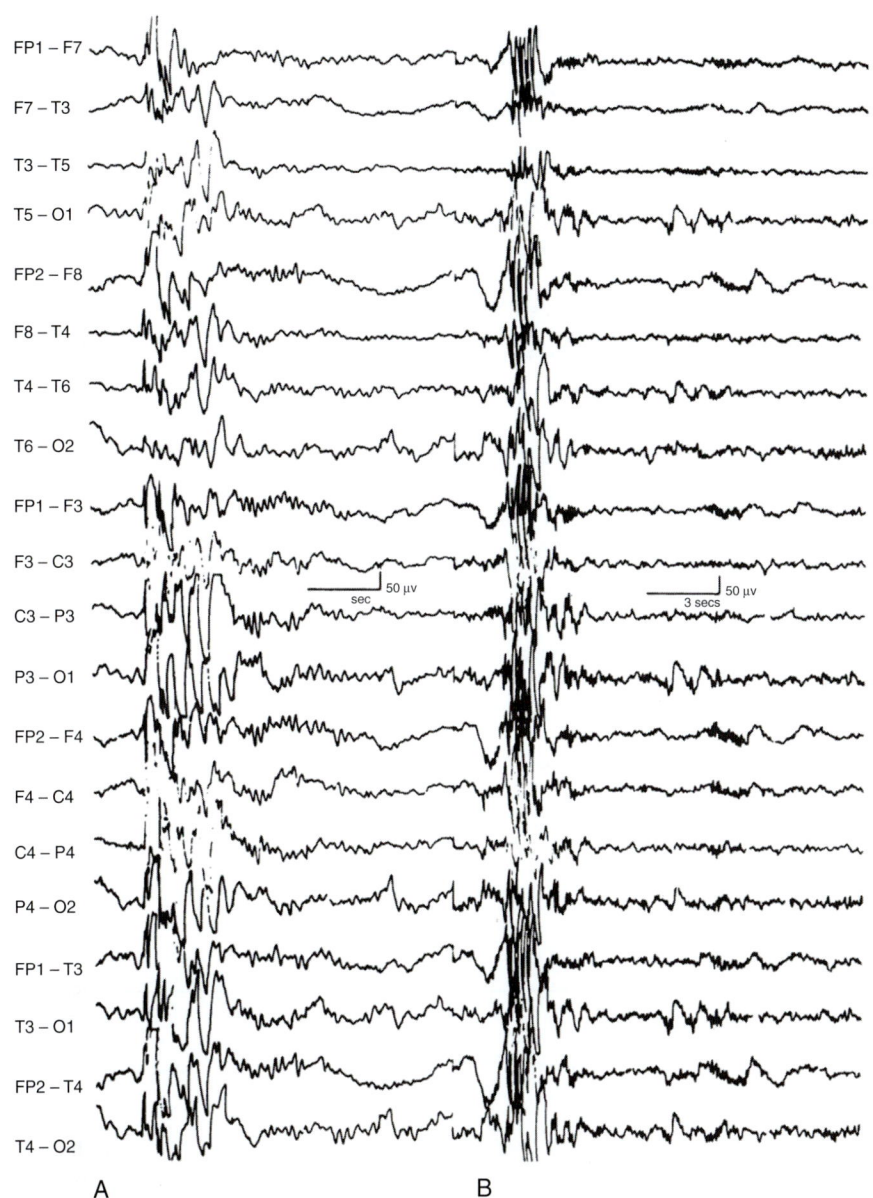

Fig. 56.12 EEG showing generalized interictal epileptiform discharges on photic stimulation as seen in juvenile myoclonic epilepsy. Generalized spike-wave discharge, erupts suddenly from a normal background. The typical spike or poly-spike discharges in JME are 3.5 to 4 Hz in frequency. *(Source: Reproduced from Sudhansu Chokroverty, Robert Thomas. Atlas of Sleep Medicine, Second Edition, Electroencephalography for the Sleep Specialist, Figure 2.30, St. Louis, Saunders, 2014. (Credit Line - (From Chokroverty S, Montagna P. Sleep and epilepsy. In Chokroverty S, ed. Sleep Disorders Medicine: Basic Science, Technical Considerations, and Clinical Aspects. 3rd ed. Philadelphia: Saunders/Elsevier, 2009:49-529.)*

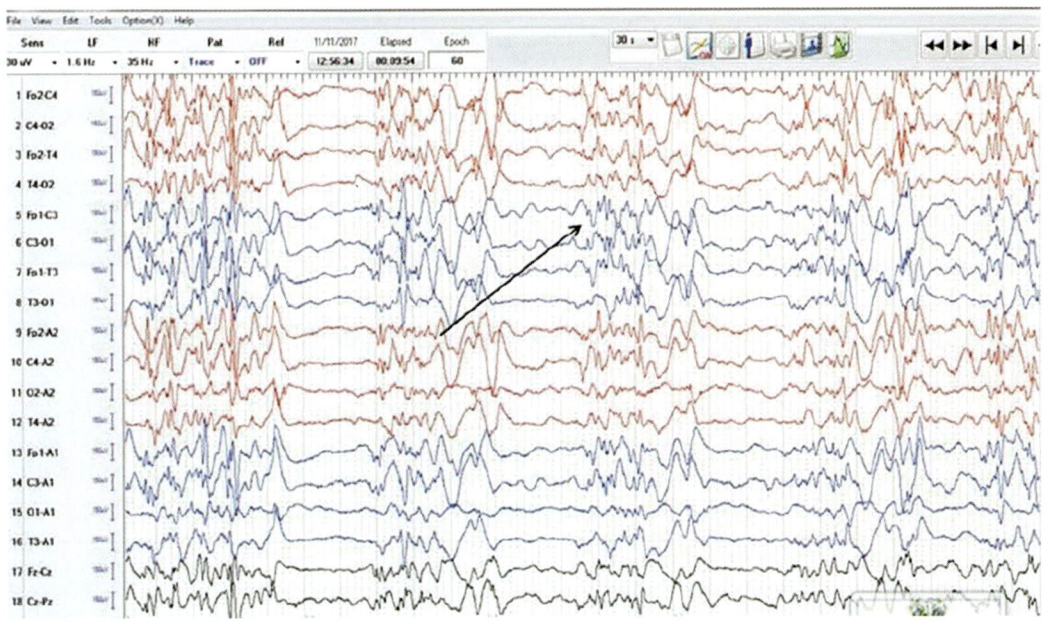

Fig. 56.13 EEG showing burst suppression pattern. *(Source: Clinical Pediatric Neurology by Gerald M. Fenichel.)*

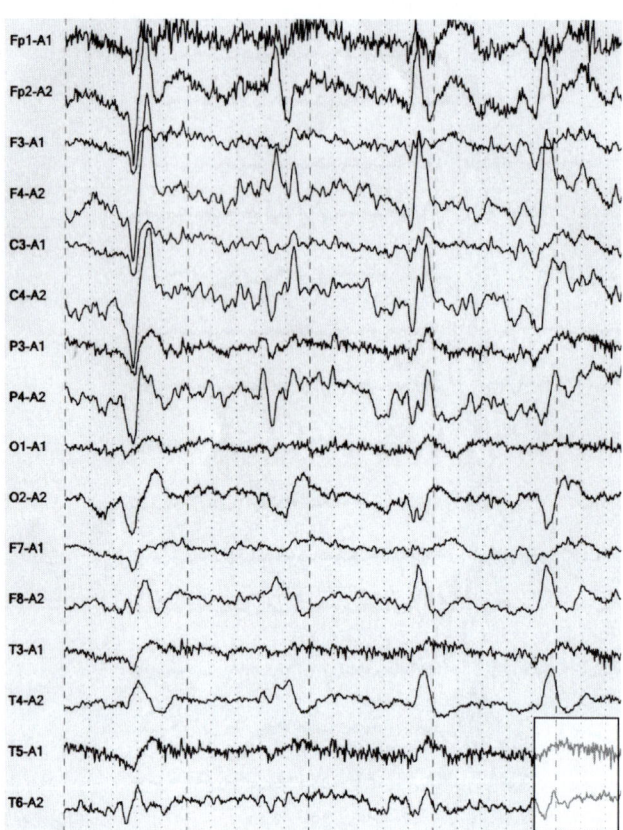

Fig. 56.14 EEG unilateral and sharp-wave complexes that appear periodically in the left hemisphere suggestive of PLEDS. *(Source:* Reproduced from Koushun Matsuo, Makoto Saburi, Hiroki Ishikawa et al. *Journal of the Neurological Sciences.* Sjögren syndrome presenting with encephalopathy mimicking Creutzfeldt–Jakob disease 326(1-2);100-103;2013.)

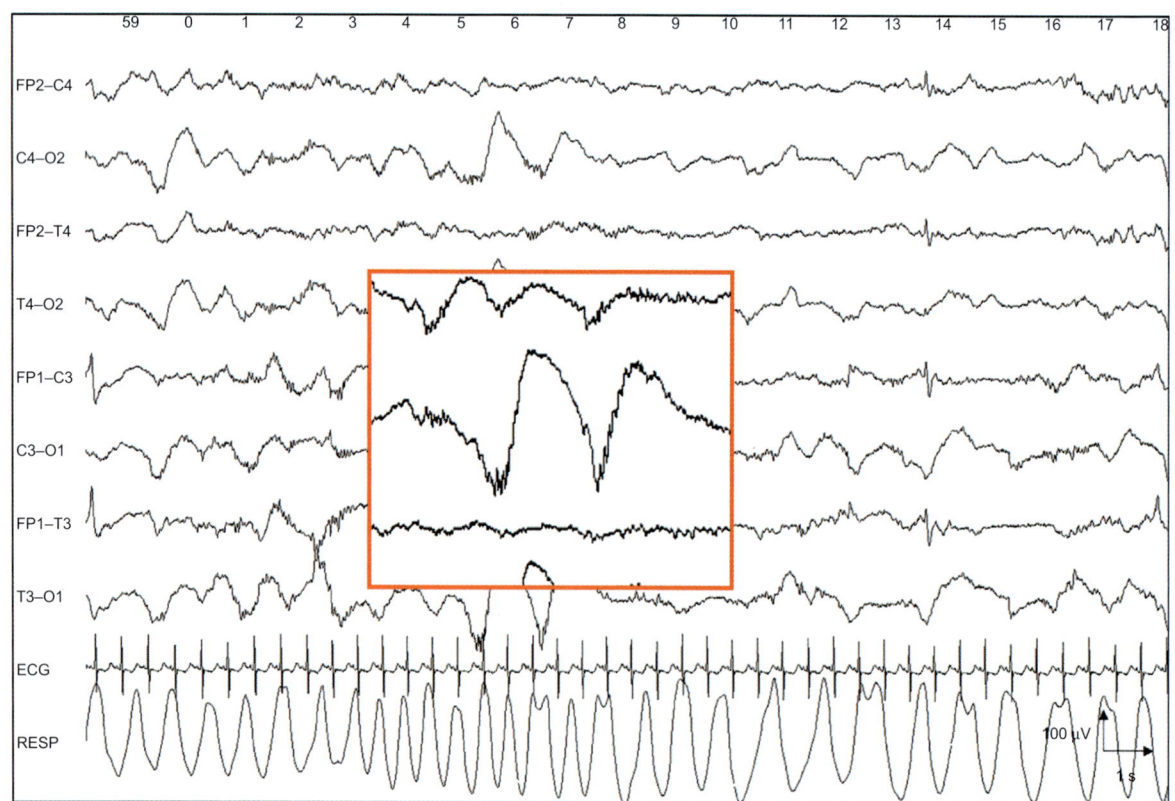

Fig. 56.15 EEG showing extreme delta brush pattern in left occipital area. *(Source:* Reproduced from Kerry Levin, Patrick Chauvel. *Clinical Neurophysiology: Basis and Technical Aspects,* Child EEG (and maturation), Fig. 8.2, Chennai, Elsevier BV, 2019.)

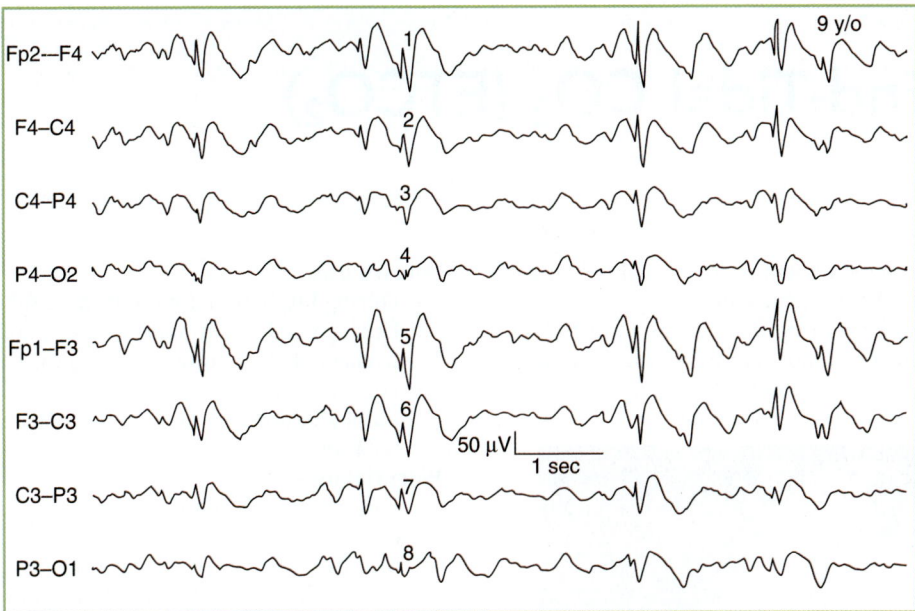

Fig. 56.16   EEG showing multiple spike and slow waves in Lennox–Gastaut syndrome. (*Source:* Reproduced from Nancy Newman, Joseph Jankovic, John Mazziotta et al. *Bradley and Daroff's Neurology in Clinical Practice*, Eighth Edition, Electroencephalography and Evoked Potentials, Fig. 35.8, Philadelphia, Elsevier Inc., 2022.)

End-Tidal CO_2 (ETCO$_2$)

Capnography

Capnography is the measurement of the partial pressure of carbon dioxide (CO_2) in exhaled air.

Capnogram is a waveform of expired CO_2 as a function of time, and capnometer as shown in fig 57.1 is a monitoring device that measures and numerically displays the concentration of carbon dioxide in exhaled air.

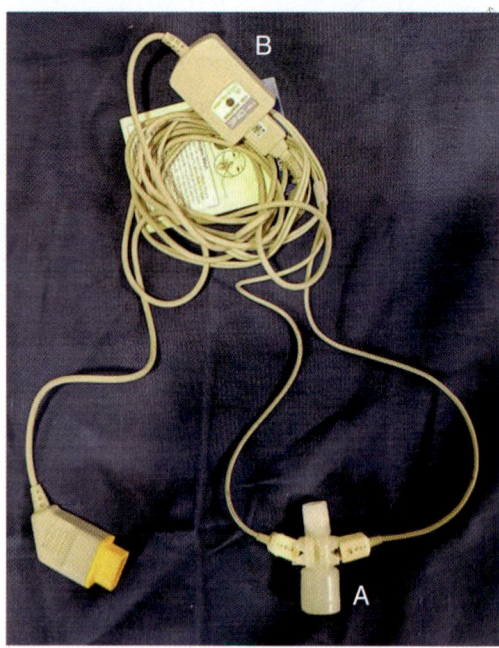

Fig. 57.1 Capnometer (A- Patient interface and B-Infra red sensor). (Source: Camp-M Mainstream Capnography ETCO$_2$ Sensor (Module) with Lemon Connector, Compatible with Masimo, Respironics and Mindary: Amazon.com: Industrial & Scientific)

Normal Capnograms
Four phases:
   Phase 1: Inspiratory baseline
   Phase 2: Expiratory upstroke (steep slope)
   Phase 3: Expiratory plateau (nearly horizontal, flat only if all alveoli have same PCO_2)
   Phase 4: Expiratory downstroke
Two angles:
Alpha angle: Between phase 2 and phase 3
Beta angle: Between phase 3 and phase 4
ETCO2: End of inspiration (point marked by arrow); normal value: 35–40 mm Hg

Standard uses:
1. During intubation, for confirming tube placement.
2. During Cardiopulmonary resuscitation (CPR), to asses effectiveness of chest compression in cardiac arrest.
3. For monitoring of ventilated patients in ICU, during procedural sedation and in operation theatre during procedural sedation.

Potential uses:
1. For dynamic monitoring in patients with acute respiratory distress.
2. May help identify septic patients: In sepsis, lactic acidosis leads to hyperventilation, thereby lowering of ETCO$_2$ values.
3. Other potential uses: In diabetic ketoacidosis (DKA), trauma, pulmonary embolism, as a triage vital sign in Emergency department.

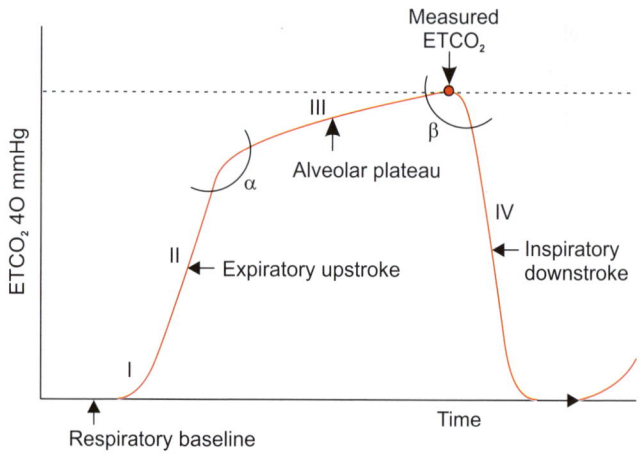

Fig. 57.2 Normal capnogram.

Abnormal Capnograms

- **Bronchospasm**
  - Can be seen in asthma
  - Obstruction in the expiratory limb of the ventilator
  - Foreign body in upper airway
  - Kinking/occlusion of the ET tube

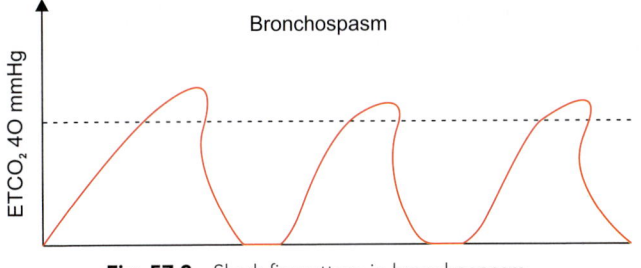

Fig. 57.3   Shark fin pattern in bronchospasm.

- **Increasing ETCO$_2$** (hypoventilation)
  - Decrease in respiratory rate/tidal volume
  - Increase in metabolic rate
  - Hyperthermia

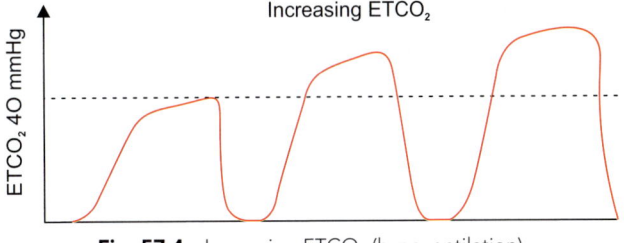

Fig. 57.4   Increasing ETCO$_2$ (hypoventilation).

- **Decreasing ETCO$_2$** (hyperventilation)
  - Increase in respiratory rate/tidal volume
  - Metabolic acidosis
  - Hypothermia

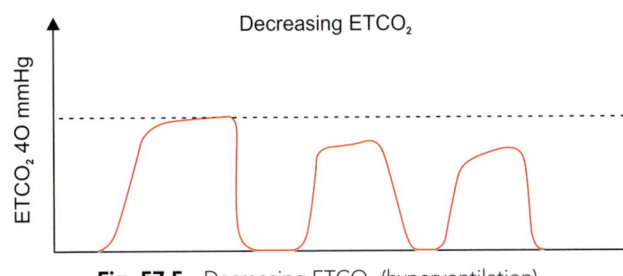

Fig. 57.5   Decreasing ETCO$_2$ (hyperventilation).

- **Rebreathing CO$_2$**
  - Faulty expiratory valve
  - Inadequate inspiratory flow
  - Partial rebreathing
  - Insufficient expiratory time

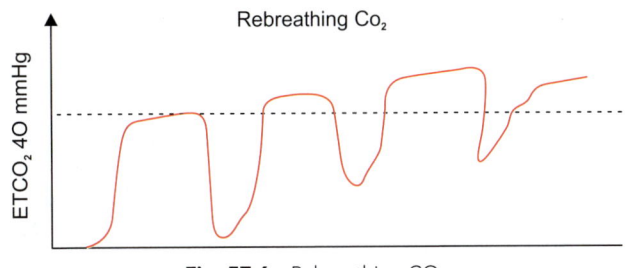

Fig. 57.6   Rebreathing CO$_2$.

- **Curare cleft**
  - Depth of cleft is proportional to degree of muscle relaxation
  - Cleft indicates return of spontaneous respiration from muscle relaxants

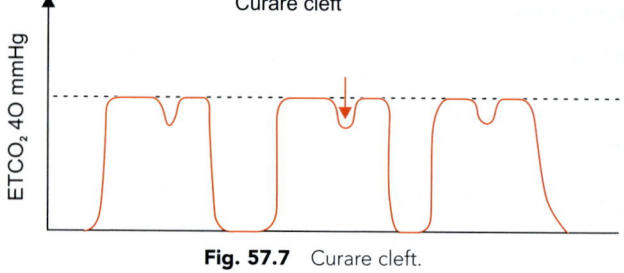

Fig. 57.7   Curare cleft.

- **Cardiac arrest during CPR**
  - $ETCO_2 > 20$ mm Hg is considered optimal for effective chest compressions
  - $ETCO_2 < 10$–15mmHg – suboptimal

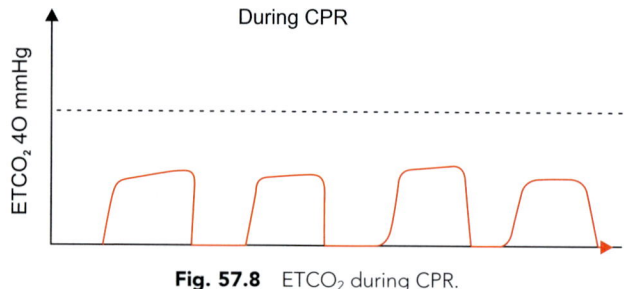

Fig. 57.8 $ETCO_2$ during CPR.

- **Return of spontaneous circulation (ROSC)**
  - An abrupt increase in $ETCO_2$ is an early indicator of ROSC

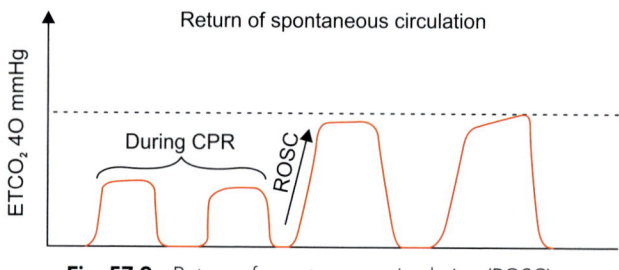

Fig. 57.9   Return of spontaneous circulation (ROSC).

- **Sudden loss of waveform**
  - Seen in tube displacement

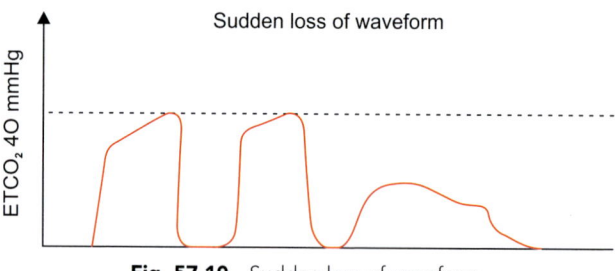

Fig. 57.10   Sudden loss of waveform.

58 Ventilator Graphics

Definition of Terms

Terminologies

Terminologies	Definition
PIP (Peak inspiratory pressure)	Highest pressure reached during inspiration
PEEP (Positive end -expiratory pressure)	Pressure at the end of expiration (to prevent alveolar collapse)
Auto-PEEP	Measured during expiratory hold applied in volume-controlled ventilator (the baseline of PT curve rises to show auto-PEEP)
Pplat	Measured during an inspiratory hold/pause in volume-controlled ventilator (i.e., pressure applied to smaller airway and alveoli)
FiO_2	Fraction of oxygen in inspired air
Delta P	Change in pressure from highest to the lowest (PIP − PEEP)
Ti	Time allowed for inflow of gas
Te	Time allowed for outflow of gas
Variables	Pressure, volume, and flow are variables of time (depending on the mode, one of the variables is independent and the other two are dependent)
Flow variables	• Flow is filling-in of the airway • Flow is a variable which depends on compliance, resistance, and patient effort • Flow depends on type of breath and **flow pattern** as shown in Fig. 58.1 (constant flow [square], ascending ramp, descending ramp, sinusoidal, exponential rise and exponential decay) • Ascending and descending ramp are same as exponential rise and decay • Sinusoidal waves represent spontaneous breathing • Flow rate in ventilator – usually kept as 2–5 times of minute volume

Phase variables (variables that determine the various phases of respiration – inspiration, inspiration to expiration, and expiration)	There are three phase variables
	1. Trigger: Variable that helps in initiating inspiration (three types of trigger)
	  a. Time trigger – preset time
	  b. Pressure trigger – preset pressure
	  c. Flow trigger – constant flow rate
	2. Sensitivity: Amount of negative pressure below the end expiratory pressure required to trigger ventilator
	3. Cycle variable: A variable that is measured to terminate inspiration and begin expiration (i.e., the cycle is terminated or cycle off when it has reached preset value – pressure, volume flow, or preset time)

Time constant	Airway resistance × compliance (how quickly lung can inhale or exhale out or how long it takes for the pressure to reach the alveoli from proximal airways – maximum possible alveolar volume)
Compliance	Change in volume per unit change in pressure (indicates stiffness of the lung/chest wall) represented by delta volume/delta pressure
Airway resistance	Impedance to airflow (lung/chest wall)

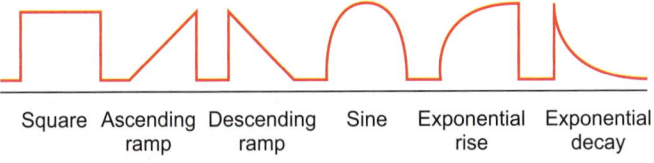

Square   Ascending ramp   Descending ramp   Sine   Exponential rise   Exponential decay

Fig. 58.1 Type of flow pattern.

Terminologies	Definition
Tidal volume	• Volume of air that goes in and out of the chest • VT = Compliance × delta P (PIP − PEEP)
Minute ventilation	Tidal volume × ventilator rate
Mean airway pressure (Paw)	Average pressure in the respiratory passage during ventilation $$\frac{(PIP \times Ti) + (PEEP \times Te)}{Ti + Te}$$
Oxygenation	Depends on Mean airway pressure (MAP) and FiO_2
Ventilation	CO_2 washout (RR × MV)

Ventilator Graphics

Ventilator Waveforms

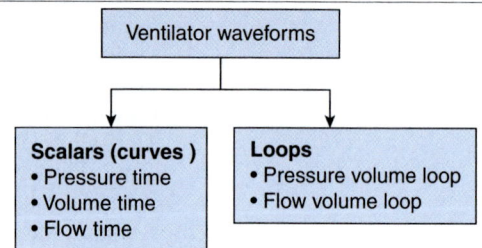

Scalars (curves)

• In choosing the modes of ventilator, one variable becomes dependent and the other variable becomes independent

• For example, Fig. 58.2 shows X-axis representing time (s) and Y-axis may be pressure (cm H_2O), volume (mL/min), and flow-control (L/min) variable, respectively

• **Pressure–time curve:**
  • In pressure-control mode, shape of the PT scalar will be square or rectangular, indicating that the pressure remains constant
  • The baseline of PT scalar increases when PEEP is added
  • In volume-control mode, PT scalar will be ascending ramp/exponential rise

• **Flow–time curve:**
  • In flow–time curve, inspiratory arm is active in nature, which depends on ventilator flow settings and mode of ventilation
  • Expiratory arm is passive, depending on elastic recoil and lung resistance
  • In pressure-control mode, inspiratory arm shows descending ramp pattern and in volume-control mode inspiratory arm shows square wave pattern

• **Volume–time scalar**
  • Volume is not measured directly
  • Derived from the flow measurement – area under the flow–time curve
  • The waveform will have a mountain peak appearance at the top

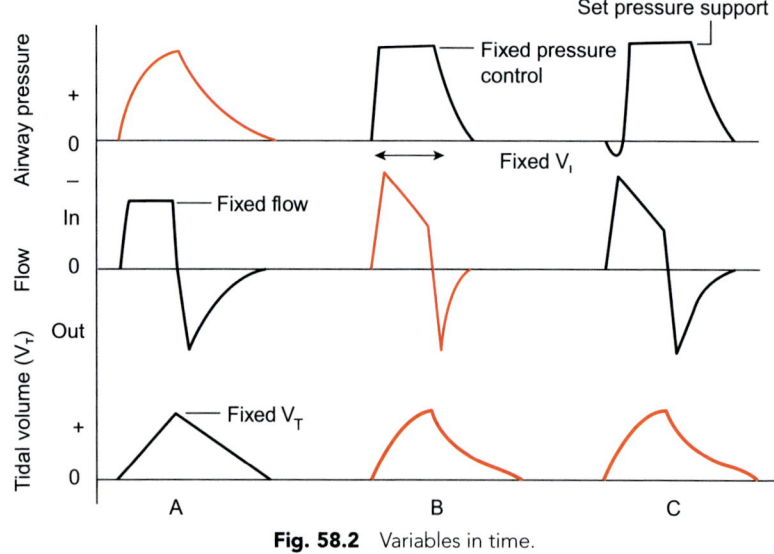

Fig. 58.2   Variables in time.

Ventilator Waveforms

Loops

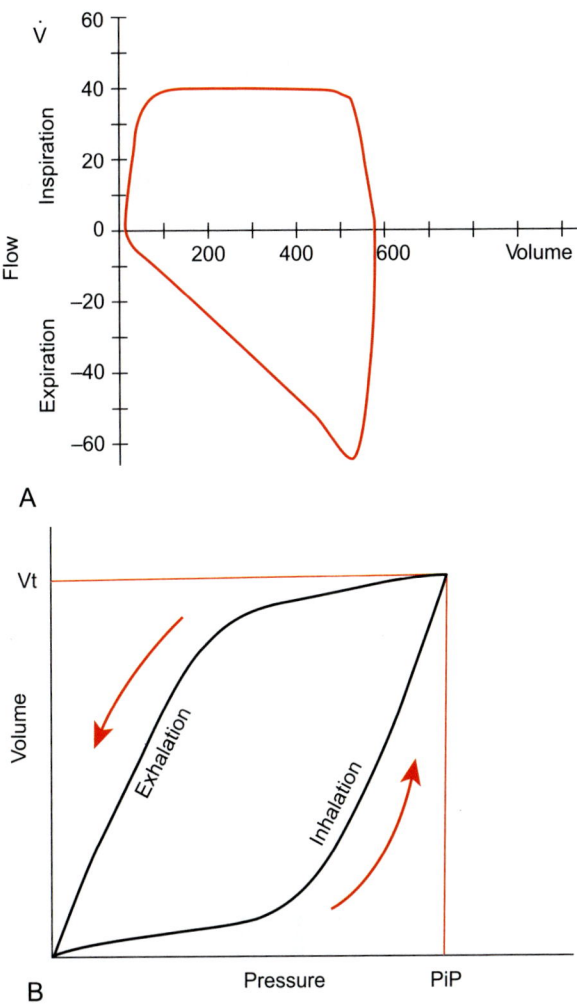

- Fig. 58.3A and B shows two variables (flow and pressure) plotted against volume
- **Flow—volume loop** (important for bronchodilator therapy)
- X-axis represents volume (mL/min) and Y-axis represents flow (L/min)
- Fig. 58.3B represents **pressure—volume loop**
- X-axis represents pressure (cm H_2O) and Y-axis represents volume (mL/min)

Fig. 58.3 (A) Flow—volume loop. (B) Pressure—volume loop.

Modes of Ventilation

Modes	Parameters
Pressure control	• Pressure guarantee • Set – PIP, PEEP, Ti, rate, FiO_2 • *Monitor tidal volume*
Volume control	• Volume guarantee • Set – VT, PEEP, I:E ratio, rate, FiO_2 • *Monitor PIP*
Pressure support	• Set – inspiratory assist pressure (preset airway pressure), PEEP, FiO_2
Synchronized intermittent mandatory ventilation (SIMV)	• Set – SIMV rate, VT or PIP, PEEP, sensitivity, FiO_2 • *Monitor tidal volume, Ti, and rate*
Spontaneous (CPAP-Continuous positive airway pressure)	• Used only when there is adequate spontaneous respiratory effort • Baseline PEEP is maintained to prevent alveolar collapse

Types of Breath

Types of breath
Usually seen in pressure−time ventilation

a. Controlled breath: Here, the ventilator controls the initiation (triggering), limit and, the termination (cycling) of each breath
b. Assisted breath: Combination of both mandatory and spontaneous breath; breath may be initiated, limited, or cycled by either ventilator or patient
c. Spontaneous breath: Patient-controlled triggering/cycling but limit may be patient or ventilator controlled

Figs 58.4 and 58.5 show the **type of breath in pressure−time scalar and pressure−volume loop**

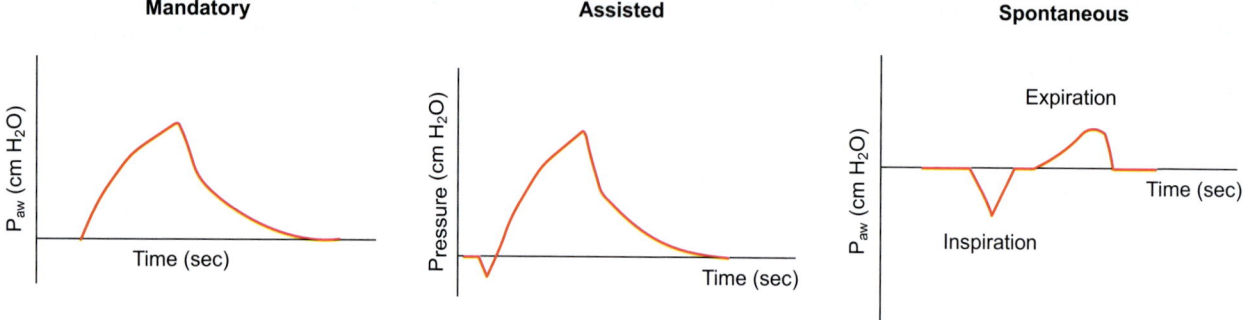

Fig. 58.4   Types of breath in pressure−time scalar.

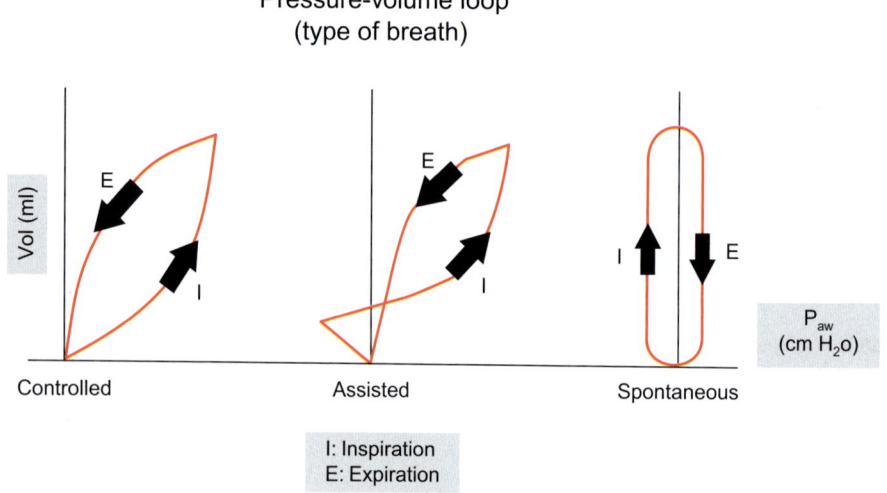

I: Inspiration
E: Expiration

Fig. 58.5   Types of breath in pressure−volume loop.

Normal Graphics

Normal pressure–time curve

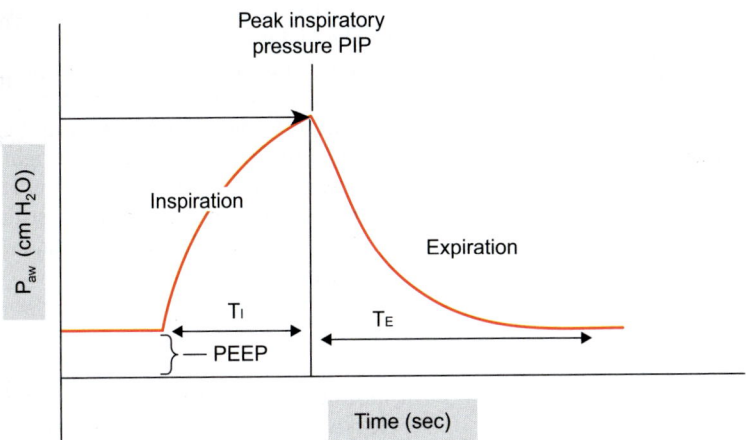

Fig. 58.6   Pressure–time curve.

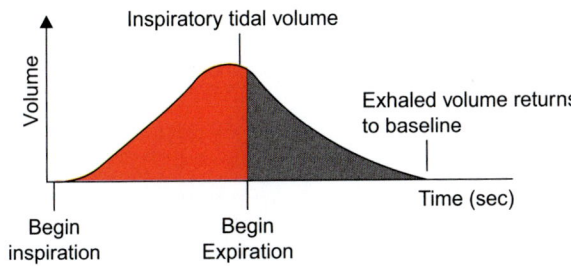

Fig. 58.7   Volume–time curve.

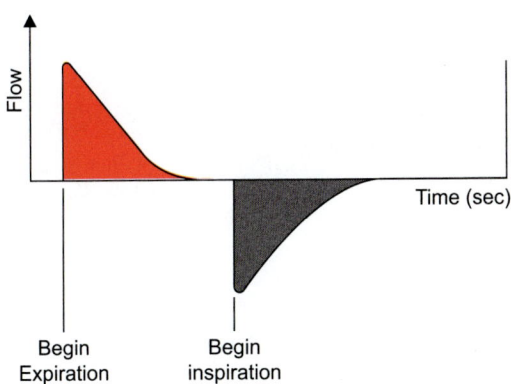

Fig. 58.8   Flow–time curve.

In a **pressure–time curve** (Fig. 58.6):
- X-axis = time (s)
- Y-axis = pressure (cm H_2O)
- Ti = inspiratory time
- Te = expiratory time

Volume–time curve (Fig. 58.7):
- Mountain peak at the top (if an inspiratory hold maneuver is applied, it can have a flattened area at the peak)

Flow–time curve (Fig. 58.8):
- X-axis = time (s)
- Y-axis = flow – descending ramp showing inspiration and expiration

Normal pressure–volume loop

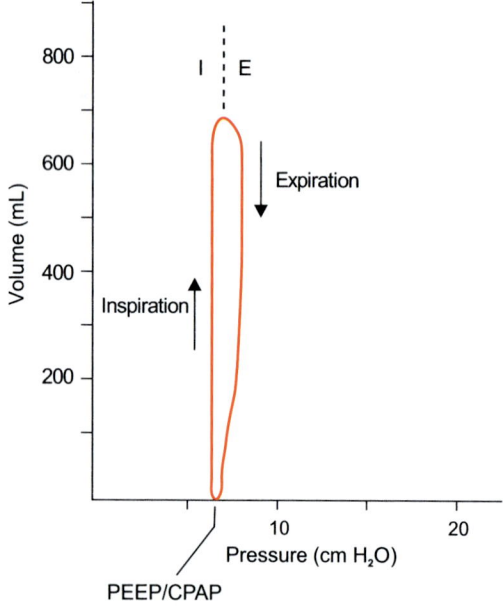

Fig. 58.9 (A) Pressure–volume loop.

In a **pressure–volume loop** (Fig. 58.9A):
- Pressure on X-axis is plotted against tidal volume on Y-axis
- The ascending curve is the inspiration and the descending curve is the expiration
- The highest point reached on the Y-axis is the tidal volume and highest point on the X-axis is the peak inspiratory pressure
- If an imaginary line is drawn in the middle of the loop, the area to the right represents inspiratory resistance and area to the left represents expiratory resistance (Palv, peak alveolar volume; Pta, transairway pressure)

In **spontaneous breathing**, inspiration goes clockwise and expiration goes counterclockwise as shown in Fig. 58.9B

Fig. 58.10 shows **flow–volume loop**

Volume on X-axis and flow (L/min) on Y-axis

Fig. 58.9, cont'd (B) Pressure–volume loop of spontaneous breath. See the curve is in clockwise direction.

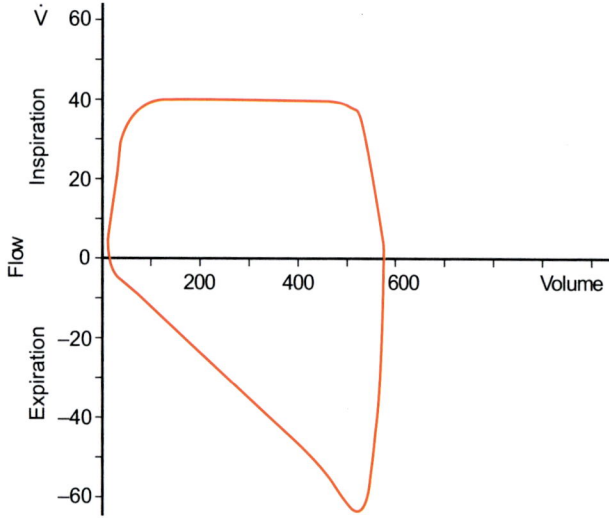

Fig. 58.10 Flow–volume loop.

Abnormal Graphics

The following types of abnormalities should be noted in curves/loops.

Curves/Loops	Type of Abnormalities to Be Noted
Pressure−time curve	Transairway pressure
	Pplat, PIP, transairway pressure
	Auto-PEEP
	Any trigger asynchrony
Volume−time curve	Air leak

Curves/Loops	Type of Abnormalities to Be Noted
Flow−time curve	Airway expiratory disease (bronchospasm)
	Auto-PEEP
Pressure–volume loop	Compliance
	Air leak
	Auto-PEEP
	Airway secretion
	Inflection points
Flow−volume loop	Air leak
	Airway secretion
	Auto-PEEP

Examples of Abnormal Graphics (Loops)

Condition	Pressure−Volume	Flow−Volume
Air leak Causes: ET leak Circuit leak Sensor not in place	In the pressure–volume loop, expiratory limb does not reach the baseline which indicates **air leak** (circuit, Endotracheal Tube (ETT)) (Fig. 58.11A)	In the flow–volume loop, expiratory limb does not reach the baseline, indicating **air leak** (Fig. 58.11B)

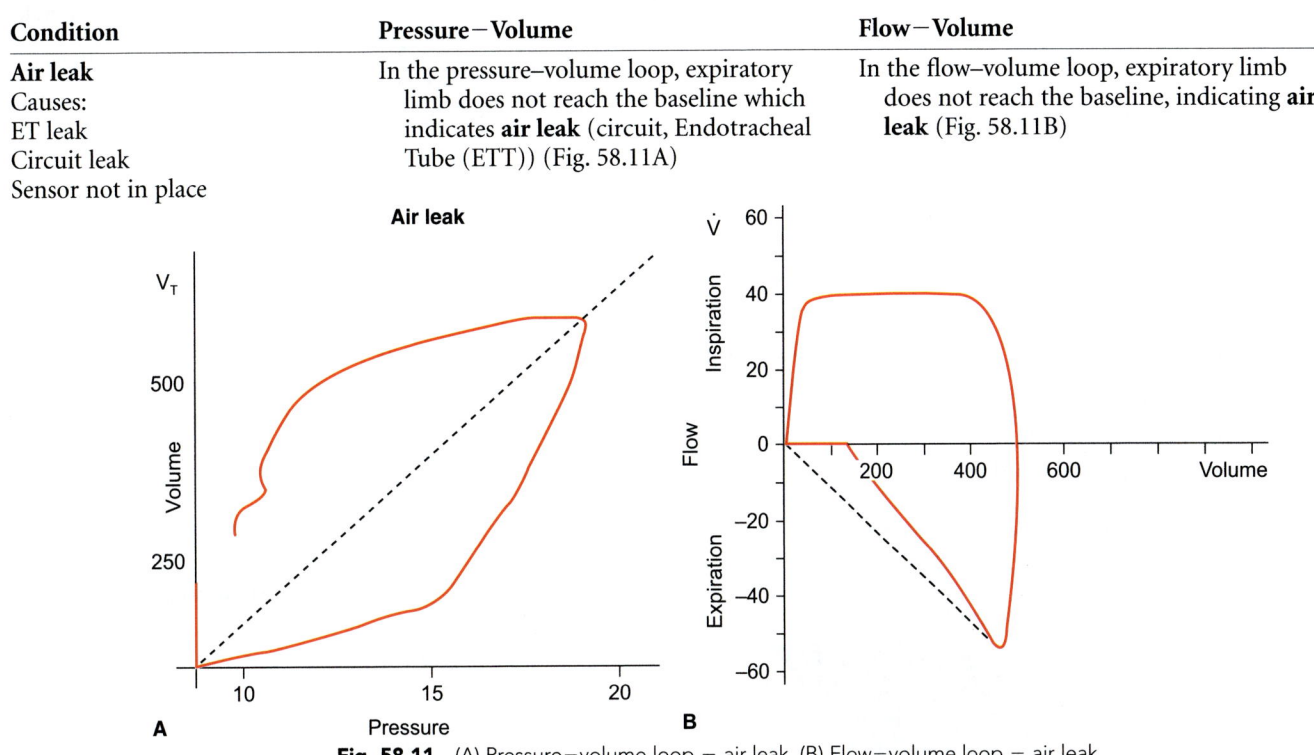

Fig. 58.11 (A) Pressure−volume loop − air leak. (B) Flow−volume loop − air leak.

Condition	Pressure–Volume	Flow–Volume

Auto-PEEP (Fig. 58.12)
Causes:
  a. Increased resistance (small ETT, secretion)
  b. Asthma
  c. ARDS (Acute Respiratory Distress Syndrome)
	Fig 58.12A Pressure volume loop showing inadequate PEEP.
	  1. Total PEEP = Intrinsic PEEP + Extrinsic PEEP
	  2. PEEP = Extrinsic PEEP and is preselected
	  3. Auto PEEP = Total PEEP - Extrinsic PEEP = Intrinsic PEEP
		Fig 58.12B Flow volume loop showing air trapping where expiratory limb terminates well before Y-axis

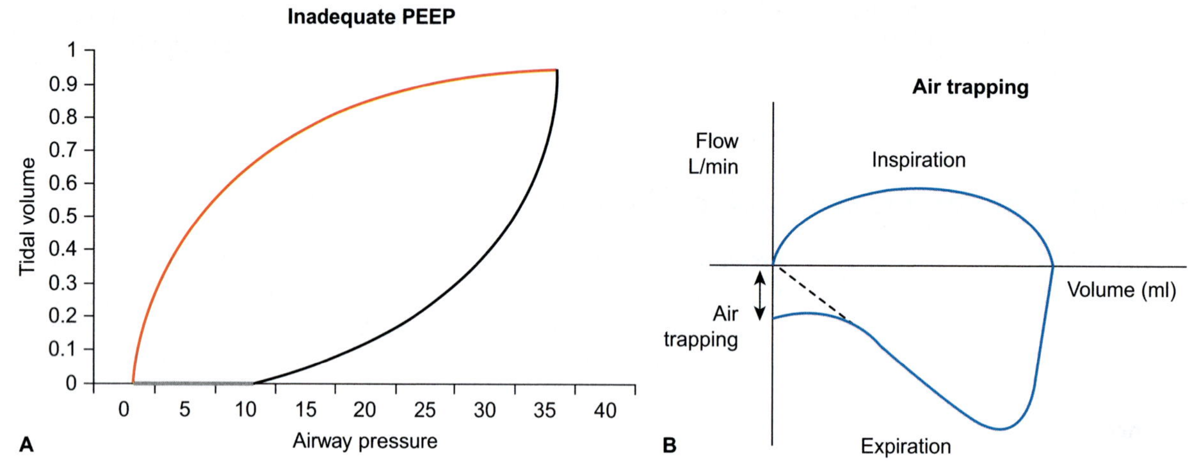

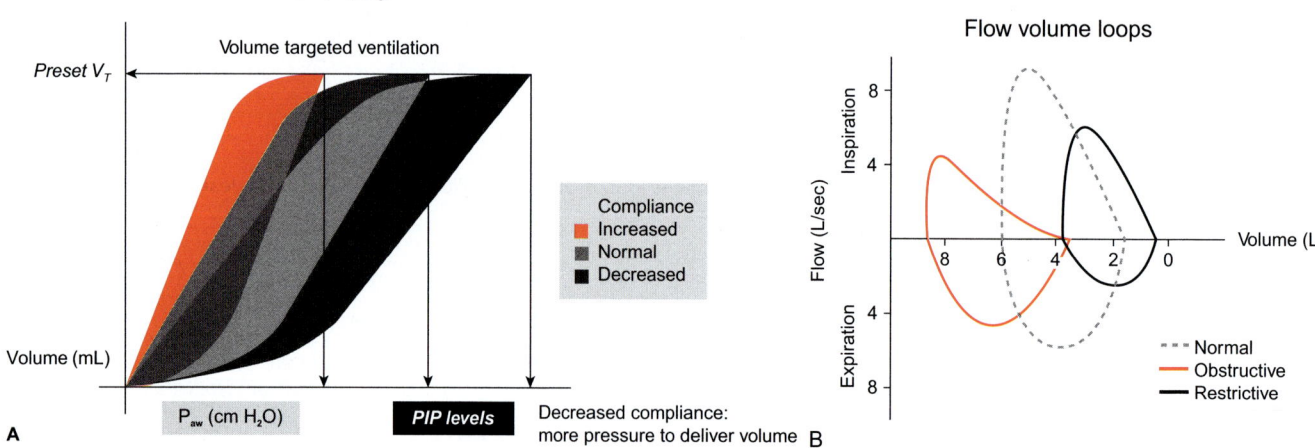

Fig. 58.12 (A) Pressure–volume loop (inadequate PEEP). (B) Flow–volume loop (auto-PEEP). In the flow–volume loop, expiratory limb terminates well before the Y-axis, indicating air trapping.

Compliance Causes: Respiratory distress syndrome (RDS) in newborn/ARDS Consolidation, pleural effusion	Pressure-volume loop (Fig 58.13A) - Lung compliance changes.	Flow–volume loop (Fig. 58.13B)

Fig. 58.13 (A) Pressure–volume loop (lung compliance). (B) Flow–volume loop in obstructive airway disease with preserved lung volume and restrictive airway disease with reduced lung volume.

Condition	Pressure–Volume	Flow–Volume
Airway secretion Cause: Secretions in the tubings, secretion in the circuit	Serrated appearance of the loop indicates secretion in the tubings or ET secretion (Fig. 58.14A)	Serrated appearance of the loop indicates secretion in the tubings or ET secretion (Fig. 58.14B)

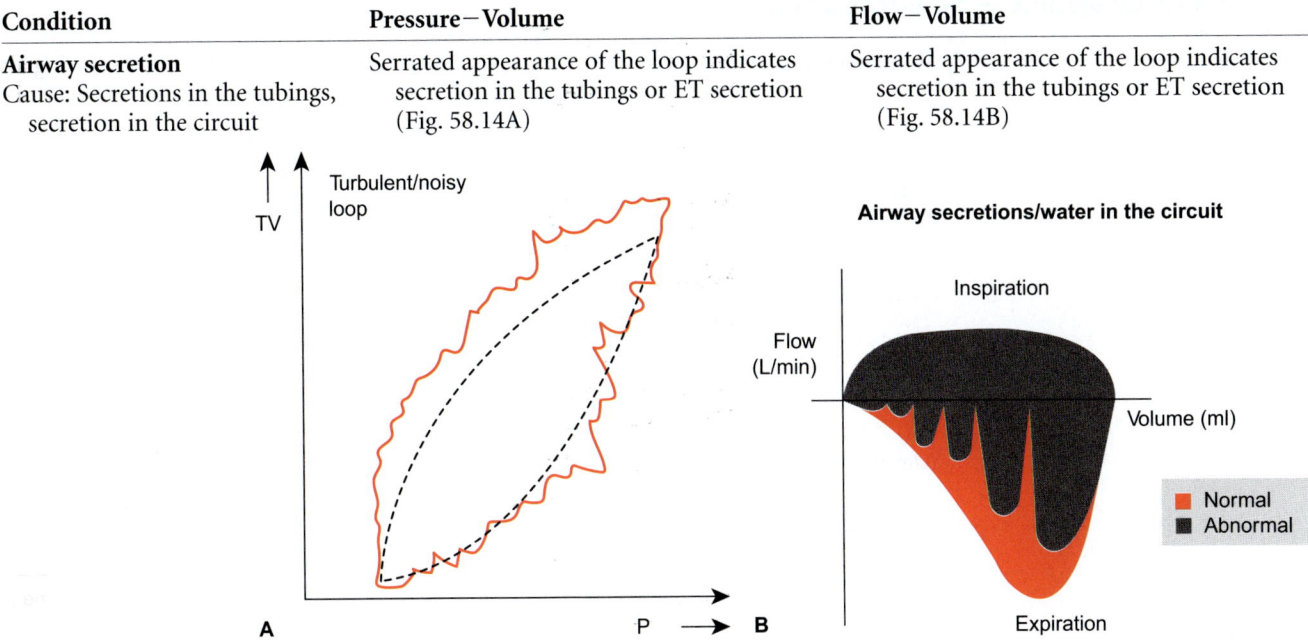

Fig. 58.14   (A) Pressure–volume loop (airway secretion). (B) Flow–volume loop (airway secretion).

Increased airway resistance
   (Fig. 58.15)
Causes:
Bronchospasm (asthma, emphysema) ETT obstruction
Expiratory valve malfunctioning

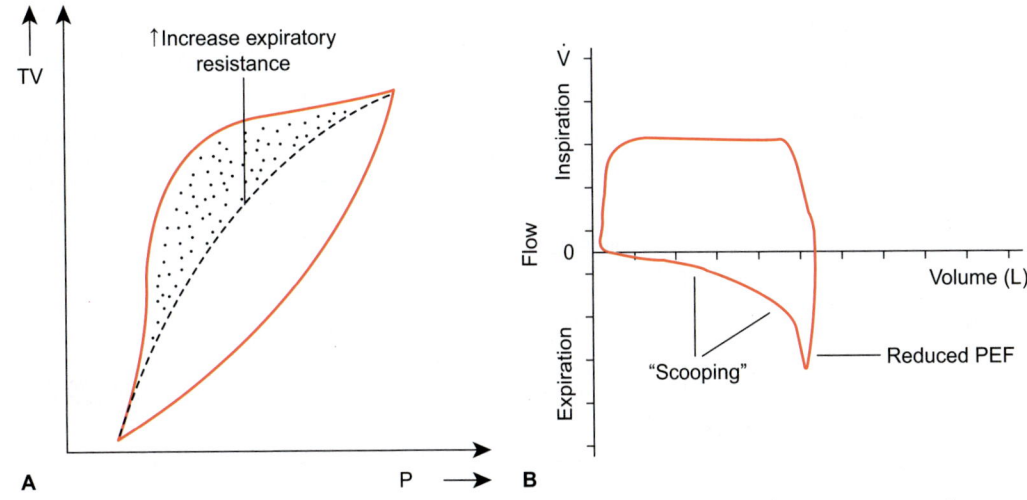

Fig. 58.15   (A) Pressure volume loop showing increased airway resistance. (B) Showing scooping of expiratory curve suggestive of smaller airway obstruction.

Abnormal Graphics – Scalar/Curve

Condition	Abnormality
Air leak (Fig. 58.16)	

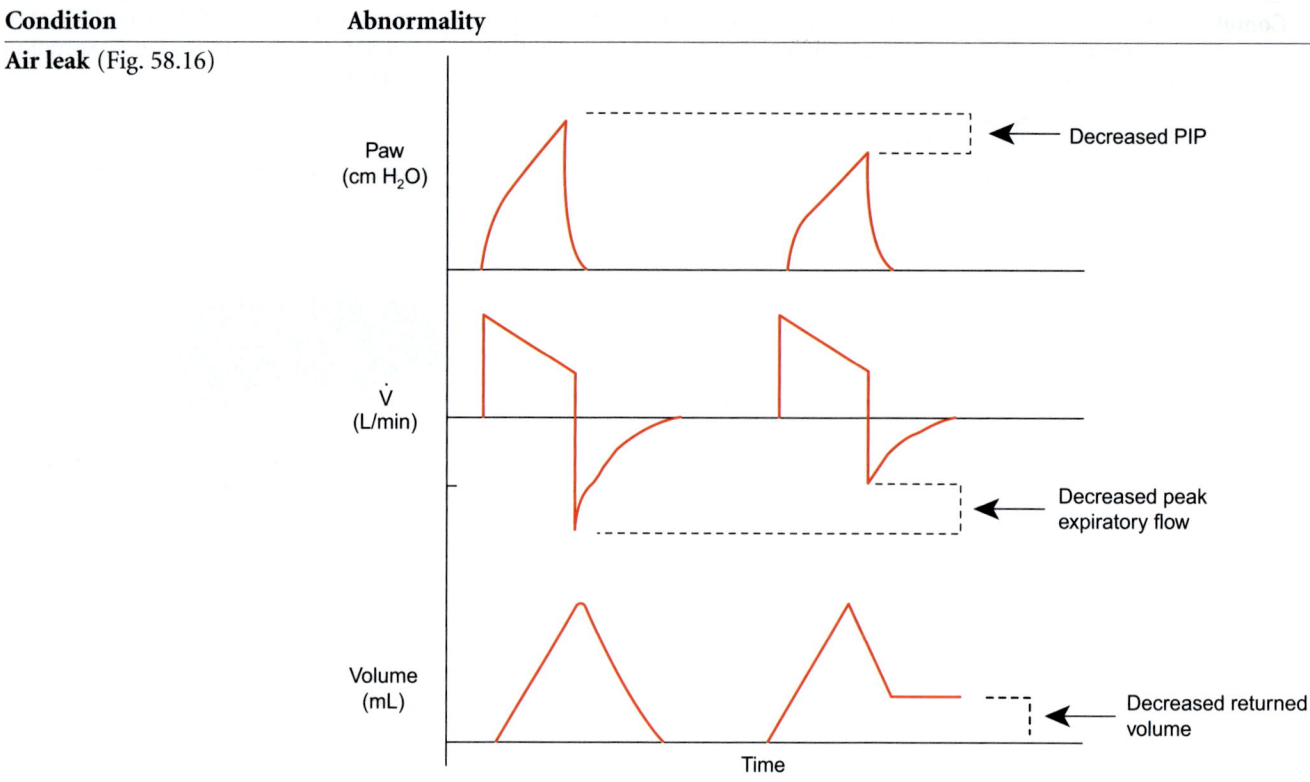

Fig. 58.16 Air leak in pressure–time, flow–time, and volume–time curves.

Auto-PEEP (Fig. 58.17)

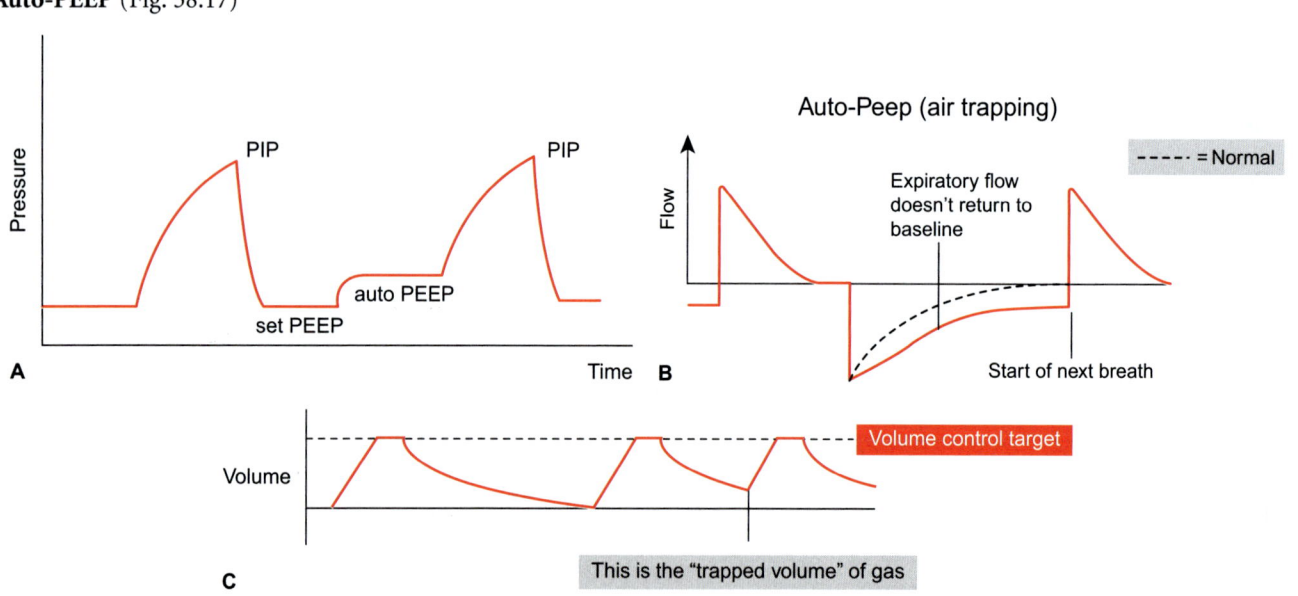

Fig. 58.17 (A) Pressure–time curve: Identification of auto-PEEP when expiratory hold is applied (red arrow). (B) Flow–time scalar (auto-PEEP). (C) -Volume–time scalar – arrow shows trapped volume of gas.

Condition	Abnormality

Compliance (Fig. 58.18)

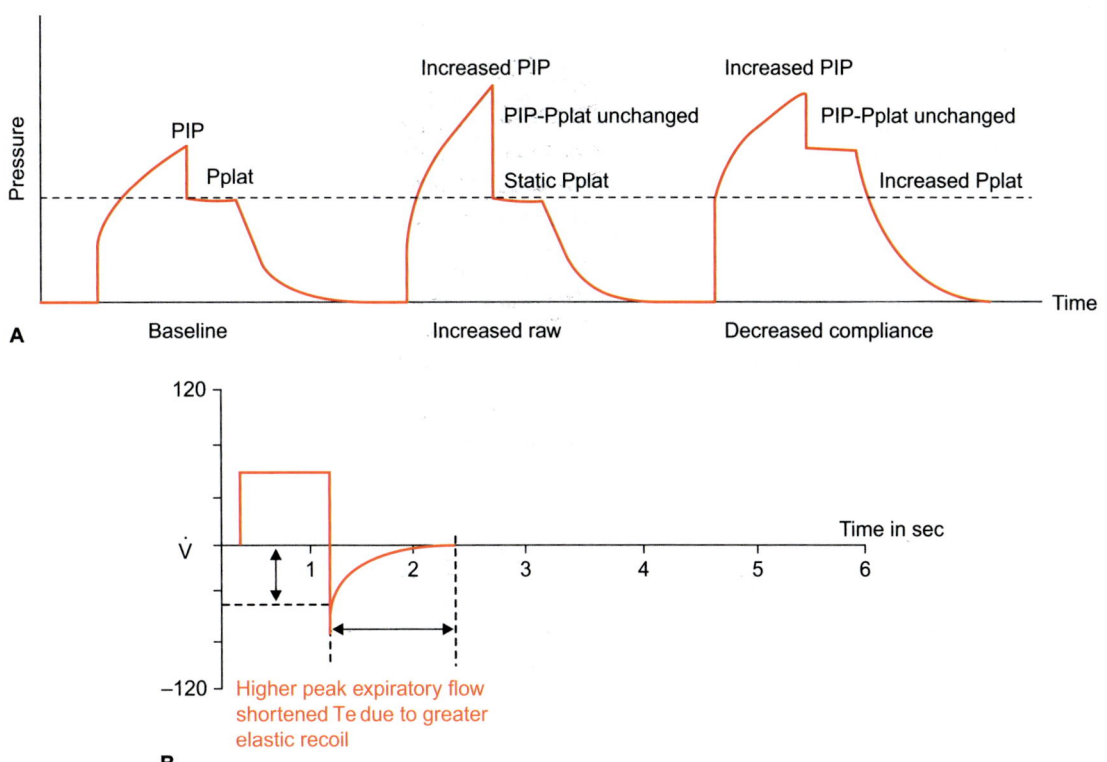

Fig. 58.18   (A) Pressure—time scalar — increased airway resistance and decreased compliance. (B) Flow—time scalar — low compliance.

Troubleshooting in Ventilation

Condition	Intervention
Sudden deterioration	Rule out DOPE: D: Displacement O: Obstruction P: Pneumothorax E: Equipment failure
Low tidal volume (volume control)	Check PIP If low VT + high PIP: 1. Airway (secretion/bronchospasm) 2. Bad lung If low VT + low PIP = circuit leak
Low tidal volume (pressure control)	Check spontaneous breath Low VT + spontaneous breath = asynchronous respiration (sedate or paralyze) Low VT + no spontaneous respiration: 1. Airway (secretions/bronchospasm) 2. Bad lung 3. Outside (chest wall problem/abdominal distension)
High pressure	Check ETT = block, secretion, kinking Check for Pplat If Pplat increased = decreased compliance of the lung (bad lung) If Pplat is normal = increased resistance in the airway (airway problem)

Condition	Intervention
High rate	Step 1: Check tidal volume Step 2: High rate + normal tidal volume = pain, fever, neurogenic cause Step 3: High rate + low tidal volume = increased PIP; if no improvement, suspect air leak, secretions

Asynchrony
Whenever there is discrepancy between patient's demand/efforts and ventilator, asynchrony occurs
	Types of asynchrony
	  Three types
	    • Rate asynchrony
	    • Flow asynchrony
	    • Trigger asynchrony

Rate asynchrony	Air hunger (reduced flow – due to high inspiratory time or decreased flow rate) Seen as dip in inspiratory or expiratory limb

Flow asynchrony as shown in Fig. 58.19
Patient demand outweighs the ventilator flow delivery system probably due to low VT, high inspiratory time, trigger set too high

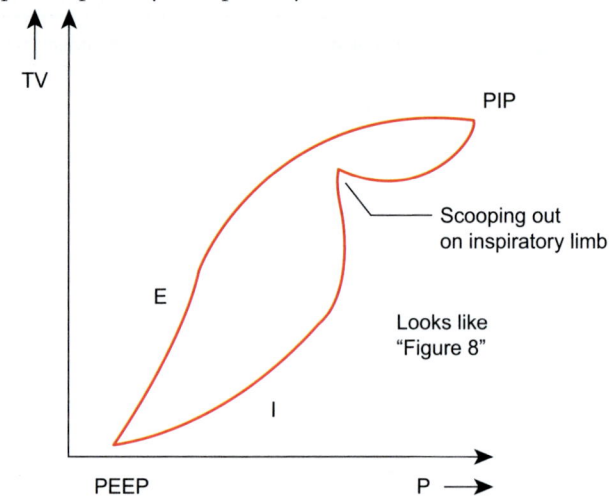

Fig. 58.19   Pressure–volume loop flow (asynchrony).

Trigger asynchrony
During expiration, the child tries to take in breath seen as positive deflection as shown in Fig. 58.20

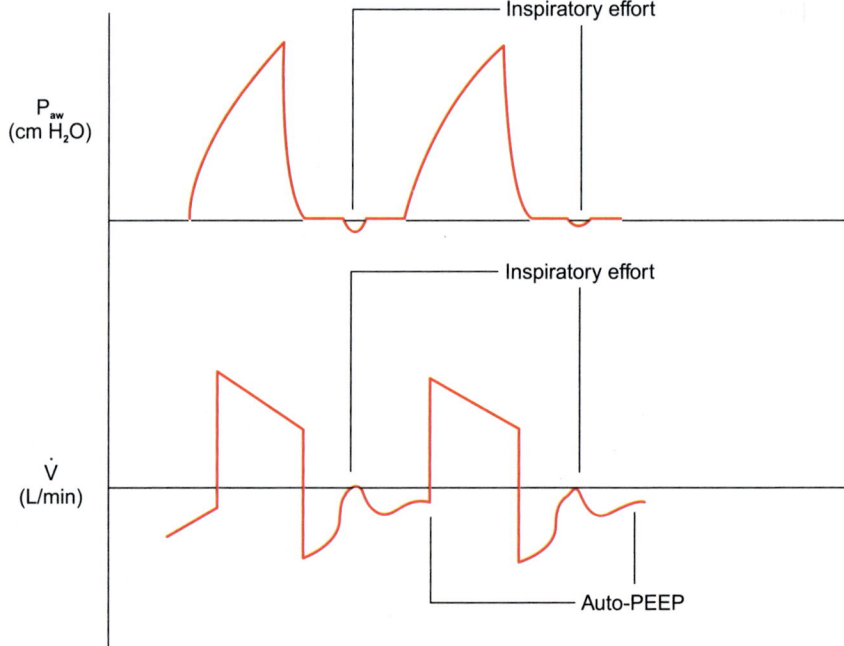

Fig. 58.20   Pressure–time and flow–time – trigger asynchrony.

Condition	Intervention

Beaking of wave (overdistension)
Due to high pressure or high tidal volume
Beaking — pressure continues to rise with
   little or no change in volume creating a
   "bird beak" and can be fixed by reducing
   the amount of tidal volume delivered as
   shown in Fig. 58.21

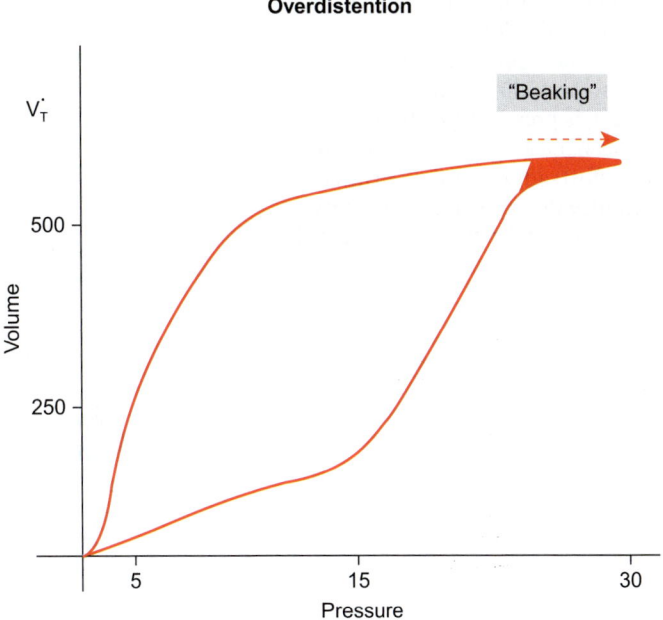

Fig. 58.21   Pressure−volume loop – overdistension.

Fig. 58.22 shows pressure−volume loop −
   upper and lower inflection points
Upper inflection point − lung maximum
   volume is reached after which overdistension occurs
Lower inflection points − alveoli begin to
   fill rapidly and alveolar recruitment
   begins

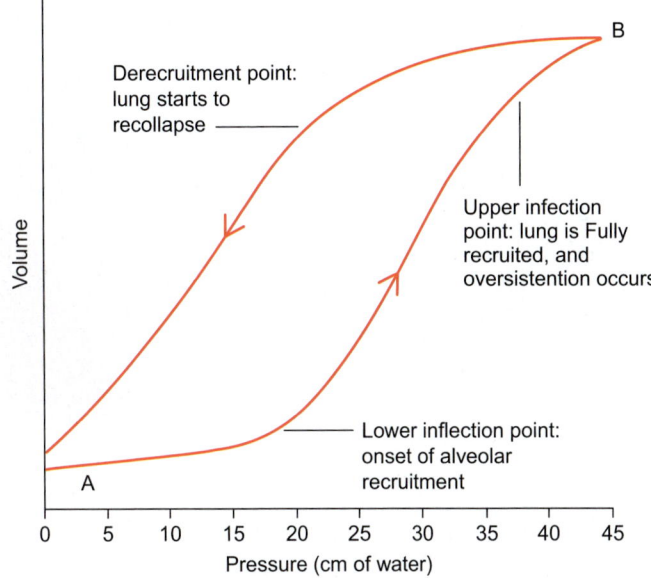

Fig. 58.22   Inflection points.

Condition	Intervention

Fig. 58.23 shows pressure−volume loop −
inadequate sensitivity

Pressure−volume loop normally traces a
counterclockwise direction; if a clockwise tracing is present prior to the initiation of mechanical breath, this indicates
patient's effort; adjusting the sensitivity
can minimize this effort; if the sensitivity is not adjusted, it results in increased
work of breathing for the patient

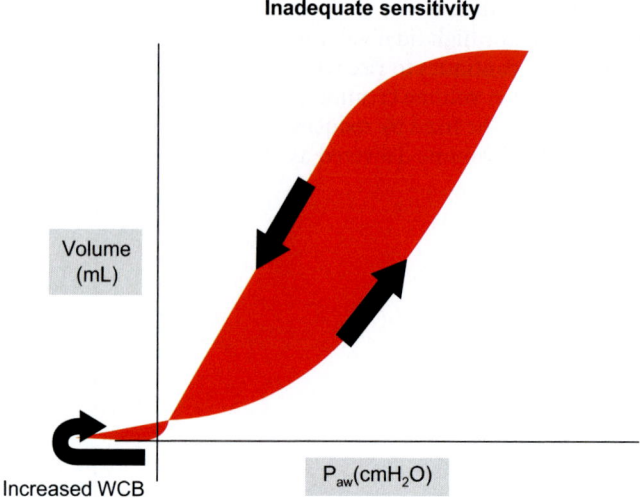

Fig. 58.23   Pressure−volume loop − inadequate sensitivity.

Fig. 58.24 shows pressure−volume loop −
hysteresis

As the airway resistance increases, the loop
will become wider

An increase in expiratory resistance is more
commonly seen; increased inspiratory
resistance is usually from a kinked ETT
or patient biting

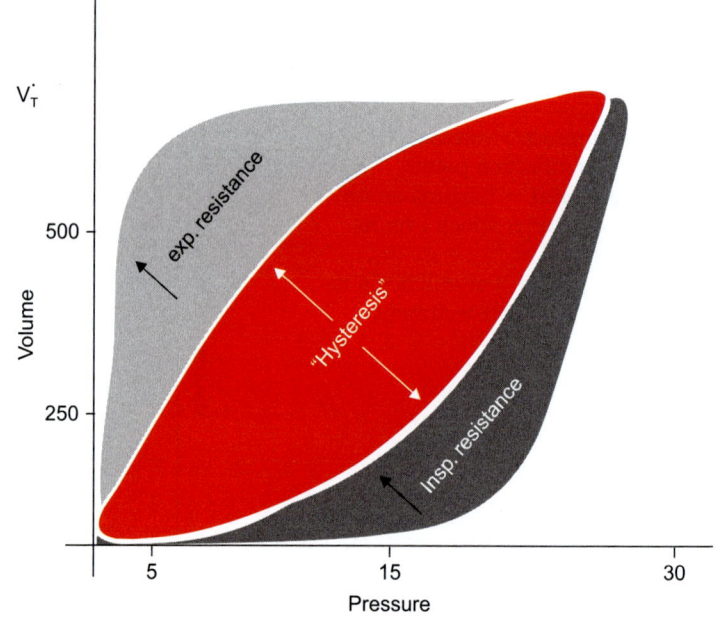

Fig. 58.24   Hysteresis.

Disease-Specific Ventilation

The following table shows disease-specific ventilation strategies.

Disease Type	Ventilation Strategy
ARDS	a. Preferred mode = pressure control b. Low tidal volume (4–8 mL/kg) c. Pplat < 28 cm H_2O if volume control Ppeak < 28 cm H_2O if pressure-controlled ventilation d. Modest PEEP e. Permissive hypercapnia ($PaCO_2$ up to 90, pH − >7.15) f. Permissive hypoxemia g. PaO_2 55−80 mm Hg (minimal tolerable FiO_2 − 0.5–0.6 with optimal PEEP), SpO_2 − 88%–95% h. Rate – 10–35/min i. I:E ratio − 1:1 to 1:3
Asthma	a. Preferred mode – no specific mode is superior; may be pressure control b. Tidal volume = 5–8 mL/kg c. Pplat = minimum PIP (<25) and MAP d. PEEP – minimum (equivalent to auto-PEEP) e. FiO_2 = 0.5–0.7, SpO_2 = 92%–97% f. Respiratory rate – low RR for age (15–20) g. I:E ratio 1:3 (high expiratory time for exhalation) h. Permissive hypoventilation (pH > 7.2) i. Permissive hypercapnia – pCO_2 – 70
Neurologically ill patient (raised ICP)	a. PaO_2 > 90 mm Hg b. Optimum pCO_2 – avoid pCO_2 < 30 c. MAP < 30 cm H_2O
Meconium aspiration syndrome	a. High PIP – 30–35 cm H_2O b. Large tidal volume c. High minute volume d. Low PEEP = 4–6 cm H_2O e. High rate = 40–60/min f. Low inspiratory time = 0.2
Respiratory distress syndrome	a. Low PIP = 20–25 cm H_2O b. Low PEEP = 4–6 cm H_2O c. Low rate = 25–30/min d. Inspiratory time = 0.3–0.4 s

59

Counseling

Counsel this mother of a 2-day-old newborn who received BCG, hepatitis B, and OPV 0 dose, regarding the vaccination in the future up to 1 year in your office practice.

1. Introduce, greet
2. Tell her what are the diseases against which the vaccinations are given now
3. Tell her about the next schedule of primary vaccines at 6, 10, and 14 weeks (DPT, Hib, hepatitis B as single injection, bOPV, and IPV)
4. IAP-recommended vaccines along with the primary vaccines (rotaviral, pneumococcal) and their cost
5. Hepatitis B and OPV at 6th month
6. Influenza vaccine after 6th month (two doses at 4 weeks interval)
7. MMR and OPV at completion of 9 months
8. Conjugate typhoid (TCV) at 9–12 months
9. Tell about the importance of all these vaccines (prevent/cause less serious infections) and need to administer them at the appropriate age
10. Tell about the availability of the primary vaccines and other vaccines which will be available in government hospital
11. Tell about the minor side effects in a nonthreatening manner
12. Give her the expected date of vaccinations and when she should come for the next due vaccination
13. Ask her whether she has any doubts and thank her

A 12-year-old boy is presenting with stage 5 CKD (Chronic Kidney Disease)/ESRD (End Stage Renal Disease) needing renal replacement therapy – kindly explain the counseling procedure.

1. Involve in the discussion both the parents and the person who is going to spend money
2. Involve the child to a reasonable extent as he or she should know the details of what is being done
3. Discuss the financial aspects
4. Obtain consent
5. Preparation of the patient – sterile precautions
6. Explain (Intermittent peritoneal dialysis) IPD, (continuous ambulatory peritoneal dialysis) CAPD, and Hemodialysis (HD) as per the choice of the parents
7. Discuss common complications of the procedure
8. Stress on the ongoing expenditure
9. Emphasize the follow-up labs and their expenditure
10. Remember anti-infective steps
11. Explore future transplant potential
12. Be definitive but supportive to the family
13. Involve the pediatrician incharge of the patient
14. Stress on the immunization completion

Counseling for intubation in a child with refractory status epilepticus

1. Introduce yourself
2. Explain about the critical nature of child's illness — about status epilepticus
3. Explain about the need for intubation
4. Explain the procedure of intubation
5. Explain about rapid sequence intubation (RSI) and the drugs
6. Discuss the complications of the procedure
7. Ask whether the parents have any doubts

Counsel the mother of a child with spinal muscular atrophy (SMA).

1. Introduce yourself to the mother and form a rapport with her
2. Appraise her regarding the genetic and progressive nature of the illness her baby had; discuss the possibility of recurrences in the next pregnancy
3. Explain the various prenatal diagnostic options available, and if possible, tell her where the tests are available
4. Discuss the treatment options for her present child
5. Thank the mother

Counsel this mother who is 8 weeks pregnant now for the second time, whose first child is diagnosed with Down syndrome.

1. Introduce yourself; greet the patient; determine which language the patient is comfortable with; ensure that the husband (any other relative) is accompanying if the patient wishes
2. Convey your wishes for their parenthood
3. Ask whether they have undergone any genetic testing for both of them after their first child was diagnosed with trisomy 21 and any details have been informed about the carrier state and translocation
4. Explain the risk of recurrence based on their result if they know (de novo — 1% risk; 13/21, 14/21, 15/21 — mother carrier — 10%–15%, father carrier — 5%; 21/21 either father or mother is carrier — 100%) or if results are not known, discuss the general risk for recurrence
5. Perform blood test and ultrasound (βhCG, Pregnancy-associated plasma protein- A (PAPPA) and nuchal translucency) in the first trimester
6. Perform triple test and quad screen in the second trimester
7. Discuss the possibility of finding external markers and major anomalies by USG in the second trimester
8. Perform amniocentesis/CVS if any findings are suggestive of trisomy in USG
9. Explain the advantage of (Chorionic Villus Sampling) CVS over amniocentesis
10. Tell about the latest noninvasive cell-free DNA in maternal serum which has good yield

Pediatric Cardiac Arrest

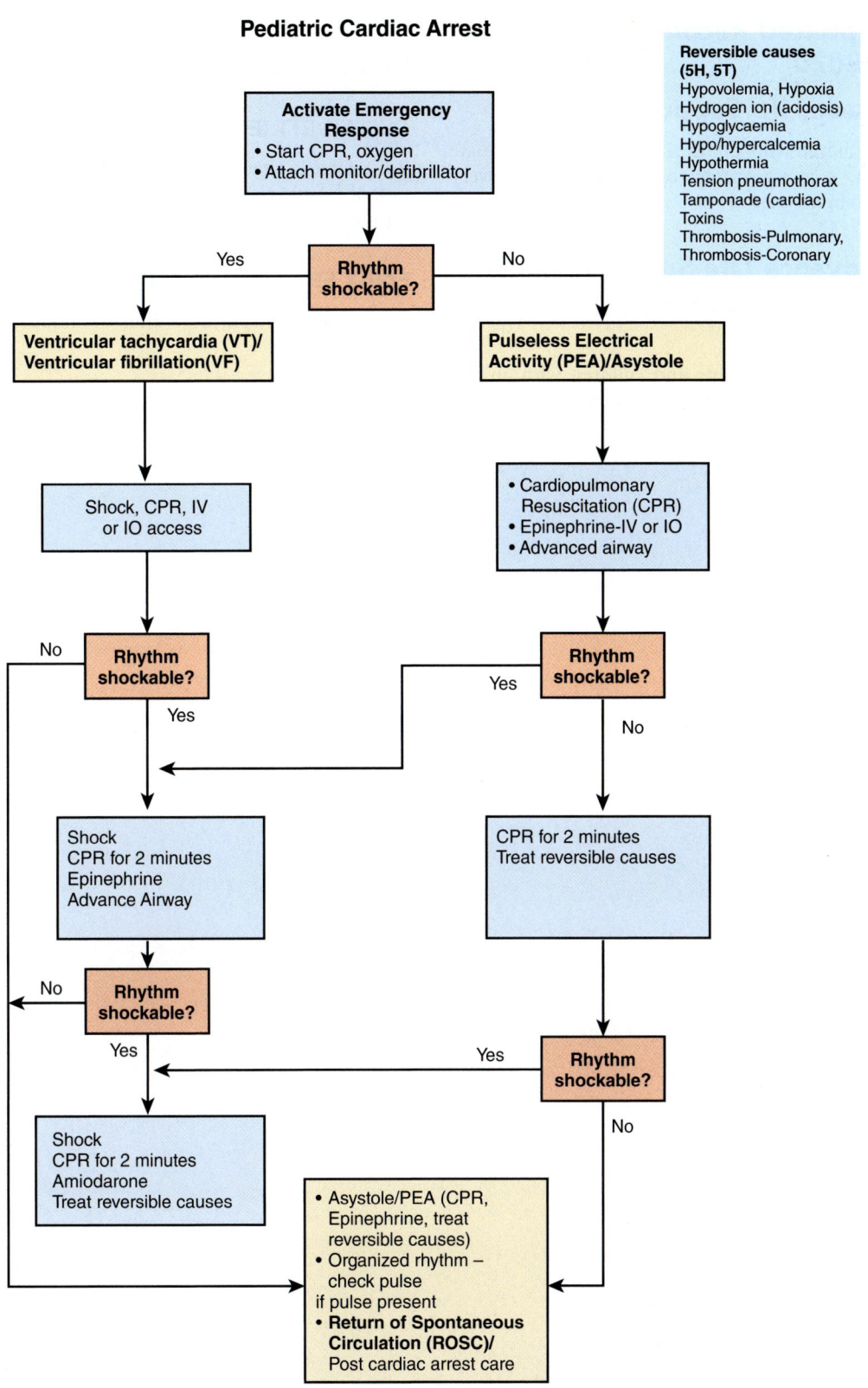

Reversible causes (5H, 5T)
Hypovolemia, Hypoxia
Hydrogen ion (acidosis)
Hypoglycaemia
Hypo/hypercalcemia
Hypothermia
Tension pneumothorax
Tamponade (cardiac)
Toxins
Thrombosis-Pulmonary,
Thrombosis-Coronary

Activate Emergency Response
• Start CPR, oxygen
• Attach monitor/defibrillator

Rhythm shockable?

Yes — **Ventricular tachycardia (VT)/ Ventricular fibrillation(VF)**

No — **Pulseless Electrical Activity (PEA)/Asystole**

Shock, CPR, IV or IO access

• Cardiopulmonary Resuscitation (CPR)
• Epinephrine-IV or IO
• Advanced airway

Rhythm shockable?

Rhythm shockable?

Yes

No

Yes

No

Shock
CPR for 2 minutes
Epinephrine
Advance Airway

CPR for 2 minutes
Treat reversible causes

Rhythm shockable?

No

Yes

Yes

Rhythm shockable?

No

Shock
CPR for 2 minutes
Amiodarone
Treat reversible causes

• Asystole/PEA (CPR, Epinephrine, treat reversible causes)
• Organized rhythm – check pulse if pulse present
• **Return of Spontaneous Circulation (ROSC)/** Post cardiac arrest care

New and Updated Recommendations in BLS/PALS (2020)

Pediatric Basic Life Support (PBLS)

For infants and children with a pulse, but absent or inadequate respiratory effort, it is reasonable to give one breath every 2-3 second (20-30 breaths/min)

Pediatric Advance Life Support (PALS)

VENTILATION RATE DURING CPR WITH AN ADVANCED AIRWAY

When performing CPR in infants and children with an advanced airway, reasonable target respiratory range is 1 breath every 2 to 3 seconds (20 - 30/min)

CRICOID PRESSURE DURING INTUBATION

Routine cricoid pressure not recommended during intubation

CUFFED ETT (ENDOTRACHEAL TUBE)

Reasonable to choose cuffed ETT over uncuffed ETT for intubation of infants and children (Attention to be paid for ETT size, position and cuff inflation pressures- usually (20-25 cm H_2O)

EARLY EPINEPHRINE ADMINISTRATION

Administer epinephrine within 5 minutes of start of chest compression

IMNCI

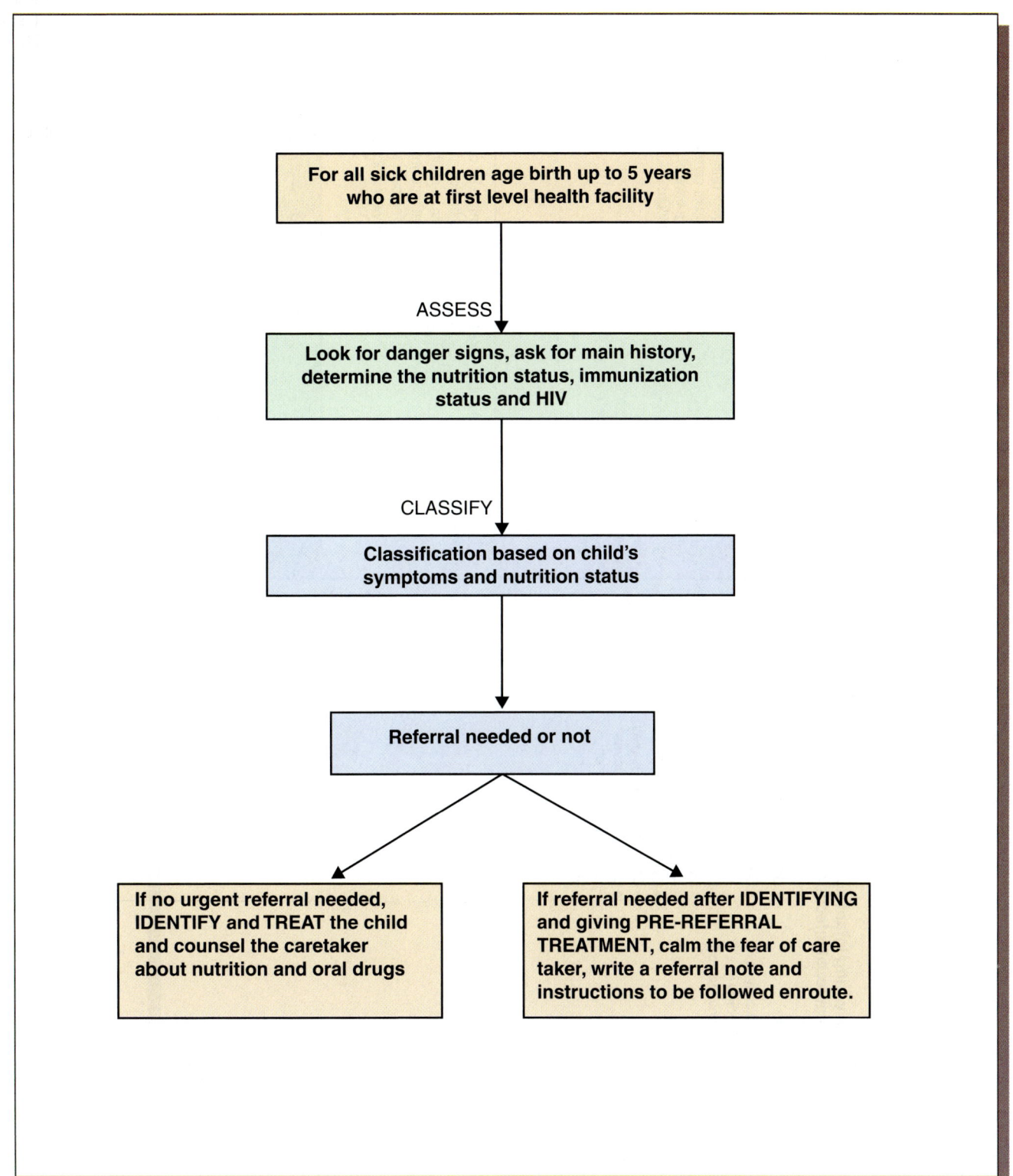

Source- Integrated Management of Newborn and Childhood Illness Module: 15. Synthesis of IMNCI for a Sick Child up to Five Years: Assess and Classify: View as single page (open.edu)

Sick young infant age up to 2 months for bacterial infection:

ASK:
- Difficulty in feeding?
- Convulsions?

LOOK, LISTEN, FEEL:
- Count breath for 1 minute.
- Look for chest indrawing
- Axillary temperature
- Examine the umbilicus
- Check for skin pustules
- See if the child moves spontaneously or on stimulation

Classify →

Any of the following signs:	**PINK** Vere severe	• Give first dose antibiotics • Treat low blood sugar • Urgent referral • Instruct caregiver to take care of infant enroute
• Not taking feed • Convulsions • Fast breathing (>60 per minute) • Severe chest retractions • Fever (>37.5°C) or hypothermia (<35.5°c) • No movement or when stimulation		
• Umbilicus red or with pus • Skin pustules	**YELLOW** Local bacterial infection	• Administer oral antibiotics • Instruct mother to treat local infection • Home care advise • Review in 2 days
• No warning signs	**GREEN** Severe disease unlikely	• Home care advise

Check for Jaundice:

If jaundice present ASK:
- Onset

LOOK and FEEL
- Yellowish discoloration
- Examine palms and soles

Classify

Any of the following signs:	*PINK* Severe disease	- Treat low sugar - Urgent referral - Instruct care giver to provide warmth enroute
- any jaundice in < 24 hours - palms and soles involved at any age		
- Jaundice appearing after 24 hours of age - Palms and soles not involved	*YELLOW* Jaundice	- Home care advice - Review immediately if palms and soles are yellow - If age > 14 days refer for evaluation - Review in 1 day
- No jaundice	*GREEN* No Jaundice	- Home care advice

Ask for Diarrhoea?

LOOK and FEEL

- Look if child is moving – no movement, moves on stimulation or irritable
- Check sunken eyes
- Skin pinch slowly or very slowly > 2 seconds

Classify

	Signs	Classify	Action
PINK Severe disease	**2 of the below:** • Moves on stimulation or no movement • Sunken eyes • Skin pinch very slowly goes back	**PINK** Severe disease	• If child has no other severe disease condition, give fluid correction – PLAN C is started If other severe disease exists • Urgent referral • Instruct mother to breastfeed and give sips of ORS
YELLOW Some dehydration	• 2 of the following Restless and irritable Sunken eyes Skin pinch goes back slowly	**YELLOW** Some dehydration	• Home care advice PLAN B fluid and breast milk • Follow up in 2 days
GREEN No dehydration	• No enough signs as some or severe dehydration	**GREEN** No dehydration	• Home care advice • Continue breast feeding and fluid correction (PLAN A) for diarrhea • Follow up in 2 days

ASK
- Has the mother and/or young infant had checked HIV status?

If YES
- What is the mother's serology HIV status?
- Infant's virology and serology status?

IF MOTHER HAS HIV BUT CHILD IS NEGATIVE
- Is the child taking breastfeed?
- Breastfeeding was continued at the time of testing or before it?
- Is the mother and infant taking ARV prophylaxis to prevent parent to child transmission?

UNKNOWN
- Mother and infant status not known

Classify

	Signs	Classify	Treatment
	Virology test is positive in infant	**YELLOW** Confirmed HIV infection	• Give cotrimoxazole prophylaxis from age 4–6 weeks • Give HIV ART and care • Advice the mother on home care • Follow up regularly
	• Mother HIV POSITIVE and negative in breast-feeding infant or completed breastfeeding 6 weeks ago • Mother positive and test not done in infant • Infant serologically positive	**YELLOW** Exposed to HIV	• Give cotrimoxazole prophylaxis from age 4–6 weeks • Start or Continue ARV prophylaxis • Virology test at 4–6 weeks and then 6 weeks after completely stopping breastmilk • Home care advice • Follow up
	Mother ad infant Negative	**GREEN** HIV infection unlikely	Treat, advice home care follow-up regularly

Check for feeding problem or LBW except HIV EXPOSED infants not on breastfeeding

ASK
- Is infant taking breastfeed?
- How many times being breastfed in a day?
- Any other food or drink given– how many times a day and what is given?

LOOK, LISTEN, FEEL
- Weight for age
- Examine for oral thrush or patch
- Breastfeeding assessment

ASK MOTHER TO FEED AND ASSESS FOR 4 MINUTES
- Attachment good or not well attached
- Suckling is effective?
- Any nasal block?

Classify feeding		
- Not well attached - No sucking - < 8 feed in a day - Receives other food - Weight for age is low - oral ulcer or thrush	**YELLOW** Feeding problem or low weight	- Correct position and attachment - Increase breastfeeding frequency in a day - Increase breastfeeding and reduce other feeds - Advice home care - Follow-up in 2 days for feeding difficulties or oral ulcer - Follow-up in 14 days for low weight for age
No low weight for age and no signs of inadequate feed	**GREEN**	- Appreciate mother for feeding well Advice home care

Check for feeding problem or low weight for age in non-breastfed infant (HIV exposed non breastfed and child who does not need referral)

ASK

- What milk is being given?
- How frequent child is fed?
- What quantity given?
- How milk is being prepared- ask mother to show how she prepares and feeds the child?
- Is breastmilk being given?
- What additional food is given instead?
- How is milk given- cup or bottle?
- How is the bottle or cup being washed?

LOOK LISTEN FEEL

- Weight for age
- Oral ulcers

Classify feeding

	Classification	Treatment
Milk not given appropriately Prepared without hygiene Replacement food inappropriate Feeding bottle used Low weight for age Oral thrush HIV mother giving mixed feed before 6 months	**YELLOW** Feeding problem or low weight	• Advice about feeding practices • Safe replacement feeding • Advice cup feeding and not with bottle • Increase breastfeeding and reduce other feeds • Advice home care • Follow-up in 2 days for feeding difficulties or oral ulcer And In 14 days for low weight
No low weight for age and no signs of inadequate feed	**GREEN** No feeding problem	• Appreciate mother for feeding well Advice home care

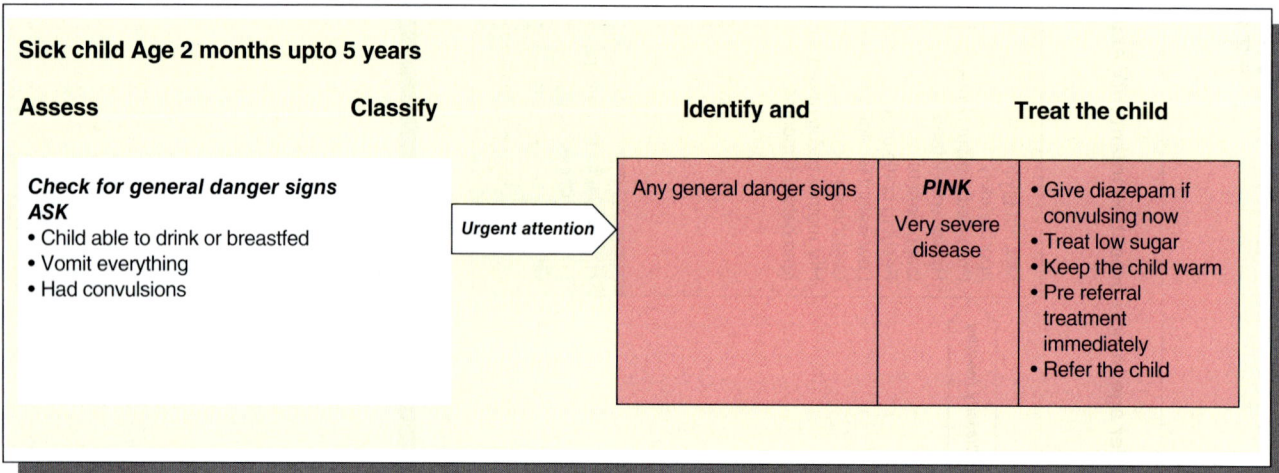

Sick child Age 2 months upto 5 years

Assess	Classify	Identify and	Treat the child

Check for general danger signs ASK
- Child able to drink or breastfed
- Vomit everything
- Had convulsions

Urgent attention

Any general danger signs

PINK

Very severe disease

- Give diazepam if convulsing now
- Treat low sugar
- Keep the child warm
- Pre referral treatment immediately
- Refer the child

Child has cough or difficulty in breathing?

ASK

For How long?

LOOK LISTEN FEEL
- Count the breath for 1 minute
- Chest indrawing?
- Look or listen for stridor?
- Look for wheezing?
- If wheeze present with fast breathing or chest indrawing- give trial inhaled bronchodilator 3 times 15 minutes apart.
- If spo2 < 90 refer

Classify cough or difficulty breathing

Signs	Classify	Treatment
Danger sign stridor	**PINK** Severe pneumonia or very severe disease	• first dose antibiotics • refer urgently
Chest indrawing Or fast breathing	**YELLOW** Pneumonia	• Give oral antibiotics 5 days • If wheezing is there bronchodilator for 5 days • If HIV EXPOSED child give amoxicillin and refer • Soothe the throat and give safe remedy • If cough > 2 weeks suspect Tuberculosis • FOLLOW-UP IN 3 DAYS
NO signs of severe disease	**GREEN** Cough or cold	• If wheezing, give inhaled bronchodilator for 5 days • If HIV exposed child, give amoxicillin and refer • Soothe the throat and give safe remedy • If cough > 2 weeks suspect Tuberculosis • FOLLOW-UP IN 5 DAYS

Child has diarrhoea

ASK

How long?

Blood in stools?

LOOK LISTEN FEEL
- Look for general condition?
- Lethargic or irritable?
- Sunken eyes?
- Child drinks fluids eagerly or thirsty or not taking fluids?
- Pinch skin goes slowly or very slowly (> 2 seconds)

> *Classify diarrhoea*

2 of following • Lethargy or unconsciousness • Sunken eyes • Does not drink • Skin pinch goes back very slowly	**PINK** Severe dehydration	*If child has no other danger signs* • Fluid as plan C • If other danger signs present refer urgently • If > 2 years, cholera in your area give antibiotics • Continue breastfeeds

2 of the following
• Restless irritable
  Sunken eyes
  Skin pinch goes back slowly
	YELLOW
	Some dehydration
		• Give fluids, zinc supplements
		• Follow Plan B
		• If other danger signs present refer urgently
		• Continue breastfeeds
		• Follow up in 5 days

NO signs of severe disease	**GREEN** NO dehydration	• Give fluids • Zinc fluids as PLAN A • Continue breast feeds • Follow up in 5 days

If diarrhea > 14 days

Dehydration present	**PINK** Severe persistent diarrhea	• Treat dehydration before referral • If any other danger sign is present refer urgently
No dehydration	**YELLOW** Persistent diarrhea	• Advice mother on feeding • Give micronutrients supplements for 14 days • Follow up in 5 days

If blood in stools

Blood in stools	**YELLOW** Dysentery	• Give ciprofloxacin • Follow up in 3 days

Child has fever? (feels hot or temperature more than 37.5°C)

If yes malaria high risk or low?

ASK

How long?
If more than 7 days, fever present everyday?
Child had measles in last 3 months

LOOK LISTEN FEEL
• Look or feel for stiff neck
• Runny nose
• Any bacterial focus for fever
  Any signs of measles

Test for malaria
If high risk area
No obvious cause of fever is present

Classify fever →

Any danger sign Stiff neck	**PINK** Severe febrile disease	• Give first dose artesunate or quinine • Give first dose antibiotics • Give one dose of paracetamol Refer urgently
Malaria test positive	**YELLOW** Malaria	• Give antimalarial as protocol • Give one dose paracetamol • Start antibiotic for bacterial infection • Advice on feed • Follow-up in 3 days If fever > 7 days refer for further evaluation
Malaria negative Other cause of fever present	**GREEN** Fever No malaria	• Give one dose paracetamol • Start antibiotic for bacterial infection • Advice on feed • Follow-up in 3 days

If no malaria risk or any significant travel history

Any danger sign Stiff neck	**PINK** Very severe febrile disease	• Give first dose antibiotics • Treat child for low sugar if there • Give one dose of paracetamol • Refer urgently
No Any danger sign No Stiff neck	Yellow Green fever	• Give one dose paracetamol • Start antibiotic for bacterial infection • Advice on feed • Follow-up in 3 days If fever > 7 days refer for further evaluation

If measles now or last 3 months

Any danger sign Clouding of cornea Deep mouth ulcer	**PINK** Very complicated measles	• Give vitamin A treatment • First dose antibiotic • If pus draining from eye give tetracycline eye drops - Refer urgently
Clouding of cornea Deep mouth ulcer	**YELLOW** Measles with eye or mouth complication	• Give vitamin A treatment • First dose antibiotic • If pus draining from eye give tetracycline eye drops • For mouth gentian violet • Follow-up in 3 days
Measles now or last 3 months	**GREEN** Measles	• Vitamin A treatment

ASSESSMENT	SIGNS, CLASSIFICATION AND TREATMENT
Does the child have an ear problem? If yes, ask: Is there ear pain?; Is there ear discharge?, if yes for how long? **Look and feel:** Look for pus draining from the ear; feel for tender swelling behind the ear. **Classify ear problem →**	Tender swelling behind the ear → **MASTOIDITIS** → Give first dose of injectable chloramphenicol (If not possible give oral amoxycillin); give first dose of paracetamol for pain; refer URGENTLY to hospital.
	Pus is seen draining from the ear and discharge is reported for less than 14 days or ear pain → **ACUTE EAR INFECTION** → Give cotrimoxazole for five days; give paracetamol for pain; dry the ear by wicking; follow-up in 5 days.
	Pus is seen draining from the ear and discharge is reported for 14 days or more → **CHRONIC EAR INFECTION** → Dry the ear by wicking; follow-up in 5 days.
	No ear pain and no pus seen draining from the ear → **NO EAR INFECTION** → No additional treatment.
Then check for malnutrition: **Look and feel:** Look for visible severe wasting, oedema of both feet and determine weight for age. **Classify nutritional status →**	Visible severe wasting or oedema of both feet → **SEVERE MALNUTRITION** → Give single dose of vitamin A; prevent low blood sugar; refer URGENTLY to hospital; while referral is being organized, warm the child; keep the child warm on the way to hospital.
	Very low weight for age → **VERY LOW WEIGHT** → Assess and counsel for feeding; advise the mother when to return immediately; follow-up in 30 days.
	Not very low weight for age and no other signs of malnutrition → **NOT VERY LOW WEIGHT** → If child is less than 2 years old, assess the child's feeding and counsel the mother on feeding, if feeding problem, follow-up in 5 days. Advise the mother when to return immediately.
Then check for Anaemia: **Look:** Look for palmar pallor, Is it severe palmar pallor or some palmar pallor? **Classify Anaemia →**	Severe palmar pallor → **SEVERE ANAEMIA** → Refer URGENTLY to hospital.
	Some palmar pallor → **ANAEMIA** → Give IFA therapy for 14 days; assess the child's feeding and counsel the mother on feeding, if feeding problem, follow-up in 5 days; advise the mother when to return immediately; follow-up in 14 days.
	No palmar pallor → **NO ANAEMIA** → Give prophylactic IFA if child is 6 months or older.
Then check for child's immunization, prophylactic vitamin A and IFA supplementation status. Assess other problems.	

Source: Modified from Rajkumar Patil. *Community Medicine: Practical Manual*, Details of specific clinicosocial cases, Figure 18.6, New Delhi, Elsevier India, 2018. (Credit line -Source: IMNCI wall charts, MOHFW, India. http://www.nhm.gov.in/nrhmcomponnets/reproductive-child-health/child-health.html?start=10.).

Reference Charts

Growth Charts

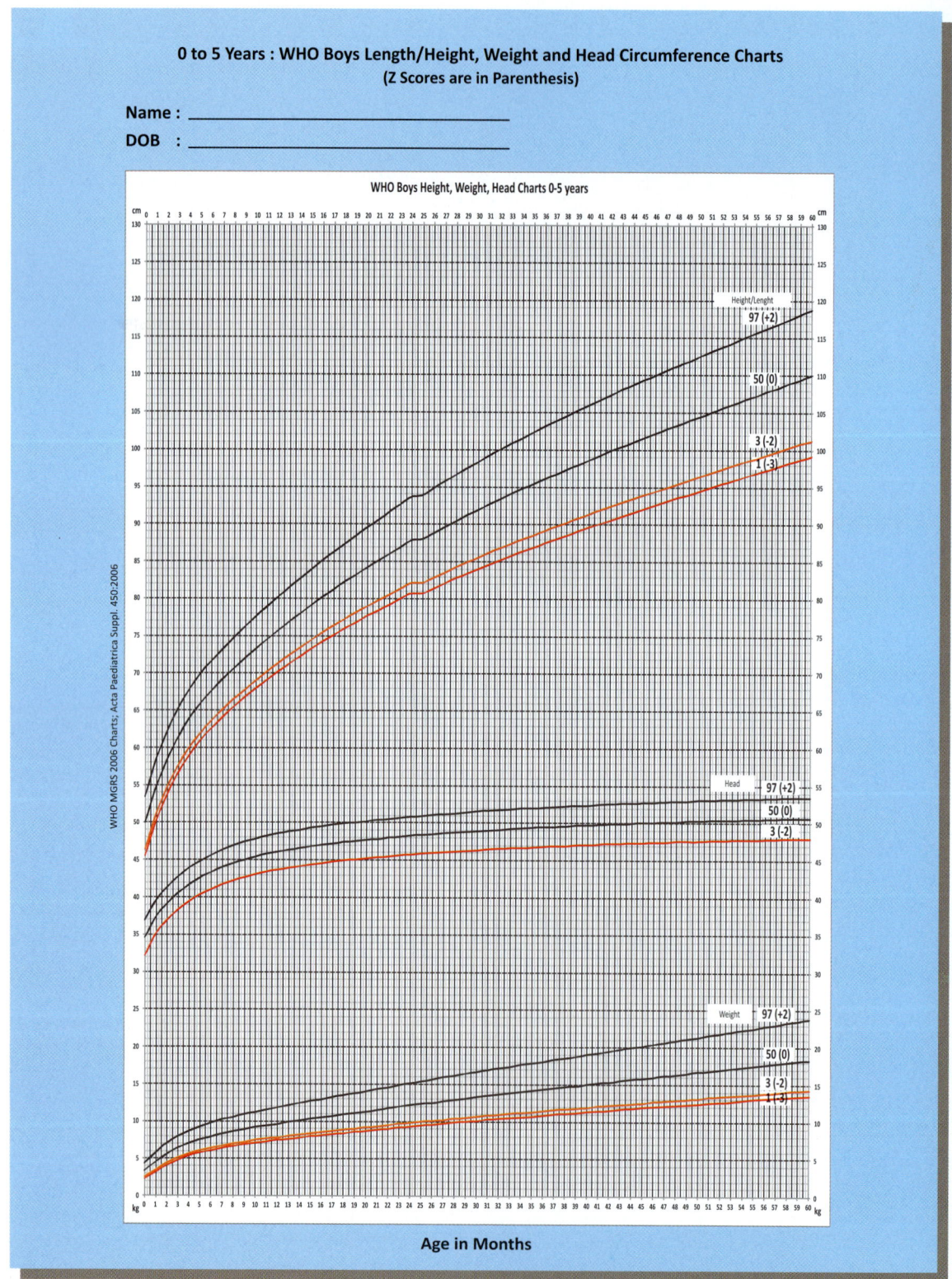

0 to 5 Years : WHO Boys Length/Height, Weight and Head Circumference Charts
(Z Scores are in Parenthesis)

Name : _____

DOB : _____

WHO Boys Height, Weight, Head Charts 0-5 years

Height/Lenght
97 (+2)
50 (0)
3 (-2)
1 (-3)

Head
97 (+2)
50 (0)
3 (-2)

Weight
97 (+2)
50 (0)
3 (-2)
1 (-3)

WHO MGRS 2006 Charts; Acta Paediatrica Suppl. 450:2006

Age in Months

WHO Boys Weight for Height/Length Charts
(Z Scores are in Parenthesis)

Name : _____

DOB : _____

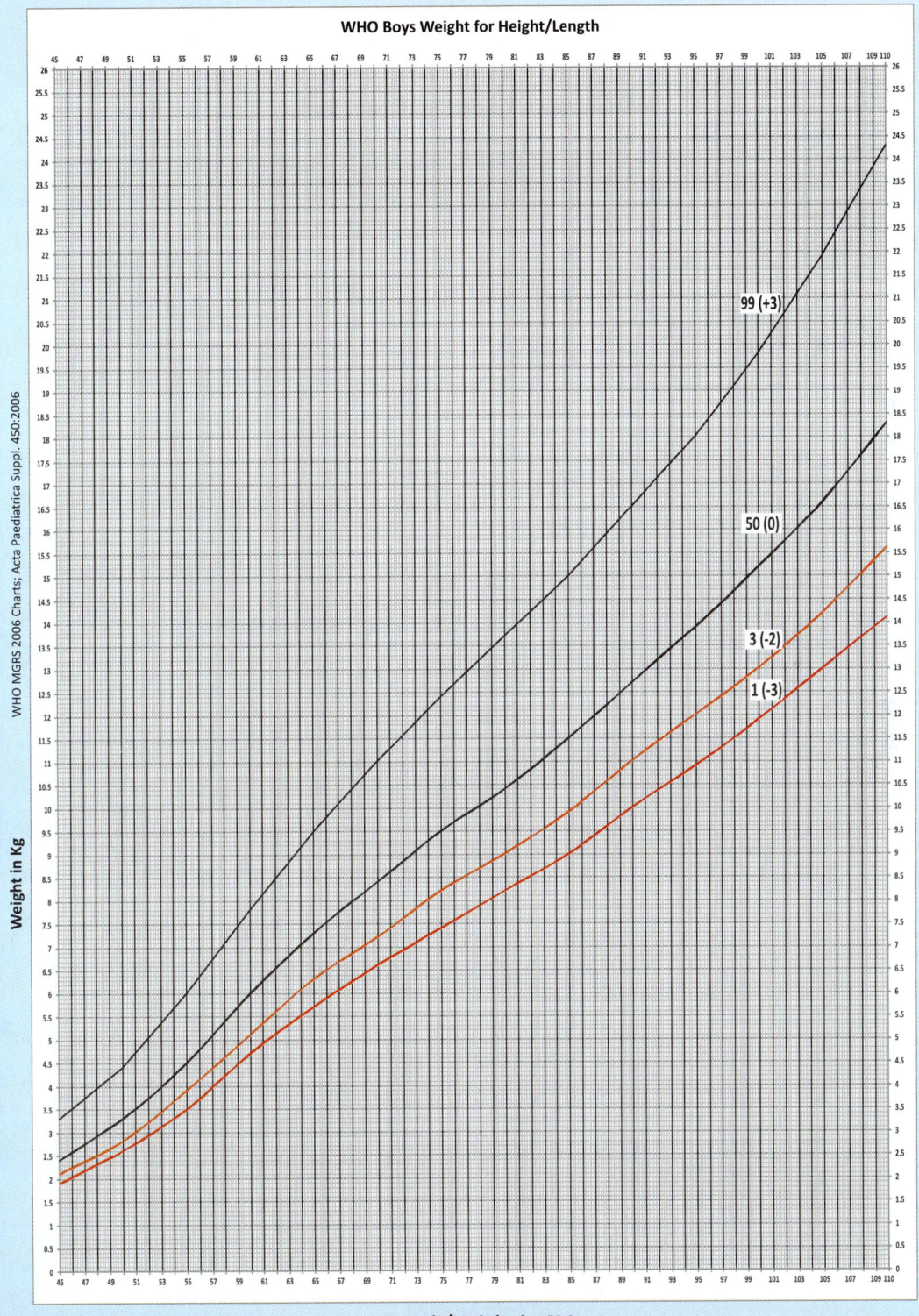

WHO Boys Weight for Height/Length

WHO MGRS 2006 Charts; Acta Paediatrica Suppl. 450:2006

Weight in Kg

99 (+3)

50 (0)

3 (-2)

1 (-3)

Length/Height in CM

0 to 5 Years : WHO Girls Length/Height, Weight and Head Circumference Charts
(Z Scores are in Parenthesis)

Name : _____

DOB : _____

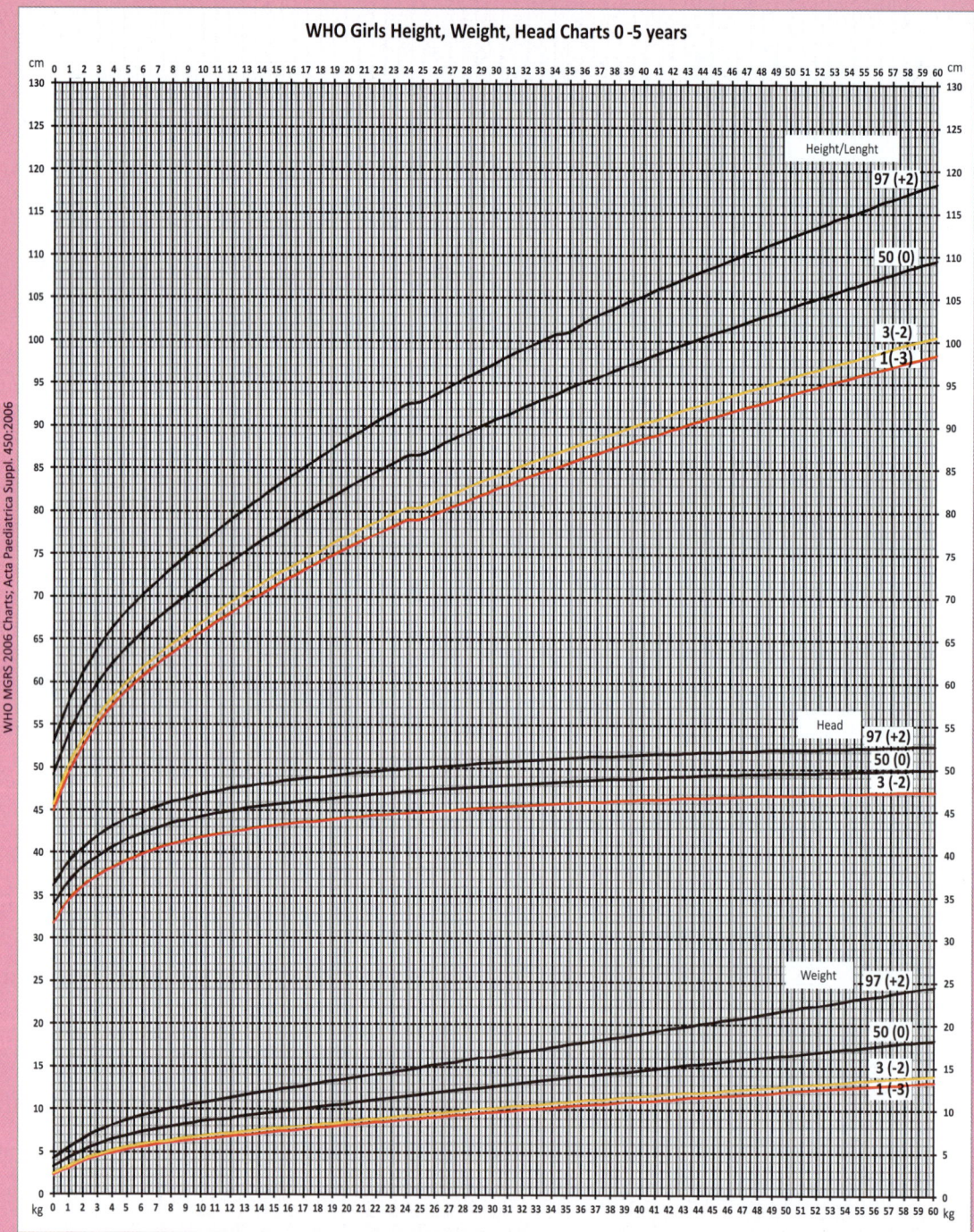

WHO Girls Height, Weight, Head Charts 0 -5 years

WHO MGRS 2006 Charts; Acta Paediatrica Suppl. 450:2006

Age in Months

WHO Girls Weight for Height/Length Charts
(Z Scores are in Parenthesis)

Name : _____

DOB : _____

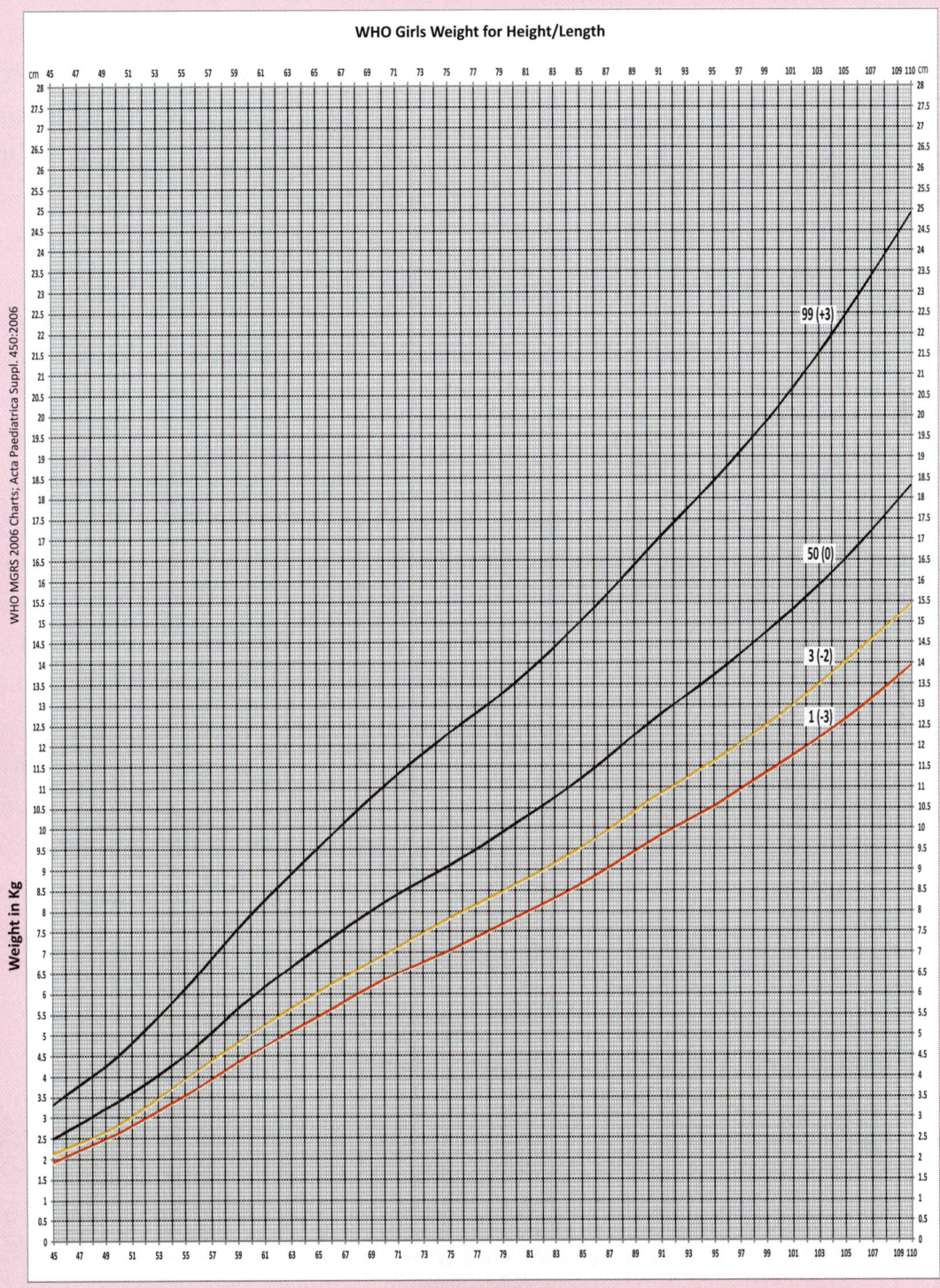

WHO Girls Weight for Height/Length

WHO MGRS 2006 Charts; Acta Paediatrica Suppl. 450:2006

Weight in Kg

99 (+3)

50 (0)

3 (-2)

1 (-3)

Length/Height in CM

Father's Height_____, Mother's Height_____, Target Height_____

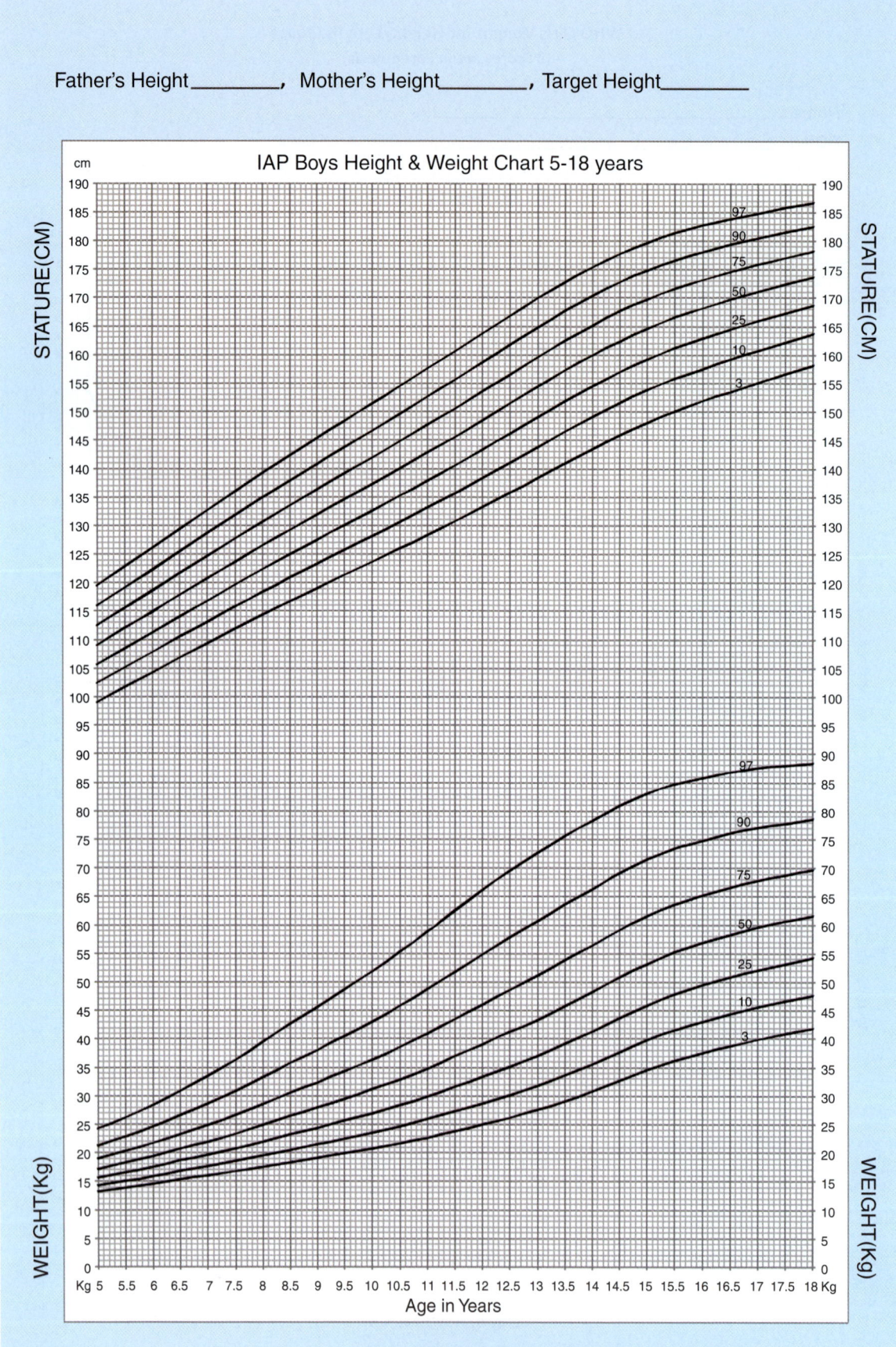

IAP Boys Height & Weight Chart 5-18 years

Source: Reproduced from Harish Pemde, Vikram Datta, Kamlesh Harish. *Clinical and Practical Paediatrics*, Second Edition, Annexurel 2 l - Growth charts, New Delhi, Elsevier India, 2020.

Name _____

DOB _____

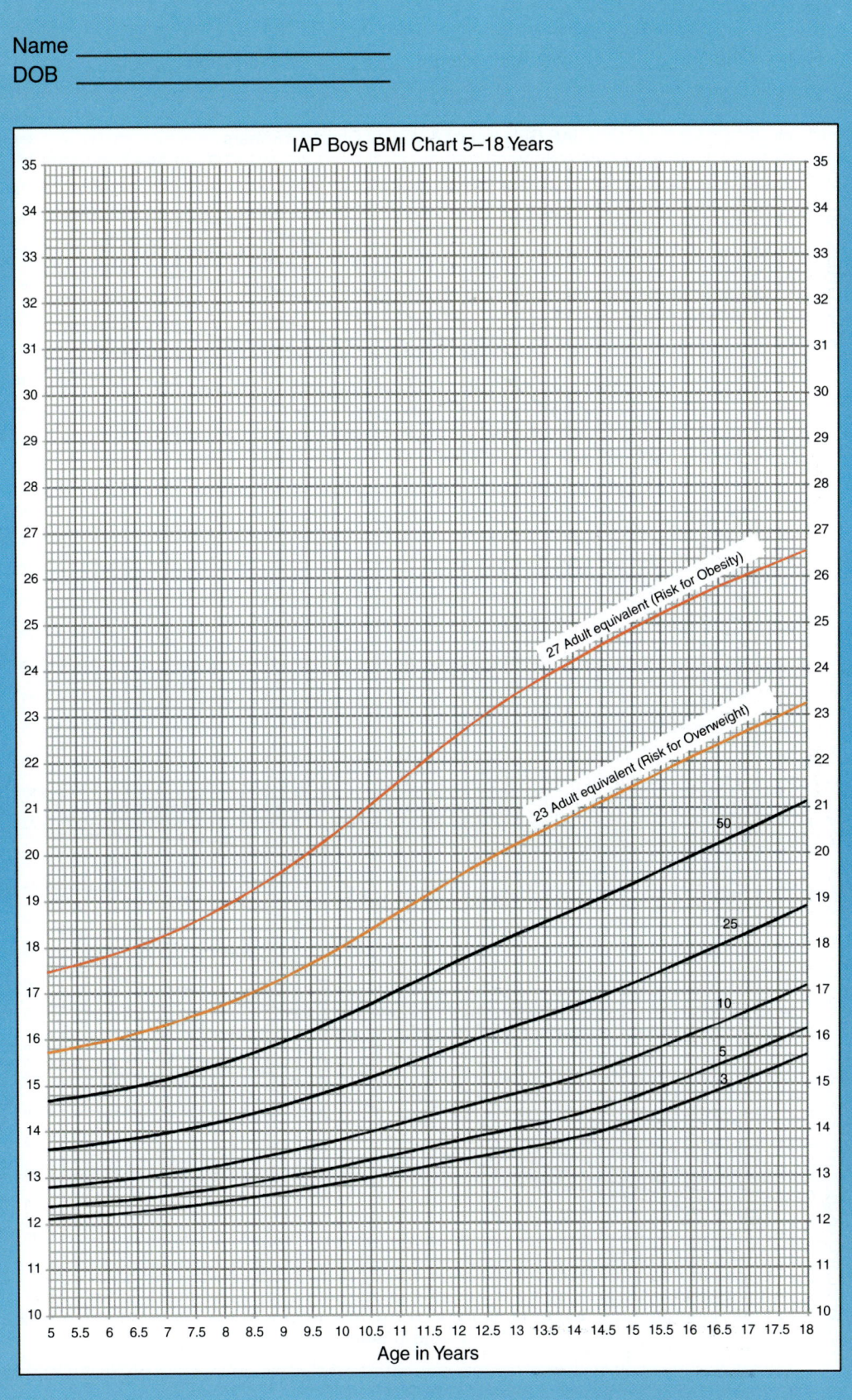

IAP Boys BMI Chart 5–18 Years

Age in Years

Source: Reproduced from Harish Pemde, Vikram Datta, Kamlesh Harish. *Clinical and Practical Paediatrics,* Second Edition, Annexurel 2 I - Growth charts, New Delhi, Elsevier India, 2020

Father's Height _____, Mother's Height _____, Target Height _____

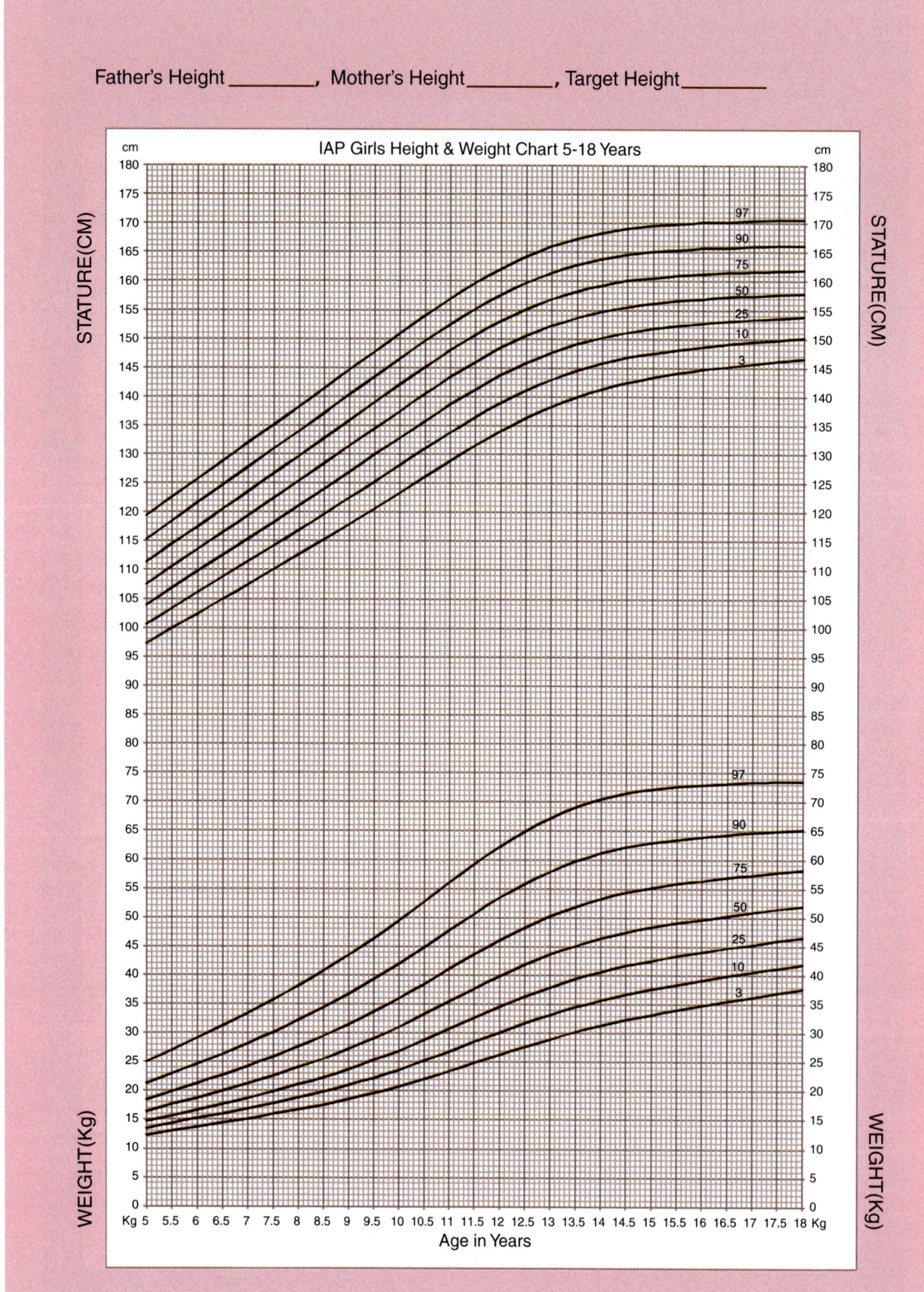

IAP Girls Height & Weight Chart 5-18 Years

Source: Reproduced from Harish Pemde, Vikram Datta, Kamlesh Harish. *Clinical and Practical Paediatrics*, Second Edition, Annexurel 2 I - Growth charts, New Delhi, Elsevier India, 2020

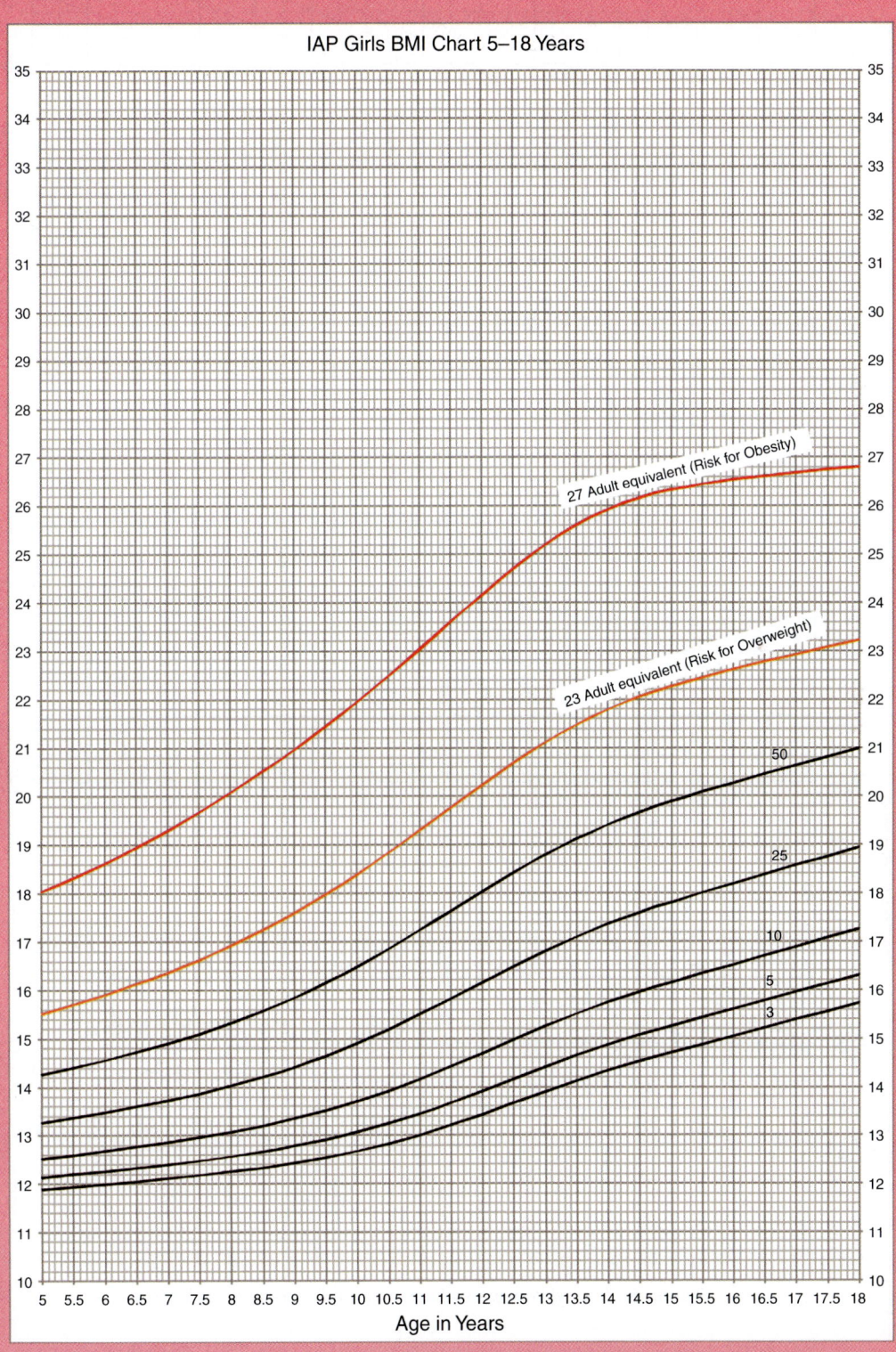

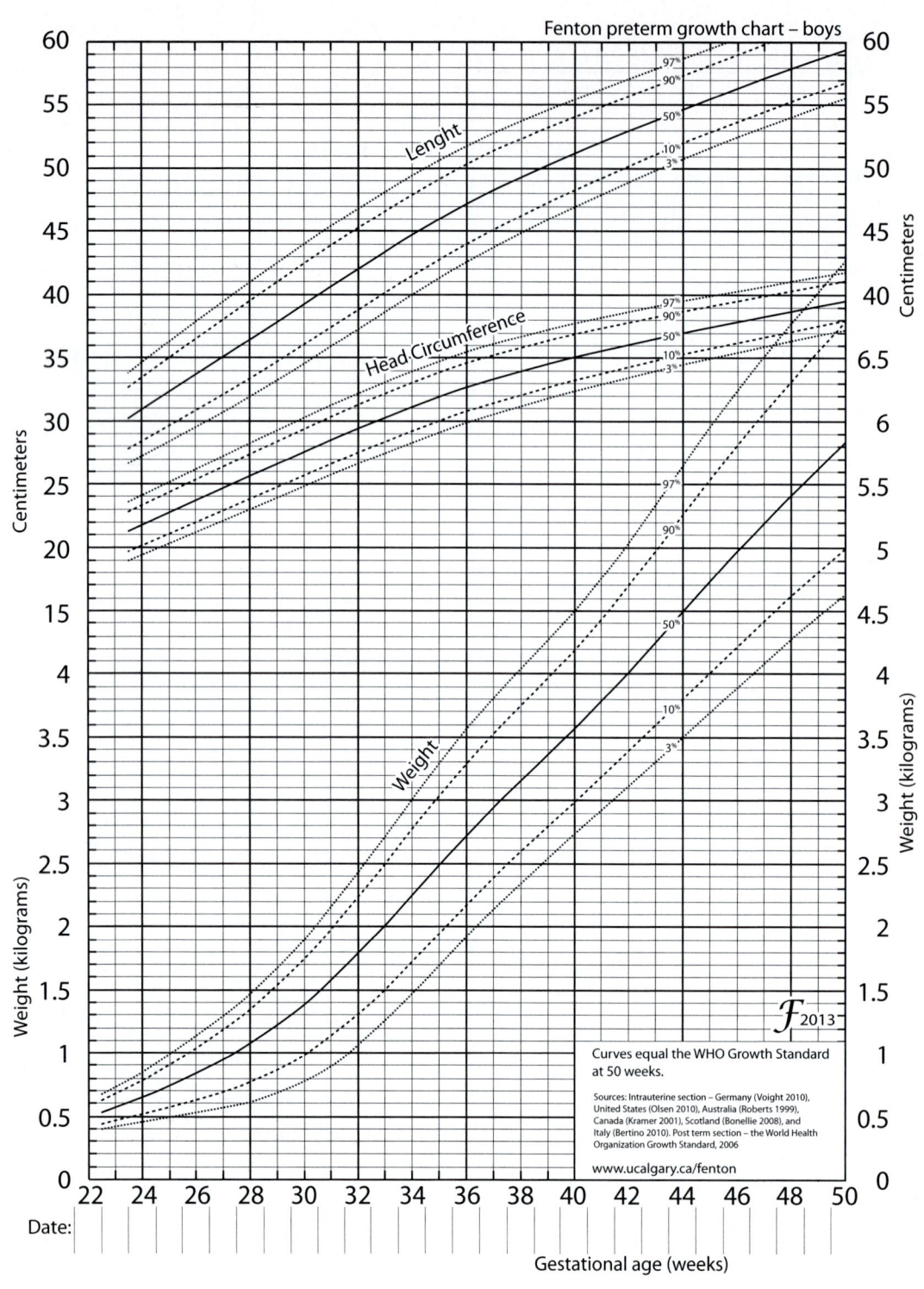

Rycina 3. Zmodyfikowane siatki centylowe Fentona dla chłopców

Source: Intrauterine section – Germany (Voight 2010), United States (Olsen 2010), Australia (Roberts 1999), Canada (Kramer 2001), Scotland (Bonellie 2008), and Italy (Bertino 2010). Post term section – the World Health Organization Growth Standard, 2006. www.ucalgary.ca/fenton

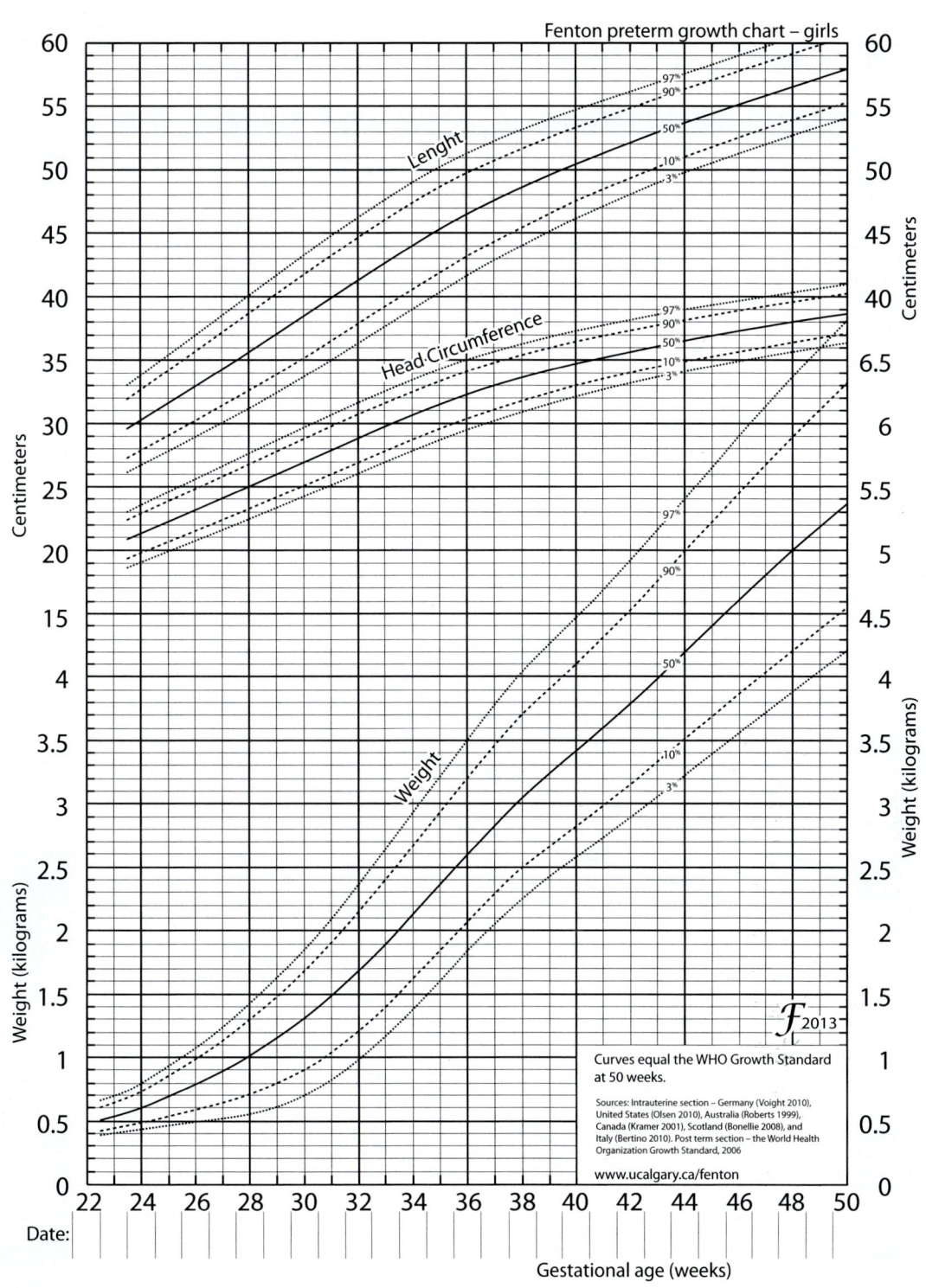

Rycina 2. Zmodyfikowane siatki centylowe Fentona dla dziewczynek

Source: Intrauterine section – Germany (Voight 2010), United States (Olsen 2010), Australia (Roberts 1999), Canada (Kramer 2001), Scotland (Bonellie 2008), and Italy (Bertino 2010). Post term section – the World Health Organization Growth Standard, 2006. www.ucalgary.ca/fenton

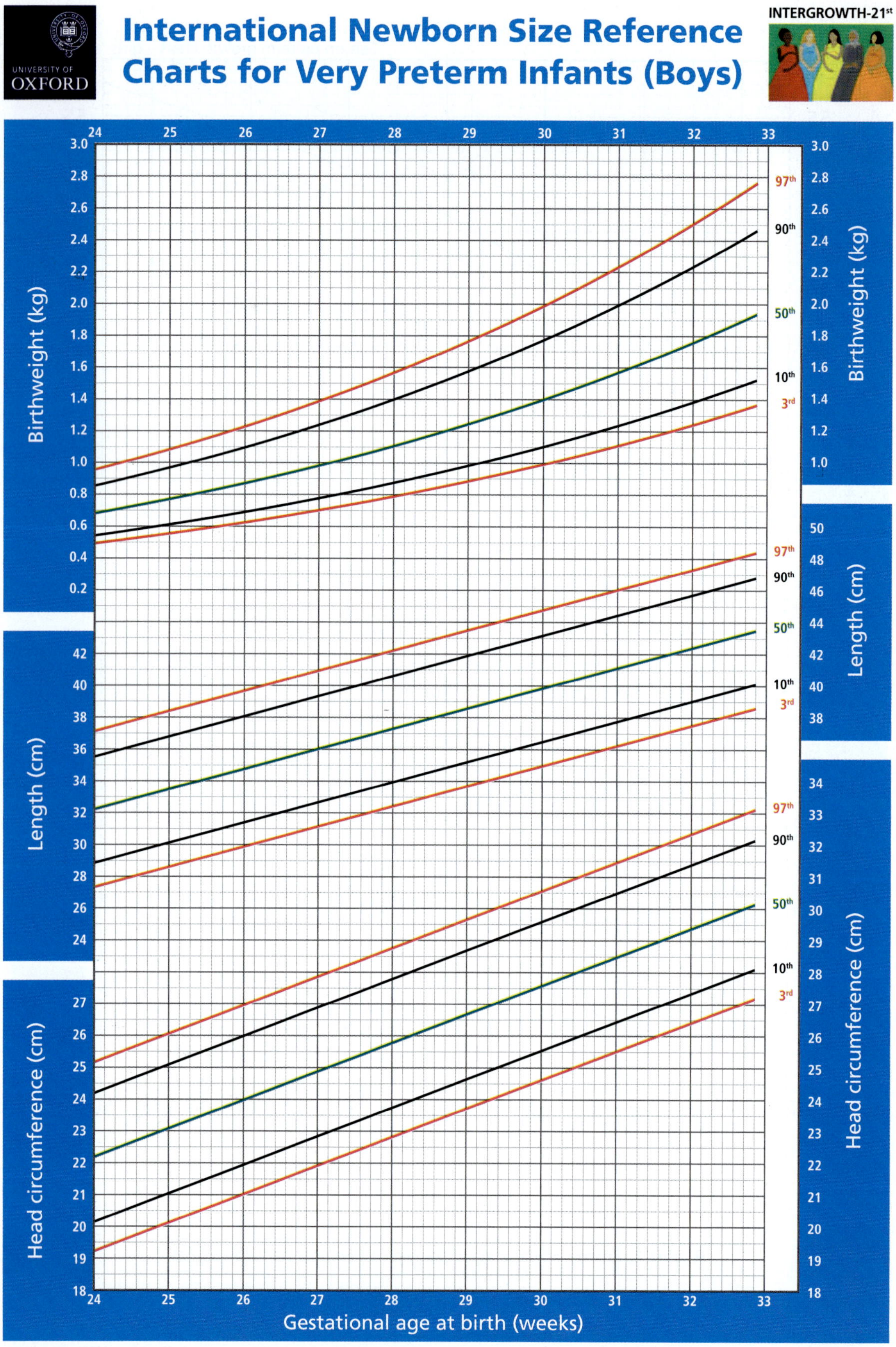

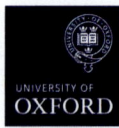

International Newborn Size Reference Charts for Very Preterm Infants (Boys)

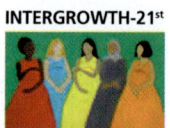

INTERGROWTH-21st

Villar et al. *Lancet* 2016;387:844-5

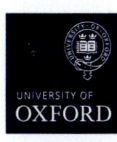

International Newborn Size Standards (Boys)

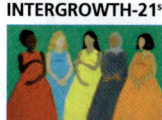

INTERGROWTH-21st

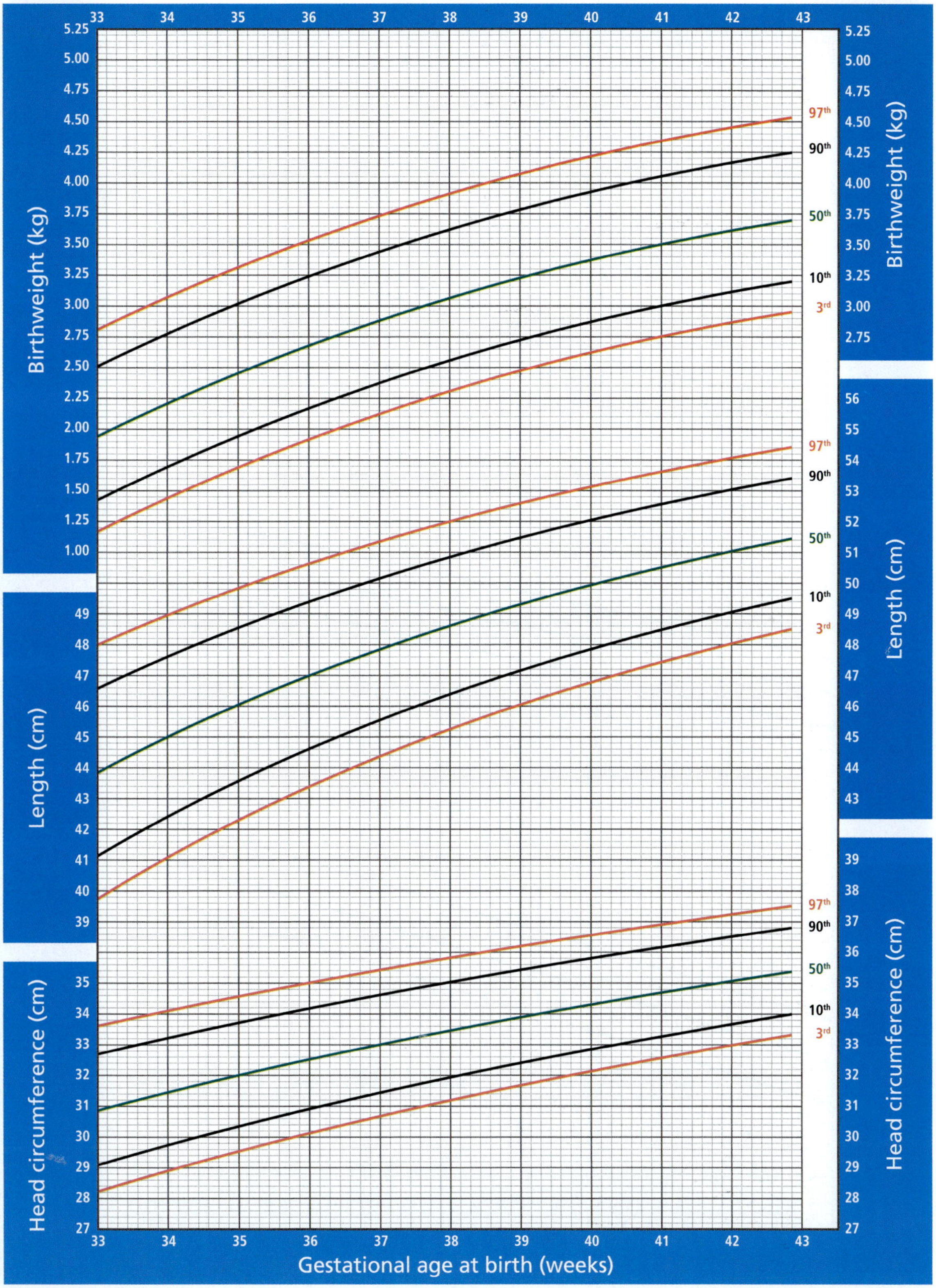
Birthweight (kg)
Length (cm)
Head circumference (cm)
Gestational age at birth (weeks)
97th
90th
50th
10th
3rd
33
34
35
36
37
38
39
40
41
42
43

Villar et al. *Lancet* 2014;384:857-68

UNIVERSITY OF OXFORD

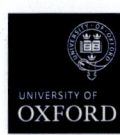

International Newborn Size Reference Charts for Very Preterm Infants (Boys)

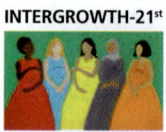

INTERGROWTH-21st

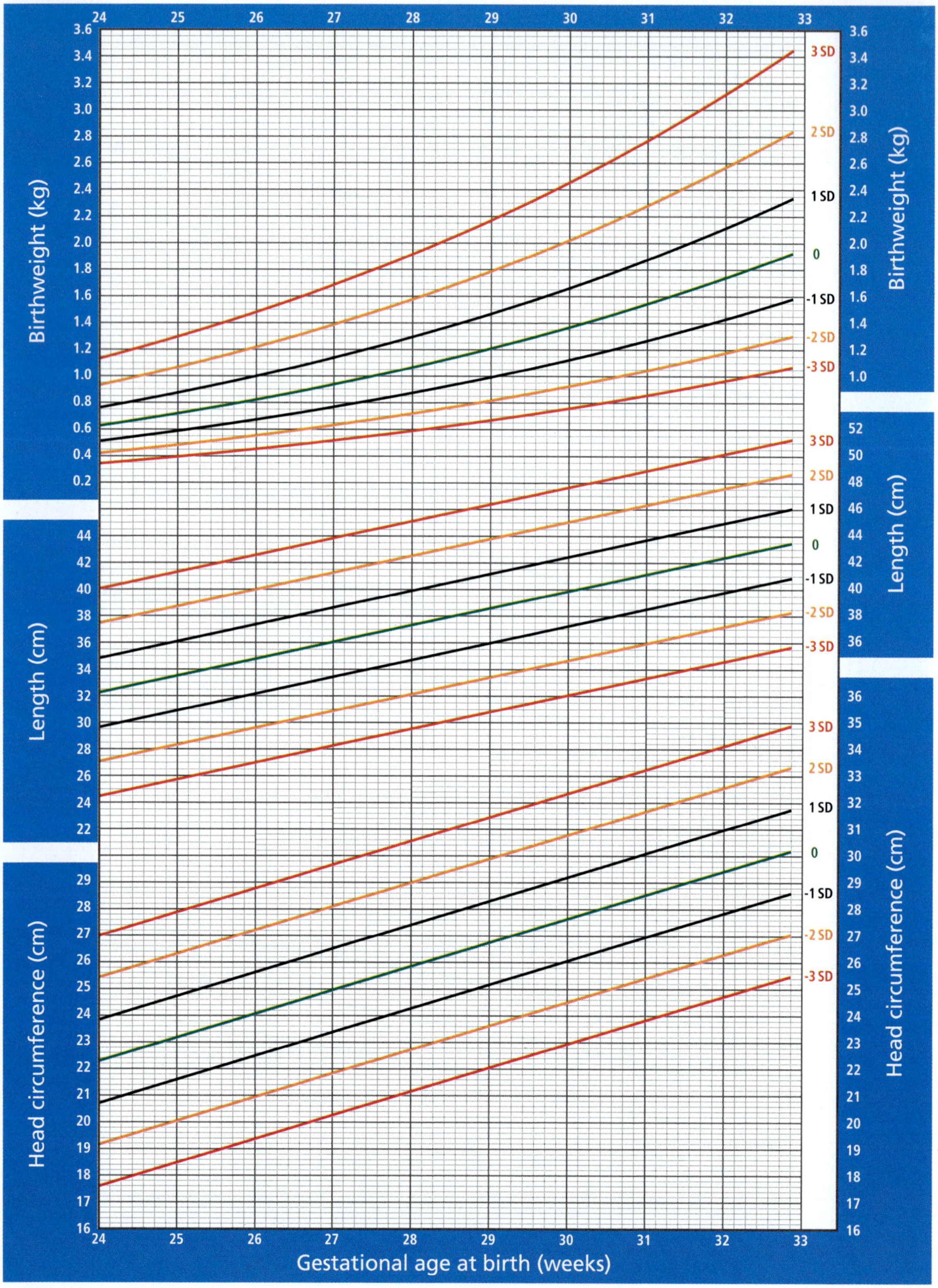

Birthweight (kg)
Length (cm)
Head circumference (cm)
Gestational age at birth (weeks)
24
25
26
27
28
29
30
31
32
33
3 SD
2 SD
1 SD
0
-1 SD
-2 SD
-3 SD

Villar et al. *Lancet* 2016;387:844-5

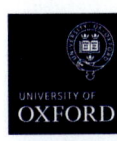

International Newborn Size Standards (Boys)

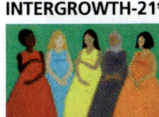

INTERGROWTH-21st

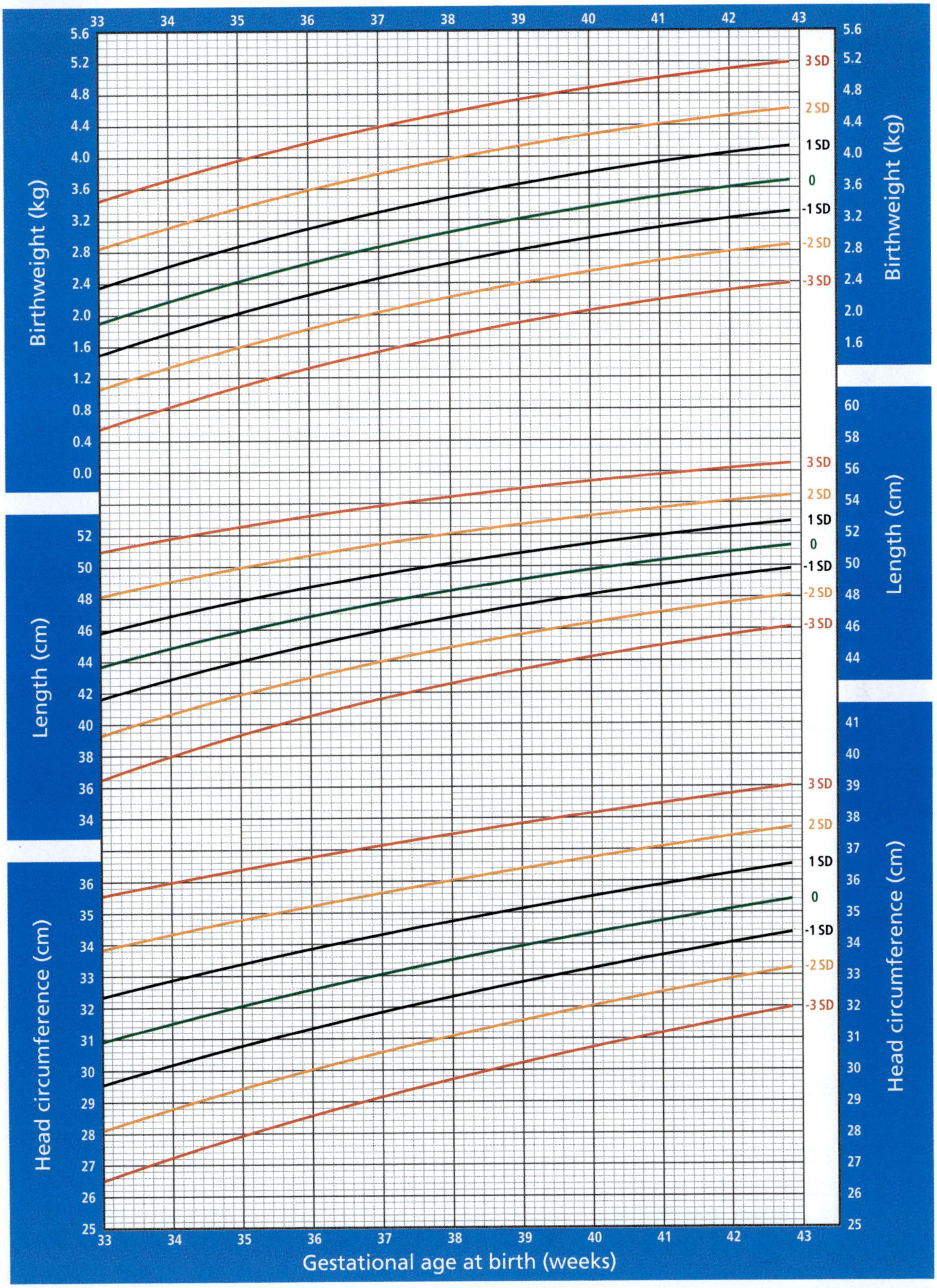

Birthweight (kg)

| 3 SD |
| 2 SD |
| 1 SD |
| 0 |
| -1 SD |
| -2 SD |
| -3 SD |

Length (cm)

| 3 SD |
| 2 SD |
| 1 SD |
| 0 |
| -1 SD |
| -2 SD |
| -3 SD |

Head circumference (cm)

| 3 SD |
| 2 SD |
| 1 SD |
| 0 |
| -1 SD |
| -2 SD |
| -3 SD |

Gestational age at birth (weeks)

Villar et al. *Lancet* 2014;384:857-68

INTERGROWTH-21st

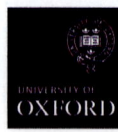

International Newborn Size Reference Charts for Very Preterm Infants (Girls)

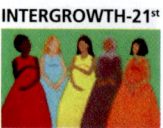

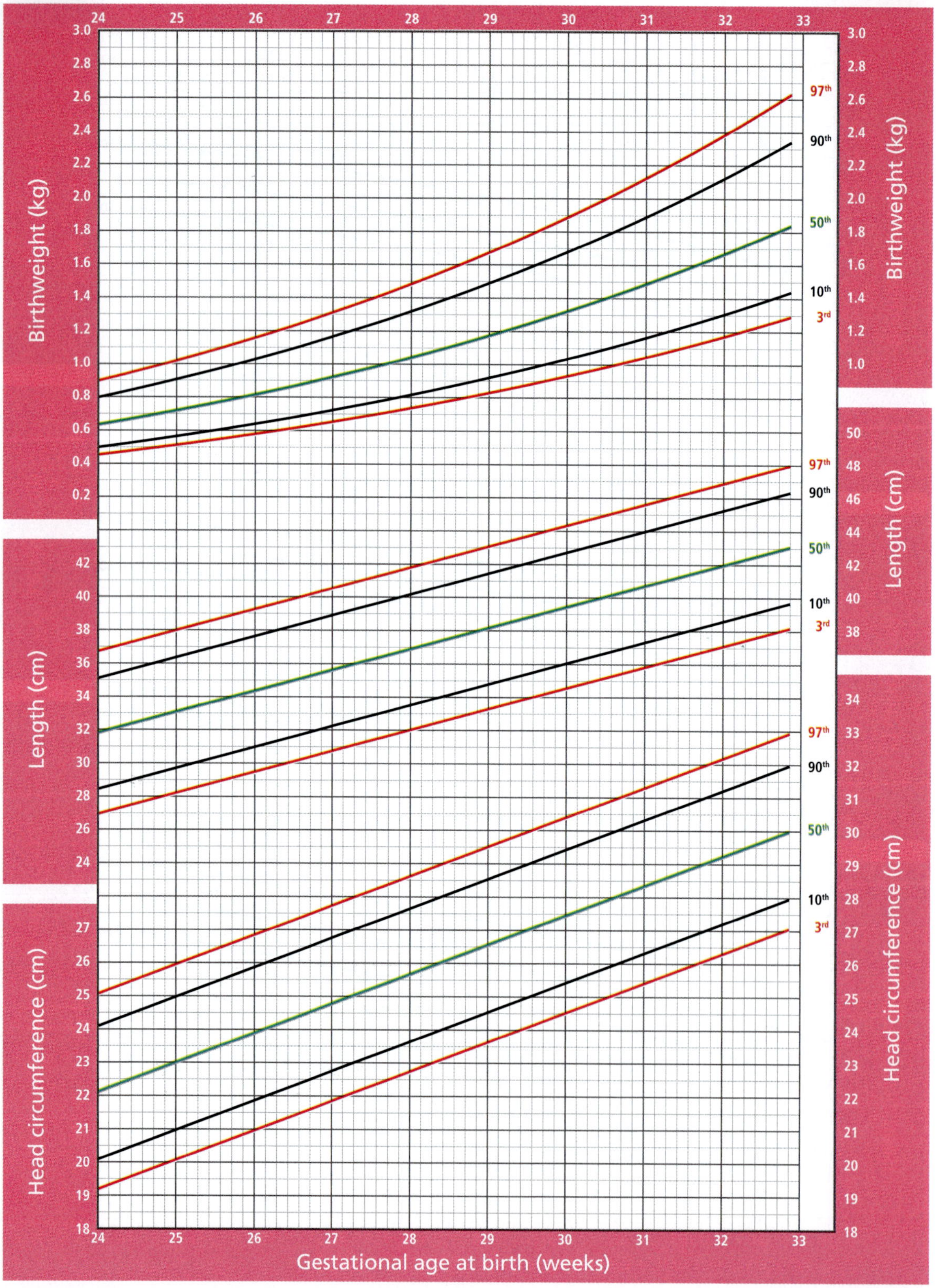
Birthweight (kg)
Length (cm)
Head circumference (cm)
Gestational age at birth (weeks)
24
25
26
27
28
29
30
31
32
33
97th
90th
50th
10th
3rd

Villar et al. *Lancet* 2016;387:844-5

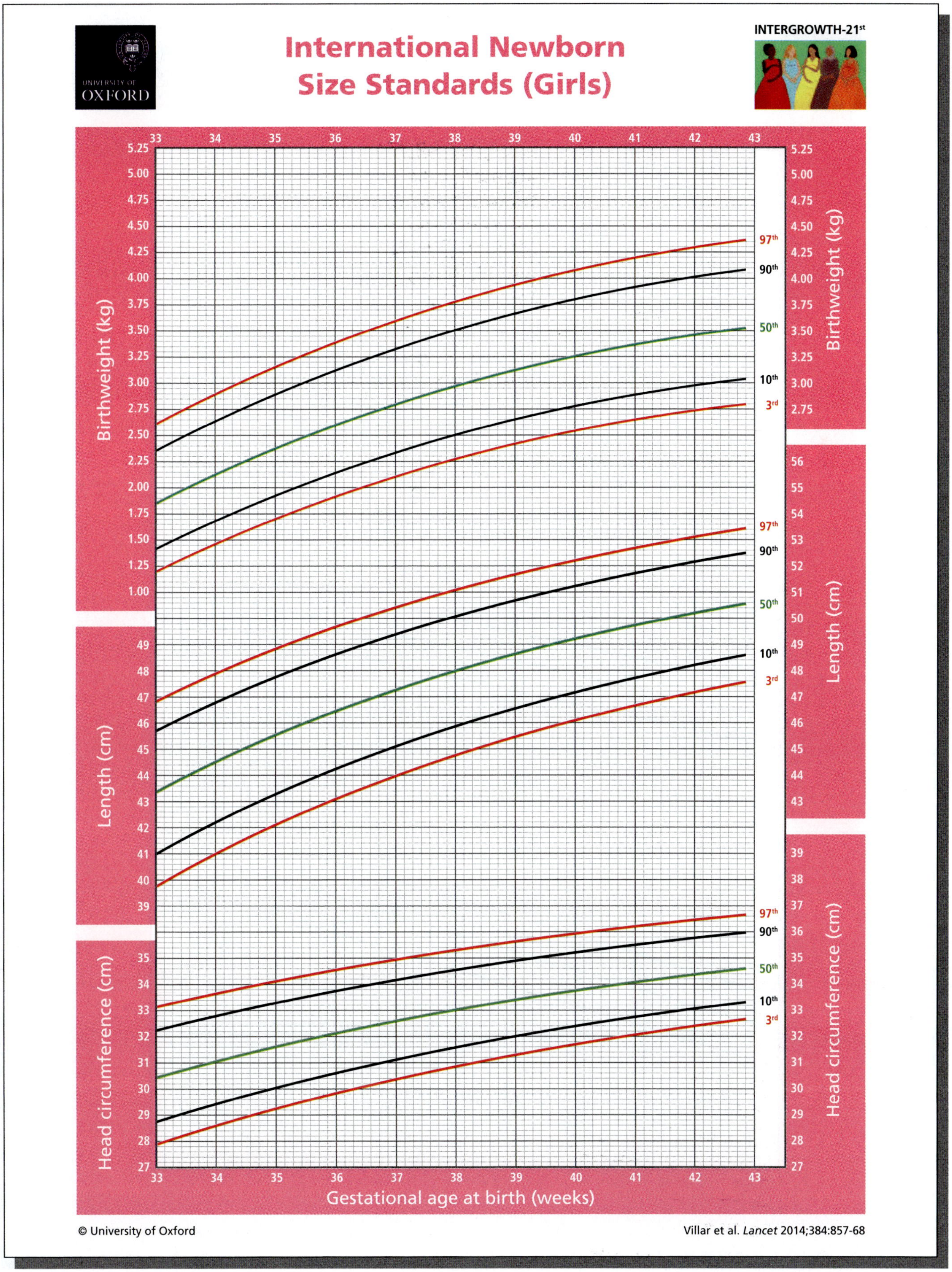

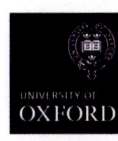

International Newborn Size Standards (Girls)

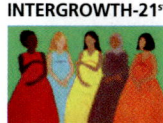

INTERGROWTH-21st

Gestational age at birth (weeks)

Birthweight (kg) — 97th, 90th, 50th, 10th, 3rd

Length (cm) — 97th, 90th, 50th, 10th, 3rd

Head circumference (cm) — 97th, 90th, 50th, 10th, 3rd

Villar et al. *Lancet* 2014;384:857-68

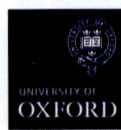

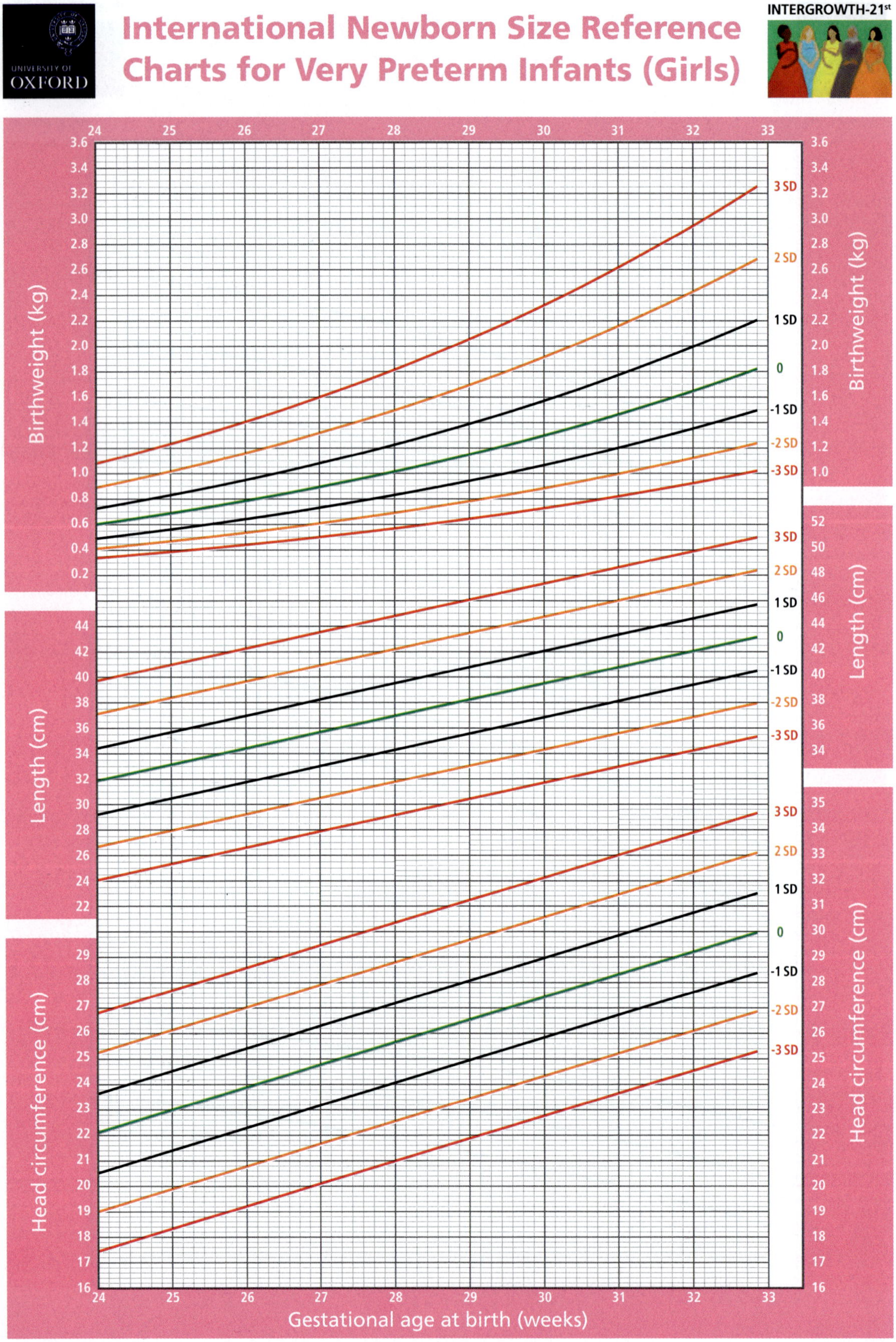
UNIVERSITY OF OXFORD
International Newborn Size Reference Charts for Very Preterm Infants (Girls)
INTERGROWTH-21st
Birthweight (kg)
Length (cm)
Head circumference (cm)
3 SD
2 SD
1 SD
0
-1 SD
-2 SD
-3 SD
Gestational age at birth (weeks)

Villar et al. *Lancet* 2016;387:844-5

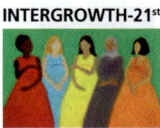

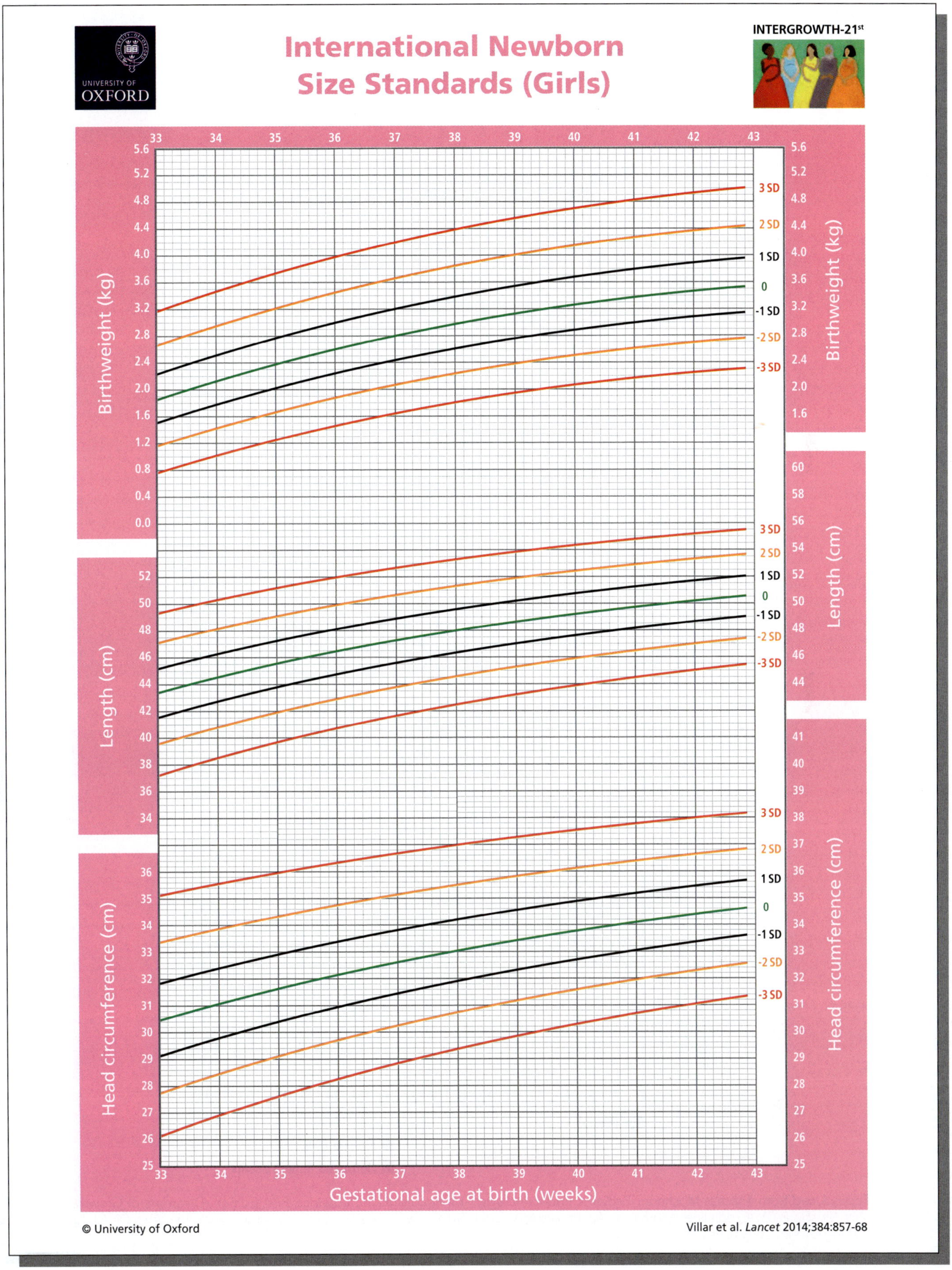

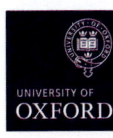

International Newborn Size Standards (Girls)

INTERGROWTH-21st

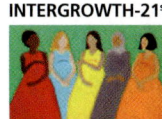

Gestational age at birth (weeks)

Birthweight (kg)

| | 3 SD |
| 2 SD |
| 1 SD |
| 0 |
| -1 SD |
| -2 SD |
| -3 SD |

Length (cm)

| 3 SD |
| 2 SD |
| 1 SD |
| 0 |
| -1 SD |
| -2 SD |
| -3 SD |

Head circumference (cm)

| 3 SD |
| 2 SD |
| 1 SD |
| 0 |
| -1 SD |
| -2 SD |
| -3 SD |

Villar et al. *Lancet* 2014;384:857-68

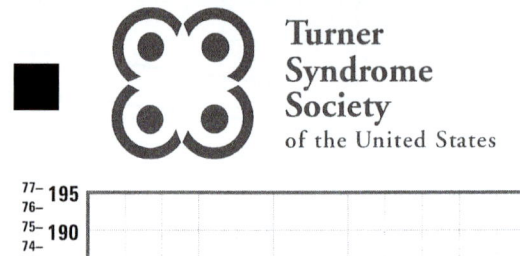

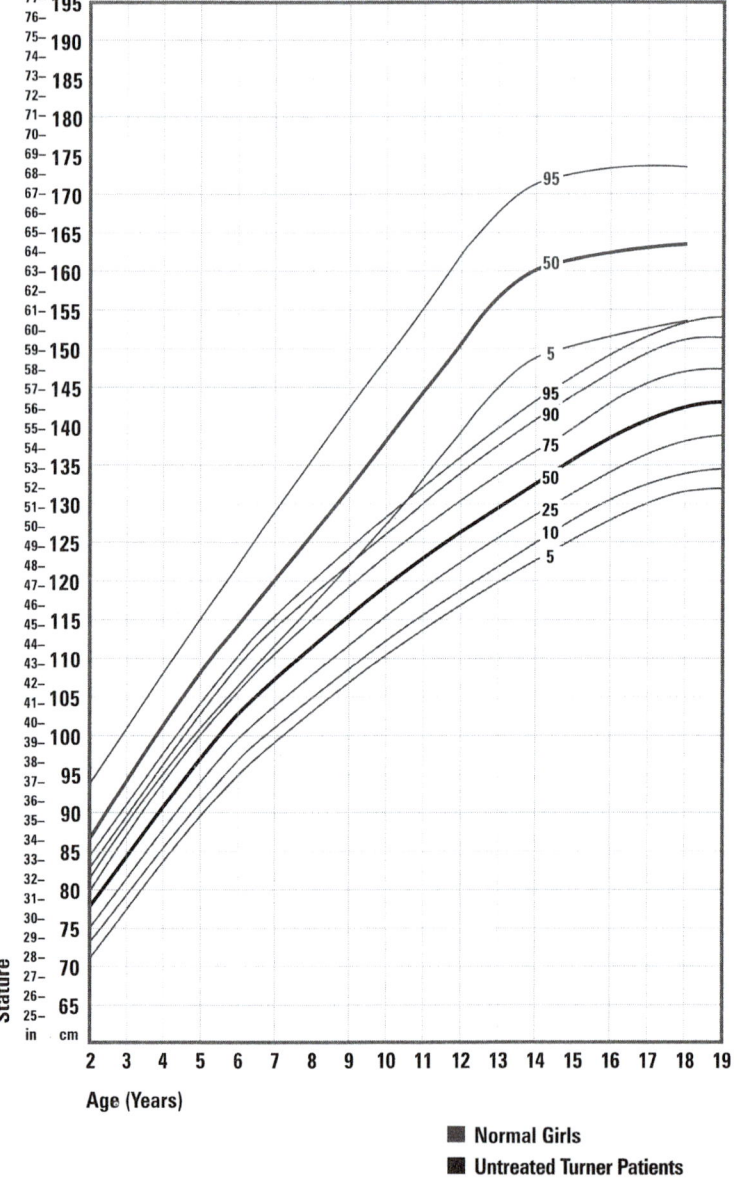

Turner Growth Chart

Source: Reproduced from Thomas Moshang. *Pediatric Endocrinology: The Requisites in Pediatrics,* First Edition, Disorders of Growth, Figure 8-11, Philadelphia, Mosby, 2005. (Credit line - From Lyon AJ, Preece MA, Grant DB: Growth curve for girls with Turner syndrome. Arch Dis Child 1985;60:932, BMJ Publishing Group, copyright 1985.).

ACHONDROPLASIA—HEIGHT, MALES

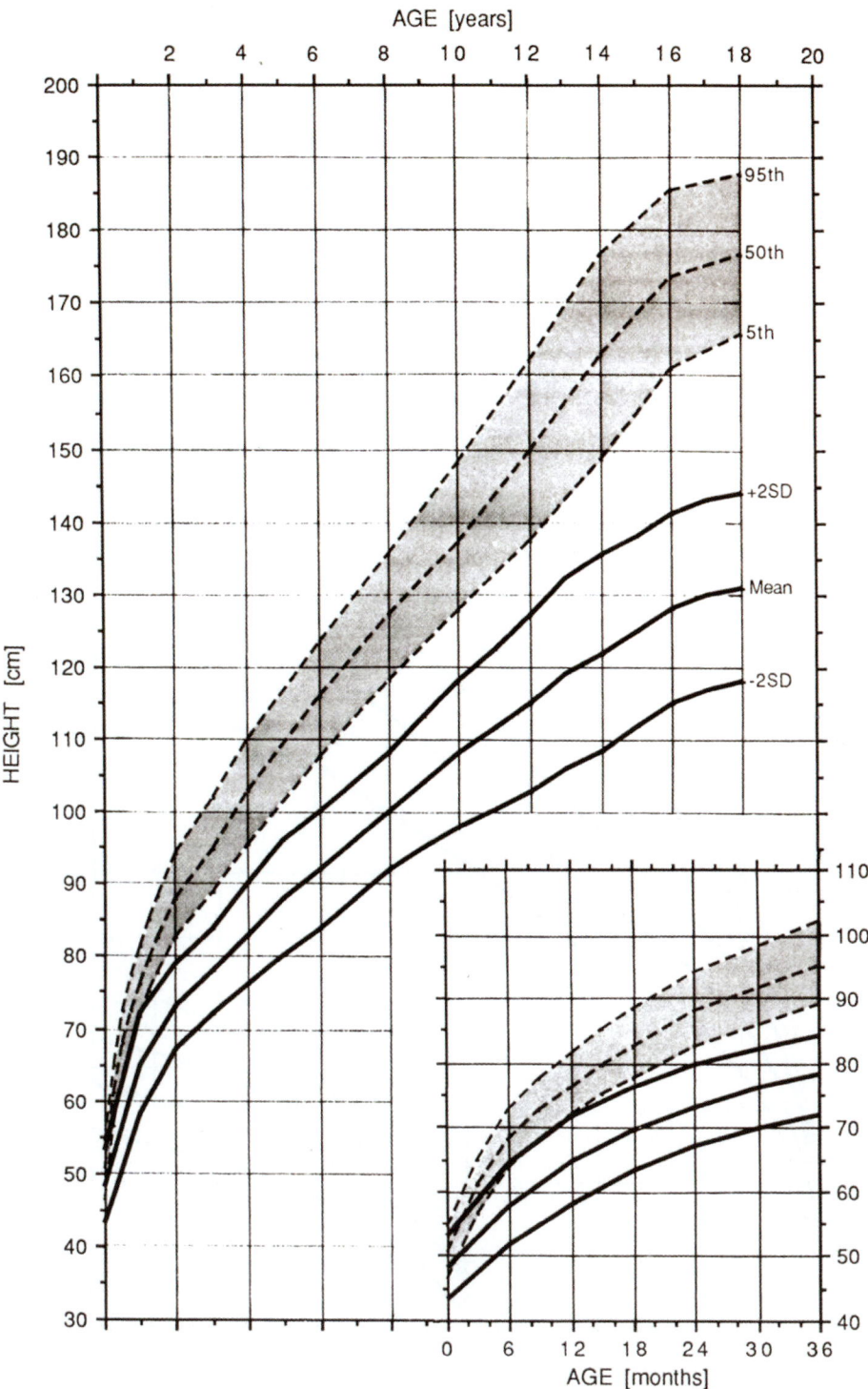

Height for males with achondroplasia (mean ± 2 S.D.) compared to normal standard curves. Graph derived from 189 males. Horton WA et al: J Pediatr 93:435, 1978.

ACHONDROPLASIA–HEIGHT, FEMALES

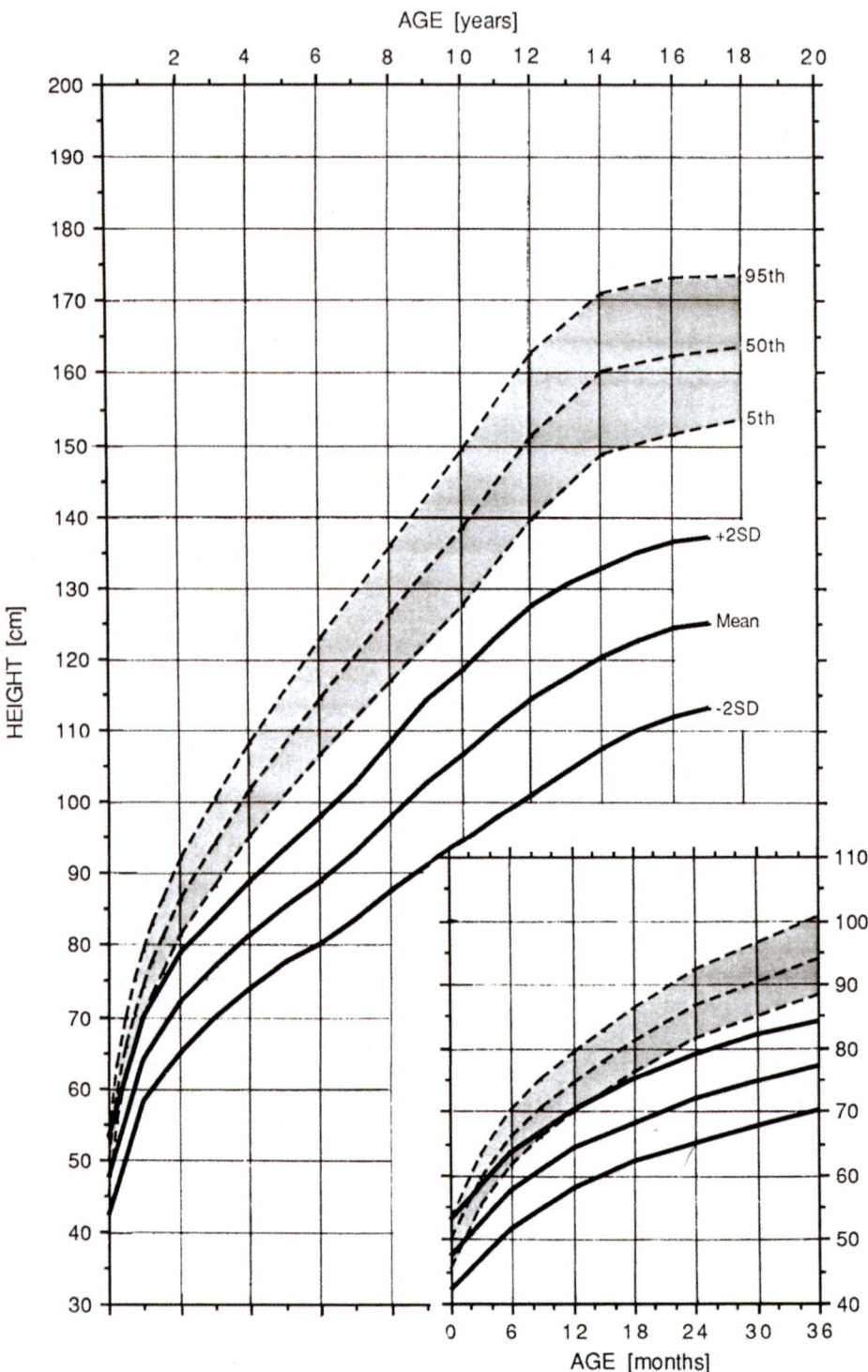

Height for females with achondroplasia (mean ± 2 S.D.) compared to normal standard curves. Graph derived from 214 females.
Horton WA et al: J Pediatr 93:435, 1978.

Growth Charts for Children with Down Syndrome
Birth to 36 months: Boys
Head circumference-for-age percentiles

Name _____

Record _____

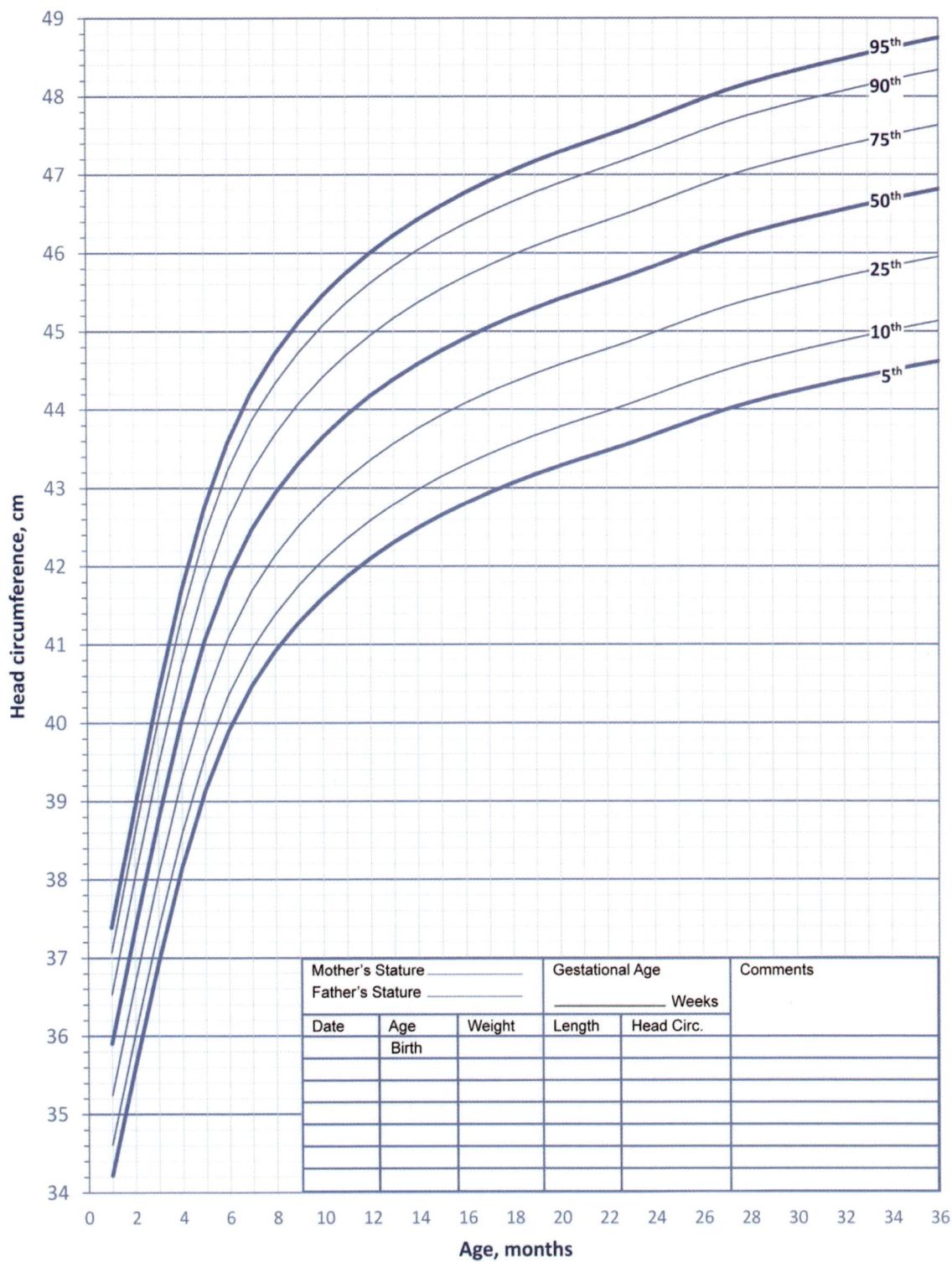

Published October 2015.
Source: Zemel BS, Pipan M, Stallings VA, Hall W, Schgadt K, Freedman DS, Thorpe P. Growth Charts for Children with Down Syndrome in the U.S. Pediatrics, 2015.
CS260242-A

Growth Charts for Children with Down Syndrome
Birth to 36 months: Boys
Length-for-age percentiles

Name _____

Record _____

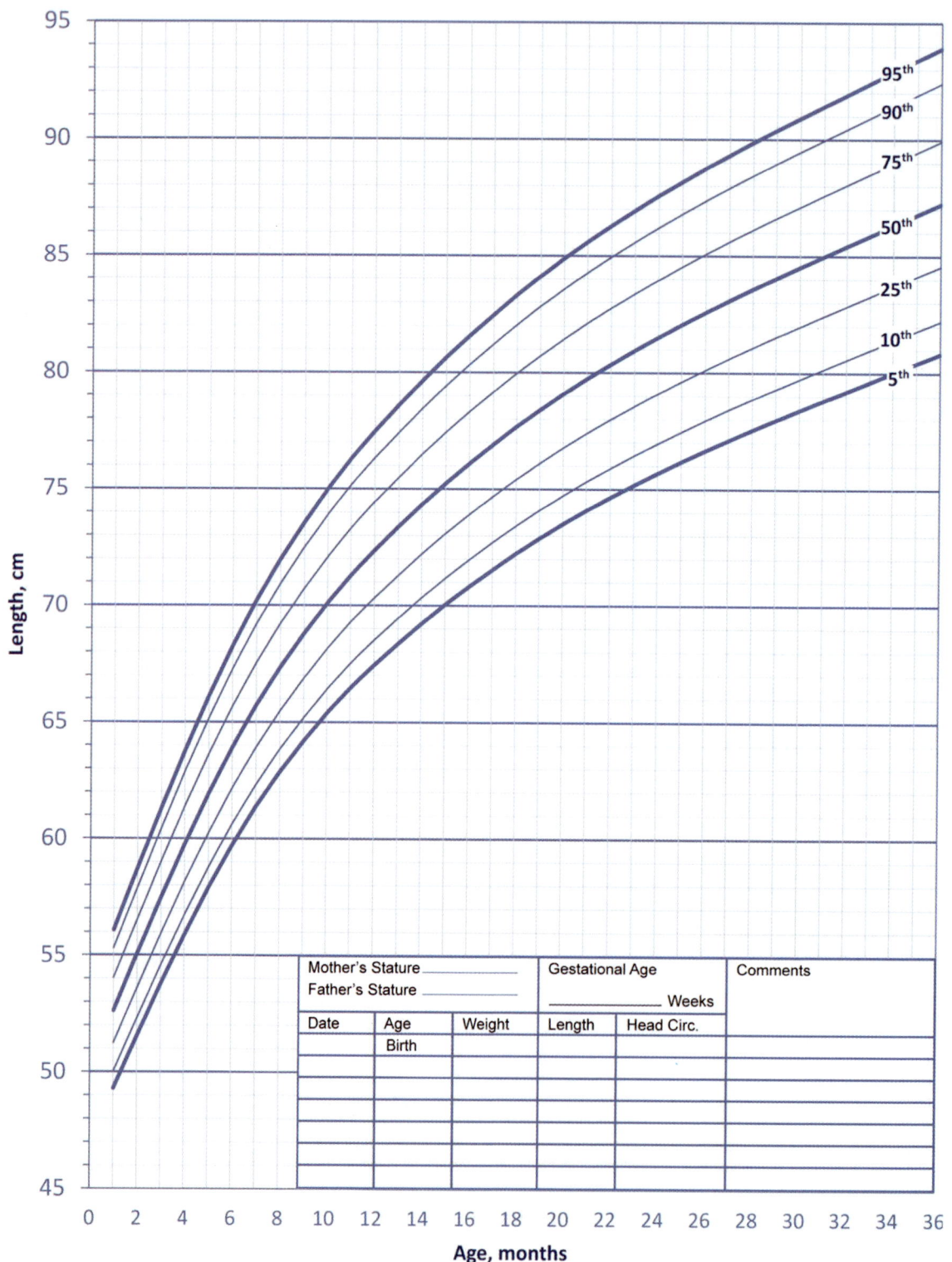

Published October 2015.
Source: Zemel BS, Pipan M, Stallings VA, Hall W, Schgadt K, Freedman DS, Thorpe P. Growth Charts for Children with Down Syndrome in the U.S. Pediatrics, 2015.
CS260242-A

Growth Charts for Children with Down Syndrome
0 to 36 months: Boys
Weight-for-length percentiles

Name _____

Record _____

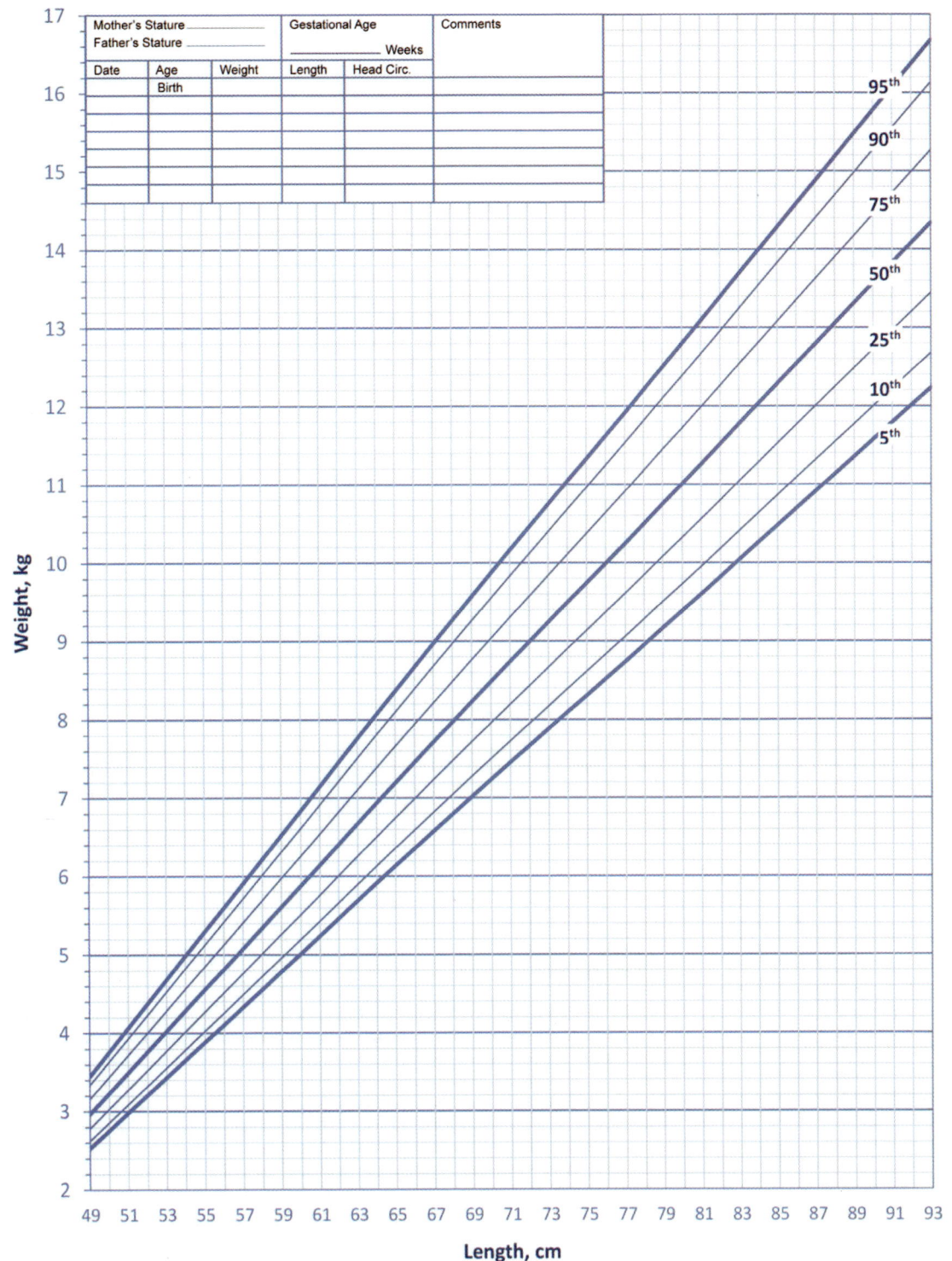

Published October 2015.
Source: Zemel BS, Pipan M, Stallings VA, Hall W, Schgadt K, Freedman DS, Thorpe P. Growth Charts for Children with Down Syndrome in the U.S. Pediatrics, 2015.
CS260242-A

Growth Charts for Children with Down Syndrome
Birth to 36 months: Boys
Weight-for-age percentiles

Name _____

Record _____

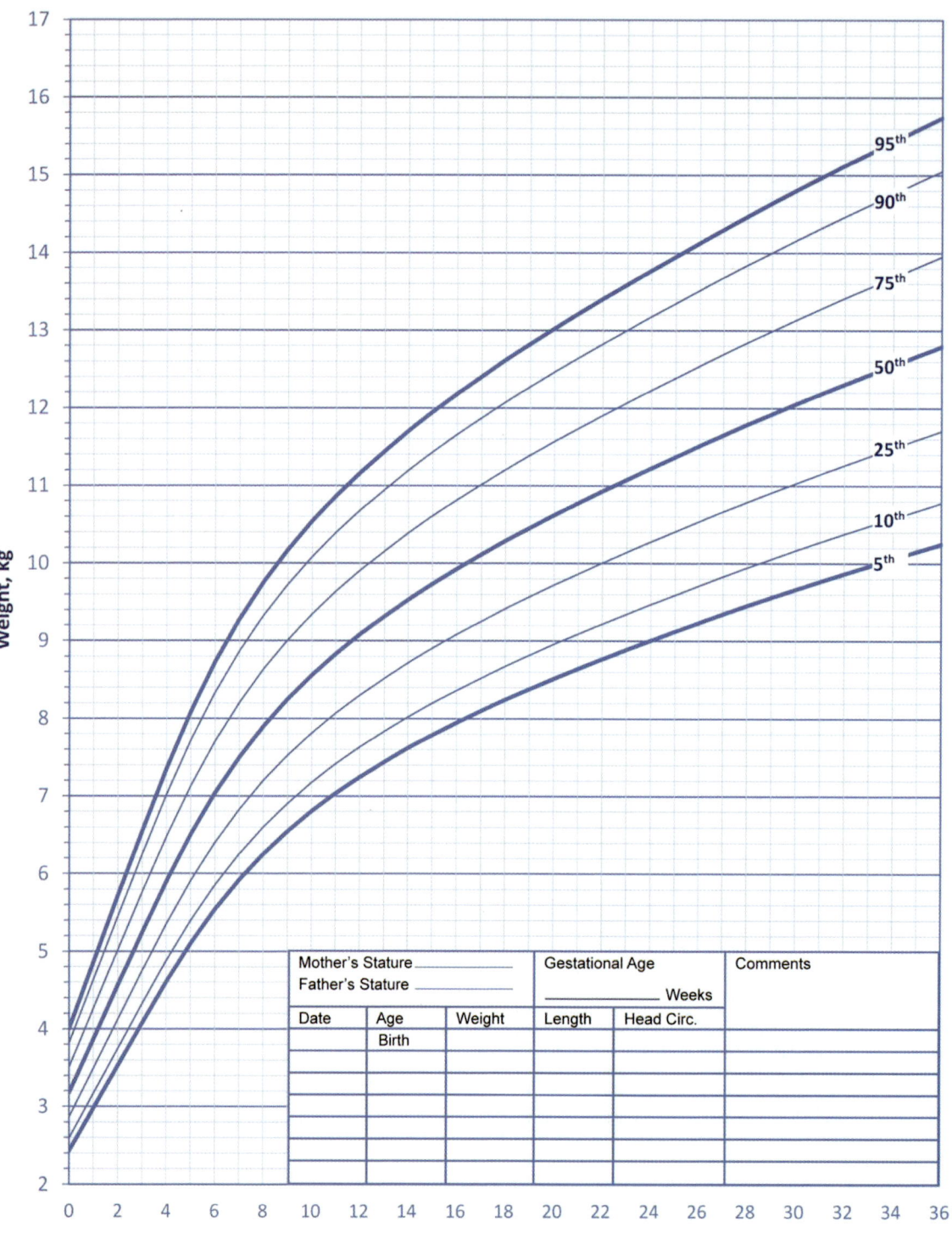

Published October 2015.
Source: Zemel BS, Pipan M, Stallings VA, Hall W, Schgadt K, Freedman DS, Thorpe P. Growth Charts for Children with Down Syndrome in the U.S. Pediatrics, 2015.
CS260242-A

Growth Charts for Children with Down Syndrome
2 to 20 years: Boys
Head circumference-for-age percentiles

Name _____

Record _____

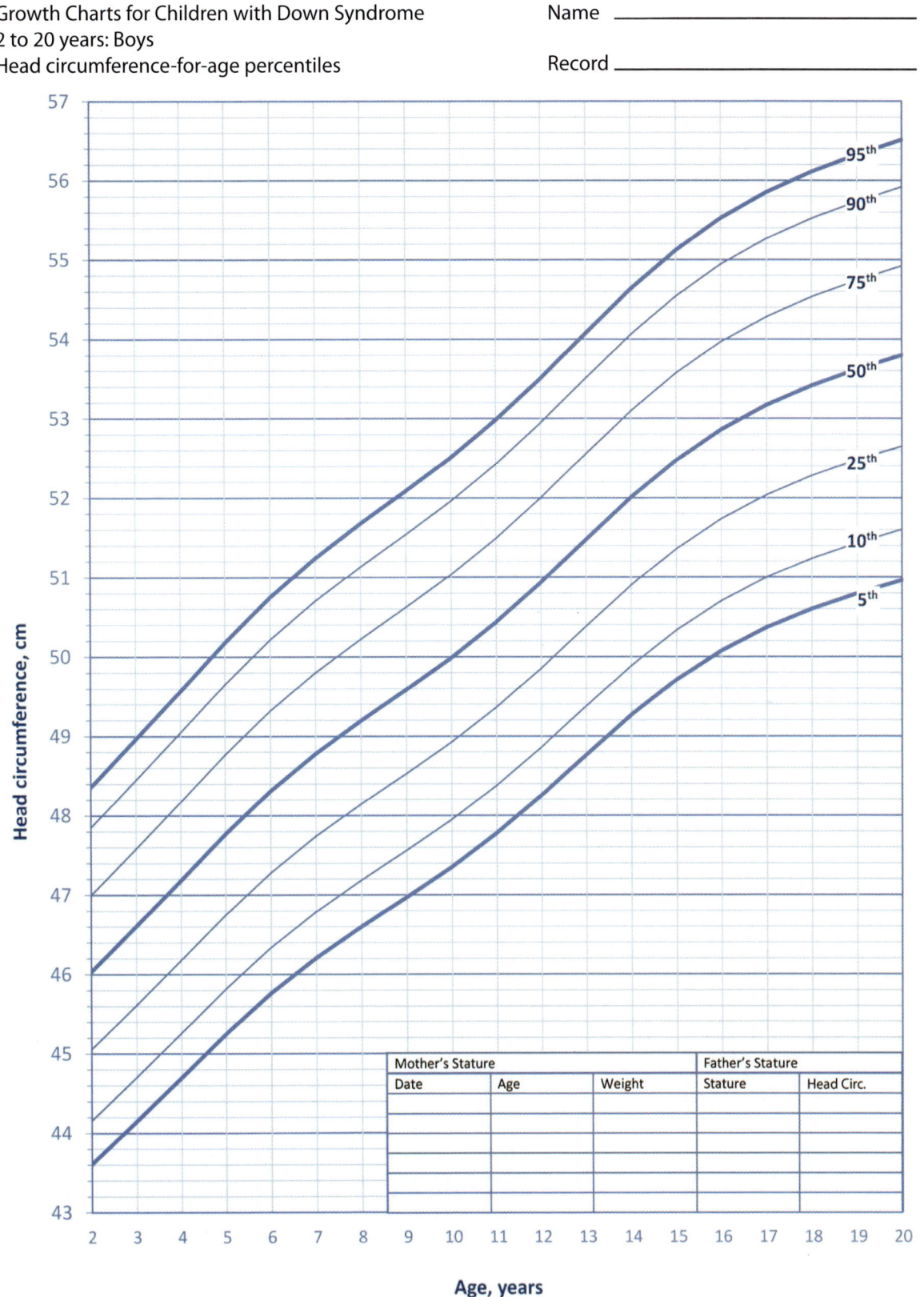

Mother's Stature			Father's Stature	
Date	Age	Weight	Stature	Head Circ.

Age, years

Published October 2015.
Source: Zemel BS, Pipan M, Stallings VA, Hall W, Schgadt K, Freedman DS, Thorpe P. Growth Charts for Children with Down Syndrome in the U.S. Pediatrics, 2015.
CS260242-A

Growth Charts for Children with Down Syndrome
2 to 20 years: Boys
Height-for-age percentiles

Name _____

Record _____

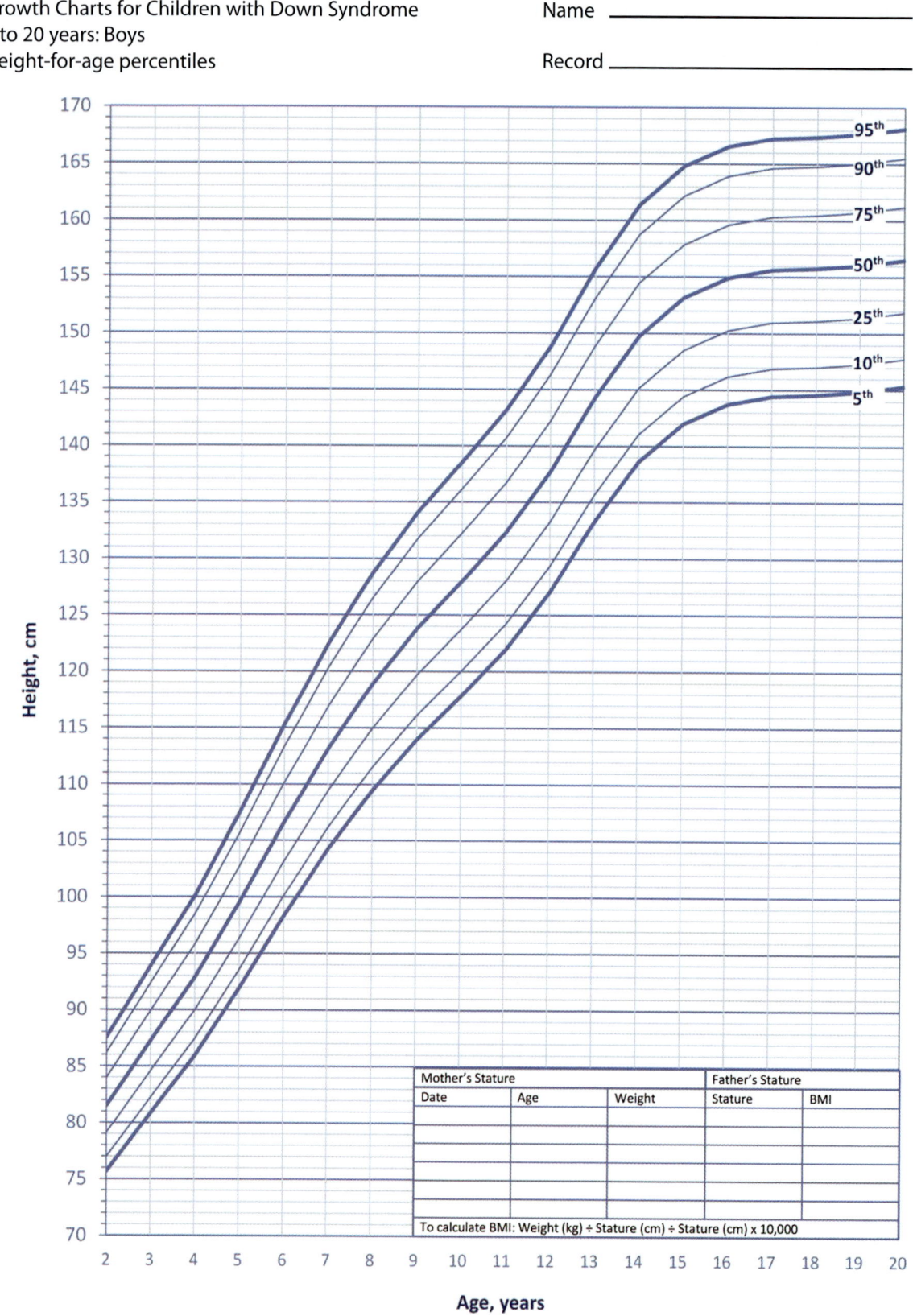

Published October 2015.
Source: Zemel BS, Pipan M, Stallings VA, Hall W, Schgadt K, Freedman DS, Thorpe P. Growth Charts for Children with Down Syndrome in the U.S. Pediatrics, 2015.

CS260242-A

Growth Charts for Children with Down Syndrome
2 to 20 years: Boys
Weight-for-age percentiles

Name _____

Record _____

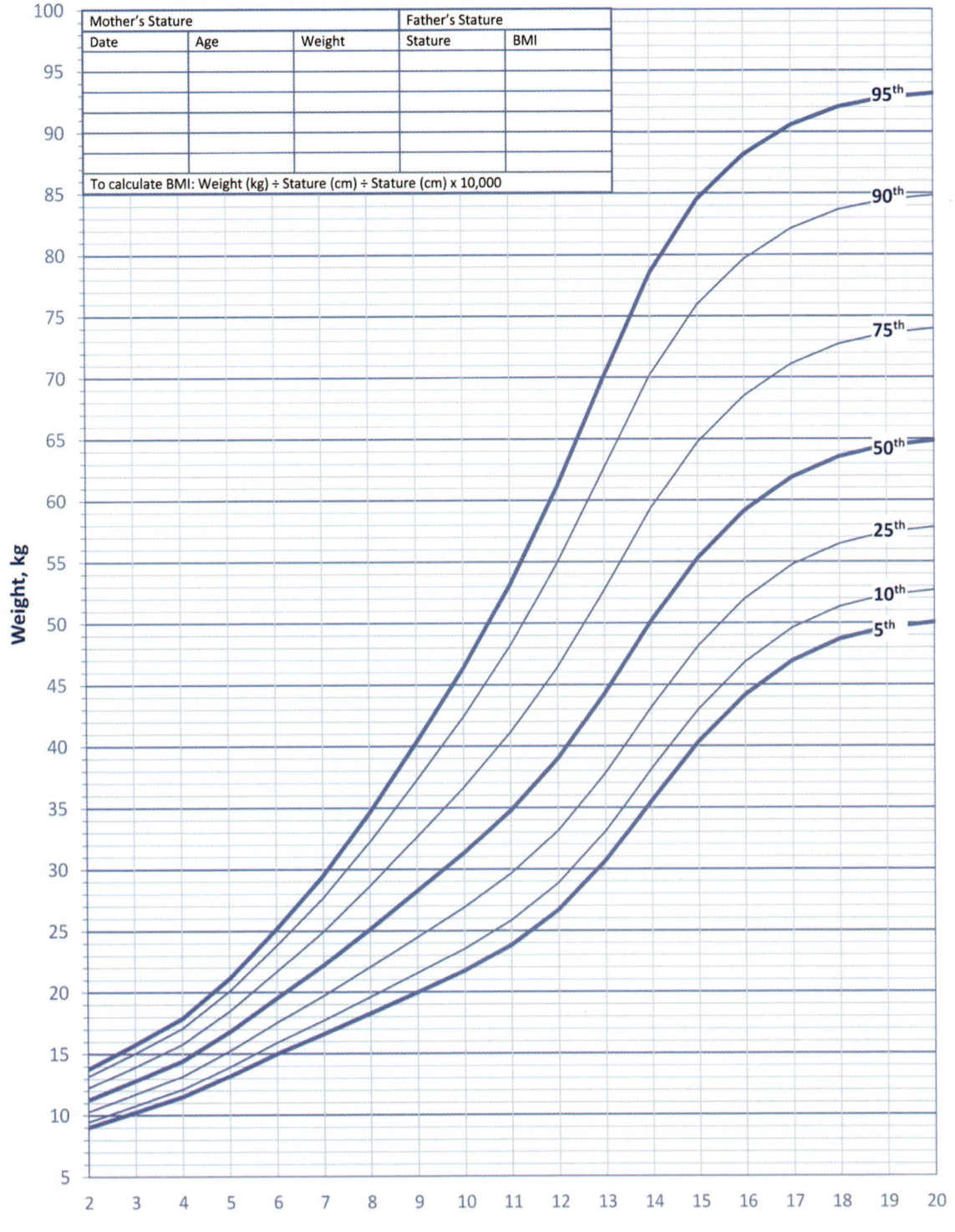

Mother's Stature			Father's Stature	
Date	Age	Weight	Stature	BMI
To calculate BMI: Weight (kg) ÷ Stature (cm) ÷ Stature (cm) x 10,000				

Weight, kg

Age, years

Published October 2015.
Source: Zemel BS, Pipan M, Stallings VA, Hall W, Schgadt K, Freedman DS, Thorpe P. Growth Charts for Children with Down Syndrome in the U.S. Pediatrics, 2015.

CS260242-A

Growth Charts for Children with Down Syndrome
Birth to 36 months: Girls
Head circumference-for-age percentiles

Name _____

Record _____

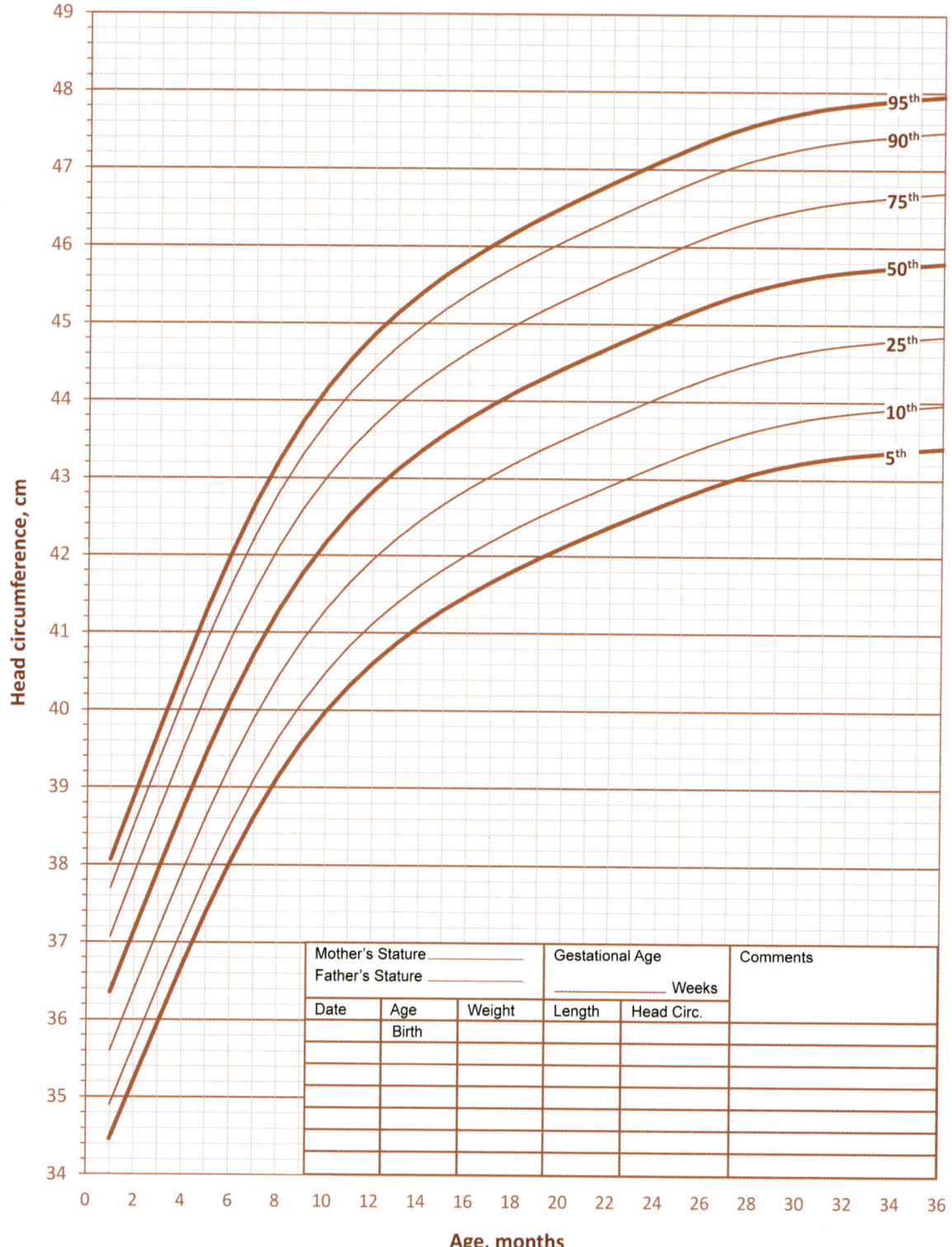

Published October 2015.
Source: Zemel BS, Pipan M, Stallings VA, Hall W, Schgadt K, Freedman DS, Thorpe P. Growth Charts for Children with Down Syndrome in the U.S. Pediatrics, 2015.

CS260242-B

Growth Charts for Children with Down Syndrome
Birth to 36 months: Girls
Length-for-age percentiles

Name _____

Record _____

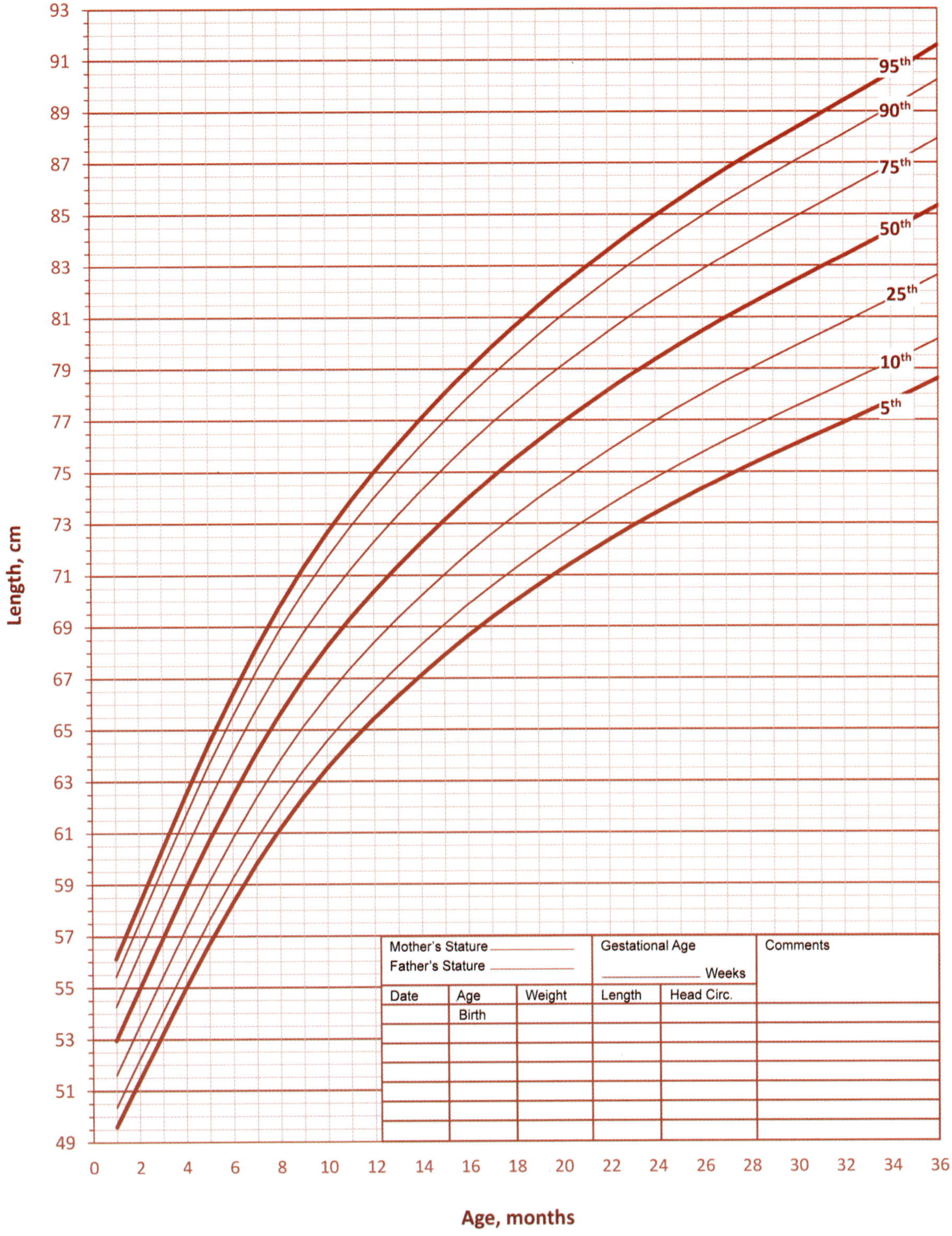

Length, cm

93
91
89
87
85
83
81
79
77
75
73
71
69
67
65
63
61
59
57
55
53
51
49

95th
90th
75th
50th
25th
10th
5th

Age, months

0 2 4 6 8 10 12 14 16 18 20 22 24 26 28 30 32 34 36

| Mother's Stature _____ | Gestational Age _____ Weeks | Comments |
| Father's Stature _____ | | |

Date	Age	Weight	Length	Head Circ.	
	Birth				

Published October 2015.
Source: Zemel BS, Pipan M, Stallings VA, Hall W, Schgadt K, Freedman DS, Thorpe P. Growth Charts for Children with Down Syndrome in the U.S. Pediatrics, 2015.

CS260242-B

Growth Charts for Children with Down Syndrome
0 to 36 months: Girls
Weight-for-length percentiles

Name _____

Record _____

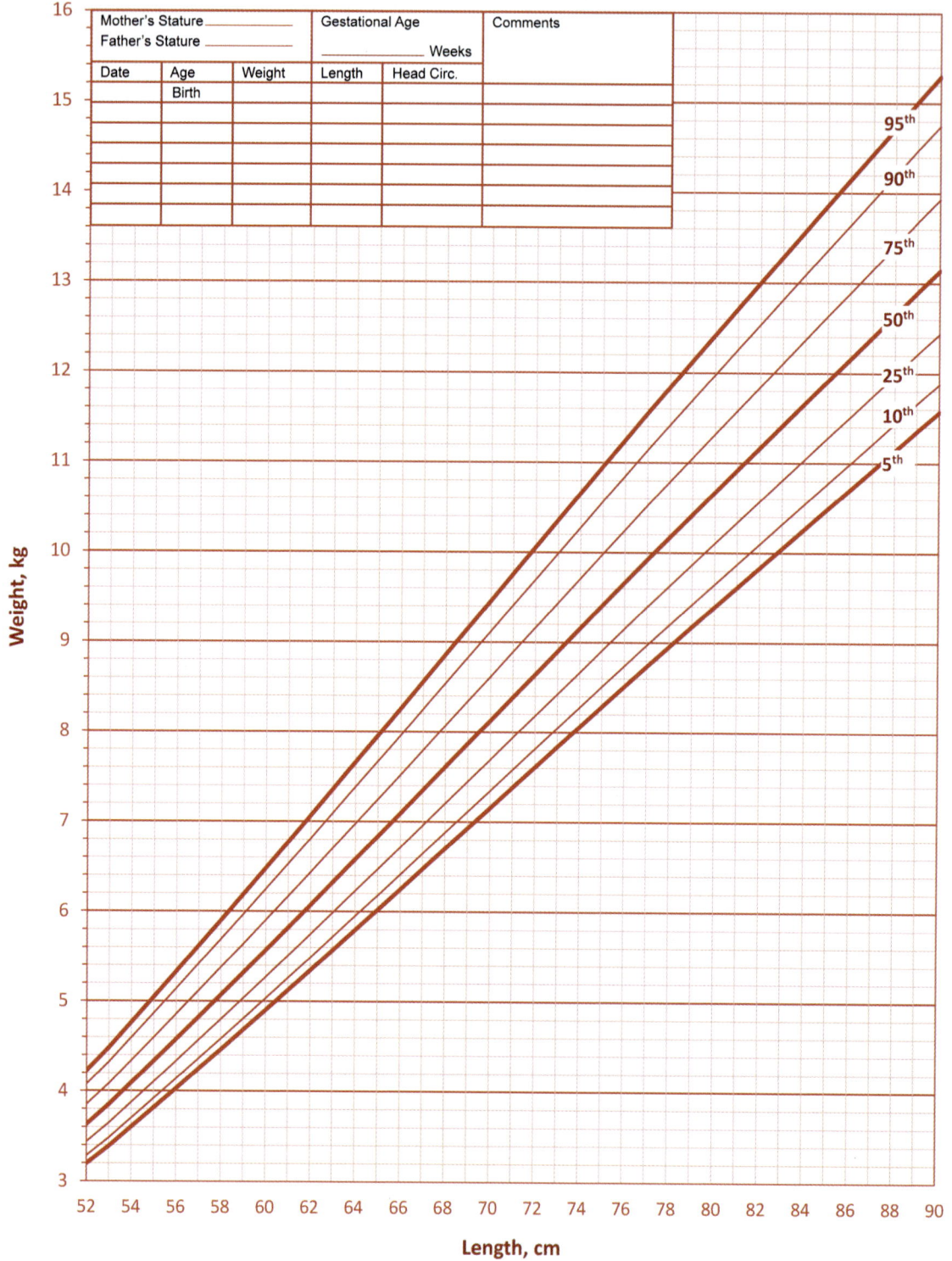

Mother's Stature _____			Gestational Age		Comments	
Father's Stature _____			_____ Weeks			
Date	Age	Weight	Length	Head Circ.		
	Birth					

95th
90th
75th
50th
25th
10th
5th

Weight, kg

Length, cm

Published October 2015.
Source: Zemel BS, Pipan M, Stallings VA, Hall W, Schgadt K, Freedman DS, Thorpe P. Growth Charts for Children with Down Syndrome in the U.S. Pediatrics, 2015.

CS260242-B

Growth Charts for Children with Down Syndrome
Birth to 36 months: Girls
Weight-for-age percentiles

Name _____

Record _____

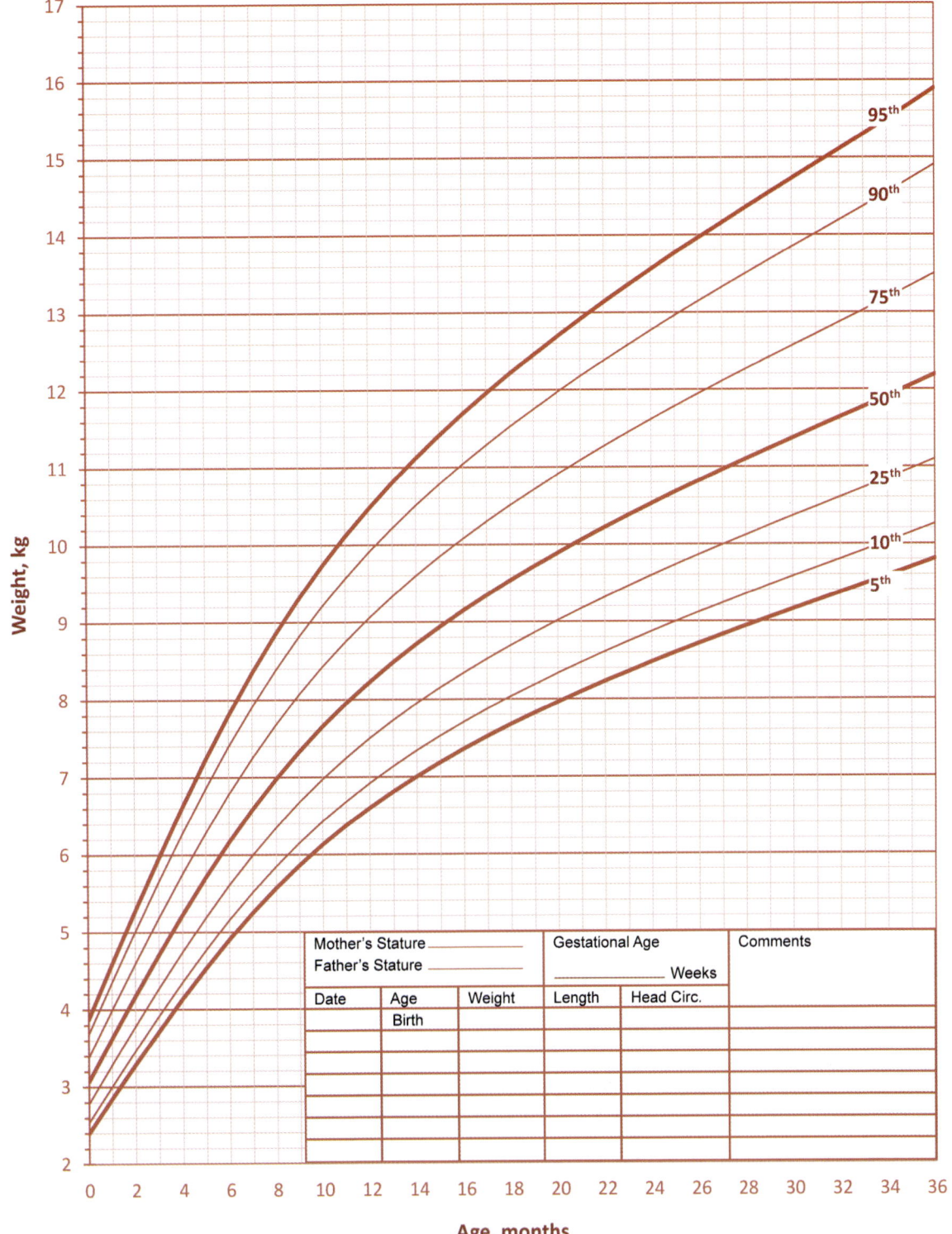

Published October 2015.
Source: Zemel BS, Pipan M, Stallings VA, Hall W, Schgadt K, Freedman DS, Thorpe P. Growth Charts for Children with Down Syndrome in the U.S. Pediatrics, 2015.

CS260242-B

Growth Charts for Children with Down Syndrome
2 to 20 years: Girls
Head circumference-for-age percentiles

Name —————————————

Record —————————————

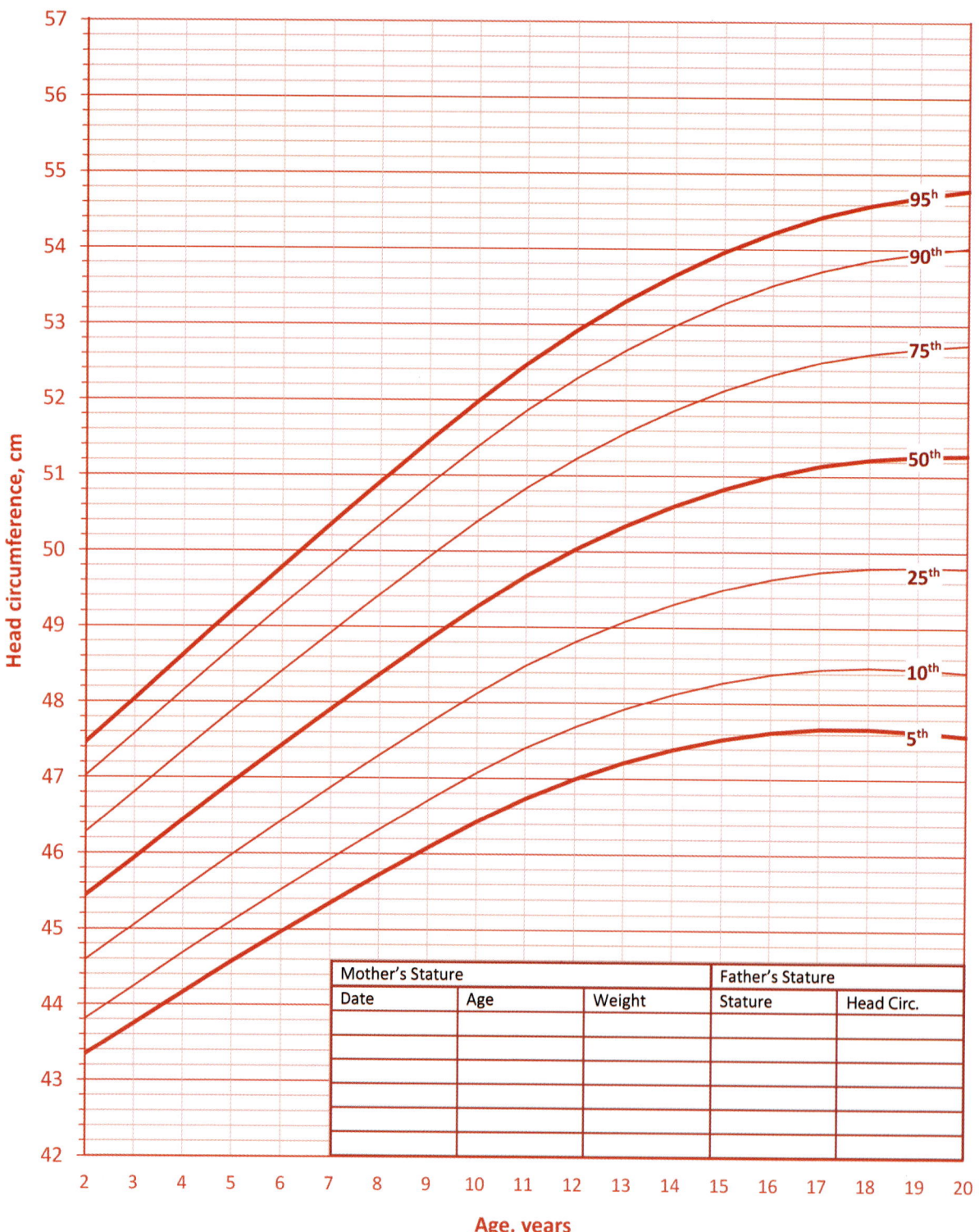

Published October 2015.
Source: Zemel BS, Pipan M, Stallings VA, Hall W, Schgadt K, Freedman DS, Thorpe P. Growth Charts for Children with Down Syndrome in the U.S. Pediatrics, 2015.

CS260242-B

Growth Charts for Children with Down Syndrome
2 to 20 years: Girls
Height-for-age percentiles

Name _____

Record _____

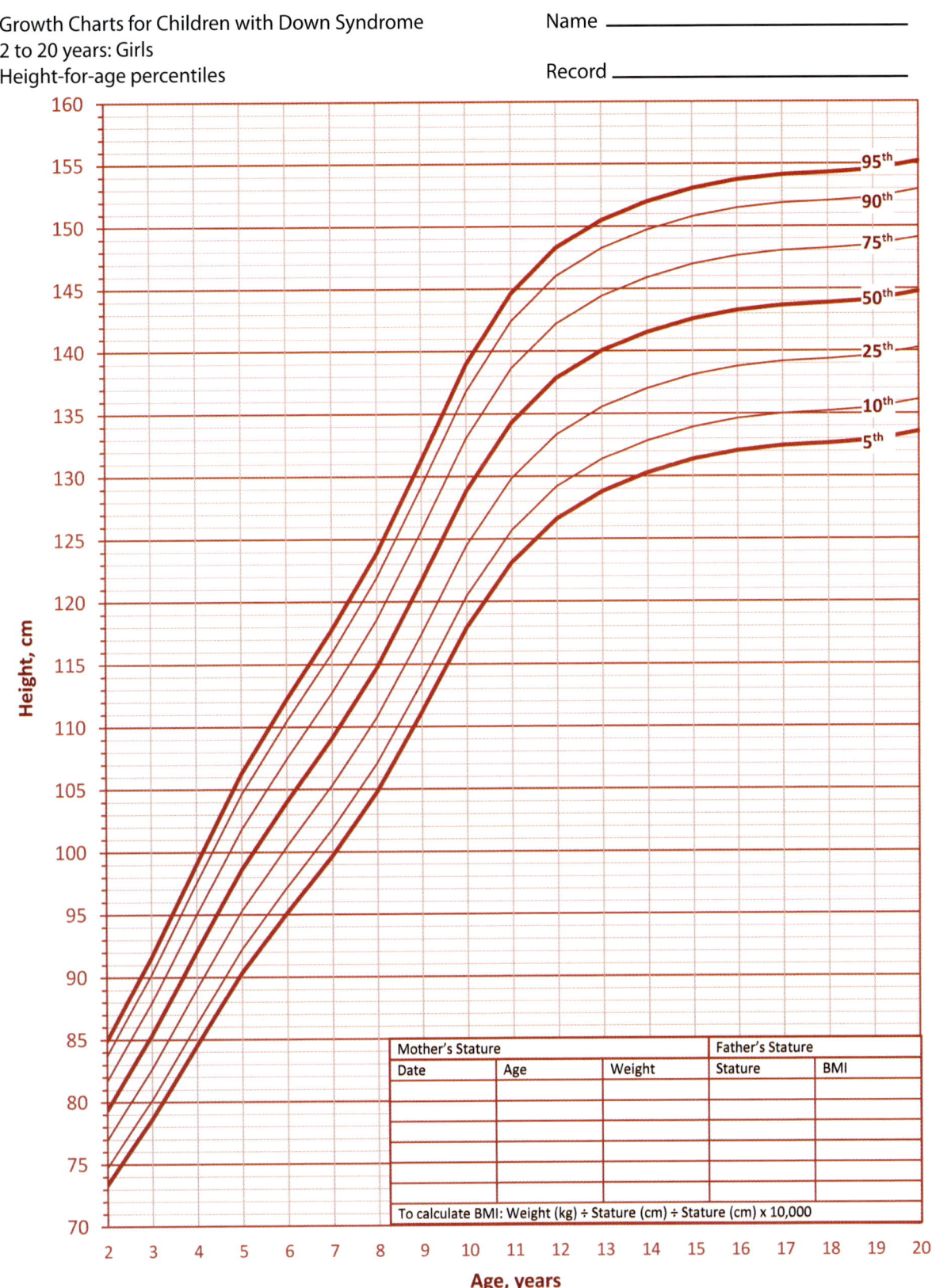

To calculate BMI: Weight (kg) ÷ Stature (cm) ÷ Stature (cm) x 10,000

Published October 2015.
Source: Zemel BS, Pipan M, Stallings VA, Hall W, Schgadt K, Freedman DS, Thorpe P. Growth Charts for Children with Down Syndrome in the U.S. Pediatrics, 2015.
CS260242-B

Growth Charts for Children with Down Syndrome
2 to 20 years: Girls
Weight-for-age percentiles

Name _____

Record _____

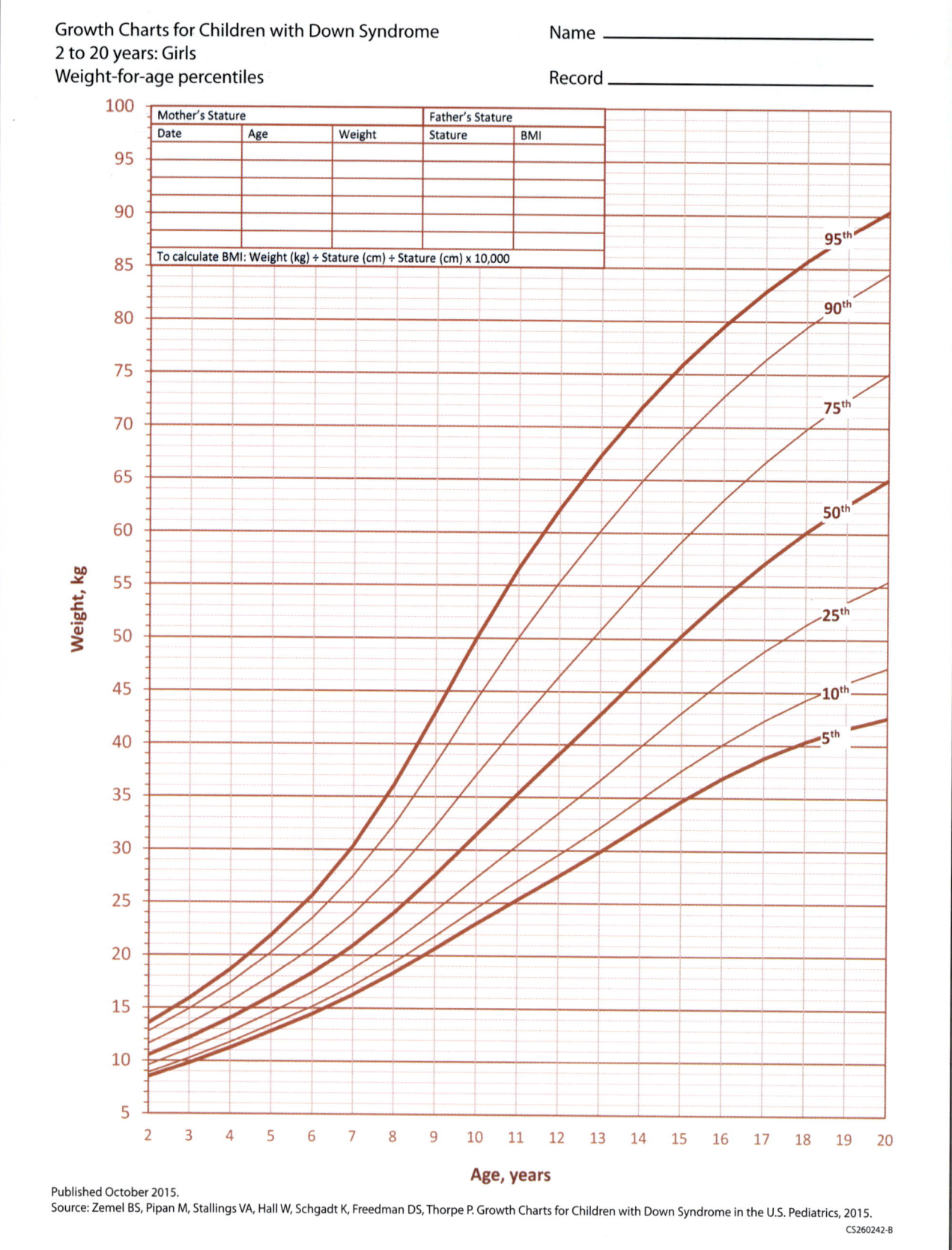

Published October 2015.
Source: Zemel BS, Pipan M, Stallings VA, Hall W, Schgadt K, Freedman DS, Thorpe P. Growth Charts for Children with Down Syndrome in the U.S. Pediatrics, 2015.

CS260242-B

Further reading: Growth chart for Children with Cerebral palsy https://www.lifeexpectancy.org/articles/GrowthCharts.shtml

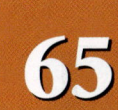

65

RDA Reference Chart for Indian Children

Age	Energy (kcal/day)	Protein (g/dl)	Calcium (mg/dl)	Magnesium (mg/dl)	Iron (mg/dl)	Iodine (micg/dl)	Zinc (mg/dl)	Folate (micg/dl)	VitB12 (micg/dl)	Vit C (mg/dl)	Vit A	Vit D (IU/d)
Infants												
0–6 months	92 kcal/ kg/day	1.16 g/ kg/day	500	–	–	–	–	25	0.2	25	–	400
6–12 months	80 kcal/ kg/day	1.69 g/ kg/day	600	–	2	130	2	71	1	25	170	400
1–3 years	960	16.7	600	73	6	65	2.8	97	1	24	180	400
4–6 years	1200	20.1	600	104	8	80	3.7	111	1	27	240	400
7–9 years	1680	29.5	600	144	10	80	4.9	142	2	36	290	400
10–12 years												
Boys	2220	27	800	199	12	100	7	180	2	45	360	400
Girls	2060	27	800	207	16	100	7	186	2	44	370	400

| TABLE 65.2 | **Acceptable Macronutrients Distribution Range by Age and Physiological Group as Percent of Energy (%E)** |

AGE GROUP			
Nutrients	1-2 Years	3-18 Years	Pregnant Ad Lactating Mother
Protein energy (PE ratio)	5–15	5–15	5–15
Total Fat	30–40	25–35	20–35
Carbohydrate	40–60	45–65	45–65

| TABLE 65.3 | **Summary of Recommended Intakes of Minerals and Trace Elements** |

Mineral/Trace Elements	Recommended Intake Per Day
Phosphorous	800-1000 mg/day
Sodium	2000 mg/dl
Potassium	3500 mg/dl
Copper	2 mg
Chromium	10 mg
Selenium	100 mg
Fluoride	1-5 mg
Molybdenum	200-500 mg

Tips for Students

Checklist for Practical Examination

PRE-EXAMINATION CHECKLIST

Ballard scoring
BP chart
Calory chart
Color object or wool
Cotton (ear buds)
Crayons/notebook/colorbook
Growth charts: Intergrowth preterm growth charts; WHO (0–5 years)
  – weight, height, head circumference, weight-for-height charts;
  IAP (Indian Academy of Pediatrics) – 5–18 years weight, height,
  BMI charts
Knee hammer
Log book/thesis
Measuring tape

Modified Kuppuswamy scale
Protractor and divider/goniometer
Pulse oximeter
Red ring/thread
Shapes
Snellen, Jagger color chart
Stethoscope
Test tube
Thermometer
Torch light
Toy
Tuning fork – 128 Hz and 526 Hz
Wooden block

67

Tips for the Candidates

1. Dress confidently and wear a white coat.
2. Behave professionally.
3. Be smart and courteous in your gestures (never be over-confident).
4. Precheck and take all the necessary equipment to the examination hall.
5. Respect your patients and be very gentle when examining (respect their privacy).
6. Examine methodically so that you do not miss anything.
7. Observe carefully.
8. Listen to the question completely and then answer. Do not hesitate to revise your diagnosis if required.
9. Speak boldly, precise, and clearly.
10. Do not commit on what you have not examined or you are not aware of.
11. Always answer in order of frequency – most common to less common.
12. Do not argue with the examiner.
13. Preparation is the key to get through the examination. Practice to create a rapport with the patient, observe the child while you ask history from the parents, and follow a systematic approach.
14. Take some toys to divert the attention of the child.
15. Finally, stay calm.